BIOMEDICAL ETHICS

SEVENTH EDITION

BIOMEDICAL ETHICS

DAVID DeGRAZIA
George Washington University

THOMAS A. MAPPES
Frostburg State University

JEFFREY BRAND-BALLARD
George Washington University

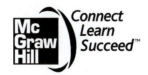

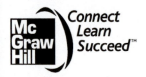

Connect
Learn
Succeed™

BIOMEDICAL ETHICS, SEVENTH EDITION

Published by McGraw-Hill Higher Education, an imprint of The McGraw-Hill Companies, Inc., 1221 Avenue of the Americas, New York, NY 10020. Copyright © 2011 by The McGraw-Hill Companies, Inc. All rights reserved. Previous editions © 2006, 2001 and 1996. No part of this publication may be reproduced or distributed in any form or by any means, or stored in a database or retrieval system, without the prior written consent of The McGraw-Hill Companies, Inc., including, but not limited to, in any network or other electronic storage or transmission, or broadcast for distance learning.

Some ancillaries, including electronic and print components, may not be available to customers outside the United States.

This book is printed on acid-free paper.

6 7 8 9 10 11 QVS/QVS 23 22 21 20 19

ISBN 978-0-07-340745-6
MHID 0-07-340745-3

Vice President & Editor-in-Chief: *Michael Ryan*
Vice President EDP/Central Publishing Services: *Kimberly Meriwether David*
Publisher: *Beth Mejia*
Sponsoring Editor: *Mark Georgiev*
Managing Editor: *Nicole Bridge*
Marketing Manager: *Pamela S. Cooper*
Senior Project Manager: *Lisa A. Bruflodt*
Buyer: *Laura Fuller*
Design Coordinator: *Margarite Reynolds*
Compositor: *Aptara®, Inc.*
Typeface: *10/12 Times Roman*
Cover Image Photo Credit: *C. Borland/PhotoLink/Getty Images*
Cover Designer: *Mary-Presley Adams*

All credits appearing on page or at the end of the book are considered to be an extension of the copyright page.

Library of Congress Cataloging-in-Publication Data

Biomedical ethics / [edited by] David DeGrazia, Jeffrey Brand-Ballard. — 7th ed.
  p. cm.
Includes bibliographical references and index.
ISBN 978-0-07-340745-6 (alk. paper)
1. Medical ethics. 2. Bioethics. I. DeGrazia, David. II. Brand-Ballard, Jeffrey.
R724.B49 2010
174.2—dc22

                                    2010011980

www.mhhe.com

ABOUT THE
AUTHORS

DAVID DeGRAZIA   earned a B.A. from the University of Chicago, an M.Stud. from Oxford University, and a Ph.D. from Georgetown University, all in philosophy. He is professor of philosophy at George Washington University, where he has taught since 1989. His publications include *Taking Animals Seriously* (Cambridge University Press, 1996) and *Human Identity and Bioethics* (Cambridge University Press, 2005), and his research has been supported by major fellowships from the National Endowment for the Humanities, the American Council of Learned Societies, and the National Institutes of Health.

THOMAS A. MAPPES   holds a B.S. in chemistry from the University of Dayton and a Ph.D. in philosophy from Georgetown University. He is professor emeritus of philosophy at Frostburg State University, where he taught from 1973 until his retirement in 2008. He is coeditor (with Jane S. Zembaty) of *Social Ethics: Morality and Social Policy* (McGraw-Hill, 7th ed., 2007), and his published work appears in journals such as *American Philosophical Quarterly* and *Kennedy Institute of Ethics Journal*.

JEFFREY BRAND-BALLARD   holds an A.B. from Vassar College, a J.D. from the University of Michigan Law School, and a Ph.D. in philosophy from the University of Michigan. He is associate professor of philosophy at George Washington University, where he has taught since 2002. His publications include *Limits of Legality: The Ethics of Lawless Judging* (Oxford University Press, 2010) and articles in journals such as *Ethics, Utilitas, Legal Theory,* and *Kennedy Institute of Ethics Journal*.

For our students

CONTENTS

PREFACE

This seventh edition of *Biomedical Ethics,* like its predecessors, is designed to provide an effective teaching instrument for courses in biomedical ethics. Although the basic character of the book remains unchanged, it has been substantially revised and updated. Almost one-third of the book's readings are new to this edition. We have added a new chapter on "Contested Therapies and Biomedical Enhancement" (Chapter 3), featuring thirteen articles on such topics as cosmetic surgery, cochlear implants for hearing-impaired children, the "Octomom" case, surgical remedies for achondroplasia (a kind of "dwarfism"), elective amputation, the use of pharmaceuticals such as Prozac to enhance cognitive functioning and personality, and other types of neuroenhancement. Chapter 9 has also been extensively updated, with new articles on health-care reform in Canada, Great Britain, Germany, and France. The chapter also includes recent scholarship on health-care reform in the United States, addressing tax credit incentives, single-payer proposals, voucher plans, and managed competition.

We have revised the other chapters, as well. The General Introduction (Chapter 1) and its bibliography have been updated. We have added to Chapter 4 new readings on research ethics, including research in developing countries and the use of animals as research subjects. Chapter 5 features cutting-edge literature on the definition and determination of death and a new paper on the "dead donor rule" that governs organ transplantation. We have added to Chapter 6 a new section on the Groningen Protocol, a decision framework developed in The Netherlands regarding active euthanasia of severely impaired infants. Chapter 7 includes discussion of the latest Supreme Court case on "partial-birth" abortion, an overview of new developments in stem cell research, and a recent article on the ethics of embryonic stem cell research.

In this seventh edition we have retained the various structural features that made earlier editions of the book effective teaching instruments. We have maintained the comprehensive character of the text, have once again organized the subject matter so that it unfolds in an effective and natural fashion, and have retained helpful editorial features such as the argument sketches that precede each selection and the annotated bibliographies at the end of each chapter. The bibliographies have been revised to incorporate recent literature.

We have also retained and updated the appendix of case studies. Finally, inasmuch as the value of any textbook anthology is largely dependent upon the quality of its readings, we have once again assembled a set of readings characterized by high-quality analysis and, to the greatest extent possible, clarity of writing style. As in the past, we have also taken care to choose readings that reflect diverse viewpoints with regard to the leading issues in biomedical ethics.

The introductions to each chapter of this book provide one of its most important editorial features. In the introductions we explicitly identify the central issues in each chapter and scan the various positions on these issues together with their supporting argumentation. Whenever possible, we draw out the relationship between the arguments that appear in a certain chapter and the ethical concepts and approaches discussed in the General Introduction. Whenever necessary, we also provide background conceptual clarification and factual information. In this vein, as a matter of course, we explicate the meaning of technical biomedical terms and introduce relevant biomedical information. The purpose of the chapter introductions is to enhance the effectiveness of the book as a teaching instrument. This same central purpose is shared by the book's other editorial features, which include the argument sketches preceding each selection and the annotated bibliographies at the end of each chapter. The annotated bibliographies provide substantial guidance for further reading and research. The various entries in the bibliographies, like the various readings in each chapter, reflect diverse viewpoints.

The first three editions of *Biomedical Ethics* were developed through the joint efforts of Thomas A. Mappes and Jane S. Zembaty. The fourth, fifth, and sixth editions were developed through the joint efforts of Thomas A. Mappes and David DeGrazia. For this edition, a new co-editor, Jeffrey Brand-Ballard, joined the team. Although David and Jeff shared the task of editing the seventh edition, Tom's contributions to the conception and content of the book are so substantial that they warrant his continued credit as co-editor. The present editors also want to acknowledge their extensive indebtedness to Jane Zembaty for numerous passages, analyses, organizational structures, and insights originally embodied in earlier editions and carried over to later editions.

We wish to thank George Washington University for its support of this project. We also thank Frostburg State University for its support of Tom Mappes's editorial work through six editions. In addition, the Kennedy Institute of Ethics, Georgetown deserves acknowledgement for providing to the public various bioethics databases; we took advantage of some of these in our online researches. Special thanks also to Nicole Bridge Caddigan, our project manager at McGraw-Hill, for her encouragement and assistance on several fronts. Finally, we would like to thank the external reviewers of the sixth edition, who provided us with valuable feedback as we began work on the seventh edition:

Jason Bernsten, Xavier University of New Orleans
Drew Chaisten, Xavier University of New Orleans
Ann Christensen, Pima Community College
Bill Kabasenche, Washington State University
Stuart Rachels, University of Alabama
Sophie Rietti, University of Ottowa
Andrew Sneddon, University of Ottawa
Leslie Whetstine, Walsh University

David DeGrazia
Jeffrey Brand-Ballard

CHAPTER 1

GENERAL
INTRODUCTION

A number of ethical issues can be identified as associated with the practice of medicine, the pursuit of biomedical research, or both. This set of ethical issues constitutes the subject matter of biomedical ethics. The proper task of biomedical ethics is to advance reasoned analysis in an effort to clarify and resolve such issues. What we term "biomedical ethics" is also commonly termed "bioethics." Although both terms are very well established and can be used interchangeably, *biomedical ethics* has the virtue of making more explicit the concern with issues associated with the practice of medicine. In any case, it is necessary in this context to understand *the practice of medicine* in an inclusive way, as referring not only to the professional activities of physicians but also to the distinctive activities of other health-care professionals.

THE NATURE OF BIOMEDICAL ETHICS

In order to situate biomedical ethics properly as a subdiscipline within the more general discipline of ethics, it is necessary to consider the nature of ethics as a philosophical discipline. *Ethics,* understood as a philosophical discipline, can be conveniently defined as the "*philosophical* study of morality." As such, it must be immediately distinguished from the *scientific* study of morality, often called "descriptive ethics." The goal of descriptive ethics is to attain empirical knowledge about morality. The practitioner of descriptive ethics is dedicated to describing existing moral views and, subsequently, explaining such views by advancing an account of their causal origin. Moral views, no less than other aspects of human experience, provide behavioral and social scientists a range of phenomena that stand in need of explanation. For example, why does a certain individual have such a Victorian view of sexual morality? A Freudian psychologist might attempt an explanation in terms of basic Freudian categories and early childhood experience. Why does a particular group of people manifest such a high incidence of moral advocacy for physician-assisted suicide? A sociologist might study the group in question and ultimately suggest an explanation based on factors such as the following: Many members of the group have seen loved ones die only after extensive suffering. Many members of the group identify themselves as nonreligious.

Ethics as a philosophical discipline stands in contrast to descriptive ethics. (Hereafter, the expression *ethics* is used to designate the philosophical discipline, as distinct from descriptive ethics.) Philosophers commonly subdivide ethics into (1) normative ethics and (2) metaethics, although the precise relationship of these two branches is a matter of some dispute. In normative ethics, philosophers attempt to determine what is morally right and what is morally wrong with regard to human action.[1] In metaethics, philosophers are concerned with tasks such as analyzing the nature of moral judgments and specifying appropriate methods for the justification of particular moral judgments and theoretical systems. It seems plausible to maintain that deliberations in normative ethics are to some extent dependent upon and cannot be completely detached from metaethical considerations. Whatever the precise relationship between normative ethics and metaethics, it is important to see that *normative ethics* is logically distinct from *descriptive ethics*. Whereas descriptive ethics attempts to describe (and explain) those moral views that in fact *are accepted*, normative ethics attempts to establish which moral views are *justifiable* and thus *ought to be accepted*. In *general* normative ethics, the task is to advance and provide a reasoned justification of an overall theory of moral obligation, thereby establishing an ethical theory that provides a general answer to the question, "What is morally right and what is morally wrong?" In *applied* normative ethics, as opposed to general normative ethics, the task is to resolve particular moral problems—for example, the issue of whether abortion can be morally justified, and, if so, under what conditions.

In light of the distinctions just made, it is now possible to identify biomedical ethics as one branch of applied (normative) ethics.[2] The task of biomedical ethics is to resolve ethical problems associated with the practice of medicine and/or the pursuit of biomedical research. Clearly, since there are ethical problems associated with other aspects of life, there are other branches of applied ethics. Business ethics, for example, is concerned with the ethical problems associated with the transaction of business. Importantly, in all branches of applied ethics, the particular issues under discussion are *normative* in character. Is this particular practice right or wrong? Is it morally justifiable? In applied ethics, the concern is not to establish which moral views people do, in fact, have. That is a descriptive matter. The concern in applied ethics, as in general normative ethics, is to establish which moral views are justifiable.

Questions such as the following are raised in biomedical ethics: Is a physician morally obligated to tell a terminally ill patient that he or she is dying? Are breaches of medical confidentiality ever morally defensible? Can euthanasia be morally justified? Is surrogate motherhood morally justified? Normative ethical questions such as these are concerned with the morality of certain acts and practices. Other questions in biomedical ethics focus on the ethical justifiability of laws. For example, is society justified in having laws that restrict the availability of abortion? Should we have laws that prohibit physician-assisted suicide? Should we have laws that prohibit research on human cloning or embryonic stem cells? The appearance of questions of this latter type shows that deliberations in biomedical ethics are intertwined not only with deliberations in general normative ethics, but also with deliberations in social-political philosophy and the philosophy of law. In these latter disciplines, a central theoretical question concerns the justifiable limits of law. Strictly speaking, if biomedical ethics is a type of applied ethics, ethics must be broadly understood as overlapping with social-political philosophy and the philosophy of law.

Although many of the ethical issues falling within the scope of biomedical ethics have historical roots, especially insofar as they are related to various codes of medical ethics, biomedical ethics did not crystallize into a full-fledged discipline until somewhat recently. Only since about 1970 have the various trappings of a relatively autonomous discipline become manifest. Numerous centers for research in biomedical ethics now exist. Four of the most prominent are the Hastings Center (Garrison, New York), the Joseph and Rose Kennedy Institute of Ethics, Georgetown University (Washington, D.C.), the Center for Bioethics, University of Pennsylvania (Philadelphia), and the Department of Bioethics, National Institutes of Health (Bethesda, Maryland). New journals continue to appear, conferences abound, and the field has its own encyclopedia, *The Encyclopedia of Bioethics,* first published in 1978. An increasing number of philosophers, theologians, lawyers, and other professionals now identify biomedical ethics as an area of specialization.

If, as is clear, many of the ethical issues falling within the scope of biomedical ethics have historical precedents, why has the field emerged as a vigorous and highly visible discipline only somewhat recently? Two cultural developments are at the root of the contemporary prominence of biomedical ethics: (1) the awesome advance of biomedical research as attended by the resultant development of biomedical technology and (2) the practice of medicine in an increasingly complicated institutional setting.

Consider first the impact of recent biomedical research. It has been responsible not only for creating historically unprecedented ethical problems, but also for adding new dimensions to old problems and making the resolution of those old problems a matter of greater urgency. Some developments—for example, those associated with reproductive technologies such as in vitro fertilization and, more recently, cloning—seem to present us with ethical problems that are genuinely unprecedented. More commonly, however, the advance of biomedical research has simply added complexity to old problems and created a sense of urgency with regard to their solution. Euthanasia is not a new problem; however, our ability to save the lives of severely impaired newborns who would have died in the past and our ability to sustain the biological processes of permanently unconscious patients have added new dimensions and, surely, a new urgency. Abortion is not a new problem, but the development of various techniques of prenatal diagnosis has created the new possibility of abortion based on genetic information. Indeed, the many successes of biomedical research in our own time, as manifested in the associated technological developments, call attention to the value of systematic biomedical research on human subjects and thus occasion reexamination of ethical constraints with regard to human experimentation.

The practice of medicine in an increasingly complicated institutional setting is, along with the advance of biomedical research, largely responsible for the contemporary prominence of biomedical ethics. In the past, the practice of medicine was largely confined within the bounds of the physician-patient relationship. Now, however, hospitals and other health-care institutions are intimately intertwined with physicians and allied personnel in the delivery of medical care. We have also witnessed an extension of the consumer rights movement into the health-care arena, a heightened emphasis on the legal requirements of informed consent, and an accompanying escalation of concern within the health-care community about legal liability. As a result, health-care professionals and institutions now find it necessary to pay closer attention to the interplay among medical, legal, and ethical considerations. Moreover, as a society we have become increasingly conscious of possible tensions between social justice and economic constraints—tensions that are acutely felt in confronting the general question of whether there is a right to health care, as well as specific problems of allocation such as those associated with managed care.

It is frequently said that biomedical ethics is an interdisciplinary field, and some explication of its interdisciplinary character might prove helpful. First, biomedical ethics is interdisciplinary within philosophy itself, inasmuch as deliberations in biomedical ethics are intertwined not only with deliberations in general normative ethics, but also with deliberations in social-political philosophy and the philosophy of law. Second, biomedical ethics is interdisciplinary precisely because the issues under discussion are frequently approached not only from the vantage point of moral philosophy (the principal vantage point in the collection of readings in this text) but also from the vantage point of moral theology. Whereas philosophical arguments are constructed without presupposing the truth of any religious claims, that is, without reliance on religious *faith,* theological arguments are generally constructed within a faith framework. There is yet a third—and most significant—way in which biomedical ethics is interdisciplinary, and that is by reference to the disciplines of medicine and biology. Medical judgments and the findings of biology often play a crucial role in ethical deliberations. (The findings of the social sciences can be relevant as well.) It is also important to recognize that the *experience* of health-care professionals and biomedical researchers is often essential to ensure that ethical discussions retain firm contact with the concrete realities that permeate the practice of medicine and the pursuit of biomedical research.

Although the issues of biomedical ethics are essentially normative, they are intertwined with both conceptual issues and factual (i.e., empirical) issues. For example, suppose we are concerned with the ethical acceptability of intervention for the sake of preventing a person from committing suicide. Our basic concern is with a normative question; however, we must face the problem of clarifying the nature of suicide, a conceptual issue. For example, if a Jehovah's Witness, on the basis of religious principle, refuses a life-saving blood transfusion, is the resultant death to be classified as a suicide? In addition to facing conceptual perplexities, we are also faced with an important factual question: Do those who typically attempt suicide really want to die? Presumably, psychologists have important things to tell us on this score. In the end, of course, we want to reach an ethical conclusion. However, ethical deliberations must proceed in the light of conceptual structures and factual beliefs. In the case of some issues in biomedical ethics, underlying factual issues are especially prominent. For example, in addressing the normative question of whether it is ever morally permissible to use children as research subjects, it is important to consider a factual question: To what extent can therapeutic techniques be developed for children in the absence of research employing children as research subjects? In the case of other issues in biomedical ethics, associated conceptual issues command special attention. For example, one could hardly discuss the normative issue of whether it is appropriate to transplant vital organs from brain-dead patients without closely examining the concept of death.

It is helpful to approach the literature of biomedical ethics with an eye toward distinguishing conceptual, factual, and normative issues. Furthermore, with regard to normative issues, which are the central issues of biomedical ethics, one cannot hope to situate argumentation in biomedical ethics properly without some awareness of the various types of ethical theory developed in general normative ethics. Such theories provide the frameworks within which many of the arguments in biomedical ethics are formulated.

RECENTLY DOMINANT ETHICAL THEORIES

An ethical theory provides a framework that can be used to determine what is morally right and morally wrong regarding human action in general, or what is morally good and morally bad regarding human character in general. The discussion of ethical theories in this section is restricted in two ways. First, consideration is limited to theories of right and wrong action, as opposed to theories of good and bad character (which fall naturally under the heading of virtue ethics, an approach that is explicated in a later section of this chapter). Second, consideration is limited to those theories of right and wrong action that commanded the most attention in the twentieth century. These recently dominant theories are frequently reflected in arguments advanced in biomedical ethics.

An ethical theory—as discussed in this section—provides an ordered set of moral standards (in some cases, simply one ultimate moral principle) that is to be used in assessing what is morally right and what is morally wrong regarding human action in general. A proponent of any such theory puts it forth as a framework with which a person can correctly determine, on any given occasion, what he or she (morally) ought to do.[3]

THE CRITICAL ASSESSMENT OF COMPETING ETHICAL THEORIES

Since a number of competing ethical theories may be identified, the question that immediately arises is what criteria are relevant to an assessment of these competing theories. There is no easy way to answer this very fundamental and very controversial question, but let us start with those considerations whose relevance is unlikely to be disputed. Any theory in any field is rightly expected to be internally consistent. Thus, a theory can be faulted on the basis of inconsistency. In a similar vein, any theory is surely flawed to the extent that it is either unclear or incomplete. In addition, a theory should be as simple as it can be without entailing a failure to satisfy other relevant criteria, such as clarity and completeness.

If the above considerations are relevant to a critical assessment of theories in any field, we must yet identify considerations relevant to our particular concern, the critical assessment of (normative) ethical theories. Responsive to this task, it is suggested that the following criteria embody the two most important considerations: (1) The implications of an ethical theory must be largely reconcilable with our experience of the moral life. (2) An ethical theory must provide effective guidance where it is most needed, that is, in those situations where substantial moral considerations can be advanced on both sides of an issue. In embracing the priority of criteria 1 and 2, we are saying that an adequate ethical theory must achieve two major goals. An adequate ethical theory must accord with the moral life as we experience it, and it must function heuristically by guiding us when we are confronted with moral perplexity. An ethical theory should, on the one hand, make sense out of the moral life by exhibiting the basic features of our ordinary moral thinking. On the other hand, it should illuminate our moral judgment precisely where it is experienced to falter—in the face of moral dilemmas.

There is certainly no suggestion here that the standards embodied in criteria 1 and 2 can be applied in some mechanical fashion to assess the relative adequacy of a proposed ethical theory. Intellectual judgments on these matters are necessarily complex and subtle. In saying, for example, that an adequate ethical theory must accord with our experience of the moral life, we certainly do not want to insist that each and every divergence from the verdict of "commonsense morality" must be interpreted as counting against an ethical theory. Perhaps we would be better advised to revise our moral judgment in light of the theory. (In empirical science, fact-theory mismatches are sometimes resolved not by modifying the theory, but by reinterpreting the facts in the light of the theory.) In embracing criterion 1 we undoubtedly commit ourselves to a point of view incompatible with the acceptance of an ethical theory that implies that *all* commonsense morality is mistaken, but we do not commit ourselves to the view that commonsense morality is sacrosanct. If an ethical theory successfully captures the basic features of our ordinary moral thinking, it will, of course, be true that its implications in large measure accord with our ordinary moral thinking. If the theory, however, cannot be reconciled with a relatively smaller range of our ordinary moral judgments, we may decide to interpret this disharmony as the product of some inadequacy in "commonsense morality" rather than as an inadequacy in the proposed theory.

CONSEQUENTIALIST VERSUS DEONTOLOGICAL THEORIES

With the introduction of criteria 1 and 2, we are now prepared to undertake a survey of alternative ethical theories. Our immediate concern is the identification, articulation, and critical consideration of those ethical theories that are the most prominent theories in general normative ethics—commanding the most attention in the twentieth century—and frequently reflected in argumentation advanced in biomedical ethics. In a later section, under the heading of "Alternative Directions and Methods," some additional theoretical perspectives that are important in biomedical ethics are presented.

In contemporary discussions, ethical theories are often grouped into two basic, and mutually exclusive, classes—*consequentialist* and *deontological.* Any ethical theory that claims that the rightness and wrongness of human action is *exclusively* a function of the goodness and badness of the consequences resulting directly or indirectly from that action is a consequentialist theory. Consequences are all-important here. A deontological theory maintains, in contrast, that the rightness and wrongness of human action is *not exclusively* (in the extreme case, not at all) a function of the goodness and badness of consequences. Accordingly, a theory is deontological (rather than consequentialist) if it places limits on the relevance of consequentialist considerations. Thus, an ethical theory in which the moral rightness and wrongness of human action is construed as totally independent of the goodness and badness of consequences would be only one kind, albeit the strongest or most extreme kind, of deontological theory.

The most prominent consequentialist ethical theory is the theory known as "utilitarianism." The adequacy of utilitarianism and the issue of its proper explication continue to be significant concerns in contemporary discussions of ethical theory. For this reason, and especially because much argumentation in biomedical ethics is based on utilitarian reasoning, utilitarianism warrants our detailed attention. However, it should first be noted that utilitarianism is not the only ethical theory that is correctly categorized as consequentialist. One other notable consequentialist theory is the theory known as "ethical egoism." The basic principle of ethical egoism can be phrased as follows: *A person ought to act so as to promote his or her own self-interest.* An action is morally right if, when compared with possible alternatives, its consequences are such as to generate the greatest balance of good over evil *for the agent.* (The impact of the action on other people is irrelevant except as it may indirectly affect the agent.) Ethical egoism is a consequentialist theory, in this broad sense, precisely because, by the terms of the theory, the rightness and wrongness of human action are exclusively a function of the goodness and badness of consequences.

Ethical egoism is an enormously problematic theory, one whose implications seem to be intensely at odds with our ordinary moral thinking. Under certain conditions, ethical egoism leads us to the conclusion that it is a person's moral obligation to perform an action that is flagrantly antisocial in nature. Consider this example. Mr. A loves to set buildings on fire; nothing makes him happier than watching a building burn. He recognizes that arson destroys property and subjects human life to serious risk, but he happens to be a thoroughly unsympathetic person, one whose well-being is not negatively affected by the misfortune of others. Of course, it is not in A's self-interest (and thus would not be A's moral obligation) to burn down a building if there is a good chance that he will be caught. (The punishment for arson is severe.) However, if A is very clever and if it is virtually certain that he will not be caught, ethical egoism seems to imply that arson is the morally right thing for him to do.

Another problematic feature of ethical egoism is that it cannot be publicly advocated without inconsistency. Suppose that Ms. B embraces ethical egoism. Accordingly, she considers it her moral obligation always to act in such a way as to promote her individual self-interest. Should she now publicly advocate ethical egoism, that is, encourage others to adopt the view that each person's moral obligation is to act in such a way as to promote his or her individual self-interest? No. Since it is to *her* advantage that others *not* act egoistically, it follows that it would be immoral for her to publicly advocate ethical egoism.

In reducing morality to considerations of personal prudence, it can be argued, ethical egoism destroys the very sense behind morality. Morality, it would seem, functions (at least in part) to restrict the pursuit of personal self-interest. It is not that morality prohibits the pursuit of personal self-interest; rather, it places limits on this pursuit. In "collapsing" morality into prudence, ethical egoism does not accord with a commonly experienced phenomenon of the moral life, the tension between self-interest and morality, between "what would be best for me" and "what is the morally right thing."

In fairness to ethical egoism, it must be noted that its proponents have sometimes devised ingenious arguments in an attempt to minimize the sort of difficulties just discussed. However, ethical egoism is not widely defended in contemporary discussions of ethical theory, and it surely plays an insignificant role in discussions of biomedical ethics. It has been introduced primarily as a notable instance of a consequentialist yet nonutilitarian theory. Attention will now be focused on utilitarianism.

In its classical formulation, utilitarianism is found most prominently in the works of two English philosophers, Jeremy Bentham (1748–1832) and John Stuart Mill (1806–1873). In contemporary discussions, a distinction is made between two kinds of utilitarianism—*act-utilitarianism* and *rule-utilitarianism*. Although it is somewhat controversial whether a significant distinction can be maintained between these two versions of utilitarianism, it is presumed for the sake of exposition that two distinct utilitarian ethical theories can indeed be articulated.[4]

ACT-UTILITARIANISM

Human action typically takes place within the fabric of our social existence. Thus, an action performed by one person often affects not only the agent but also the lives of many others. Consider a man who refuses to stop smoking even though he suffers from emphysema. He will not be the only one to suffer the consequences; certainly those who care about him will also. His refusal to give up smoking, since it has the effect of further damaging his health, also produces a higher level of anxiety among the members of his family. Among the other detrimental consequences of his continuing to smoke is the negative impact on any nonsmokers in the vicinity when he smokes: annoyance, displeasure, and the like.

However, the various consequences of a single action are seldom uniformly good or uniformly bad. In addition to the bad consequences already indicated, there are also a number of good consequences that result from the refusal to stop smoking. Most notably, the emphysema patient continues to derive the satisfaction associated with cigarette smoking. In addition, it is likely that his continuing to smoke will make him less irritable around others. When the various consequences of a single action are fully analyzed, more often than not we find ourselves confronted with a mixture of good and bad. For example, if a person throws a late-night party, it is true that those in attendance may have a very good time, but it is also true that the neighbors may lose out on some much-needed sleep.

The basic principle of act-utilitarianism can be stated as follows: *A person ought to act so as to produce the greatest balance of good over evil, everyone considered.* Act-utilitarianism stands in vivid contrast to ethical egoism, which directs a person always to act so as to produce the greatest balance of good over evil *for oneself* (i.e., the agent). The act-utilitarian is committed to the proposition that the interests of everyone affected by an action are to be weighed in the balance along with the interests of the agent. Everyone's interests are entitled to an impartial consideration. According to the act-utilitarian, an action is morally right if, when compared with possible alternatives, its likely consequences are such as to generate the greatest balance of good over evil, everyone considered. If we refer to the net balance of good over evil (everyone considered) that is likely to be produced by a certain action as its (overall) *utility,* then we can say that act-utilitarianism directs a person always to choose that alternative that has the greatest utility. Thus, we can express the basic principle of act-utilitarianism as follows: A person ought to act so as to maximize utility.

For the act-utilitarian, calculation is a paramount element in the moral assessment of action. The question is always this: What is the utility of each of my alternatives in this particular set of circumstances? However, any system of utilitarian calculation must ultimately be anchored in some conception of intrinsic value (i.e., that which is good or desirable in and of itself). The act that will maximize utility (by our definition) is the act that is likely to produce the greatest balance of good over evil, everyone considered. However, what is to count as "good" and what as "evil" in our calculations? The answers provided within the framework of classical utilitarianism reflect a so-called hedonistic theory of intrinsic value. According to Bentham, only pleasure (understood broadly to include any type of satisfaction or enjoyment) has intrinsic value; only pain (understood broadly to include any dissatisfaction, frustration, or displeasure) has intrinsic disvalue. According to Mill, only happiness has intrinsic value; only unhappiness has intrinsic disvalue. To what extent there is substantive disagreement between Bentham and Mill on this matter is a complex question that cannot be dealt with here. It should be mentioned, however, that many contemporary utilitarian thinkers have embraced more elaborate and nonhedonistic theories of intrinsic value.[5] Nevertheless, for the sake of exposition, we shall presume that a hedonistic theory of intrinsic value, in the spirit of Bentham and Mill, underlies utilitarian calculation.

In the spirit of act-utilitarianism, in order to determine what I should do in a certain situation, I must first attempt to delineate alternative paths of action. Next, I attempt to foresee the consequences (sometimes numerous and far-reaching) of each alternative action. Then I attempt, in each case, to evaluate the consequences and to weigh the good against the bad, considering the impact of my action on everyone whom it is likely to affect. Such a reckoning will reveal the act that is likely to produce the greatest balance of good over evil, and this act is the morally right act for me in my particular circumstances. (If it appears likely that two competing actions would produce the same balance of good over evil, then either action will qualify as morally correct.) In some situations, it is true that no matter what I do, more evil (pain or unhappiness) will come into the world than good (pleasure or happiness). In such unfortunate situations, according to the act-utilitarian, the morally right act is the one that will bring the least unfavorable balance of evil and good into the world.

Act-utilitarianism can rightly be understood as a form of "situation ethics." The act-utilitarian has no sympathy for the notion that certain kinds of actions are intrinsically wrong, that is, wrong by their very nature. Rather, a certain kind of action (e.g., lying) may be wrong in one set of circumstances yet right in another. The circumstances in which an action is to be performed are relevant to its morality (i.e., its rightness or wrongness) because the consequences of the action will vary depending upon the circumstances. Thus, the morality of action is a function of the situation confronting the agent—"situation ethics."

The situational character of act-utilitarianism is reflected in the act-utilitarian attitude toward moral rules. Among the "commonsense rules of morality" are the following: "do not kill," "do not injure," "do not steal," "do not lie," "do not break promises." According to the act-utilitarian, these rules are to be understood merely as rules of thumb. They are, for the most part, reliable guides for human action, especially relevant when time constraints undermine the possibility of careful calculation. In most circumstances, acting in accordance with a moral rule is the way to maximize utility, but in some cases this is not so. In these latter cases, whenever there is good reason to believe that breaking a moral rule will produce a greater balance of good over evil (everyone considered), the right thing to do is to break it. In such a case, it would be wrong to follow the rule. Lying is usually wrong, breaking promises is usually wrong, killing is usually wrong; however, whenever circumstances are such that there is good reason to believe that breaking a certain moral rule will maximize utility, the rule should be broken. Of course, the act-utilitarian insists, one must be cautious in concluding that any given exception to a moral rule is indeed justified. One must be wary of rationalization and not allow one's own interests to weigh more heavily than the interests of others in the utilitarian calculation. Most importantly, one must not be simpleminded in a consideration of the likely consequences of breaking a moral rule. Indirect and long-term consequences must be considered as well as direct and short-term consequences. Lying on a certain occasion may seem to promote most effectively the interests of those immediately involved, but perhaps the lie will provide a bad example for less reflective people, or perhaps it will contribute to a general breakdown of trust among human beings. In this same vein, one prominent contemporary act-utilitarian emphasizes the significance of the long-term, indirect consequences of promise breaking, while at the same time exhibiting the underlying act-utilitarian attitude toward moral rules:

> The rightness or wrongness of keeping a promise on a particular occasion depends only on the goodness or badness of the consequences of keeping or of breaking the promise on that particular occasion. Of course part of the consequences of breaking the promise, and a part to which we will normally ascribe decisive importance, will be the weakening of faith in the institution of promising. However, if the goodness of the consequences of breaking the rule is *in toto* greater than the goodness of the consequences of keeping it, then we must break the rule . . . .[6]

Act-utilitarianism has often been criticized on the grounds that, due to the extensive sort of calculations it seems to demand, it cannot function as a useful guide for human action. In the spirit of this criticism, the following questions are asked: How can I possibly predict all the consequences of my actions? How am I to assign weights to the various kinds of human satisfactions—for example, the pleasure of eating a candy bar versus the aesthetic enjoyment of the ballet? How am I to weigh the anxiety of one person against the inconvenience of another? Besides, how am I supposed to have time to do these extensive calculations? Act-utilitarians, in response to such questions, usually appeal rather directly to "common sense." They say, typically, that there is no escape from a consideration of probabilities in rational decision making; predict as best you can and weigh as best you can, considering the time you have available for deliberation. All that can be expected is that you come to grips with the likely consequences of your alternatives in a serious-minded, sensible way and then act accordingly. Utilitarians, they may add, are not the only ones who need to predict the future and who require simplifying devices and heuristics to that end.

Examples of Act-Utilitarian Reasoning in a Biomedical Context   The following examples are provided in an effort to exhibit act-utilitarian reasoning as it might arise in a biomedical context. It is not claimed that an act-utilitarian must necessarily reach the conclusion suggested in each case. It is claimed only that an act-utilitarian might plausibly reach the stated conclusion.

(1) A severely impaired newborn, believed to have no realistic chance of surviving more than a few weeks, has contracted pneumonia. (The treatment of impaired newborns is discussed in Chapter 6.) A physician, in conjunction with the parents of the infant, must decide whether to fight off the pneumonia with antibiotics, thereby prolonging the life of the infant. The alternative is simply to allow the infant to die. It seems clear that the interests of all those immediately involved are best served by deciding not to treat the pneumonia. Surely the infant has nothing to gain, and something to lose, by a slight extension of a pain-filled life. The parents, whose suffering cannot be eradicated whatever action is taken, nevertheless will find some relief knowing that their child's suffering has ended. In addition, hospital resources can be better utilized than by prolonging the dying process of an infant who cannot benefit from further treatment. However, there may be decisive consequences of allowing death to occur that are indirect and long-term. Perhaps allowing this infant to die will contribute to a breakdown of protective attitudes toward infants in general. No, the risk of this untoward consequence seems minimal. Withholding antibiotics, thereby allowing the infant to die, is the right thing to do in this case.

(2) A biomedical researcher, on the basis of animal studies she has conducted, believes that a certain drug therapy has great promise for the treatment of a particular kind of cancer in human beings. (The use of animals in research is discussed in Chapter 4.) At present, however, her primary concern is to establish an appropriate dosage level for human beings; there have been several troublesome side effects exhibited by the animals who received large doses of the drug. Over the years, the researcher has found that students at her university are very willing to volunteer as research subjects in experiments that can be identified as presenting only minimal risks to themselves. They are, however, understandably reluctant to volunteer for experiments that seem to present more substantial risks. The researcher in this case cannot honestly say that there are no substantial risks for research subjects. She expects, in particular, that perhaps 30 to 40 percent of the research subjects will have to contend with very prolonged nausea. However, if she is honest in conveying this information to potential research subjects, it is unlikely that they will volunteer in sufficient numbers. (The ethics of experimentation on human subjects is discussed in Chapter 4.) Perhaps, she reasons, it is justifiable in this case to withhold information about the risk of very

prolonged nausea. After all, it is very likely that numerous people will eventually derive great benefit from the therapeutic technique under study. Surely this likely benefit far outweighs the short-term discomfort of a much smaller number. But consider the very real possibility that the deception would come to light. If those who routinely volunteer as research subjects are given a reason to distrust those conducting the experiments, the overall research effort on campus will be negatively affected. Moreover, publicity about the deception would create a major public relations scandal for the university, forcing it to devote valuable time, energy, and money to repairing its reputation. These seem to be decisive considerations. In this case, then, deception would be wrong. (If there were no realistic chance of the deception's being discovered, it seems that the conclusion would be different.)

(3) The setting is in the 1960s, when kidney dialysis machines are scarce, and it is not possible for all who need them to be given access. A hospital administrator or perhaps a committee has been charged with the responsibility of deciding, in essence, whose lives will be saved. (Such decisions are often referred to as "microallocation decisions.") On a particular occasion, when there is room for one more patient, there are two candidates in great need. One of the candidates, a civic-minded woman of 40, is married and the mother of four children. The other candidate, an unmarried man of the same age, is known to be a drifter and an alcoholic. It seems clear, at first glance, that the consequences of saving the woman's life are far superior to those of saving the man's life. Her husband, her children, and the community in general would be negatively affected in very substantial ways by her death. However, is it not problematic to accord a person access to a scarce medical resource on the basis of his or her social role? If a precedent of this sort is set, will not those whose lives are less "socially useful" become somewhat anxious and fearful? On the other hand, perhaps this negative consequence will be balanced by a positive consequence; that is, people will be more inclined to become "socially useful." It still seems clear that the woman in this case should have priority over the man.

Critical Assessment of Act-Utilitarianism   Act-utilitarianism arguably fares poorly when measured against a previously identified standard: The implications of an ethical theory must be largely reconcilable with our experience of the moral life. In a number of ways, it can be argued, act-utilitarianism clashes with our experience of the moral life. This perceived failure to accord with our ordinary moral thinking is reflected in the following well-known objections to act-utilitarianism.

(1) Act-Utilitarianism Confronts Individuals with an Overly Demanding Moral Standard. We are accustomed to thinking that at least some of our decisions are matters of "mere prudence," rightly decided on the basis of "what is best for me." Which major a college student should choose is a good example of a choice that we are inclined to consider essentially a nonmoral matter, a matter of "mere prudence." According to the act-utilitarian, however, a person is continually under a moral obligation to produce the greatest balance of good over evil, everyone considered. Whereas ethical egoism seems to wrongly "collapse" morality into prudence, it would seem that act-utilitarianism "expands" morality so as to destroy the realm of prudence. No aspect of a person's life can be considered merely a matter of prudence. Every decision is a moral decision, to be made on the basis of utilitarian calculation. However, no matter how noble it might be for a college student to decide his or her major on the basis of a utilitarian calculation, it would seem that one is certainly not under an obligation to proceed in this manner. Doing so, we would ordinarily say, is not one's duty but, rather, is something "above and beyond the call of duty." Act-utilitarianism, in directing a

person always to act so as to maximize utility, seems problematically to imply that it is one's duty to act in a way that we ordinarily consider "above and beyond the call of duty."

(2) Act-Utilitarianism Does Not Accord with Our Experience of Particular, Morally Significant Relationships. In our experience of the moral life, we are continually aware of highly particular, morally significant relationships that exist between ourselves and others. We are related to particular individuals in a host of morally significant ways, such as spouse to spouse, parent to child, creditor to debtor, promisor to promisee, employer to employee, teacher to student, physician or nurse to patient. In view of such relationships, it is ordinarily thought, we have special obligations—obligations that restrict the effort to maximize utility. Parents, we are strongly inclined to say, are obligated to care for their children even if there is good reason to think that the time and energy necessary for this task would maximize utility if redirected to some other task. In the same way, by virtue of the special relationship that exists between a physician and a patient, would it not be wrong for a physician to make decisions regarding a patient's treatment in the manner of an act-utilitarian? For a physician to compromise the interests of an individual patient in an effort to maximize utility surely seems wrong. W. D. Ross, who has vigorously pressed this overall line of criticism against act-utilitarianism, asserts that the "essential defect of the . . . theory is that it ignores, or at least does not do full justice to, the highly personal character of duty."[7]

(3) Act-Utilitarianism Does Not Accord with Our Conviction That Individuals Have Rights. The notion of rights plays an important part in our ordinary moral thinking, but act-utilitarianism seems incapable of accommodating this notion. Moreover, in certain circumstances, the action that would maximize utility (and thus the right action, according to the act-utilitarian) is one that we are inclined to consider seriously immoral precisely because it entails the violation of some person's right. For example, it seems that act-utilitarianism would allow an innocent person to be unjustly punished, as long as circumstances were such as to make this line of action the one that would generate the greatest balance of good over evil. Suppose extreme social unrest has been created by a wave of unsolved crimes. The enraged crowd will violently erupt, bringing massive evil into the world, unless the authorities punish someone (anyone) in an effort to appease the appetite for vengeance. So act-utilitarianism seems to allow the unjust treatment of a person as a scapegoat, as a mere means to a social end. But surely an innocent person has a right not to be punished, and it is by reference to this right that the wrongness of scapegoating is most naturally understood. Similarly, "the common moral opinion that painless undetected murders of old unhappy people are wicked, no matter what benefits result"[8] can be thought to rest on the contention that people, however old and unhappy, nevertheless have a *right* to life. It is often asserted against act-utilitarianism that it is a defective theory because it allows "the end to justify the means." At least part of the sense behind this charge can be made out in reference to the notion of rights. Certain means of achieving a desirable social end are simply wrong because they entail the violation of a person's right. Contrary to act-utilitarianism, such means cannot be justified by the end.

Act-utilitarians have responded in two ways to the overall claim that the theory cannot be reconciled with our ordinary moral thinking. Some say, in essence, "so much the worse for our ordinary moral thinking." In their view, we must simply overhaul our collective moral consciousness and embrace the mind-set of the act-utilitarian. Most act-utilitarians, however, do not adopt this revisionary stance. Rather, they seek to demonstrate that the clash between act-utilitarianism and our ordinary moral thinking is not nearly so severe as the above criticisms suggest. They argue that, when act-utilitarianism is properly applied, when all the significant long-term, indirect consequences are taken into account, the theory does not give rise to conclusions that seem so patently objectionable. It is very doubtful, however, that this strategy of argument can completely rescue act-utilitarianism from its difficulties.

Perhaps act-utilitarianism fares better when measured against the second of our previously identified standards: An ethical theory must provide effective guidance where it is most needed. At the very least, it must be said in favor of act-utilitarianism that it provides a reasonably clear decision procedure, a sense of direction, for the resolution of moral dilemmas. In the face of moral considerations that incline our judgment in conflicting ways, act-utilitarianism counsels us to analyze the likely consequences of alternative actions in order to determine the alternative that will maximize utility. Still, however well act-utilitarianism might be thought to fare with regard to our second standard—and even that is debatable—it seems to encounter significant problems when measured against our first standard. Indeed, in contemporary times, most utilitarian thinkers have rejected act-utilitarianism in favor of a theory known as rule-utilitarianism.[9]

RULE-UTILITARIANISM

The basic principle of act-utilitarianism has previously been formulated as follows: A person ought to act so as to produce the greatest balance of good over evil, everyone considered. In contrast, the basic principle of rule-utilitarianism can be formulated as follows: *A person ought to act in accordance with the rule that, if generally followed, would produce the greatest balance of good over evil, everyone considered.* If the demand to produce the greatest balance of good over evil, everyone considered, is referred to as the principle (standard) of utility, then the principle of utility is the basic ethical principle in both the act-utilitarian and the rule-utilitarian systems. However, in the act-utilitarian system, determining the morally correct action is a matter of assessing alternative actions directly against the standard of utility, whereas in the rule-utilitarian system determining the morally correct action involves an *indirect* appeal to the principle of utility. In the spirit of rule-utilitarianism, a moral code is first established by reference to the principle of utility. That is, a set of valid moral rules is established by determining which rules (as opposed to conceivable alternatives), if generally followed, would produce the greatest balance of good over evil. In rule-utilitarianism, individual actions are morally right if they are in accord with those rules.

The difference between act-utilitarian reasoning and rule-utilitarian reasoning can be represented schematically as follows:

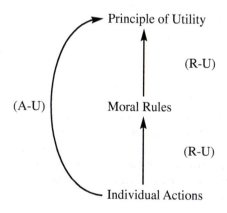

Act-utilitarian reasoning embodies a single-stage procedure; rule-utilitarian reasoning, a two-stage procedure. Act utilitarians assess individual actions strictly on the basis of utilitarian considerations. Rule utilitarians develop a moral code (a set of moral rules) on the basis of utilitarian considerations and then assess individual actions, not on the basis of utilitarian considerations but on the basis of the moral rules that have been established.

For the act-utilitarian, moral rules have a very subordinate status. They are merely "rules of thumb," providing some measure of practical guidance. For the rule-utilitarian, moral rules assume a much more fundamental status, indeed a theoretical primacy. Only in reference to established moral rules can the moral assessment of individual actions be carried out. Thus, the first and most crucial step for the rule-utilitarian is the articulation of a set of moral rules, themselves justified on the basis of utilitarian considerations. Underlying this task is the question of which rules (as opposed to conceivable alternatives), if generally followed, would produce the greatest balance of good over evil, everyone considered. That is, which rules, if adopted or recognized in our moral code, would maximize utility?

As a first approximation of a set of moral rules that could be justified on the basis of utilitarian considerations, consider the "commonsense rules of morality," such as "do not kill," "do not steal," "do not lie," "do not break promises." It is not difficult to think of such rules as resting upon a utilitarian foundation. Surely the consequences of the adoption of the rule "do not kill" are dramatically better than the consequences of the adoption of the rule "kill whenever you want." If the latter rule were generally followed, society would give way to anarchy. Similarly, the consequences of the adoption of the rule "do not steal" are dramatically better than the consequences of the adoption of the rule "steal whenever you want." If the former rule is generally followed, individuals will enjoy an important measure of personal security. If the latter rule were adopted by a society, anxiety and tension would dominate social existence. As for lying and promise breaking, if people felt free to engage in such behavior, the numerous advantages that derive from human trust and cooperation would evaporate. However, the rules thus far exhibited as having a utilitarian foundation are essentially prohibitions. Are there not also rules of a more positive sort that could also be justified on the basis of utilitarian considerations? It would seem so. Consider rules such as "come to the aid of people in distress" and "prevent innocent people from being harmed." It surely seems that human welfare would be enhanced by the adoption of such rules as part of the overall fabric of our moral code.

According to the rule-utilitarian, an individual action is morally right when it accords with the rules or moral code established on a utilitarian basis. However, the account of moral rules thus far presented is too simplistic. In order to be plausible, the rules that constitute the moral code must be understood as incorporating certain exceptions. The need to recognize justified exceptions is perhaps most apparent when we remember that moral rules, if stated unconditionally, can easily come into conflict with each other. When an obviously agitated person waves a gun and inquires as to the whereabouts of a third party, it may not be possible to act in accordance with both the rule "do not lie" and the rule "prevent innocent people from being harmed." Indeed, it is precisely this sort of situation that inclines us to consider incorporating an exception into our rule against lying. Suppose we say, "Do not lie *except* when necessary to prevent an innocent person from being seriously harmed." When the possibility of a justified exception is raised, the rule-utilitarian employs the following decision procedure. The question is posed, "Would the adoption of the rule with the exception have better consequences than the adoption of the rule without the exception?" If so, the exception is a justified one; the rule incorporating the exception has greater utility than the rule without the exception. In the face of our proposed exception to the rule against lying, the rule-utilitarian would probably conclude that it does constitute a justified exception. The adoption of the rule "do not lie *except* when necessary to protect an innocent person from being seriously harmed" would seem to preserve essentially all the social benefits provided by the adoption of the rule "do not lie," while bringing about an additional social benefit, an increased measure of personal security for potential victims of assault.

Examples of Rule-Utilitarian Reasoning in a Biomedical Context (1) A substantial problem in biomedical ethics (discussed in Chapter 2) is whether it is ever right for a physician to lie to a patient, saying that the patient's illness is not terminal when it is believed to be so. The rule-utilitarian would conceptualize this issue as raising the possibility of a justified exception to the rule against lying. (Notice that an act-utilitarian, in contrast, would insist on assessing every individual case on its own utilitarian merits.) Suppose we consider incorporating into the rule against lying an exception to this effect: "*except* when in the judgment of a physician it would be better for a patient not to know that his or her illness is believed to be terminal." Would the adoption of the rule incorporating this exception have better consequences than the adoption of the rule without the exception? The correct answer to this question is perhaps arguable, but it would seem that the rule-utilitarian would conclude that the proposed exception is an unjustified one. It is perhaps true that adoption of a rule incorporating the proposed exception would result in many patients' being spared (at least temporarily) the distress that accompanies knowledge of one's impending death. On the other hand, it seems that this gain would be dwarfed by the distress and anxiety that would emerge from the erosion of trust within the confines of the physician-patient relationship. Whether a more limited exception could be formulated to a rule-utilitarian's satisfaction remains an open question.

(2) Another substantial problem in biomedical ethics (discussed in Chapter 6) has to do with the morality of mercy killing. Suppose a terminally ill patient, in great pain, requests that a physician terminate his or her life by administering a lethal dose of a drug. Such a case raises the issue of voluntary (active) euthanasia. The rule-utilitarian would conceptualize this issue (and other issues, such as suicide and abortion) as raising the possibility of a justified exception to our rule against killing. Notice that at least one exception to our rule against killing is relatively uncontroversial. Killing in self-defense is justifiable, according to the rule-utilitarian, because although the adoption of the rule "do not kill" has dramatically better consequences than the adoption of the rule "kill whenever you want," adoption of the rule "do not kill *except* in self-defense" has still better consequences. As for voluntary (active) euthanasia, perhaps we should say that strong rule-utilitarian arguments can be advanced on both sides of the issue. Rule-utilitarian proponents of voluntary (active) euthanasia emphasize that social acceptance of this practice would result in great benefits— the primary one being that many dying people would be able to escape an extension of an anguished dying process. On the other side of the issue, however, we find, among a number of important concerns, insistence that availability of the lethal dose would create a climate of fear and anxiety among the elderly. Will dying people not come to feel that their families, to whom they have become a burden, expect them to ask for the lethal dose?

(3) A final illustration of rule-utilitarian reasoning in a biomedical context can be presented in reference to the principle of medical confidentiality (discussed in Chapter 2). This principle, which has an obvious basis in a rule-utilitarian structure, demands that information

revealed within the context of a therapeutic relationship be held confidential. If patients could not rely on this expectation, they would be reluctant to communicate information that is essential to their proper treatment. Still, are there not justifiable exceptions to the principle of medical confidentiality? Suppose, for example, a patient reveals to his or her therapist an intention to kill or injure a third party. Is it not incumbent upon the therapist to break medical confidentiality in an effort to ensure protection for the third party? The situation just described is the basis of the *Tarasoff* case considered in Chapter 2, and rule-utilitarian arguments on both sides of the issue can be found in the judicial opinions presented. There is an obvious benefit associated with the recognition of an exception to medical confidentiality based on the interests of innocent third parties; namely, threatened people will sometimes be saved from injury and death. On the other hand, it is argued, emotionally disturbed patients are likely to become more inhibited in communicating with therapists; thus, their treatment will be inhibited, and a greater incidence of violence against innocent people will result.

Critical Assessment of Rule-Utilitarianism Rule-utilitarianism, it would seem, goes some distance toward alleviating the perceived difficulties of act-utilitarianism. Although act-utilitarians have charged rule-utilitarians with "superstitious rule-worship,"[10] it is act-utilitarianism rather than rule-utilitarianism that seems to clash with our ordinary moral thinking on this score. Rule-utilitarianism seems to fare at least somewhat better than act-utilitarianism when measured against the standard that the implications of an ethical theory must be largely reconcilable with our experience of the moral life.

Whereas act-utilitarianism seems to confront individuals with an overly demanding moral standard, placing each of us under a continuing obligation to maximize utility with each of our actions, rule-utilitarianism may prove to be far less demanding of individuals. It requires only that individuals conform their actions to the rules that constitute a utilitarian-based moral code, which may not include any rules that prove overly demanding. Rule-utilitarianism also seems to accord reasonably well with our experience of particular, morally significant relationships. We commonly perceive ourselves as having special obligations arising out of our various morally significant relationships, and we think of these obligations as incompatible with functioning in the manner of an act-utilitarian. For example, parents have a special obligation to care for their children, physicians have a special obligation to act in the interests of their patients, and so forth. Such special obligations can be understood as having a rule-utilitarian foundation, as deriving from rules that, if generally followed, would maximize utility. Thus, rule-utilitarianism seems to remedy another perceived difficulty of act-utilitarianism.

It is less clear that rule-utilitarianism is capable of providing a complete remedy for another perceived difficulty of act-utilitarianism, that is, its inability to provide an adequate theoretical foundation for individual rights. Surely rule-utilitarianism does not lead us as easily as does act-utilitarianism to conclusions that are incompatible with our ordinary moral thinking about the rights of individuals. For example, in suggesting that the painless murder of an old, unhappy (but not suicidal) person is the right thing as long as it can be done in complete secrecy, act-utilitarianism seems to clash violently with our conviction that such an action is patently objectionable, inasmuch as it constitutes a violation of a person's right to life. Rule-utilitarianism, in contrast, would never lead us to the conclusion that this sort of killing is morally legitimate. Surely the consequences of adopting the rule "do not kill *except* in the case of old, unhappy people who can be killed in complete secrecy" are dramatically worse than the consequences of adopting the rule without such an exception. If the rule with the exception were adopted, the lives of elderly people would be filled with anxiety and fear; moreover, people attempting to follow such a rule would no doubt sometimes kill old, *happy* people, mistakenly believing them to be unhappy. In addition to rescuing utilitarian thinking from such obvious clashes with our ordinary moral thinking, rule-utilitarianism suggests a way of accommodating the notion of individual rights. Just as our special obligations can be understood as deriving from rules in a utilitarian-based moral code, so, too, can an individual's rights be understood in this fashion. A person's right to life, for example, can be understood as a correlate of our utilitarian-based rule against killing. Of course, whatever exceptions are properly incorporated into our rule against killing will factor out as limitations on a person's right to life. Whether rule-utilitarianism in this manner can provide an adequate theoretical foundation for individual rights is a very controversial matter. Its critics charge that it cannot.

Closely related to the claim that rule-utilitarianism does not provide an adequate theoretical foundation for individual rights is the somewhat broader claim that rule-utilitarianism fails to provide an adequate theoretical grounding for what we take to be the obligations of justice. This broader criticism, which is also vigorously advanced against act-utilitarianism, is perhaps the principal residual difficulty confronting rule-utilitarianism. Critics of rule-utilitarianism allege, for example, that the theory is compatible with the blatant injustice of enslaving one segment of a society's population or at least discriminating against this segment. The idea is that social rules discriminating against an explicitly identified minority group might maximize utility by bringing about more happiness in the advantaged majority than unhappiness in the disadvantaged minority. Rule-utilitarians are inclined to argue in response to this line of criticism that, when the consequences of adopting "unjust rules" are completely analyzed, it is never true that their adoption can be justified on utilitarian grounds. Rather, the rule-utilitarian contends, "the rules of justice" rest on a secure utilitarian foundation. Whether rule-utilitarianism, in this manner, can adequately be reconciled with the perceived obligations of justice is a matter of contemporary debate.

Rule-utilitarianism also seems to fare reasonably well when measured against the second of our suggested standards: An ethical theory must provide effective guidance where it is most needed. In a dilemma, where one moral rule, or principle, inclines us one way and another moral rule, or principle, inclines us another way, the rule-utilitarian instructs us to establish relative priority by considering the consequences of incorporating appropriate exceptions into the rules that are in conflict. The dilemma is to be resolved by adoption of a rule that will maximize utility. Although this decision procedure sometimes entails very complex factual analysis and deliberation, it does seem to provide us a substantial measure of explicit guidance. Since rule-utilitarianism also seems to be reasonably harmonious with our ordinary moral thinking, it is an ethical theory that cannot easily be dismissed.

KANTIAN DEONTOLOGY

The most prominent of the classical deontological theories is that developed by German philosopher Immanuel Kant (1724–1804). Kantian deontology continues to command substantial attention in contemporary discussions of ethical theory and, importantly, is the underlying framework of much argumentation in biomedical ethics. In both of these respects, Kantian deontology is similar to utilitarianism and, like utilitarianism, warrants our detailed attention.

Kant sees utilitarianism as embodying a radically wrong approach in ethical theory. He emphasizes the need to avoid the "serpent-windings" of utilitarian thinking and refers to the principle of utility as "a wavering and uncertain standard." There is indeed a single, fundamental principle that is the basis of all moral obligation, but this fundamental principle is *not* the principle of utility. The supreme principle of morality, the principle from which all of our various duties derive, Kant calls the "categorical imperative."

Although our present objective is an exposition of Kantian deontology, the enormous complexity of Kant's moral philosophy is a formidable obstacle to any concise exposition of the structure of Kant's ethical system. In particular, we are faced with the problem that Kant formulated the basic principle of his system, the categorical imperative, in a number of different ways. Although Kant insists that his various formulations are all equivalent, this contention is explicitly denied by his contemporary expositors and critics. Thus, if we are to provide a coherent account of Kantian deontology, mindful of the need to provide an account that is especially useful in dealing with issues in biomedical ethics, it seems advisable to settle on a favored formulation of the categorical imperative. Since two of Kant's formulations of the categorical imperative are especially prominent, it will suffice for our purposes to choose a favored formulation from these two.

According to what we will call the "first formulation," the categorical imperative tells us: "Act only on that maxim through which you can at the same time will that it should become a universal law."[11] According to what we will call the "second formulation," the categorical imperative tells us: "Act in such a way that you always treat humanity, whether in your own person or in the person of any other, never simply as a means, but always at the same time as an end."[12] The first formulation of the categorical imperative has often been compared to the Golden Rule ("Do unto others as you would have them do unto you"), and it may be true that these principles, when suitably interpreted, have roughly the same implications. At any rate, Kant apparently considered the first formulation to be the most basic of all his formulations, yet despite this fact, and despite the fact that ethical theorists have tended to pay more attention to the first formulation than the second, it is the second formulation that we take to have greater promise for the task at hand. Two major reasons can be advanced for choosing to exhibit the structure of Kant's ethical system in reference to the second formulation of the categorical imperative. First, the second formulation embodies a central notion—respect for persons—that is somewhat easier to grasp and apply than the more formalistic notion of universalizability, which is the core element of the first formulation. Second, when argumentation in biomedical ethics reflects a Kantian viewpoint, it is almost always couched in terms of the second formulation rather than the first.

Kantian deontology is an ethics of respect for persons. In Kant's view, every person, by virtue of his or her humanity (i.e., rational nature) has an inherent dignity. All persons, as rational creatures, are entitled to respect, not only from others but from themselves as well. Thus, the categorical imperative directs each of us to "act in such a way that you always treat humanity, whether in your own person or in the person of any other, never simply as a means, but always at the same time as an end." From this fundamental principle, according to Kant, a host of particular duties can be derived. The resultant system of duties includes duties to self as well as duties to others. In each of these cases, "perfect duties" must be distinguished from "imperfect duties," thus generating a fourfold classification of duties: (1) perfect duties to self, (2) imperfect duties to self, (3) perfect duties to others, and (4) imperfect duties to others. Although the distinction between perfect and imperfect duties is not a transparent one, its structural importance in the Kantian system is hard to overemphasize. Perfect duties require that we do or abstain from certain acts. *There are no legitimate exceptions to a perfect duty.* Such duties are binding in all circumstances, because certain kinds of action are simply incompatible with respect for persons, hence strictly impermissible. Imperfect duties, by contrast, require us to pursue or promote certain goals (e.g., the welfare of others). However, action in the name of these goals must never be at the expense of a perfect duty. One of Kant's most prominent commentators relates the distinction between perfect and imperfect duties to the categorical imperative in the following way: "We transgress perfect duties by treating any person *merely* as a means. We transgress imperfect duties by failing to treat a person as an end, even though we do not actively treat him as a means."[13]

Our discussion of Kant's fourfold classification of duties begins with a consideration of perfect duties to others. A transgression in this category of duty occurs whenever one person treats another person merely as a means. It is strictly impermissible for person A to treat person B merely as a means because such treatment is incompatible with respect for B as a person. Notice that Kant does not claim that it is morally wrong for one person to use another as a means. His claim is that it is morally wrong for one person to use another *merely* as a means. In the ordinary course of life, it is surely unavoidable (and morally unproblematic) that each of us in numerous ways uses others as means to achieve our various ends. A college teacher uses students as a means to achieve his or her livelihood. A college student uses instructors as a means of gaining knowledge and skills. Such human interactions, presumably based on the voluntary participation of the respective parties, are quite compatible with a principle of respect for persons. However, respect for persons entails that each of us recognizes the rightful authority of other persons (as rational beings) to conduct their individual lives as they see fit. We may legitimately recruit others to participate in the satisfaction of our personal ends, but they are used merely as a means whenever we undermine the voluntary or informed character of their consent to interact with us in some desired way. Person A coerces person B at knifepoint to hand over $200. A uses B merely as a means. If A had requested of B a gift of $200, leaving B free to determine whether or not to make the gift, A would have proceeded in a manner compatible with respect for B as a person. Person C deceptively rolls back the odometer of a car and thereby manipulates person D's decision to buy the car. C uses D merely as a means. C has acted in a way that is strictly incompatible with respect for D as a person.

In the Kantian system, among the most notable of our perfect duties to others are (1) the duty not to kill an innocent person, (2) the duty not to lie, and (3) the duty to keep promises. Murdering an innocent person, lying, and promise breaking are actions that are intrinsically wrong. However beneficial the consequences of such an action might be in a given circumstance, the action is strictly impermissible. (Notice the anti-utilitarian character of Kant's thinking.) The murderer exhibits obvious disrespect for the person of the victim. The liar, in misinforming another person, violates the respect due to that person as a rational creature with a fundamental interest in the truth. A person who makes a promise issues a guarantee upon which the recipient of the promise is entitled to rely in his or her future planning. The person who breaks a promise shows disrespect for another by undermining the effort to conduct the affairs of one's life. By murdering, lying, or breaking a promise, an agent uses another person merely as a means to the agent's own ends.

According to Kant, each person has not only perfect duties to others but also perfect duties to self. The categorical imperative demands that no person (including oneself) be treated merely as a means. It is no more permissible to manifest disrespect for one's own person than to do so for the person of another. Kant insists, for example, that each person has a perfect duty to self to avoid drunkenness. Since drunkenness undermines a person's rational capacities, it is incompatible with respect for oneself as a rational creature. Kant believes that individuals debase themselves in the effort to achieve pleasure via inebriation. Inebriates treat themselves merely as a means (to the end of pleasure). Few modern Kantians share Kant's staunch opposition to getting drunk. They are more divided about the foremost example of a perfect duty to self in the Kantian system: the duty not to commit suicide. To terminate one's own life, Kant insists, is strictly incompatible with respect for oneself as a person. In eradicating one's very existence as a rational creature, a person treats oneself merely as a means (ordinarily to the end of avoiding discomfort or distress). Suicide is an action that is intrinsically wrong, and there are no circumstances in which it is morally permissible.

In addition to the notion of perfect duties (both to self and others), the Kantian system also incorporates the notion of imperfect duties. Whereas perfect duties require, in essence, strict abstention from those actions that involve using a person merely as a means, imperfect duties have a very different underlying sense. Imperfect duties require the promotion of certain goals. In broad terms, there are two such goals—an agent's personal perfection (i.e., development) and the happiness or welfare of others. Respect for oneself as a person requires commitment to the development of one's capacities as a rational being. Thus Kant spoke of an imperfect duty to self to develop one's talents. The sense of this duty is that, by and large, it is up to each individual to decide which talents to cultivate and which to deemphasize. But a person is not free to abandon the goal of personal development. Although the duty to develop one's talents requires no *specific* actions, it does require each individual to formulate a plan of life that embodies a commitment to the goal of personal development.

Before discussing Kant's final category of duty, imperfect duty to others, it will prove helpful to introduce the notion of *beneficence*.[14] If one acts in such a way as to further the happiness or welfare of another, then one acts beneficently. (A benevolent person is one who is inclined to act beneficently.) Beneficence may be contrasted with *nonmaleficence,* which is ordinarily understood as the noninfliction of harm on others. One who harms ("does evil" to) another acts in a maleficent fashion. One who *refrains* from harming others acts in a nonmaleficent fashion. One who acts, in a more positive way, to contribute to the welfare of others acts in a beneficent fashion. Beneficence is a generic notion that can best be understood as including the following types of activity: (1) preventing evil or harm from befalling someone, (2) removing an evil that is presently afflicting someone, and (3) providing benefits ("doing good") for someone. Although it is sometimes difficult to decide which of these categories is the most appropriate classification for a particular beneficent action, the following examples seem relatively straightforward. Pushing someone out of the path of an oncoming car is an example of the first type of activity. Curing a patient's disease is an example of the second. Giving someone a $100 gift is an example of the third.

According to Kant, respect for other persons requires not only that we avoid using them merely as a means (by the observance of our perfect duties to others), but also that we commit ourselves in some general way to furthering their happiness or welfare. Thus, Kant considers what we will call the "duty of beneficence" to be an imperfect duty to others. As with the duty to develop our talents, an imperfect duty to self, the duty of beneficence requires no *specific* actions. One does not violate the duty of beneficence by refusing to act beneficently in any individual case where the opportunity arises. What is required instead of specific actions is that each person incorporate into his or her lifeplan a commitment to promote the well-being of others. Individuals are free to choose the sorts of actions they will embrace in an effort to further the well-being of others (e.g., contributing to the relief of famine victims); they are not free to abandon the general goal of furthering the well-being of others.

Since the duty of beneficence is an imperfect duty in the Kantian system, action in the name of beneficence must never be taken at the expense of a perfect duty. For example, it is impermissible to lie or break a promise in an effort to save a third party from harm. The same is true with regard to the imperfect duty to develop one's talents. For example, if one has resolved (quite properly) to develop one's creative powers, it is nevertheless impermissible to do so by "creatively" defrauding others.

The Kantian Framework in a Biomedical Context With our exposition of Kantian deontology now complete, we are in a position to exhibit some of the more important implications of this ethical theory in the realm of biomedical ethics. To begin with, the theory has an obvious relevance to the much-discussed problem of whether or not a physician may justifiably lie to a patient (an issue discussed in Chapter 2). Since every person has a perfect duty to others not to lie, a straightforward implication of Kantian deontology is that a physician may *never* lie to a patient. If a patient diagnosed as terminally ill by a physician inquires about his or her prognosis, the physician may be much inclined to lie, motivated by a desire to protect the patient from the psychological turmoil that would accompany knowledge of his or her true condition; however, action in the name of beneficence (an imperfect duty) may never be at the expense of a perfect duty. This same analysis is relevant to the use of placebos by physicians. Sometimes a patient becomes psychologically dependent on a certain medication. When the medication is discontinued, because the physician is convinced it is no longer needed and because its continued use represents a threat to health, the patient complains of the reemergence of symptoms. If such a patient is given a placebo, that is, a therapeutically inert but harmless substance, misrepresented as a medication, the patient may feel fine. Nevertheless, despite the fact that placebos may be capable of enhancing patient welfare, their use is morally impermissible, at least in cases involving an explicit lie.

Kantian deontology has some very important and very direct implications for the ethics of experimentation with human subjects (a topic discussed in Chapter 4). Since it is morally wrong for any person to use any other person merely as a means, it follows that it is morally wrong for a biomedical researcher to use a human research subject merely as a means. From this consideration it is but a short step to the requirement of voluntary informed consent as a basic principle of research ethics. If a researcher is engaged in a study that involves human subjects, we may presume that the immediate "end" being sought by the researcher is the successful completion of the study. But notice that the researcher may desire this particular end for any number of reasons: the speculative understanding it will provide; the technology it will make possible; the eventual benefit to humankind; personal recognition in the eyes of the scientific community; a raise in pay; and so forth. This mixture of self-centered and benevolent motivations may be considered the researcher's less immediate ends. If researchers are to avoid using their research subjects merely as means (to the ends of the researchers), surely they must refrain from coercing the participation of their subjects and must provide information about the research project (most notably, risks to the subjects) sufficient for the subjects to make a rational decision with regard to their personal participation.

Thus, respect for persons demands that researchers honor the requirement of voluntary informed consent.

Suppose a researcher explains to a potential research subject how important it is that he or she consent to participate. There is no question but that the research project at issue, if brought to a successful conclusion, will provide substantial benefit to humankind. Does the potential subject have a moral obligation to participate? Surely not. Within the framework of Kantian deontology, the duty of beneficence is an imperfect duty. A person must on occasion act beneficently, but there is no obligation to perform any *specific* beneficent action.

Critical Assessment of Kantian Deontology Are the implications of Kantian deontology largely reconcilable with our experience of the moral life? Can this theory provide effective guidance in the face of perceived moral dilemmas? These two questions reflect the criteria suggested earlier as most central to the assessment of the relative adequacy of an ethical theory.

Before indicating some of the ways in which Kantian deontology can be thought to be at odds with our ordinary moral thinking, it is important to emphasize that the theory does successfully account for crucial aspects of our experience of the moral life. To begin with, Kantian deontology provides an obvious foundation for the "commonsense rules of morality." The wrongfulness of actions that fly in the face of these rules—actions such as killing, injuring, stealing, lying, breaking promises—can very plausibly be understood as flowing from the categorical imperative. The Kantian deontologist maintains that these actions are wrong because they involve treating another person merely as a means, and there is something very compelling about the notion of respect for persons as the core notion of morality.

Kantian deontology also seems to provide a secure foundation for the notion of individual rights, a notion that is very prominent in our ordinary moral thinking. Individual rights, in the Kantian system, are to be understood as the correlates of our perfect duties to others. (Imperfect duties, in contrast, do not generate rights.) For example, each of us has a perfect *duty* not to kill an innocent person; thus, every innocent person has a *right* not to be killed. More generally, every person has a right not to be used by another merely as a means. An innocent person has a right not to be punished, no matter how socially desirable the consequences might be in a certain set of circumstances. A potential research subject has a right not to be coerced or deceived into participation, even if the satisfactory completion of the study promises great benefit for humankind. In its insistence that individual rights cannot be overridden by "utilitarian" considerations, Kantian deontology achieves accord with our firmly entrenched (if somewhat vague) conviction that the end does not justify the means.

However, there are aspects of Kantian deontology that cannot be easily reconciled with our experience of the moral life. One very prominent difficulty has to do with the Kantian contention that keeping promises and not lying are both duties of perfect obligation. We are quite at home, in our ordinary moral thinking, with both a duty to keep promises and a duty not to lie, but it is the exceptionless character of these duties in the Kantian system that we find troublesome. Surely in extreme cases, we are inclined to say, these duties must yield to more weighty moral considerations. For example, if a person breaks a rather trivial promise (say, to return a book at a certain time) in order to respond to the needs of a person in serious distress, surely he or she has not acted immorally. Or again, if a person lies to a would-be murderer about the whereabouts of the intended victim, surely the liar has not (all things considered) acted immorally. The Kantian deontologist sees in such examples a clash between a perfect duty and the imperfect duty of beneficence, and the Kantian teaching is that the former may never yield to the latter. But it would seem that a theory with such implausible implications stands in need of revision. Perhaps the problem is not only that Kantian deontology overstates the significance of certain "perfect" duties, but also that it understates the significance of the duty of beneficence, at least that aspect of beneficence that has to do with preventing serious harm from befalling another or alleviating the serious distress of another.

In our everyday existence as moral agents, we are accustomed to the idea that we have a number of important duties to others. It is less clear that the Kantian notion of duties to self can be satisfactorily reconciled with our experience of the moral life. This is difficult territory. For one thing, the issue of suicide (discussed in Chapter 6) seems to confound our moral "common sense" in a way that blatant wrongs such as murder, rape, and slavery do not. Still, despite significant disagreement, suicide is considered by many to be morally wrong. But the issue is this: Do those who consider suicide morally wrong experience the duty not to commit suicide as a duty to self? It seems more likely that this duty is experienced as a duty to others (who may be negatively affected by one's suicide) or, in the case of religious believers, as a duty to God. (Whether a similar argument would be persuasive with regard to the imperfect duty to develop one's talents is unclear.)

It cannot be denied that Kantian deontology, to a substantial degree, is reconcilable with our experience of the moral life. On the other hand, it appears that the theory is attended with some significant and unresolved difficulties. How does Kantian deontology fare when measured against the second of our standards, the requirement that an ethical theory provide effective guidance in the face of moral dilemmas? Once again, it seems, the verdict is somewhat mixed.

It might be argued that Kantian deontology, by sorting our various duties into the categories of perfect and imperfect and assigning priority to perfect duties, provides us with a structure in terms of which moral dilemmas can be resolved. This is perhaps true to the extent that our perplexity can be analyzed in terms of perfect duties marshaled against imperfect duties, but even here it is difficult to overlook the fact that the priority of perfect over imperfect duties is itself a somewhat problematic feature of Kantian deontology. One is tempted to say that, even if the theory provides reasonably *clear* guidance, it sometimes fails to provide *correct* guidance.

W. D. ROSS'S THEORY OF PRIMA FACIE DUTIES

In a book entitled *The Right and the Good* (1930), English philosopher W. D. Ross proposed a deontological theory that has received considerable attention among ethical theorists. The point of departure for the development of Ross's theory is his concern to provide a defensible account of "cases of conscience," that is, situations that confront us with a conflict of duties. One perceived line of obligation pulls us in one direction; another perceived line of obligation pulls us in a contrary direction. We find ourselves unsettled and uncertain but cannot avoid a choice. Which duty takes precedence over the other? The parent of a young child has promised to attend a community meeting, but the child seems to need special attention. Since our social existence is complex, conflict-of-duty situations are a recurrent feature of our daily life. In the biomedical context, such situations are pervasive.

For understandable reasons, Ross maintains that neither the Kantian nor the utilitarian can provide an account of conflict-of-duty situations that harmonizes with what he calls "ordinary moral consciousness." We have just considered the relevant deficiency in the Kantian approach. It is implausible to maintain that the duty of beneficence can never take precedence over the duty to keep promises or the duty not to lie. As for the utilitarian approach (and here it is clear that Ross has act-utilitarianism in mind), this theory's insistence that in reality we have only the one duty of maximizing utility clashes with our conviction that we have distinct lines of obligation to distinct people. In order to provide an adequate account of conflict-of-duty situations, Ross maintains, it is essential to introduce the notion of "prima facie duty." The Latin phrase *prima facie,* now commonplace in moral philosophy, literally means "at first glance." But the word *conditional* best expresses the sense of the phrase as Ross intends it. A prima facie duty is a conditional duty. A prima facie duty (as opposed to an absolute duty) can be overridden by another prima facie duty that in a particular set of circumstances is more stringent.

According to Ross, there are no absolute, or unconditional, duties (such as "Never lie"), only prima facie duties. But what is the basis of our prima facie duties? Both the utilitarian and the Kantian assert that our various duties have a unitary basis in a fundamental principle of morality. The utilitarian believes that our various duties can be derived from the principle of utility. The Kantian believes that our various duties can be derived from the categorical imperative. Ross, in vivid contrast, maintains that our various prima facie duties have no unitary basis. Rather, they emerge out of our numerous "morally significant relations," relations such as promisee to promiser, creditor to debtor, spouse to spouse, child to parent, friend to friend, citizen to the state, fellow human being to fellow human being. "Each of these relations is the foundation of a *prima facie* duty, which is more or less incumbent on me according to the circumstances of the case."[15]

In unproblematic circumstances, where we are bound by only one prima facie duty, this particular prima facie duty is our *actual* duty. In conflict-of-duty situations, where two (or more) prima facie duties compete for priority, only one of these duties, the more stringent one in the circumstances, can be our actual duty. We have, for example, both a prima facie duty to keep promises and a prima facie duty to assist those who are in need. According to Ross, when these two duties come into conflict, it is clear (in terms of our "ordinary moral consciousness") that the duty to keep promises is usually more incumbent upon us than the duty to assist those who are in need. However, if the promise is relatively trivial and the need of another is compelling—a matter of serious distress—then it is equally clear that the priority is reversed. In the difficult cases, Ross maintains, there is in principle no hard-and-fast rule to apply. In his view, the best anyone can do is to make a reflective, "considered decision" as to which of the competing prima facie duties has the priority in any given situation.

According to Ross, "there is nothing arbitrary about [our] *prima facie* duties. Each rests on a definite circumstance which cannot seriously be held to be without moral significance."[16] Accordingly, he proposes the following division of our prima facie duties.

(1) *Duties of fidelity* include keeping promises, honoring contracts and agreements, and telling the truth. Duties in this class rest on a person's previous acts. In giving one's word to do something, a person creates the duty to do so. (Ross thinks that by entering a conversation, a person implicitly agrees to tell the truth.) Notice that a person's so-called role responsibilities can be identified as an important subclass of duties of fidelity. For example, a teacher has certain responsibilities as a teacher, a physician certain responsibilities as a physician, and a nurse certain responsibilities as a nurse. In taking on a certain social role, a person brings into existence various duties of fidelity. In addition, further duties of fidelity arise out of agreements (both explicit and implicit) that a person enters into while functioning in a professional capacity.

(2) *Duties of reparation* also rest on a person's previous acts. Any person, by wrongfully treating someone else, creates the duty to rectify the wrong that has been perpetrated. For example, if A steals a certain amount of money from B, A thereby brings into existence the duty to repay this amount. (3) *Duties of gratitude* rest upon previous acts of other persons, namely, beneficial services provided by them. If A has provided a good service for B when B was in need, B thereby stands under a duty to provide a good service for A when A is in need.

(4) *Duties of beneficence* "rest on the mere fact that there are other beings in the world whose condition we can make better."[17] (5) *Duties of nonmaleficence* rest on the complementary fact that we can also make the condition of other beings worse. The duties in this category, which Ross recognizes as especially stringent, can be summed up under the heading of "not injuring others." The duty not to kill is an obvious example.

(6) *Duties of justice* "rest on the fact or possibility of a distribution of pleasure or happiness (or of the means thereto) which is not in accordance with the merit of the persons concerned."[18] Benefits are to be distributed in accordance with personal merit, and existing unjust patterns of distribution are to be rectified. (7) *Duties of self-improvement* "rest on the fact that we can improve our own condition."[19]

Prima Facie Duties in a Biomedical Context Ross's framework of prima facie duties is helpful for conceptualizing many of the moral dilemmas that arise in a biomedical context. In analyzing such dilemmas as they arise from the point of view of health-care professionals, the category of duties of fidelity is especially important. Consider, for example, the physician-patient relationship (a topic discussed in Chapter 2). The social understanding or implicit agreement that underlies this relationship undoubtedly includes a number of important provisions. Among these are the provision that the physician is to act in the best medical interest of the patient and the provision that the physician is to keep confidential any personal information that comes to light within the context of the physician-patient relationship. In the very act of accepting a patient for treatment, a physician thereby incurs a number of important prima facie duties of fidelity.

Suppose a physician is convinced that lying to a patient is in the best medical interest of the patient. In Ross's scheme, the prima facie duty not to lie, itself a duty of fidelity, comes into conflict with another duty of fidelity, the prima facie duty to act in the best medical interest of the patient. Since neither duty is unconditional, in one case the duty not to lie might be more incumbent upon the physician, whereas in another case the duty to act in the best interest of the patient might be the more stringent duty. Suppose, in a different case, a physician is treating a patient suffering from a condition that renders the patient in his or her occupation a danger to others. In addition, suppose that the patient is a bus driver subject to blackouts. The patient is desperate to keep his or her job and refuses to divulge the problem to his or her employer. Should the physician break medical confidentiality and notify the patient's employer in an effort to ensure the public safety? In this case, the prima facie duty of beneficence comes into conflict with a duty of fidelity, the prima facie duty to keep medical confidentiality. (Justifiable exceptions to the duty to keep medical confidentiality are discussed in Chapter 2.)

Among the explicit role responsibilities of a typical hospital nurse is the obligation to follow a physician's orders in the treatment of patients. By the simple act of accepting employment in the hospital setting, a nurse thereby incurs, among other numerous duties of fidelity, the prima facie duty to obey a physician's orders. An important moral dilemma for the hospital nurse arises when, in the judgment of the nurse, following a physician's order would be detrimental to the patient. (This dilemma is discussed in Chapter 2.) Thinking in terms of Ross's theory, we can structure the dilemma as follows. The prima facie duty to follow a physician's orders comes into conflict with two other prima facie duties. First, there is a relevant duty of nonmaleficence. A nurse should not act in a way that would, in effect, injure another person. Second, there is another relevant duty of fidelity, deriving from the fact that a nurse has an implicit contract or agreement with the patient to act in his or her best medical interest. Is the collective force of these two prima facie duties more incumbent upon the nurse than the prima facie duty to follow a physician's orders? Since the duty of nonmaleficence is recognized by Ross (and "ordinary moral consciousness") as especially stringent, it seems that, in most cases, at least where the potential harm to patients is significant, the nurse must conclude that it would be wrong to follow the physician's order.

Abstracting from any relevant role responsibilities on the part of health-care professionals, the issue of the moral justifiability of active euthanasia (discussed in Chapter 6) might be conceptualized, in accordance with Ross's scheme, as a moral dilemma involving the conflict between a duty of beneficence and a duty of nonmaleficence. A terminally ill person suffering unbearable pain could be understood to benefit from an immediate and painless death. Thus, we have on one hand a duty of beneficence—the prima facie duty to come to the assistance of a person in serious distress—and on the other hand a duty of nonmaleficence—the prima facie duty not to kill.

Critical Assessment of Ross's Theory Since Ross developed his theory of prima facie duties explicitly in reference to the promptings of "ordinary moral consciousness," it would be surprising if his theory could not be reconciled with our experience of the moral life. Indeed, let us put aside whatever worries might be expressed on this score, for there is a much more obvious deficiency in Ross's theory. Recall that we have asked not only that an ethical theory be largely reconcilable with our experience of the moral life but also that it provide us with effective guidance where it is most needed, in the face of moral dilemmas. And despite the fact that Ross's theory provides us with a helpful framework for conceptualizing our moral dilemmas, it provides us with virtually no substantive guidance for resolving them.

In the difficult cases, where two prima facie duties come into strong conflict, Ross holds that there are no principles we can appeal to in an effort to make an appropriate decision. The most we can do, in his view, is render a "considered decision" as to which duty is more incumbent upon us in a certain situation. Although it is fine to be told to make a considered decision, what exactly is worthy of consideration in reaching a decision? At this point, there is a strong argument for moving beyond Ross's theory. One plausible approach would identify *considerations of coherence* (within our overall system of moral convictions) as the relevant standard. (See the discussion "Reflective Equilibrium and Appeals to Coherence" later in this chapter.) If Ross's theory were supplemented with a coherence-based decision procedure, the advantages of thinking in terms of prima facie duties could be combined with a plausible methodology for mediating among conflicting duties.

THE PRINCIPLES OF BIOMEDICAL ETHICS

One prominent approach to problems in biomedical ethics has been articulated by Tom Beauchamp and James Childress in *Principles of Biomedical Ethics,* originally published in 1979. The basic idea is that problems can be appropriately identified, analyzed, and resolved by reference to a set of four principles, each of which corresponds to a prima facie (i.e., conditional) obligation. The four principles, tailored specifically to be relevant in the field of biomedical ethics, are as follows: the principle of respect for autonomy, the principle of nonmaleficence, the principle of beneficence, and the principle of justice.

This distinctive principle-based approach has much in common with W. D. Ross's theory of prima facie duties, which can also be understood as a principle-based approach. In each case, we are dealing with several prima facie principles of obligation. So in each case, it is common for the principles of the system to conflict, thus requiring a judgment as to which principle has overriding weight or significance in any particular set of circumstances.[20]

Frequent references to "the principles of biomedical ethics," both individually and collectively, can be found in the literature of biomedical ethics (including the readings collected in this textbook). As presented by Beauchamp and Childress, each of the principles must ultimately be understood by reference to numerous distinctions and clarifications. For our purposes, however, it is useful to identify a central (if less than complete) meaning for each principle. The *principle of respect for autonomy* requires that health-care professionals not interfere with the effective exercise of patient autonomy. (A suggested analysis of the concept of autonomy is presented in a later section of this chapter.) The *principle of nonmaleficence* requires that health-care professionals not act in ways that entail harm or injury to patients. The *principle of beneficence* requires that health-care professionals act in ways that promote patient welfare. (The closely related concepts of beneficence and nonmaleficence are briefly explicated in our earlier discussion of Kantian deontology.) The *principle of justice* requires that social benefits (e.g., health-care services) and social burdens (e.g., taxes) be distributed in accordance with the demands of justice. Although this articulation of the principle of justice is somewhat uninformative, it is impossible to give the principle any clearer content without considering questions that are at issue in competing theories of distributive justice. These theories are discussed in the introduction to Chapter 9.

ALTERNATIVE DIRECTIONS AND METHODS

By the 1990s a challenge was well under way both to recently dominant ethical theories (that is, those theories—discussed earlier—that commanded the most attention in the twentieth century) and to the idea that these theories can simply be *applied* to generate satisfactory solutions to concrete problems. In biomedical ethics, criticisms have increasingly been directed at two broad approaches to ethical reasoning. These approaches are known as *deductivism* and *principle-based ethics* (also called "principlism"). A deductivist theory, such as utilitarianism or Kantianism, features a single foundational principle that supposedly provides a basis for all ethical justification.[21] According to this approach, correct ethical judgments can, in principle, be derived from the foundation, given relevant factual information (e.g., concerning the consequences of possible actions, in utilitarianism). As we saw in the previous section, principle-based ethics features a framework of several principles, rules, or duties, none of which takes absolute priority over any other. In principle-based ethics, as it is commonly understood,[22] one considers whatever principles, rules, or duties are relevant in the circumstances, settling conflicts by determining which seems more weighty.[23] Specific criticisms of deductivism and principle-based ethics will emerge in the discussions of leading alternative approaches.

VIRTUE ETHICS

An emphasis on the moral evaluation of *actions* is common both to deductivist theories and to principle-based ethics. These approaches offer principles or rules of conduct as their main source of moral guidance. One is directed to maximize utility, never to treat persons as mere means to one's ends, or the like. Sometimes principles or rules are expressed in the language of rights and duties. For example, it is said that competent adults have a right to refuse medical treatment and health-care professionals have a duty to respect the decision making of competent adults. In contrast, virtue ethics, the tradition of Plato and Aristotle, gives *virtuous character* a preeminent place. For our purposes, virtues may be understood as character traits that are morally valued, such as truthfulness, courage, compassion, and sincerity. In virtue ethics, agents—those performing the actions—are the focus. Whereas the principal concern in an action-based approach to ethics is with the right thing to do, the principal concern in a virtue-based approach is with what kind of person to be.

In recent years there has been a significant revival of virtue ethics, a development affecting bioethics. Some theorists have argued that mainstream theories have overemphasized action-guides to the neglect of issues of character. What is needed, they maintain, is a *supplementation* of action-based ethics with virtue ethics. Other theorists have defended the more radical thesis that the neglect of virtue has caused action-based ethical theories to be *importantly misconceived* (so that merely supplementing them is insufficient). Among these theorists, some have argued for a robust *integration* of action-based ethics and virtue ethics (without giving priority to either), while others have gone further, calling for the *replacement* of action-based ethics by virtue ethics.

What arguments can be advanced in favor of virtue ethics? One difficulty with theories that are solely action-based is that they seem to neglect the fact that we often morally judge people's motivations and character, not just their actions. For example, in praising someone's kindness or criticizing a person's meanness, our evaluation makes no explicit reference to actions. Sometimes we even fault a person who acts rightly but with questionable motivation or attitude. For example, consider a person who gives to charities only when seeking public office, or a surgeon who only begrudgingly solicits a patient's informed consent to surgery. Conversely, sometimes we temper our blame of a person who has acted wrongly if, in doing so, admirable motives and character traits were displayed. For example, we might moderate our criticism of someone who lied to assuage another's feelings, even if we think lying was the wrong choice.

Another argument addresses what is most useful in guiding moral choice. It is claimed that principles, rules, and codes are of little use in actual decision making (e.g., in biomedical contexts). Such action-guides are too abstract to provide practical guidance. Moreover, they often conflict. (The suggestion that conflicts can be effectively resolved by appeal to an ethical theory immediately confronts the problem that there is such extensive disagreement on which theory is most adequate.) A more effective approach, according to this argument, is to cultivate enduring traits (such as competence, attentiveness, honesty, compassion, and loyalty) through education, the influence of role models, and habitual exercise of those traits. Such virtues, it is claimed, are a more reliable basis, in practice, for morally correct action than is knowledge of principles, rules, or codes.

The arguments surveyed so far are compatible with the program of supplementing action-based theories with virtue ethics. Even the idea that virtues are more useful in practice is consistent with these claims: (1) Ethics is more centrally concerned with what people should do (virtues being generally reliable means for doing the right thing); (2) right action, in principle, can be characterized without reference to virtue. However, the following arguments are more radical. They suggest that virtue is often at least as morally important or fundamental as right action and that sometimes the latter cannot even be characterized independently of virtue.

First, several philosophers have argued that in many cases right action cannot be described in an illuminating way without referring to virtue. Consider the idea that we should help those who are suffering. (This idea expresses a principle of action.) Truly helping someone often requires keen attention to the subtleties of the situation at hand to determine whether, and what sort of, intervention is called for. Would calling a particular student aside, telling him or her an anecdote, and offering advice be helpful, or would it be intrusive and condescending? One cannot reliably perform acts that are helpful (as opposed to intrusive or condescending) without exercising a capacity for discernment, which involves such virtues as emotional attunement and sympathetic insightfulness.[24] Since being helpful in such circumstances involves being virtuous, the proper conclusion is that virtue partly constitutes right action.

Second, the manner in which we act—what we express in our action—can matter as much as, or more than, what we do. (We might even say that our manner of acting is part of what we do.) Suppose Earl borrows money from his brother, Jake, and promises to repay him within a month. Four weeks later Jake gently reminds Earl of his promise. If Earl later storms into his brother's house, slams down the money, and marches off in resentment and anger, he has fulfilled his duty to keep a promise, but he has not acted well. A full account of how Earl should have conducted himself would include a description of the manner in which he should have acted (perhaps courteously). Here, again, the conclusion is that virtue partly constitutes right action.

Moreover, sometimes emotional responses, which can reveal a person's character, are of paramount moral importance (a point suggested in the last example). This is especially evident in situations in which no particular action is morally called for. For example, a social worker might be deeply affected by another social worker's detailed account of a patient who lost his job and committed suicide. If the two work at different hospitals, there is probably nothing the first social worker can do about the tragedy. However, her pain at a stranger's plight reveals virtue; complete indifference arguably would reveal a moral deficiency.[25]

While the previous arguments probably succeed in showing the need to integrate virtue ethics and action-based ethics, there are compelling reasons to resist the stronger thesis that virtue ethics should *replace* action-based approaches. First, while action-guides such as principles and rules are not exhaustive of what is important in the moral life, neither is virtue. One can be well motivated and have a good character yet act wrongly; conversely, acting without virtue does not *always* mean doing the wrong thing. (This is consistent with the view that virtue sometimes partly constitutes right action.) Morally, we are concerned with both action and character, doing and being.

Second, the specificity of such action-guides as rules, codes, and rights-claims often provides an attractive form of bottom-line moral protection. Rules such as those requiring informed consent for medical interventions and prohibiting psychotherapists from having sexual relations with psychiatric patients provide an important bedrock of action require-ments. In fact, such rules can often help professionals establish relationships with patients in which certain virtues can be exercised more naturally.

Similarly, it seems unlikely that any specification of virtues would be sufficient to guide conduct. In bioethics we are interested in such questions as "Is it ever right for a psy-chotherapist to violate patient confidentiality, and, if so, when?" Such a question probably cannot be answered by appeal to virtue alone. In conclusion, it would seem that an adequate portrait of the moral life would include action-guides such as principles, rules, and rights-claims—not just virtues. The question we are left with, then, is not whether both virtues and action-guides have important places in ethical theory and bioethics but, rather, how to un-derstand in greater detail their roles and relationship to one another.

How might virtues play a role in biomedical ethics? Here is one example. A physician has just received test results strongly suggesting that her thirty-year-old patient has inopera-ble ovarian cancer. Neither of them expected such a calamity. The physician knows that she has an obligation to inform her patient of the results. However, in reflecting on how to broach and discuss this matter with her, the physician finds such principles as beneficence and non-maleficence too general to be useful; no helpful rules of conduct come to mind, either. The physician keeps coming back to such ideas as *compassion, sensitivity,* and *honesty.* Although these words describe virtues, we could say that "Be compassionate," "Be sensitive," and "Be honest" are rules of action. Nevertheless, such instructions do not really tell the physician how to handle her delicate predicament. To handle it well, she will have to *be* compassion-ate, sensitive, and honest, and no set of rules can explain how to be that way. The physician, in other words, will have to manifest virtue. She might find it useful to model her behavior on that of a mentor or colleague whom she identifies as having the desired qualities.

THE ETHICS OF CARE AND FEMINIST ETHICS

The ethics of care and feminist ethics represent further challenges to recently dominant ethi-cal theories, to deductivism, and to principle-based ethics. While the ethics of care and feminist ethics both stem importantly from the moral experience of women, they represent overlapping—but certainly not identical—sets of concerns.

Like virtue ethics, the ethics of care pays considerable attention to affective compo-nents of the moral life, but with special emphasis on empathy and concern for the needs of others, that is, on caring. Like casuistry (an approach discussed in the next section), the ethics of care emphasizes the particularities and context of moral judgment. It also under-scores the moral importance of relationships and the responsibilities to which they give rise.

Perhaps more than any other work, Carol Gilligan's study of gender differences in ethi-cal thinking has brought the ethics of care into the mainstream of philosophical discussion.[26] In a study of responses to moral conflicts, Gilligan finds that females often focus on details about the relationships among the persons involved and seek innovative solutions that pro-tect everyone's interests. In contrast, males typically try to identify and apply a relevant prin-ciple or rule (which they take to be universal or valid from an impartial perspective), even if doing so means sacrificing someone's interests. Gilligan calls the former approach an *ethic of care* (or responsibility) and the latter (which includes recently dominant ethical theories) an *ethic of justice.* She notes in her study that the empirical correlations are far from per-fect; males sometimes work from the care perspective and women fairly often use the jus-tice approach. In any event, the tendencies she notes are striking, for they suggest that traditional approaches to ethics have been more responsive to the moral experience of males than to that of females. Gilligan concludes that there is no reason to consider the care perspective inferior and that an ideal ethics would incorporate both approaches.

As originally characterized by Gilligan and now generally understood, the ethics of care downplays rights and allegedly universal principles and rules in favor of an emphasis on caring, interpersonal relationships, and context. Numerous specific criticisms of recently dominant ethical theories have been developed in the ethics of care literature. A summary of several critical arguments follows.

To begin with, there is a problematic presumption underlying theories such as utilitarianism and Kantianism. The presumption is that impartiality is a fundamental aspect of moral thinking. In reality, impartiality is a demand reflective of male thinking; the partiality that comes with caring relationships is no less legitimate. Indeed, certain relationships merit special weight. For example, in many contexts, a father should favor his own children's interests over those of other children.[27] Moreover, the abstract principles of traditional theories have very limited practical use; contextualization and attention to detail are needed for problem solving in ethics. In many complex situations involving ethical conflicts, such principles as "Respect all persons as ends in themselves" and "Maximize utility" simply provide inadequate guidance.

Furthermore, ethical theories featuring abstract principles tend to neglect affective components of the moral life. Caring responsiveness to others' needs is often morally preferable to detached, dispassionate moral evaluation. For example, the ethics of care would strongly affirm a health-care professional's heartfelt dedication to a patient, without conditioning its value on good consequences or respect for persons. The abstract nature of recently dominant theories also tends to cover up certain morally salient experiences—such as being a woman, a parent, a minority, or a professional who has particular working relationships with other professionals.

A health-care professional working within the spirit of the ethics of care would bear in mind (or internalize) considerations such as these: (1) the individualized needs, both physical and psychological, of the patient; (2) how to respond in a caring, personalized manner to those needs; (3) the likely impact of various options on the quality of the relationships among the involved persons, including the patient and professional, but also other members of the health-care team and any involved family members; and (4) how to attain or maintain the best possible relationships among those persons. Suppose a nurse faces a conflict between loyalty to a patient and loyalty to the attending physician, who refuses to disclose certain medical options to the patient. The "justice" approach might view the dilemma in terms of overall utility, conflicting rights, or the like. In contrast, the ethics of care would emphasize the lived relationships and the responsibilities inherent in them, the impact of possible responses on those relationships, and the prospects for conflict resolution.

The relationship between *feminist ethics* and the ethics of care is a complex one, and this complexity is reflected in the different ways that various feminists have responded to the emergence and widespread discussion of the ethics of care. Some feminists have celebrated the reception accorded the ethics of care and feel validated by the recognition of a distinctly female moral perspective. Others, however, have reacted negatively to at least certain aspects of the ethics of care.

Feminist ethics can be initially characterized in the following ways. (1) As with the ethics of care, it is firmly committed to the view that the moral experience of women must be taken seriously (but often with a critical eye to the role that the subordination of women may play in shaping that experience). (2) It is deeply committed to the overriding moral importance of ending oppression—with special emphasis on the subordination of women.

These features of feminist ethics together motivate a redirection of focus to women (and, to an important extent, minorities and other historically disadvantaged groups). This focus includes both an emphasis on the importance of women's interests and special attention to issues that especially concern or affect women. Thus, in bioethics, feminist ethics urges careful examination of the interests of women in matters of reproduction and as the almost exclusive participants in the profession of nursing. Special attention is also given, for example, to the distinctive needs of women in the area of medical research, to the moral complexities of surrogate motherhood, and to arguably sexist undercurrents in the promotion of in vitro fertilization and in various medical practices surrounding childbirth.

In feminist ethics, a critical eye is turned toward practices and institutions that may perpetuate and legitimate forms of oppression. Some of these practices and institutions, feminists argue, are so deeply embedded in our culture that they go unnoticed. Accordingly, some feminists have charged proponents of the ethics of care with naïveté for accepting women's moral experiences at face value—without questioning the oppressive practices and attitudes that may have helped make certain experiences and ways of thinking typical for women. Perhaps women's proficiency at caring is related to their subordinate status.[28] In fact, nurturing, caring, and the disposition to preserve relationships at almost any cost may simply be the survival skills of an oppressed group; it has been noted that such dispositions are also found among persons of both genders who are members of groups that have been subjected to slavery or colonization.[29] Some feminists also argue that the value of mothering, so affirmed in the ethics of care, may be tied to the norm of the nuclear family—a norm that can be seen as discounting the perspectives of homosexuals, persons in single-parent families, and others who remain legally unmarried. They point out that caring has led some women to direct nearly all of their energies to others' needs, without adequately attending to their own. While caring is an admirable trait in many circumstances, these feminists maintain, it is sometimes better withheld when a focus on rights and autonomy is necessary. In general, they conclude, we must not valorize the traits that tend to perpetuate women's subordinate status.[30]

How might we assess the ethics of care and feminist ethics as alternatives to recently dominant theories and to the idea that these theories can simply be applied in order to resolve concrete problems? The care perspective's emphasis on relationships and the affective components of the moral life merits careful attention; arguably, the traditional theories greatly understate their significance. (Ross's theory, which highlights morally significant relationships, is a partial exception.) The critical-minded attention of feminist ethics to oppression, inequalities, and issues pertaining to women and other disadvantaged groups is surely valuable. In addition, the feminist caution about gender stereotyping is well taken. Uncritical acceptance of traditionally feminine and masculine qualities may lead too easily to the assignment of people to "appropriate" roles (such as women to midnight infant feedings and men to aggressive professional pursuits).

However, the distance between the perspectives presently under discussion, on the one hand, and recently dominant theories, on the other, can easily be overdrawn. Utilitarians, for example, should be firmly dedicated to the eradication of oppression (given all of its bad consequences). Kantian respect for persons, while perhaps vague and abstract, is at least compatible with caring and special relationships (the validity of which could be impartially recognized). Caring attention to particularities might even provide a useful way of specifying or supplementing abstract but worthy principles. A sophisticated Kantian, for example, will attend to concrete particulars and relationships in moral deliberation, even if these details are often missing from simplified, textbook discussions.

In the end, Gilligan argues that "care" and "justice" are both only parts of a broader ethics, and few proponents of the care perspective propose that it monopolize ethics. In a pluralistic spirit, one might adopt a similar attitude toward feminist ethics, concentrating on whatever insight and illumination this perspective brings to ethics. Following is a concluding suggestion from feminist philosopher Susan Sherwin:

> I do not envision feminist ethics to be a comprehensive . . . theory that can be expected to resolve every moral question with which it is confronted. It is a theoretical perspective that must be combined with other considerations to address the multitude of moral dilemmas that confront human beings. . . . Although very little of the literature in ethics addresses the issue of sexism or any other form of systematic oppression, surely the responsibility to do so in one's moral evaluations is implicit. Feminist ethics has assumed leadership in pursuing such analysis.[31]

CASUISTRY: CASE-BASED REASONING IN HISTORICAL CONTEXT

Casuistry, which has received a great deal of attention in recent years, is a method of moral reasoning that was reawakened from three centuries of slumber with the publication of *The Abuse of Casuistry,* by Albert Jonsen and Stephen Toulmin.[32] Following Aristotle and other philosophers as well as theologians throughout the ages, the authors contend that the "top-down" reasoning inherent in deductivism and principle-based ethics (as they understand it) is entirely inadequate for the resolution of concrete problems, such as those that arise in bioethics. (Jonsen and Toulmin never clearly distinguish deductivism and principle-based ethics. While some of their criticisms concern both approaches, others concern only deductivism.)

First, according to the casuists, no simple, unified ethical theory can capture the great diversity of our moral ideas, a consideration that helps to account for the fact that there is such extensive disagreement about ethical theories. Second, our actual moral thinking does not typically consist of straightforward deductive reasoning (deriving an ethical judgment from a supreme principle). *Practical wisdom* is required to determine which of various norms (principles or rules) applies in a complicated or ambiguous case. For example, if a patient awaiting admission to a fully occupied intensive care unit better fulfills admission criteria than someone already admitted, would it ever be right to admit the waiting patient if doing so would be detrimental to the one who would be displaced? Casuists doubt that the answers to such questions can be derived from a traditional ethical theory, such as utilitarianism or Kantianism, or from a set of abstract principles. Third, such approaches miss the fact that moral certainty, where it exists, concerns particular cases. For example, that a particular person acts wrongly in torturing for sadistic pleasure is far more certain than any full-blown ethical theory could be.

The alternative of casuistry is a form of case-based reasoning. It begins with clear "paradigm" cases in which some *maxim* (a relatively specific principle or rule) is clearly relevant and indicates the right action or judgment. For example, if we learn that a man stole a car just for a thrill, we know he acted wrongly. From this and similar cases we can extract a maxim, "Stealing is wrong," which holds in the absence of unusual circumstances. The paradigm cases illuminate other cases by way of analogy. Maxims are refined as new cases are confronted in which the norms apply ambiguously (for example, if someone finds an expensive watch in a classroom and does not attempt to locate its owner) or in conflict (for example, if someone believes that temporarily appropriating a bicycle is the only way to save an innocent person's life). Often, the refinements involve stating exceptions.

In order to reach a defensible moral judgment in any particular case, we must first determine which paradigms are relevant. Difficulties arise, of course, when paradigms fit only ambiguously or when two or more paradigms fit in conflicting ways. Jonsen and Toulmin see the history of moral practice as revealing an ongoing clarification of the use of paradigms and of admitted exceptions. This brings us to an important point.

Moral reasoning about cases cannot proceed without reference to actual moral traditions. Casuists assert the priority of *practice* over theory. Moral norms are to be found in practice; practice is not to be justified (or condemned) by absolute moral principles, because there are none. In rejecting the idea of a timeless, rationally required ethical theory, the casuists have important allies in such American pragmatists as William James (1842–1910) and John Dewey (1859–1952). But the emphasis on practice is not simply a broad historicism, grounding our understanding of morality in the developing Western moral tradition. Also crucial are the specific institutions and practices (such as those of American medicine) that provide the context for any set of ethical problems. To illustrate their method, casuists point to case law—including, in bioethics, classic cases such as *Quinlan, Conroy,* and *Cruzan,* which have greatly illuminated the ethics of terminating life-sustaining treatment.[33]

For an example of casuistry in action, consider the question of whether Jehovah's Witness parents have the right to refuse a blood transfusion for their young child who will die without one. Rather than appealing to an ethical theory or to general principles such as beneficence or respect for autonomy, a casuist would try to reason by analogy from cases about which we have relatively settled opinions. The casuist would cite various cases that support (1) the right of competent adults to refuse medical treatment for themselves and (2) the right of parents to make decisions for their children. Regarding the second right, we let parents send their children to private religious schools, for example. On the other hand, society tends to limit parental discretion if choices amount to serious neglect. Thus, while parents have much discretion over where to send their children to school, they may not keep them out of school (using the term broadly to include home schooling). The choice to keep them out of school is regarded as seriously detrimental to children's well-being. Similarly, a casuist might argue that because refusing a blood transfusion would ensure the child's death, such a choice would be seriously neglectful and therefore beyond the bounds of parental discretion. Unlike the parents, the child has not autonomously chosen to be a Jehovah's Witness. If and when the child becomes an adult, he or she may choose or reject this value system and make medical and other decisions accordingly.

How viable is casuistry as an alternative to recently dominant theories and top-down methods of ethical reasoning? It certainly avoids the remoteness from concrete problems that arguably plagues utilitarianism and Kantianism. Indeed, it seems to capture the way much of our ethical reasoning actually proceeds. Moreover, casuistry is capable of producing consensus even when people disagree about ethical theories. Furthermore, the casuists are surely right that at least some specific moral judgments are more certain than any ethical theory.

At the same time, a number of problems confront casuistry. Some concern the work of its currently leading proponents, Jonsen and Toulmin. For example, while they identify casuistry as an alternative to top-down approaches represented in the theories already described, they never clearly distinguish their primary targets: deductivism and principle-based ethics. This omission is significant, because some of their criticisms can be validly made against at most one of these approaches. For instance, while some specific moral judgments are more certain than any *complete ethical theory,* it is far from clear that such judgments are more certain than any *principle.* Since principle-based ethics involves the use of principles (as opposed to the use of a complete ethical theory), the casuists' point about the locus of ethical certainty may only constitute an advantage over deductivism.

One might therefore wonder whether casuistry is so different from principle-based ethics. Casuists claim that moral certainty is to be found in particular cases. However, giving priority to the particular over the general may be undermined by the following possibility: *Grasping the ethical significance of a case is indistinguishable from grasping a prima facie principle or rule that applies to that case.* We can grasp that a man beating a child is wrong. However, in order to make this judgment, we must also grasp the prima facie wrongness of some kind of action, such as harming the innocent or hurting children, for it is something about the man's action that is understood to make it wrong. There seems to be no reason to claim that judgments about particular cases are more certain than judgments about prima facie principles or rules relevant to such cases. Indeed, it is not clear that the two kinds of judgments can be completely separated.

Another possible charge against casuistry is that it is overly "intuitionistic" in resolving difficult cases. Suppose we start with the established view that a competent adult patient may refuse medical treatment. May such a patient also refuse all nutrition and hydration? If so, what makes this second kind of case *relevantly similar* to the first, such that the maxim guiding the first (respecting competent adult patients' refusals) applies also to the second? Where matters are debatable, how does one *justify* particular judgments? At this point, the casuist is likely to vest decision-making authority in community judgment. Such a judgment becomes incorporated into the community's evolving traditions and practices. For example, our society has judged that food and water can be thought of, in medical settings, as similar to medical care, so a competent adult patient may refuse them.

While casuistry can respond to the charge of being overly intuitionistic by appealing to traditions and practices, it must then confront the charge of being too *accepting* of the latter. Why take at face value the ethical convictions woven into our cultural traditions and professional practices? American medical practice, for instance, may embody a vision of the physician-nurse relationship that is elitist and sexist. Therefore, is it not unsound, as contemporary feminists would insist, to appeal to established medical practice in considering issues concerning the interactions of physicians and nurses? To take another example, arguably neither broad cultural traditions nor the professional practice of researchers has sufficient critical "edge" to confront squarely the question of whether animals should be used in biomedical research and, if so, with what restrictions.

Finally, by focusing so exclusively on cases, casuistry risks (1) being unable to make progress with especially controversial issues and (2) missing very general and fundamental issues, the resolution of which may be relevant to specific cases. As an example of problem (1), case analysis is almost certainly insufficient to illuminate the moral status of animals. In our society today there is fundamental disagreement about animals' moral status, so people are likely to have widely varying responses to individual cases. Regarding (2), fundamental issues can be missed because of excessive faith in precedents (judgments about previous cases). How do we know our precedents are right? For example, the fact that

Medicare covers renal dialysis and kidney transplants, open-heart surgery, and certain other treatments may seem to weigh in favor of funding heart transplants. But perhaps we never should have funded those other treatments in the first place.[34]

In conclusion, while casuistry embodies important insights about ethical reasoning, it faces significant challenges. Contrary to the claims of recent defenders, casuistry may be compatible with principle-based ethics. Further reflection on its strengths and weaknesses may suggest that casuistry is best regarded as part of a more comprehensive model of ethical reasoning.

REFLECTIVE EQUILIBRIUM AND APPEALS TO COHERENCE

Recently dominant approaches (whether deductivist or principle-based) are sometimes criticized for viewing ethical justification as essentially "downward"; that is, *theories or principles,* assumed to be firmly established, are thought to justify our judgments about particular cases. On the other hand, casuistry may oversimplify the nature of ethical reasoning in the opposite direction. Casuists claim that ethical certainty lies in *cases,* the study of which allows us to identify maxims to be used and revised in exploring new cases. Arguably, each of these models is excessively rigid in giving priority to one level of ethical conviction: general norms (theories or principles) or particular cases. Perhaps our ethical insights and reasoning lack any such exclusive foundation.

According to the model of *reflective equilibrium,* formulated by John Rawls, no level of ethical conviction deserves such priority.[35] Justification occurs at all levels of generality: (1) theories, (2) principles and rules of differing degrees of specificity, and (3) judgments about cases. Judgments that seem especially compelling at any level can be used to revise less certain judgments at any other level.

The reflective-equilibrium model directs us to start with *considered judgments,* that is, those judgments about which we have a high degree of confidence after careful and extensive consideration. These judgments differ in some ways from the paradigm case judgments of casuistry. First, considered judgments may be of any level of generality. Some may be specific case judgments (as in casuistry); others may be rules such as a prohibition of rape; still others may be principles such as the principle of respect for autonomy. Second, a judgment counts as a considered judgment only if it is reasonably believed not to have resulted from bias. (Casuistry, again, ties its paradigm case judgments so closely to accepted practices that many such judgments may be suspected of bias.) Considered judgments serve as a basis for revising other ethical beliefs or judgments that one may hold, in an effort to achieve a more coherent overall set of beliefs. (What coherence involves is described later in this section.)

For example, one might initially believe it appropriate to deceive prospective participants in an important biomedical study if deception seems necessary to attract a sufficient number of participants. But Kant's principle that we should not treat persons merely as means casts doubt on this initial judgment. Prospective participants are not treated as ends in themselves unless they are given full information about what their participation would involve. This revision of judgments moves "downward" (from principle to case), but in the present model one may also revise "upward." For example, in consideration of a case in which a psychiatric patient threatens to kill an identified third party, we might revise a principle of patient confidentiality to allow exceptions in this sort of case.

One point stressed by defenders of the reflective-equilibrium model is that revisions are never considered final; we must always admit the possibility that our ethical convictions (sometimes even considered judgments) will require modification in light of further considerations. Thus, while we strive, through continual reflection, for a state of equilibrium in our total set of ethical convictions (hence the model's name), we are never finished with moral inquiry. New problems arise, and fresh information and novel insights make us question old judgments. As in casuistry, moral reasoning is viewed as dynamic and is not expected to produce a final, rationally necessary theory.

But how do we know which judgments or norms should get revised when there is a conflict? In the cases previously mentioned, why not (1) reject or revise the prohibition against treating persons merely as means, or (2) retain confidentiality as an exceptionless principle, instead of the other way around in each case? How can we *justify* any particular resolution of conflicts? In brief, conflicts are to be settled by making revisions that seem to produce the greatest *coherence* in our overall system of ethical convictions.

Appeals to coherence may be understood, more specifically, to include requirements of logical consistency, argumentative support, and plausibility (reconcilability with our moral experience).[36] *Logical consistency* is simply the avoidance of outright contradiction. For example, it is logically inconsistent to hold that killing an innocent person is always wrong, yet hold that it would be right to grant this person's request to be killed on grounds of mercy. *Argumentative support* is the giving of reasons that back up one's ethical views (reasons that, of course, must be consistent with one's reasoning about other ethical issues). Thus, if one favors paternalistically prohibiting the use of certain drugs but opposes paternalistic seat belt laws, one must provide a reason that supports the claim that paternalism is justified in one case but not in the other. (Paternalism will be discussed in detail later in this chapter.) Wherever there is ethical controversy, lack of argumentative support for a particular position suggests dogmatism and invites reasonable doubts that the position is really justified. The third requirement for selecting from among alternative viewpoints is *plausibility.* Suppose someone argues that no actions are ethically right or wrong (a logically consistent position) and gives as a reason (argumentative support) for this view the fact that ethical judgments are subject to seemingly endless dispute. This view is utterly implausible. It implies that it is not wrong to commit genocide out of sheer racial hatred. Thus, in the present model one seeks logically consistent judgments, supported by ethical reasons or arguments, that are largely plausible upon reflection.[37]

The reflective-equilibrium model, involving appeals to coherence, appears to be gaining support as more theorists and professionals question the adequacy of more traditional approaches. The model is especially favored by those contemporary philosophers who identify with the spirit of the early American pragmatists (who saw ethical reasoning as dynamic and rejected claims of an absolute foundation for morality). The model incorporates the case-based reasoning of casuistry, as well as the downward argumentation associated with principle-based ethics.[38] It concedes to deductivism that sometimes theoretical thinking is needed to check our particular judgments. Depending upon how it is developed, the model can also include many insights and elements of virtue theory as well as the ethics of care and feminist ethics. Overall, it may seem to offer a flexible and balanced approach to moral reasoning.

Nevertheless, the model of reflective equilibrium has its difficulties. Arguably, it buys flexibility and freedom from dogmatism at the cost of vagueness and lack of structure. By contrast, deductivism, which identifies a single principle as a basis for ethical justification, provides a framework or method that may be easier to conceptualize. And casuistry, by focusing on concrete cases, may provide a clearer method for approaching some issues.

A critic could argue that, in the reflective-equilibrium model, one might not know where to start or how to proceed. A defender of the model might respond as follows. Theoretically, we start with considered judgments; in practice, we often simply start wherever we have ethical concern, and we use various tools of reasoning as we work toward more coherent positions. While this model is receiving increasing attention in bioethics and appears to have many strengths, it may be premature to judge its overall adequacy as an alternative to casuistry and recently dominant approaches.

CONFRONTING ETHICAL RELATIVISM

In critically examining various ethical theories and methodologies in this introduction, we have implicitly assumed that there can be right and wrong answers to moral questions, reasonable and unreasonable moral positions, better and worse ways of addressing ethical issues. Naturally, this assumption underlies the theories and methodologies themselves, as each represents an effort to provide the most adequate approach to addressing moral questions. Moreover, the articles reprinted in this volume also seem to rely on this assumption in defending particular positions on issues in biomedical ethics. Indeed, the assumption that there can be right and wrong answers to moral questions is so fundamental that it is implicit in the very act of making a moral judgment. To judge, for example, that genocide is wrong is equivalent to believing that this judgment is *correct* and that someone who denies that genocide is wrong is *mistaken.* Unless we believe that moral judgments can be correct or incorrect, reasonable or unreasonable, there seems to be little point in discussing and debating ethical issues: If all moral judgments are *equally* correct or reasonable, why bother trying to persuade anyone of your position on some ethical issue? Our everyday practices of moral discussion assume that some moral answers are more adequate and defensible than others.

Nevertheless, many people wonder whether there are any *universal* moral judgments—that is, any moral judgments whose legitimacy or authority extends *across cultural boundaries.* Perhaps, as *ethical relativism* claims, moral judgments are justified only relative to one's culture and upbringing. Today ethical relativism is casually asserted by many students, faculty members, and other individuals in our culture (although by very few ethicists and moral philosophers). Why is ethical relativism so commonly asserted? The following considerations may provide part of the answer.

We are encouraged today to become better informed about cultures in other countries—as well as distinct cultures within our own (e.g., those of different ethnic groups)—and to be respectful of their traditions, values, and beliefs. When one adopts such a multicultural attitude and appreciates differences among cultures in their moral practices and traditions, one might find it natural to think that no moral values are common to all human cultures. Moreover, since it is obvious that an individual's upbringing (e.g., one's religious education and the political values espoused by one's parents) and broader culture (e.g., secular, Western, democratic values) profoundly affect his or her moral outlook, one might infer that a person's moral judgments make sense only within this framework of values. For these and other reasons, increasingly many people appear to be attracted to ethical relativism.

Nevertheless, we find ethical relativism deeply problematic. Moreover, discussions in biomedical ethics usually assume that ethical relativism is not a viable option, an assumption reflected in this book as a whole. Before outlining our reasons for rejecting this view, we must clarify that we are not rejecting certain important ideas that are sometimes associated with ethical relativism. First, we are not claiming that whenever two cultures approach a moral issue differently, one culture must be wrong. For example, in balancing the values of (1) individual autonomy and (2) familial closeness and solidarity, in cases where the two seem to conflict, one culture may tend to give greater weight to the first value while another culture places greater importance on the second—without either culture's priorities being unreasonable or even less reasonable than the other. How to set priorities among conflicting values is often a matter of reasonable disagreement. On the other hand, it might be unreasonable to place *no* value on individual autonomy or *no* value on familial closeness.

Second, to reject ethical relativism is not to claim that moral principles and rules are *absolute* in the sense of never having exceptions and never being justifiably overridden by other principles or rules. Our discussion of recently dominant ethical theories suggested that general principles and most rules must sometimes be overridden by other principles or rules and sometimes admit of exceptions. Rather than implying that moral principles and rules are absolute, the rejection of relativism implies that some of these norms are binding across cultures. For example, all persons, regardless of culture, have prima facie obligations to respect other people, to communicate truthfully and keep promises, and to refrain from harming others. Third, in rejecting ethical relativism in favor of some universal norms, we are not claiming that *our* society's prevailing values are always correct. On the contrary, we are convinced that they are not always correct. For example, many Americans believe in a basic moral right to obtain firearms easily and inexpensively. We disagree.

Interestingly, one consideration that is sometimes thought to support ethical relativism proves, upon close examination, to undermine it. Lately increasing emphasis has been placed on the importance of *tolerance,* the attitude that we should not be too quick to judge negatively those who have beliefs, traditions, and values that differ from our own. Thus, for example, people who are comfortable in mainstream twenty-first century American or Canadian society should not dismiss the value systems and ways of life that have characterized Native American societies. Note that this is an ethical judgment, which implies that it would be wrong or inappropriate to dismiss these alternative cultural practices out of hand. But tolerance, which is a component of respecting persons more generally, is presumably a value that all persons ought to recognize. One who urges tolerance is very unlikely to think rabid intolerance is just fine as long as one's own culture and upbringing favor intolerance. One is likely to think, rather, that a society that executes people for having particular religious beliefs is profoundly wrong to do so.

This example suggests another important point: While tolerance seems to set appropriate standards for behavior across cultures, it also has limits insofar as we need not tolerate or accept *all* differences among people and cultures. The imagined society's violent intolerance of particular religious beliefs is beyond the pale of reasonable differences—and in that sense intolerable. Similarly, we are hardly obligated to tolerate rape, slavery, genocide, racism, or any other flagrant abuse of human beings (or animals) anywhere. What we should tolerate, generally, are cultural differences that do not involve extensive and unambiguous harm or violation of human rights. This principle of tolerance, it seems, is valid across cultures, providing our first argument against ethical relativism.

Another reason to reject ethical relativism is the sheer implausibility of some of its implications. Suppose a society's values are such that the systematic rape, torture, and killing of a despised minority are judged by the overwhelming majority to be appropriate. If ethical relativism were correct, then we would have no basis for claiming that the majority's brutality toward the minority is wrong. Yet we do not think, "Well, we have our liberal, more gentle ways of treating minorities, they have their way of treating minorities, and neither approach is morally better or worse." Instead, we condemn the brutality. In doing so, and in making similar cross-cultural moral judgments (e.g., condemning slavery or apartheid), we reveal our deep conviction that some moral standards ought to be recognized as binding on everyone.

Now consider the fact that, when a particular culture changes morally, the change often impresses people within that culture as being an improvement. For example, it is widely believed today that greater equality among the races and sexes over the years represents *moral progress,* as does growing tolerance of and respect for gay people. But, if ethical relativism were true, there could be no such thing as moral progress. On this view, we lack any basis for saying that when most Americans accepted slavery, this was unenlightened or unjustified; the only values by which their practice could be appropriately judged are their own (racist) values of the time, and by these values slavery was justified. Those who believe moral progress is a meaningful concept should reject ethical relativism.

Finally, consider individuals who challenge currently prevailing values within their culture. Abolitionists did so during the time of slavery; today's animal rights activists furnish another example. If ethical relativism were correct, then the moral position of these reformers—their conviction that some current practice is unjustified—would often be hard to understand. According to ethical relativism, moral judgments are justified only relative to a culture. That means the reformers would be claiming, in effect, that their culture's practice (which they are criticizing) is inconsistent with the culture's values (the only possible basis for criticism). But frequently moral reformers are advancing a more fundamental criticism that targets some of their culture's basic values, such as unequal regard for different races or unequal consideration for different species. In such cases, reformers contend that some of their culture's prevailing values are wrong—a claim that would make no sense if relativism were true. One need not agree with the reformer's moral agenda to appreciate this argument against relativism; one need only grant that the reformer's moral claim is intelligible.

For all of these reasons, then, we do not believe that ethical relativism is a viable option for biomedical ethics. At the same time, we endorse some aspects of *multiculturalism.* We understand multiculturalism, roughly, as an appreciation of the often differing values and traditions of different cultures, an openness to learning important practical lessons from other cultures, and a rejection of the assumption that our own culture's values are always superior and deserving of emulation by other cultures. Multiculturalism, so understood, does not imply ethical relativism. Indeed, the recognition that our culture is not beyond reproach and that we may learn valuable moral lessons from other cultures implies that some moral standards are so reasonable they deserve to be embraced by all persons across cultures.

FUNDAMENTAL CONCEPTS AND PRINCIPLES

The concepts of autonomy and paternalism are of fundamental importance in biomedical ethics. Closely associated with these concepts is a set of principles called "liberty-limiting principles," which are often invoked in order to justify limitations on individual liberty. This section provides an examination of these concepts and principles.

AUTONOMY

Many discussions in biomedical ethics presume the importance of individual autonomy, stressing the right of autonomous decision makers to determine for themselves what will be done to their bodies. This "right of self-determination" is said to limit what physicians, nurses, and other health-care professionals can justifiably do to patients. In fact, this right is often taken so seriously that professionals who act against their patients' wishes, even to save their patients' lives, are condemned as morally blameworthy and leave themselves open to charges of battery. In view of all this, it is useful to discuss the following questions, the first a conceptual question and the second an ethical one. (1) What sense of autonomy is operative in the widespread presumption that individual autonomy is an important value? (2) What is the ethical basis for the value accorded to individual autonomy?

The Concept of Autonomy Autonomy is typically defined as self-governance or self-determination. Individuals are said to act autonomously when they, and not others, make the decisions that affect their lives and act on the basis of these decisions. This general characterization needs to be explicated, however, because autonomy is a complex notion. In fact, different ways of conceptualizing autonomy may be appropriate in different contexts. In this section we attempt to elucidate the sense of autonomy or self-determination that is most prominent in biomedical ethics, one that squares with our ethical ideas about respect for autonomy. Although one may meaningfully talk about individuals' lives and political states as autonomous, we will focus on the nature of *autonomous action* (including *autonomous choice,* choice being a kind of action), because whether a certain action is autonomous is often a central question in biomedical ethics; secondarily, we will also refer to autonomous *agents*. It is widely agreed that for an action to qualify as autonomous, it must be (1) intentional, (2) based on sufficient understanding, (3) sufficiently free of external constraints, and (4) sufficiently free of internal constraints.[39] A brief elaboration of these conditions should both clarify the concept of autonomous action and illustrate various ways in which action can be less than fully autonomous.

Intentionality Imagine a patient, Mark, who has just been admitted to the psychiatric unit of a hospital to receive treatment for depression. The day after his admission, a staff psychiatrist talks to him for an extended period of time, during which Mark is highly distracted. The psychiatrist then requests Mark's signature, which Mark provides, believing that he is consenting to remain in the hospital for several days. Suppose, however, that the paper Mark signs has nothing to do with remaining in the hospital. As the psychiatrist had attempted to explain, the paper is a consent form authorizing Mark's participation in a study of patients with a particular form of depression.

In this scenario, Mark intentionally signs a piece of paper and, in doing so, formally consents to participate in a study. But Mark does not *intentionally consent to participate;* his intention is to authorize an extended stay in the hospital. Clearly, Mark's consenting to participate is not an autonomous action. To perform an action autonomously, one must, as a first condition, intentionally perform that action. But one must also satisfy other conditions.

Understanding Imagine a second depressed patient, Judy, who is also approached about possible participation in a biomedical study. Suppose that Judy, unlike Mark, does intentionally consent to participate in the study described to her. But despite the psychiatrist's best efforts to explain clearly what the study would entail, Judy is confused by the long presentation of details. She very much hopes to receive the promising new medication whose effectiveness the study is designed to determine. Due to a number of factors—this hope, her belief that researchers would not ask her to participate in a study that could be contrary to her interests, and her difficulty absorbing large amounts of information in a single presentation—Judy misses one very salient detail: There is a 50 percent chance that she will be one of a group of patients who will receive an established medication with which Judy has had very unpleasant experiences in the past. Indeed, if she were to grasp that she might receive this medication, she would refuse to participate in the study.

In this example, Judy intentionally consents to participate in a study, but since she does so with *insufficient understanding* of what participation entails, her decision cannot count as autonomous. Sometimes insufficient understanding results from blameworthy actions of others. For example, if a physician lies, misleads, or presents significantly incomplete information to a patient, the patient's understanding of his or her options may be insufficient for an autonomous decision. In other cases, insufficient understanding is the result of a person's lacking the mental capacities needed for understanding. Although there are exceptions to the following generalization, children are ordinarily presumed to lack the mental capacities required for a sufficient understanding of the options involved in medical decision making. If we define *autonomous agents* as individuals who are generally capable of acting autonomously, we may restate the point by saying that children are ordinarily presumed to be *nonautonomous* agents.

It is important to recognize that understanding, however it comes about, is a matter of degree. Rarely, if ever, does one *perfectly* understand the implications and likely consequences of one's various options when confronted with an important decision. Because understanding is a matter of degree, autonomous action may also be conceptualized as being a matter of degree. Thus, on this way of thinking about autonomy, one may act more or less autonomously, making it sensible to say that adolescents and even children can act autonomously to some degree.

At the same time, certain purposes favor thinking of autonomy in terms of a threshold—or cut-off point—so that a given action either qualifies as autonomous or does not. Thinking of autonomy in this way requires that its conditions have cut-off points. Thus, we identify *sufficient* understanding as a condition for autonomous action (although we recognize that in practice it will sometimes be difficult to determine whether this somewhat vaguely stated threshold has been met). One purpose that favors a threshold conception of autonomous action is the need to determine whether a patient's consent to receive medical treatment qualifies as "informed consent"—which implies that the patient's act of decision making has been autonomous. If the patient's consent counts as informed consent, it is ordinarily respected; if it does not qualify as informed consent, the decision is viewed as problematic, and a proxy decision maker may need to be involved in the decision-making process. In this practical context, there is little or no room for thinking of consent as a matter of degree. Thus, there are pragmatic reasons, in some contexts, to conceptualize autonomous action as a threshold concept and not as a matter of degree. Accordingly, we identify sufficient understanding of what is at stake—of the implications and likely consequences of one's action, and those of available alternatives—as a condition of autonomous action.

Freedom from External Constraints   Think of Rhee, a medical student, who is attending a concert the night before her final exam in anatomy class. She is free to leave anytime she chooses. Her actions result from her conscious intention to listen to a concert, and she clearly understands what she is doing and the implications of her choice—including the risk of doing substandard work on the final. Importantly, Rhee's choice to remain at the concert is also voluntary in the sense that it is free from external constraints.

External constraints may be understood as including physical barriers deliberately imposed by other individuals and different forms of coercion. (Although in a sense a person is "constrained" by the laws of physics from high-jumping to the moon, such impersonal constraints are not relevant to the present conception of autonomy.) Prisoners are constrained by the physical barriers of locked doors and prison walls. If they attempt to escape from prison and are detected in the process, they are likely to encounter coercion from prison guards. Coercion involves the deliberate use of force or the threat of harm. The coercer's purpose is to get the person being coerced to do something that he or she would not otherwise be willing to do (in the present case, submit to continued incarceration). "Occurrent" coercion involves the use of physical force. "Dispositional" coercion involves the threat of harm.[40] An unscrupulous medical researcher, for example, might literally force individuals to participate as research subjects, as was done in Nazi Germany. This is occurrent coercion. The researcher might also bring about the desired participation by threatening reluctant patients with some harm, such as the withdrawal of care essential for their recovery. This is dispositional coercion. Moreover, regarding the threat of harm, individuals can coerce others either directly or by enacting laws that threaten them with harm. Laws as well as individuals can be coercive. For example, a physician is constrained from actively killing patients by laws that threaten harm (in the form of punishment) to those who do so.

Let us revise the story of Rhee the concert-goer in a way that makes the voluntariness of her actions more questionable. Suppose that her decision regarding what to do that evening is based mainly on strong pressure from her family members, who want Rhee to watch her father perform in the concert. Rhee, as it happens, comes from a culture in which family loyalty is prized very highly and paternal authority is generally respected. While it would seem exaggerated to say that Rhee is coerced into attending the concert, she clearly faces some external pressure. (There may be a point at which external pressure shades into coercion.) This suggests that freedom from external constraints is really a matter of degree—reinforcing the idea, suggested earlier in our discussion of understanding, that autonomy itself may be thought of as something that comes in degrees. In the present scenario, Rhee's decision to attend the concert might be considered less than fully autonomous but more autonomous than some actions (such as when coercion or physical barriers deliberately imposed by others constrain one's options).

In contexts where there is good reason to think of autonomy as a threshold concept, such that one's action either is autonomous or is not, the present condition may be stated this way: An autonomous action must be *sufficiently free of external constraints*. If an adult patient's choice to undergo surgery is largely her own choice, it can be considered sufficiently free of external constraints for her decision to count as autonomous, even if she feels slight pressure from her family or physician to consent.[41]

Freedom from Internal Constraints Imagine now a classmate of Rhee's, Salvator, who on the night before the final exam is imbibing beer at a fast pace in a pub near campus. Having had several beers, Salvator faces a choice: He can go home and open his anatomy textbook or he can stay at the pub and order another beer. He decides on the latter course. His decision is intentional, and he fully understands his options and their likely consequences. Furthermore, no one is coercing him to stay and party. Nor are there physical barriers, such as locked doors, that prevent him from leaving the pub. Is his choice to stay and have another beer autonomous? That depends on further detail.

Suppose Salvator has a severe case of alcoholism. Once he begins to drink, he feels an uncontrollable urge to keep drinking—*even though he thinks doing so is contrary to his best interests*—and this urge typically continues to exert its force until he passes out. Perhaps Salvator's going to the pub, ordering a drink, and beginning to imbibe were autonomous actions. (People might reasonably disagree about this, even if all the details of the case are provided.) But surely the uncontrollable urge to continue drinking, once drinking commences, that characterizes severe alcoholism, creates an *internal constraint* that substantially reduces the autonomy of one's subsequent actions. A person who is driven by such an urge is, in an important sense, "out of control" and no longer self-determining.

As an alternative, suppose that Salvator is not an alcoholic but is a schizophrenic. (Schizophrenia is a mental illness characterized by disorganized and delusional thinking and, very frequently, auditory and visual hallucinations.) He generally functions well when he takes antipsychotic medications—indeed, well enough to attend medical school—but for some reason he stopped taking them several days ago. Now, the night before the final, he hears "voices" ("command" auditory hallucinations) telling him that he must go to the pub and drink heavily. He is terrified of these "voices" and unwilling to disobey them. He goes to the pub, orders a drink, and begins imbibing. He is thinking clearly enough to understand that this course of action is likely to lead to inebriation and places him at risk of doing poorly on the final.[42] No external constraints control his actions, but internal constraints—the "voices" and his terror at the thought of disobeying them—do control his actions. Salvator's actions are substantially nonautonomous.

While the unleashed urges of severe alcoholism and the power of "command" hallucinations are dramatic examples of internal constraints on action, there are also more common internal phenomena that, to some degree, constrain our actions and choices. Intense fears, acute pain or persistent discomfort, and strong emotions such as rage and grief sometimes influence us to make choices that represent departures from our stable values and usual priorities; that is, these phenomena sometimes cause us to act out of character with the result that we later feel that we were "not ourselves" in doing what we did.[43] Sometimes, however, these internal phenomena simply make it more difficult to behave as one normally would. Clearly, then, one can be *more or less* free of internal constraints. In contexts where it is helpful to think of autonomy as involving a threshold, this final condition may be stated as follows: One acts autonomously only if one's action is *sufficiently free of internal constraints*.

Let us bring together the conditions we have discussed. First, autonomy may be conceived of in terms of a threshold: One acts autonomously only if one acts intentionally, with sufficient understanding of what is at stake, and one's action is sufficiently free of external and internal constraints. Second, conceptualizing autonomous action as a matter of degree, we may say that one acts autonomously *to the extent* that one acts intentionally, with understanding, and freely of external and internal constraints.

Both in biomedical contexts and in social life generally, it is an especially important fact that, even when people are capable of acting autonomously, the actions of others often prevent them from doing so. A person's autonomy can be infringed upon, limited, or usurped by others in many ways. For example, lying, practicing other forms of deception, and failing to supply needed information all can undermine another person's understanding of his or her options. By contrast, coercion and the deliberate imposition of physical barriers can undermine a person's autonomy by constraining his or her *liberty of action.*[44] In each of these ways of undermining autonomy, one individual interferes in some way with the effective exercise of another's capacity to act autonomously, and this is incompatible with the ethical principle of respect for autonomy.

The Value of Autonomy What is the basis for the moral value accorded to individual autonomy? The strongest claims regarding its moral primacy come from Kant and from certain other deontologists. In Kant's view, persons, unlike things, must always be accorded respect as self-determining subjects. They must be treated as ends in themselves and never merely as objects. For Kant, the fundamental principle of morality, respect for persons as moral agents, entails respect for personal autonomy. Such respect is due them as a right— autonomous agents are entitled to respect. If persons were not taken to be autonomous agents, there would be no basis for the moral responsibility we have toward other human beings, which precludes our using them—as we do cattle, chickens, rocks, land, and trees— simply to serve our own ends. But how does Kant understand autonomy?

Kant's primary focus is on the autonomy of the will. For Kant, "Autonomy of the will is the property the will has of being a law to itself."[45] What Kant calls the "dignity of man as a rational creature" is based on human beings possessing just that property that enables them to govern their own actions in accordance with rules of their own choosing. Putting aside many complexities in Kant's own thinking, a Kantian position central in biomedical ethics describes autonomy in terms of self-control, self-direction, or self-governance. The individual capable of acting on the basis of effective deliberation, guided by reason, and neither driven by emotions or compulsions nor manipulated or coerced by others, is, on a Kantian position, the model of autonomy.

For utilitarians, autonomy is an important value. John Stuart Mill, who speaks of individuality rather than autonomy, argues, for example, that liberty of action and thought is essential in developing both the intellectual and character traits necessary for truly human happiness:

> The human faculties of perception, judgment, discriminative feeling, mental activity, and even moral preference, are exercised only in making a choice. He who does anything because it is the custom makes no choice. He gains no practice either in discerning or in desiring what is best. The mental and moral, like the muscular powers, are improved by being used. . . .
>
> He who lets the world, or his own portion of it, choose his plan of life for him, has no need of any other faculty than the ape-like one of imitation. He who chooses his plan for himself employs all his faculties. He must use observation to see, reasoning and judgment to foresee, activity to gather materials for decision, discrimination to decide, and when he has decided, firmness and self-control to hold to his deliberate decision. . . .
>
> Where, not the person's own character, but the traditions or customs of other people are the rule of conduct, there is wanting one of the principal ingredients of human happiness.[46]

For Mill, persons possessing "individuality" are autonomous in a very strong sense, reflectively choosing their own plans of life, making their own decisions without coercion or manipulation by others, and exercising firmness and self-control in acting on their decisions.

Despite the high value placed on autonomy by utilitarians, their interest in autonomy differs from the Kantian one. On a Kantian view, respect for the autonomy of rational agents is entailed by the fundamental principle of morality, which serves as a limiting criterion for all moral conduct. That is, it places limits on what one individual can do to another without acting immorally. As noted earlier, one person can never use another as a subject in a medical experiment without his or her consent, no matter what potential good consequences for society as a whole might result. For a utilitarian such as Mill, respect for individual autonomy has utility value. A society that fosters respect for persons as autonomous agents will be a more progressive and, on balance, a happier society because its citizens will have the opportunities to develop their capacities to act as rational, responsible moral agents. If it could be shown that respect for individual autonomy does not have sufficient utility value, the utilitarian might have no good grounds for objecting to practices that infringe upon that autonomy.

LIBERTY-LIMITING PRINCIPLES

Since autonomy is accorded such great moral value, a moral justification must be given for any infringement upon or limitation or usurpation of autonomy. Many discussions in biomedical ethics explore such *proposed* justifications. The following exposition centers on the most general kinds of reasons advanced in these discussions.

Six suggested general reasons, most frequently considered when limitations of liberty are at issue, are embodied in the following six principles, often called "liberty-limiting principles."[47] (Liberty, or freedom from external constraints, is one aspect or component of autonomy.) It is important to note at the outset that while some writers advance these principles as legitimate liberty-limiting principles, others argue against the legitimacy of many, or even most, of them.

1. A person's liberty is justifiably restricted to prevent that person from harming others (the harm principle).[48]
2. A person's liberty is justifiably restricted to prevent that person from offending others (the offense principle).
3. A person's liberty is justifiably restricted to prevent that person from harming himself or herself (the principle of paternalism).
4. A person's liberty is justifiably restricted to benefit that person (the principle of extreme paternalism).
5. A person's liberty is justifiably restricted to prevent that person from acting immorally (the principle of legal moralism).
6. A person's liberty is justifiably restricted to benefit others (the social welfare principle).

These liberty-limiting principles are most frequently discussed when questions arise about the justification of coercive laws, such as laws limiting access to hallucinogenic drugs. But the considerations they embody are also pertinent when applied to individual acts and practices that infringe upon or limit others' autonomy. It should also be noted that more than one of these principles might be advanced to justify a proposed limitation or infringement.

The harm principle is the most widely accepted liberty-limiting principle. Few will dispute that the law is within its proper bounds when it constrains individuals from performing acts that will seriously harm other persons or will seriously impair important institutional practices. Laws that threaten thieves, murderers, and the like with punishment, for example, are usually perceived as a necessary part of any social system. Individual acts of coercion whose intent is to prevent individuals from harming others are also usually considered morally permissible. A bystander, for example, who prevents a terrorist from killing or wounding someone is praised and not blamed for interfering with the terrorist's action. Aside from the harm principle, however, the moral legitimacy of the liberty-limiting principles under discussion here is a matter of dispute.

According to the offense principle, the law may justifiably be invoked to prevent offensive behavior in public. "Offensive" behavior may be understood as behavior that causes shame, embarrassment, or discomfort to onlookers. In an example of the relevance of the offense principle to biomedical ethics, individuals who behaved offensively in public were sometimes, in the past, involuntarily committed to psychiatric hospitals, even though their behavior did not pose a serious threat of harm to themselves or others. Committing individuals to psychiatric hospitals simply because their behavior was considered offensively eccentric involved at least an implicit appeal to the offense principle. Attacks on the use of such grounds to deprive individuals of much of their liberty are attacks on the legitimacy of the offense principle.

According to the principle of legal moralism, liberty may justifiably be limited to prevent immoral behavior or, as it is often expressed, to "enforce morals." Acts such as kidnapping, murder, and fraud are undoubtedly immoral, but the principle of legal moralism does not have to be invoked to justify laws against them. An appeal to the harm principle already provides a widely accepted independent justification. The principle of legal moralism usually comes to the fore only when so-called victimless crimes are at issue. Is it justifiable to legislate against homosexual acts, gambling, or prostitution simply on the grounds that such activities are thought by some to be morally unacceptable? In biomedical ethics, the principle of legal moralism is sometimes invoked, at least implicitly, when it is argued that suicide is an immoral act and that, therefore, it is justifiable to act to prevent suicide, even if the decision to take one's own life is the result of careful deliberation. Many do not accept the principle of legal moralism as a legitimate liberty-limiting principle, however. Mill holds, for example, that to accept the principle is tantamount to permitting a "tyranny of the majority."

The social welfare principle also has some relevance in biomedical ethics. According to this principle, individual liberty can justifiably be restricted to benefit others. Such justifications are sometimes attempted in discussions of funding for certain public health-care programs, such as Medicaid in the United States. These programs are funded by tax revenues. Since individual taxpayers are not given the option not to pay that amount of their taxes that is directed toward these programs—which benefit others—the liberty of taxpayers is restricted in a way that might be justified by appeal to the social welfare principle.

The liberty-limiting principles that are most prominent in the literature of biomedical ethics are the paternalistic principles. Disagreements about the legitimacy of paternalistic justifications affect the resolution of a number of important issues in biomedical ethics. Physicians or nurses, for example, who lie to patients in order to spare them pain are often accused of acting paternalistically and therefore wrongly. The paternalistic justifications offered for certain laws that are of special concern in biomedical ethics are also frequently attacked. Among such laws are those that allow courts to commit individuals to psychiatric hospitals either in order to keep them from harming themselves or in order to force them to receive beneficial treatment. Because of the centrality of paternalism in biomedical ethics, it is essential to examine the concept of paternalism as well as some of the arguments offered both for and against paternalistic actions and practices.

PATERNALISM

One widely cited definition of *paternalism* is Gerald Dworkin's: "[Paternalism is] the interference with a person's liberty of action justified by reasons referring exclusively to the welfare, good, happiness, needs, interests, or values of the person being coerced."[49] When paternalism in the legal system is at issue, this definition is acceptable, since laws, backed by force or the threat of harm, are by nature coercive and therefore restrictive of liberty. However, many of the actions considered paternalistic in biomedical ethics do not fit this definition. Consider the following examples:

(1) A patient has frequently asserted that he would immediately commit suicide if he were ever diagnosed with Alzheimer's disease, and his physician believes he is serious. The patient says that Alzheimer's disease is antithetical to everything he values in life. The physician has now arrived at a diagnosis of Alzheimer's disease, but she lies to the patient about the diagnosis. She does so because she believes that a premature death is incompatible with the patient's best interests.

(2) A physician believes that surgery is the best available treatment for a patient's cancer. The physician does not disclose significant information about nonsurgical alternatives because he believes that the patient would be inclined to choose one of these alternatives, and he wants to ensure that the patient consents to the treatment that the physician believes to be in the patient's best interests.

Note that neither of these cases involves coercion or interference with a person's liberty of action, yet both can be correctly described as involving paternalism. In both cases, the physicians have infringed upon or limited the patients' autonomy. In both, the physicians have denied the patients information vital to effective deliberation and have done so for the patients' own good. The physicians have treated the patients as individuals incapable of making the correct judgments about their own best interests. In doing so, each physician has effectively usurped a patient's decision-making power, substituting his or her judgment for the patient's. While it is difficult to capture this sense of paternalism in a precise definition, a rough definition can be given as follows: *Paternalism* is the interference with, limitation of, or usurpation of individual autonomy justified by reasons referring exclusively to the welfare or needs of the person whose autonomy is being interfered with, limited, or usurped. (The sense of autonomy employed in this definition is autonomy as a matter of degree. Thus, our definition will cover both cases of strong paternalism and cases of weak paternalism, a distinction explained later in this discussion.)

Is such paternalistic behavior ever morally justified? If the answer is yes, under what conditions do paternalistic grounds constitute good reasons, either for using coercion or for effectively taking decisions out of individuals' hands for their own good? In considering the justifiability of paternalistic actions, it may be helpful to keep in mind the difference between the principle of paternalism and the principle of extreme paternalism. The latter applies to paternalistic actions whose intent is to benefit individuals, whereas the former applies to paternalistic actions whose intent is to keep individuals from harm.

In the framework of Kantian ethical theory, the moral centrality of individual autonomy seems to prohibit any paternalistic actions when the individuals affected are capable of self-governance or self-determination. It would always be morally wrong, for example, for physicians to withhold information about surgical procedures from patients simply because the physicians believed that their patients would refuse to undergo potentially beneficial procedures if informed of all the risks. Charles Fried, an ethicist (and former solicitor general) who adopts a Kantian approach to paternalism in the medical context, maintains that patients must never be denied relevant information. By withholding it, physicians treat patients as mere means to the end of improving their own health. In Fried's view, patients may never be treated simply as means to ends, even when the ends in question are their own ends (e.g., their restored health).[50]

John Stuart Mill provides the classic utilitarian statement on the illegitimacy of paternalistic actions. This statement is sometimes cited in court opinions concerning the right of self-determination in medical matters. Mill argues:

> [O]ne very simple principle [is] entitled to govern absolutely the dealings of society with the individual in the way of compulsion and control, whether the means used be physical force in the form of legal penalties, or the moral coercion of public opinion. That principle is, that the sole end for which mankind are warranted, individually or collectively, in interfering with the liberty of action of any of their number, is self-protection. That the only purpose for which power can be rightfully exercised over any member of a civilized community, against his will, is to prevent harm to others. His own good, either physical or moral, is not sufficient warrant. He cannot rightfully be compelled to do or forbear because it will be better for him to do so, because it will make him happier, because, in the opinion of others, to do so would be wise, or even right.[51]

In this statement, Mill asserts that while prevention of harm to others is sometimes sufficient justification for interfering with another's autonomy, the individual's own good never is. Mill rejects paternalistic interventions because of the high utility value that he assigns to individual autonomy. In assigning it this value, he assumes that individuals are, on the whole, better judges of their own interests than anyone else, so that minimizing paternalistic interventions will maximize human happiness. However, Mill himself qualifies his rejection of paternalism in the following way:

> [T]his doctrine is meant to apply only to human beings in the maturity of their faculties. We are not speaking of children, or of young persons below the age which the law may fix as that of manhood or womanhood. Those who are still in a state to require being taken care of by others, must be protected against their own actions as well as external injury.[52]

In the kinds of cases he cites, Mill assumes that people are justified in acting paternalistically because they are better judges of an individual's interest than the individual himself or herself. Arguing in this way, Mill seems to open the door for the justification of paternalism in the case of individuals who may not be able to identify and advance their own interests correctly because they lack the required level of ability for effective deliberation—and in particular for sufficiently understanding their options and the likely consequences of specific choices. Such individuals, often described as having diminished autonomy insofar as they lack the necessary abilities or capacities for self-determination, include young children and the severely mentally retarded. It is important to see that the paternalistic restrictions Mill would allow in this regard do typically amount to restrictions on individual autonomy—at least in a certain sense. To the extent that an individual is subject to coercion, individual liberty of action is restricted, and liberty of action may be understood as one aspect of individual autonomy. However, the paternalistic restrictions at issue here do not limit autonomy in the sense central to Mill's, as well as Kant's, moral position, since those whose liberty would be limited are substantially lacking in autonomy to begin with. (They are nonautonomous where autonomy is thought of as having a threshold.)

Many contemporary attempts to justify *some* paternalistic actions adopt an approach similar to Mill's, stressing the apparently diminished autonomy of those who are treated paternalistically. If their autonomy were not so compromised, the argument runs, they would want the benefits involved and would want to avoid harm. Those who argue in this way must deal with an underlying conceptual issue. They must identify the criteria that should be used in determining whether a person's autonomy is sufficiently diminished to justify paternalism. In light of our earlier discussion of autonomy, it seems plausible to hold the following view regarding diminished autonomy. When a person's ability to act autonomously is significantly constrained by intellectual deficits (e.g., lack of reasoning ability or ignorance of relevant facts) and cannot be easily augmented (e.g., by providing needed information), it is sufficiently impaired to justify paternalistic acts, especially when necessary to prevent serious, irrevocable harm. Two examples may be helpful here. People under the influence of hallucinogenic drugs who decide to leap from twentieth-floor windows in order to get home more quickly, believing that they (like Superman) can fly, are hardly acting in an autonomous manner. Their decisions are grossly inconsistent with available inductive evidence regarding what happens to human beings who leap out of windows and are therefore *irrational* in a familiar sense of the term. Severely retarded individuals who decide to go out alone in a busy city but are incapable of understanding traffic signals would also seem to be acting in a significantly nonautonomous way. They are unaware of the kind of risk they would be running by going out alone. In both cases, there is good reason to assume that the individuals are incapable, whether temporarily or permanently, of the level of understanding required for sufficiently autonomous decision making. Thus, paternalistic interventions seem to be justified.

Does the fact that a decision will result in death or some other serious, irrevocable harm *always* provide sufficient grounds for the claim that autonomy is so severely diminished that paternalism is justified? Some especially problematic cases involve decisions to attempt suicide. Many suicide attempts are the result of temporary disorientation associated with drugs, alcohol, or extreme, but reversible, depression. Decisions to attempt suicide in these cases are apparently due to insufficient understanding of one's situation and options—or perhaps internal constraints that impede effective deliberation—and can therefore be considered nonautonomous. Indeed, cases involving individuals who are so constrained in their reasoning that they are temporarily or permanently incapable of identifying the probable (severely harmful) consequences of their acts would seem to provide clear instances of autonomy that is sufficiently diminished to justify paternalism. However, some decisions to end or risk life may be based on carefully thought-out reasons and may be consistent with the person's own long-held conception of a satisfying or meaningful life or the result of a new but reflective reassessment of ultimate values and priorities. It would beg the question to assume—in an effort to justify paternalistic interventions— that all decisions to end or risk life are irrational (due to being based on insufficient understanding and/or insufficient freedom from internal constraints) and therefore nonautonomous. But perhaps in the case of those outcomes that are usually considered highly undersirable (e.g., death or severe injury) it should be presumed that the individual's choice is irrational and therefore nonautonomous. This presumption would justify, at best, temporarily constraining someone from certain acts in order to establish the rationality or irrationality of the choice.

In summary, it can plausibly be maintained that paternalistic interventions can be justified either (1) when intervention is responsive to the welfare of an individual whose autonomy is significantly diminished or (2) when temporary constraint is necessary to prevent a person from acting in a self-harming and *presumably* nonautonomous manner until it can be determined whether the individual is, in fact, acting autonomously. Paternalism in accordance with these two conditions is often called "weak paternalism," and it is entirely consistent with Mill's criticism of paternalism (which is essentially a rejection of so-called "strong paternalism"). The interventions that are characteristic of weak paternalism do not show a lack of respect for individual autonomy. In the first case, an individual is simply incapable of acting in a significantly autonomous manner. In the second, the point of the intervention is to ensure that an individual will not harm himself or herself while acting nonautonomously. Thus, the legitimacy of weak paternalism is widely accepted. In contrast, the legitimacy of strong paternalism is a hotly disputed issue. Strong paternalism is characterized by interventions that go beyond the limits set by conditions 1 and 2. Advocates of strong paternalism maintain that paternalistic interference with autonomous actions and choice can sometimes be justified.

Is strong paternalism ever justified? One defense of strong paternalism rests on a prudential argument that itself appeals to the importance of autonomy. We are aware that we are often tempted to act in ways that are likely to frustrate our long-term interests. Indeed, we may do ourselves serious irreversible harm of a sort that would severely diminish our autonomy. We should be willing, therefore, to accept those paternalistic acts, laws, and practices whose intent is to protect individual autonomy from being severely diminished. This argument is advanced in order to justify both (1) laws, such as those against the sale of seriously mind-altering drugs, that protect us against our own weakness of will and (2) laws that allow courts and psychiatrists to commit the mentally ill to institutions against their will in order to keep them from the kind of self-harm that might reduce their autonomy. The same sort of prudential argument is sometimes invoked to justify paternalistic acts by physicians when these acts are performed to prevent serious deterioration of the patient's autonomy. However, some of the constraining interventions that seem to be justified by this line of argument are very problematic. Some individuals, for example, might prefer to give in to temptations, weighing the pleasures of using seriously mind-altering drugs more highly than its risks (including that of diminished autonomy). The appropriateness of involuntary civil commitment of the mentally ill is, of course, also quite disputable in cases involving strong paternalism (i.e., in cases in which the mental illness in question has not destroyed the person's capacity to make autonomous decisions).

NOTES

1 Efforts to determine what is morally good and what is morally bad with regard to human character also fall under the heading of normative ethics. This aspect of normative ethics is of central importance in a school of thought known as *virtue ethics*. A discussion of virtue ethics is presented later in Chapter 1.

2 Some scholars prefer to identify biomedical ethics as a type of *practical ethics,* rather than *applied* ethics. Their underlying concern is to avoid any suggestion that particular moral problems can be effectively resolved simply by "applying" ethical theories or principles. We continue to employ the commonly used category of applied ethics, but in no way do we mean to imply the appropriateness of any mechanical "application" model. (See the section "Alternative Directions and Methods.")

3 Ethical theories are also used to evaluate the conduct of other people. The best standards to use for evaluating the conduct of others might or might not be the best standards for real-time decision making under the pressures and constraints of real life. Ethicists consider both the "first-person" decision making and "third-person" judging perspectives.

4 In what follows, the two versions of utilitarianism are articulated in ways intended to emphasize a contrast between them. There are alternative ways of articulating both act-utilitarianism and rule-utilitarianism, and some of these articulations bring the two versions of utilitarianism much closer than our account suggests.

5 Possibly a majority of contemporary utilitarians take the satisfaction of preferences to constitute intrinsic value. See, for example, Jonathan Glover, ed., *Utilitarianism and Its Critics* (New York: Macmillan, 1990), Part 2.

6 J. J. C. Smart, "Extreme and Restricted Utilitarianism," in Michael D. Bayles, ed., *Contemporary Utilitarianism* (New York: Doubleday, 1968), p. 100.

7 W. D. Ross, *The Right and the Good* (Oxford: Clarendon Press, 1930), p. 22.

8 Alan Donagan, "Is There a Credible Form of Utilitarianism?" in *Contemporary Utilitarianism,* p. 189. Donagan's point is that act-utilitarianism is "monstrous" and "incredible" because it seems to recommend such murders.

9 The distinction between act-utilitarianism and rule-utilitarianism is a distinction that has become prominent only in contemporary times. Accordingly, the writings of Bentham and Mill are somewhat ambiguous with regard to these categories. Although Bentham is probably rightly understood as an act-utilitarian, a very strong case can be made for interpreting Mill as a rule-utilitarian. See, for example, J. O. Urmson, "The Interpretation of the Moral Philosophy of J. S. Mill," in *Contemporary Utilitarianism,* pp. 13–24. Some contemporary philosophers offer theories that cut across the distinction between act and rule utilitarianism. See, e.g., Shelly Kagan, *Normative Ethics* (Boulder, CO.: Westview, 1997).

10 Smart, "Extreme and Restricted Utilitarianism," p. 107. For a response to the charge of rule-worship see Brad Hooker, *Ideal Code, Real World: A Rule-Consequentialist Theory of Morality* (Oxford: Oxford University Press, 2000).

11 Immanuel Kant, *Groundwork of the Metaphysic of Morals,* trans. H. J. Paton (New York: Harper & Row, 1964), p. 88.

12 *Ibid.,* p. 96.

13 H. J. Paton, *The Categorical Imperative: A Study in Kant's Moral Philosophy* (Chicago: University of Chicago Press, 1948), p. 172.

14 The account of beneficence suggested here reflects an analysis originally presented by Tom L. Beauchamp and James F. Childress in Chapters 4 and 5 of *Principles of Biomedical Ethics* (New York: Oxford University Press, 1979).

15 Ross, *The Right and the Good,* p. 19.

16 *Ibid.,* p. 20.

17 *Ibid.,* p. 21.

18 *Ibid.*

19 *Ibid.*

20 Beauchamp and Childress, *Principles of Biomedical Ethics,* 6th ed. (New York: Oxford University Press, 2008), Chapter 1.

21 Such a foundational principle might have a complex structure (unlike that of utilitarianism or Kantianism). For example, a foundational principle might consist of two or more simpler principles arranged in a strict hierarchy.

22 But see the section "Reflective Equilibrium and Appeals to Coherence" later in the chapter.

23 We have noted that Beauchamp and Childress, *Principles of Biomedical Ethics,* is an influential work of principle-based ethics in biomedical ethics. Another is National Commission for the Protection of Human Subjects of Biomedical and Behavioral Research, *The Belmont Report: Ethical Principles and Guidelines for Research Involving Human Subjects* (Washington, DC: Government Printing Office, 1979).

24 Arguments of this sort can be found in, for example, Iris Murdoch, *The Sovereignty of Good* (London: Routledge and Kegan Paul, 1970); and Martha Nussbaum, *Love's Knowledge* (New York: Oxford University Press, 1990).

25 The last three paragraphs have benefited from ideas in Alisa L. Carse, "Rules of Conduct and the Uncodifiability of Virtue" (unpublished manuscript).

26 Carol Gilligan, *In a Different Voice: Psychological Theory and Women's Moral Development* (Cambridge, MA: Harvard University Press, 1982).

27 Modern Kantians, however, generally accept this idea. They allow a father to provide for his own children rather than other children. They merely forbid him to violate the rights of others in order to benefit his own.

28 Susan Sherwin, *No Longer Patient: Feminist Ethics and Health Care* (Philadelphia: Temple University Press, 1992), p. 50.

29 See, e.g., Allison M. Jaggar, "Feminist Ethics: Projects, Problems, Prospects," in Claudia Card, ed., *Feminist Ethics* (Lawrence: University of Kansas Press, 1991), p. 89.

30 See Sherwin, *No Longer Patient,* pp. 49–51. Cf. Sara Ruddick, "Remarks on the Sexual Politics of Reason," in Eva Feder Kittay and Diana T. Meyers, eds., *Women and Moral Theory* (Savage, MD: Rowman & Littlefield, 1987), p. 246; John M. Broughton, "Women's Rationality and Men's Virtues: A Critique of Gender Dualism in Gilligan's Theory of Moral Development," in Mary Jeanne Larrabee, ed., *An Ethic of Care: Feminist and Interdisciplinary Perspectives* (New York: Routledge, 1993), p. 134; and Zella Luria, "A Methodological Critique," in Larrabee, *An Ethic of Care,* pp. 202–203.

31 Sherwin, *No Longer Patient,* p. 57. Feminist ethics has, indeed, flourished since Sherwin wrote these words.

32 Albert R. Jonsen and Stephen Toulmin, *The Abuse of Casuistry: A History of Moral Reasoning* (Berkeley: University of California Press, 1988). For a distinct version of casuistry, see Baruch Brody, *Taking Issue: Pluralism and Casuistry in Bioethics* (Washington, DC: Georgetown University Press, 2003).

33 See *In re Quinlan,* 70 N.J. 10 (1976); *In re Conroy,* 486 A. 2d 1209 (N.J. 1985); and *Cruzan v. Director,* 110 S. Ct. 2841 (1990).

34 John D. Arras, "Getting Down to Cases: The Revival of Casuistry in Bioethics," *Journal of Medicine and Philosophy* 16 (1991), p. 46.

35 See "Outline for a Decision Procedure for Ethics," *Philosophical Review* 60 (1951), pp. 177–197; and *A Theory of Justice* (Cambridge, MA: Harvard University Press, 1971).

36 Strictly speaking, coherence involves other theoretical virtues as well, such as simplicity and clarity. Moreover, any proponent of this model—in fact, of any model or theory—must seek not only coherence among ethical beliefs but also coherence between ethical beliefs and empirical beliefs. Thus, the claim that surgery without anesthesia on dogs is morally appropriate because dogs are incapable of suffering is undermined by evidence showing that dogs, in fact, can suffer.

37 A commonly cited distinction pertaining to the present model is that between "narrow" and "wide" reflective equilibrium. See, for example, Norman Daniels, "Wide Reflective Equilibrium and Theory Acceptance in Ethics," *Journal of Philosophy* 76 (1979), pp. 256–282; and Margaret Holmgren, "The Wide and Narrow of Reflective Equilibrium," *Canadian Journal of Philosophy* 19 (1989), pp. 43–60.

38 Indeed, contrary to its reputation as an exclusively top-down form of reasoning, principle-based ethics may be best understood as a version of reflective equilibrium that emphasizes principles. See David DeGrazia, "Moving Forward in Bioethical Theory: Theories, Cases, and Specified Principlism," *Journal of Medicine and Philosophy* 17 (1992), pp. 511–539.

39 Authors writing on the nature of autonomous action present analyses that differ at the level of details, but leading contributions seem to agree that the conditions just stated are at least necessary for autonomous action. For example, the analysis of Beauchamp and Childress (*Principles of Biomedical Ethics,* 4th ed. [1994], p. 123) is close to the present analysis (and, in fact, significantly influenced it). Some authors, however, suggest—controversially—that the four conditions just stated are insufficient for autonomous action. According to these authors, autonomous action involves the exercise of the capacity to form higher-order values or desires about the desires (to do certain things) that are involved in intentional action. See, e.g., Harry G. Frankfurt, "Freedom of the Will and the Concept of a Person," *Journal of Philosophy* 68 (1971), pp. 5–20; Gerald Dworkin, *The Theory and Practice of Autonomy* (Cambridge: Cambridge University Press, 1988), Chapter 1; and David DeGrazia, "Autonomous Action and Autonomy-Subverting Psychiatric Conditions," *Journal of Medicine and Philosophy* 19 (1994), pp. 279–297.

40 The distinction between occurrent and dispositional coercion is made by Michael D. Bayles in "A Concept of Coercion," in J. Roland Pennock and John D. Chapman, eds., *Coercion: Nomos XIV* (Chicago: Aldine-Atherton, 1972), pp. 16–29.

41 Some may find it plausible to understand freedom from external constraints as including *freedom of choice,* which is constrained by actions and policies that narrow the range of options that one can reasonably expect to be available to one. This understanding of freedom from external constraints is very broad (and controversial) because it implies that the *nonprovision* of certain goods or services can count as an external constraint, as well as disrespectful of autonomy. For example, excluding Medicaid coverage for a procedure that was previously funded—and that the poor can reasonably expect to be covered—would narrow some indigent persons' range of medical options and would therefore count as disrespectful of their autonomy.

42 Perhaps he does not sufficiently understand the alternative of studying; perhaps he thinks studying puts him in some kind of danger. In any case, his capacity to act autonomously is clearly compromised by the constraint described in the case.

43 Because nonautonomous action is often inconsistent with one's usual values and priorities—and is, therefore, in a sense less authentically "one's own"—autonomy is sometimes conceptualized as involving *authenticity.*

44 There are some situations in which constraining someone's liberty is compatible with respecting his or her autonomy. For example, suppose Salvator asks Danny to take away Salvator's car keys if the latter drinks too much at a party; Salvator does not trust himself to exercise good judgment while drunk. If, hours later, Salvator has imbibed excessively, Danny would not show disrespect for Salvator's autonomy by snatching away his car keys, thereby restricting his liberty at that moment. Or, to cite a famous example, if you see a man who is about to walk onto a seriously faulty bridge, you might grab him—much to his annoyance—and prevent his walking farther until you are sure that he knows the risks. Since not knowing the risks undermines the man's understanding of his options, this minor interference with his liberty is consistent with respecting his autonomy.

45 Kant, *Groundwork,* p. 108.

46 John Stuart Mill, *Utilitarianism, On Liberty, Essay on Bentham,* ed. Mary Warnock (New York: New American Library, 1962), pp. 185, 187. All quotations in this chapter are from this edition of *On Liberty.*

47 Joel Feinberg's discussion of such principles served as a guide for the formulations adopted here. See Joel Feinberg, *Social Philosophy* (Englewood Cliffs, NJ: Prentice-Hall, 1973), Chapter 2.

48 "Harm principle" often denotes Mill's view that *only* harm to others justifies restrictions on liberty. See the section on "Paternalism," below.

49 Gerald Dworkin, "Paternalism," *The Monist* 56 (1972), p. 65.

50 Charles Fried, *Medical Experimentation: Personal Integrity and Social Policy* (New York: American Elsevier, 1974), p. 101.

51 Mill, *On Liberty,* p. 135.

52 *Ibid.*

ANNOTATED BIBLIOGRAPHY

Beauchamp, Tom L., and James F. Childress: *Principles of Biomedical Ethics,* 6th ed. (New York: Oxford University Press, 2008). The authors defend and deploy a principle-based approach in biomedical ethics.

Blustein, Jeffrey: *Care and Commitment: Taking the Personal Point of View* (New York: Oxford University Press, 1991). Blustein argues for a synthesis of insights from recently dominant ethical theories, the ethics of care, and recent philosophical work on personal integrity into a unified moral outlook.

Brand-Ballard, Jeffrey: "Consistency, Common Morality, and Reflective Equilibrium," *Kennedy Institute of Ethics Journal* 13 (September 2003), pp. 231–58. Brand-Ballard argues that an adequate ethical theory may involve revising some of our confidently held moral convictions.

Brody, Baruch: *Taking Issue: Pluralism and Casuistry in Bioethics* (Washington, DC: Georgetown University Press, 2003). Brody defends a unique variant of casuistry before employing it in exploring various issues in biomedical ethics.

Carse, Alisa L., and Hilde Lindemann Nelson: "Rehabilitating Care," *Kennedy Institute of Ethics Journal* 6 (March 1996), pp. 19–35. The authors identify four major criticisms that are commonly directed against the ethics of care, and they argue that the ethics of care can respond adequately to those criticisms.

Childress, James F.: *Who Should Decide? Paternalism in Health Care* (New York: Oxford University Press, 1982). In this extended discussion of paternalism, Childress examines the metaphors and principles underlying the disputes about professional paternalism in health care.

Christman, John, ed.: *The Inner Citadel: Essays on Individual Autonomy* (New York: Oxford University Press, 1989). This anthology provides a collection of articles on the nature and value of individual autonomy.

DeGrazia, David: "Moving Forward in Bioethical Theory: Theories, Cases, and Specified Principlism," *Journal of Medicine and Philosophy* 17 (October 1992), pp. 511–539. After challenging several leading methodologies in ethics, DeGrazia defends a "specified" principlism.

Dworkin, Gerald: *The Theory and Practice of Autonomy* (Cambridge: Cambridge University Press, 1988). In Part 1, Dworkin examines the nature and value of autonomy. In Part 2, he applies the general framework developed in Part 1 to various moral questions.

Foot, Philippa: *Virtues and Vices* (Oxford: Blackwell, 1978). Foot argues that virtue is more central, morally, than obligation; the paradigm moral person is one who is disposed by character to be rightly motivated.

Gert, Bernard, Charles M. Culver, and K. Danner Clouser: *Bioethics: A Systematic Approach*, 2nd ed. (New York: Oxford University Press, 2006). The authors of this philosophical introduction to bioethics defend a unified approach that proceeds from the common morality: a set of moral beliefs held by all rational persons. They defend their approach against competitors in bioethical theory. Topics covered include mental illness, informed consent, paternalism, death, and euthanasia.

Glover, Jonathan, ed.: *Utilitarianism and Its Critics* (New York: Macmillan, 1990). The various selections in this anthology incorporate both objections to utilitarianism and attempts to defend utilitarianism against the objections.

Jonsen, Albert R., and Stephen Toulmin: *The Abuse of Casuistry: A History of Moral Reasoning* (Berkeley: University of California Press, 1988). After examining the history of casuistry and the criticism it has received, the authors argue for its revival.

Journal of Medicine and Philosophy 15 (April 1990). The articles included in this issue appear under the heading of "Philosophical Critique of Bioethics." Various methodological issues are considered, and several of the articles develop criticisms of the principle-based approach associated with Beauchamp and Childress in *Principles of Biomedical Ethics*.

Kant, Immanuel: *Groundwork of the Metaphysic of Morals,* translated and analyzed by H. J. Paton (New York: Harper & Row, 1964). In this work, a basic reference point, Kant offers an overall statement and defense of his ethical theory.

Korsgaard, Christine M.: *Creating the Kingdom of Ends* (Cambridge: Cambridge University Press, 1996). This collection of the author's essays represents a leading attempt to defend, refine, and engage Kant's moral philosophy.

Larrabee, Mary Jeanne, ed.: *An Ethic of Care: Feminist and Interdisciplinary Perspectives* (New York: Routledge, 1993). This anthology focuses on Carol Gilligan's work and its implications. Special attention is given to debates in moral philosophy, empirical claims in psychology about alleged gender differences in moral reasoning, and challenges to Gilligan's work that claim it excludes African American and other cultures.

MacIntyre, Alasdair: *After Virtue: A Study in Moral Theory,* 2nd ed. (Notre Dame, IN: University of Notre Dame Press, 1984). Advancing the disquieting thesis that contemporary moral language consists of the fragmented remnants of a worldview no longer accepted in the secular West, MacIntyre advocates a return to Aristotelean virtue ethics.

Mill, John Stuart: *Utilitarianism, On Liberty, Essay on Bentham,* edited by Mary Warnock (New York: New American Library, 1962). In his famous essay "Utilitarianism," Mill offers a classic statement of the utilitarian position. In his equally well-known essay "On Liberty," he defends the classic liberal view regarding the limitation of individual liberty.

O'Neill, Onora: *Autonomy and Trust in Bioethics* (Cambridge: Cambridge University Press, 2002). A distinguished Kantian who has been involved in bioethics policy in the United Kingdom addresses tensions between the values of trust and autonomy in biomedical ethics, focusing especially on reproductive autonomy.

Rawls, John: *A Theory of Justice* (Cambridge, MA: Harvard University Press, 1971). In this classic work, Rawls presents and defends his theory of justice as an alternative to utilitarian theory. In doing so, he also argues for and uses the method of reflective equilibrium.

Sartorius, Rolf, ed.: *Paternalism* (Minneapolis: University of Minnesota Press, 1983). The various articles in this collection deal with the nature and justifiability of paternalism.

Sumner, L. W.: *Welfare, Happiness, and Ethics* (Oxford: Clarendon, 1996). Sumner defends an updated version of the theory that happiness constitutes an individual's good or well-being and argues that utilitarianism is the most promising approach to ethical and political theory.

Tong, Rosemarie: *Feminist Approaches to Bioethics: Theoretical Reflections and Practical Applications* (Boulder, CO: Westview, 1997). Tong articulates feminist and nonfeminist approaches to bioethics, defends the former, and explores implications for medical issues related to procreation.

Wolf, Susan, ed.: *Feminism & Bioethics: Beyond Reproduction* (New York: Oxford University Press, 1996). This anthology takes feminist theory beyond reproductive issues, tackling such problems as euthanasia, AIDS, the physician-patient relationship, and health-care reform.

APPENDIX: SELECTED REFERENCE SOURCES IN BIOMEDICAL ETHICS

PRINT RESOURCES

Craig, Edward, ed.: *The Routledge Encyclopedia of Philosophy* (New York: Routledge, 1998). This ten-volume resource contains articles on all major topics in philosophy including many in ethics.

Kennedy Institute of Ethics, Georgetown University: Scope Note series. This series provides extensive annotated bibliographies on a wide variety of issues in biomedical ethics. Currently Scope Notes are available on more than forty topics. They can be ordered toll-free by telephone at 800-MED-ETHX or by e-mail at bioethics@georgetown.edu.

Lineback, Richard H., ed.: *The Philosopher's Index* (Bowling Green, OH: Philosophers' Information Center). This reference source, updated quarterly, is "a current, comprehensive and easy-to-use subject and author index" to philosophical articles, books, anthologies, and contributions to anthologies. The subject index identifies useful material on virtually all major topics in biomedical ethics. A bibliography follows each article, and article abstracts are usually available.

Post, Stephen G., ed. in chief: *Encyclopedia of Bioethics,* 3rd ed. (New York: Macmillan, 2003). This five-volume set is a basic reference source in biomedical ethics, containing entries on virtually all major topics in biomedical ethics. Each article is followed by a selected bibliography.

Walters, LeRoy, and Tamar Joy Kahn, eds.: *Bibliography of Bioethics* (Washington, DC: Kennedy Institute of Ethics, Georgetown University). With volumes listed annually, this bibliography is exceptionally comprehensive.

WEB RESOURCES

Bioethics net (http://ajobonline.com). This resource is provided by the Center for Bioethics, University of Pennsylvania. It contains links to journals in biomedical ethics, updates and editorials on current issues, and a listing of jobs in the field. The center's online *American Journal of Bioethics* is accessible by subscription.

ETHX on the Web (http://bioethics.georgetown.edu/databases/ETHXWeb/basice.htm). Sponsored by the Kennedy Institute of Ethics, Georgetown University, this source permits visitors to search for journal articles, book chapters, bills, laws, court decisions, books, and news articles pertaining to biomedical ethics and other types of professional ethics.

Locator Plus (http://locatorplus.gov). Sponsored by the National Library of Medicine, this resource allows visitors to search for books, journals, and audiovisuals, including many in biomedical ethics, in the National Library of Medicine collection.

PubMed (http://www.ncbi.nlm.nih.gov/pubmed). A service of the National Library of Medicine, PubMed includes more than 14 million citations for articles in medicine and the life sciences, including articles in biomedical ethics. This resource also provides links to sites that provide full text articles.

Stanford Encyclopedia of Philosophy (http://plato.stanford.edu). Peer-reviewed, dynamic entries, including many on ethics.

THE PROFESSIONAL-PATIENT RELATIONSHIP

INTRODUCTION

What moral rules should health professionals observe in dealing with patients? What qualities of character will a virtuous professional exhibit? Will the rules and virtues appropriate to a health professional differ depending on whether one is a physician or a nurse (the two types of health professional considered in this chapter)? Are physicians in particular ever morally justified in acting paternalistically toward their patients? Are physicians or nurses ever morally justified in withholding information from their patients, lying to them, overriding the presumption of patient confidentiality, or treating patients without their consent? And what does valid consent involve? When a nurse experiences a conflict between advocacy for a patient and loyalty to the health-care team with a physician as its leader, what are the nurse's primary responsibilities? What is his or her proper role? How should physicians and nurses negotiate the complexities of a multicultural environment, in which patients sometimes embrace values that differ significantly from those of the professional and his or her culture? This chapter confronts these and other fundamental moral issues associated with the professional-patient relationship and, therefore, with many of the other issues taken up in this book.

PHYSICIANS' OBLIGATIONS AND VIRTUES

The Hippocratic Oath, reprinted in this chapter, reflects the traditional paternalism of the medical profession. The oath requires physicians to act so as to benefit the sick and "keep them from harm," but says nothing about patients' rights. Until fairly recently, the codes of ethics developed by the American Medical Association revealed a similar approach. They articulated rules and virtues that should guide physicians in their professional relationships with

58

patients and others but remained silent on patients' rights. For example, physicians were expected to promote their patients' well-being, but nothing was said about a patient's right to define his or her own "well-being"—or to participate in decisions affecting it. By contrast, the discussions that have taken place over the past three decades in biomedical ethics have frequently emphasized patients' rights, especially their right of self-determination. This emphasis reflects, among other factors, a growing change in lay attitudes toward physicians.

For a long time physicians were viewed as selfless individuals who could be expected to do everything in their power to benefit their patients. Patients, by contrast, were viewed as dependent individuals with an obligation to trust their physicians. It was often taken for granted that doctors—because of their presumed wisdom, objectivity, skill, and benevolence—were best positioned to decide what was in their patients' best interests. Professional codes of medical ethics reflected this view of the physician-patient relationship, affirming that physicians would act to benefit, and not exploit, the often vulnerable patients over whom they frequently held great influence and power.

Current attitudes toward physicians are somewhat different due to many factors. First among them, the physician-patient relationship has become increasingly impersonal as the growth of medical knowledge and technology has made medicine more complex. Growing complexity has led to increased specialization and the growth of large, depersonalized medical institutions. Second, the rise of "iatrogenic harm," illnesses and injuries resulting from medical interventions, has sometimes raised doubts about the skills and judgment of physicians. Third, it is commonly thought that many physicians engage in practices that compromise patients' interests either for the sake of physicians' financial gain or to protect the financial interests of an insurance company or program. In an article reprinted in this chapter, Edmund D. Pellegrino argues that physician virtue is of paramount importance in situations in which altruism and self-interest appear to conflict.

In keeping with such changing attitudes toward physicians, many recent discussions of medical ethics have attempted to expose and criticize the extensive paternalism embodied in traditional codes of medical ethics. Numerous authors have criticized professional codes that sanction paternalistic justifications for medical practices—such as lying for a patient's "own good"—that violate a patient's right to self-determination. But in several recent statements, including "Fundamental Elements of the Patient-Physician Relationship,"[1] the American Medical Association, for example, acknowledges numerous patient rights, including the right to receive information relevant to one's medical care.

PATERNALISM AND RESPECT FOR PATIENT AUTONOMY

Is fostering a patient's well-being, in accordance with the traditional commitment, always compatible with respecting patient autonomy? In their analysis of several models—or metaphors—of the physician-patient relationship, James F. Childress and Mark Siegler suggest in this chapter that these two goals are not always compatible. The paternalism model, which emphasizes the traditional commitment to serve patient well-being, is usually inadequate in today's world, according to the authors. Physicians and patients may disagree in their health-related values (for example, if only the physician considers addiction to cigarettes a disease); or they may disagree about the relative value of health in comparison with other values (as when a Jehovah's Witness refuses a blood transfusion, knowing that death will inevitably result, while the patient's physician considers the transfusion necessary). As the authors put it, paternalism "tends to concentrate on care rather than respect, patients' needs rather than their rights, and physicians' discretion rather than patients' autonomy or self-determination."

That is not to say that paternalism is never justified, however. Childress and Siegler defend the commonly accepted form of paternalism (identified in Chapter 1 as *weak* paternalism) in which a patient is incompetent, or substantially lacking in decision-making capacity, and at risk of harm. Moreover, the authors ultimately recommend, for many physician-patient interactions in which the patient is competent, the metaphor of *negotiation*. This metaphor illuminates two important aspects of medical relationships: (1) the autonomy of both parties (where autonomy is construed not as a goal that in some cases might be imposed on a patient, but as a constraint on permissible interactions between autonomous persons), and (2) the ongoing nature of the relationship. The metaphor of negotiation invites both patient and physician to determine what they consider acceptable terms for continuing the relationship. Those terms may involve one or more of the models Childress and Siegler discuss—even paternalism, for a patient might autonomously decide to turn the medical decision-making reins over to a physician willing to take them.

As presented in Chapter 1, paternalism is the interference with, limitation of, or usurpation of individual autonomy justified by reasons referring exclusively to the welfare or needs of the person whose autonomy is being interfered with, limited, or usurped. In acting paternalistically, physicians in effect act as if they, and not their patients, can best identify what is in their patients' best interests as well as the best means to advance those interests. Many commentators contend that paternalism and respect for patient autonomy are incompatible. But Terrence F. Ackerman argues in this chapter that genuine respect for autonomy may require physicians to override patients' treatment-related preferences (suggesting at least weak paternalism) in order to help them regain some of the autonomy lost due to the constraining effects of illness. While affirming the importance of honesty and respect for patients' rights, Ackerman criticizes the interpretation of respect for autonomy that takes it to be essentially a principle of *noninterference*. To understand his concern, it is helpful to discuss two kinds of cases in which the values perceived as fundamental in physician-patient interactions—promotion of patient well-being and respect for patient autonomy—appear to conflict.

First, a patient's abilities to reason and deliberate may be so severely constrained by illness (e.g., high fever, delirium) that autonomous decisions are virtually impossible and apparent decisions may be inconsistent with the patient's history of decisions and values. In such cases, the promotion of a patient's well-being may require acting against his or her wishes as currently expressed. This would appear to violate the principle of respect for autonomy. But the conflict between the two values may be illusory. If the patient's autonomy is severely diminished and the desires expressed are inconsistent with the patient's history and values, the principle of respect for autonomy would not even seem to apply. When there are compelling reasons to believe that a patient's decisions are not autonomous and that as a result the patient cannot exercise the right of self-determination, no paternalistic violation of that right—no *strong* paternalism—is involved when a physician makes decisions for the patient.

Second, a patient and physician may disagree about just what constitutes the patient's well-being (a point noted by Childress and Siegler). A physician, for example, might insist on continuing aggressive treatment for a cancer patient, even though past treatment has brought no positive results. The patient might have a strong desire to discontinue the recommended therapy and die without the additional discomforts caused by the therapy. To foster the patient's well-being, then, the physician might think it necessary to override the patient's decision paternalistically. Here the physician may see a conflict between two obligations: an obligation to promote the patient's well-being, as understood from an objective medical standpoint, and an obligation to respect the patient's right of self-determination. The physician may believe that virtually any chance of prolonging life justifies continuing treatment. But while the prolongation of life is generally regarded as a good, and premature death a harm, the paternalistic model itself does not commit one to the prolongation of life irrespective of the harms the patient might incur. Thus, the physician's belief that this life must be prolonged, whatever the discomfort to the patient and no matter how brief the extension of life, is apparently due to the physician's own values rather than to some indisputably objective medical values. The patient, meanwhile, may believe that a few extra days or weeks of uncomfortable in-hospital life, with an extremely small chance of further prolonging life, are not worth the price. If the patient's decision is the result of reflection and is in keeping with his or her history of decisions and values, respect for autonomy would seem to require acting in accord with the *patient's* conception of his or her well-being. If the patient's decision is not in accord with his or her history of decisions and values but is the result of a careful, reflective revision of those values, respect for autonomy would again seem to require acting in accord with the patient's choices. The conflict here is not between an obligation to respect autonomy and an obligation to promote patient well-being, but between two different conceptions of well-being. The conflict arises because what constitutes a person's well-being is, at least to some extent, a subjective or personal judgment.

The problematic cases that concern Ackerman arise because of the constraining effects illness has on autonomy. In relation to the first kind of case, for example, it is sometimes difficult to judge to what extent a patient's capacity for clear-headed deliberation is undermined. In the face of such uncertainty, does the physician's obligation to promote the patient's well-being entail an obligation to act so as to "restore the patient's autonomy" to the greatest extent possible, even if this involves some measure of paternalism? Ackerman holds that the physician's obligation is to act to restore autonomy—suggesting (in Childress and Siegler's terms) that autonomy is a goal to be sought when it is absent or diminished, not just a constraint on physician-patient interactions when the patient is already considered autonomous. Ackerman gives examples intended to show how psychological states, such as depression, or social factors, such as family influence, can constrain a patient's decision making. He argues that physicians have an obligation to act in ways that will offset the effects of these constraints to make the patient more autonomous. It is not clear that all of Ackerman's examples involve paternalism, since they do not all involve the usurpation of patients' decision making. In any event, physicians who act as Ackerman recommends run the danger exemplified by the second kind of case, when they fail to see that a disagreement with a patient about some course of treatment may be due, not to the constraining effects of illness on autonomy, but to a disagreement about values.

THE ROLE AND RESPONSIBILITIES OF NURSES

Nurses face moral problems similar to those faced by physicians as well as moral problems uniquely related to their professional role. Like physicians, nurses must sometimes choose between doing what they believe will promote patients' well-being and respecting patients' self-determination. Various models of the nurse-patient relationship are possible, including a paternalistic model and a very different contracted-clinician model, which respects both a patient's right of self-determination and a nurse's right of conscientious refusal.[2]

But nurses also face dilemmas that physicians do not face. These dilemmas result from the nurse's position within the system or unit in which nurses work—which may be regarded as a *hierarchy* or as a *team,* depending on which features are emphasized. Nurses in hospitals care for patients and supervise others providing care. Usually, they are directly responsible both for patient care and implementing therapy. At the same time, nurses often have little influence in decision making regarding patients. Furthermore, they are generally regarded as subordinate to doctors, who make diagnoses and issue orders that nurses are expected to carry out. Under these circumstances, nurses are sometimes confronted with situations in which their obligations to patients seem to conflict with their obligations to physicians. The following questions exemplify the kinds of problems nurses face: Should nurses follow physicians' orders when nurses have good reason to believe that the orders are mistaken, the physicians refuse to admit that they might be mistaken, and following orders seems likely to jeopardize patients' safety? What should nurses do if they have good reason to believe that physicians are violating one or more of their patients' rights? For example, what should a nurse do when a physician lies to or withholds important information from a patient?

Developing themes emphasized in feminist ethics (as discussed in Chapter 1), some commentators have emphasized the difficulties nurses face when protecting patients' interests requires them to "buck" the system. Joy Kroeger-Mappes, for example, underscores the hierarchical nature of this system and attributes a large part of the difficulty to classist and sexist forces in society.[3] She defends the increasingly prominent ideal of the nurse as an autonomous professional who is prepared, under some circumstances, to challenge physicians' authority in advocating for patients' interests.

In response to this emerging ideal, Lisa H. Newton, in an article reprinted in this chapter, defends the traditional ideal of the nurse, whose role requires submission to the authority of physicians. In defending the traditional nurse, Newton argues that hospitals can function properly only if professionals' roles are clearly recognized; since only physicians have the training required to deal with many medical situations, their authority must be respected. (Her arguments suggest viewing the doctor much as a quarterback. From this perspective, a player who questions and interferes with the quarterback's play calling is unlikely to help the team.) Moreover, hospital patients have emotional needs that are best met by nurses, who in their traditional role can act as surrogate mothers to patients.

Helga Kuhse in this chapter directly challenges the claim that the nature of nursing demands submission and subservience, rebutting a variety of arguments—including some advanced by Newton—that have been offered in support of this claim. For example, according to Kuhse, the idea that nurses' subservience is required for efficient handling of patients' medical needs rests on two dubious assumptions: that most or all medical decision making is characterized by great urgency and that maximal efficiency is achieved by nurses' adopting an absolute rule (as opposed to a presumption) of following doctors' orders. She also contends that the surrogate mother role for nurses would be unnecessary and condescending to many patients, demoralizing to nurses, and overly deferential to physicians' views about the goals of treatment. She concludes that the proper role for nurses is one of advocacy for patients rather than subservience to physicians. Indeed, in her view, subservience would harm patients more than it would benefit them.

TRUTH TELLING

Traditional codes of medical ethics have little to say about lying, other forms of deception, or truth telling. Yet some of the most widely disputed issues in biomedical ethics center on physicians' obligation to be truthful with patients. Until fairly recently, it was not unusual for physicians to lie to patients about their illnesses for paternalistic reasons. Nor was it unusual for physicians to prescribe alternating injections of sterilized water with injections of painkilling drugs for patients who were told that all the injections contained an opiate. In the first kind of case, physicians often argued that patients did not want to know the truth or that the truth could seriously harm patients. In the second kind of case, physicians often argued that the deceptive practices were justified because water can have a psychotherapeutic effect but is much less dangerous to the patient than overly frequent injections of opiates.[4] Are physicians ever morally justified in paternalistic lies or deceptive practices? If so, under what conditions?

One way to approach these questions is to begin with more general questions. Is it always morally wrong to lie? Is it always right to tell the truth? If it is *always* wrong to lie or to deceive others, then it is wrong for anyone, including physicians, to do so. If lies and intentional deception are *sometimes* morally acceptable, we should attempt to specify the conditions that make them acceptable. Once these conditions are determined, we can then explore the particular physician-patient encounter to see if it satisfies them.

Rule-utilitarians, for example, faced with deciding under what conditions, if any, lies and deceptive practices are justified, would have to consider the possible consequences of adopting and following a particular rule. In the medical context, they would ask, "What would be the effect on the physician-patient relationship if physicians followed the rule, 'Lie to your patients whenever you believe that doing so is in the patient's best interests'?" In weighing the potential consequences of following such a rule, they would have to account for the erosive effect that following it would have on patients' trust of physicians.

Suppose a physician argued as follows: Physicians ought to lie to patients because (1) it is extremely difficult to convey the technical facts and uncertainties inherent in a medical situation to persons who lack medical training, (2) most patients do not want to know the truth, and (3) the truth can harm patients. In responding to this argument, a rule-utilitarian would have to examine the three factual claims underpinning this view, a task carried out by Roger Higgs in this chapter (though without special reference to rule-utilitarianism). In response to (1), Higgs argues that (a) while communicating the patient's medical situation to the patient may be difficult, it is generally not impossible, and (b) the admission "'I do not know' can be a major piece of honesty." In response to (2), Higgs cites studies suggesting that most patients *do* want the truth. In response to (3), Higgs contends the following: (a) While the truth can sometimes harm patients, such cases are less common than physicians have claimed; (b) the manner of disclosure is crucial to the likelihood of harm; and (c) lying can also be harmful by preventing a patient from being able to plan appropriately for the future and by weakening patient trust of physicians.

The rule-utilitarian who agreed with Higgs's findings would still have to determine whether exceptions should be built into a rule against lying to patients. These exceptions would probably be designed to cover cases with strong evidence to show that a patient does not want to know or would be seriously harmed by knowing. The rule-utilitarian would then have to determine whether the harm done to these patients would be outweighed by the overall good consequences of following a rule that prohibits all lying to patients.

Deontologists, of course, take a different approach. Immanuel Kant, whose deontological position is discussed in Chapter 1, is usually read as defending an "absolutist" position: All lies, including those told out of altruistic motives, are wrong. Not all deontologists agree with this absolutist position. As noted in Chapter 1, W. D. Ross maintains, for example, that there is a prima facie obligation not to lie or intentionally deceive, but that this obligation can sometimes be overridden by some other prima facie obligation. In medicine, the overriding obligation might sometimes be the physician's duty to promote the patient's medical well-being.

In the end, perhaps the kind of situation in which it is most plausible to argue that physicians may lie or deceive is one in which truthfulness seems likely to destroy a patient's hope. An example is that of a critically ill patient who might be devastated by the disclosure that her cancer is inoperable; without hope, she might quickly succumb to her disease. But we must not assume prematurely that truthful disclosure would have this effect, because hope may prove to be highly resilient. Moreover, it has been argued that disclosing the truth is usually compatible with inspiring hope, by responding to important patient concerns other than survival—such as the patient's hope that death will be relatively painless, the hope that he or she will not be abandoned before death, and the hope that loved ones will maintain contact in the time remaining.[5]

The question of whether physicians may ever lie or otherwise deceive their patients represents one aspect of the more general issue of what truth telling requires of physicians. Another aspect of this general issue concerns *nondisclosure* as opposed to active deception. Is it ever morally acceptable for a physician not to disclose a patient's diagnosis to him or her? There is broad agreement that, in emergencies, patients may receive medical treatment without prior disclosure of their condition and without other elements of informed consent (as discussed in a later section). But, after the emergency has passed, is it ever acceptable not to disclose information about the patient's medical condition, information that may have emerged for the first time during the emergency?

Or suppose, in another sort of case, that a patient's family insists, for reasons related to their cultural background, that a patient not be informed of his or her diagnosis. The patient, let us suppose, has inoperable colon cancer. Her family insists that, in their culture, treatment decisions are left to family members and physicians while medical "death sentences" are withheld from unknowing patients. Such a scenario is likely to create a dilemma for the physician (or at least for any physician working in a culture where truthful disclosure is the prevailing norm). On the one hand, the physician recognizes that the patient has a right to truthful disclosure about his or her medical condition. On the other hand, the physician appreciates the value of respecting other cultures and their moral practices. This dilemma is taken up in the final section of this chapter.

CONFIDENTIALITY AND CONFLICTING OBLIGATIONS

Among patients' rights, in addition to the right to truthful disclosure, the rights to privacy and confidentiality deserve special discussion along with the ethical principle of confidentiality. This chapter focuses on confidentiality rather than privacy. However, a clear understanding of confidentiality is best achieved in view of the distinction between confidentiality and privacy.

A person enjoys *privacy* when other individuals do not without permission invade what may be called his or her "sphere of privacy": a realm of intimate or sensitive information about the person that he or she generally does not wish to share with others or wishes to share with only a small circle of persons. Thus, sensitive medical information about Mr. Ramirez lies within his sphere of privacy. Since he would approve of his attending physician and other health professionals closely involved in his care learning details of his medical history, Mr. Ramirez would not consider their examining his medical record a violation of his privacy. By contrast, if another patient examined Mr. Ramirez's medical record without his permission, Mr. Ramirez would no doubt regard this intrusion as a violation of his privacy (an unauthorized entering of his sphere of privacy). To take another example, how Ms. Robbins appears while undressed lies within her sphere of privacy. Thus, if a stranger goes to great lengths to peer through Ms. Robbins's bedroom window while she is undressing, Ms. Robbins would almost certainly consider this unauthorized viewing an invasion of her privacy.

While privacy involves others not entering a person's sphere of privacy without permission, *confidentiality* involves those who have legitimate access to private information not bringing it out of that sphere and sharing it with others without permission. Thus, a doctor may legitimately enter (or access) large segments of a patient's sphere of privacy: his or her medical history, the appearance of his or her naked body if a physical examination or other procedure requires undressing, aspects of the patient's social history that bear directly on the patient's medical situation (e.g., concerning a history of alcoholism), and so on. If a doctor lacking permission discloses sensitive information to individuals other than health professionals who are closely involved with the patient's care, such disclosure constitutes a breach of confidentiality.

The importance of the principle of confidentiality in medicine has long been recognized. It is affirmed in the Hippocratic Oath as well as in more recent professional codes and statements such as those of the American Medical Association and the American Hospital Association. It is also recognized by the ethical codes of medical record librarians and social workers. The law further recognizes, in two ways, the importance of the patient's right to control information held by health professionals. First, physicians and psychotherapists are subject to legal sanctions if they reveal confidential information about patients. Second, physicians and psychotherapists are ordinarily exempt from giving testimony about their patients before a court of law. Most discussions of the moral significance of the principle of confidentiality in health care stress either respect for patient autonomy or the importance of protecting the trust undergirding the professional-patient relationship.

While the importance of medical confidentiality is broadly appreciated, some commentators hold that the duty to respect confidentiality is a prima facie one—that is, one that is sometimes justifiably overridden in conflicts with other moral duties. In this chapter the opinions in *Tarasoff v. Regents of the University of California* focus on the moral dilemmas posed for health-care professionals when such conflicts arise. Some of these conflicts take graphic form in the case (with commentaries) about HIV and confidentiality included in this chapter. The general issue this case provokes is, "Under what conditions, if any, may health-care professionals disclose confidential information about patients infected with HIV, in order to prevent harm to others?" In the *Tarasoff* case, the conflict at issue was between a psychologist's duty to respect the confidence of a patient, Prosenjit Poddar, and the psychologist's possible duty to warn a young woman, Tatiana Tarasoff, that Poddar might try to kill her. He did not warn the woman or her family, and Poddar did kill her. Did the psychologist have a duty to warn someone who was not his patient? If he did, should this duty have taken precedence over his duty to respect Poddar's confidences? The contrast between the majority and the dissenting opinions in the case serves to heighten awareness of the moral dilemmas raised for the professional who must choose between violating confidentiality and failing to perform an act that might save the life of another human being or otherwise prevent serious harm.

INFORMED CONSENT

It is now widely accepted that competent adult patients have a moral and legal right not to be subjected to medical interventions without their informed and voluntary consent.[6] But lying to patients or withholding information from them can seriously undermine their ability to make informed decisions and, therefore, to give informed consent. To be able to give such consent, and thereby exercise their right of self-determination, patients must have access to relevant information, and physicians are usually in the best position to supply it. Judge Spotswood W. Robinson III affirms this point in a judicial opinion, *Canterbury v. Spence*, when he argues that physicians have a duty to "satisfy the vital informational needs of the patient."[7]

The informed consent requirement is a relatively recent addition to the recognized ethical constraints governing the physician-patient relationship. Traditional codes of medical ethics recognize no physician obligation to inform patients about their diagnoses and the risks and benefits of alternative treatments. There is some controversy about when exactly the doctrine of informed consent was introduced into case law. But the 1972 *Canterbury* decision firmly established the doctrine and language of informed consent (even if the doctrine was introduced earlier), and great attention has been given in biomedical ethics to informed consent since that time. For example, Congress assigned the task of determining the ethical and legal implications of the informed consent requirement to the President's Commission for the Study of Ethical Problems in Medicine and Biomedical and Behavioral Research. In its 1982 report, a selection from which is reprinted here, the commission describes informed consent "as an ethical obligation that involves a process of shared decisionmaking based upon the mutual respect and participation ([of patients and health-care professionals])"[8] and identifies two values as providing the ethical foundation of the requirement: respect for the patient's autonomy, or self-determination, and promotion of the patient's well-being.

Much of the literature on informed consent focuses on several difficulties that affect the application of the requirement. (1) Who is *competent* to give consent? (2) When is consent *informed*? That is, how much information must a patient receive and understand before his or her consent is considered adequately informed? (3) When is consent *voluntary*? Each of these questions will be briefly examined in order to show some of the difficulties that affect the application of the requirement. It is important to note that the problems here are both conceptual and empirical. The meaning of the concepts *competent*, *informed*, and *voluntary* must be explicated so that it can be determined just what counts as voluntary and informed consent. Then in a particular case, it must be determined whether the individual in question is, in fact, capable of giving voluntary and informed consent and actually does so.

(1) Who is *competent* to give consent? At a general conceptual level, we might say that *to be competent to give consent is to be capable of consenting autonomously*. In view of the analysis of autonomous action presented in Chapter 1, a patient who is capable of consenting autonomously would be capable of consenting intentionally, with sufficient understanding of what consent entails in the circumstances, and with sufficient freedom from internal and external constraints. A sick patient in a hospital or institution may not be functioning normally enough to be competent. Patients who are under great emotional stress, who are frightened or in severe pain, are often incapable of making important decisions autonomously.

Recent work on competence stresses that it is not "all or nothing." Still, for practical purposes in medical decision making, some threshold must be used to determine who counts as competent and who does not. The commission's report maintains that individuals should be judged incapable of decision making only when they lack the ability to make decisions that promote their well-being in keeping with their own previously expressed values and preferences.

(2) How much *information* must patients receive—and understand—before their consent is informed? Suppose a patient suffering from breast cancer agrees to have a radical mastectomy. But she has not been told that studies indicate that this radical surgery is no more effective, in circumstances like hers, than much less radical surgery. Presumably, the patient has not been given sufficient information for her decision to count as an informed one. But what general criteria must the physician use in determining when sufficient information has been given? And is more information always better than less? Studies have shown that patients receiving long, detailed explanations of the risks and purposes of a procedure may understand and retain little of the significant information. In contrast, those who are given less detailed information may be able to comprehend and retain more of the important information.[9]

(3) When is consent really *voluntary*, or sufficiently free of internal and external constraints? It is often argued that it is easy to manipulate even clearly competent patients into giving consent when someone in a position of authority makes the request. For example, it has been shown that physicians, whose patients sometimes see them as "god" figures, and psychiatrists, whose judgments patients generally trust, find it easy to get the consent they request. When patients are influenced in this way, is their consent sufficiently voluntary? How about patients who are strongly pressured by family members to consent to treatment?

In consideration of these criteria for informed consent, leading work on this topic, such as that of the President's Commission, stresses the importance of the process of communication and of the patient's information processing. Studies have been undertaken both to understand and to improve the procedures used to get consent.[10] For genuine informed consent, it is often insufficient simply to transmit information to patients via a form or a short conversation listing possible risks and alternatives; it may be necessary to assess the degree of patient understanding, and perhaps some of the other factors that may affect the patient's decision, such as concern about a physician's reaction to a refusal.

Take the example of a terminally ill, diabetic, cancer-ridden patient who, after repeatedly rejecting amputation of his gangrenous left foot, suddenly consented. His consent appeared both voluntary and informed. However, given his history and the staff's knowledge of his values, an ethics consultant was called in to determine the reasons for the patient's change of mind. After a long conversation with the patient, the consultant learned that the patient had consented to the amputation only because he erroneously believed that without his consent the physician and the hospital would refuse to continue their care—raising questions about how informed and voluntary his decision was. Once the patient understood that this belief was incorrect, he withdrew his consent to the amputation. This case illustrates that informed consent requires more than forms and cursory rituals. It also shows the need for medical professionals to have insight into the communication processes they use to achieve informed consent.

But what extent, or quality, of communication can be reasonably expected, legally and morally, as a standard of informed consent? Whatever the answer, is it compatible with good medical practice? In one of this chapter's readings, Howard Brody criticizes the prevailing legal standards of informed consent for encouraging the impression that informed consent is separate from, and even interferes with, sound medical care. In his view, part of the problem stems from the fact that most physician-patient encounters occur in the context of primary care, whereas the courts and many commentators appear to take surgery and other risky procedures as the paradigm of such encounters. Brody discusses the advantages of a "conversation" standard of informed consent (which is illustrated in the case described previously), but argues that this demanding standard is probably not feasible legally. As a compromise between prevailing legal standards and the conversation standard, Brody recommends a "transparency" standard: A physician has provided adequate disclosure when his or her essential thinking about the medical situation has been made transparent to the patient.

THE PRACTICE OF MEDICINE IN A MULTICULTURAL SOCIETY

A cluster of issues regarding the physician-patient relationship may be somewhat loosely collected together under the term *multicultural*. The physician-patient encounter often brings together individuals who come from different countries with distinct cultures (or different subcultures within the same country) and who may speak different languages. For this reason, a physician and patient may have different cultural understandings of ethically appropriate practices and even different views about the governance of the universe (e.g., a universe governed by natural, causal laws versus one featuring the supernatural effects of spirit or magic).

A physician and patient who have different cultural perspectives may disagree significantly on *ethical* matters. For example, they may have different views regarding who possesses legitimate decision-making authority, the importance of truth telling in medical practice, the role of family in decisions primarily affecting a patient, and the proper treatment of children.

A physician and patient associated with different cultural traditions may also differ on *factual or metaphysical* questions that bear on patient care. A patient may, for example, believe that discussing the possibility of negative medical outcomes—such as succumbing to cancer—increases the likelihood of these possibilities coming to pass; or a patient may believe that rituals that cause great pain to children are necessary to eradicate evil spirits from their bodies. With a different view of causation, a Western physician may consider such beliefs irrational and potentially harmful if taken seriously—yet may feel ethically conflicted due to an awareness of the importance of respecting patients' cultural beliefs and traditions. In a reading reprinted in this chapter, Ruth Macklin explores several types of conflicts that can arise for physicians in multicultural settings and recommends ways of resolving some of these conflicts.

NOTES

1 Council on Ethical and Judicial Affairs, American Medical Association, "Fundamental Elements of the Patient-Physician Relationship," *Code of Medical Ethics: Current Opinions with Annotations* (2008–2009 edition), Opinion 10.01.

2 Sheri Smith, "Three Models of the Nurse-Patient Relationship," in Stuart F. Spicker and Sally Gadow (eds.), *Nursing: Images and Ideals* (New York: Springer, 1980). pp. 176–188.

3 Joy Kroeger-Mappes, "Ethical Dilemmas for Nurses: Physicians' Orders Versus Patients' Rights" (originally published in Thomas A. Mappes and Jane S. Zembaty, eds., *Biomedical Ethics* [New York: McGraw-Hill, 1981], pp. 75–102).

4 See, e.g., J. Slice, "Letter to the Editor," *Lancet* 2 (1972), p. 651.

5 This viewpoint is forcefully articulated in Howard Brody, "Hope," *JAMA* 246 (September 25, 1981), pp. 1411–1412.

6 Some commentators prefer the language of "decision-making capacity" to that of "competence" outside of legal contexts, but we are not persuaded that "competence" is exclusively a legal term.

7 *Canterbury* v. *Spence,* U.S. Court of Appeals, District of Columbia Circuit; May 19, 1972. 464 Federal Reporter, 2nd Series, 772.

8 President's Commission for the Study of Ethical Problems in Medicine and Biomedical and Behavioral Research, *Making Health Care Decisions: The Ethical and Legal Implications of Informed Consent in the Patient-Practitioner Relationship,* Vol. 1: *Report* (Washington, DC: U.S. Government Printing Office, 1982), p. 2.

9 On this point, see Ralph J. Alfidi, "Controversy, Alternatives, and Decisions in Complying with the Legal Doctrine of Informed Consent," *Radiology* 114 (January 1975), pp. 231–234.

10 Barrie R. Cassileth et al., "Informed Consent—Why Are Its Goals Imperfectly Realized?" *New England Journal of Medicine* 302 (1980), pp. 896–900; and T. M. Grundner, "On the Readability of Surgical Consent Forms," *ibid*, pp. 900–902.

PHYSICIANS' OBLIGATIONS AND VIRTUES

THE HIPPOCRATIC OATH

Little is known about the life of Hippocrates, a Greek physician born about 460 B.C. A collection of documents known as the *Hippocratic Writings* (largely written from the fifth to the fourth century B.C.) is believed to represent the remains of the Hippocratic school of medicine. Some of the works in this collection are credited to Hippocrates. The oath reprinted here, however, is believed to have been written by a philosophical sect known as the Pythagoreans in the latter part of the fourth century B.C. For the Middle Ages and later centuries, the Hippocratic Oath embodied the highest aspirations of the physician. It sets forth two sets of duties: (1) duties to the patient and (2) duties to the other members of the guild (profession) of medicine. In regard to the patient, it includes a set of absolute prohibitions (e.g., against abortion and euthanasia) as well as a statement of the physician's obligation to help and not to harm the patient.

I swear by Apollo Physician and Asclepius and Hygieia and Panaceia and all the gods and goddesses, making them my witnesses, that I will fulfill according to my ability and judgment this oath and this covenant:

To hold him who has taught me this art as equal to my parents and to live my life in partnership with him, and if he is in need of money to give him a share

Reprinted with permission of the publisher from *Ancient Medicine: Selected Papers of Ludwig Edelstein*, edited by Owsei Temkin and C. Lilian Temkin, p. 6. Copyright © 1967 by the Johns Hopkins Press: Baltimore.

of mine, and to regard his offspring as equal to my brothers in male lineage and to teach them this art—if they desire to learn it—without fee and covenant; to give a share of precepts and oral instruction and all the other learning to my sons and to the sons of him who has instructed me and to pupils who have signed the covenant and have taken an oath according to the medical law, but to no one else.

I will apply dietetic measures for the benefit of the sick according to my ability and judgment; I will keep them from harm and injustice.

I will neither give a deadly drug to anybody if asked for it, nor will I make a suggestion to this effect. Similarly I will not give to a woman an abortive remedy. In purity and holiness I will guard my life and my art.

I will not use the knife, not even on sufferers from stone, but will withdraw in favor of such men as are engaged in this work.

Whatever houses I may visit, I will come for the benefit of the sick, remaining free of all intentional injustice, of all mischief and in particular of sexual relations with both female and male persons, be they free or slaves.

What I may see or hear in the course of the treatment or even outside of the treatment in regard to the life of men, which on no account one must spread abroad, I will keep to myself holding such things shameful to be spoken about.

If I fulfill this oath and do not violate it, may it be granted to me to enjoy life and art, being honored with fame among all men for all time to come; if I transgress it and swear falsely, may the opposite of all this be my lot.

THE VIRTUOUS PHYSICIAN AND THE ETHICS OF MEDICINE
Edmund D. Pellegrino

Pellegrino defends a vision of medical ethics in which virtue ethics and duty-based ethics are each essential components. Citing several important codes of medical ethics, including the Hippocratic Oath, Pellegrino argues for a three-tiered system of obligations incumbent upon physicians. In "ascending order of ethical sensitivity," they are (1) obedience to the law, (2) the observance of moral rights and fulfillment of moral duties, and (3) the practice of virtue. According to Pellegrino, physicians' practice of virtue distinguishes itself less in the avoidance of clearly unethical actions than in the avoidance of actions at the ambiguous margin of moral responsibility, where altruism is pitted against self-interest. Examples of practices at this moral margin include investing in for-profit hospitals, selling services for whatever the market will bear, and making referrals on the basis of friendship and reciprocity rather than skill.

. . . In most professional ethical codes, virtue and duty-based ethics are intermingled. The Hippocratic Oath, for example, imposes certain duties like protection of confidentiality, avoiding abortion, not harming the patient. But the Hippocratic physician also pledges: ". . . in purity and holiness I will guard

From *Virtue and Medicine: Explorations in the Character of Medicine*, edited by Earl E. Shelp, pp. 248–253. © 1985 by D. Reidel Publishing Company. Reprinted by permission of Kluwer Academic Publishers.

my life and my art." This is an exhortation to be a good person and a virtuous physician, in order to serve patients in an ethically responsible way.

Likewise, in one of the most humanistic statements in medical literature, the first century A.D. writer, Scribonius Largus, made *humanitas* (compassion) an essential virtue. It is thus really a role-specific duty. In doing so he was applying the Stoic doctrine of virtue to medicine [1, 5].

The latest version (1980) of the AMA 'Principles of Medical Ethics' similarly intermingles duties, rights, and exhortations to virtue. It speaks of 'standards of behavior,' 'essentials of honorable behavior,' dealing 'honestly' with patients and colleagues and exposing colleagues 'deficient in character.' The *Declaration of Geneva*, which must meet the challenge of the widest array of value systems, nonetheless calls for practice 'with conscience and dignity' in keeping with 'the honor and noble traditions of the profession.' Though their first allegiance must be to the Communist ethos, even the Soviet physician is urged to preserve 'the high title of physician,' 'to keep and develop the beneficial traditions of medicine' and to 'dedicate' all his 'knowledge and strength to the care of the sick.'

Those who are cynical of any protestation of virtue on the part of physicians will interpret these excerpts as the last remnants of a dying tradition of altruistic benevolence. But at the very least, they attest to the recognition that the good of the patient cannot be fully protected by rights and duties alone. Some degree of supererogation is built into the nature of the relationship of those who are ill and those who profess to help them.

This too may be why many graduating classes, still idealistic about their calling, choose the Prayer of Maimonides (not by Maimonides at all) over the more deontological Oath of Hippocrates. In that 'prayer' the physician asks: ". . . may neither avarice nor miserliness, nor thirst for glory or for a great reputation engage my mind; for the enemies of truth and philanthropy may easily deceive me and make me forgetful of my lofty aim of doing good to thy children." This is an unequivocal call to virtue and it is hard to imagine even the most cynical graduate failing to comprehend its message.

All professional medical codes, then, are built of a three-tiered system of obligations related to the special roles of physicians in society. In the ascending order of ethical sensitivity they are: observance of the laws of the land, then observance of rights and fulfillment of duties, and finally the practice of virtue.

A legally based ethic concentrates on the minimum requirements—the duties imposed by human laws which protect against the grosser aberrations of personal rights. Licensure, the laws of torts and contracts, prohibitions against discrimination, good Samaritan laws, definitions of death, and the protection of human subjects of experimentation are elements of a legalistic ethic.

At the next level is the ethics of rights and duties which spells out obligations beyond what law defines. Here, benevolence and beneficence take on more than their legal meaning. The ideal of service, of responsiveness to the special needs of those who are ill, some degree of compassion, kindliness, promise-keeping, truth-telling, and non-maleficence and specific obligations like confidentiality and autonomy, are included. How these principles are applied, and conflicts among them resolved in the patient's best interests, are subjects of widely varying interpretation. How sensitively these issues are confronted depends more on the physician's character than his capability at ethical discourse or moral casuistry.

Virtue-based ethics goes beyond these first two levels. We expect the virtuous person to do the right and the good even at the expense of personal sacrifice and legitimate self-interest. Virtue ethics expands the notions of benevolence, beneficence, conscientiousness, compassion, and fidelity well beyond what strict duty might require. It makes some degree of supererogation mandatory because it calls for standards of ethical performance that exceed those prevalent in the rest of society [6].

At each of these three levels there are certain dangers from over-zealous or misguided observance. Legalistic ethical systems tend toward a justification for minimalistic ethics, a narrow definition of benevolence or beneficence, and a contract-minded physician-patient relationship. Duty- and rights-based ethics may be distorted by too strict adherence to the letter of ethical principles without the modulations and nuances the spirit of those principles implies. Virtue-based ethics, being the least specific, can more easily lapse into self-righteous paternalism or an unwelcome over-involvement in the personal life of the patient. Misapplication of any moral system even with good intent converts benevolence into maleficence. The virtuous person might be expected to be more sensitive to these aberrations than someone whose ethics is more deontologically or legally flavored.

The more we yearn for ethical sensitivity the less we lean on rights, duties, rules, and principles, and the more we lean on the character traits of the moral agent. Paradoxically, without rules, rights, and duties specifically spelled out, we cannot predict what form a particular person's expression of virtue will take. In a pluralistic society, we need laws, rules, and principles to assure a dependable minimum level of moral conduct. But that minimal level is insufficient in the complex and often unpredictable circumstances of decision-making, where technical and value desiderata intersect so inextricably.

The virtuous physician does not act from unreasoned, uncritical intuitions about what feels good. His dispositions are ordered in accord with that 'right reason' which both Aristotle and Aquinas considered essential to virtue. Medicine is itself ultimately an exercise of practical wisdom—a right way of acting in difficult and uncertain circumstances for a specific end, i.e., the good of a particular person who is ill. It is when the choice of a right and good action becomes more difficult, when the temptations to self-interest are most insistent, when unexpected nuances of good and evil arise and no one is looking, that the differences between an ethics based in virtue and an ethics based in law and/or duty can most clearly be distinguished.

Virtue-based professional ethics distinguishes itself, therefore, less in the avoidance of overtly immoral practices than in avoidance of those at the margin of moral responsibility. Physicians are confronted, in today's morally relaxed climate, with an increasing number of new practices that pit altruism against self-interest. Most are not illegal, or, strictly speaking, immoral in a rights- or duty-based ethic. But they are not consistent with the higher levels of moral sensitivity that a virtue-ethics demands. These practices usually involve opportunities for profit from the illness of others, narrowing the concept of service for personal convenience, taking a proprietary attitude with respect to medical knowledge, and placing loyalty to the profession above loyalty to patients.

Under the first heading, we might include such things as investment in and ownership of for-profit hospitals, hospital chains, nursing homes, dialysis units, tie-in arrangements with radiological or laboratory services, escalation of fees for repetitive, high-volume procedures, and lax indications for their use, especially when third party payers 'allow' such charges.

The second heading might include the ever decreasing availability and accessibility of physicians, the diffusion of individual patient responsibility in group practice so that the patient never knows whom he will see or who is on call, the itinerant emergency room physician who works two days and skips three with little commitment to hospital or community, and the growing over-indulgence of physicians in vacations, recreation, and 'self-development.'

The third category might include such things as 'selling one's services' for whatever the market will bear, providing what the market demands and not necessarily what the community needs, patenting new procedures or keeping them secret from potential competitor-colleagues, looking at the investment of time, effort, and capital in a medical education as justification of 'making it back,' or forgetting that medical knowledge is drawn from the cumulative experience of a multitude of patients, clinicians, and investigators.

Under the last category might be included referrals on the basis of friendship and reciprocity rather than skill, resisting consultations and second opinions as affronts to one's competence, placing the interest of the referring physician above those of the patients, looking the other way in the face of incompetence or even dishonesty in one's professional colleagues.

These and many other practices are defended today by sincere physicians and even encouraged in this era of competition, legalism, and self-indulgence. Some can be rationalized even in a deontological ethic. But it would be impossible to envision the physician committed to the virtues assenting to these practices. A virtue-based ethics simply does not fluctuate with what the dominant social mores will tolerate. It must interpret benevolence, beneficence, and responsibility in a way that reduces self interest and enhances altruism. It is the only convincing answer the profession can give to the growing perception clearly manifest in the legal commentaries in the FTC ruling that medicine is nothing more than business and should be regulated as such.

A virtue-based ethic is inherently elitist, in the best sense, because its adherents demand more of themselves than the prevailing morality. It calls forth that extra measure of dedication that has made the best physicians in every era exemplars of what the human spirit can achieve. No matter to what depths a society may fall, virtuous persons will always be the beacons that light the way back to moral sensitivity; virtuous physicians are the beacons that show the way back to moral credibility for the whole profession.

Albert Jonsen, rightly I believe, diagnoses the central paradox in medicine as the tension between self-interest and altruism [4]. No amount of deft juggling of rights, duties, or principles will suffice to resolve that tension. We are all too good at rationalizing what we want to do so that personal gain can be converted from vice to virtue. Only a character formed by the virtues can feel the nausea of such intellectual hypocrisy.

To be sure, the twin themes of self-interest and altruism have been inextricably joined in the history of medicine. There have always been physicians who reject the virtues or, more often, claim them falsely. But, in addition, there have been physicians, more often than the critics of medicine would allow, who have been truly virtuous both in intent and act. They have been, and remain, the leaven of the profession and the hope of all who are ill. They form the sea-wall that will not be eroded even by the powerful forces of commercialization, bureaucratization, and mechanization inevitable in modern medicine.

We cannot, need not, and indeed must not, wait for a medical analogue of MacIntyre's 'new St. Benedict' to show us the way. There is no new concept of virtue waiting to be discovered that is peculiarly suited to the dilemmas of our own dark age. We must recapture the courage to speak of character, virtue, and perfection in living a good life. We must encourage those who are willing to dedicate themselves to a "higher standard of self effacement" [2].

We need the courage, too, to accept the obvious split in the profession between those who see and feel the altruistic imperatives in medicine, and those who do not. Those who at heart believe that the pursuit of private self-interest serves the public good are very different from those who believe in the restraint of self-interest. We forget that physicians since the beginnings of the profession have subscribed to different values and virtues. We need only recall that the Hippocratic Oath was the Oath of physicians of the Pythagorean school at a time when most Greek physicians followed essentially a craft ethic [3]. A perusal of the Hippocratic Corpus itself, which intersperses ethics and etiquette, will show how differently its treatises deal with fees, the care of incurable patients, and the business aspects of the craft.

The illusion that all physicians share a common devotion to a high-flown set of ethical principles has done damage to medicine by raising expectations that some members of the profession could not, or will not, fulfill. Today, we must be more forthright about the differences in value commitment among physicians. Professional codes must be more explicit about the relationships between duties, rights, and virtues. Such explicitness encourages a more honest relationship between physicians and patients and removes the hypocrisy of verbal assent to a general code, to which an individual physician may not really subscribe. Explicitness enables patients to choose among physicians on the basis of their ethical commitments as well as their reputations for technical expertise.

Conceptual clarity will not assure virtuous behavior. Indeed, virtues are usually distorted if they are the subject of too conscious a design. But conceptual clarity will distinguish between motives and provide criteria for judging the moral commitment one can expect from the profession and from its individual members. It can also inspire those whose virtuous inclinations need reinforcement in the current climate of commercialization of the healing relationship.

To this end the current resurgence of interest in virtue-based ethics is altogether salubrious. Linked to a theory of patient good and a theory of rights and duties, it could provide the needed groundwork for a reconstruction of professional medical ethics as that work matures. Perhaps even more progress can be made if we take Shakespeare's advice in *Hamlet*: "Assume the virtue if you have it not. . . . For use almost can change the stamp of nature."

BIBLIOGRAPHY

[1] Cicero: 1967, *Moral Obligations,* J. Higginbotham (trans.), University of California Press, Berkeley and Los Angeles.
[2] Cushing, H.: 1929, *Consecratio Medici and Other Papers,* Little, Brown and Co., Boston.

[3] Edelstein, L.: 1967, "The Professional Ethics of the Greek Physician," in O. Temkin (ed.), *Ancient Medicine: Selected Papers of Ludwig Edelstein,* Johns Hopkins University Press, Baltimore.

[4] Jonsen, A.: 1983, "Watching the Doctor," *New England Journal of Medicine* 308: 25, 1531–1535.

[5] Pellegrino, E.: 1983, "Scribonius Largus and the Origins of Medical Humanism," address to the American Osler Society.

[6] Reader, J.: 1982, "Beneficence, Supererogation, and Role Duty," in E. Shelp (ed.), *Beneficence and Health Care,* D. Reidel, Dordrecht, Holland, pp. 83–108.

PHYSICIAN-PATIENT MODELS AND PATIENT AUTONOMY

METAPHORS AND MODELS OF DOCTOR-PATIENT RELATIONSHIPS: THEIR IMPLICATIONS FOR AUTONOMY

James F. Childress and Mark Siegler

Childress and Siegler examine five models, or metaphors, for the physician-patient relationship: (1) *paternalism* (the physician as caring parent, the patient as child); (2) *partnership* (both parties as collaborating in pursuit of the shared goal of the patient's health); (3) *contract* (physician and patient as related to each other by specific contracts, detailing their obligations and rights); (4) *friendship* (physician and patient as intimately related due to the highly personal nature of health); and (5) *technical assistance* (the physician as technician, the patient as customer). The authors then explore the relative advantages and disadvantages of regarding the physician-patient relationship as a relationship between *intimates* or as one between *strangers,* before examining the implications of each for patient autonomy. They conclude by developing the metaphor of *negotiations* as a way to understand many interactions between physicians and patients.

INTRODUCTION

Many metaphors and models have been applied to relationships between patients and physicians. One example is an interpretation of physician-patient relationships as paternalistic. In this case, the physician is regarded as a parent and the patient is regarded as a child. Opponents of such a paternalistic view of medicine rarely reject the use of metaphors to interpret medical relationships; rather, they simply offer alternative metaphors, for example, the physician as partner or the patient as rational contractor. Metaphors may operate even when patients and physicians are unaware of them. Physician-patient conflicts may arise if each party brings to their encounter

Theoretical Medicine, vol. 5 (1984), pp. 17–30. © 1984 by D. Reidel Publishing Company. Reprinted by permission of Kluwer Academic Publishers.

a different image of medicine, as, for example, when the physician regards a paternalistic model of medicine as appropriate, but the patient prefers a contractual model.

As these examples suggest, metaphors involve seeing something as something else, for example, seeing a lover as a red rose, human beings as wolves, or medical therapy as warfare. Metaphors highlight some features and hide other features of their principal subject.[1] Thus, thinking about a physician as a parent highlights the physician's care for dependent others and his or her control over them, but it conceals the patient's payment of fees to the physician. Metaphors and models may be used to describe relationships as they exist, or to indicate what those relationships ought to be. In either the descriptive or the prescriptive use of metaphors, this highlighting and hiding occurs, and it must be considered in determining the adequacy of various metaphors. When metaphors are used to describe roles, they can be criticized if they distort more features than they illuminate. And when they are used to direct roles, they can be criticized if they highlight one moral consideration, such as care, while neglecting others, such as autonomy.

Since there is no single physician-patient relationship, it is probable that no single metaphor can adequately describe or direct the whole range of relationships in health care, such as open heart surgery, clinical research, and psychoanalysis. Some of the most important metaphors that have shaped health care in recent years include: parent-child, partners, rational contractors, friends, and technician-client. We want to determine the adequacy of these metaphors to describe and to direct doctor-patient relationships in the real world. In particular, we will assess them in relation to patient and physician autonomy.

METAPHORS AND MODELS OF RELATIONSHIPS IN HEALTH CARE

(1) The first metaphor is *paternal* or *parental,* and the model is paternalism. For this model, the locus of decision-making is the health care professional, particularly the physician, who has 'moral authority' within an asymmetrical and hierarchical relationship. (A variation on these themes appear in a model that was especially significant earlier—the priest-penitent relationship.)

Following Thomas Szasz and Marc Hollender, we can distinguish two different versions of paternalism, based on two different prototypes.[2] If we take the *parent-infant relationship* as the prototype, the physician's role is active, while the patient's role is passive. The patient, like the infant, is primarily a dependent recipient of care. This model is applied easily to such clinical situations as anesthesia and to the care of patients with acute trauma, coma, or delirium. A second version takes the *parent-adolescent child* relationship as the prototype. Within this version, the physician guides the patient by telling him or her what to expect and what to do, and the patient co-operates to the extent of obeying. This model applies to such clinical situations as the outpatient treatment of acute infectious diseases. The physician instructs the patient on a course of treatment (such as antibiotics and rest), but the patient can either obey or refuse to comply.

The paternalist model assigns moral authority and discretion to the physician because good health is assumed to be a value shared by the patient and the physician and because the physician's competence, skills, and ability place him or her in a position to help the patient regain good health. Even if it was once the dominant model in health care and even if many patients and physicians still prefer it, the paternalist model is no longer adequate to describe or to direct all relationships in health care. Too many changes have occurred. In a pluralistic society such as ours, the assumption that the physician and patient have common values about health may be mistaken. They may disagree about the *meaning* of health and disease (for example, when the physician insists that cigarette smoking is a disease, but the patient claims that it is merely a nasty habit) or about the *value* of health relative to other values (for example, when the physician wants to administer a blood transfusion to save the life of a Jehovah's Witness, but the patient rejects the blood in order to have a chance of heavenly salvation).

As a normative model, paternalism tends to concentrate on care rather than respect, patients' needs rather than their rights, and physicians' discretion rather than patients' autonomy or self-determination. Even though paternalistic actions can sometimes be justified, for example, when a patient is not competent to make a decision and is at risk of harm, not all paternalistic actions can be justified.[3]

(2) A second model is one of *partnership,* which can be seen in Eric Cassell's statement: "Autonomy for the sick patient cannot exist outside of a good and properly functioning doctor-patient relation. And the relation between them is inherently a *partnership.*"[4] The language of collegiality, collaboration, association, co-adventureship, and covenant is also used. This model stresses that health care professionals and their patients are partners or colleagues in the pursuit of the shared value of health. It is similar to the paternalist model in that it emphasizes the shared general values of the enterprise in which the participants are involved. But what makes this model distinctive and significant is its

emphasis on the equality of the participants' interpretations of shared values such as health, along with respect for the personal autonomy of all the participants.[5] The theme of equality does not, however, cancel a division of competence and responsibility along functional lines within the relationship.

Szasz and Hollender suggest that the prototype of the model of 'mutual participation' or partnership is the adult-adult relationship. Within this model the physician helps the patient to help himself, while the patient uses expert help to realize his (and the physician's) ends. Some clinical applications of this model appear in the care of chronic diseases and psychoanalysis. It presupposes that "the participants (1) have approximately equal power, (2) be mutually interdependent (i.e., need each other), and (3) engage in activity that will be in some ways satisfying to both." Furthermore, "the physician does not know what is best for the patient. The search for this becomes the essence of the therapeutic interaction. The patient's own experiences furnish indispensable information for eventual agreement, under otherwise favorable circumstances, as to what 'health' might be for him."[6]

Although this model describes a few practices, it is most often offered as a normative model, indicating the morally desirable and even obligatory direction of practice and research.[7] As a normative model, it stresses the equality of value contributions and the autonomy of both professionals and other participants, whether sick persons or volunteers for research.

(3) A third model is that of *rational contractors.* Health care professionals and their patients are related or should be related to each other by a series of specific contracts. The prototype of this model is the specific contract by which individuals agree to exchange goods and services, and the enforcement of such contracts by governmental sanctions. According to Robert Veatch, one of the strongest proponents of the contractual model in health care, this model is the best compromise between the *ideal of partnership,* with its emphasis on both equality and autonomy, and the *reality* of medical care, where mutual trust cannot be presupposed. If we could realize mutual trust, we could develop partnerships. In the light of a realistic assessment of our situation, however, we can only hope for contracts. The model

of rational contracts, according to Veatch, is the only realistic way to share responsibility, to preserve both equality and autonomy under less than ideal circumstances, and to protect the integrity of various parties in health care (e.g., physicians are free not to enter contracts that would violate their consciences and to withdraw from them when they give proper notice).[8]

Such a model is valuable but problematic both descriptively and normatively. It neglects the fact that sick persons do not view health care needs as comparable to other wants and desires, that they do not have sufficient information to make rational contracts with the best providers of health services, and that current structure of medicine obstructs the free operation of the marketplace and of contracts.[9] This model may also neglect the virtues of benevolence, care, and compassion that are stressed in other models such as paternalism and friendship.

(4) A fourth attempt to understand and direct the relationships between health care professionals and patients stresses *friendship.* According to P. Lain Entralgo,

> Insofar as man is a part of nature, and health an aspect of this nature and therefore a natural and objective good, the *medical relation* develops into comradeship, or association for the purpose of securing this good by technical means. Insofar as man is an individual and his illness a state affecting his personality, the medical relation ought to be more than mere comradeship—in fact it should be a friendship. All dogma apart, a good doctor has always been a friend to his patient, to all his patients.[10]

For this version of 'medical philia,' the patient expresses trust and confidence in the physician while the doctor's "friendship for the patient should consist above all in a desire to give effective technical help—benevolence conceived and realised in technical terms."[11] Technical help and generalized benevolence are 'made friendly' by explicit reference to the patient's personality.

Charles Fried's version of 'medical philia' holds that physicians are *limited, special-purpose friends* in relation to their patients. In medicine as well as in other professional activities such as law, the client may have a relationship with the professional that is analogous to friendship. In friendship and in these relationships, one person assumes the interests of another. Claims in both sets of relationships are intense and demanding, but medical friendship is more limited in scope.[12]

Of course, this friendship analogy is somewhat strained, as Fried recognizes, because needs (real and felt) give rise to medical relationships, even if professionals are free not to meet them unless they are emergencies, because patients pay professionals for their 'personal care,' and because patients do not have reciprocal loyalties. Nevertheless, Fried's analysis of the medical relationship highlights the equality, the autonomy, and the rights of both parties—the 'friend' and the 'befriended.' Because friendship, as Kant suggested, is "the union of two persons through equal and mutual love and respect," the model of friendship has some ingredients of both paternalism (love or care) and anti-paternalism (equality and respect).[13] It applies especially well to the same medical relationships that fit partnership; indeed, medical friendship is very close to medical partnership, except that the former stresses the intensity of the relationship, while the latter stresses the emotional reserve as well as the limited scope of the relationship.

(5) A fifth and final model views the health care professional as a *technician*. Some commentators have referred to this model as plumber, others as engineer; for example, it has been suggested that with the rise of scientific medicine the physician was viewed as "the expert engineer of the body as a machine."[14] Within this model, the physician 'provides' or 'delivers' technical service to patients who are 'consumers.' Exchange relations provide images for this interpretation of medical relations.

This model does not appear to be possible or even desirable. It is difficult to imagine that the health care professional as technician can simply present the 'facts' unadorned by values, in part because the major terms such as health and disease are not value-free and objective. Whether the 'technician' is in an organization or in direct relation to clients, he or she serves some values. Thus, this model may collapse into the contractual model or a bureaucratic model (which will not be discussed in this essay). The professional may be thought to have only technical authority, not moral authority. But he or she remains a moral agent and thus should choose to participate or not in terms of his or her own commitments, loyalties, and integrity. One shortcoming of the paternalist and priestly models, as Robert Veatch notes, is the patient's "moral abdication," while one shortcoming of the technician model is the physician's "moral abdication."[15] The technician model offers autonomy to the patient, whose values dominate (at least in some settings) at the expense of the professional's moral agency and integrity. In other models such as contract, partnership, and friendship, moral responsibility is shared by all the parties in part because they are recognized, in some sense, as equals.

RELATIONS BETWEEN INTIMATES AND BETWEEN STRANGERS

The above models of relationships between physicians and patients move between two poles: intimates and strangers.[16] In relations of intimacy, all the parties know each other very well and often share values, or at least know which values they do not share. In such relations, formal rules and procedures, backed by sanctions, may not be necessary; they may even be detrimental to the relationships. In relations of intimacy, trust rather than control is dominant. Examples include relationships between parents and children and between friends. Partnerships also share some features of such relationships, but their intimacy and shared values may be limited to a specific set of activities.

By contrast, in relations among strangers, rules and procedures become very important, and control rather than trust is dominant.[17] Of course, in most relations there are mixtures of trust and control. Each is present to some degree. Nevertheless, it is proper to speak about relations between strangers as structured by rules and procedures because the parties do not know each other well enough to have mutual trust. Trust means confidence in and reliance upon the other to act in accord with moral principles and rules or at least in accord with his or her publicly manifested principles and rules, whatever they might be. But if the other is a stranger, we do not know whether he or she accepts what we would count as moral principles and rules. We do not know whether he or she is worthy of trust. In the absence of intimate knowledge, or of shared values, strangers resort to rules and procedures in order to establish some control. Contracts between strangers, for example, to supply certain goods, represent instances of attempted control. But contractual relations do not only depend on legal sanctions; they also presuppose confidence in a shared structure of rules and procedures. As Talcott Parsons has noted, "transactions are actually entered into in accordance with a body of binding rules which are not part of the ad hoc agreement of the parties."[18]

Whether medicine is now only a series of encounters between strangers rather than intimates, medicine is increasingly regarded by patients and doctors, and by analysts of the profession—such as philosophers, lawyers, and sociologists—as a practice that is best understood and regulated *as if it were* a practice among strangers rather than among intimates. Numerous causes can be identified: first, the pluralistic nature of our society; second, the decline of close, intimate contact over time among professionals and patients and their families; third, the decline of contact with the 'whole person,' who is now parcelled out to various specialists; fourth, the growth of large, impersonal, bureaucratically structured institutions of care, in which there is discontinuity of care (the patient may not see the same professionals on subsequent visits).[19]

In this situation, Alasdair MacIntyre contends, the modern patient "usually approaches the physician as stranger to stranger: and the very proper fear and suspicion that we have of strangers extends equally properly to our encounters with physicians. We do not and cannot know what to expect of them . . . ."[20] He suggests that one possible response to this situation is to develop a rule-based bureaucracy in which "we can confront *any* individual who fills a given role with exactly the same expectation of exactly the same outcomes . . .". Our encounters with physicians and other health care professionals are encounters between strangers precisely because of our pluralistic society: several value systems are in operation, and we do not know whether the physicians we encounter share our value systems. In such a situation, patient autonomy is "a solution of last resort" rather than "a central moral good." Finally patients have to decide for themselves what will be done to them or simply delegate such decisions to others, such as physicians.

Just as MacIntyre recognizes the value of patient autonomy in our pluralistic society, so John Ladd recognizes the value of the concept of rights among strangers.[21] He notes that a legalistic, rights-based approach to medicine has several important advantages because rules and rights "serve to define our relationships with strangers as well as with people whom we know . . . In the medical context . . . we may find ourselves in a hospital bed in a strange place, with strange company, and confronted by a strange physician and staff. The strangeness of the situation makes the concept of rights, both legal and moral, a very useful tool for defining our relationship to those with whom we have to deal."

Rules and rights that can be enforced obviously serve as ways to control the conduct of others when we do not know them well enough to be able to trust them. But all of the models of health care relationships identified above depend on some degree of trust. It is too simplistic to suppose that contracts, which can be legally enforced, do away with trust totally. Indeed, as we have argued, a society based on contracts depends to a very great extent on trust, precisely because not everything is enforceable at manageable cost. Thus, the issue is not simply whether trust or control is dominant, but, in part, the basis and extent of trust. Trust, at least limited trust, may be possible even among strangers. There may be a presumption of trust, unless the society is in turmoil. And there may be an intermediate notion of 'friendly strangers.' People may be strangers because of differences regarding values or uncertainty regarding the other's values; they may be friendly because they accept certain rules and procedures, which may ensure that different values are respected. If consensus exists in a pluralistic society, it is primarily about rules and procedures, some of which protect the autonomy of agents, their freedom to negotiate their own relationships.

PHYSICIAN-PATIENT INTERACTIONS AS NEGOTIATIONS

It is illuminating, both descriptively and prescriptively, to view some encounters and interactions between physicians and patients as negotiations. The metaphor of negotiation has its home in discussions to settle matters by mutual agreement of the concerned parties. While it frequently appears in disputes between management and labor and between nations, it does not necessarily presuppose a conflict of interests between the parties. The metaphor of negotiation may also illuminate processes of reaching agreement regarding the terms of continuing interaction even when the issue is mainly the determination of one party's interests and the means to realize those interests. This metaphor captures two important characteristics of medical relationships: (1) it accents the autonomy of both patient and physician, and (2) it suggests a process that occurs over time rather than an event which occurs at a particular moment.

The model of negotiation can both explain what frequently occurs and identify what ought to occur in physician-patient interactions. An example can make this point: A twenty-eight-year-old ballet dancer suffered from moderately severe asthma. When she moved from New York to Chicago, she changed physicians and placed herself in the hands of a famed asthma specialist. He initiated aggressive steroid therapy to control her asthma, and within several months he had managed to control her wheezing. But she was distressed because her dancing had deteriorated. She suspected that she was experiencing muscle weakness and fluid accumulation because of the steroid treatment. When she attempted to discuss her concerns with the physician, he maintained that "bringing the disease under complete control—achieving a complete remission of wheezes—will be the best thing for you in the long run." After several months of unhappiness and failure to convince the physician of the importance of her personal goals as well as her medical goals, she sought another physician, insisting that she didn't live just to breathe, but breathed so that she could dance.[22]

As in this case—and despite the claims of several commentators—people with medical needs generally do not confront physicians as strangers and as adversaries in contemporary health care. As we suggested earlier, even if they can be viewed as strangers in that they often do not know each other prior to the encounter, both parties may well proceed with a presumption of trust. Patients may approach physicians with some trust and confidence in the medical profession, even though they do not know the physicians

before them. Indeed, codes of medical ethics have been designed in part to foster this trust by indicating where the medical profession stands and by creating a climate of trust. Thus, even if patients approach individual physicians as strangers, they may have some confidence in these physicians as members of the profession as they negotiate the particular terms of their relationship. At the other extreme, some patients may approach physicians as adversaries or opponents. But for negotiation to proceed, some trust must be present, even if it is combined with some degree of control, for example, through legal requirements and the threat of legal sanctions.

The general public trust in the medical profession's values and skills provides the presumptive basis for trust in particular physicians and can facilitate the process of negotiation. But, as we noted earlier, in a pluralistic society, even people who are strangers, i.e., who share very few substantive values, may be 'friendly' if they share procedural values. Certain procedural values may provide the most important basis for the trust that is necessary for negotiation; indeed, procedural principles and rules should structure the negotiation in order to ensure equal respect for the autonomy of all the parties.

First, the negotiation should involve adequate disclosure by both parties. In this process of communication—much broader and richer than most doctrines of informed consent recognize—both parties should indicate their values as well as other matters of relevance. Without this information, the negotiation cannot be open and fair. Second, the negotiation should be voluntary, i.e., uncoerced. Insofar as critical illness can be viewed as 'coercing' individuals through the creation of fear, etc., it may be difficult to realize this condition for patients with certain problems. However, for the majority of patients this condition is achievable. Third, the accommodation reached through the negotiation should be mutually acceptable.[23]

What can we say about the case of the ballet dancer in the light of these procedural requirements for negotiation? It appears that the relationship foundered not because of inadequate disclosure at the outset, or along the way, but because of the patient's change in or clarification of her values and the physician's inability to accommodate these other values. The accommodation reached at the outset was mutually acceptable for a time. Initially their values and their metaphors for their relationship were the same. The physician regarded himself as a masterful scientist who was capable technically of controlling a patient's symptoms of wheezing. In fact, he remarked on several occasions: "I have never met a case of asthma I couldn't help." The patient, for her part, selected the physician initially for the same reasons. She was unhappy that her wheezing persisted, and she was becoming discouraged by her chronic health problem. Because she wanted a therapeutic success, she selected an expert who would help her achieve that goal. Both the patient and the physician made several voluntary choices. The patient chose to see *this* physician and to see him for several months, and the physician chose to treat asthma aggressively with steroids.

In a short time, the patient reconsidered or clarified her values, discovering that her dancing was even more important to her than the complete remission of wheezing, and she wanted to renegotiate her relationship so that it could be more mutual and participatory. But her new metaphor for the relationship was incompatible with the physician's nonnegotiable commitment to his metaphor—which the patient had also accepted at the outset. Thus, the relationship collapsed. This case illustrates both the possibilities and the limitations of the model of negotiation. Even when the procedural requirements are met, the negotiation may not result in a satisfactory accommodation over time, and the negotiation itself may proceed in terms of the physician's and the patient's metaphors and models of the relationships, as well as the values they affirm.

Autonomy constrains and limits the negotiations and the activities of both parties: Neither party may violate the autonomy of the other or use the other merely as a means to an end. But respecting autonomy as a constraint and a limit does not imply seeking it as a *goal* or praising it as an *ideal*.[24] This point has several implications. It means, for example, that patients may exercise their autonomy to turn their medical affairs completely over to physicians. A patient may instruct the physician to do whatever he or she deems appropriate: "You're the doctor; whatever you decide is fine." This relation-

ship has been characterized as "paternalism with permission,"[25] and it is not ruled out by autonomy as a constraint or a limit. It might, however, be ruled out by a commitment to autonomy as an ideal. Indeed, commitment to autonomy as an ideal can even be paternalistic in a negative sense; it can lead the health care professional to try to force the patient to be free and to live up to the ideal of autonomy. But our conception of autonomy as a constraint and a limit prevents such actions toward competent patients who are choosing and acting voluntarily. Likewise, maintenance, restoration, or promotion of the patient's autonomy may be, and usually is, one important goal of medical relationships. But its importance can only be determined by negotiation between the physician and the patient. The patient may even subordinate the goal of autonomy to various other goals, just as the ballet dancer subordinated freedom from wheezing to the power to dance.

This view of autonomy as a limit or a constraint, rather than an ideal or a goal, permits individuals to define the terms of their relationship. Just as it permits the patient to acquiesce in the physician's recommendations, it permits the physician to enter a contract as a mere technician to provide certain medical services, as requested by the patient. In such an arrangement, the physician does *not* become a mere means or a mere instrument to the patient's ends. Rather, the physician exercises his or her autonomy to enter into the relationship to provide technical services. Such actions are an expression of autonomy, not a denial of autonomy. If, however, the physician believes that an action requested by the patient—for example, a specific mode of therapy for cancer or a sterilization procedure—is not medically indicated, or professionally acceptable, or in the patient's best interests, he or she is not obligated to sacrifice autonomy and comply. In such a case, the professional refuses to be an instrument of or to carry out the patient's wishes. When the physician cannot morally or professionally perform an action (not legally prohibited by the society) he or she may have a duty to inform the patient of other physicians who might be willing to carry out the patient's wishes. A refusal to be an instrument of another's wishes is very different from trying to prevent another from realizing his or her goals.

Negotiation is not always possible or desirable. It is impossible, or possible only to a limited extent, in certain clinical settings in which the conditions for a fair, informed, and voluntary negotiation are severely limited, often because one party lacks some of the conditions for autonomous choices. First, negotiation may be difficult if not impossible with some types of patients, such as the mentally incompetent. Sometimes paternalism may be morally legitimate or even morally obligatory when the patient is not competent to negotiate and is at risk. In such cases, parents, family members, or others may undertake negotiation with the physician, for example, regarding defective newborns or comatose adults. But health care professionals and the state may have to intervene in order to protect the interests of the patient who cannot negotiate directly. Second, the model of negotiation does not fit situations in which patients are forced by law to accept medical interventions such as compulsory vaccination, involuntary commitment, and involuntary psychiatric treatment. In such situations, the state authorizes or requires treatment against the wishes of the patient; the patient and the physician do not negotiate their relationship. Third, in some situations physicians have dual or multiple allegiances, some of which may take priority over loyalty to the patient. Examples include military medicine, industrial medicine, prison medicine, and university health service. The physician is not free in such settings to negotiate in good faith with the patient, and the patient's interests and rights may have to be protected by other substantive and procedural standards and by external control. Fourth, negotiation may not be possible in some emergencies in which people desperately need medical treatment because of the risk of death or serious bodily harm. In such cases, the physician may *presume* consent, apart from a process of negotiation, if the patient is unable to consent because of his/her condition or if the process of disclosing information and securing consent would consume too much time and thus endanger the patient. Finally, procedural standards are important for certain types of patients, such as the poor, the uneducated, or those with 'unattractive medical problems' (e.g., drug addiction, obesity, and hypochondriasis). In such cases, there is a tendency—surely not a universal one—to limit the degree of negotiation with the patient because of social stigmatization. A patient advocate may even be appropriate.

In addition to the procedural requirements identified earlier, there are societal constraints and limits on negotiation. Some actions may not be negotiable. For example, the society may prohibit 'mercy killing,' even when the patient requests it and the physician is willing to carry it out.[26] Such societal rules clearly limit the autonomy of both physicians and patients, but some of these rules may be necessary in order to protect important societal values. However, despite such notable exceptions as 'mercy killing,' current societal rules provide physicians and patients with considerable latitude to negotiate their own relationship and actions within that relationship.

If negotiation is a process, its accommodations at various points can often be characterized in terms of the above models—parent-child, friends, partners, contractors, and technician-consumer. Whatever accommodation is reached through the process of negotiation is not final or irrevocable. Like other human interactions, medical relationships change over time. They are always developing or dissolving. For example, when a patient experiencing anginal chest pain negotiates a relationship with a cardiologist, he may not have given or even implied consent to undergo coronary angiography or cardiac surgery if the cardiologist subsequently believes that it is necessary. Medical conditions change, and people change, often clarifying or modifying their values over time. In medical relationships either the physician or the patient may reopen the negotiation as the relationship evolves over time and may even terminate the relationship. For example, the ballet dancer in the case discussed above elected to terminate the relationship with the specialist. That particular relationship had not been fully negotiated in the first place. But even if it had been fully negotiated, she could have changed her mind and terminated it. Such an option is essential if the autonomy of the patient is to be protected over time. Likewise, the physician should have the option to renegotiate or to withdraw from the relationship (except in emergencies), as long as he or she gives adequate notice so that the patient can find another physician.

NOTES

1 On metaphors, see George Lakoff and Mark Johnson, *Metaphors We Live By* (Chicago: University of Chicago Press, 1980).

2 See Thomas S. Szasz and Marc H. Hollender, 'A contribution to the philosophy of medicine: The basic models of the doctor-patient relationship,' *Archives of Internal Medicine* 97, (1956) 585–92; see also, Thomas S. Szasz, William F. Knoff, and Marc H. Hollender, 'The doctor-patient relationship and its historical context,' *American Journal of Psychiatry* 115, (1958) 522–28.

3 For a fuller analysis of paternalism and its justification, see James F. Childress, *Who Should Decide?: Paternalism in Health Care* (New York: Oxford University Press, 1982).

4 Eric Cassell, 'Autonomy and ethics in action,' *New England Journal of Medicine* 297, (1977) 333–34. Italics added. Partnership is only one of several images and metaphors Cassell uses, and it may not be the best one to express his position, in part because he tends to view autonomy as a goal rather than as a constraint.

5 According to Robert Veatch, the main focus of this model is "an equality of dignity and respect, an equality of value contributions". Veatch, 'Models for ethical medicine in a revolutionary age,' *Hastings Center Report* 2, (June 1972) 7. Contrast Eric Cassell who disputes the relevance of notions of "equality" and "inequality." *The Healer's Art: A New Approach to the Doctor-Patient Relationship* (Philadelphia: J. B. Lippincott Company, 1976), pp. 193–94.

6 Thomas S. Szasz and Marc H. Hollender, 'A contribution to the philosophy of medicine: The basic models of the doctor-patient relationship,' pp. 586–87. (See Note 2.)

7 See, for example, Paul Ramsey, 'The ethics of a cottage industry in an age of community and research medicine,' *New England Journal of Medicine* 284, (1971) 700–706; *The Patient as Person: Explorations in Medical Ethics* (New Haven: Yale University Press, 1970), esp. Chap. 1; and Hans Jonas, 'Philosophical reflections on experimenting with human subjects,' Ethical Aspects of Experimentation with Human Subjects, *Daedalus* 98, (1969) 219–47.

8 Robert Veatch, 'Models for ethical medicine in a revolutionary age,' p. 7. (See Note 5.)

9 See Roger Masters, 'Is contract an adequate basis for medical ethics?,' *Hastings Center Report* 5, (December 1975) 24–28. See also May, 'Code and covenant or philanthropy and contract?' in *Ethics in Medicine: Historical Perspectives and Contemporary Concerns*, ed. by Stanley Joel Reiser, Arthur J. Dyck, and William J. Curran (Cambridge, Mass.: The MIT Press, 1977), pp. 65–76.

10 P. Lain Entralgo, *Doctor and Patient*, trans. from the Spanish by Frances Partridge (New York: McGraw-Hill Book Co., World University Library, 1969), p. 242.

11 *Ibid.*, p. 197.

12 See Charles Fried, *Medical Experimentation: Personal Integrity and Social Policy* (New York: American Elsevier Publishing Co., Inc., 1974), p. 76. Our discussion of Fried's position is drawn from that work, *Right and Wrong* (Cambridge, Mass.: Harvard University Press, 1978), Chap. 7, and 'The lawyer as friend: The moral foundations of the lawyer-client relation,' *The Yale Law Journal* 85, (1976) 1060–89.

13 Immanuel Kant, *The Doctrine of Virtue*, Part II of *The Metaphysic of Morals*, trans. by Mary J. Gregor (New York: Harper and Row, Harper Torchbook, 1964), p. 140.

14 Thomas S. Szasz, William F. Knoff, and Marc H. Hollender, 'The doctor-patient relationship and its historical context,' p. 525. See also Robert Veatch, 'Models for ethical medicine in a revolutionary age,' p. 5, and Leon Kass, 'Ethical dilemmas in the care of the ill: I. What is the physician's service?' *Journal of the American Medical Association* 244, (1980) 1815 for criticisms of the technical model (from very different normative positions).

15 Veatch, 'Models for ethical medicine in a revolutionary age,' p. 7.

16 See Stephen Toulmin, 'The tyranny of principles,' *Hastings Center Report* 11, (December 1981) 31–39.

17 On trust and control, see James F. Childress, 'Non-violent resistance: Trust and risk-taking,' *Journal of Religious Ethics* 1, (1973) 87–112.

18 Talcott Parsons, *The Structure of Social Action* (New York: The Free Press, 1949), p. 311.

19 On the factors in the decline of trust, see Michael Jellinek, 'Erosion of patient trust in large medical centers,' *Hastings Center Report* 6, (June 1976) 16–19.

20 Alasdair MacIntyre, 'Patients as agents,' in *Philosophical Medical Ethics: Its Nature and Significance*, ed. by Stuart F. Spicker and H. Tristram Engelhardt, Jr. (Boston: D. Reidel Publishing Co., 1977).

21 John Ladd, 'Legalism and medical ethics,' *The Journal of Medicine and Philosophy* 4, (March 1979) 73.

22 This case has been presented in Mark Siegler, 'Searching for moral certainty in medicine: A proposal for a new model of the doctor-patient encounter,' *Bulletin of the New York Academy of Medicine* 57, (1981) 56–69.

23 See *ibid.* for a discussion of negotiation. Other proponents of a model of negotiation include Robert A. Burt, *Taking Care of Strangers: The Rule of Law in Doctor-Patient Relations* (New York: Free Press, 1979) and Robert J. Levine, *Ethics and Regulation of Clinical Research* (Baltimore: Urban and Schwarzenberg, 1981).

24 See the discussion in Childress, *Who Should Decide?*, Chap. 3.

25 Alan W. Cross and Larry R. Churchill, 'Ethical and cultural dimensions of informed consent,' *Annals of Internal Medicine* 96, (1982) 110–13.

26 See Oscar Thorup, Mark Siegler, James Childress, and Ruth Roettinger, 'Voluntary exit: Is there a case of rational suicide?' *The Pharos* 45, (Fall 1982) 25–31.

WHY DOCTORS SHOULD INTERVENE

Terrence F. Ackerman

Ackerman criticizes the notion of respect for autonomy that identifies it with noninterference. He argues that noninterference fails to respect patient autonomy because it does not take account of the transforming effects of illness. Ackerman's major contention is that the autonomy of those who are ill is limited by all kinds of constraints—physical, cognitive, emotional, and social. Ackerman argues in favor of sometimes overriding patients' treatment-related preferences, maintaining that real respect for the autonomy of patients requires physicians actively to attempt to neutralize the impediments that interfere with patients' choices, helping them restore control over their lives.

Patient autonomy has become a watchword of the medical profession. According to the revised 1980 AMA Principles of Medical Ethics,[1] no longer is it permissible for a doctor to withhold information from a patient, even on grounds that it may be harmful. Instead, the physician is expected to "deal honestly with patients" at all times. Physicians also have a duty to respect the confidentiality of the doctor-patient relationship. Even when disclosure to a third party may be in the patient's interests, the doctor is instructed to release information only when required by law. Respect for the autonomy of patients has given rise to many specific patient rights—among them the right to refuse treatment, the right to give informed consent, the right to privacy, and the right to competent medical care provided with "respect for human dignity."

While requirements of honesty, confidentiality, and patients' rights are all important, the underlying moral vision that places exclusive emphasis upon these factors is more troublesome. The profession's notion of respect for autonomy makes noninterference its essential feature. As the Belmont Report has described it, there is an obligation to "give weight to autonomous persons' considered opinions and choices while refraining from obstructing their actions unless they are clearly detrimental to others."[2] Or, as Tom Beauchamp and James Childress have suggested, "To respect autonomous agents is to recognize with due appreciation their own considered value judgments and outlooks even when it is believed that their judgments are mistaken." They argue that people "are entitled to autonomous determination without limitation on their liberty being imposed by others."[3]

When respect for personal autonomy is understood as noninterference, the physician's role is dramatically simplified. The doctor need be only an honest and good technician, providing relevant information and dispensing professionally competent care. Does noninterference really respect patient autonomy? I maintain that it does not, because it fails to take account of the transforming effects of illness.

"Autonomy," typically defined as self-governance, has two key features. First, autonomous behavior is governed by plans of action that have been formulated through deliberation or reflection. This deliberative activity involves processes of both information gathering and priority setting. Second, autonomous behavior issues, intentionally and voluntarily, from choices people make based upon their own life plans.

But various kinds of constraints can impede autonomous behavior. There are physical constraints—confinement in prison is an example—where internal or external circumstances bodily prevent a person from deliberating adequately or acting on life plans. Cognitive constraints derive from either a lack of information or an inability to understand that information. A consumer's ignorance regarding the merits or defects of a particular product fits the description. Psychological constraints, such as anxiety or depression, also inhibit adequate deliberation. Finally,

Reprinted with permission of the author and the publisher from *Hastings Center Report*, vol. 12 (August 1982), pp. 14–17.

there are social constraints—such as institutional-ized roles and expectations ("a woman's place is in the home," "the doctor knows best") that block con-sidered choices.

Edmund Pellegrino suggests several ways in which autonomy is specifically compromised by illness:

> In illness, the body is interposed between us and reality—it impedes our choices and actions and is no longer fully responsive. . . . Illness forces a reap-praisal and that poses a threat to the old image; it opens up all the old anxieties and imposes new ones—often including the real threat of death or dras-tic alterations in life-style. This ontological assault is aggravated by the loss of . . . freedoms we identify as peculiarly human. The patient. . .lacks the knowl-edge and skills necessary to cure himself or gain re-lief of pain and suffering. . . . The state of being ill is therefore a state of "wounded humanity," of a person compromised in his fundamental capacity to deal with his vulnerability.[4]

The most obvious impediment is that illness "interposes" the body or mind between the patient and reality, obstructing attempts to act upon cher-ished plans. An illness may not only temporarily ob-struct long-range goals; it may necessitate permanent and drastic revision in the patient's major activities, such as working habits. Patients may also need to set limited goals regarding control of pain, alter-ation in diet and physical activity, and rehabilitation of functional impairments. They may face consider-able difficulties in identifying realistic and produc-tive aims.

The crisis is aggravated by a cognitive con-straint—the lack of "knowledge and skills" to over-come their physical or mental impediment. Without adequate medical understanding, the patient cannot assess his or her condition accurately. Thus the choice of goals is seriously hampered and subse-quent decisions by the patient are not well founded.

Pellegrino mentions the anxieties created by ill-ness, but psychological constraints may also include denial, depression, guilt, and fear. I recently visited an eighteen-year-old boy who was dying of a cancer that had metastasized extensively throughout his ab-domen. The doctor wanted to administer further chemotherapy that might extend the patient's life a few months. But the patient's nutritional status was poor, and he would need intravenous feedings prior to chemotherapy. Since the nutritional therapy might also encourage tumor growth, leading to a blockage of the gastrointestinal tract, the physician carefully explained the options and the risks and benefits sev-eral times, each time at greater length. But after each explanation, the young man would say only that he wished to do whatever was necessary to get better. Denial prevented him from exploring the alternatives.

Similarly, depression can lead patients to make choices that are not in harmony with their life plans. Recently, a middle-aged woman with a history of ovarian cancer in remission returned to the hospital for the biopsy of a possible pulmonary metastasis. Complications ensued and she required the use of an artificial respirator for several days. She became se-verely depressed and soon refused further treatment. The behavior was entirely out of character with her previous full commitment to treatment. Fully sup-porting her overt wishes might have robbed her of many months of relatively comfortable life in the midst of a very supportive family around which her activities centered. The medical staff stalled for time. Fortunately, her condition improved.

Fear may also cripple the ability of patients to choose. Another patient, diagnosed as having a cere-bral tumor that was probably malignant, refused life-saving surgery because he feared the cosmetic effects of neurosurgery and the possibility of neuro-logical damage. After he became comatose and new evidence suggested that the tumor might be benign, his family agreed to surgery and a benign tumor was removed. But he later died of complications related to the unfortunate delay in surgery. Although while competent he had agreed to chemotherapy, his fears (not uncommon among candidates for neuro-surgery) prevented him from accepting the medical intervention that might have secured him the health he desired.

Social constraints may also prevent patients from acting upon their considered choices. A recent case involved a twelve-year-old boy whose rhab-domyosarcoma had metastasized extensively. Since all therapeutic interventions had failed, the only remaining option was to involve him in a phase 1 clinical trial. (A phase 1 clinical trial is the initial testing of a drug in human subjects. Its primary purpose is to identify toxicities rather than to evaluate therapeutic effectiveness.) The patient's course had been very stormy, and he privately expressed to the staff his desire to quit further therapy and return home. However, his parents denied the hopelessness of his condition, remaining steadfast in their belief that God would save their child. With deep regard for his parents' wishes, he refused to openly object to their desires and the therapy was administered. No antitumor effect occurred and the patient soon died.

Various social and cultural expectations also take their toll. According to Talcott Parsons, one feature of the sick role is that the ill person is obligated ". . . to seek *technically competent* help, namely, in the most usual case, that of a physician and to *cooperate* with him in the process of trying to get well."[5] Parsons does not describe in detail the elements of this cooperation. But clinical observation suggests that many patients relinquish their opportunity to deliberate and make choices regarding treatment in deference to the physician's superior educational achievement and social status ("Whatever you think, doctor!"). The physical and emotional demands of illness reinforce this behavior.

Moreover, this perception of the sick role has been socially taught from childhood—and it is not easily altered even by the physician who ardently tries to engage the patient in decision making. Indeed, when patients are initially asked to participate in the decision-making process, some exhibit considerable confusion and anxiety. Thus, for many persons, the institutional role of patient requires the physician to assume the responsibilities of making decisions.

Ethicists typically condemn paternalistic practices in the therapeutic relationship, but fail to investigate the features that incline physicians to be paternalistic. Such behavior may be one way to assist persons whose autonomous behavior has been impaired by illness. Of course, it is an open moral question whether the constraints imposed by illness ought to be addressed in such a way. But only by coming to grips with the psychological and social dimensions of illness can we discuss how physicians can best respect persons who are patients.

RETURNING CONTROL TO PATIENTS

In the usual interpretation of respect for personal autonomy, noninterference is fundamental. In the medical setting, this means providing adequate information and competent care that accords with the patient's wishes. But if serious constraints upon autonomous behavior are intrinsic to the state of being ill, then noninterference is not the best course, since the patient's choices will be seriously limited. Under these conditions, real respect for autonomy entails a more inclusive understanding of the relationship between patients and physicians. Rather than restraining themselves so that patients can exercise whatever autonomy they retain in illness, physicians should actively seek to neutralize the impediments that interfere with patients' choices.

In *The Healer's Art*, Eric Cassell underscored the essential feature of illness that demands a revision in our understanding of respect for autonomy:

> If I had to pick the aspect of illness that is most destructive to the sick, I would choose the loss of control. Maintaining control over oneself is so vital to all of us that one might see all the other phenomena of illness as doing harm not only in their own right but doubly so as they reinforce the sick person's perception that he is no longer in control.[6]

Cassell maintains, "The doctor's job is to return control to his patient." But what is involved in "returning control" to patients? Pellegrino identifies two elements that are preeminent duties of the physician: to provide technically competent care and to fully inform the patient. The noninterference approach emphasizes these factors, and their importance is clear. Loss of control in illness is precipitated by a physical or mental defect. If technically competent therapy can fully restore previous health, then the patient will again be in control. Consider a patient who is treated with antibiotics for a routine throat infection of streptococcal origin. Similarly, loss of control is fueled by lack of knowledge—not knowing what is the matter, what it portends for life and limb, and how it might be dealt with. Providing information that will enable the patient to make decisions and adjust goals enhances personal control.

If physical and cognitive constraints were the only impediments to autonomous behavior, then

Pellegrino's suggestions might be adequate. But providing information and technically competent care will not do much to alter psychological or social impediments. Pellegrino does not adequately portray the physician's role in ameliorating these.

How can the doctor offset the acute denial that prevented the adolescent patient from assessing the benefits and risk of intravenous feedings prior to his additional chemotherapy? How can he deal with the candidate for neurosurgery who clearly desired that attempts be made to restore his health, but feared cosmetic and functional impairments? Here strategies must go beyond the mere provision of information. Crucial information may have to be repeatedly shared with patients. Features of the situation that the patient has brushed over (as in denial) or falsely emphasized (as with acute anxiety) must be discussed in more detail or set in their proper perspective. And the physician may have to alter the tone of discussions with the patient, emphasizing a positive attitude with the overly depressed or anxious patient, or a more realistic, cautious attitude with the denying patient, in order to neutralize psychological constraints.

The physician may also need to influence the beliefs or attitudes of other people, such as family members, that limit their awareness of the patient's perspective. Such a strategy might have helped the parents of the dying child to conform with the patient's wishes. On the other hand, physicians may need to modify the patient's own understanding of the sick role. For example, they may need to convey that the choice of treatment depends not merely upon the physician's technical assessment, but on the quality of life and personal goals that the patient desires.

Once we admit that psychological and social constraints impair patient autonomy, it follows that physicians must carefully assess the psychological and social profiles and needs of patients. Thus, Pedro Lain-Entralgo insists that adequate therapeutic interaction consists in a combination of "objectivity" and "cooperation." Cooperation "is shown by psychologically reproducing in the mind of the doctor, insofar as that is possible, the meaning the patient's illness has for him."[7] Without such knowledge, the physician cannot assist patients in restoring control over their lives. Ironically, some critics have insisted that physicians are not justified in acting for the well-being of patients because they possess no "expertise" in securing the requisite knowledge about the patient.[8] But knowledge of the patient's psychological and social situation is also necessary to help the patient to act as a fully autonomous person.

BEYOND LEGALISM

Current notions of respect for autonomy are undergirded by a legal model of doctor-patient interaction. The relationship is viewed as a typical commodity exchange—the provision of technically competent medical care in return for financial compensation. Moreover, physicians and patients are presumed to have an equal ability to work out the details of therapy, *provided that* certain moral rights of patients are recognized. But the compromising effects of illness, the superior knowledge of physicians, and various institutional arrangements are also viewed as giving the physician an unfair power advantage. Since the values and interests of patients may conflict with those of the physician, the emphasis is placed upon noninterference.[9]

This legal framework is insufficient for medical ethics because it fails to recognize the impact of illness upon autonomous behavior. Even if the rights to receive adequate information and to provide consent are secured, affective and social constraints impair the ability of patients to engage in contractual therapeutic relationships. When people are sick, the focus upon equality is temporally misplaced. The goal of the therapeutic relationship is the "development" of the patient—helping to resolve the underlying physical (or mental) defect, and to deal with cognitive, psychological, and social constraints in order to restore autonomous functioning. In this sense, the doctor-patient interaction is not unlike the parent-child or teacher-student relationship.

The legal model also falls short because the therapeutic relationship is not a typical commodity exchange in which the parties use each other to accomplish mutually compatible goals, without taking a direct interest in each other. Rather, the status of patients as persons whose autonomy is compromised constitutes the very stuff of therapeutic art. The physician is attempting to alter the fundamental ability of patients to carry through their life plans. To accomplish this delicate task requires a personal knowledge about and interest in the patient. If we accept these points, then we must reject the narrow focus of medical ethics upon noninterference and emphasize patterns of interaction that free patients from constraints upon autonomy.

I hasten to add that I am criticizing the legal model only as a *complete* moral framework for therapeutic interaction. As case studies in medical ethics suggest, physicians and patients *are* potential adversaries. Moreover, the disability of the patient and various institutional controls provide physicians with a distinct "power advantage" that can be abused. Thus, a legitimate function of medical ethics is to formulate conditions that assure noninterference in patient decision making. But various positive interventions must also be emphasized, since the central task in the therapeutic process is assisting patients to reestablish control over their own lives.

In the last analysis, the crucial matter is how we view the patient who enters into the therapeutic relationship. Cassell points out that in the typical view "... the sick person is seen simply as a well person with a disease, rather than as qualitatively different, not only physically but also socially, emotionally, and even cognitively." In this view, "... the physician's role in the care of the sick is primarily the application of technology ... and health can be seen as a commodity."[10] But if, as I believe, illness renders sick persons "qualitatively different," then respect for personal autonomy requires a therapeutic interaction considerably more complex than the noninterference strategy.

Thus the current "Principles of Medical Ethics" simply exhort physicians to be honest. But the crucial requirement is that physicians tell the truth in a way, at a time, and in whatever increments are necessary to allow patients to effectively use the information in adjusting their life plans.[11] Similarly, respecting a patient's refusal of treatment maximizes autonomy only if a balanced and thorough deliberation precedes the decision. Again, the "Principles" suggest that physicians observe strict confidentiality. But the more complex moral challenge is to use confidential information in a way that will help to give the patient more freedom. Thus, the doctor can keep a patient's report on family dynamics private, and still use it to modify attitudes or actions of family members that inhibit the patient's control.

At its root, illness is an evil primarily because it compromises our efforts to control our lives. Thus, we must preserve an understanding of the physician's art that transcends noninterference and addresses this fundamental reality.

REFERENCES

1 American Medical Association, *Current Opinions of the Judicial Council of the American Medical Association* (Chicago, Illinois: American Medical Association, 1981), p. ix. Also see Robert Veatch, "Professional Ethics: New Principles for Physicians?," *Hastings Center Report* 10 (June 1980), 16–19.

2 The National Commission for the Protection of Human Subjects of Biomedical and Behavioral Research, *The Belmont Report: Ethical Principles and Guidelines for the Protection of Human Subjects of Research* (Washington, D.C.: U.S. Government Printing Office, 1978), p. 58.

3 Tom Beauchamp and James Childress, *Principles of Biomedical Ethics* (New York: Oxford University Press, 1980), p. 59.

4 Edmund Pellegrino, "Toward a Reconstruction of Medical Morality: The Primacy of the Act of Profession and the Fact of Illness," *The Journal of Medicine and Philosophy* 4 (1979), 44–45.

5 Talcott Parsons, *The Social System* (Glencoe, Illinois: The Free Press, 1951), p. 437.

6 Eric Cassell, *The Healer's Art* (New York: Lippincott, 1976), p. 44. Although Cassell aptly describes the goal of the healer's art, it is unclear whether he considers it to be based upon the obligation to respect the patient's autonomy or the duty to enhance the well-being of the patient. Some parts of his discussion clearly suggest the latter.

7 Pedro Lain-Entralgo, *Doctor and Patient* (New York: McGraw-Hill, 1969), p. 155.

8 See Allen Buchanan, "Medical Paternalism," *Philosophy and Public Affairs* 7 (1978), 370–90.

9 My formulation of the components of the legal model differs from, but is highly indebted to, John Ladd's stimulating analysis in "Legalism and Medical Ethics," in John Davis et al, editors, *Contemporary Issues in Biomedical Ethics* (Clifton, N.J.: The Humana Press, 1979), pp. 1–35. However, I would not endorse Ladd's position that the moral principles that define our duties in the therapeutic setting are of a different logical type from those that define our duties to strangers.

10 Eric Cassell, "Therapeutic Relationship: Contemporary Medical Perspective," in Warren Reich, editor, *Encyclopedia of Bioethics* (New York: Macmillan, 1978), p. 1675.

11 Cf. Norman Cousins, "A Layman Looks at Truth-telling," *Journal of the American Medical Association* 244 (1980), 1929–30. Also see Howard Brody, "Hope," *Journal of the American Medical Association* 246 (1981), pp. 1411–12.

IN DEFENSE OF THE TRADITIONAL NURSE
Lisa H. Newton

Newton counters the emerging ideal of the nurse as an autonomous professional who is prepared to challenge doctors' authority and advocate for patients' interests. In its place she urges "the traditional ideal of the skilled and gentle caregiver, whose role in health care requires submission to authority as an essential component." In defending the traditional nurse, Newton argues the following: (1) to run properly, hospital bureaucracies require clear roles and lines of authority; (2) only physicians are properly trained to handle serious medical situations that arise without warning; and (3) the vulnerable, compromised situation of hospital patients gives rise to emotional needs that can be met only by nurses, who serve (in some respects) as surrogate mothers. After exploring limits of the nurse-mother analogy, Newton responds to objections motivated by a feminist perspective. In this discussion, she emphasizes that being an autonomous person is compatible with choosing a nonautonomous professional role, such as that of the nurse, and that support for men's participation in nursing would be liberating for them.

When a truth is accepted by everyone as so obvious that it blots out all its alternatives and leaves no respectable perspectives from which to examine it, it becomes the natural prey of philosophers, whose essential activity is to question accepted opinion. A case in point may be the ideal of the "autonomous professional" for nursing. The consensus that this ideal and image are appropriate for the profession is becoming monolithic and may profit from the presence of a full-blooded alternative ideal to replace the cardboard stereotypes it routinely condemns. That alternative, I suggest, is the traditional ideal of the skilled and gentle caregiver, whose role in health care requires submission to authority as an essential component. We can see the faults of this traditional ideal very clearly now, but we may perhaps also be able to see virtues that went unnoticed in the battle to displace it. It is my contention that the image and ideal of the traditional nurse contain virtues that can be found nowhere else in the health care professions, that perhaps make an irreplaceable contribution to

Reprinted from *Nursing Outlook,* vol. 29 (June 1981), pp. 348–354, with permission from Mosby-Year Book, Inc.

the care of patients, and that should not be lost in the transition to a new definition of the profession of nursing. . . .

ROLE COMPONENTS

The first task of any philosophical inquiry is to determine its terminology and establish the meanings of the key terms for its own purposes. To take the first term, a *role* is a norm-governed pattern of action undertaken in accordance with social expectations. The term is originally derived from the drama, where it signifies a part played by an actor in a play. In current usage, any ordinary job or profession (physician, housewife, teacher, postal worker) will do as an example of a social role; the term's dramatic origin is nonetheless worth remembering, as a key to the limits of the concept.

Image and ideal are simply the descriptive and prescriptive aspects of a social role. The *image* of a social role is that role as it is understood to be in fact, both by the occupants of the role and by those with whom the occupant interacts. It describes the character the occupant plays, the acts, attitudes, and expectations normally associated with the role. The *ideal* of a role is a conception of what that role could or should be—that is, a conception of the norms that should govern its work. It is necessary to distinguish between the private and public aspects of image and ideal.

Since role occupants and the general public need not agree either on the description of the present operations of the role or on the prescription for its future development, the private image, or self-image of the role occupant, is therefore distinct from the public image or general impression of the role maintained in the popular media and mind. The private ideal, or aspiration of the role occupant, is distinct from the public ideal or normative direction set for the role by the larger society. Thus, four role-components emerge, from the public and private, descriptive and prescriptive, aspects of a social role. They may be difficult to disentangle in some cases, but they are surely distinct in theory, and potentially in conflict in fact.

TRANSITIONAL ROLES

In these terms alone we have the materials for the problematic tensions within transitional social roles. Stable social roles should exhibit no significant disparities among images and ideals: what the public generally gets is about what it thinks it should get; what the job turns out to require is generally in accord with the role-occupant's aspirations; and public and role-occupant, beyond a certain base level of "they-don't-know-how-hard-we-work" grumbling, are in general agreement on what the role is all about. On the other hand, transitional roles tend to exhibit strong discrepancies among the four elements of the role during the transition; at least the components will make the transition at different times, and there may also be profound disagreement on the direction that the transition should take. . . .

BARRIERS TO AUTONOMY

The first contention of my argument is that the issue of autonomy in the nursing profession lends itself to misformulation. A common formulation of the issue, for example, locates it in a discrepancy between public image and private image. On this account, the public is asserted to believe that nurses are ill-educated, unintelligent, incapable of assuming responsibility,

and hence properly excluded from professional status and responsibility. In fact they are now prepared to be truly autonomous professionals through an excellent education, including a thorough theoretical grounding in all aspects of their profession. Granted, the public image of the nurse has many favorable aspects—the nurse is credited with great manual skill, often saintly dedication to service to others, and, at least below the supervisory level, a warm heart and gentle manners. But the educational and intellectual deficiencies that the public mistakenly perceives outweigh the "positive" qualities when it comes to deciding how the nurse shall be treated, and are called upon to justify not only her traditionally inferior status and low wages, but also the refusal to allow nursing to fill genuine needs in the health care system by assuming tasks that nurses are uniquely qualified to handle. For the sake of the quality of health care as well as for the sake of the interests of the nurse, the public must be educated through a massive educational campaign to the full capabilities of the contemporary nurse; the image must be brought into line with the facts. On this account, then, the issue of nurse autonomy is diagnosed as a public relations problem: the private ideal of nursing is asserted to be that of the autonomous professional and the private image is asserted to have undergone a transition from an older subservient role to a new professional one but the public image of the nurse ideal is significantly not mentioned in this analysis.

An alternative account of the issue of professional autonomy in nursing locates it in a discrepancy between private ideal and private image. Again, the private ideal is that of the autonomous professional. But the actual performance of the role is entirely slavish, because of the way the system works—with its tight budgets, insane schedules, workloads bordering on reckless endangerment for the seriously ill, bureaucratic red tape, confusion, and arrogance. Under these conditions, the nurse is permanently barred from fulfilling her professional ideal, from bringing the reality of the nurse's condition into line with the self-concept she brought to the job. On this account, then, the nurse really is not an autonomous professional, and total reform of the power structure of the health care industry will be necessary in order to allow her to become one.

A third formulation locates the issue of autonomy in a struggle between the private ideal and an altogether undesirable public ideal: on this account, the public does not want the nurse to be an autonomous professional, because her present subservient status serves the power needs of the physicians; because her unprofessional remuneration serves the monetary needs of the entrepreneurs and callous municipalities that run the hospitals; and because the low value accorded her opinions on patient care protects both physicians and bureaucrats from being forced to account to the patient for the treatment he receives. On this account, the nurse needs primarily to gather allies to defeat the powerful interest groups that impose the traditional ideal for their own unworthy purposes, and to replace that degrading and dangerous prescription with one more appropriate to the contemporary nurse.

These three accounts, logically independent, have crucial elements of content in common. Above all, they agree on the objectives to be pursued: full professional independence, responsibility, recognition, and remuneration for the professional nurse. And as corollary to these objectives, they agree on the necessity of banishing forever from the hospitals and from the public mind that inaccurate and demeaning stereotype of the nurse as the Lady with the Bedpan: an image of submissive service, comforting to have around and skillful enough at her little tasks, but too scatterbrained and emotional for responsibility.

In none of the interpretations above is any real weight given to a public ideal of nursing, to the nursing role as the public thinks it ought to be played. Where public prescription shows up at all, it is seen as a vicious and false demand imposed by power alone, thoroughly illegitimate and to be destroyed as quickly as possible. The possibility that there may be real value in the traditional role of the nurse, and that the public may have good reasons to want to retain it, simply does not receive any serious consideration on any account. It is precisely that possibility that I take up in the next section.

DEFENDING THE "TRADITIONAL NURSE"

As Aristotle taught us, the way to discover the peculiar virtues of any thing is to look to the work that it accomplishes in the larger context of its environment. The first task, then, is to isolate those factors of need or demand in the nursing environment that require the nurse's work if they are to be met. I shall concentrate, as above, on the hospital environment, since most nurses are employed in hospitals.

The work context of the hospital nurse actually spans two societal practices or institutions: the hospital as a bureaucracy and medicine as a field of scientific endeavor and service. Although there is enormous room for variation in both hospitals bureaucracies and medicine, and they may therefore interact with an infinite number of possible results, the most general facts about both institutions allow us to sketch the major demands they make on those whose function lies within them.

To take the hospital bureaucracy first: its very nature demands that workers perform the tasks assigned to them, report properly to the proper superior, avoid initiative, and adhere to set procedures. These requirements are common to all bureaucracies, but dramatically increase in urgency when the tasks are supposed to be protective of life itself and where the subject matter is inherently unpredictable and emergency prone. Since there is often no time to re-examine the usefulness of a procedure in a particular case, and since the stakes are too high to permit a gamble, the institution's effectiveness, not to mention its legal position, may depend on unquestioning adherence to procedure.

Assuming that the sort of hospital under discussion is one in which the practice of medicine by qualified physicians is the focal activity, rather than, say, a convalescent hospital, further contextual requirements emerge. Among the prominent features of the practice of medicine are the following: it depends on esoteric knowledge, which takes time to acquire and which is rapidly advancing; and, because each patient's illness is unique, it is uncertain. Thus, when a serious medical situation arises without warning, only physicians will know how to deal with it (if their licensure has any point), and they will not always be able to explain or justify their actions to nonphysicians, even those who are required to assist them in patient care.

If the two contexts of medicine and the hospital are superimposed, three common points can be seen. Both are devoted to the saving of life and health; the atmosphere in which that purpose is carried out is inevitably tense and urgent; and, if the purpose is to be accomplished in that atmosphere, all participating activities and agents must be completely subordinated to the medical judgments of the physicians. In short, those, other than physicians, involved in medical procedures in a hospital context have no right to insert their own needs, judgments, or personalities into the situation. The last thing we need at that point is another autonomous professional on the job, whether a nurse or anyone else.

PATIENT NEEDS: THE PRIME CONCERN

From the general characteristics of hospitals and medicine, that negative conclusion for nursing follows. But the institutions are not, after all, the focus of the endeavor. If there is any conflict between the needs of the patient and the needs of the institutions established to serve him, his needs take precedence and constitute the most important requirements of the nursing environment. What are these needs?

First, because the patient is sick and disabled, he needs specialized care that only qualified personnel can administer, beyond the time that the physician is with him. Second, and perhaps most obviously to the patient, he is likely to be unable to perform simple tasks such as walking unaided, dressing himself, and attending to his bodily functions. He will need assistance in these tasks, and is likely to find this need humiliating; his entire self-concept as an independent human being may be threatened. Thus, the patient has serious emotional needs brought on by the hospital situation itself, regardless of his disability. He is scared, depressed, disappointed, and possibly, in reaction to all of these, very angry. He needs reassurance, comfort, someone to talk to. The person he really needs, who would be capable of taking care of all these problems, is obviously his mother, and the first job of the nurse is to be a mother surrogate.

That conclusion, it should be noted, is inherent in the word "nurse" itself: it is derived ultimately from the Latin *nutrire,* "to nourish or suckle"; the first meaning of "nurse" as a noun is still, according to *Webster's New Twentieth Century Unabridged Dictionary* "one who suckles a child not her own." From the outset, then, the function of the nurse is identical with that of the mother, to be exercised when the mother is unavailable. And the meanings proceed in logical order from there: the second definitions given for both noun and verb involve caring for children, especially young children, and the third, caring for those who are childlike in their dependence—the sick, the injured, the very old, and the handicapped. For all those groups—infants, children, and helpless adults—it is appropriate to bring children's caretakers, surrogate mothers, nurses, into the situation to minister to them. It is especially appropriate to do so, for the sake of the psychological economies realized by the patient: the sense of self, at least for the Western adult, hangs on the self-perception of independence. Since disability requires the relinquishing of this self-perception, the patient must either discover conditions excusing his dependence somewhere in his self-concept, or invent new ones, and the latter task is extremely difficult. Hence the usefulness of the maternal image association: it was, within the patient's understanding of himself "all right" to be tended by mother; if the nurse is (at some level) mother, it is "all right" to reassume that familiar role and to be tended by her.

LIMITS ON THE "MOTHER" ROLE

The nurse's assumption of the role of mother is therefore justified etymologically and historically but most importantly by reference to the psychological demands of and on the patient. Yet the maternal role cannot be imported into the hospital care situation without significant modification—specifically, with respect to the power and authority inherent in the role of mother. Such maternal authority includes the right and duty to assume control over children's lives and make all decisions for them; but the hospital patient most definitely does not lose adult status even if he is sick enough to want to. The ethical legitimacy as well as the therapeutic success of his treatment depend on his voluntary and active cooperation in it and on his deferring to some forms of power and authority—the hospital rules and the physician's sapiential authority, for example. But these very partial, conditional, restraints are nowhere near the threat to patient autonomy that the real presence of a mother would be; maternal authority, total, diffuse, and unlimited, would be incompatible with the retention of moral freedom. And it is just this sort of total authority that the patient is most tempted to attribute to the nurse, who already embodies the nurturant component of the maternal role. To prevent serious threats to patient autonomy, then, the role of nurse must be from the outset, as essentially as it is nurturant, unavailable for such attribution of authority. Not only must the role of nurse not include authority; it must be incompatible with authority: essentially, a subservient role.

The nurse role, as required by the patient's situation, is the nurturant component of the maternal role and excludes elements of power and authority. A further advantage of this combination of maternal nurturance and subordinate status is that, just as it permits the patient to be cared for like a baby without threatening his autonomy, it also permits him to unburden himself to a sympathetic listener of his doubts and resentments, about physicians and hospitals in general, and his in particular, without threatening the course of his treatment. His resentments are natural, but they lead to a situation of conflict, between the desire to rebel against treatment and bring it to a halt (to reassert control over his life), and the desire that the treatment should continue (to obtain its benefits). The nurse's function speaks well to this condition: like her maternal model, the nurse is available for the patient to talk to (the physician is too busy to talk), sympathetic, understanding, and supportive; but in her subordinate position, the nurse can do absolutely nothing to change his course of treatment. Since she has no more control over the environment than he has, he can let off steam in perfect safety, knowing that he cannot do himself any damage.

The norms for the nurse's role so far derived from the patient's perspective also tally, it might be noted, with the restrictions on the role that arise from the needs of hospitals and medicine. The patient does not need another autonomous professional at his bedside, any more than the physician can use one or the hospital bureaucracy contain one. The conclusion so far, then, is that in the hospital environment, the traditional (nurturant and subordinate) role of the nurse seems more adapted to the nurse function than the new autonomous role.

PROVIDER OF HUMANISTIC CARE

So far, we have defined the hospital nurse's function in terms of the specific needs of the hospital, the physician, and the patient. Yet there is another level of function that needs to be addressed. If we consider the multifaceted demands that the patient's family, friends, and community make on the hospital once the patient is admitted, it becomes clear that this concerned group cannot be served exclusively by attending to the medical aspect of care, necessary though that is. Nor is it sufficient for the hospital-as-institution to keep accurate and careful records, maintain absolute cleanliness, and establish procedures that protect the patient's safety, even though this is important. Neither bureaucracy nor medical professional can handle the human needs of the human beings involved in the process.

The general public entering the hospital as patient or visitor encounters and reacts to that health care system as an indivisible whole, as if under a single heading of "what the hospital is like." It is at this level that we can make sense of the traditional claim that the nurse represents the "human" as opposed to "mechanical" or "coldly professional" aspect of health care, for there is clearly something terribly missing in the combined medical and bureaucratic approach to the "case": they fail to address the patient's fear for himself and the family's fear for him, their grief over the separation, even if temporary, their concern for the financial burden, and a host of other emotional components of hospitalization.

The same failing appears throughout the hospital experience, most poignantly obvious, perhaps, when the medical procedures are unavailing and the patient dies. When this occurs, the physician must determine the cause and time of death and the advisability of an autopsy, while the bureaucracy must record the death and remove the body; but surely this is not enough. The death of a human being is a rending of the fabric of human community, a sad and fearful time; it is appropriately a time of bitter regret, anger, and weeping. The patient's family, caught up in the institutional context of the hospital, cannot assume alone the burden of discovering and expressing the emotions appropriate to the occasion; such expression, essential for their own regeneration after their loss, must originate somehow within the hospital context itself. The hospital system must, somehow, be able to share pain and grief as well as it makes medical judgments and keeps records.

The traditional nurse's role addresses itself directly to these human needs. Its derivation from the maternal role classifies it as feminine and permits ready assumption of all attributes culturally typed as "feminine": tenderness, warmth, sympathy, and a tendency to engage much more readily in the expression of feeling than in the rendering of judgment. Through the nurse, the hospital can be concerned, welcoming, caring, and grief-stricken; it can break through the cold barriers of efficiency essential to its other functions and share human feeling.

The nurse therefore provides the in-hospital health care system with human capabilities that would otherwise be unavailable to it and hence unavailable to the community in dealing with it. Such a conclusion is unattractive to the supporters of the autonomous role for the nurse, because the tasks of making objective judgments and of expressing emotion are inherently incompatible; and since the nurse shows grief and sympathy on behalf of the system, she is excluded from decision-making and defined as subordinate.

However unappealing such a conclusion may be, it is clear that without the nurse role in this function, the hospital becomes a moral monstrosity, coolly and mechanically dispensing and disposing of human life and death, with no acknowledgment at all of the individual life, value, projects, and relationships of the persons with whom it deals. Only the nurse makes the system morally tolerable. People in pain deserve sympathy, as the dead deserve to be grieved; it is unthinkable that the very societal institution to which we generally consign the suffering and the dying should be incapable of sustaining sympathy and grief. Yet its capability hangs on the presence of nurses willing to assume the affective functions of the traditional nursing role, and the current attempt to banish that role, to introduce instead an autonomous professional role for the nurse, threatens to send the last hope for a human presence in the hospital off at the same time.

THE FEMINIST PERSPECTIVE

From this conclusion it would seem to follow automatically that the role of the traditional nurse should be retained. It might be argued, however, that the value of autonomy is such that any nonautonomous role ought to be abolished, no matter what its value to the current institutional structure.

Those who aimed to abolish black slavery in the United States have provided a precedent for this argument. They never denied the slave's economic usefulness; they simply denied that it could be right to enslave any person and insisted that the nation find some other way to get the work done, no matter what the cost. On a totally different level, the feminists of our own generation have proposed that the traditional housewife and mother role for the woman, which confined women to domestic life and made them subordinate to men, has been very useful for everyone except the women trapped in it. All the feminists have claimed is that the profit of others is not a sufficient reason to retain a role that demeans its occupant. As they see it, the "traditional nurse" role is analogous to the roles of slave and housewife—it is derived directly, in fact, as we have seen, from the "mother" part of the latter role—exploitative of its occupants and hence immoral by its very nature and worthy of abolition.

But the analogy does not hold. A distinction must be made between an autonomous person—one who, over the course of adult life, is self-determining in all major choices and a significant number of minor ones, and hence can be said to have chosen, and to be responsible for, his own life—and an autonomous *role*—a role so structured that its occupant is self-determining in all major and most minor role-related choices. An autonomous person can certainly take on a subordinate role without losing his personal autonomy. For example, we can find examples of slaves (in the ancient world at least) and housewives who have claimed to have, and shown every sign of having, complete personal integrity and autonomy with their freely chosen roles.

Furthermore, slave and housewife are a very special type of role, known as "life-roles." They are to be played 24 hours a day, for an indefinite period of time; there is no customary or foreseeable respite from them. Depending on circumstances, there may be de facto escapes from these roles, permitting their occupants to set up separate personal identities (some of the literature from the history of American slavery suggests this possibility), but the role-definitions do not contemplate part-time occupancy. Such life-roles are few in number; most roles are the part-time "occupational roles," the jobs that we do eight hours a day and have little to do with the structuring the rest of the twenty-four. An autonomous person can, it would seem, easily take up a subordinate role of this type and play it well without threat to personal autonomy. And if there is excellent reason to choose such a role—if, for example, an enterprise of tremendous importance derives an essential component of its moral worth from that role—it would seem to be altogether rational and praiseworthy to do so. The role of "traditional nurse" would certainly fall within this category.

But even if the traditional nurse role is not inherently demeaning, it might be argued further, it should be abolished as harmful to the society because it preserves the sex stereotypes that we are trying to overcome. "Nurse" is a purely feminine role, historically derived from "mother," embodying feminine attributes of emotionality, tenderness, and nurturance, and it is subordinate—thus reinforcing the link between femininity and subordinate status. The nurse role should be available to men, too, to help break down this unfavorable stereotype.

This objective to the traditional role embodies the very fallacy it aims to combat. The falsehood we know as sexism is not the belief that some roles are autonomous, calling for objectivity in judgment, suppression of emotion, and independent initiative in action, but discouraging independent judgment and action and requiring obedience to superiors; the falsehood is the assumption that only men are eligible for the first class and only women are eligible for the second class.

One of the most damaging mistakes of our cultural heritage is the assumption that warmth, gentleness, and loving care, such as are expected of the nurse, are simply impossible for the male of the species, and that men who show emotion, let alone those who are ever known to weep, are weaklings, "sissies," and a disgrace to the human race. I suspect that this assumption has done more harm to the culture than its more publicized partner, the assumption that women are (or should be) incapable of objective judgment or executive function. Women will survive without leadership roles, but it is not clear that a society can retain its humanity if all those eligible for leadership are forbidden, by virtue of that eligibility, to take account of the human side of human beings: their altruism, heroism, compassion, and grief, their fear and weakness, and their ability to love and care for others.

In the words of the current feminist movement, men must be liberated as surely as women. And one of the best avenues to such liberation would be the encouragement of male participation in the health care system, or other systems of the society, in roles like the traditional nursing role, which permit, even require, the expressive side of the personality to develop, giving it a function in the enterprise and restoring it to recognition and respectability.

CONCLUSIONS

In conclusion, then, the traditional nurse role is crucial to health care in the hospital context; its subordinate status, required for its remaining features, is neither in itself demeaning nor a barrier to its assumption by men or women. It is probably not a role that everyone would enjoy. But there are certainly many who are suited to it, and should be willing to undertake the job.

One of the puzzling features of the recent controversy is the apparent unwillingness of some of the current crop of nursing school graduates to take on the assignment for which they have ostensibly been prepared, at least until such time as it shall be redefined to accord more closely with their notion of professional. These frustrated nurses who do not want the traditional nursing role, yet wish to employ their skills in the health care system in some way, will clearly have to do something else. The health care industry is presently in the process of very rapid expansion and diversification, and has created significant markets for those with a nurse's training and the capacity, and desire, for autonomous roles. Moreover, the nurse in a position which does not have the "nurse" label, does not need to combat the "traditional nurse" image and is ordinarily accorded greater freedom of action. For this reason alone it would appear that those nurses intent on occupying autonomous roles and tired of fighting stereotypes that they find degrading and unworthy of their abilities, should seek out occupational niches that do not bear the label, and the stigma, of "nurse."

I conclude, therefore: that much of the difficulty in obtaining public acceptance of the new "autonomous professional" image of the nurse may be due, not to public ignorance, but to the opposition of a vague but persistent public ideal of nursing; that the ideal is a worthy one, well-founded in the hospital context in which it evolved; and that

the role of traditional nurse, for which that ideal sets the standard, should therefore be maintained and held open for any who would have the desire and the personal and professional qualifications, to assume it. Perhaps the current crop of nursing school graduates do not desire it, but there is ample room in the health care system for the sort of "autonomous professional" they wish to be, apart from the hospital nursing role. Wherever we must go to fill this role, it is worth going there, for the traditional nurse is the major force remaining for humanity in a system that will turn into a mechanical monster without her.

ADVOCACY OR SUBSERVIENCE FOR THE SAKE OF PATIENTS?
Helga Kuhse

Kuhse addresses the question of whether nurses, whose primary professional obligation is to serve the interests of patients, should conduct themselves as patient advocates or assume a role of subservience to physicians (as Newton argues). Against the claim that the role of the nurse is *naturally* subservient to the doctor's role, Kuhse argues that professional roles evolve over time and have no fixed essences (natures); moreover, there is considerable overlap between contemporary nursing functions and the functions traditionally performed by physicians. She next casts doubt, with a variety of arguments, on the thesis that, because nursing and medicine have fundamentally different philosophical commitments, nurses should accept a subservient role. Taking up specific arguments advanced by Newton, Kuhse contends (1) that the claim that nurses' subservience is required for proper handling of serious medical situations is based on dubious assumptions and (2) that there are several good reasons to reject the surrogate mother role for nurses. She concludes that nurses' subservience to physicians would likely harm patients more than it would help them.

. . . The view that doctors were gods whose commands must always be obeyed was beginning to be seriously questioned in the 1960s and 1970s. There had always been courageous nurses who had occasionally challenged orders,[1] but it is almost as if nurses needed a new metaphor to capture their new

Reproduced with permission of Blackwell Publishers Ltd. from Helga Kuhse, *Caring: Nurses, Women and Ethics* (1997), pp. 35–36, 41–53, 58–60. Copyright © Helga Kuhse, 1997.

understanding of their role before they could finally attempt to free themselves from the shackles of the past. This new focus was provided by the metaphor of the nurse as patient advocate. Whereas the old metaphors had focused attention on such virtues as submissiveness and unquestioning obedience and loyalty to those in command, the new metaphor of patient advocate highlighted the virtues of assertiveness and courage, and marked a revolutionary shift in the self-perception of nurses and their role. The nurse's first loyalty, the metaphor suggested, is owed not to the doctor but to the patient. In thus focusing on the nurse's responsibilities to patients, that is, on the *recipients* rather than the *providers* of medical care, the metaphor of the nurse as patient advocate made it possible for nurses to see themselves as *professionals.* No longer were they, as the old metaphors had suggested, the loyal handmaidens of medical men: they were professionals whose primary responsibility—like that of all professionals—was to their clients or patients.[2] . . .

NURSING—A NATURALLY SUBSERVIENT PROFESSION?

. . . Our first question must be this: *should* nurses reject their traditional largely subservient role and act as patient advocates? . . .

. . . I shall, without argument, assume that a profession such as medicine or nursing does not exist for the sole or even primary purpose of benefiting its members. This view is widely shared and is implicit in most if not all professional codes;[3] it is also regarded as one of the necessary conditions for an organization to claim professional status.[4] For the purposes of our discussion, then, I shall assume that both nursing and medicine are professions which are, or ought to be, aiming at the welfare of others, where those others are patients or clients.

This raises the question of the relationship between medicine and nursing, and between doctors and nurses. Might it not be the case that the subordinate role of nurses has its basis not in objectionable sexism but rather in a natural hierarchy between the professions, a hierarchy that serves patients best?

Robert Baker is among those who have pointed out that we cannot simply assume that the nurse's subservient role has a sexist basis. He does not deny that sexism exists or that the subservient nursing role has traditionally been seen as a feminine one; but, he writes,

> it is not at all clear whether the role of the nurse is seen as dependent because it is filled by females, who are held to be incapable of independent action by a male-dominated, sexist society . . . *or* whether females have been channelled into nursing because the profession, *by its very nature,* requires its members to play a dependent and subservient role (i.e., the traditional female role in a sexist society).[5]

In other words, the facts that almost all nurses are women, that the traditional nurse's role has been a subservient one and that most societies were and are male-dominated and sexist, cannot lead us to the conclusion that the nurse's role necessarily rests on objectionable sexism. The nurse's role may, 'by its very nature,' be a subservient one. But is nursing 'by its very nature' subservient to medicine—is it a naturally subservient profession?

There is clearly something odd about speaking of the 'natural subservience' of nursing to medicine, or for that matter of 'the natural subservience' of any profession in relation to another. To speak of 'natural subservience' suggests that the subservient or dominant character of the relevant profession is somehow naturally given and in that sense fixed and largely unchangeable. But is this view correct? . . . [N]ursing has developed in a very particular social and historical context, in response to the then prevailing goals and purposes of medicine on the one hand and the social roles of women and men on the other. Would this not make it more appropriate to view the character of the two health-care professions, and the tasks and privileges that attach to them, as a historically contingent accident or social construct, rather than as a compelling natural necessity?[6]

It seems to me the answer must be 'yes.' There are no natural professional hierarchies that exist independently of human societies, and we should reject the idea that professions have fixed natures and instead view them as changing and changeable social institutions. When looking at professions in this way we may, of course, still want to think of them as having particular characteristics by which they can be defined ('social natures,' if you like), but we would now view these characteristics as socially constructed, in much the same way as the institution itself is a social and historical construct.

How, then, might one go about capturing the 'social nature' or characteristics of a profession? One might do this in one of two ways: either by focusing on the functions or roles performed by members of the profession or by focusing on the profession's philosophical presuppositions or goals.

Function or Role What is the function or role of a nurse? What is a nurse? The clear and neat boundaries and distinctions presupposed by our everyday language and by the terms we use rarely accord with the real world.[7] We often speak of 'the role' or 'the function' of the nurse, or of 'the role' or 'the function' of the doctor. These terms are problematical because nurses and doctors working in different areas of health care perform very different functions and act in many different roles, and there is a considerable degree of overlap between the changeable and changing functions performed by members of the two professions.

The expansion of knowledge, of nursing education, and of medical science and technology has resulted in the redefinition and scope of nursing practice. Nurses now carry out a range of procedures that were formerly exclusively performed by doctors. Some nurses give injections, take blood samples, administer medication, perform diagnostic procedures, do physical examinations, respond to medical emergencies and so on.

Take diagnosis and medical treatment. The diagnosis and treatment of medical problems had always been regarded as the realm solely of doctors. But, as H. Tristram Engelhardt notes, if one looks closely at the diagnostic activities performed by nurses, it is difficult to see them as essentially different from medical diagnoses. Nursing diagnoses such as ' "Airway clearance, ineffective;" "Bowel elimination, alteration in: Diarrhoea;" "Cardiac output, alteration in, decrease;" "Fluid volume deficit," ' Engelhardt points out, all have their medical equivalents; and the diagnosis of psychological or psychiatric disturbances, such as ' "Coping, ineffective individual," or "Thought processes, alteration in" can be given analogues in the *Diagnostic and Statistical Manual of Mental Disorders* of the American Psychiatric Association.'[8]

Nurses are not permitted by law to perform any 'medical acts,' but in practice the line between medical and nursing acts has become rather blurred[9] and is, in any case, the result of social and historical choice. Moreover, as nurses have become more assertive and conscious of their own knowledge and expertise, there has been a broadening of the definitions of nursing practice. In 1981 the American Nursing Association thus produced a model definition of nursing practice, which included 'diagnosis . . . in the promotion and maintenance of health.' By 1984, 23 US states had included [nursing] diagnoses, or similar terms, in their nursing practice acts.[10]

To conclude, then, the fact that nurses work in very different areas of health care, where they perform very different functions, and the fact that there are considerable overlaps between contemporary nursing functions and the functions traditionally performed by doctors makes it difficult to see how it would be possible to define nursing in terms of a particular function or role performed by nurses. If we thus think of 'the nature' of nursing in terms of some specific function or role performed by all nurses, this suggests not only that nursing lacks a particular nature, but also makes it difficult to claim that nursing is 'naturally subservient' to medicine.

It is true, of course, that nurses frequently work under the direction of doctors, and that control over many of the functions performed by them is retained by the medical profession. It is also true that only doctors may, by law, perform operations, prescribe medical treatments and authorize access to certain drugs. This might lead one to the conclusion that nursing and medicine can be distinguished by the range of socially and legally sanctioned tasks and privileges that members of one but not of the other profession may lawfully engage in. Such a distinction would, of course, be possible. But it is not a distinction that allows one to infer anything about the subservient or dominant 'nature' of either one of the two professions. The distribution of socially and legally sanctioned privileges and powers between medicine and nursing is itself a historically contingent fact, and there is nothing to suggest that the current distribution of powers and privileges is either natural or that it is the one that we should, upon reflection, adopt.[11] . . .

Philosophical Commitment Is it possible to distinguish the two professions by their philosophical commitment, that is, by the philosophical presuppositions that guide their respective health-care endeavours? It is, again, not easy to see how this might be done. Someone intent on rejecting the view that nursing is naturally subservient to medicine might point out that there is no essential difference between the philosophical commitment of the two professions that would allow one to speak of one of them as being subservient to the other. Both nursing and medicine are other-directed and committed to the welfare of clients or patients; members of both professions have a similar understanding of pain and of suffering, of well-being and of health, and both accept the same scientific presuppositions. If there are differences between individual doctors and nurses, these are no more pronounced than those found between individuals from the same professions. Hence, one might conclude, nursing does not have a nature which is different from that of medicine and can therefore not be said to be naturally subservient to medicine.

Another, diametrically opposed avenue is sometimes chosen by those writing in the field to prove wrong the claim that the nurse's role is a naturally subservient one. Rather than trying to show that the nurse's role is—either functionally or in terms of its philosophical commitment—*indistinguishable* from that of doctors, this second group of nurses claims that the nursing commitment is fundamentally *different* from that of medicine. In other words, those who take this approach start with the premise that medicine and nursing have different philosophical commitments or 'natures,' and then go on to deny that this will necessarily lead to the conclusion that nursing ought to be playing a subservient role to medicine.[12]

This is generally done in one of two ways. The first involves drawing a distinction in terms of a commitment to 'care' and to 'cure.' Whereas medicine is said to be directed at 'cure,' the therapeutic commitment or moral end of nursing is identified as 'care.' Medicine and doctors, it is said, often focus on treating or curing the patient's medical condition; nursing, on the other hand, is based on holistic care, where patients are treated as complex wholes. . . . The second way of attempting to draw a distinction between nursing and medicine involves an appeal to two different ethics. Whereas medicine is said to be based on principles and rules (a so-called [male] ethics of justice), nursing is said to be based on relational caring (a so-called [female] ethics of care).

This means, very roughly, that doctors will put ethical principles or rules before the needs or wants of individual patients, whereas nurses regard the needs or wants of individual patients as more important than adherence to abstract principles or rules.

These two views do not deny that nursing is context-dependent or that nurses perform very different functions in different health-care settings; they also acknowledge that nurses and doctors sometimes perform very similar or identical functions and act in very similar roles. Nonetheless, those who take this view assume that nursing is different from medicine because it has a different philosophical commitment or end—that of care. 'Care'—the nurture, the physical care, and the emotional support provided by nurses to preserve the 'human face' of medicine and the dignity of the patient—cannot, the suggestion is, 'be absent if nursing is present.'[13]

There are a number of reasons why I am pessimistic about the endeavour of distinguishing nursing from medicine and nurses from doctors in this way. . . . Here the following [summary] will suffice: it seems very difficult, in a straightforward and practical sense, to make philosophical commitments, such as the commitment to care, the defining characteristic of a profession. Such a definition would presumably include all nurses who have this commitment, but would exclude all those who do not. A registered nurse, who has all the relevant professional knowledge and expertise, who performs her nursing functions well, but—let us assume—subscribes to 'the scientific medical model' or to an 'ethics of justice' would now, presumably, no longer *be* a nurse. Would her philosophical commitment make her a doctor? And would a doctor who subscribes to 'care' now more appropriately be described as a nurse?

The problem is raised particularly poignantly in settings, such as intensive care units (ICUs), where the emphasis is on survival and 'cure.' After Robert Zussman, a sociologist, had observed doctors and nurses in two American ICUs for some time, he reached the conclusion that ICU nurses were not 'gentle carers' but technicians. Zussman does not deny that other nurses may well be differently motivated, but in the ICU, he says, they are 'mini-interns.' 'They are not patient advocates. They are not "angels of mercy." Like physicians, they have become technicians.'[14] ...

... Even if a sound distinction in the philosophical or ethical commitments of nursing and medicine could be drawn, this would not settle the question of whether nursing is or is not a naturally subservient profession. The fact (if it is a fact) that medicine has one philosophical commitment or nature and nursing another is quite independent of the further question of whether one of the professions is, or ought to be, subservient to the other. Further argument would be needed to show that, for nothing of substance follows from establishing that one thing, or one profession, is different from another.

SUBSERVIENCE FOR THE SAKE OF LIFE OR LIMB?

What arguments could be provided to show that nurses and nursing ought to adopt a subservient role to doctors and medicine? In accordance with our assumption that nursing is an other-directed profession, a profession that primarily aims at the good of patients, such arguments would have to show that nurses' subservience would benefit patients more than nurses' autonomy. ...

... [O]ur main focus will be hospital-based nurses. Most nurses work in hospitals, and it is part of their role to carry out the treatment plans of doctors. Here a powerful argument is sometimes put that, regardless of what is true for other nurses, it is essential that nurses who work in acute-care settings adopt a subservient role. Those who take this view do not necessarily deny that it may be quite appropriate for some nurses, in some contexts, to play an autonomous role; but, they insist, when we are talking about hospitals, matters are different.[15]

Hospitals are bureaucratic institutions and bureaucratic institutions, so a typical argument goes, rely for efficient functioning on vertical structures of command, on strict adherence to procedure and on avoidance of initiative by those who have been charged with certain tasks. While this is true of all bureaucratic institutions, strict adherence to rules and to chains of command becomes critically important when we are focusing on hospitals. In such a setting much is at stake. A patient's health, and even her life, will often depend on quick and reliable responses by members of the health-care team to the directions of the person in charge.[16]

Let us accept that efficiency will often depend on some of the central criteria identified above. This does not, however, answer questions regarding the proper relationship between nurses and doctors. Take the notion of a bureaucratic hierarchy. A simple appeal to that notion does not tell us how the bureaucratic hierarchy should be arranged.[17] Here it is generally assumed that it is appropriate for doctors to be in charge and appropriate for nurses to follow the doctors' orders. But why should this be so? Why is it so widely assumed that doctors should perform the role of 'captain of the ship'[18] and nurses those of 'members of the crew'?

The Argument from Expertise The reason most commonly given for this type of arrangement is that doctors, but not nurses, have the relevant medical knowledge and expertise to deal with the varied and often unique medical conditions that afflict patients, and the different emergencies that might arise. Just as it would not do to put crewmembers with only a limited knowledge of navigation in charge of a ship traversing unpredictable and potentially dangerous waters, so it would not do to put nurses with only a limited knowledge of medicine in charge of the treatment plans of patients. Many a ship and many a patient would be lost as a result of such an arrangement. Hence, if we want ships and patients to be in good hands, it follows that those with expertise—doctors and captains—must be in charge.

Such an argument is put by Lisa H. Newton, a vocal critic of nursing's quest for autonomy. If the purpose of saving life and health is to be accomplished in an atmosphere which is often tense and urgent, then, Newton argues,

> all participating activities and agents must be completely subordinated to the medical judgements of the physician ... [T]hose other than physicians, involved in medical procedures in a hospital context, have no right to insert their own needs, judgements, or personalities into the situation. The last thing we need at that point is another autonomous professional on the job, whether a nurse or anyone else.[19]

There is something right and something wrong about the above kind of argument. To see this, the argument needs untangling.

Shared Goals, Urgency and Medical Authority
In her argument Newton implicitly assumes that the therapeutic goals of doctors are morally worthy ones, and that the ethical question of whether a doctor should, for example, prolong a patient's life or allow her to die is not in dispute. This assumption is inherent in her observation that the tasks at hand are, or ought to be 'protective of life itself.'[20] While we know that this very question is frequently in dispute, let us, for the purpose of our initial discussion, accept and work with that assumption. We shall question it later.

There is no doubt that doctors have special medical expertise that is relevant to the achievement of various therapeutic goals, including the goal of saving or prolonging life. Extensive medical studies and registration or licensing procedures ensure that doctors are experts in medical diagnosis and medical therapy. Their education equips them well to act quickly and decisively in complicated and unforeseen medical circumstances. As a general rule (but only as a general rule—there could be exceptions to this rule) doctors would thus be better equipped than nurses to respond to a range of medical emergencies. In emergency situations, then, where urgent action is required, it is likely that the best outcome for patients as a whole will be achieved if doctors are in charge. Moreover, since the outcome of medical measures in such contexts often depends crucially on the practical assistance of nurses, it is important that nurses will, as a general rule, quickly and unquestioningly respond to the doctor's orders. . . .

In addition to those cases where urgent action by a medical expert is required to achieve the desired therapeutic goal, there are also some other specialized contexts, such as the operating room, where it is appropriate for doctors to exercise and for nurses to recognize medical authority. . . . There is a connection, then, between the possession of particular expertise and authority. Expertise can be crucial to the achievement of goals and, provided the goals are shared, it will frequently be appropriate for people who are authorities in a particular field to also be *in* authority.

If we accept this argument, it follows that doctors ought, other things being equal, to be in charge in medical emergencies and in other specialized contexts that are characterized by an element of urgency. They ought to be in charge because this arrangement best ensures that the therapeutic goal will be reached.

Acceptance of this view has, however, less far-reaching consequences than might be assumed. First, even if particular therapeutic treatment goals are most likely to be achieved if a single medically trained person is in charge *during,* for example, operations or resuscitation procedures, this does not entail that the doctor should have overall authority as far as the patient's treatment is concerned. The authority to decide on an operation or on the desirability of implementing resuscitation procedures might, for example, rest with the patient or her relatives, and the nurse could conceivably be in charge of the overall treatment plan of the patient.[21]

Second, it does not follow that nurses must, even during emergency procedures, *blindly* follow a doctor's order. Doctors, like the rest of us, are fallible human beings and sometimes make mistakes. This means that the nurse's obligation to follow a doctor's order, even in these specialized contexts, cannot be absolute and may at times be overridden by other considerations, such as the avoidance of harm to patients. . . .

. . . Given, then, that doctors will occasionally make mistakes and that nurses frequently have the professional knowledge to detect them, it will be best if nurses do not understand their duty to follow a doctor's order as an absolute and exceptionless one. If the doctor's order is, in the nurse's professional judgement, clearly wrong, then the nurse must bring her 'professional intelligence' into play and question it. . . .

Does a nurse who subscribes to the general proposition or rule that there are times when it will best serve the interests of patients that she accept the authority of doctors thereby necessarily adopt a subservient or non-autonomous role? Does she abrogate her autonomy? I think not. As long as a nurse does not *surrender* her autonomy or judgement, that is, does not blindly follow every order she is given, but rather *decides,* after reflection, to adopt a general rule that it will be best to accept and act on the doctor's authority under certain circumstances, then she is not a subservient tool in the doctor's hands. She is not, as was once proposed, simply 'an intelligent machine.'[22] She is a moral agent who, in distinction from a mere machine, *chooses* to act in one way rather than another.

To sum up, then: the argument that nurses should—for the sake of achieving certain worthy therapeutic goals such as the saving of life—adopt a subservient role to doctors typically rests on at least two rather dubious assumptions. The first assumption is that all or most decision-making is characterized by great urgency. The second assumption is that the therapeutic goal is best achieved by nurses adopting an absolute rather than a prima facie rule to carry out the doctor's orders. But, as we have seen, both assumptions must be rejected, on the grounds outlined above. . . .

DO PATIENTS NEED SUBSERVIENT MOTHER SURROGATES?

A different kind of argument is sometimes put to show that nurses should, for the sake of patients, adopt a subservient role to doctors. Only then, the argument asserts, will nurses be able to meet the emotional needs of patients. To examine that claim, we shall once again focus on an argument provided by Lisa H. Newton. In her defence of the traditional role of the nurse, Newton appeals to an argument based on the patient's needs. Because a patient may not be able to take care of himself, Newton points out,

> his entire self-concept of an independent human being may be threatened . . . He needs comfort, reassurance, someone to talk to. The person he really needs, who would be capable of taking care of all these problems, is obviously his mother, and the first job of the nurse is to be a mother surrogate.[23]

But, Newton continues her argument, mothers are not only figures of considerable authority; it is also ordinarily part of the mother's role to take control of various aspects of her dependent children's lives, and to make important decisions for them. Patients are, however, not children. Their autonomy must be protected from the threatening authority of the mother surrogate. This requires, Newton asserts, that

the role of the nurse must be from the outset, as essentially as it is nurturant, unavailable for such attribution of authority. Not only must the role of the nurse not include authority; it must be incompatible with authority: essentially, a subservient role.[24]

This non-threatening caring function, performed by the nurse, would not only permit the patient 'to be cared for like a baby,' but would also allow patients to unburden themselves and to express their doubts and resentments about doctors and the treatments prescribed by them. Patients, Newton notes, may sometimes be torn between the desire to discontinue treatment (to reassert control over their lives) and a desire to continue treatment (to reap its benefits). The nurse will be there as a sympathetic listener 'but in her subordinate position . . . can do absolutely nothing to change the course of treatment,' that is, both nurse and patient are subject to what she calls the 'sapiential authority' of the physician.[25]

The traditional subordinate role of the nurse is thus justified by the needs of patients. Patients, Newton holds, need the emotional support of a mother surrogate but, to protect the patient's autonomy and to ensure compliance with the medical treatment plan, the nurse must completely surrender her autonomy.

Should we accept this type of argument? The first point to be noted is this: Newton's claims about humiliating treatment, about strong emotional needs and about the threatened loss of the patient's self-concept as an independent human being, while undoubtedly correct in some cases, do not apply to all patients and in all circumstances. Many patients enter hospital for relatively minor treatments or observations and do not feel that their self-concept is threatened in any way by their status of patient. They do not need or want a mother surrogate. Rather, their needs are much more likely to be met by a nurse who not only provides them with professional nursing care, but who also refuses to surrender her professional intelligence and autonomy to the doctor to protect the patient from potential harm.

Then there are the patients who are seriously ill and whose self-concept may indeed be threatened by the medical treatment they are receiving or by their incapacitated state. Many of these patients will undoubtedly benefit from the presence of a caring and sympathetic nurse, who will listen to them with warmth and understanding. But would they want the subservient nurse Newton holds in store for them? Would their emotional needs really be satisfied by talking to a self-effacing health-care professional who, afraid of either posing a threat to the patient's autonomy or the 'sapiential authority' of the doctor, would be making sympathetic clucking noises, but would not engage with the patient in any meaningful way? I doubt it very much. By refusing to engage with patients in a meaningful way, she would be signalling to them that she does not take their concerns seriously, no more seriously than a well-meaning mother would take the incoherent babbling of her sick baby. This would not only be extremely upsetting to many patients, but would also enforce their sense of powerlessness, the feeling that they have lost control over their lives—as indeed they may have. . . .

As we noted above, Newton recognizes that a patient may wish to discontinue treatment so as to 'reassert control over his life.'[26] Would supporting the patient in this desire—assuming that it is a reasonable one—really threaten his autonomy? And is not the nurse's refusal ever to take the patient's desire seriously tantamount to abandoning him to another authority—the authority of the doctor? While we should not ignore the possibility that a powerful mother figure might pose a threat to the patient's autonomy, why should we assume that a powerful father figure—that of the doctor—might not pose a similar or a greater threat?

Newton simply assumes that the therapeutic success of treatment presupposes that the patient defer to the 'physician's sapiential authority.' What she does not explain, however, is why the physician's ends or goals—therapeutic success or prolongation of life, for example—should count for more than, say, the judgement of the patient or the nurse. In other words, we are not told where the doctor's moral authority comes from or why we should regard his decisions as sound. . . .

The adoption by nurses of a subservient role of the kind envisaged by Newton would most likely harm patients more than it would benefit them; it would also be an utterly demoralizing role for many contemporary nurses, even if it would be compatible with some understanding of autonomy. Nurses would be required to stand by, doing nothing, while doctors make the occasional mistake, or provide treatment to unwilling but disempowered patients. To conclude, then, I can see no good reason why nurses should adopt a subservient mother surrogate role for the sake of patients. On the contrary, there are a number of strong reasons why nurses should reject it. . . .

NOTES

[1] See, for example, 'Where does loyalty to the physician end?' (editorial), *American Journal of Nursing*, 10 (Jan. 1910), pp. 230–1; 'Where does loyalty to the physician end?' (letters), *American Journal of Nursing*, 10 (Jan. 1910), pp. 274, 276. (I owe these reference to Gerald R. Winslow, 'From loyalty to advocacy: a new metaphor for nursing,' *Hastings Center Report*, 14 (June 1984), p. 34.)

[2] Parts of this chapter have greatly benefited from Gerald R. Winslow, 'From loyalty to advocacy.'

[3] See, for example, the 1973 International Council of Nurses *Code for Nurses,* which holds that '[t]he nurse's primary responsibility is to those people who require nursing care.' See also the 1980 report on revisions to the Principles of Medical Ethics endorsed by the American Medical Association, which states that '[t]he profession does not exist for itself; it exists for a purpose and increasingly that purpose will be defined by society.' (As quoted by Robert M. Veatch, 'Medical ethics: an introduction,' in R. M. Veatch (ed.), *Medical Ethics* (1989), p. 22.)

[4] See, for example, Carolla A. Quinn and Michael D. Smith, *The Professional Commitment: Issues and ethics in nursing* (1987), ch. 1.

[5] Robert Baker, 'Care of the sick and cure of the disease: comment on "The Fractured Image," ' in Stuart F. Spicker and Sally Gadow (eds), *Nursing: Images and ideals—Opening dialogue with the humanities* (1980), pp. 42–3. See also James L. Muyskens, *Moral Problems in Nursing: A philosophical investigation* (1982), pp. 31ff.

[6] On this point, see also H. Tristram Engelhardt, Jr, 'Physicians, patients, health care institutions—and the people in between: nurses,' in Anne Bishop and John R. Scudder, Jr, *Caring, Curing, Coping* (1985), p. 63.

[7] Ibid., p. 62.

[8] American Psychiatric Association, *Diagnostic and Statistical Manual of Mental Disorders*, 3rd edn (1980), as cited by Engelhardt, ibid., p. 71.

[9] See Martin Benjamin and Joy Curtis, *Ethics in Nursing*, 3rd edn (1992), pp. 91–5.

[10] Ibid., p. 92.

[11] H. Tristram Engelhardt, Jr, 'Physicians, patients, health care institutions—and the people in between: nurses,' pp. 62–79.

[12] See, for example, Jean Watson, 'Introduction: an ethic of caring/curing/nursing *qua* nursing,' in *The Ethics of Care and the Ethics of Cure: Synthesis in Chronicity*, ed. Jean Watson and Marilyn A. Ray (1988), pp. 1–3.

[13] James L. Muyskens, *Moral Problems in Nursing*, p. 36.

[14] Robert Zussman, *Intensive Care: Medical ethics and the medical profession* (1992), ch. 5, at p. 80.

[15] Lisa Newton, 'In defense of the traditional nurse,' *Nursing Outlook*, 29 (June 1981), pp. 348–54. See also Lisa H. Newton, 'A vindication of the gentle sister: comment on "The Fractured Image,"' in Stuart F. Spicker and Sally Gadow (eds), *Nursing: Images and ideals*, pp. 34–40.

[16] Lisa H. Newton, 'In defense of the traditional nurse,' p. 350.

[17] Of course, it also leaves open the question of whether bureaucratic, hierarchical structures are the ones we should adopt in the first place. While I believe that there might well be other and more satisfactory arrangements, I will set this question aside and not discuss it any further.

[18] As H. Tristram Engelhardt, Jr, notes ('Physicians, patients, health care institutions' p. 68), the now famous phrase by which doctors were construed as 'captain of the ship,' was used in the case of *McConnel* v. *Williams*, 361 Pa. 355, 65 A. 2nd 243 (1959).

[19] Lisa H. Newton, 'In defense of the traditional nurse,' p. 351.

[20] Ibid.

[21] This point is made by Andrew Jameton, *Nursing Practice: The ethical issues*, p. 46. There might, however, be some advantage in having doctors—on account of their expertise—in charge of the treatment plans of emergency-prone patients *if* the agreed goal is to save life. This would ensure that the person most qualified to conduct the relevant procedure would not have to defer to the authority in charge of the overall treatment plan before implementing a procedure.

[22] Sarah Dock, 'The relation of the nurse to the doctor and the doctor to the nurse,' *American Journal of Nursing*, 17 (1917), p. 394.

[23] Lisa H. Newton, 'In defense of the traditional nurse,' p. 351.

[24] Ibid., p. 352.

[25] Ibid.

[26] Ibid.

TRUTH TELLING AND CONFIDENTIALITY

ON TELLING PATIENTS THE TRUTH
Roger Higgs

Higgs argues for the paramount importance of physicians' telling patients the truth, before taking on the complex issue of whether this rule has exceptions. He considers and rejects most of the arguments commonly offered to justify lying to patients or otherwise deceiving them. In the end, he maintains, "there are *some* circumstances in which the health professions are probably exempted from society's general requirement for truthfulness," but these are very rare circumstances in which there are clearly no acceptable alternatives.

... [T]hose with experience, either as patients or professionals, will immediately recognize the situation. Although openness is increasingly practised, there is still uncertainty in the minds of many doctors or nurses faced with communicating bad news; as for instance when a test shows up an unexpected

Reprinted from Michael Lockwood, ed., *Moral Dilemmas in Modern Medicine* (1985), pp. 187–191, 193–202, by permission of Oxford University Press. © Roger Higgs 1985.

and probably incurable cancer, or when meeting the gaze of a severely ill child, or answering the questions of a mother in mid-pregnancy whose unborn child is discovered to be badly handicapped. What should be said? There can be few who have not, on occasions such as these, told less than the truth. Certainly the issue is a regular preoccupation of nurses and doctors in training. Why destroy hope? Why create anxiety, or something worse? Isn't it 'First, do no harm'?[1]

The concerns of the patient are very different. For many, fear of the unknown is the worst disease of all, and yet direct information seems so hard to obtain. The ward round goes past quickly, unintelligible words are muttered—was I supposed to hear and understand? In the surgery the general practitioner signs his prescription pad and clearly it's time to be gone. Everybody is too busy saving lives to give explanations. It may come as a shock to learn that it is policy, not just pressure of work, that prevents a patient learning the truth about himself. If truth is the first casualty, trust must be the second. 'Of course they wouldn't say, especially if things were bad,' said the elderly woman just back from outpatients, 'they've got that Oath, haven't they?' She had learned to expect from doctors, at the best, silence; at the worst, deception. It was part of the system, an essential ingredient, as old as Hippocrates. However honest a citizen, it was somehow part of the doctor's job not to tell the truth to his patient. . . .

[I]t is easier to decide what to do when the ultimate outcome is clear. It may be much more difficult to know what to say when the future is less certain, such as in the first episode of what is probably multiple sclerosis, or when a patient is about to undergo a mutilating operation. But even in work outside hospital, where such dramatic problems arise less commonly, whether to tell the truth and how much to tell can still be a regular issue. How much should this patient know about the side effects of his drugs? An elderly man sits weeping in an old people's home, and the healthy but exhausted daughter wants the doctor to tell her father that she's medically unfit to have him back. The single mother wants a certificate to say that she is unwell so that she can stay at home to look after her sick child. A colleague is often drunk on duty, and is making mistakes. A husband with venereal disease wants his wife to be treated without her knowledge. An outraged father demands to know if his teenage daughter has been put on the pill. A mother comes in with a child to have a boil lanced. 'Please tell him it won't hurt.' A former student writes from abroad needing to complete his professional experience and asks for a reference for a job he didn't do.[2] Whether the issue is large or small, the truth is at stake. What should the response be?

Discussion of the apparently more dramatic situations may provide a good starting point. Recently a small group of medical students, new to clinical experience, were hotly debating what a patient with cancer should be told. One student maintained strongly that the less said to the patient the better. Others disagreed. When asked whether there was any group of patients they could agree should never be told the truth about a life-threatening illness, the students chose children, and agreed that they would not speak openly to children under six. When asked to try to remember what life was like when they were six, one student replied that he remembered how his mother had died when he was that age. Suddenly the student who had advocated non-disclosure became animated. 'That's extraordinary. My mother died when I was six too. My father said she'd gone away for a time, but would come back soon. One day he said she was coming home again. My younger sister and I were very excited. We waited at the window upstairs until we saw his car drive up. He got out and helped a woman out of the car. Then we saw. It wasn't mum. I suppose I never forgave him—or her, really.'[3]

It is hard to know with whom to sympathize in this sad tale. But its stark simplicity serves to highlight some essential points. First, somehow more clearly than in the examples involving patients, not telling the truth is seen for what it really is. It is, of course, quite possible, and very common in clinical practice, for doctors (or nurses) to engage in deliberate deceit without actually *saying* anything they believe to be false. But, given the special responsibilities of the doctor, and the relationship of trust that exists between him and his patient, one could hardly argue that this was morally any different from telling outright lies. Surely it is the *intention* that is all important. We may be silent, tactful, or reserved, but if we intend to deceive, what we are doing is tantamount to lying. The debate in ward or surgery is suddenly stood on its head. The question is no longer 'Should we tell the truth?' but 'What justification is there for telling a lie?' This relates to the second important point, that medical ethics are part of general morality, and not a separate field of their own with their own rules. Unless there are special justifications, health-care professionals are working within the same moral constraints as lay people. A lie is a lie wherever told and whoever tells it.

But do doctors have a special dispensation from the usual principles that guide the conduct of our society? It is widely felt that on occasion they do, and such a dispensation is as necessary to all doctors as freedom from the charge of assault is to a surgeon. But if it is impossible to look after ill patients and always be open and truthful, how can we balance this against the clear need for truthfulness on all other occasions? If deception is like a medicine to be given in certain doses in certain cases, what guidance exists about its administration?

. . . Although the writer of the 'Decorum' in the Hippocratic corpus advises physicians of the danger of telling patients about the nature of their illness '. . . for many patients through this cause have taken a turn for the worse,'[4] the Oath itself is completely silent on this issue. This extraordinary omission is continued through all the more modern codes and declarations. The first mention of veracity as a principle is to be found in the American Medical Association's 'Principles of Ethics' of 1980, which states that the physician should 'deal honestly with patients and colleagues and strive to expose those physicians deficient in character or competence, or who engage in fraud and deception.'[5] Despite the difficulties of the latter injunction, which seems in some way to divert attention from the basic need for honest communication with the patient, here at last is a clear statement. This declaration signally fails, however, to provide the guidance that we might perhaps have expected for the professional facing his or her individual dilemma.

The reticence of these earlier codes is shared, with some important exceptions, by medical writing elsewhere. Until recently most of what had been usefully said could be summed up by the articles of medical writers such as Thomas Percival, Worthington Hooker, Richard Cabot, and Joseph Collins, which show a wide scatter of viewpoints but do at least confront the problems directly.[6] There is, however, one widely quoted statement by Lawrence Henderson, writing in the *New England Journal of Medicine* in 1935.[7] 'It is meaningless to speak of telling the truth, the whole truth and nothing but the truth to a patient . . . because it is . . . a sheer impossibility . . . Since

telling the truth is impossible, there can be no sharp distinction between what is true and what is false.' . . .

But we must not allow ourselves to be confused, as Henderson was, and as so many others have been, by a failure to distinguish between truth, the abstract concept, of which we shall always have an imperfect grasp, and *telling* the truth, where the intention is all important. Whether or not we can ever fully grasp or express the whole picture, whether we know ultimately what the truth really is, we must speak truthfully, and intend to convey what we understand, or we shall lie. In Sissela Bok's words 'The moral question of whether you are lying or not is not *settled* by establishing the truth or falsity of what you say. In order to settle the question, we must know whether you *intend your statement to mislead*.'[8] . . .

Most modern thinkers in the field of medical ethics would hold that truthfulness is indeed a central principle of conduct, but that it is capable of coming into conflict with other principles, to which it must occasionally give way. On the other hand, the principle of veracity often receives support from other principles. For instance, it is hard to see how a patient can have autonomy, can make a free choice about matters concerning himself, without some measure of understanding of the facts as they influence the case; and that implies, under normal circumstances, some open, honest discussion with his advisers.[9] . . .

Once the central position of honesty has been established, we still need to examine whether doctors and nurses really do have, as has been suggested, special exemption from being truthful because of the nature of their work, and if so under what circumstances. . . . It may finally be decided that in a crisis there is no acceptable alternative, as when life is ebbing and truthfulness would bring certain disaster. Alternatively, the moral issue may appear so trivial as not to be worth considering (as, for example, when a doctor is called out at night by a patient who apologizes by saying, 'I hope you don't mind me calling you at this time, doctor,' and the doctor replies, 'No, not at all.'). However, . . . occasions of these two types are few, fewer than those in which deliberate deceit would generally be regarded as acceptable in current medical practice, and should regularly be debated 'in public' if abuses are to be avoided.[10] To this end it is necessary now to examine critically the arguments commonly used to defend lying to patients.

First comes the argument that it is enormously difficult to put across a technical subject to those with little technical knowledge and understanding, in a situation where so little is predictable. A patient has bowel cancer. With surgery it might be cured, or it might recur. Can the patient understand the effects of treatment? The symptom she is now getting might be due to cancer, there might be secondaries, and they in turn might be suppressible for a long time, or not at all. What future symptoms might occur, how long will she live, how will she die—all these are desperately important questions for the patient, but even for her doctor the answers can only be informed guesses, in an area where uncertainty is so hard to bear.

Yet to say we do not know anything is a lie. As doctors we know a great deal, and *can* make informed guesses or offer likelihoods. The whole truth may be impossible to attain, but truthfulness is not. 'I do not know' can be a major piece of honesty. To deprive the patient of honest communication because we cannot know everything is, as we have seen, not only confused thinking but immoral. Thus deprived, the patient cannot plan, he cannot choose. If choice is the crux of morality, it may also, as we have argued elsewhere, be central to health. If he cannot choose, the patient cannot ever be considered to be fully restored to health.[11]

This argument also raises another human failing—to confuse the difficult with the unimportant. Passing information to people who have more restricted background, whether through lack of experience or of understanding, can be extremely difficult and time-consuming, but this is no reason why it should be shunned. Quite the reverse. Like the difficult passages in a piece of music, these tasks should be practiced, studied, and techniques developed so that communication is efficient and effective. For the purposes of informed consent, the patient must be given the information he needs, as a reasonable person, to make a reasoned choice.

The second argument for telling lies to patients is that no patient likes hearing depressing or frightening news. That is certainly true. There must be few who do. But in other walks of life no professional would normally consider it his or her duty to suppress information simply in order to preserve happiness. No accountant, foreseeing bankruptcy in his client's affairs, would chat cheerfully about the budget or a temporarily reassuring credit account. Yet such suppression of information occurs daily in wards or surgeries throughout the country. Is this what patients themselves want?

In order to find out, a number of studies have been conducted over the past thirty years.[12] In most studies there is a significant minority of patients, perhaps about a fifth, who, if given information, deny having been told. Sometimes this must be pure forgetfulness, sometimes it relates to the lack of skill of the informer, but sometimes with bad or unwelcome news there is an element of what is (perhaps not quite correctly) called 'denial.' The observer feels that at one level the news has been taken in, but at another its validity or reality has not been accepted. This process has been recognized as a buffer for the mind against the shock of unacceptable news, and often seems to be part of a process leading to its ultimate acceptance.[13] But once this group has been allowed for, most surveys find that, of those who have had or who could have had a diagnosis made of, say, cancer, between two-thirds and three-quarters of those questioned were either glad to have been told, or declared that they would wish to know. Indeed, surveys reveal that most *doctors* would themselves wish to be told the truth, even though (according to earlier studies at least) most of those same doctors said they would not speak openly to their patients—a curious double standard! Thus these surveys have unearthed, at least for the present, a common misunderstanding between doctors and patients, a general preference for openness among patients, and a significant but small group whose wish not to be informed must surely be respected. We return once more to the skill needed to detect such differences in the individual case, and the need for training in such skills.

Why doctors have for so long misunderstood their patients' wishes is perhaps related to the task itself. Doctors don't want to give bad news, just as patients don't want it in abstract, but doctors have the choice of withholding the information, and in so doing protecting themselves from the pain of telling, and from the blame of being the bearer of bad news. In addition it has been suggested that doctors are particularly fearful of death and illness. Montaigne suggested that men have to think about death and be prepared to accept it, and one would think that doctors would get used to death. Yet perhaps this very familiarity has created an obsession that amounts to fear. Just as the police seem over-concerned with violence, and firemen with fire, perhaps doctors have met death in their professional training only as the enemy, never as something to come to terms with, or even as a natural force to be respected and, when the time is ripe, accepted or even welcomed. . . .

. . . Paternalism may be justifiable in the short term, and to 'kid' someone, to treat him as a child because he is ill, and perhaps dying, may be very tempting. Yet true respect for that person (adult or child) can only be shown by allowing him allowable choices, by granting him whatever control is left, as weakness gradually undermines his hold on life. If respect is important then at the very least there must be no acceptable or effective alternative to lying in a particular situation if the lie is to be justified.

. . . However, a third argument for lying can be advanced, namely, that truthfulness can actually do harm. 'What you don't know can't hurt you' is a phrase in common parlance (though it hardly fits with concepts of presymptomatic screening for preventable disease!). However, it is undeniable that blunt and unfeeling communication of unpleasant truths can cause acute distress, and sometimes long-term disability. The fear that professionals often have of upsetting people, of causing a scene, of making fools of themselves by letting unpleasant emotions flourish, seems to have elevated this argument beyond its natural limits. It is not unusual to find that the fear of creating harm will deter a surgical team from discussing a diagnosis gently with a patient, but not deter it from performing radical and mutilating surgery. Harm is a very personal concept. Most medical schools have, circulating in the refectory, a story about a patient who was informed that he had cancer and then leapt to his death. The intended moral for the medical student is, keep your mouth shut and do no harm. But that may not be the correct

lesson to be learned from such cases (which I believe, in any case, to be less numerous than is commonly supposed). The style of telling could have been brutal, with no follow-up or support. It may have been the suggested treatment, not the basic illness, that led the patient to resort to such a desperate measure. Suicide in illness is remarkably rare, but, though tragic, could be seen as a logical response to an overwhelming challenge. No mention is usually made of suicide rates in other circumstances, or the isolation felt by ill and warded patients, or the feelings of anger uncovered when someone takes such precipitate and forbidden action against himself. What these cases do, surely, is argue, not for no telling, but for better telling, for sensitivity and care in determining how much the patient wants to know, explaining carefully in ways the patient can understand, and providing full support and 'after-care' as in other treatments.

But even if it is accepted that the short-term effect of telling the truth may sometimes be considerable psychological disturbance, in the long term the balance seems definitely to swing the other way. The effects of lying are dramatically illustrated in 'A Case of Obstructed Death?'[14] False information prevented a woman from returning to healthy living after a cancer operation, and robbed her of six months of active life. Also, the long-term effect of lies on the family and, perhaps most importantly, on society, is incalculable. If trust is gradually corroded, if the 'wells are poisoned,' progress is hard. Mistrust creates lack of communication and increased fear, and this generation has seen just such a fearful myth created around cancer.[15] Just how much harm has been done by this 'demonizing' of cancer, preventing people coming to their doctors, or alternatively creating unnecessary attendances on doctors, will probably never be known.

There are doubtless many other reasons why doctors lie to their patients; but these can hardly be used to justify lies, even if we should acknowledge them in passing. Knowledge is power, and certainly doctors, though usually probably for reasons of work-load rather than anything more sinister, like to remain 'in control.' Health professionals may, like others, wish to protect themselves from confrontation, and may find it easier to coerce or manipulate than to gain permission. There may be a desire to avoid any pressure for change. And there is the constant problem of lack of time. . . .

If the importance of open communication with the patient is accepted, [however,] we need to know when to say what. If a patient is going for investigations, it may be possible at that time, before details are known, to have a discussion about whether he would like to know the details. A minor 'contract' can be made. 'I promise to tell you what I know, if you ask me.' Once that time is past, however, it requires skill and sensitivity to assess what a patient wants to know. Allowing the time and opportunity for the patient to ask questions is the most important thing, but one must realize that the patient's apparent question may conceal the one he really wants answered. 'Do I have cancer?' may contain the more important questions 'How or when will I die?' 'Will there be pain?' The doctor will not necessarily be helping by giving an extended pathology lesson. The informer may need to know more: 'I don't want to avoid your question, and I promise to answer as truthfully as I can, but first . . .' It has been pointed out that in many cases the terminal patient will tell the doctor, not vice versa, if the right opportunities are created and the style and timing is appropriate. Then it is a question of not telling but listening to the truth.[16]

If in spite of all this there still seems to be a need to tell lies, we must be able to justify them. That the person is a child, or 'not very bright,' will not do. Given the two ends of the spectrum of crisis and triviality, the vast middle range of communication requires honesty, so that autonomy and choice can be maintained. If lies are to be told, there really must be no acceptable alternative. . . . If we break an important moral principle, that principle still retains its force, and its 'shadow' has to be acknowledged. As professionals we shall have to ensure that we follow up, that we work through the broken trust or the disillusionment that the lie will bring to the patient, just as we would follow up and work through bad news, a major operation, or a psychiatric 'sectioning.' This follow-up may also be called for in our relationship with our colleagues if there has been major disagreement about what should be done.

In summary, there are *some* circumstances in which the health professions are probably exempted from society's general requirement for truthfulness. But not telling the truth is usually the same as telling a lie, and a lie requires strong justification. Lying must be a last resort, and we should act as if we were to be called upon to defend the decision in public debate, even if our duty of confidentiality does not allow this in practice. We should always aim to respect the other important principles governing interactions with patients, especially the preservation of the patient's autonomy. When all is said and done, many arguments for individual cases of lying do not hold water. Whether or not knowing the truth is essential to the patient's health, telling the truth is essential to the health of the doctor-patient relationship.

NOTES

1 *Primum non nocere*—this is a latinization of a statement which is not directly Hippocratic, but may be derived from the *Epidemics* Book 1 Chapter II: 'As to diseases, make a habit of two things—to help, or at least do no harm.' *Hippocrates,* 4 Vols. (London: William Heinemann, 1923–31), Vol. I. Translation W. H. S. Jones.

2 Cases collected by the author in his own practice.

3 Case collected by the author.

4 Quoted in Reiser, Dyck, and Curran (eds), *Ethics in Medicine, Historical Perspectives and Contemporary Concerns* (Cambridge, Mass.: MIT Press, 1977).

5 American Medical Association, 'Text of the American Medical Association New Principles of Medical Ethics.' *American Medical News* (August 1–8, 1980), 9.

6 To be found in Reiser *et al.*, op. cit. (see n. 4 above).

7 Lawrence Henderson, 'Physician and Patient as a Social System,' *New England Journal of Medicine,* 212 (1935).

8 Sissela Bok, *Lying: Moral Choice in Public and Private Life* (London: Quartet, 1980).

9 Alastair Campbell and Roger Higgs, *In That Case* (London: Darton, Longman and Todd, 1982).

10 John Rawls, *A Theory of Justice* (Cambridge, Mass.: Harvard University Press, Belknap Press, 1971).

11 Op. cit. (see n. 9 above).

12 Summarized well in Robert Veatch, 'Truth-telling I' in Warren T. Reich (ed.), *Encyclopaedia of Bioethics* (New York: Free Press, 1978).

13 The five stages of reacting to bad news, or news of dying, are described in *On Death and Dying* by Elizabeth Kübler-Ross (London: Tavistock, 1970). Not everyone agrees with her model. For another view see a very stimulating article 'Therapeutic Uses of Truth' by Michael Simpson in E. Wilkes (ed.), *The Dying Patient* (Lancaster: MTP Press, 1982). 'In my model there are only two stages—the stage when you believe in the Kübler-Ross five and the stage when you do not.'

14 Roger Higgs, 'Truth at the Last—A Case of Obstructed Death?', *Journal of Medical Ethics*, 8 (1982), 48–50, and Roger Higgs, 'Obstructed Death Revisited,' *Journal of Medical Ethics,* 8 (1982), pp. 154–56.

15 Susan Sontag, *Illness as Metaphor* (New York: Farrar, Straus and Giroux, 1978).

16 Cicely Saunders, 'Telling Patients,' *District Nursing* (now *Queens Nursing Journal*) (September 1963), pp. 149–50, 154.

MAJORITY OPINION IN *TARASOFF V. REGENTS OF THE UNIVERSITY OF CALIFORNIA*

Justice Mathew O. Tobriner

Tatiana Tarasoff was murdered by Prosenjit Poddar, who was a patient of psychotherapists employed by the University of California Hospital. Her parents brought an action against the university regents, doctors, and campus police. The Tarasoffs complained that the doctors and police had failed to warn them that their daughter was in danger from Poddar. In finding for the Tarasoffs, Justice Tobriner argues that a doctor or psychotherapist treating a mentally ill patient has a duty to warn third parties of threatened dangers arising out of the patient's violent intentions. Responding to the defendants' appeal to the important role played by the principle of confidentiality in the psychotherapeutic situation, Tobriner argues that the public interest in safety from violent assault must be weighed against the patient's right to privacy.

On October 27, 1969, Prosenjit Poddar killed Tatiana Tarasoff. Plaintiffs, Tatiana's parents, allege that two months earlier Poddar confided his intention to kill Tatiana to Dr. Lawrence Moore, a psychologist employed by the Cowell Memorial Hospital at the University of California at Berkeley. They allege that on Moore's request, the campus police briefly detained Poddar, but released him when he appeared rational. They further claim that Dr. Harvey Powelson, Moore's superior, then directed that no further action be taken to detain Poddar. No one warned plaintiffs of Tatiana's peril. . . .

We shall explain that defendant therapists cannot escape liability merely because Tatiana herself was not their patient. When a therapist determines, or pursuant to the standards of his profession should determine, that his patient presents a serious danger of violence to another, he incurs an obligation to use

California Supreme Court; July 1, 1976. 131 California Reporter 14. Reprinted with permission of West Publishing Co.

reasonable care to protect the intended victim against such danger. The discharge of this duty may require the therapist to take one or more of various steps, depending upon the nature of the case. Thus it may call for him to warn the intended victim or others likely to apprise the victim of the danger, to notify the police, or to take whatever other steps are reasonably necessary under the circumstances. . . .

PLAINTIFFS' COMPLAINTS

. . . Plaintiffs' first cause of action, entitled "Failure to Detain a Dangerous Patient," alleges that on August 20, 1969, Poddar was a voluntary outpatient receiving therapy at Cowell Memorial Hospital. Poddar informed Moore, his therapist, that he was going to kill an unnamed girl, readily identifiable as Tatiana, when she returned home from spending the summer in Brazil. Moore, with the concurrence of Dr. Gold, who had initially examined Poddar, and Dr. Yandell, assistant to the director of the department of psychiatry, decided that Poddar should be committed for observation in a mental hospital. Moore orally notified Officers Atkinson and Teel of the campus police that he would request commitment. He then sent a letter to Police Chief William Beall requesting the assistance of the police department in securing Poddar's confinement.

Officers Atkinson, Brownrigg, and Halleran took Poddar into custody, but, satisfied that Poddar was rational, released him on his promise to stay away from Tatiana. Powelson, director of the department of psychiatry at Cowell Memorial Hospital, then asked the police to return Moore's letter, directed that all copies of the letter and notes that Moore had taken as therapist be destroyed, and "ordered no action to place Prosenjit Poddar in 72-hour treatment and evaluation facility."

Plaintiffs' second cause of action, entitled "Failure to Warn on a Dangerous Patient," incorporates the allegations of the first cause of action, but adds the assertion that defendants negligently permitted Poddar to be released from police custody without "notifying the parents of Tatiana Tarasoff that their daughter was in grave danger from Prosenjit Poddar." Poddar persuaded Tatiana's brother to share an apartment with him near Tatiana's residence; shortly after her return from Brazil, Poddar went to her residence and killed her.

Plaintiffs' third cause of action, entitled "Abandonment of a Dangerous Patient," seeks $10,000 punitive damages against defendant Powelson. Incorporating the crucial allegations of the first cause of action, plaintiffs charge that Powelson "did the things herein alleged with intent to abandon a dangerous patient, and said acts were done maliciously and oppressively."

Plaintiffs' fourth cause of action, for "Breach of Primary Duty to Patient and the Public," states essentially the same allegations as the first cause of action, but seeks to characterize defendants' conduct as a breach of duty to safeguard their patient and the public. Since such conclusory labels add nothing to the factual allegations of the complaint, the first and fourth causes of action are legally indistinguishable. . . .

. . . We direct our attention . . . to the issue of whether Plaintiffs' second cause of action can be amended to state a basis for recovery.

PLAINTIFFS CAN STATE A CAUSE OF ACTION AGAINST DEFENDANT THERAPISTS FOR NEGLIGENT FAILURE TO PROTECT TATIANA

The second cause of action can be amended to allege that Tatiana's death proximately resulted from defendants' negligent failure to warn Tatiana or others likely to apprise her of her danger. Plaintiffs contend that as amended, such allegations of negligence and proximate causation, with resulting damages, establish a cause of action. Defendants, however, contend that in the circumstances of the present case they owed no duty of care to Tatiana or her parents and that, in the absence of such duty, they were free to act in careless disregard of Tatiana's life and safety.

In analyzing this issue, we bear in mind that legal duties are not discoverable facts of nature, but merely conclusory expressions that, in cases of a particular type, liability should be imposed for damage done. "The assertion that liability must . . . be denied because defendant bears no 'duty' to plaintiff 'begs the essential question—whether the plaintiff's interests are entitled to legal protection against the defendant's conduct. . . . [Duty] is not sacrosanct in itself, but only an expression of the sum total of those considerations of policy which lead the law to say that the particular plaintiff is entitled to protection.' "

In the landmark case of *Rowland v. Christian* (1968), Justice Peters recognized that liability should be imposed "for an injury occasioned to another by his want of ordinary care or skill" as expressed in section 1714 of the Civil Code. Thus, Justice Peters, quoting from *Heaven v. Pender* (1883) stated: "Whenever one person is by circumstances placed in such a position with regard to another . . . that if he did not use ordinary care and skill in his own conduct . . . he would cause danger of injury to the person or property of the other, a duty arises to use ordinary care and skill to avoid such danger.' "

We depart from "this fundamental principle" only upon the "balancing of a number of considerations"; major ones "are the foreseeability of harm to the plaintiff, the degree of certainty that the plaintiff suffered injury, the closeness of the connection between the defendant's conduct and the injury suffered, the moral blame attached to the defendant's conduct, the policy of preventing future harm, the extent of the burden to the defendant and consequences to the community of imposing a duty to exercise care with resulting liability for breach, and the availability, cost and prevalence of insurance for the risk involved."

The most important of these considerations in establishing duty is foreseeability. As a general principle, a "defendant owes a duty of care to all persons who are foreseeably endangered by his conduct, with respect to all risks which make the conduct unreasonably dangerous." As we shall explain, however, when the avoidance of foreseeable harm requires a defendant to control the conduct of another person, or to warm of such conduct, the common law has traditionally imposed liability only if the defendant bears some special relationship to the dangerous person or to the potential victim. Since the relationship between a therapist and his patient satisfies this requirement, we need not here decide whether foreseeability alone is sufficient to create a duty to exercise reasonable care to protect a potential victim of another's conduct.

Although, as we have stated above, under the common law, as a general rule, one person owed no duty to control the conduct of another nor to warn those endangered by such conduct, the courts have carved out an exception to this rule in cases in which the defendant stands in some special relationship to either the person whose conduct needs to be controlled or in a relationship to the foreseeable victim of that conduct. Applying this exception to the present case, we note that a relationship of defendant therapists to either Tatiana or Poddar will suffice to establish a duty of care; as explained in section 315 of the Restatement Second of Torts, a duty of care may arise from either "(a) a special relation . . . between the actor and the third person which imposes a duty upon the actor to control the third person's conduct, or (b) a special relation . . . between the actor and the other which gives to the other a right of protection."

Although Plaintiffs' pleadings assert no special relation between Tatiana and defendant therapists, they establish as between Poddar and defendant therapists the special relation that arises between a patient and his doctor or psychotherapist. Such a relationship may support affirmative duties for the benefit of third persons. Thus, for example, a hospital must exercise reasonable care to control the behavior of a patient which may endanger other persons. A doctor must also warn a patient if the patient's condition or medication renders certain conduct, such as driving a car, dangerous to others.

Although the California decisions that recognize this duty have involved cases in which the defendant stood in a special relationship *both* to the victim and to the person whose conduct created the danger, we do not think that the duty should logically be constricted to such situations. Decisions of other jurisdictions hold that the single relationship of a doctor to his patient is sufficient to support the duty to exercise reasonable care to protect others against dangers emanating from the patient's illness. The courts hold that a doctor is liable to persons infected by his patient if he negligently fails to diagnose a contagious disease, or having diagnosed the illness, fails to warn members of the patient's family.

Since it involved a dangerous mental patient, the decision in *Merchants Nat. Bank & Trust Co. of Fargo v. United States* (1967) comes closer to the issue. The Veterans Administration arranged for the patient to work on a local farm, but did not inform the farmer of the man's background. The farmer consequently permitted the patient to come and go freely during non-working hours; the patient borrowed a car, drove to his wife's residence and killed her. Notwithstanding the lack of any "special relationship" between the Veterans Administration and the wife, the court found the Veterans Administration liable for the wrongful death of the wife.

In their summary of the relevant rulings Fleming and Maximov conclude that the "case law should dispel any notion that to impose on the therapists a duty to take precautions for the safety of persons threatened by a patient, where due care so requires, is in any way opposed to contemporary ground rules on the duty relationship. On the contrary, there now seems to be sufficient authority to support the conclusion that by entering into a doctor-patient relationship the therapist becomes sufficiently involved to assume some responsibility for the safety, not only of the patient himself, but also of any third person whom the doctor knows to be threatened by the patient." [Fleming & Maximov, *The Patient or His*

Victim: The Therapist's Dilemma (1974) 62 Cal. L. Rev. 1025, 1030.]

Defendants contend, however, that imposition of a duty to exercise reasonable care to protect third persons is unworkable because therapists cannot accurately predict whether or not a patient will resort to violence. In support of this argument amicus representing the American Psychiatric Association and other professional societies cites numerous articles which indicate that therapists, in the present state of the art, are unable reliably to predict violent acts; their forecasts, amicus claims, tend consistently to overpredict violence, and indeed are more often wrong than right. Since predictions of violence are often erroneous, amicus concludes, the courts should not render rulings that predicate the liability of therapists upon the validity of such predictions.

The role of the psychiatrist, who is indeed a practitioner of medicine, and that of the psychologist who performs an allied function, are like that of the physician who must conform to the standards of the profession and who must often make diagnoses and predictions based upon such evaluations. Thus the judgment of the therapist in diagnosing emotional disorders and in predicting whether a patient presents a serious danger of violence is comparable to the judgment which doctors and professionals must regularly render under accepted rules of responsibility.

We recognize the difficulty that a therapist encounters in attempting to forecast whether a patient presents a serious danger of violence. Obviously we do not require that the therapist, in making the determination, render a perfect performance; the therapist need only exercise "that reasonable degree of skill, knowledge, and care ordinarily possessed and exercised by members of [that professional specialty] under similar circumstances." Within the broad range of reasonable practice and treatment in which professional opinion and judgment may differ, the therapist is free to exercise his or her own best judgment without liability; proof, aided by hindsight, that he or she judged wrongly is insufficient to establish negligence.

In the instant case, however, the pleadings do not raise any question as to failure of defendant therapists to predict that Poddar presented a serious danger of violence. On the contrary, the present complaints allege that defendant therapists did in fact predict that Poddar would kill, but were negligent in failing to warn.

Amicus contends, however, that even when a therapist does in fact predict that a patient poses a serious danger of violence to others, the therapist should be absolved of any responsibility for failing to act to protect the potential victim. In our view, however, once a therapist does in fact determine, or under applicable professional standards reasonably should have determined, that a patient poses a serious danger of violence to others, he bears a duty to exercise reasonable care to protect the foreseeable victim of that danger. While the discharge of this duty of due care will necessarily vary with the facts of each case, in each instance the adequacy of the therapist's conduct must be measured against the traditional negligence standard of the rendition of reasonable care under the circumstances. As explained in Fleming and Maximov, *The Patient or His Victim: The Therapist's Dilemma* (1974), ". . . the ultimate question of resolving the tension between the conflicting interests of patient and potential victim is one of social policy, not professional expertise. . . . In sum, the therapist owes a legal duty not only to his patient, but also to his patient's would-be victim and is subject in both respects to scrutiny by judge and jury. . . ."

The risk that unnecessary warnings may be given is a reasonable price to pay for the lives of possible victims that may be saved. We would hesitate to hold that the therapist who is aware that his patient expects to attempt to assassinate the President of the United States would not be obligated to warn the authorities because the therapist cannot predict with accuracy that his patient will commit the crime.

Defendants further argue that free and open communication is essential to psychotherapy; that "unless a patient . . . is assured that . . . information [revealed by him] can and will be held in utmost confidence, he will be reluctant to make the full disclosure upon which diagnosis and treatment . . . depends." The giving of a warning, defendants contend, constitutes a breach of trust which entails the revelation of confidential communications.

We recognize the public interest in supporting effective treatment of mental illness and in protecting the rights of patients to privacy and the consequent public importance of safeguarding the confidential character of psychotherapeutic communication. Against this interest, however, we must weigh the public interest in safety from violent assault. The Legislature has undertaken the difficult task of balancing the countervailing concerns. In Evidence Code section 1014, it established a broad rule of privilege to protect confidential communications between patient and psychotherapist. In Evidence Code section 1024, the Legislature created a specific and limited exception to the psychotherapist-patient privilege: "There is no privilege . . . if the psychotherapist has reasonable cause to believe that the patient is in such mental or emotional condition as to be dangerous to himself or to the person or property of another and that disclosure of the communication is necessary to prevent the threatened danger."

We realize that the open and confidential character of psychotherapeutic dialogue encourages patients to express threats of violence, few of which are ever executed. Certainly a therapist should not be encouraged routinely to reveal such threats; such disclosures could seriously disrupt the patient's relationship with his therapist and with the persons threatened. To the contrary, the therapist's obligations to his patient require that he not disclose a confidence unless such disclosure is necessary to avert danger to others, and even then that he do so discreetly, and in a fashion that would preserve the privacy of his patient to the fullest extent compatible with the prevention of the threatened danger.

The revelation of a communication under the above circumstances is not a breach of trust or a violation of professional ethics; as stated in the Principles of Medical Ethics of the American Medical Association (1957), section 9: "A physician may not reveal the confidence entrusted to him in the course of medical attendance . . . *unless he is required to do so by law or unless it becomes necessary in order to protect the welfare of the individual or of the community.*" (Emphasis added.) We conclude that the public policy favoring protection of the confidential character of patient-psychotherapist communications must yield to the extent to which disclosure is essential to avert danger to others. The protective privilege ends where the public peril begins.

Our current crowded and computerized society compels the interdependence of its members. In this risk-infested society we can hardly tolerate the further exposure to danger that would result from a concealed knowledge of the therapist that his patient was lethal. If the exercise of reasonable care to protect the threatened victim requires the therapist to warn the endangered party or those who can reasonably be expected to notify him, we see no sufficient societal interest that would protect and justify concealment. The containment of such risks lies in the public interest. For the foregoing reasons, we find that Plaintiffs' complaints can be amended to state a cause of action against defendants Moore, Powelson, Gold, and Yandell and against the Regents as their employer, for breach of a duty to exercise reasonable care to protect Tatiana. . . .

DISSENTING OPINION IN *TARASOFF V. REGENTS OF THE UNIVERSITY OF CALIFORNIA*
Justice William P. Clark

Justice Clark, dissenting from Justice Tobriner's majority opinion, argues that confidentiality in the psychiatrist-patient relationship must be assured for three reasons. (1) Without the promise of such confidentiality, people needing treatment will be deterred from seeking it. (2) Effective therapy requires the patient's full disclosure of his or her innermost thoughts. Without the assurance that the thoughts disclosed will not be revealed by the therapist, the patient could not overcome the psychological barriers standing in the way of such revelations. (3) Successful treatment itself requires a relationship of trust between psychiatrist and patient. In light of these three reasons, Clark argues that if a duty to warn is imposed on psychiatrists, the result will be an increase in violent acts by persons who either don't seek help or whose therapy is unsuccessful. Furthermore, Clark holds, imposing such a duty on psychiatrists will result in an increase in the involuntary civil commitment of patients.

Until today's majority opinion, both legal and medical authorities have agreed that confidentiality is essential to effectively treat the mentally ill, and that imposing a duty on doctors to disclose patient threats to potential victims would greatly impair treatment. Further, recognizing that effective treatment and society's safety are necessarily intertwined, the Legislature has already decided effective and confidential treatment is preferred over imposition of a duty to warn.

The issue whether effective treatment for the mentally ill should be sacrificed to a system of warnings is, in my opinion, properly one for the Legislature, and we are bound by its judgment. Moreover, even in the absence of clear legislative direction, we must reach the same conclusion because imposing the majority's new duty is certain to result in a net increase in violence. . . .

COMMON LAW ANALYSIS

Entirely apart from the statutory provisions, the same result must be reached upon considering both general tort principles and the public policies favoring effective treatment, reduction of violence, and justified commitment.

Generally, a person owes no duty to control the conduct of another. Exceptions are recognized only in limited situations where (1) a special relationship exists between the defendant and injured party, or (2) a special relationship exists between defendant and the active wrongdoer, imposing a duty on defendant to control the wrongdoer's conduct. The majority does not contend the first exception is appropriate to this case.

Policy generally determines duty. Principal policy considerations include foreseeability of harm,

certainty of the plaintiff's injury, proximity of the defendant's conduct to the plaintiff's injury, moral blame attributable to defendant's conduct, prevention of future harm, burden on the defendant, and consequences to the community.

Overwhelming policy considerations weigh against imposing a duty on psychotherapists to warn a potential victim against harm. While offering virtually no benefit to society, such a duty will frustrate psychiatric treatment, invade fundamental patient rights and increase violence.

The importance of psychiatric treatment and its need for confidentiality have been recognized by this court. "It is clearly recognized that the very practice of psychiatry vitally depends upon the reputation in the community that the psychiatrist will not tell." [Slovenko, *Psychiatry and a Second Look at the Medical Privilege* (1960) 6 Wayne L. Rev. 175, 188.]

Assurance of confidentiality is important for three reasons.

Deterrence from Treatment First, without substantial assurance of confidentiality, those requiring treatment will be deterred from seeking assistance. It remains an unfortunate fact in our society that people seeking psychiatric guidance tend to become stigmatized. Apprehension of such stigma—apparently increased by the propensity of people considering treatment to see themselves in the worst possible light—creates a well-recognized reluctance to seek aid. This reluctance is alleviated by the psychiatrist's assurance of confidentiality.

Full Disclosure Second, the guarantee of confidentiality is essential in eliciting the full disclosure necessary for effective treatment. The psychiatric patient approaches treatment with conscious and unconcious inhibitions against revealing his innermost thoughts.

California Supreme Court; July 1, 1976. 131 California Reporter 14.
Reprinted with permission of West Publishing Co.

"Every person, however well-motivated, has to overcome resistances to therapeutic exploration. These resistances seek support from every possible source and the possibility of disclosure would easily be employed in the service of resistance." (Goldstein & Katz, *Psychiatrist-Patient Privilege: The GAP Proposal and the Connecticut Statute,* 36 Conn. Bar J., 175, 179; see also, 118 Am. J. Psych. 734, 735.) Until a patient can trust his psychiatrist not to violate their confidential relationship, "the unconscious psychological control mechanism of repression will prevent the recall of past experiences." [Butler, *Psychotherapy and Griswold: Is Confidentiality a Privilege or a Right?* (1971) 3 Conn. L. Rev. 599, 604.]

Successful Treatment Third, even if the patient fully discloses his thoughts, assurance that the confidential relationship will not be breached is necessary to maintain his trust in his psychiatrist—the very means by which treatment is effected. "[T]he essence of much psychotherapy is the contribution of trust in the external world and ultimately in the self, modelled upon the trusting relationship established during therapy" (Dawidoff, *The Malpractice of Psychiatrists,* 1966 Duke L. J. 696, 704). Patients will be helped only if they can form a trusting relationship with the psychiatrist. All authorities appear to agree that if the trust relationship cannot be developed because of collusive communication between the psychiatrist and others, treatment will be frustrated.

Given the importance of confidentiality to the practice of psychiatry, it becomes clear the duty to warn imposed by the majority will cripple the use and effectiveness of psychiatry. Many people, potentially violent—yet susceptible to treatment—will be deterred from seeking it; those seeking it will be inhibited from making revelations necessary to effective treatment; and, forcing the psychiatrist to violate the patient's trust will destroy the interpersonal relationship by which treatment is effected.

VIOLENCE AND CIVIL COMMITMENT

By imposing a duty to warn, the majority contributes to the danger to society of violence by the mentally ill and greatly increases the risk of civil commitment—the total deprivation of liberty—of those who should not be confined. The impairment of treatment and risk of improper commitment resulting from the new duty to warn will not be limited to a few patients but will extend to a large number of the mentally ill. Although under existing psychiatric procedures only a relatively few receiving treatment will ever present a risk of violence, the number making threats is huge, and it is the latter group—not just the former—whose treatment will be impaired and whose risk of commitment will be increased.

Both the legal and psychiatric communities recognize that the process of determining potential violence in a patient is far from exact, being fraught with complexity and uncertainty.[1]

In fact, precision has not even been attained in predicting who of those having already committed violent acts will again become violent, a task recognized to be of much simpler proportions.

This predictive uncertainty means that the number of disclosures will necessarily be large. As noted above, psychiatric patients are encouraged to discuss all thoughts of violence, and they often express such thoughts. However, unlike this court, the psychiatrist does not enjoy the benefit of overwhelming hindsight in seeing which few, if any, of his patients will ultimately become violent. Now, confronted by the majority's new duty, the psychiatrist must instantaneously calculate potential violence from each patient on each visit. The difficulties researchers have encountered in accurately predicting violence will be heightened for the practicing psychiatrist dealing for brief periods in his office with heretofore nonviolent patients. And, given the decision not to warn or commit must always be made at the psychiatrist's civil peril, one can expect most doubts will be resolved in favor of the psychiatrist protecting himself.

Neither alternative open to the psychiatrist seeking to protect himself is in the public interest. The warning itself is an impairment of the psychiatrist's ability to treat, depriving many patients of adequate treatment. It is to be expected that after disclosing their threats, a significant number of patients, who would not become violent if treated according to existing practices, will engage in violent conduct as a result of unsuccessful treatment. In short, the majority's duty to warn will not only impair treatment of many who would never become violent but worse, will result in a net increase in violence.[2]

The second alternative open to the psychiatrist is to commit his patient rather than to warn. Even in the absence of threat of civil liability, the doubts of psychiatrists as to the seriousness of patient threats have led psychiatrists to overcommit to mental institutions. This overcommitment has been authoritatively documented in both legal and psychiatric studies. This practice is so prevalent that it has been estimated that "as many as twenty harmless persons are incarcerated for every one who will commit a violent act." [Steadman & Cocozza, *Stimulus/Response: We Can't Predict Who Is Dangerous* (Jan. 1975) 8 Psych. Today 32, 35.]

Given the incentive to commit created by the majority's duty, this already serious situation will be worsened. . . .

NOTES

1 A shocking illustration of psychotherapists' inability to predict dangerousness . . . is cited and discussed in Ennis, *Prisoners of Psychiatry: Mental Patients, Psychiatrists, and the Law* (1972): "In a well-known study, psychiatrists predicted that 989 persons were so dangerous that they could not be kept even in civil mental hospitals, but would have to be kept in maximum security hospitals run by the Department of Corrections. Then, because of a United States Supreme Court decision, those persons were transferred to civil hospitals. After a year, the Department of Mental Hygiene reported that one-fifth of them had been discharged to the community, and over half had agreed to remain as voluntary patients. During the year, only 7 of the 989 committed or threatened any act that was sufficiently dangerous to require retransfer to the maximum security hospital. Seven correct predictions out of almost a thousand is not a very impressive record.

"Other studies, and there are many, have reached the same conclusion: psychiatrists simply cannot predict dangerous behavior." (*Id.* at p. 227.)

2 The majority concedes that psychotherapeutic dialogue often results in the patient expressing threats of violence that

are rarely executed. The practical problem, of course, lies in ascertaining which threats from which patients will be carried out. As to this problem, the majority is silent. They do, however, caution that the therapist certainly "should not be encouraged routinely to reveal such threats; such disclosures could seriously disrupt the patient's relationships, with his therapist and with the persons threatened."

Thus, in effect, the majority informs the therapists that they must accurately predict dangerousness—a task recognized as extremely difficult—or face crushing civil liability. The majority's reliance on the traditional standard of care for professionals that "therapist need only exercise 'that reasonable degree of skill, knowledge, and care ordinarily possessed and exercised by members of [that professional specialty] under similar circumstances' " is seriously misplaced. This standard of care assumes that, to a large extent, the subject matter of the specialty is ascertainable. One clearly ascertainable element in the psychiatric field is that the therapist cannot accurately predict dangerousness, which, in turn, means that the standard is inappropriate for lack of a relevant criterion by which to judge the therapist's decision. The inappropriateness of the standard the majority would have us use is made patent when consideration is given to studies, by several eminent authorities, indicating that "[t]he chances of a second psychiatrist agreeing with the diagnosis of a first psychiatrist 'are barely better than 50–50; or stated differently, there is about as much chance that a different expert would come to some different conclusion as there is that the other would agree.' " (Ennis & Litwack, *Psychiatry and the Presumption of Expertise: Flipping Coins in the Courtroom,* 62 Cal. L. Rev. 693, 701, quoting Ziskin, Coping with Psychiatric and Psychological Testimony, 126.) The majority's attempt to apply a normative scheme to a profession which must be concerned with problems that balk at standardization is clearly erroneous.

In any event, an ascertainable standard would not serve to limit psychiatrist disclosure of threats with the resulting impairment of treatment. However compassionate, the psychiatrist hearing the threat remains faced with potential crushing civil liability for a mistaken evaluation of his patient and will be forced to resolve even the slightest doubt in favor of disclosure or commitment.

PLEASE DON'T TELL!: A CASE ABOUT HIV AND CONFIDENTIALITY

(with commentaries by Leonard Fleck and Marcia Angell)

The case features a 21-year-old Hispanic male, Carlos, who is about to end his hospital stay for gunshot wounds and receive nursing care at home from his sister, Consuela. Secretly homosexual and concerned about disgrace within his family, Carlos pleads with the attending physician not to inform his sister that he (Carlos) is HIV-positive. Yet not informing Consuela would seem to increase her risk of contracting HIV while attending to his wounds. The case ends with the question of whether Carlos's physician would be justified in breaching confidentiality on the grounds that he has a "duty to warn."

In the first commentary, Fleck states his assumption that breaches of confidentiality are justified only when there is an imminent threat of serious, irreversible harm; there is no alternative way to avert that threat; and the harm that would thereby be averted is proportionate to the harm associated with breaching confidentiality. Citing a very remote risk of Carlos's infecting Consuela and identifying an alternative to informing her, Fleck argues that breaching confidentiality would be unjustified. In the second commentary, Angell argues that Consuela should be neither deceived nor further exploited by a health-care system that is encouraging her to provide a service it would otherwise be responsible for. Angell concludes that the doctor should give Carlos the choice of either telling his sister that he is HIV-positive or forfeiting her nursing care.

The patient, Carlos R., was a twenty-one-year-old Hispanic male who had suffered gunshot wounds to the abdomen in gang violence. He was uninsured. His stay in the hospital was somewhat shorter than might have been expected, but otherwise unremarkable. It was felt that he could safely complete his recovery at home. Carlos admitted to his attending physician that he was HIV-positive, which was confirmed.

At discharge the attending physician recommended a daily home nursing visit for wound care. However, Medicaid would not fund this nursing visit because a caregiver lived in the home who could adequately provide this care, namely, the patient's twenty-two-year-old sister Consuela, who in fact was willing to accept this burden. Their mother had died almost ten years ago, and Consuela had been a mother to Carlos and their younger sister since then. Carlos had no objection to Consuela's providing this care, but he insisted absolutely that she was not to know his HIV status. He had always been on good terms with Consuela, but she did not know he was actively homosexual. His greatest fear, though, was that his father would learn of his homo-

sexual orientation, which is generally looked upon with great disdain by Hispanics.

Would Carlos's physician be morally justified in breaching patient confidentiality on the grounds that he had a "duty to warn"?

COMMENTARY

By Leonard Fleck If there were a home health nurse to care for this patient, presumably there would be no reason to breach confidentiality since the expectation would be that she would follow universal precautions. Of course, universal precautions could be explained to the patient's sister. In an ideal world this would seem to be a satisfactory response that protects both Carlos's rights and Consuela's welfare. But the world is not ideal.

We know that health professionals, who surely ought to have the knowledge that would motivate them to take universal precautions seriously, often fail to take just such precautions. It is easy to imagine that Consuela could be equally casual or careless, especially when she had not been specifically warned that her brother was HIV-infected. Given this possibility, does the physician have a duty to warn that would justify breaching confidentiality? I shall argue that he may not breach confidentiality but he must be reasonably attentive to Consuela's safety. Ordinarily the conditions that must be met to

Reprinted with permission of the authors and the publisher from *Hastings Center Report*, vol. 21 (November–December 1991), pp. 39–40.

invoke a duty to warn are: (1) an imminent threat of serious and irreversible harm, (2) no alternative to averting that threat other than this breach of confidentiality, and (3) proportionality between the harm averted by this breach of confidentiality and the harm associated with such a breach. In my judgment, none of these conditions are satisfactorily met.

No one doubts that becoming HIV-infected represents a serious and irreversible harm. But, in reality, is that threat imminent enough to justify breaching confidentiality? If we were talking about two individuals who were going to have sexual intercourse on repeated occasions, then the imminence condition would likely be met. But the patient's sister will be caring for his wound for only a week or two, and wound care does not by itself involve any exchange of body fluids. If we had two-hundred and forty surgeons operating on two-hundred and forty HIV-infected patients, and if each of those surgeons nicked himself while doing surgery, then the likelihood is that only one of them would become HIV-infected. Using this as a reference point, the likelihood of this young woman seroconverting if her intact skin comes into contact with the blood of this patient is very remote at best.

Moreover, in this instance there are alternatives. A frank and serious discussion with Consuela about the need for universal precautions, plus monitored, thorough training in correct wound care, fulfills what I would regard as a reasonable duty to warn in these circumstances. Similar instructions ought to be given to Carlos so that he can monitor her performance. He can be reminded that this is a small price for protecting his confidentiality as well as his sister's health. It might also be necessary to provide gloves and other such equipment required to observe universal precautions.

We can imagine easily enough that there might be a lapse in conscientiousness on Consuela's part, that she might come into contact with his blood. But even if this were to happen, the likelihood of her seroconverting is remote at best. This is where proportionality between the harm averted by the breach and the harm associated with it comes in. For if confidentiality were breached and she were informed of his HIV status, this would likely have very serious consequences for Carlos. As a layperson with no

professional duty to preserve confidentiality herself, Consuela might inform other family members, which could lead to his being ostracized from the family. And even if she kept the information confidential, she might be too afraid to provide the care for Carlos, who might then end up with no one to care for him.

The right to confidentiality is a right that can be freely waived. The physician could engage Carlos in a frank moral discussion aimed at persuading him that the reasonable and decent thing to do is to inform his sister of his HIV status. Perhaps the physician offers assurances that she would be able to keep that information in strict confidence. The patient agrees. Then what happens? It is easy to imagine that Consuela balks at caring for her brother, for fear of infection.

Medicaid would still refuse to pay for home nursing care because a caregiver would still be in the home, albeit a terrified caregiver. Consuela's response may not be rational, but it is certainly possible. If she were to react in this way it would be an easy "out" to say that it was Carlos who freely agreed to the release of the confidential information so now he'll just have to live with those consequences. But the matter is really more complex than that. At the very least the physician would have to apprise Carlos of the fact that his sister might divulge his HIV status to some number of other individuals. But if the physician impresses this possibility on Carlos vividly enough, Carlos might be even more reluctant to self-disclose his HIV status to Consuela. In that case the physician is morally obligated to respect that confidentiality.

COMMENTARY

By Marcia Angell It would be wrong, I believe, to ask this young woman to undertake the nursing care of her brother and not inform her that he is HIV-infected.

The claim of a patient that a doctor hold his secrets in confidence is strong but not absolute. It can be overridden by stronger, competing claims. For example, a doctor would not agree to hold in confidence a diagnosis of rubella, if the patient were planning to be in the presence of a pregnant woman without warning her. Similarly, a doctor would be justified in acting on knowledge that a patient planned to commit a crime. Confidentiality should, of course, be honored when the secret is entirely personal, that is, when it could have no substantial impact on anyone else. On the other hand, when it would pose a major threat to others, the claim of confidentiality must be overridden. Difficulties arise when the competing claims are nearly equal in moral weight.

In this scenario, does Consuela have any claims on the doctor? I believe she does, and that her claims are very compelling. They stem, first, from her right to have information she might consider relevant to her decision to act as her brother's nurse, and, second, from the health care system's obligation to warn of a possible risk to her health. I would like to focus first on whether Consuela has a right to information apart from the question of whether there is in fact an appreciable risk. I believe that she has such a right, for three reasons.

First, there is an element of deception in *not* informing Consuela that her brother is HIV-infected. Most people in her situation would want to know if their "patient" were HIV-infected and would presume that they would be told if that were the case. (I suspect that a private nurse hired in a similar situation would expect to be told—and that she would be.) At some level, perhaps unconsciously, Consuela would assume that Carlos did not have HIV infection because no one said that he did. Thus, in keeping Carlos's secret, the doctor implicitly deceives Consuela—not a net moral gain, I think.

Second, Consuela has been impressed to provide nursing care in part because the health system is using her to avoid providing a service it would otherwise be responsible for. This fact, I believe, gives the health care system an additional obligation to her, which includes giving her all the information that might bear on her decision to accept this responsibility. It might be argued that the information about her brother's HIV infection is not relevant, but it is patronizing to make this assumption. She may for any number of reasons, quite apart from the risk of transmission, find it important to know that he is HIV-infected.

Finally, I can't help feeling that this young woman has already been exploited by her family and that the health care system should not collude in doing so again. We are told that since she was twelve, she has acted as "mother" to a brother only one year younger, presumably simply because she is female, since she is no more a mother than he is. Now she is being asked to be a nurse, as well as a mother, again presumably because she is female. In this context, concerns about the sensibilities of the father or about Carlos's fear of them are not very compelling, particularly when they are buttressed by stereotypes about Hispanic families. Furthermore, both his father and his sister will almost certainly learn the truth eventually.

What about the risk of transmission from Carlos to Consuela? Many would—wrongly, I believe—base their arguments solely on this question. Insofar as they did, they would have very little to go on. The truth is that no one knows what the risk would be to Consuela. To my knowledge, there have been no studies that would yield data on the point. Most likely the risk would be extremely small, particularly if there were no blood or pus in the wound, but it would be speculative to say how small. We do know that Consuela has no experience with universal precautions and could not be expected to use them diligently with her brother unless she had some sense of why she might be doing so. In any case, the doctor has no right to decide for this young woman that she should assume a risk, even if he believes it would be remote. That is for her to decide. The only judgment he has a right to make is whether *she* might consider the information that her brother is HIV-infected to be relevant to her decision to nurse him, and I think it is reasonable to assume she might.

There is, I believe, only one ethical way out of this dilemma. The doctor should strongly encourage Carlos to tell his sister that he is HIV-infected or offer to do it for him. She could be asked not to tell their father, and I would see no problem with this. I would have no hesitation in appealing to the fact that Carlos already owes Consuela a great deal. If Carlos insisted that his sister not be told, the doctor should see to it that his nursing needs are met in some other way. In sum, then, I believe the doctor should pass the dilemma to the patient: Carlos can decide to accept Consuela's generosity—in return for which he must tell her he is HIV-infected (or ask the doctor to tell her)—or he can decide not to tell her and do without her nursing care.

THE VALUES UNDERLYING INFORMED CONSENT

President's Commission for the Study of Ethical Problems
in Medicine and Biomedical and Behavioral Research

The Commission identifies and discusses two values that should guide decision making in the health-care provider/patient relationship: the promotion of a patient's well-being and respect for a patient's self-determination. The Commission locates the ethical foundation of informed consent in the promotion of these two values and makes recommendations intended to ensure that these values are respected and enhanced. In making its recommendations, the Commission rejects the idea that obtaining informed consent is simply a matter of reciting the contents of a form and getting a signature. It sees ethically valid consent as a *process* of shared decision making based on mutual respect and participation. Although stressing the importance of self-determination, the commission recognizes that some people may be permanently incapable of making their own decisions and that others may be temporarily unable to exercise their right of self-determination. It, therefore, provides some recommendations about making decisions for those unable to do so.

What are the values that ought to guide decision-making in the provider-patient relationship or by which the success of a particular interaction can be judged? The Commission finds two to be central: promotion of a patient's well-being and respect for a patient's self-determination.

SERVING THE PATIENT'S WELL-BEING

Therapeutic interventions are intended first and foremost to improve a patient's health. In most circumstances, people agree in a general way on what "improved health" means. Restoration of normal functioning (such as the repair of a fractured limb) and avoidance of untimely death (such as might occur without the use of antibiotics to control life-threatening infections in otherwise healthy persons) are obvious examples. Health care is, in turn, usually a means of promoting patients' well-being. The connection between a particular health care decision and an individual's well-being is not perfect, however. First, the definition of health can be quite controversial: does wrinkled skin or uncommonly short stature constitute impaired health, such that surgical repair or growth hormone is appropriate? Even more substantial variation can be found in ranking the importance of health with other goals in an individual's life. For some, health is a paramount value; for others—citizens who volunteer in time of war, nurses who care for patients with contagious diseases, hang-glider enthusiasts who risk life and limb—a different goal sometimes has primacy.

Absence of Objective Medical Criteria Even the most mundane case—in which there is little if any disagreement that some intervention will promote health—may well have no objective medical criteria that specify a single best way to achieve the goal. A fractured limb can be repaired in a number of ways; a life-threatening infection can be treated with a variety of antibiotics; mild diabetes is subject to control by diet, by injectable natural insulin, or by oral synthetic insulin substitutes. Health care professionals often reflect their own value preferences when they favor one alternative over another; many are matters of choice, dictated neither by biomedical principles or data nor by a single, agreed-upon professional standard.

In the Commission's survey it was clear that professionals recognize this fact: physicians maintained that decisional authority between them and their patients should depend on the nature of the decision at hand. Thus, for example, whether a pregnant woman over 35 should have amniocentesis was viewed as largely a patient's decision, whereas the decision of which antibiotic to use for strep throat was seen as primarily up to the doctor. Furthermore, on the question of whether to continue aggressive treatment for a cancer patient with metastases in whom such treatment had already failed, two-thirds of the physicians felt it was not a scientific, medical decision, but one that turned principally on personal values. And the same proportion felt the decision should be made jointly (which 64% of the doctors claimed it usually was).

Patients' Reasonable Subjective Preferences Determining what constitutes health and how it is best promoted also requires knowledge of patients' subjective preferences. In pursuit of the other goals and interests besides health that society deems legitimate, patients may prefer one type of medical intervention to another, may opt for no treatment at all, or may even request some treatment when a practitioner would prefer to follow a more conservative course that involved, at least for the moment, no medical intervention. For example, a slipped disc may be treated surgically or with medications and bed rest. Which treatment is better can be unclear, even to a physician. A patient may prefer surgery because, despite its greater risks, in the past that individual has spent considerable time in bed and become demoralized and depressed. A person with an injured knee, when told that surgery has about a 30% chance of reducing pain but almost no chance of eliminating it entirely, may prefer to leave the condition untreated. And a baseball pitcher with persistent inflammation of the elbow may prefer to take cortisone on a continuing basis even though the doctor suggests that a new position on the team would eliminate the inflammation permanently. In each case the goals and interests of particular patients incline them in different directions not only as to how, but even as to whether, treatment should proceed.

Given these two considerations—the frequent absence of objective medical criteria and the legitimate subjective preferences of patients—ascertaining whether a health care intervention will, if successful, promote a patient's well-being is a matter of individual judgment. Societies that respect personal freedom usually reach such decisions by leaving the judgment to the person involved.

The Boundaries of Health Care This does not mean, however, that well-being and self-determination are really just two terms for the same value. For example, when an individual (such as a newborn baby) is unable to express a choice, the value that guides health care decisionmaking is the promotion of well-being—not necessarily an easy task but also certainly not merely a disguised form of self-determination.

Moreover, the promotion of well-being is an important value even in decisions about patients who can speak for themselves because the boundaries of the interventions that health professionals present for consideration are set by the concept of well-being. Through societal expectations and the traditions of the professions, health care providers are committed to helping patients and to avoiding harm. Thus, the well-being principle circumscribes the range of alternatives offered to patients: informed consent does not mean that patients can insist upon anything they might want. Rather, it is a choice among medically accepted and available options, all of which are believed to have some possibility of promoting the patient's welfare, including always the option of no further medical interventions, even when that would not be viewed as preferable by the health care providers.

In sum, promotion of patient well-being provides the primary warrant for health care. But, as indicated, well-being is not a concrete concept that has a single definition or that is solely within the competency of health care providers to define. Shared decisionmaking requires that a practitioner seek not only to understand each patient's needs and develop reasonable alternatives to meet those needs but also to present the alternatives in a way that enables patients to choose one they prefer. To participate in this process, patients must engage in a dialogue with the practitioner and make their views on well-being clear. The majority of physicians (56%) and the public (64%) surveyed by the Commission felt that increasing the patient's role in medical decision-making would improve the quality of health care.[1]

Since well-being can be defined only within each individual's experience, it is in most circumstances congruent to self-determination, to which the Report now turns.

RESPECTING SELF-DETERMINATION

Self-determination (sometimes termed "autonomy") is an individual's exercise of the capacity to form, revise, and pursue personal plans for life. Although it clearly has a much broader application, the relevance of self-determination in health care decisions seems undeniable. A basic reason to honor an individual's choices about health care has already emerged in this Report: under most circumstances the outcome that will best promote the person's well-being rests on a subjective judgment about the individual. This can be termed the instrumental value of self-determination.

More is involved in respect for self-determination than just the belief that each person knows what's best for him- or herself, however. Even if it could be shown that an expert (or a computer) could do the job better, the worth of the individual, as acknowledged in Western ethical traditions and especially in Anglo-American law, provides an independent—and more important—ground for recognizing self-determination as a basic principle in human relations, particularly when matters as important as those raised by health care are at stake. This noninstrumental aspect can be termed the intrinsic value of self-determination.

Intrinsic Value of Self-Determination The value of self-determination readily emerges if one considers what is lost in its absence. If a physician selects a treatment alternative that satisfies a patient's individual values and goals rather than allowing the patient to choose, the absence of self-determination has not interfered with the promotion of the patient's well-being. But unless the patient has requested this course of conduct, the individual will not have been shown proper respect as a person nor provided with adequate protection against arbitrary, albeit often well-meaning, domination by others. Self-determination can thus be seen as both a shield and a sword.

Freedom from Interference Self-determination as a shield is valued for the freedom from outside control it is intended to provide. It manifests the wish to be an instrument of one's own and "not of other men's acts of will."[2] In the context of health care, self-determination overrides practitioner-determination even if providers were able to demonstrate that they could (generally or in a specific instance) accurately assess the treatment an informed patient would choose. To permit action on the basis of a professional's assessment rather than on a patient's choice would deprive the patient of the freedom not to be forced to do something—whether or not that person would agree with the choice. Moreover, denying self-determination in this way risks generating the frustration people feel when their desires are ignored or countermanded. . . .

SUMMARY OF CONCLUSIONS AND RECOMMENDATIONS

. . . The ethical foundation of informed consent can be traced to the promotion of two values: personal well-being and self-determination. To ensure that these values are respected and enhanced, the Commission finds that patients who have the capacity to make decisions about their care must be permitted to do so voluntarily and must have all relevant information regarding their condition and alternative treatments, including possible benefits, risks, costs, other consequences, and significant uncertainties surrounding any of this information. This conclusion has several specific implications:

1. Although the informed consent doctrine has substantial foundations in law, it is essentially an ethical imperative.

2. Ethically valid consent is a process of shared decisionmaking based upon mutual respect and participation, not a ritual to be equated with reciting the contents of a form that details the risks of particular treatments.

3. Much of the scholarly literature and legal commentary about informed consent portrays it as a highly rational means of decisionmaking about health care matters, thereby suggesting that it may only be suitable for and applicable to well-educated,

articulate, self-aware individuals. Whether this is what the legal doctrine was intended to be or what it has inadvertently become, it is a view the Commission unequivocally rejects. Although subcultures within American society differ in their views about autonomy and individual choice and about the etiology of illness and the roles of healers and patients,[3] a survey conducted for the Commission found a universal desire for information, choice, and respectful communication about decisions.[4] Informed consent must remain flexible, yet the process, as the Commission envisions it throughout this Report, is ethically required of health care practitioners in their relationships with all patients, not a luxury for a few.

4. Informed consent is rooted in the fundamental recognition—reflected in the legal presumption of competency—that adults are entitled to accept or reject health care interventions on the basis of their own personal values and in furtherance of their own personal goals. Nonetheless, patient choice is not absolute.

- Patients are not entitled to insist that health care practitioners furnish them services when to do so would violate either the bounds of acceptable practice or a professional's own deeply held moral beliefs or would draw on a limited resource on which the patient has no binding claim.

- The fundamental values that informed consent is intended to promote—self-determination and patient well-being—both demand that alternative arrangements for health care decisionmaking be made for individuals who lack substantial capacity to make their own decisions. Respect for self-determination requires, however, that in the first instance individuals be deemed to have decisional capacity, which should not be treated as a hurdle to be surmounted in the vast majority of cases, and that incapacity be treated as a disqualifying factor in the small minority of cases.

- Decisionmaking capacity is specific to each particular decision. Although some people lack this capacity for all decisions, many are incapacitated in more limited ways and are capable of making some decisions but not others. The concept of capacity is best understood and applied in a functional manner. That is, the presence or absence of capacity does not depend on a person's status or on the decision reached, but on that individual's actual functioning in situations in which a decision about health care is to be made.

- Decisionmaking incapacity should be found to exist only when people lack the ability to make decisions that promote their well-being in conformity with their own previously expressed values and preferences.

- To the extent feasible people with no decisionmaking capacity should still be consulted about their own preferences out of respect for them as individuals.

5. Health care providers should not ordinarily withhold unpleasant information simply because it is unpleasant. The ethical foundations of informed consent allow the withholding of information from patients only when they request that it be withheld or when its disclosure per se would cause substantial detriment to their well-being. Furthermore, the Commission found that most members of the public do not wish to have "bad news" withheld from them.

6. Achieving the Commission's vision of shared decisionmaking based on mutual respect is ultimately the responsibility of individual health care professionals. However, health care institutions such as hospitals and professional schools have important roles to play in assisting health care professionals in this obligation. The manner in which health care is provided in institutional settings often results in a fragmentation of responsibility that may neglect the human side of health care. To assist in

guarding against this, institutional health care providers should ensure that ultimately there is one readily identifiable practitioner responsible for providing information to a particular patient. Although pieces of information may be provided by various people, there should be one individual officially charged with responsibility for ensuring that all the necessary information is communicated and that the patient's wishes are known to the treatment team.

7. Patients should have access to the information they need to help them understand their conditions and make treatment decisions. To this end the Commission recommends that health care professionals and institutions not only provide information but also assist patients who request additional information to obtain it from relevant sources, including hospital and public libraries.

8. As cases arise and new legislation is contemplated, courts and legislatures should reflect this view of ethically valid consent. Nevertheless, the Commission does not look to legal reforms as the primary means of bringing about changes in the relationship between health care professionals and patients.

9. The Commission finds that a number of relatively simple changes in practice could facilitate patient participation in health care decisionmaking. Several specific techniques—such as having patients express, orally or in writing, their understanding of the treatment consented to—deserve further study. Furthermore, additional societal resources need to be committed to improving the human side of health care, which has apparently deteriorated at the same time there have been substantial gains in health care technology. The Department of Health and Human Services, and especially the National Institutes of Health, is an appropriate agency for the development of initiatives and the evaluation of their efficacy in this area.

10. Because health care professionals are responsible for ensuring that patients can participate effectively in decisionmaking regarding their care, educators have a responsibility to prepare physicians and nurses to carry out this obligation. The Commission therefore concludes that:

- Curricular innovations aimed at preparing health professionals for a process of mutual decisionmaking with patients should be continued and strengthened, with careful attention being paid to the development of methods for evaluating the effectiveness of such innovations.

- Examinations and evaluations at the professional school and national levels should reflect the importance of these issues.

- Serious attention should be paid to preparing health professionals for team practice in order to enhance patient participation and well-being.

11. Family members are often of great assistance to patients in helping to understand information about their condition and in making decisions about treatment. The Commission recommends that health care institutions and professionals recognize this and judiciously attempt to involve family members in decisionmaking for patients, with due regard for the privacy of patients and for the possibilities for coercion that such a practice may entail.

12. The Commission recognizes that its vision of health care decisionmaking may involve greater commitments of time on the part of health professionals. Because of the importance of shared decisionmaking based on mutual trust, not only for the promotion of patient well-being and self-determination but also for the therapeutic gains that can be realized, the Commission recommends that all medical and surgical interventions be thought of as including appropriate discussion with patients. Reimbursement to the professional should

therefore take account of time spent in discussion rather than regarding it as a separate item for which additional payment is made.

13. To protect the interests of patients who lack decisionmaking capacity and to ensure their well-being and self-determination, the Commission concludes that:

- Decisions made by others on patients' behalf should, when possible, attempt to replicate the ones patients would make if they were capable of doing so. When this is not feasible, decisions by surrogates on behalf of patients must protect the patients' best interests. Because such decisions are not instances of personal self-choice, limits may be placed on the range of acceptable decisions that surrogates make beyond those that apply when a person makes his or her own decisions.

- Health care institutions should adopt clear and explicit policies regarding how and by whom decisions are to be made for patients who cannot decide.

- Families, health care institutions, and professionals should work together to make health care decisions for patients who lack decisionmaking capacity. Recourse to courts should be reserved for the occasions when concerned parties are unable to resolve their disagreements over matters of substantial import, or when adjudication is clearly required by state law. Courts and legislatures should be cautious about requiring judicial review of routine health care decisions for patients who lack capacity.

- Health care institutions should explore and evaluate various informal administrative arrangements, such as "ethics committees," for review and consultation in nonroutine matters involving health care decisionmaking for those who cannot decide.

- As a means of preserving some self-determination for patients who no longer possess decisionmaking capacity, state courts and legislatures should consider making provision for advance directives through which people designate others to make health care decisions on their behalf and/or give instructions about their care.

The Commission acknowledges that the conclusions contained in this Report will not be simple to achieve. Even when patients and practitioners alike are sensitive to the goal of shared decisionmaking based on mutual respect, substantial barriers will still exist. Some of these obstacles, such as long-standing professional attitudes or difficulties in conveying medical information in ordinary language, are formidable but can be overcome if there is a will to do so. Others, such as the dependent condition of very sick patients or the ever-growing complexity and subspecialization of medicine, will have to be accommodated because they probably cannot be eliminated. Nonetheless, the Commission's vision of informed consent still has value as a measuring stick against which actual performance may be judged and as a goal toward which all participants in health care decisionmaking can strive. . . .

NOTES

1 Many physicians and patients said they believed an increased patient role would give the patient a better understanding of the medical condition and treatment, would improve physician performance in terms of the honesty and scope of discussion, and would generally improve the doctor-patient relationship. However, a number of physicians claimed that greater patient involvement would improve the quality of care because it would improve compliance and would make patients more cooperative and willing to accept the doctor's judgment.

2 Isaiah Berlin, "Two Concepts of Liberty," in *Four Essays on Liberty*, Clarendon Press, Oxford (1969) at 118–38.

3 Robert A. Hahn, *Culture and Informed Consent: An Anthropological Perspective* (1982), Appendix F, in Volume Three of this Report.

4 The Commission's survey of the public broke down these responses on the basis of variables such as age, gender, race, education, and income.

TRANSPARENCY: INFORMED CONSENT IN PRIMARY CARE
Howard Brody

Brody argues that accepted legal standards of informed consent, as commonly employed by the courts, give physicians the unhelpful message that informed consent is essentially a legalistic exercise intruding upon good medical care—an impression especially likely in the context of primary-care medicine. An alternative that would send physicians the right message, a "conversation" standard, is probably not legally workable, according to the author. Brody contends that a compromise, the "transparency" standard, sets reasonable obligations for physicians and permits courts to review appropriately. According to this standard, disclosure is considered adequate when the physician's basic thinking has been made transparent to the patient.

While the patient's right to give informed consent to medical treatment is now well-established both in U.S. law and in biomedical ethics, evidence continues to suggest that the concept has been poorly integrated into American medical practice, and that in many instances the needs and desires of patients are not being well met by current policies.[1] It appears that the theory and the practice of informed consent are out of joint in some crucial ways. This is particularly true for primary care settings, a context typically ignored by medical ethics literature, but where the majority of doctor-patient encounters occur. Indeed, some have suggested that the concept of informed consent is virtually foreign to primary care medicine where benign paternalism appropriately reigns and where respect for patient autonomy is almost completely absent.[2]

It is worth asking whether current legal standards for informed consent tend to resolve the problem or to exacerbate it. I will maintain that accepted legal standards, at least in the form commonly employed by courts, send physicians the wrong message about what is expected of them. An alternative standard that would send physicians the correct message, a conversation standard, is probably unworkable legally. As an alternative, I will propose a transparency standard as a compromise that gives physicians a doable task and allows courts to review

appropriately. I must begin, however, by briefly identifying some assumptions crucial to the development of this position even though space precludes complete argumentation and documentation.

CRUCIAL ASSUMPTIONS

Informed consent is a meaningful ethical concept only to the extent that it can be realized and promoted within the ongoing practice of good medicine. This need not imply diminished respect for patient autonomy, for there are excellent reasons to regard respect for patient autonomy as a central feature of good medical care. Informed consent, properly understood, must be considered an essential ingredient of good patient care, and a physician who lacks the skills to inform patients appropriately and obtain proper consent should be viewed as lacking essential medical skills necessary for practice. It is not enough to see informed consent as a nonmedical, legalistic exercise designed to promote patient autonomy, one that interrupts the process of medical care.

However, available empirical evidence strongly suggests that this is precisely how physicians currently view informed consent practices. Informed consent is still seen as bureaucratic legalism rather than as part of patient care. Physicians often deny the existence of realistic treatment alternatives, thereby attenuating the perceived need to inform the patient of meaningful options. While patients may be informed, efforts are seldom made to assess accurately the patient's actual need or desire for information, or what the patient then proceeds to do with

Reprinted with permission of the author and the publisher from *Hastings Center Report*, vol. 19 (September–October 1989), pp. 5–9. © The Hastings Center.

the information provided. Physicians typically under-estimate patients' desire to be informed and overestimate their desire to be involved in decision-making. Physicians may also view informed consent as an empty charade, since they are confident in their abilities to manipulate consent by how they discuss or divulge information.[3]

A third assumption is that there are important differences between the practice of primary care medicine and the tertiary care settings that have been most frequently discussed in the literature on informed consent. The models of informed consent discussed below typically take as the paradigm case something like surgery for breast cancer or the performance of an invasive and risky radiologic procedure. It is assumed that the risks to the patient are significant, and the values placed on alternative forms of treatment are quite weighty. Moreover, it is assumed that the specialist physician performing the procedure probably does a fairly limited number of procedures and thus could be expected to know exhaustively the precise risks, benefits, and alternatives for each.

Primary care medicine, however, fails to fit this model. The primary care physician, instead of performing five or six complicated and risky procedures frequently, may engage in several hundred treatment modalities during an average week of practice. In many cases, risks to the patient are negligible and conflicts over patient values and the goals of treatment or non-treatment are of little consequence. Moreover, in contrast to the tertiary care patient, the typical ambulatory patient is much better able to exercise freedom of choice and somewhat less likely to be intimidated by either the severity of the disease or the expertise of the physician; the opportunities for changing one's mind once treatment has begun are also much greater. Indeed, in primary care, it is much more likely for the full process of informed consent to treatment (such as the beginning and the dose adjustment of an anti-hypertensive medication) to occur over several office visits rather than at one single point in time.

It might be argued that for all these reasons, the stakes are so low in primary care that it is fully appropriate for informed consent to be interpreted only with regard to the specialized or tertiary care setting.

I believe that this is quite incorrect for three reasons. First, good primary care medicine ought to embrace respect for patient autonomy, and if patient autonomy is operationalized in informed consent, properly understood, then it ought to be part and parcel of good primary care. Second, the claim that the primary care physician cannot be expected to obtain the patient's informed consent seems to undermine the idea that informed consent could or ought to be part of the daily practice of medicine. Third, primary care encounters are statistically more common than the highly specialized encounters previously used as models for the concept of informed consent.[4]

ACCEPTED LEGAL STANDARDS

Most of the literature on legal approaches to informed consent addresses the tension between the community practice standard and the reasonable patient standard, with the latter seen as the more satisfactory, emerging legal standard.[5] However, neither standard sends the proper message to the physician about what is expected of her to promote patient autonomy effectively and to serve the informational needs of patients in daily practice.

The community practice standard sends the wrong message because it leaves the door open too wide for physician paternalism. The physician is instructed to behave as other physicians in that specialty behave, regardless of how well or how poorly that behavior serves patients' needs. Certainly, behaving the way other physicians behave is a task we might expect physicians to readily accomplish; unfortunately, the standard fails to inform them of the end toward which the task is aimed.

The reasonable patient standard does a much better job of indicating the centrality of respect for patient autonomy and the desired outcome of the informed consent process, which is revealing the information that a reasonable person would need to make an informed and rational decision. This standard is particularly valuable when modified to include the specific informational and decisional needs of a particular patient.

If certain things were true about the relationship between medicine and law in today's society, the reasonable patient standard would provide acceptable guidance to physicians. One feature would be that physicians esteem the law as a positive force in guiding their practice, rather than as a threat to their well-being that must be handled defensively. Another element would be a prospective consideration by the law of what the physician could reasonably have been expected to do in practice, rather than a retrospective review armed with the foreknowledge that some significant patient harm has already occurred.

Unfortunately, given the present legal climate, the physician is much more likely to get a mixed or an undesirable message from the reasonable patient standard. The message the physician hears from the reasonable patient standard is that one must exhaustively lay out all possible risks as well as benefits and alternatives of the proposed procedure. If one remembers to discuss fifty possible risks, and the patient in a particular case suffers the fifty-first, the physician might subsequently be found liable for incomplete disclosure. Since lawsuits are triggered when patients suffer harm, disclosure of risk becomes relatively more important than disclosure of benefits. Moreover, disclosure of information becomes much more critical than effective patient participation in decision making. Physicians consider it more important to document what they said to the patient than to document how the patient used or thought about that information subsequently.

In specialty practice, many of these concerns can be nicely met by detailed written or videotaped consent documents, which can provide the depth of information required while still putting the benefits and alternatives in proper context. This is workable when one engages in a limited number of procedures and can have a complete document or videotape for each.[6] However, this approach is not feasible for primary care, when the number of procedures may be much more numerous and the time available with each patient may be considerably less. Moreover, it is simply not realistic to expect even the best educated of primary care physicians to rattle off at a moment's notice a detailed list of significant risks attached to any of the many drugs and therapeutic modalities they recommend.

This sets informed consent apart from all other aspects of medical practice in a way that I believe is widely perceived by nonpaternalistic primary care physicians, but which is almost never commented upon in the medical ethics literature. To the physician obtaining informed consent, *you never know when you are finished.* When a primary care physician is told to treat a patient for strep throat or to counsel a person suffering a normal grief reaction from the recent death of a relative, the physician has a good sense of what it means to complete the task at hand. When a physician is told to obtain the patient's informed consent for a medical intervention, the impression is quite different. A list of as many possible risks as can be thought of may still omit some significant ones. A list of all the risks that actually have occurred may still not have dealt with the patient's need to know risks in relation to benefits and alternatives. A description of all benefits, risks, and alternatives may not establish whether the patient has understood the information. If the patient says he understands, the physician has to wonder whether he really understands or whether he is simply saying this to be accommodating. As the law currently *appears* to operate (in the perception of the defensively minded physician), there never comes a point at which you can be certain that you have adequately completed your legal as well as your ethical task.

The point is not simply that physicians are paranoid about the law; more fundamentally, physicians are getting a message that informed consent is very different from any other task they are asked to perform in medicine. If physicians conclude that informed consent is therefore not properly part of medicine at all, but is rather a legalistic and bureaucratic hurdle they must overcome at their own peril, blame cannot be attributed to paternalistic attitudes or lack of respect for patient autonomy.

THE CONVERSATION MODEL

A metaphor employed by Jay Katz, informed consent as conversation, provides an approach to respect for patient autonomy that can be readily integrated within primary care practice.[7] Just as the specific needs of an individual patient for information, or the meaning that patient will attach to the information as it is presented, cannot be known in advance, one cannot always tell in advance how a conversation is going to turn out. One must follow the process along and take one's cues from the unfolding conversation itself. Despite the absence of any formal rules for carrying out or completing a conversation on a specific subject, most people have a good intuitive grasp of what it means for a conversation to be finished, what it means to change the subject in the middle of a conversation, and what it means to later reopen a conversation one had thought was completed when something new has just arisen. Thus, the metaphor suggests that informed consent consists not in a formal process carried out strictly by protocol but in a conversation designed to encourage patient participation in all medical decisions to the extent that the patient wishes to be included. The idea of informed consent as physician-patient conversation could, when properly developed, be a useful analytic tool for ethical issues in informed consent, and could also be a powerful educational tool for highlighting the skills and attitudes that a physician needs to successfully integrate this process within patient care.

If primary care physicians understand informed consent as this sort of conversation process, the idea that exact rules cannot be given for its successful management could cease to be a mystery. Physicians would instead be guided to rely on their own intuitions and communication skills, with careful attention to information received from the patient, to determine when an adequate job had been done in the informed consent process. Moreover, physicians would be encouraged to see informed consent as a genuinely mutual and participatory process, instead of being reduced to the one-way disclosure of information. In effect, informed consent could be demystified, and located within the context of the everyday relationships between physician and patient, albeit with a renewed emphasis on patient participation.[8]

Unfortunately, the conversation metaphor does not lend itself to ready translation into a legal standard for determining whether or not the physician has satisfied her basic responsibilities to the patient. There seems to be an inherently subjective element to conversation that makes it ill-suited as a legal standard for review of controversial cases. A conversation in which one participates is by its nature a very different thing from the same conversation described to an outsider. It is hard to imagine how a jury could be instructed to determine in retrospect whether or not a particular conversation was adequate for its purposes. However, without the possibility for legal review, the message that patient autonomy is an important value and that patients have important rights within primary care would seem to be severely undermined. The question then is whether some of the important strengths of the conversation model can be retained in another model that does allow better guidance.

THE TRANSPARENCY STANDARD

I propose the transparency standard as a means to operationalize the best features of the conversation model in medical practice. According to this standard, adequate informed consent is obtained when a reasonably informed patient is allowed to participate in the medical decision to the extent that patient wishes. In turn, "reasonably informed" consists of two features: (1) the physician discloses the basis on which the proposed treatment, or alternative possible treatments, have been chosen; and (2) the patient is allowed to ask questions suggested by the disclosure of the physician's reasoning, and those questions are answered to the patient's satisfaction.

According to the transparency model, the key to reasonable disclosure is not adherence to existing standards of other practitioners, nor is it adherence to a list of risks that a hypothetical reasonable patient would want to know. Instead, disclosure is adequate when the physician's basic thinking has been rendered transparent to the patient. If the physician arrives at a recommended therapeutic or diagnostic intervention only after carefully examining a list of risks and benefits, then rendering the physician's thinking transparent requires that those risks and benefits be detailed for the patient. If the physician's thinking has not followed that route but has reached its conclusion by other considerations, then what needs to be disclosed to the patient is accordingly different. Essentially, the transparency standard requires the physician to engage in the typical patient-management thought process, only to *do it out loud in language understandable to the patient.*[9]

To see how this might work in practice, consider the following as possible general decision-making strategies that might be used by a primary physician:

1. The intervention, in addition to being presumably low-risk, is also routine and automatic. The physician, faced with a case like that presented by the patient, almost always chooses this treatment.

2. The decision is not routine but seems to offer clear benefit with minimal risk.

3. The proposed procedure offers substantial chances for benefit, but also very substantial risks.

4. The proposed intervention offers substantial risks and extremely questionable benefits. Unfortunately, possible alternative courses of action also have high risk and uncertain benefit.

The exact risks entailed by treatment loom much larger in the physician's own thinking in cases 3 and 4 than in cases 1 and 2. The transparency standard would require that physicians at least mention the various risks to patients in scenarios 3 and 4, but would not necessarily require physicians exhaustively to describe risks, unless the patient asked, in scenarios 1 and 2.

The transparency standard seems to offer some considerable advantages for informing physicians what can legitimately be expected of them in the promotion of patient autonomy while carrying out the activities of primary care medicine. We would hope that the well-trained primary care physician generally thinks before acting. On that assumption, the physician can be told exactly when she is finished obtaining informed consent—first, she has to share her thinking with the patient; secondly, she has to encourage and answer questions; and third, she has to discover how participatory he wishes to be and facilitate that level of participation. This seems a much more reasonable task within primary care than an exhaustive listing of often irrelevant risk factors.

There are also considerable advantages for the patient in this approach. The patient retains the right to ask for an exhaustive recital of risks and alternatives. However, the vast majority of patients, in a primary care setting particularly, would wish to supplement a standardized recital of risks and benefits of treatment with some questions like, "Yes, doctor, but what does this really mean for me? What meaning am I supposed to attach to the information that you've just given?" For example, in scenarios 1 and 2, the precise and specific risk probabilities and possibilities are very small considerations in the thinking of the physician, and reciting an exhaustive list of risks would seriously misstate just what the physician was thinking. If the physician did detail a laundry list of risk factors, the patient might very well ask, "Well, doctor, just what should I think about what you have just told me?" and the thoughtful and concerned physician might well reply, "There's certainly a small possibility that one of these bad things will happen to you; but I think the chance is extremely remote and in my own practice I have never seen anything like that occur." The patient is very likely to give much more weight to that statement, putting the risks in perspective, than he is to the listing of risks. And that emphasis corresponds with an understanding of how the physician herself has reached the decision.

The transparency standard should further facilitate and encourage useful questions from patients. If a patient is given a routine list of risks and benefits and then is asked "Do you have any questions?" the response may well be perfunctory and automatic. If the patient is told precisely the grounds on which the physician has made her recommendation, and then asked the same question, the response is much more likely to be individualized and meaningful.

There certainly would be problems in applying the transparency standard in the courtroom, but these do not appear to be materially more difficult than those encountered in applying other standards; moreover, this standard could call attention to more important features in the ethical relationship between physician and patient. Consider the fairly typical case, in which a patient suffers harm from the occurrence of a rare but predictable complication of a procedure, and then claims that he would not have consented had he known about that risk. Under the present "enlightened" court standards, the jury would examine whether a reasonable patient would have needed to know about that risk factor prior to making a decision on the proposed intervention. Under the transparency standard, the question would instead be whether the physician thought about that risk factor as a relevant consideration prior to recommending the course of action to the patient. If the physician did seriously consider that risk factor, but failed to reveal that to the patient, he was in effect making up the patient's mind in advance about what risks were worth accepting. In that situation, the physician could easily be held liable. If, on the other hand, that risk was considered too insignificant to play a role in determining which intervention ought to be performed, the physician may still have rendered his thinking completely transparent to the patient even though that specific risk factor was not mentioned. In this circumstance, the physician would be held to have done an adequate job of disclosing information.[10] A question would still exist as to whether a competent physician ought to have known about that risk factor and ought to have considered it more carefully prior to doing the procedure. But that question raises the issue of negligence, which is where such considerations properly belong, and removes the problem from the context of informed consent. Obviously, the standard of informed consent is misapplied if it is intended by itself to prevent the practice of negligent medicine.

TRANSPARENCY IN MEDICAL PRACTICE

Will adopting a legal standard like transparency change medical practice for the better? Ultimately only empirical research will answer this question. We know almost nothing about the sorts of conversations primary care physicians now have with their patients, or what would happen if these physicians routinely tried harder to share their basic thinking about therapeutic choices. In this setting it is possible to argue that the transparency standard will have deleterious effects. Perhaps the physician's basic thinking will fail to include risk issues that patients, from their perspective, would regard as substantial. Perhaps how physicians think about therapeutic choice will prove to be too idiosyncratic and variable to serve as any sort of standard. Perhaps disclosing basic thinking processes will impede rather than promote optimal patient participation in decisions.

But the transparency standard must be judged, not only against ideal medical practice, but also against the present-day standard and the message it sends to practitioners. I have argued that that message is, "You can protect yourself legally only by guessing all bad outcomes that might occur and warning each patient explicitly that he might suffer any of them." The transparency standard is an attempt to send the message, "You can protect yourself legally by conversing with your patients in a way that promotes their participation in medical decisions, and more specifically by making sure that they see the basic reasoning you used to arrive at the recommended treatment." It seems at least plausible to me that the attempt is worth making.

The reasonable person standard may still be the best way to view informed consent in highly specialized settings where a relatively small number of discrete and potentially risky procedures are the daily order of business. In primary care settings, the best ethical advice we can give physicians is to view informed consent as an ongoing process of conversation designed to maximize patient participation after adequately revealing the key facts. Because the conversation metaphor does not by itself suggest measures for later judicial review, a transparency standard, or something like it, may be a reasonable way to operationalize that concept in primary care practice. Some positive side-effects of this might be more focus on good diagnostic and therapeutic decision-making on the physician's part, since it will be understood that the patient will be made aware of what the physician's reasoning process has been like, and better documentation of management decisions in the patient record. If these occur, then it will be clearer that the standard of informed consent has promoted rather than impeded high quality patient care.

ACKNOWLEDGMENTS

I plan to develop these ideas at somewhat greater length, with special emphasis on the duty to disclose remote risks, in a volume to be titled *The Healer's Power* (in preparation). I am grateful to Margaret Wallace and Stephen Wear for their insightful comments during the preparation of this manuscript.

REFERENCES

1 Charles W. Lidz *et al.*, "Barriers to Informed Consent," *Annals of Internal Medicine* 99:4 (1983), 539–43.

2 Tom L. Beauchamp and Laurence McCullough, *Medical Ethics: The Moral Responsibilities of Physicians* (Englewood Cliffs, NJ: Prentice-Hall, 1984).

3 For a concise overview of empirical data about contemporary informed consent practices, see Ruth R. Faden and Tom L. Beauchamp, *A History and Theory of Informed Consent* (New York: Oxford University Press, 1986), 98–99 and associated footnotes.

4 For efforts to address ethical aspects of primary care practice, see Ronald J. Christie and Barry Hoffmaster, *Ethical Issues in Family Medicine* (New York: Oxford University Press, 1986); and Harmon L. Smith and Larry R. Churchill, *Professional Ethics and Primary Care Medicine* (Durham, NC: Duke University Press, 1986).

5 Faden and Beauchamp, *A History and Theory of Informed Consent,* 23–49 and 114–50. I have also greatly benefited from an unpublished paper by Margaret Wallace.

6 For a specialty opinion to the contrary, see W. H. Coles *et al.*, "Teaching Informed Consent," in *Further Developments in Assessing Clinical Competence,* Ian R. Hart and Ronald M. Harden, eds. (Montreal: Can-Heal Publications, 1987), 241–70. This paper is interesting in applying to specialty care a model very much like the one I propose for primary care.

7 Jay Katz, *The Silent World of Doctor and Patient* (New York: Free Press, 1984).

8 Howard Brody, *Stories of Sickness* (New Haven: Yale University Press, 1987), 171–81.

9 For an interesting study of physicians' practices on this point, see William C. Wu and Robert A. Pearlman, "Consent in Medical Decisionmaking: The Role of Communication," *Journal of General Internal Medicine* 3:1 (1988), 9–14.

10 A court case that might point the way toward this line of reasoning is *Precourt v. Frederick,* 395 Mass. 689 (1985). See William J. Curran, "Informed Consent in Malpractice Cases: A Turn Toward Reality," *New England Journal of Medicine* 314:7 (1986), 429–31.

THE PRACTICE OF MEDICINE IN A MULTICULTURAL SOCIETY

ETHICAL RELATIVISM IN A MULTICULTURAL SOCIETY
Ruth Macklin

Macklin explores ethical problems that sometimes arise when a physician and a patient come from different cultural backgrounds. Respect for cultural diversity requires physicians to be generally tolerant or respectful of patients' differing beliefs and practices, according to Macklin. But in some cases tolerance can lead to harm of patients or their family members, while in other cases tolerance apparently conflicts with what mainstream Western ethics regards as the autonomy-based rights of the patient (e.g., the right to disclosure of medical information). In analyzing these ethical problems, Macklin attempts to determine which of the values involved are culturally relative and which are based on universal ethical principles.

Cultural pluralism poses a challenge to physicians and patients alike in the multicultural United States, where immigrants from many nations and diverse religious groups visit the same hospitals and doctors. Multiculturalism is defined as "a social-intellectual movement that promotes the value of diversity as a core principle and insists that all cultural groups be treated with respect and as equals" (Fowers and Richardson 1996, p. 609). This sounds like a value

that few enlightened people could fault, but it produces dilemmas and leads to results that are, at the least, problematic if not counterintuitive.

Critics of mainstream bioethics within the United States and abroad have complained about the narrow focus on autonomy and individual rights. Such critics argue that much—if not most—of the world embraces a value system that places the family, the community, or the society as a whole above that of the individual person. The prominent American sociologist Renée Fox is a prime example of such critics: "From the outset, the conceptual framework of bioethics has accorded paramount status to the value-complex of individualism, underscoring the principles of individual rights, autonomy, self-determination, and their legal expression in the jurisprudential notion of privacy" (Fox 1990, p. 206).

The emphasis on autonomy, at least in the early days of bioethics in the United States, was never intended to cut patients off from their families by focusing monistically on the patient. Instead, the intent was to counteract the predominant and longstanding paternalism on the part of the medical profession. In fact, there was little discussion of where the family entered in and no presumption that a family-centered approach to sick patients was somehow a violation of the patient's autonomy. Most patients want and need the support of their families, regardless of whether they seek to be autonomous agents regarding their own care. Respect for autonomy is perfectly consistent with recognition of the important role that families play when a loved one is ill. Autonomy has fallen into such disfavor among some bioethicists that the pendulum has begun to swing in the direction of families, with urgings to "take families seriously" (Nelson 1992) and even to consider the interests of family members equal to those of the competent patient (Hardwig 1990). . . .

A circumstance that arises frequently in multicultural urban settings is one that medical students bring to ethics teaching conferences. The patient and family are recent immigrants from a culture in which physicians normally inform the family rather than the patient of a diagnosis of cancer. The medical students wonder whether they are obligated to follow the family's wish, thereby respecting their cultural custom, or whether to abide by the ethical requirement at least to explore with patients their desire to receive information and to be a participant in their medical care. When medical students presented such a case in one of the conferences I co-direct with a physician, the dilemma was heightened by the demographic picture of the medical students themselves. Among the 14 students, 11 different countries of origin were represented. Those students either had come to the United States themselves to study or their parents had immigrated from countries in Asia, Latin America, Europe, and the Middle East.

The students began their comments with remarks like, "Where I come from, doctors never tell the patient a diagnosis of cancer" or "In my country, the doctor always asks the patient's family and abides by their wishes." The discussion centered on the question of whether the physician's obligation is to act in accordance with what contemporary medical ethics dictates in the United States or to respect the cultural difference of their patients and act according to the family's wishes. Not surprisingly, the medical students were divided on the answer to this question.

Medical students and residents are understandably confused about their obligation to disclose information to a patient when the patient comes from a culture in which telling a patient she has cancer is rare or unheard of. They ask: "Should I adhere to the American custom of disclosure or the Argentine custom of withholding the diagnosis?" That question is miscast, since there are some South Americans who want to know if they have cancer and some North Americans who do not. It is not, therefore, the cultural tradition that should determine whether disclosure to a patient is ethically appropriate, but rather the patient's wish to communicate directly with the physician, to leave communications to the family, or something in between. It would be a simplistic, if not unethical response on the part of doctors to reason that "This is the United States, we adhere to the tradition of patient autonomy, therefore I must disclose to this immigrant from the Dominican Republic that he has cancer."

Most patients in the United States do want to know their diagnosis and prognosis, and it has been amply demonstrated that they can emotionally and psychologically handle a diagnosis of cancer. The same may not be true, however, for recent immigrants from other countries, and it may be manifestly untrue in certain cultures. Although this, too, may change in time, several studies point to a cross-cultural difference in beliefs and practice regarding disclosure of diagnosis and informed consent to treatment.

One survey examined differences in the attitudes of elderly subjects from different ethnic groups toward disclosure of the diagnosis and prognosis of a terminal illness and regarding decision making at the end of life (Blackhall et al. 1995). This study found marked differences in attitudes between

Korean Americans and Mexican Americans, on the one hand, and African Americans and Americans of European descent, on the other. The Korean Americans and Mexican Americans were less likely than the other two groups to believe that patients should be told of a prognosis of terminal illness and also less likely to believe that the patient should make decisions about the use of life-support technology. The Korean and Mexican Americans surveyed were also more likely than the other groups to have a family-centered attitude toward these matters; they believed that the family and not the patient should be told the truth about the patient's diagnosis and prognosis. The authors of the study cite data from other countries that bear out a similar gap between the predominant "autonomy model" in the United States and the family-centered model prevalent in European countries as well as in Asia and Africa.

The study cited was conducted at 31 senior citizen centers in Los Angeles. In no ethnic group did 100 percent of its members favor disclosure or nondisclosure to the patient. Forty-seven percent of Korean Americans believed that a patient with metastatic cancer should be told the truth about the diagnosis, 65 percent of Mexican Americans held that belief, 87 percent of European Americans believed patients should be told the truth, and 89 percent of African Americans held that belief.

It is worth noting that the people surveyed were all 65-years-old or older. Not surprisingly, the Korean and Mexican American senior citizens had values closer to the cultures of their origin than did the African Americans and European Americans who were born in the United States. Another finding was that among the Korean American and Mexican American groups, older subjects and those with lower socioeconomic status tended to be opposed to truth telling and patient decision making more strongly than the younger, wealthier, and more highly educated members of these same groups. The authors of the study draw the conclusion that physicians should ask patients if they want to receive information and make decisions regarding treatment or whether they prefer that their families handle such matters.

Far from being at odds with the "autonomy model," this conclusion supports it. To ask patients

how much they wish to be involved in decision making does show respect for their autonomy: patients can then make the autonomous choice about who should be the recipient of information or the decision maker about their illness. What would fail to show respect for autonomy is for physicians to make these decisions without consulting the patient at all. If doctors spoke only to the families but not to the elderly Korean American or Mexican American patients without first approaching the patients to ascertain their wishes, they would be acting in the paternalistic manner of the past in America, and in accordance with the way many physicians continue to act in other parts of the world today. Furthermore, if physicians automatically withheld the diagnosis from Korean Americans because the majority of people in that ethnic group did not want to be told, they would be making an assumption that would result in a mistake almost 50 percent of the time.

INTOLERANCE AND OVERTOLERANCE

A medical resident in a New York hospital questioned a patient's ability to understand the medical treatment he had proposed and doubted whether the patient could grant truly informed consent. The patient, an immigrant from the Caribbean islands, believed in voodoo and sought to employ voodoo rituals in addition to the medical treatment she was receiving. "How can anyone who believes in that stuff be competent to consent to the treatment we offer?" the resident mused. The medical resident was an observant Jew who did not work, drive a car, or handle money on the sabbath and adhered to Kosher dietary laws. Both the Caribbean patient and the Orthodox Jew were devout believers in their respective faiths and practiced the accepted rituals of their religions.

The patient's voodoo rituals were not harmful to herself or to others. If the resident had tried to bypass or override the patient's decision regarding treatment, the case would have posed an ethical problem requiring resolution. Intolerance of another's religious or traditional practices that pose no threat of harm is, at least, discourteous and at worst, a prejudicial attitude. And it does fail to show respect for persons and their diverse religious and cultural practices. But it does not (yet) involve a failure to respect persons at a more fundamental level, which would occur if the doctor were to deny the patient her right to exercise her autonomy in the consent procedures.

At times, however, it is the family that interferes with the patient's autonomous decisions. Two brothers of a Haitian immigrant were conducting a conventional Catholic prayer vigil for their dying brother at his hospital bedside. The patient, suffering from terminal cancer and in extreme pain, had initially been given the pain medication he requested. Sometime later a nurse came in and found the patient alert, awake, and in excruciating pain from being undermedicated. When questioned, another nurse who had been responsible for the patient's care said that she had not continued to administer the pain medication because the patient's brothers had forbidden her to do so. Under the influence of the heavy dose of pain medication, the patient had become delirious and mumbled incoherently. The brothers took this as an indication that evil spirits had entered the patient's body and, according to the voodoo religion of their native culture, unless the spirit was exorcised it would stay with the family forever, and the entire family would suffer bad consequences. The patient manifested the signs of delirium only when he was on the medication, so the brothers asked the nurse to withhold the pain medication, which they believed was responsible for the entry of the evil spirit. The nurse sincerely believed that respect for the family's religion required her to comply with the patient's brothers' request, even if it contradicted the patient's own expressed wish. The person in charge of pain management called an ethics consultation, and the clinical ethicist said that the brothers' request, even if based on their traditional religious beliefs, could not override the patient's own request for pain medication that would relieve his suffering.

There are rarely good grounds for failing to respect the wishes of people based on their traditional religious or cultural beliefs. But when beliefs issue in actions that cause harm to others, attempts to prevent those harmful consequences are justifiable. An example that raises public health concerns is a ritual practiced among adherents of the religion known as Santería, practiced by people from Puerto Rico and other groups of Caribbean origin. The ritual involves scattering mercury around the household to ward off

bad spirits. Mercury is a highly toxic substance that can harm adults and causes grave harm to children. Shops called "botánicas" sell mercury as well as herbs and other potions to Caribbean immigrants who use them in their healing rituals.

The public health rationale that justifies placing limitations on people's behavior in order to protect others from harm can justify prohibition of the sale of mercury and penalties for its domestic use for ritual purposes. Yet the Caribbean immigrants could object: "You are interfering with our religious practices, based on your form of scientific medicine. This is our form of religious healing and you have no right to interfere with our beliefs and practices." It would not convince this group if a doctor or public health official were to reply: "But ours is a well-confirmed, scientific practice while yours is but an ignorant, unscientific ritual." It may very well appear to the Caribbean group as an act of cultural imperialism: "These American doctors with their Anglo brand of medicine are trying to impose it on us." This raises the difficult question of how to implement public health measures when the rationale is sufficiently compelling to prohibit religious or cultural rituals. Efforts to eradicate mercury sprinkling should enlist members of the community who agree with the public health position but who are also respected members of the cultural or religious group.

BELIEF SYSTEM OF A SUBCULTURE

Some widely held ethical practices have been transformed into law, such as disclosure of risks during an informed consent discussion and offering to patients the opportunity to make advanced directives in the form of a living will or appointing a health care agent. Yet these can pose problems for adherents of traditional cultural beliefs. In the traditional culture of Navajo Native Americans, a deeply rooted cultural belief underlies a wish not to convey or receive negative information. A study conducted on a Navajo Indian reservation in Arizona demonstrated how Western biomedical and bioethical concepts and principles can come into conflict with traditional Navajo values and ways of thinking (Carrese and Rhodes 1995). In March 1992, the Indian Health Service adopted the requirements of the Patient

Self-Determination Act, but the Indian Health Service policy also contains the following proviso: "Tribal customs and traditional beliefs that relate to death and dying will be respected to the extent possible when providing information to patients on these issues" (Carrese and Rhodes 1995, p. 828).

The relevant Navajo belief in this context is the notion that thought and language have the power to shape reality and to control events. The central concern posed by discussions about future contingencies is that traditional beliefs require people to "think and speak in a positive way." When doctors disclose risks of a treatment in an informed consent discussion, they speak "in a negative way," thereby violating the Navajo prohibition. The traditional Navajo belief is that health is maintained and restored through positive ritual language. This presumably militates against disclosing risks of treatment as well as avoiding mention of future illness or incapacitation in a discussion about advance care planning. Western-trained doctors working with the traditional Navajo population are thus caught in a dilemma. Should they adhere to the ethical and legal standards pertaining to informed consent now in force in the rest of the United States and risk harming their patients by "talking in a negative way"? Or should they adhere to the Navajo belief system with the aim of avoiding harm to the patients but at the same time violating the ethical requirement of disclosure to patients of potential risks and future contingencies?

The authors of the published study draw several conclusions. One is that hospital policies complying with the Patient Self-Determination Act are ethically troublesome for the traditional Navajo patients. Since physicians who work with that population must decide how to act, this problem requires a solution. A second conclusion is that "the concepts and principles of Western bioethics are not universally held" (Carrese and Rhodes 1995, p. 829). This comes as no surprise. It is a straightforward statement of the thesis of descriptive ethical relativism, the evident truth that a wide variety of cultural beliefs about morality exist in the world. The question for normative ethics endures: What follows from these particular facts of cultural relativity? A third conclusion the authors draw, in light of their findings, is that health care providers and institutions caring for Navajo patients should reevaluate their policies and procedures regarding advance care planning.

This situation is not difficult to resolve, ethically or practically. The Patient Self-Determination Act does not mandate patients to actually make an advance directive; it requires only that health care institutions provide information to patients and give them the opportunity to make a living will or appoint a health care agent. A physician or nurse working for the Indian Health Service could easily fulfill this requirement by asking Navajo patients if they wish to discuss their future care or options, without introducing any of the negative thinking. This approach resolves one of the limitations of the published study. As the authors acknowledge, the findings reflect a more traditional perspective and the full range of Navajo views is not represented. So it is possible that some patients who use the Indian Health Service may be willing or even eager to have frank discussions about risks of treatment and future possibilities, even negative ones, if offered the opportunity.

It is more difficult, however, to justify withholding from patients the risks of proposed treatment in an informed consent discussion. The article about the Navajo beliefs recounts an episode told by a Navajo woman who is also a nurse. Her father was a candidate for bypass surgery. When the surgeon informed the patient of the risks of surgery, including the possibility that he might not wake up, the elderly Navajo man refused the surgery altogether. If the patient did indeed require the surgery and refused because he believed that telling him of the risk of not waking up would bring about that result, then it would be justifiable to withhold that risk of surgery. Should not that possibility be routinely withheld from all patients, then, since the prospect of not waking up could lead other people—Navajos and non-Navajos alike—to refuse the surgery? The answer is no, but it requires further analysis.

Respect for autonomy grants patients who have been properly informed the right to refuse a proposed medical treatment. An honest and appropriate disclosure of the purpose, procedures, risks, benefits, and available alternatives, provided in terms the patient can understand, puts the ultimate decision in the hands of the patient. This is the ethical standard according to Western bioethics. A clear exception exists in the case of patients who lack decisional capacity altogether, and debate continues regarding the ethics of paternalistically overriding the refusal of marginally competent patients. This picture relies on a key feature that is lacking in the Navajo case: a certain metaphysical account of the way the world works. Western doctors and their patients generally do not believe that talking about risks of harm will produce those harms (although there have been accounts that document the "dark side" of the placebo effect). It is not really the Navajo values that create the cross-cultural problem but rather, their metaphysical belief system holding that thought and language have the power to shape reality and control events. In fact, the Navajo values are quite the same as the standard Western ones: fear of death and avoidance of harmful side effects. To understand the relationship between cultural variation and ethical relativism, it is essential to distinguish between cultural relativity that stems from a difference in values and that which can be traced to an underlying metaphysics or epistemology.

Against this background, only two choices are apparent: insist on disclosing to Navajo patients the risks of treatment and thereby inflict unwanted negative thoughts on them; or withhold information about the risks and state only the anticipated benefits of the proposed treatment. Between those two choices, there is no contest. The second is clearly ethically preferable. It is true that withholding information about the risks of treatment or potential adverse events in the future radically changes what is required by the doctrine of informed consent. It essentially removes the "informed" aspect, while leaving in place the notion that the patient should decide. The physician will still provide some information to the Navajo patient, but only the type of information that is acceptable to the Navajos who adhere to this particular belief system. True, withholding certain information that would typically be disclosed to patients departs from the ethical ideal of informed consent, but it does so in order to achieve the ethically appropriate goal of beneficence in the care of patients.

The principle of beneficence supports the withholding of information about risks of treatment from Navajos who hold the traditional belief system. But so, too, does the principle of respect for autonomy. Navajos holding traditional beliefs can act autonomously only when they are not thinking in a negative way. If doctors tell them about bad contingencies, that will lead to negative thinking, which in their view will fail to maintain and restore health. The value of both doctor and patient is to maintain and restore health. A change in the procedures regarding the informed consent discussion is justifiable based on a distinctive background condition: the Navajo belief system about the causal efficacy of thinking and talking in a certain way. The less-than-ideal version of informed consent does constitute a "lower" standard than that which is usually appropriate in today's medical practice. But the use of a "lower" standard is justified by the background assumption that that is what the Navajo patient prefers.

What is relative and what is nonrelative in this situation? There is a clear divergence between the Navajo belief system and that of Western science. That divergence leads to a difference in what sort of discussion is appropriate for traditional Navajos in the medical setting and that which is standard in Western medical practice. According to one description, "always disclose the risks as well as the benefits of treatment to patients," the conclusion points to ethical relativism. But a more general description, one that heeds today's call for cultural awareness and sensitivity, would be: "Carry out an informed consent discussion in a manner appropriate to the patient's beliefs and understanding." That obligation is framed in a nonrelative way. A heart surgeon would describe the procedures, risks, and benefits of bypass surgery in one way to a patient who is another physician, in a different way to a mathematician ignorant of medical science, in yet another way to a skilled craftsman with an eighth grade education, and still differently to a traditional Navajo. The ethical principle is the same; the procedures differ.

OBLIGATIONS OF PHYSICIANS

The problem for physicians is how to respond when an immigrant to the United States acts according to the cultural values of her native country, values that differ widely from accepted practices in American medicine. Suppose an African immigrant asks an obstetrician to perform genital surgery on her baby girl. Or imagine that a Laotian immigrant from the Iu Mien culture brings her four-month-old baby to the pediatrician for a routine visit and the doctor discovers burns on the baby's stomach. The African mother seeks to comply with the tradition in her native country, Somalia, where the vast majority of women have had clitoridectomies. The Iu Mien woman admits that she had used a traditional folk remedy to treat what she suspected was her infant's case of a rare folk illness.

What is the obligation of physicians in the United States when they encounter patients in such situations? At one extreme is the reply that in the United States, physicians are obligated to follow the ethical and cultural practices accepted here and have no obligation to comply with patients' requests that embody entirely different cultural values. At the other extreme is the view that cultural sensitivity requires physicians to adhere to the traditional beliefs and practices of patients who have emigrated from other cultures.

A growing concern on the part of doctors and public health officials is the increasing number of requests for genital cutting and defense of the practice by immigrants to the United States and European countries. A Somalian immigrant living in Houston said he believed his Muslim faith required him to have his daughters undergo the procedure; he also stated his belief that it would preserve their virginity. He was quoted as saying, "It's my responsibility. If I don't do it, I will have failed my children" (Dugger 1996, p. 1). Another African immigrant living in Houston sought a milder form of the cutting she had undergone for her daughter. The woman said she believed it was necessary so her daughter would not run off with boys and have babies before marriage. She was disappointed that Medicaid would not cover the procedure, and planned to go to Africa to have the procedure done there. A New York City physician was asked by a father for a referral to a doctor who would do the procedure on his three-year-old daughter. When the physician told him this was not done in America, the man accused the doctor of not understanding what he wanted (Dugger 1996, pp. 1, 9).

However, others in our multicultural society consider it a requirement of "cultural sensitivity" to accommodate in some way to such requests of African immigrants. Harborview Medical Center in Seattle sought just such a solution. A group of doctors agreed to consider making a ritual nick in the fold of skin that covers the clitoris, but without removing any tissue. However, the hospital later abandoned the plan after being flooded with letters, postcards, and telephone calls in protest (Dugger 1996).

A physician who conducted research with East African women living in Seattle held the same view as the doctors who sought a culturally sensitive solution. In a talk she gave to my medical school department, she argued that Western physicians must curb their tendency to judge cultural practices different from their own as "rational" or "irrational." Ritual genital cutting is an "inalienable" part of some cultures, and it does a disservice to people from those cultures to view it as a human rights violation. She pointed out that in the countries where female genital mutilation (FGM) is practiced, circumcised women are "normal." Like some anthropologists who argue for a "softer" linguistic approach (Lane and Rubinstein 1996), this researcher preferred the terminology of "circumcision" to that of "female genital mutilation."

One can understand and even have some sympathy for the women who believe they must adhere to a cultural ritual even when they no longer live in the society where it is widely practiced. But it does not follow that the ritual is an "inalienable" part of that culture, since every culture undergoes changes over time. Furthermore, to contend that in the countries where FGM is practiced, circumcised women are "normal" is like saying that malaria or malnutrition is "normal" in parts of Africa. That a human condition is statistically normal implies nothing whatever about whether an obligation exists to seek to alter the statistical norm for the betterment of those who are affected.

Some Africans living in the United States have said they are offended that Congress passed a law prohibiting female genital mutilation that appears to be directed specifically at Africans. France has also passed legislation, but its law relies on general statutes that prohibit violence against children (Dugger 1996). In a recent landmark case, a French court sent a Gambian woman to jail for having had the genitals of her two baby daughters mutilated by a midwife. French doctors report an increasing number of cases of infants who are brought to clinics hemorrhaging or with severe infections. . . .

Another case vignette describes a Laotian woman from the Mien culture who immigrated to the United States and married a Mien man. When she visited her child's pediatrician for a routine four-month immunization, the doctor was horrified to see five red and blistered quarter-inch round markings on the child's abdomen (Case Study: Culture, Healing, and Professional Obligations 1993). The mother explained that she used a traditional Mien "cure" for pain, since she thought the infant was experiencing a rare folk illness among Mien babies characterized by incessant crying and loss of appetite, in addition to other symptoms. The "cure" involves dipping a reed in pork fat, lighting the reed, and passing the burning substance over the skin, raising a blister that "pops like popcorn." The popping indicates that the illness is not related to spiritual causes; if no blisters appear, then a shaman may have to be summoned to conduct a spiritual ritual for a cure. As many as 11 burns might be needed before the end of the "treatment." The burns are then covered with a mentholated cream.

The Mien woman told the pediatrician that infection is rare and the burns heal in a week or so. Scars sometimes remain but are not considered disfiguring. She also told the doctor that the procedure must be done by someone skilled in burning, since if a burn is placed too near the line between the baby's mouth and navel, the baby could become mute or even retarded. The mother considered the cure to have been successful in the case of her baby, since the child had stopped crying and regained her appetite. Strangely enough, the pediatrician did not say anything to the mother about her practice of burning the baby, no doubt from the need to show "cultural sensitivity." She did, however, wonder later whether she should have said something since she thought the practice was dangerous and also cruel to babies. . . .

[In commentaries on these cases, one often finds] a great reluctance to criticize, scold, or take legal action against parents from other cultures who employ painful and potentially harmful rituals that have no scientific basis. This attitude of tolerance is appropriate against the background knowledge that the parents do not intend to harm the child and are simply using a folk remedy widely accepted in their own culture. But tolerance of these circumstances must be distinguished from a judgment that the actions harmful to children should be permitted to continue. What puzzles me is the notion that "cultural sensitivity" must extend so far as to refrain from providing a solid education to these parents about the potential harms and the infliction of gratuitous pain. In a variety of other contexts, we accept the role of physicians as educator of patients. Doctors are supposed to tell their patients not to smoke, to lose weight, to have appropriate preventive medical checkups such as pap smears, mammograms, and proctoscopic examinations.

Pediatricians are thought to have an even more significant obligation to educate the parents of their vulnerable patients: inform them of steps that minimize the risks of sudden infant death syndrome, tell them what is appropriate for an infant's or child's diet, and give them a wide array of other social and psychological information designed to keep a child healthy and flourishing. Are these educational obligations of pediatricians only appropriate for patients whose background culture is that of the United States or Western Europe? Should a pediatrician not attempt to educate parents who, in their practice of the Santería religion, sprinkle mercury around the house? The obligation of pediatricians to educate and even to urge parents to adopt practices likely to contribute to the good health and well being of their children, and to avoid practices that will definitely or probably cause harm and suffering, should know no cultural boundaries.

My position is consistent with the realization that Western medicine does not have all the answers. This position also recognizes that some traditional healing practices are not only not harmful but may be as beneficial as those of Western medicine. The injunction to "respect cultural diversity" could rest on the premise that Western medicine sometimes causes harm without compensating benefits (which is true) or on the equally true premise that traditional practices such as acupuncture and herbal remedies, once scorned by mainstream Western medicine, have come to be accepted side-by-side with the precepts of scientific medicine. Typically, however, respect for multicultural diversity goes well beyond these reasonable views and requires toleration of manifestly painful or harmful procedures such as the burning remedy employed in the Mien culture. We ought to be able to respect cultural diversity without having to accept every single feature embedded in traditional beliefs and rituals.

The reluctance to impose modern medicine on immigrants from a fear that it constitutes yet another instance of "cultural imperialism" is misplaced. Is it not possible to accept non-Western cultural practices side by side with Western ones, yet condemn those that are manifestly harmful and have no compensating benefit except for the cultural belief that they are beneficial? [Two] commentators who urged respect for the Mien woman's burning treatment on the grounds that it is practiced widely, the reasons for it are widely understood among the Mien, and the procedure works, from a Mien point of view [Brown and Jameton 1993, p. 17], seemed to be placing that practice on a par with practices that "work" from the point of view of Western medicine. Recall that if the skin does not blister, the Mien belief holds that the illness may be related to spiritual causes and a shaman might have to be called. Should the pediatrician stand by and do nothing, if the child has a fever of 104° and the parent calls a shaman because the skin did not blister? Recall also that the Mien woman told the pediatrician that if the burns are not done in the right place, the baby could become mute or even retarded. Must we reject the beliefs of Western medicine regarding causality and grant equal status to the Mien beliefs? To refrain from seeking to educate such parents and to not exhort them to alter their traditional practices is unjust, as it exposes the immigrant children to health risks that are not borne by children from the majority culture.

It is heresy in today's postmodern climate of respect for the belief systems of all cultures to entertain the notion that some beliefs are demonstrably false and others, whether true or false, lead to manifestly harmful actions. We are not supposed to talk about the evolution of scientific ideas or about progress in the Western world, since that is a colonialist way of thinking. If it is simply "the white man's burden, medicalized" (Morsy 1991) to urge African families living in the United States not to genitally mutilate their daughters, or to attempt to educate Mien mothers about the harms of burning their babies, then we are doomed to permit ethical relativism to overwhelm common sense.

Multiculturalism, as defined at the beginning of this paper, appears to embrace ethical relativism and yet is logically inconsistent with relativism. The second half of the definition states that multiculturalism "insists that all cultural groups be treated with respect and as equals." What does this imply with regard to cultural groups that oppress or fail to respect other cultural groups? Must the cultural groups that violate the mandate to treat all cultural groups with respect and as equals be respected themselves? It is impossible to insist that all such groups be treated with respect and as equals, and at the same time accept any particular group's attitude toward and treatment of another group as inferior. Every cultural group contains subgroups within the culture: old and young, women and men, people with and people without disabilities. Are the cultural groups that discriminate against women or people with disabilities to be respected equally with those that do not?

What multiculturalism does not say is whether all of the beliefs and practices of all cultural groups must be equally respected. It is one thing to require that cultural, religious, and ethnic groups be treated as equals; that conforms to the principle of justice as equality. It is quite another thing to say that any cultural practice whatever of any group is to be tolerated and respected equally. This latter view is a statement of extreme ethical relativism. If multiculturalists endorse the principle of justice as equality, however, they must recognize that normative ethical relativism entails the illogical consequence of toleration and acceptance of numerous forms of injustice in those cultures that oppress women and religious and ethnic minorities.

REFERENCES

Blackhall, Leslie; Murphy, Sheila T.; Frank, Gelya; Michel, Vicki; and Azen, Stanley. 1995. Ethnicity and Attitudes Toward Patient Autonomy. *Journal of the American Medical Association* 274: 820–25.

Brown, Kate, and Jameton, Andrew. 1993. Culture, Healing, and Professional Obligations: Commentary. *Hastings Center Report* 23 (4): 17.

Carrese, Joseph, and Rhodes, Lorna A. 1995. Western Bioethics on the Navajo Reservation: Benefit or Harm? *Journal of the American Medical Association* 274: 826–29.

Case Study: Culture, Healing, and Professional Obligations. 1993. *Hastings Center Report* 23 (4): 15.

Dugger, Celia W. 1996. Tug of Taboos: African Genital Rite vs. U.S. Law. *New York Times* (28 December): 1, 9.

Fowers, Blaine J., and Richardson, Frank C. 1996. Why Is Multiculturalism Good? *American Psychologist* 51: 609–21.

Fox, Renée C. 1990. The Evolution of American Bioethics: A Sociological Perspective. In *Social Science Perspectives on Medical Ethics,* ed. George Weisz, pp. 201–20. Philadelphia: University of Pennsylvania Press.

Hardwig, John. 1990. "What About the Family?" *Hastings Center Report* 20 (2): 5–10.

Lane, Sandra D., and Rubinstein, Robert A. 1996. Judging the Other: Responding to Traditional Female Genital Surgeries. *Hastings Center Report* 26 (5): 31–40.

Morsy, Soheir A. 1991. Safeguarding Women's Bodies: The White Man's Burden Medicalized. *Medical Anthropology Quarterly* 5 (1): 19–23.

Nelson, James Lindemann. 1992. Taking Families Seriously. *Hastings Center Report* 22 (4): 6–12.

ANNOTATED BIBLIOGRAPHY

Beauchamp, Tom L.: "The Promise of the Beneficence Model for Medical Ethics," *Journal of Contemporary Health Law and Policy 6* (Spring 1990), pp. 145–155. Beauchamp presents a historical and conceptual overview of the beneficence and autonomy models of the physician-patient relationship, before critically evaluating the effort of Edmund D. Pellegrino to reconcile the two in a reconstructed beneficence model.

Benjamin, Martin and Joy Curtis: *Ethics in Nursing,* 3rd ed. (New York: Oxford University Press, 1992). The purpose of this book is to introduce nursing students and nurses to the identification and analysis of ethical issues in nursing. The book includes a large number of actual cases, many of which are explored in detail.

Bok, Sissela: *Lying: Moral Choice in Public and Private Life* (New York: Random House, 1978). In this classic book, Bok provides a highly detailed examination of ethical issues connected with lying.

Buchanan, Allen E., and Dan W. Brock: *Deciding for Others: The Ethics of Surrogate Decision Making* (Cambridge: Cambridge University Press, 1989). Part I of this influential work develops a general theory of medical decision making for incompetent patients. Part II applies this theoretical framework to the distinctive problems raised by minor, elderly, and psychiatric patients.

Council on Ethical and Judicial Affairs, American Medical Association: "Conflicts of Interests: Physician Ownership of Medical Facilities," *JAMA* 267 (May 6, 1992), pp. 2366–2369. This position paper by the American Medical Association argues that physicians generally should not refer patients to medical facilities at which they do not directly provide care if they have a financial interest in the facility. An exception is made, however, for cases in which the community has a demonstrated need for the facility, and there is no alternative way to finance the facility.

Edelstein, Ludwig: *Ancient Medicine* (Baltimore, MD: Johns Hopkins, 1967). Edelstein discusses the Hippocratic Oath and identifies two distinct sets of obligations—those to the patient and those to the physician's teacher and the teacher's progeny.

Faden, Ruth R., and Tom L. Beauchamp: *A History and Theory of Informed Consent* (New York: Oxford University Press, 1986). This ambitious work spans the history, theory, and practice of informed consent in medicine, human behavioral research, philosophy, and law.

Grisso, Thomas, and Paul S. Appelbaum: *Assessing Competence to Consent to Treatment: A Guide for Physicians and Other Health Professionals* (New York: Oxford University Press, 1998). The product of an eight-year study of patients' decision-making capacities, this book describes the role of competence in the doctrine of informed consent, analyzes the elements of decision making, and shows how determinations of competence can be made in varied medical settings.

Kuhse, Helga: "Clinical Ethics and Nursing: 'Yes' to Caring, But 'No' to a Female Ethics of Care," *Bioethics* 9 (July 1995), pp. 207–219. Kuhse argues that, while care—a sensitivity and responsiveness to the particularities of a situation and to people's needs—is necessary for nursing ethics, the "ethics of care" is seriously inadequate for nursing ethics and as a general moral theory.

Lidz, Charles W., Paul S. Appelbaum, and Alan Meisel: "Two Models of Implementing Informed Consent," *Archives of Internal Medicine* 148 (June 1988), pp. 1385–1389. The authors provide detailed, contrasting descriptions of two ways of implementing the doctrine of informed consent: the event model and the process model. They argue in favor of the process model before noting some of its limitations.

Macklin, Ruth: "HIV-Infected Psychiatric Patients: Beyond Confidentiality," *Ethics & Behavior* 1 (1991), pp. 3–20. Macklin examines ethical issues concerning HIV-infected psychiatric patients. Devoting most of her analysis to professionals' conflicting obligations of confidentiality and protecting persons at risk, she defends some limits to the first obligation before turning to other kinds of ethical dilemmas.

Parens, Erik, ed.: *Enhancing Human Traits: Ethical and Social Implications* (Washington, DC: Georgetown University Press, 1998). This anthology serves as an excellent introduction to such biomedical enhancements as cosmetic surgery, antidepressants for "the worried well," and genetic enhancements. The thirteen essays explore conceptual, ethical, policy-related, and cultural issues provoked by efforts to enhance human traits with biomedical means.

Pellegrino, Edmund D.: "Managed Care at the Bedside: How Do We Look in the Moral Mirror?" *Kennedy Institute of Ethics Journal* 7 (December 1997), pp. 321–330. Focussing on ethical issues that arise at the bedside, Pellegrino argues that while managed care is morally neutral in principle, in practice it often creates significant conflicts for physicians and forces compromises in the caring dimensions of the physician-patient relationship.

Pence, Terry: "Nursing's Most Pressing Moral Issue," *Bioethics Forum* 10 (Winter 1994), pp. 3–9. In defending the thesis that nurses' appropriate role is one of advocacy for patients, Pence offers an account of the concept of advocacy, argues that advocacy's ascendance as a moral metphor was a major turning point in nursing history, and responds to leading criticisms of the advocacy model.

_____: *Making Health Care Decisions*, Vol. 2: *Appendices: Empirical Studies of Informed Consent.* This volume contains the empirical studies used by the President's Commission in formulating its conclusions.

_____: *Making Health Care Decisions*, Vol. 3: *Studies in the Foundations of Informed Consent.* Viewpoints represented in this volume are those of a psychologist, a historian, an anthropologist, a sociologist, a pediatrician-oncologist, a philosopher, and a medical student.

President's Council on Bioethics: *Beyond Therapy: Biotechnology and the Pursuit of Happiness* (Washington, DC: President's Council on Bioethics, 2003). This report investigates the potential implications of using biotechnology "beyond therapy" in seeking better children, superior individual performance, avoidance of the effects of aging, and happiness. The PCB intends with this report "to advance the nation's awareness and understanding of a critical set of bioethical issues and to bring them beyond the narrow circle of bioethics professionals into the larger public arena."

White, Becky Cox: *Competence to Consent* (Washington, DC: Georgetown University Press, 1994). In addition to offering a concise introduction to major philosophical and ethical issues involved in competence to consent, this book presents White's own theory of competence and a set of practical suggestions.

Wicclair, Mark R.: "Patient Decision-Making Capacity and Risk," *Bioethics* 5 (April 1991), pp. 91–104. Wicclair criticizes "risk-related standards" of decision-making capacity (competence). His main target is the standard defended by Allen E. Buchanan and Dan W. Brock, which requires balancing the values of (1) respecting a patient's self-determination and (2) protecting his or her well-being.

Winslow, Betty J., and Gerald R. Winslow: "Integrity and Compromise in Nursing Ethics," *Journal of Medicine and Philosophy* 16 (June 1991), pp. 307–323. The authors grapple with ethical issues that arise for nurses when they consider compromise as a means of resolving conflicts in which they are entagled. They argue that compromise is compatible with moral integrity if certain conditions are met.

CHAPTER 3

CONTESTED THERAPIES AND BIOMEDICAL ENHANCEMENT

INTRODUCTION

Chapter 2 provided a broad introduction to the professional-patient relationship. It explored the basic obligations and virtues of physicians, the role and responsibilities of nurses, respect for patient autonomy and the issue of medical paternalism, specific obligations regarding truth-telling, informed consent, and confidentiality, as well as the moral complexities that arise when health professionals work in a multicultural environment. The present chapter continues to examine the professional-patient relationship and the obligations of health professionals, especially physicians, but now with a focus on contexts in which the services offered by professionals are themselves the object of moral scrutiny. To a lesser extent, this chapter also explores the obligations of parents in making decisions regarding the use of controversial medical services for their children.

The medical services in question test the boundaries of appropriate practices by health professionals. Uncontroversial examples of appropriate medical care include primary care, pediatrics and geriatrics as they are ordinarily practiced, psychiatric services for those suffering from mental illness, emergency medicine, and certain types of surgery. Another type of intervention that is widely (though not universally) regarded as appropriate is gene therapy—or, inasmuch as this area of medicine remains in its clinical infancy, gene therapy *research* involving patients for whom established, effective therapies are unavailable. But should physicians be permitted to employ their skills in a medical setting for purposes other than the treatment or prevention of disease, impairment, or dysfunction? Or does such employment of medical expertise transgress the appropriate boundaries of medicine? And how are we to determine these boundaries? It would seem impossible to delineate them by the consensus of physicians, because no such consensus exists—as the readings of this chapter, taken together, will indicate. Do the proper boundaries of medicine, then, include the full range of services that patients want and physicians are willing to provide, as suggested by a market model of health-care delivery? Or are the normative boundaries of medical practice determined by moral values inherent in medicine—or by some other standard?

In this chapter we will consider two broad classes of boundary-challenging medical interventions. First, we will consider *contested therapies* such as limb-lengthening surgery for children with dwarfism and the implantation of multiple embryos in women undergoing in vitro fertilization. Then we will take up *biomedical enhancements* for patients who, despite having no diagnosable illness or impairment, request services in the hope of improving their bodies or minds. Such enhancements include cosmetic surgery, the enhancement of psychological and/or cognitive functioning with biomedical means, and genetic enhancement. (Chapter 8, on genetics and human reproduction, will take up ethical issues connected with the future prospect of genetic enhancement.)

Some interventions, to be sure, are ambiguous as between therapies and enhancements. Consider, for example, the amputation of one or more limbs from persons who persistently request such surgeries in the absence of any apparent medical reason for their requests. These individuals usually feel a pressing *need* for amputation, suggesting that the procedure would be therapeutic for them; yet physicians perceive no medical need for the surgery, suggesting an intervention "beyond therapy" and therefore more akin to enhancement (even though a physician may doubt that surgery would really make the patient *better off*). Although, for the purposes of this chapter, the reading that discusses elective amputations is located in the section on contested therapies, we regard the proper classification of this issue as highly uncertain. The same uncertainty about classification applies to several other issues discussed in this chapter. For example, sometimes what is classified as psychological enhancement may be ambiguous as between enhancement beyond psychological normalcy and treatment of a genuine psychological impairment.

Because contested therapies and even biomedical enhancements may be available for children and adolescents, an ethical analysis of these boundary-challenging interventions must consider the ethics of proxy decision-making. For this reason, in addition to examining the obligations of physicians in connection with controversial medical services—our primary focus—this chapter will also explore the obligations of parents in deciding for or against these services for their dependent children.

In this context, it will be helpful to consider what is perhaps the most significant breakthrough in contemporary biomedical ethics: the substantial moral authority now conferred on patients with decision-making capacity (see the introduction to Chapter 2) and sometimes, by extension, on proxies for patients lacking decision-making capacity. The contemporary emphasis on respect for patient autonomy has helped to generate a widely accepted hierarchy of medical decision-making standards. According to this hierarchy of standards, in cases where patients are competent—that is, where they have decision-making capacity—their *informed consent* is needed to justify medical interventions on them.[1] The standard of informed consent, however, does not meaningfully apply in the case of patients who are at the relevant time incompetent and therefore incapable of mature, responsible decision-making. In the case of formerly competent patients, however, if there is significant evidence supporting a particular *substituted judgment,* then that standard applies. A substituted judgment is a judgment about what a patient would have wanted for the current situation in which he or she is incompetent.[2] In the case of patients who have never been competent, such as children and some severely mentally retarded adults, and in the case of formerly competent patients for whom there is insufficient evidence regarding what they would have wanted in the present circumstance, it is apparently impossible to respect their autonomy—either past or present. Thus, medical decisions for these patients are to be guided by consideration of their *best interests*. The hierarchy of decision-making standards therefore has this structure:

1. Informed Consent
2. Substituted Judgment
3. Best Interests

The readings in this chapter concern decisions by competent adults for themselves or for minors who are presumed to lack decision-making capacity. Thus the standards of informed consent and best interests will be especially important to the issues raised here.

CONTESTED THERAPIES

Our investigation of contested medical therapies begins with the topic of cochlear implants. Cochlear implants are surgically implanted devices that can partially enable hearing and speech comprehension for many deaf individuals. It may seem obvious that it is in a deaf child's best interests to have this surgery—even though it may not prove effective in his or her case and the surgeries so far that have been considered successful have been only partially effective. After all, one might naturally assume, deafness is a major disability so we should embrace any intervention that offers a chance of reducing the effects of deafness.

Matters are not so simple, however. First, for deaf children who have undergone cochlear implant surgery, learning to recognize and produce spoken language while depending on these devices is likely to be a long, arduous process—again, with no guarantee of success. Moreover, according to some commentators, enthusiasm about this type of surgery reflects the hearing majority's prejudice against deafness. Indeed, some have argued, cochlear implants represent a threat to a unique culture: Deaf (with a capital D) culture. As Bonnie Tucker explains in a reading reprinted in this chapter, champions of Deaf culture regard deafness as a cultural identity rather than a disability. Deaf culturalists define their community partly in terms of a shared language, American Sign Language (ASL). From their perspective, cochlear implant surgery represents an effort to assimilate deaf persons into the hearing mainstream, at best devaluing Deaf culture and at worst threatening cultural genocide.

In one of this chapter's selections, Robert Crouch expresses a moderate version of this view. According to Crouch, the technology of cochlear implant surgery is currently insufficient to guarantee that children who undergo it will ever learn a spoken language. More fundamentally, he argues, for a prelinguistically deaf child to acquire a cochlear implant and join the hearing mainstream involves a significant loss: a missed opportunity for "membership in the Deaf community, a unique community with a rich history, a rich language, and a value system of its own." Because membership in this community is a substantial benefit, deaf parents of deaf children should enjoy the prerogative to forgo cochlear implant surgery. Responding to this position, Tucker, who is deaf, contends that deafness poses substantial objective disadvantages and that learning a spoken language in addition to ASL is the most promising approach to overcoming these disadvantages. Accordingly, she criticizes parents who refuse to authorize cochlear implant surgeries—a choice that, she thinks, constricts the opportunities available to deaf children—as well as Deaf culturalists who oppose the use of these devices while demanding costly accommodations for their deafness.

While the selections by Crouch and Tucker focus on the ethics of parental decision-making on behalf of their deaf children, parallel issues arise for physicians who offer cochlear implant surgeries. In view of the charge that the hearing majority underappreciates the advantages of membership in the Deaf community while exaggerating the disadvantages of deafness—and failing to notice the role that policy decisions by the hearing majority play in creating the disadvantages that do exist—what are the responsibilities of physicians who are qualified to provide these surgeries? Do they have a responsibility, in communicating with parents of deaf children, to represent the Deaf community's perspective in identifying the advantages and disadvantages of cochlear implant surgery? Might they have a responsibility to refrain from providing it altogether or, less radically, to embrace a presumption against it?

Medical and parental decisions for intersex children are no less difficult and controversial than such decisions about cochlear implant surgery. Some infants are born intersex—that is, with one of various conditions that make it difficult to determine from outward appearance whether the infants are boys or girls. Intersex conditions include a wide variety of genital anomalies, such as a very large clitoris, a very small penis, or an underdeveloped vagina or testes. The most common intersex condition is congenital adrenal hyperplasia, in which an excess of androgen in infants who are genetically female causes the genitals to appear more masculine. Whereas removal of the entire clitoris used to be common in such cases, today it is more common to trim down excess tissue while preserving nerve-rich tissue. A rarer condition is that of a genetically male infant who is born with a "micropenis." Surgically creating a larger penis is extremely complicated, so many infants with this condition have undergone surgery that created a vagina and were raised as girls. In one of this chapter's readings, Sherri A. Groveman (who later married and took the last name Morris) describes her intersex condition, Androgren Insensitivity Syndrome, which is characterized by XY (male) chromosomes and testes, but, due to an androgen receptor defect, an inability of the body to respond to testosterone in the testes and thereby acquire masculine-looking characteristics. Groveman's parents consented to a gonadectomy (removal of the testes) and female gender assignment; they also hid the truth of Groveman's condition from her, leaving her to discover the truth as an adult.

At least until recently, the standard medical approach to intersex was to perform "normalizing" surgery on the infant with a long-term strategy of shielding the growing child from the truth about his and/or her condition.[3] Lately this strategy has been challenged by many mature intersex individuals who have expressed anger and dismay at having been surgically modified before they could consent and then deceived about their condition. For the greater part, physicians have been highly paternalistic in pressuring parents to consent to the standard approach ("normalizing" surgery and gender assignment without disclosure), have known little about long-term effects of different approaches, and have arguably expressed their own discomfort about ambiguous genitalia in favoring the standard approach. According to Groveman, what parents of intersex children need are emotional support, education about intersex, and the opportunity to make well-informed, voluntary decisions for their children. While this assertion addresses the circumstances of the parents' decision-making, there remains the question of what the intersex child's best interests require. Groveman implicitly addresses this question by arguing that intersex children need the truth about their ambiguous sexuality, need social acceptance, and—at least before they can competently decide for themselves—need no more surgery than is necessary for physical health.

While intersex children have often had the truth about their intersexuality hidden from them, secrecy has not been an option for children of extremely short stature. Such diminutive height, often referred to as *dwarfism,* can result from more than 200 conditions; it is sometimes defined as stature of less than 4 feet 10 inches as an adult. More than half of all cases of dwarfism result from *achondroplasia,* a genetically inherited condition that causes limbs to be disproportionately short in comparison with the head and trunk.[4] Another common cause of dwarfism is a deficiency of human growth hormone.[5]

In one of this chapter's readings, Lisa Abelow Hedley describes her experiences as a mother confronted with a seductive medical option for her daughter, who has achondroplasia. Hedley and her husband had just decided upon surgery to prevent bowing of their daughter's legs, a surgery that would entail a summer in bed with leg casts, only to be informed of the option of gradual limb-lengthening. This option would require attaching to their daughter's legs external fixators that would incrementally open each day before the leg casts are put on, with an expected gain of several inches of height. As Hedley explains, the parents were nearly seduced by the prospect of moving their daughter towards normal height—despite the awkward tension between this plan and the parental imperative to love one's children just as they are. Ultimately, Hedley and her husband chose only the surgery to prevent leg bowing, leaving to their daughter—when she is old enough—any decision about limb-lengthening. The discussion concludes with reflections about physicians' obligation to provide appropriate guidance and parents' obligation to protect their children's best interests.

The contested therapies we have considered so far—cochlear implant surgery, various surgeries in response to intersex, and limb-lengthening surgery—have been examined in the context of surrogate decisions for children. The other contested therapies to be addressed in this chapter involve competent adults as patients. In the first of these readings, however, an adult patient makes a decision with far-reaching consequences not just for herself but also for her children—both her existing children and her future children. In a reading reprinted here, Josephine Johnston takes up the "Octomom" case, in which an unemployed single woman on public assistance, Nadya Suleman—who already had six children—had eight more babies in a single pregnancy with the help of in vitro fertilization (IVF). Having conceived her first six children using IVF, Ms. Suleman apparently demanded that her fertility doctor transfer her six remaining frozen embryos simultaneously. After cautioning her about the risks entailed by multiple pregnancies, he transferred all six embryos, two of which produced twins. Citing the position of the American Society for Reproductive Medicine, Johnston argues that Suleman's fertility doctor acted irresponsibly in acceding to her rather extreme request. Should he have refused to treat her at all—even if she had requested the transfer of only one or two embryos—in view of her situation as a single, unemployed mother of six and her dependence on public assistance? While finding much merit in the concerns behind this question, Johnston answers in the negative, contending that fertility clinics are poorly positioned to make such judgments and therefore cannot be trusted to avoid unjust discrimination.

As explained earlier in this introduction, contemporary biomedical ethics is distinguished by the moral authority conferred upon competent adults in making decisions regarding their own medical care. The same moral authority is extended to the research context insofar as competent adults are permitted to make informed, voluntary decisions about whether to participate in clinical trials for which they are eligible. (The ethics of human research is discussed in Chapter 4.) The autonomy-respecting tenor that distinguishes contemporary biomedical ethics has become so pronounced that one might find it natural to infer that competent adult patients have the right to request and expect *any* medical intervention that they believe will benefit them. Even if physicians have no obligation to provide services that conflict with their moral sensibilities—as, for example, obstetricians are presumably not obliged to provide abortions if they object to abortion—surely, one might believe, physicians *may* (ethically) provide any medical service that a competent patient requests. But what if such a patient requests an intervention that seems dramatically contrary to his or her medical best interests?

In one of this chapter's readings, Carl Elliott introduces a phenomenon that provokes this question about as powerfully as it can be provoked:

> In January 2000 British newspapers began running articles about Robert Smith, a surgeon . . . in Scotland. Smith had amputated the legs of two patients at their request, and he was planning to carry out a third amputation when the trust that runs his hospital stopped him. These patients were not physically sick. Their legs did not need to be amputated for any medical reason. Nor were they incompetent, according to the psychiatrists who examined them. They simply wanted to have their legs cut off. In fact, both the men whose limbs Smith amputated have declared in public interviews how much happier they are, now that they have finally had their legs amputated.

Would it be right for a qualified surgeon to accede to a request for elective—indeed, seemingly gratuitous—amputation?

A surgeon approached with such a request is immediately confronted with the problem of interpreting it. Why does this person, for whom there is no evident medical reason for an amputation, so intensely want one? As Elliott explains, at least some people who want to be amputees are thought to have an attraction *to the idea of being an amputee*, an attraction that may develop for a variety of reasons. According to some experts, individuals who request elective amputations suffer from a mismatch between the actual state of their bodies and their sense of how their bodies should be. Comparing this phenomenon with the self-image of presurgical transsexuals, and with a variety of psychological disorders as well as more ordinary psychological phenomena, Elliott entertains the hypothesis that elective amputation and other psycho-medical phenomena that appear to have become more common in recent years might be fueled by (1) psychiatry's growing list of recognized psychological disorders and (2) the Internet's tendency to foster a sense of group membership.

How we interpret this phenomenon of requests for elective amputation will influence our view of ethically appropriate responses to "amputee wannabes." If the latter are believed to be psychiatrically ill, psychological treatment will seem indicated. But some individuals with this desire do not respond to treatment. If psychiatry's best interventions are unable to end the suffering of such an individual, might the surgery be judged necessary as a means to ending suffering? Certainly one goal of medicine is to eliminate or ameliorate suffering, but sometimes this goal is qualified as ". . . suffering *that has a medical basis*." But what counts as a medical basis? In psychiatry and psychology, the suffering itself—or at least suffering that takes such forms as depression, acute anxiety, and the like—is deemed worthy of treatment, irrespective of its source. That might suggest that any suffering is fair game for medical treatment. But can amputation be considered a medical treatment when there is no apparent medical reason for it? But what counts as a *medical* reason? Inasmuch as psychological pain—suffering—counts as adequate grounds for professional intervention in psychiatry (a branch of medicine), should not suffering count as sufficient reason for professional intervention in other areas of medicine such as surgery? Perhaps, but one might also reply that if the symptom that requires treatment is suffering *per se*, as opposed to some physically distinguishable disorder or dysfunction that causes suffering, then the problem is, after all, one of psychiatry. In that case, the argument might continue, the only appropriate treatment is some sort of psychiatric treatment, not the severing of a limb. Needless to say, the issue of the appropriate ethical response by physicians to requests for elective amputation is far from being resolved.

Not surprisingly, the other contested treatments explored in this chapter also remain highly controversial. So, too, are the interventions grouped here under the rubric of *biomedical enhancements*.

BIOMEDICAL ENHANCEMENTS

Introduction to the Concept In discussing biomedical enhancements, we will sometimes refer to *enhancement technologies*. Let us use that term to refer to certain technologies when they are used for purposes of enhancement. Thus, the same technology—the medication Prozac, for example—will count as an enhancement technology in certain contexts (when used for enhancement purposes) but not in other contexts (when used for treatment of a psychological illness).

In biomedicine, enhancements are commonly understood as "interventions designed to improve human form or functioning beyond what is necessary to sustain or restore good health."[6] Stated another way, enhancements are interventions to improve human form or function that *do not respond to genuine medical needs*, where the latter are conceptualized (1) in terms of disease, impairment, illness, etc., (2) as deviations from normal (perhaps species-typical) functioning, or (3) by reference to prevailing medical understandings. This conception of enhancements identifies them by the goal of improvements in the absence of medical need. But sometimes enhancements are identified by reference to their *means*. Some means of self-improvement, such as exercise, impress us as natural and virtuous. By contrast, other means are regarded as artificial, as involving corrosive short-cuts, or as distorting the practice of medicine, rendering the self-improvement morally questionable and classifying it as an enhancement—for example, steroid use in sports.

As noted earlier in this introduction, the treatment/enhancement distinction can be difficult to draw. Indeed, some may question that it is a meaningful distinction at all. Consider that children who are very short due to a deficiency of growth hormone are classified as receiving *treatment* in receiving synthetic growth hormone. Meanwhile, children who have normal levels of this hormone, but are equally short simply because their parents are short, are classified as normal, with the implication that their receiving synthetic growth hormone counts as enhancement—despite their facing the same disadvantage (at least in human societies as we know them today) in being short and standing to gain equally from the drug. Later, as we consider the use of medications such as Prozac and Zoloft, particular cases may inspire doubts about the treatment/enhancement distinction. In view of someone who struggles with certain psychological issues and wants the medication, despite having no diagnosable illness or psychological condition, it may seem almost meaningless to say that providing the medication for him would be enhancement whereas providing the medication for someone who just barely satisfies clinical criteria for depression or anxiety counts as medical treatment. The relevant psychological phenomena, one might argue, exist on a *continuum* so that line-drawing on that continuum, dividing those who are "ill" from those who are not, will inevitably prove arbitrary.

While the treatment/enhancement distinction surely appears arbitrary in some contexts such as the two just considered, one might nevertheless hold that it is meaningful and compelling in most contexts, despite the gray area between treatment and enhancement. However illness may be defined, there is surely such a thing as illness—that is, there are cases in which people are obviously ill and in need of treatment; and given any reasonable understanding of illness, there are surely many cases in which individuals are obviously not ill (or injured or suffering from some dysfunction) such that their requests for biomedical interventions to improve their situation must count as enhancement. Put in this way, the argument seems almost irresistible in its logic: rather than denying that there is an arbitrary line between treatments and enhancements, the claim is simply that there are many paradigm cases of treatment and many paradigm cases of enhancement. It is with this understanding that we will consider various types of biomedical enhancement—even if some of the cases considered in the articles collected here may be ambiguous as to their proper classification.

While enhancement technologies are not new, the language designating them is newer. Clinicians and ethicists began to express concerns about enhancements in the 1980s with the impending development of gene therapy: Should society employ genetic interventions, beyond therapeutic purposes, to bring about other types of improvements such as increased height for those of ordinary stature, changes in eye and hair color, or greater mental powers for the cognitively normal? Sensing public jitters about genetic technologies in general, many clinicians thought it would be prudent to draw a clear line between genetic therapy, which the public was more likely to accept, and genetic enhancement (as explored in Chapter 8), which clinicians were willing to characterize as beyond medical acceptability.[7]

Today enhancements come in myriad varieties. We use school, educational games, and academic summer camps to enhance intellectual capabilities. Exercise, a carefully planned diet, and swimming lessons serve to improve various forms of physical functioning. Fluoride in tap water enhances our teeth's ability to fight off tooth decay, and routinely administered immunizations and vaccines enhance our immune system's ability to ward off illnesses. (Some, however, would not count fluoride and immunizations as enhancements, suggesting instead that they represent a third category: *prevention*.[8]) In order to improve our looks, we pump iron, color our hair, regrow hair with Rogaine, fight wrinkles with Botox, use makeup, and either seek or avoid sunlight in an effort to achieve a desired complexion. Many of us drink coffee not only for enjoyment but because it makes us more alert and ready to work. The range of enhancements is vast. In this chapter, of course, we focus on those involving the products or techniques of biomedicine: biomedical enhancements.

Cosmetic Surgery Cosmetic surgery is surgery whose purpose is primarily esthetic: to make someone more physically attractive. It includes breast augmentation, face-lifts, liposuction, hair transplants for balding men, most cases of nasal reconstruction, and such extreme measures as removing a couple of ribs to make a woman look more like a supermodel and reshaping one's face to make it appear more Caucasian. Cosmetic surgery does not include nasal reconstruction when the main purpose is to correct a breathing problem caused by a deviated septum in the nose, nor does it include breast reduction surgery for the purpose of relieving strain on chest and back muscles.

Is cosmetic surgery a morally problematic use of medical expertise? Addressing this question in an article reprinted here, Franklin G. Miller, Howard Brody, and Kevin C. Chung argue that clinical integrity requires adherence to an "internal morality of medicine": a moral framework determined by the proper goals of medicine, certain role-specific duties of physicians, and virtues appropriate to the profession. Emphasizing the distinct standards of professional ethics that characterize the business world and medicine, the authors contend that advertising for cosmetic surgery frequently violates the Code of Ethics for the American Society of Plastic and Reconstructive Surgeons. They go on to assert that from the perspective of the internal morality of medicine, cosmetic surgery must be viewed as ethically questionable, resting at best near the outer boundary of acceptable medical practice.

In another of this chapter's readings, Margaret Olivia Little approaches the ethics of cosmetic surgery from a different perspective. Not confining her analysis to doctors' obligations to patients, she argues that doctors must take responsibility for their relationship to the suspect social norms (e.g., sexist ones) that frequently motivate requests for cosmetic surgery; at the same time, doctors retain the responsibility to address their patients' suffering, which is sometimes best accomplished by performing cosmetic surgery. Little addresses the moral tension experienced by cosmetic surgeons who take to heart both of these responsibilities—to avoid complicity with unjust social norms and to respond adequately to their patients' suffering. The proper way to interpret the moral meaning of these surgeons' actions, she suggests, is holistic: A given action (e.g., performing a particular surgery) should be evaluated not in isolation but against the background of the doctor's moral choices over time (e.g., working against the social system that makes such surgery seem so desirable). This permits cosmetic surgeons to "sometimes perform the surgery, and always fight the system."

Cosmetic Psychopharmacology While cosmetic surgery has been available for decades, some means of biomedical enhancement are relatively new. "Cosmetic psychopharmacology," for example, emerged in the early 1990s. The term *cosmetic psychopharmacology* was coined by psychiatrist Peter Kramer in his landmark book, *Listening to Prozac*, to refer to the use of psychiatric medications for certain patients who lacked any diagnosable psychiatric illness or condition.[9] Kramer had noticed that, among the "worried well"—patients who were not clinically depressed, anxious, or obsessive, for example, but who struggled with fairly ordinary psychological issues—some not only felt better with Prozac, but also functioned more successfully at work, in relationships, and in other respects. Quite a few of these patients experienced personality changes—becoming more trusting, energetic, socially confident, and attractive in self-presentation—and welcomed these transformations. Hence the term *cosmetic psychopharmacology*. Since the publication of Kramer's book, other SSRIs (selective serotonin reuptake inhibitors) besides Prozac, such as Lexapro and Zoloft, have proved to have similar effects on some patients who lack any diagnosable disorder or illness. Naturally, the prescription of psychiatric medications for enhancement purposes tests the boundaries of appropriate medical practice. Moreover, the success of such use of medicines for enhancement purposes raises philosophical issues such as those connected with the meaning of mental illness and the continuity (or discontinuity) of human selves over time. In an excerpt from his book, reprinted in this chapter, Kramer reflects on his experiences with patients using Prozac, identifying a variety of philosophical, social, and ethical issues that are provoked by the medication's effects.

Cosmetic psychopharmacology appears to have grown massively in recent years. The qualification "appears to" is appropriate because it is much easier to find statistics on the overall use of particular medications such as Prozac—which we know, anecdotally from Kramer and others, are sometimes used in the absence of psychiatric illness—than to determine how often these medications are used for enhancement purposes. The greatly expanding use of SSRIs and the increasing number of officially recognized disorders for which they are prescribed strongly suggest an increase in cosmetic psychopharmacology. Today psychiatrists and primary care physicians prescribe antidepressants, including SSRIs, to treat not only depression but also social anxiety disorder, panic disorder, paraphilias such as exhibitionism and fetishism, sexual impulsivity, obsessive-compulsive disorder, and premenstrual dysphoric disorder.[10] The drugs' success in treating these disorders has been associated with marked increases in estimates of how often these disorders occur.[11]

Not everyone has greeted the expanding use of SSRIs—whether for enhancement purposes or for the treatment of depression, anxiety, and other disorders—with the enthusiasm that characterizes Kramer's reaction. In a reading reprinted here, Carol Freedman replies directly to Kramer's discussion of Prozac. According to Freedman, rather than regarding emotions primarily as pleasant or painful experiences—as if they were analogous to headaches (a view she attributes to Kramer)—we should conceptualize emotions as ways of understanding reality and one's situation in it. Accordingly, we should understand a particular emotional experience in terms of the *reasons why* someone has this experience rather than simply in terms of its *cause*, the latter concept encouraging an overly mechanistic approach. When we regard emotional problems as related to reasons, she continues, we are well positioned to address these problems with insight and understanding; failure to do so, by contrast, amounts to a failure to respect persons as selves and responsible agents. Responding to this and other leading concerns about the discretionary use of Prozac and similar medications, David DeGrazia, in another of this chapter's selections, argues that none of these concerns justifies a blanket moral condemnation of cosmetic psychopharmacology. Giving special attention to themes related to personal identity, DeGrazia further contends that deliberate self-transformation via Prozac can be, contrary to some critics, entirely authentic.

Other Types of Neuroenhancement The use of psychiatric medications for enhancement purposes can be seen as part of a broader category of enhancement that is sometimes called *neuroenhancement*. Let us use this term to refer to the full range of biomedical technologies that are employed in an effort to manipulate the human brain for enhancement purposes. These means can be relatively indirect as in the case of SSRIs for cosmetic psychopharmacology or the use of medications to enhance cognitive functions such as attention and memory. Some types of neuroenhancement, by contrast, operate more directly. Examples include transcranial magnetic stimulation, vagus nerve stimulation, and deep-brain stimulation (described in this chapter's selection by Martha J. Farah and Paul Root Wolpe), all of which have been used to improve mental functioning or mood in patients with psychiatric illness but can also, in principle if not yet in practice, be employed for enhancement purposes.

One trend that raises concerns about the appropriate use of medications and the boundaries of appropriate medical practice is the increasing prescription of stimulants such as Ritalin and Adderall for children. These apparently safe medications help people who have attention deficit/hyperactivity disorder (ADHD) as well as people who simply have trouble concentrating. Today, especially in the United States, these stimulants are increasingly prescribed to children—mostly boys—who have trouble focusing, sitting still, and completing assignments but may not meet clinical criteria for ADHD or any other disorder for which stimulants are normally prescribed. Are these children being drugged as an alternative to improving teacher-student ratios, making helpful changes in the home environment, or introducing other remedies to fairly normal, if inconvenient, juvenile behavior? Rather than taking stimulants on a regular basis, some children and teenagers take them to improve concentration during important exams or while completing especially taxing assignments. Is their reliance on a medication in such contexts in their long-term best interests? Is such discretionary use of stimulants fair to those children who lack access to them? Moreover, what is our society doing to childhood when pressures to behave and excel lead so many parents to seek stimulants for cognitively and behaviorally normal youngsters? These and other questions redound to a question raised earlier: Can physicians responsibly prescribe medications for patients who enjoy normal health and functioning? Claudia Mills addresses such questions as these in an article reprinted here.

In this chapter's final selection, Martha J. Farah and Paul Root Wolpe describe the use—for enhancement purposes—of such technologies as SSRIs and stimulants, transcranial magnetic stimulation, and brain-machine interfaces. Such biomedical enhancements, they argue, raise substantial concerns about safety as well as "a group of related concerns resulting from the many ways in which neuroscience-based enhancement intersects with our understanding of what it means to be a person, to be healthy and whole, to do meaningful work, and to value human life in all its imperfection."[12] Reflection on neuroenhancements and the biotechnologies that make them possible, they conclude, amplify the scientific image of human beings as part of nature while also threatening some traditional notions tied to our sense of personhood.

NOTES

1 Exceptions in the case of emergencies, in which there is insufficient time for obtaining informed consent, are generally accepted and may be justified by the assumption that patients *would* consent to interventions in such circumstances if they had the opportunity to do so. Such presumed consent may also justify other exceptions to the rule requiring (explicit) informed consent, but we need not consider them here.

2 One form of evidence that can be especially useful in attempting to determine what a formerly competent patient would have wanted in the present situation is an *advance directive* that offers some specific directions for treatment decisions. Allen E. Buchanan and Dan W. Brock have argued, however, that there are compelling reasons to conceptualize the honoring of advance directives as a distinct decision-making standard that is appropriately located between the informed-consent and substituted-judgment standards within the hierarchy under discussion. See *Deciding for Others* (Cambridge: Cambridge University Press, 1989), Chapter 2.

3 Lisa Melton, "New Perspectives on the Management of Intersex," *The Lancet* 357 (June 30, 2001), p. 2110.

4 "Dwarfism," *Medline Plus* (http://www.nlm.nih.gov/medlineplus/dwarfism.html).

5 Like intersex, dwarfism is commonly regarded as a medical condition, yet even this seemingly innocuous perception is highly questionable. While it is true that individuals of ambiguous sexuality and individuals of very short stature represent a statistical minority—and may in that sense be regarded as not normal—the perception of such individuals as abnormal in a more value-laden sense—that is, as having a problem that should, if possible, be fixed—may reflect social and cultural attitudes as much as, or more than, biological or medical realities. If no one felt disturbed by ambiguous sexuality, it is not clear what the basis would be for considering it abnormal in anything other than a statistical sense. It is true that many intersex individuals are infertile, but infertility itself is not normally regarded as a reason for invasive surgery. Nor does it seem plausible that nature divides human beings into two sexes but occasionally "goofs" by producing individuals with ambiguous sexuality. Nature has no need for the mutually exclusive and exhaustive categories for male and female as applied to human beings; the need, if it exists, derives from our attitudes. As for dwarfism, while it frequently results from a genetic or biological abnormality—in a sense involving some dysfunction (e.g., a deficiency in growth hormone)—short stature *per se* need not be problematic. Much of what is experienced as problematic in dwarfism is a function of the way furniture, stairs, and countless other cultural artifacts are constructed in view of the needs of a taller majority.

6 Eric Juengst, "What Does *Enhancement* Mean?" in Erik Parens (ed.), *Enhancing Human Traits* (Washington, DC: Georgetown University Press, 1998), p. 29.

7 French Anderson, "Human Gene Therapy: Scientific and Ethical Considerations," *Journal of Medicine and Philosophy* 10 (1985), pp. 275–291.

8 See, e.g., Erik Parens, "Is Better Always Good? The Enhancement Project," in *Enhancing Human Traits*, p. 5.

9 Peter D. Kramer, *Listening to Prozac* (New York: Viking, 1993).

10 Carl Elliott, *Better Than Well: American Medicine Meets the American Dream* (New York: Norton, 2003), p. 123.

11 David Healy, "Good Science or Good Business?" *Hastings Center Report* 30 (2) (2000), pp. 19-22.

12 These sorts of concerns are discussed with exceptional elegance in President's Council on Bioethics, *Beyond Therapy: Biotechnology and the Pursuit of Happiness* (Washington, DC: PCB, 2003).

CONTESTED THERAPIES

LETTING THE DEAF BE DEAF: RECONSIDERING THE USE OF COCHLEAR IMPLANTS IN PRELINGUISTICALLY DEAF CHILDREN

Robert A. Crouch

In this excerpt from a longer article, Crouch addresses the use of cochlear implants—devices that enable partial hearing—in children who are born deaf or who become deaf prior to any meaningful acquisition of an oral language. Contrary to the mainstream perspective that assumes that deafness is a disability (an objectively disadvantageous condition) and that it is in a prelinguistically deaf child's best interests to have these implants, Crouch advances two main arguments. First, he argues, cochlear implants often fail to achieve their objective: to enable the child not merely to hear sound, but to perceive speech well enough to be able to produce intelligible speech herself. Second, even if these technological limitations are overcome, a decision to forgo cochlear implants for one's child must be understood as conferring a tremendous advantage that mainstream, hearing society overlooks: "membership in the Deaf community, a unique community with a rich history, a rich language [American Sign Language], and a value system of its own." When the alleged disadvantages of being deaf are put into cultural perspective and the riches of membership in the Deaf community are appreciated, both individual decisions and educational policies affecting deaf children are more likely to be well-suited, rather than inimical, to their needs.

. . .

THE PROBLEM

The central concern of this paper is the problematic use of cochlear implants in "prelingually" deaf children; namely, those who are born deaf or who become deaf before any meaningful acquisition of oral language has taken place (roughly, before three or four years of age). My arguments against the use of cochlear implants do not apply to postlingually deafened adolescents and adults. And while I will be principally concerned throughout with deaf children of hearing parents, my views are equally applicable to deaf children of deaf parents.

In theory, the use of cochlear implants holds out the possibility of giving hearing to profoundly prelingually deaf children. In this regard, the use of cochlear implants in prelingually deaf children may be conceived of as an intervention that can

Reprinted with permission of the author and the publisher from *Hastings Center Report*, vol. 27 (July–August 1997), pp. 15–21. Copyright © 1997 by The Hastings Center.

determine community membership. In other words, the cochlear implant is intended to help the deaf child ultimately learn an oral language and, in so doing, to facilitate the assimilation of the implant-using child into the mainstream hearing culture. When the child receives a cochlear implant, he or she is put on a lifelong course of education and habilitation, the focus of which is the acquisition of an oral language, and ultimately, a meaningful engagement with the hearing world.

Hearing parents, not surprisingly, almost always decide that it is in their child's best interests to be "like us"; that is, to be hearing. Of course, given our predominantly hearing society, parents are also likely to believe that being hearing is objectively better than being deaf. Regardless of the parental motivation, these considerations underscore my claim that the intervention of cochlear implantation can be thought of as one that determines community membership. Struck by the otherness of the life that they imagine their child will lead—a life they imagine to be like their own lives would become if they were now suddenly to lose their hearing—parents will usually choose to provide their child with as much hearing as is medically possible either to prevent a chasm from opening up between them and their child (so that their child is in the same community as they are), or to avert what they believe will be the tragedies of a life bereft of sound (so that their child is in the "better" community).

The hope these parents have is made possible by the cochlear implant, an electronic device that consists of an externally worn speech processor and headset transmitter, and a surgically implanted receiver stimulator. Incoming speech is processed and transmitted through the skin to the implanted device, which then directly stimulates the auditory nerve of the child, thus bypassing the dysfunctional nerve endings within the deaf child's cochlea. Not all children who are born with profoundly impaired hearing, however, are potential candidates for cochlear implantation. The National Institutes of Health, in its consensus statement dealing with cochlear implants in adults and children, recently articulated a set of eligibility criteria to aid clinicians in identifying those who might reasonably be expected to benefit from a cochlear prosthetic. Prospective candidates must be older than two years of age; they must have profound bilateral sensorineural hearing loss with a hearing threshold greater than 90 dB (as a point of reference, the threshold of those without hearing loss is less than 25 dB)[1]; they must have used conventional hearing or vibrotactile aids and have received little or no benefit from such aids; the family and the child must display high motivation and appropriate expectations vis-à-vis the cochlear implant; and there must be no medical, financial, or psychosocial contraindications to implantation.[2]

Once selected and implanted, however, what can the child and the family expect from the cochlear implant? The most basic aim of the cochlear implant is to help the child perceive sound, and in this limited capacity the implant does work. Ultimately, however, the pragmatic goal of the cochlear implant is to facilitate the entrance of the previously deaf child into the hearing community. To accomplish this end, the following three conditions must obtain. First, the implant-using child must learn how to perceive, not merely *sound,* but *speech.* That is, the child must be able to identify parts of speech—for example, that the word just spoken has two syllables and that the stress is on the second syllable. And the child must be able to identify spoken words—for example, that the word just spoken was "dog." Second, once the child can identify speech and its components, she must then learn how to *produce intelligible speech* herself; if one is to function in the hearing world, one must be understood. Finally, the child must be able to *acquire an oral language,* by which I mean that the child must be able to hear and understand speech and then be able to respond intelligibly in grammatically correct speech.

Given the above three necessary conditions for the possibility of becoming a fully functional member of hearing society, the idea behind the cochlear implant is simple: the more speech a child can perceive, the easier it will be for that child to understand speech, to produce intelligible speech, and ultimately, to function in oral English. As one enthusiastic otologist claimed, "cochlear implants can drastically alter the future for most hearing-impaired children and take them into the 21st century as productive citizens in the hearing community."[3]

Has experience borne out such a proclamation? The results of longitudinal studies suggest that many deaf children who use and train with cochlear implants for extended periods of time do not improve their oral communication skills sufficiently to enable them to become functioning members of hearing society. In terms of speech recognition, the gains afforded by cochlear implantation for many prelingually deaf children are modest, especially if we recall that these children are engaged in auditory training and habilitation every day, be it at home with the parents, in the clinic, or in the school.[4] Similarly modest gains are observed when it comes to the speech production capabilities of implant-using children. A recent study showed that after five years of implant use the mean score for correct pronunciation of vowel sounds was 70 percent; although 70 percent is encouraging, this is a small benefit won only after five hard years of oral language habilitation, and a benefit that doubtfully brings the child closer to the ultimate goal of immersion in the hearing culture.[5] Moreover, in another study that measured the speech intelligibility of prelingually deaf children who had used their cochlear implants for three and a half years or more, only approximately 40 percent of the words spoken by these children were understood by a panel of three persons.[6]

Of course, there will always be success stories among implant-using prelingually deaf children. Yet such successes are so infrequent that focusing on them would misrepresent clinical reality. Despite the limited successes of the few, and despite the successes of the many on audiological tests of lesser importance, the performance of the cohort of interest on speech perception, production, and intelligibility is quite poor. The oral language acquisition skills in many implant-using children is at this stage essentially nonexistent.

The vexing clinical problem presented by prelingually deaf children is that unlike postlingually deafened children or adults, the prelingually deafened child has no solid linguistic foundation in place prior to the onset of deafness to enable the learning of an oral language. While the postlingually deafened person, once fitted with a cochlear implant, can maintain his or her present speech production capabilities and *relearn* to hear, the prelingually deaf child using a cochlear implant must be intensively taught and trained to recognize and produce each vowel and consonant sound and each word from the ground up. For the implant-using prelingually deaf child, then, the path to oral language development is a long and arduous one beset with many pitfalls, where there seems to be no guarantee that the destination will be reached.

OVERCOMING THE NARRATIVE OF DISABILLTY

The evidence suggests, then, that the benefits of cochlear implantation in many prelingually deaf children are modest. A general problem with the information available is that it has only been a little over six years since the U.S. Food and Drug Administration gave pre-market approval to implant children with the Nucleus-22 multichannel cochlear implant. Longitudinal studies with longer follow-up periods would be needed to determine more clearly what the *peak* benefits of implant use can be in this population. Nonetheless, with the available information, we might reasonably ask whether the benefits associated with the use of cochlear implants outweigh the burdens of this procedure, and whether there are other reasonable options for deaf children. Although the cochlear implant works quite well in populations of postlingually deafened persons,[7] the good results of those studies simply cannot be generalized to prelingually deafened children. I believe that given the current state of knowledge vis-à-vis cochlear implant efficacy, the burdens associated with cochlear implant use do indeed outweigh the benefits and we should rethink the policy of using implants in many prelingually deaf children and examine other options.

However, as with many newly introduced medical interventions, it is not unreasonable to expect that five to ten years hence, when more follow-up years have been observed and when possible improvements in technology have been made, otologists and audiologists will be able to claim greater successes for the cochlear implant in prelingually deaf children. Yet even if such were the case, I would invoke another, perhaps more fundamental critique. It is my contention that the predominant view of deafness—that the deaf are "merely and wholly" disabled[8]—is wrong and that we should quickly disabuse ourselves of this ill-begotten notion. Considered in the proper light, the decision to forgo cochlear implantation for one's child, far from condemning a child to a world of meaningless silence, opens the child up to membership in the Deaf community, a unique community with a rich history, a rich language, and a value system of its own.[9] Thus, contrary to popularly held beliefs, the child who is permitted to remain deaf *can* look forward to acquiring a language, namely, American Sign Language (ASL), or whatever signed language is indigenous to the child's geographical area. And when the child has acquired such a language, she thereby possesses the language of an active cultural and linguistic minority group, which can then serve as the linguistic foundations upon which new written languages can be built, thereby ensuring access to the wider hearing society. Once we conceive of the Deaf as being members of a linguistic and cultural minority, our moral landscape should be altered. My beliefs regarding the value of Deaf culture, the richness of the lives of Deaf persons, and the importance of recognizing and overcoming our cultural biases regarding the Deaf would therefore be unchanged by a dramatic improvement in implant efficacy.

What I hope to demonstrate, then, is that parents of prelingually deaf children have a reasonable basis upon which to refuse a cochlear implant for their child, either presently, because of a mix of reasons, including poor implant efficacy, the burdens associated with ineffective implant use, and the benefits of membership in the Deaf community, or at some unknown point in the future when cochlear implants might work with greatly improved efficacy, because of the benefits of membership in the Deaf community. I do not endorse the view that the only reason it is acceptable to be a member of the Deaf community is that there is no way to treat one's impaired hearing. This paper represents, then, one response to a current medical and societal state-of-affairs. I ask: Given the efficacy of cochlear implants in prelingually deaf children, and given the authentic nature of signed languages and Deaf communities, what are some of the options available for prelingually deaf children, and which option might be reasonable to choose? While many may find the terms in which the debate is presently carried out philosophically uninteresting, preferring instead to examine a possible world where cochlear implants were significantly

efficacious, the present moral problem as I see it seems sufficiently worthy of attention.

It is important at this point to understand why the goal of implantation and oral language habilitation has been pursued so aggressively. It is not, I would claim, being pursued simply because of the benefits that come with being able to hear in a predominantly hearing society, but more importantly it is also being pursued because of the perceived burdens associated with being deaf. Indeed, given the rather poor efficacy of cochlear implants in many prelingually deaf children, there seems to be an implicit belief that while implants may not work that well, surely some hearing and oral language, however rudimentary, is better than none. To take one example, supporters of cochlear implant use frequently recite the fact that by the age of five, a child with no hearing impairment will commonly have a vocabulary of between 5,000 and 26,000 words, while at the same age a deaf child will have a far inferior vocabulary of only 200 signed or spoken words.[10] The implication of this line of thought is that deaf children should be fitted with cochlear implants and that exclusive oral language instruction should be pursued aggressively so that such tragic outcomes can be avoided. While this reasoning does display its own internal logic, it shows little sensitivity to the deaf child's educational context, and to the history of the education of the deaf, which has produced generations of deaf persons who have suffered from linguistic and educational neglect.[11] Once we recognize that historically deaf children have been educated predominantly in an oral-only environment—despite their imperfect auditory systems and to the exclusion of ASL training—it should not surprise us that their vocabularies are often much smaller, and that their emotional and social development so often lags behind that of their hearing counterparts.

To be sure, the education of deaf children has improved somewhat in the last forty years, but the denial of the Deaf perspective chiefly remains. For example, legislation, in the form of the Individuals with Disabilities Education Act (IDEA-B) of 1975, mandated that the educational segregation of deaf children be stopped and that the deaf be "mainstreamed" into regular hearing classrooms so that their oral skills would improve, and with them their emotional and social skills. However, with its emphasis on educational integration, the IDEA-B purchased increased access to oral education for deaf children at the cost of a dramatic decrease in the quality of their education.[12] Often, the best that the deaf student can hope for is to be given access to an unskilled ASL interpreter, or to an interpreter in the classroom who knows no ASL and who works only in manually coded English—a manual form of English that follows the rules of English grammar, and that seems not to help deaf children learn English.[13] The life of a deaf child in such a mainstreamed educational environment can also be very difficult socially. A boy in the eighth grade who testified before the U.S. National Council on Disabilities began by declaring, "I'm not disabled, just deaf," and went on to give an account of how it feels to be forced into an educational environment where the focus is on oral English acquisition. He testified: "Learning through an interpreter is very hard; it's bad socially in the mainstream; you are always outnumbered; you don't feel like it's your school; you never know deaf adults; you don't belong; you don't feel comfortable as a deaf person." Another boy, also attempting to learn oral English at school, put it more starkly: "I hate it if people know I am deaf."[14]

The perspective *of the Deaf* in creating educational policies *for the Deaf* has mostly been ignored, and consequently, the outcome of the "education" of deaf children by means illsuited, inimical in fact, to their needs, perpetuates the stereotypical view of deaf people as disabled and slower witted than their hearing counterparts. Against such an historical background, the proper response is not to maintain that deaf people will unavoidably lead impoverished and fragmentary lives, but rather to start paying attention to the Deaf point of view and to realize that positive change can thereby be effected.

As with previous strategies for the deaf, the decision to pursue cochlear implantation and auditory habilitation for one's child also has burdens associated with it beyond the failure to achieve oral language competence. The child whose life is centered upon disability and the attempt to overcome it grows up in a context that continually reinforces this disability, despite his or her own best efforts to hear and

to speak and despite the diligent work of the educators of the deaf and hearing-impaired. These children are therefore always aware that they are outsiders, and not merely outsiders, but outsiders attempting to be on the inside. This narrative of disability within which the deaf implant-using child lives is not the only one available to her. There is an alternate narrative in reference to which the child may judge her own life and it is the one that exists within the Deaf community. Simply put, my concerns about the burdens of using cochlear implants in prelingually deaf children can be reduced to a cluster of considerations grouped under the heading of "opportunity costs." One of the main burdens of implanting a child and setting her on the course of auditory habilitation is that it deprives her of the alternate linguistic, educational, and social opportunities that the Deaf community can offer her, while (presently) offering a poor guarantee that functional membership in the hearing community will materialize.

Contrary to what many believe, the Deaf community has a distinct history, language, and value system that plays a central role in the lives of its members. Two prominent members of the American Deaf community have noted that the beliefs and practices that make up the culture of Deaf people should not be viewed simply as "a camaraderie with others who have a similar physical condition," but rather as "like many other cultures in the traditional sense of the term, historically created and actively transmitted across generations."[15] Members of the Deaf community have their own language that, far from being merely a means of communication, is also, as are other languages, a "repository of cultural knowledge and a symbol of social identity."[16] In contrast to Helmer Myklebust's claims that the manual signed languages of Deaf persons were "inferior to the verbal as a language" because they lacked "precision, subtlety, and flexibility," and that humans would not be able to achieve their "ultimate potential" through signed languages,[17] Carol Padden and Tom Humphries have argued that

> Despite the misconceptions, for Deaf people, their sign language is a creation of their history and is what allows them to fulfull the potential for which

evolution has prepared them—*to attain full human communication as makers and users of symbols.* (emphasis added) (p. 9)

Thus, the deaf child no less than the hearing child has all the requisite skills that will enable her to achieve a different, but no less human, expressive potential.

The key point is that this narrative is a *validating narrative,* it is, in other words, a socially available story to which the child may refer when building his own life and making sense of that life and the lives of those around him. As the child learns about adult members of his Deaf community, or historic Deaf figures, or the history of ASL, or Deaf poetry and theater he "gains ideas of [the] possible lives that he can lead and finds a basis for self-esteem in a [hearing] society that insists he is inferior."[18] But it does more than that: it also provides a basis for self-*respect,* that is, for the Deaf child's sense of dignity according to the community's acceptance and valorization of the Deaf way of being-in-the-world.[19] Identification with the Deaf community is important, then, because it opens up a cultural space within which the Deaf *themselves* may establish their own norms, and within which one's sense of personal dignity is thereby engendered. Access to the validating narrative of the Deaf community will thus enable Deaf children to see themselves in a more positive light, while their peers and teachers will see them in this way and relate to them as similarly situated individuals in a shared story.

The implant-using child, although nominally within hearing culture, is, as I have claimed, virtually condemned to be an outsider—not only from the perspective of the hearing world, but also from the perspective of the Deaf world, which generally looks down upon those who attempt to be, as they say, ORAL. The child who embraces Deaf culture, on the other hand, *will* have a context, he will have a milieu in which to make sense of his life, and he will be an insider.

A key component of this view involves regarding members of the Deaf community as part of a *linguistic* minority. In my discussion of the goals of cochlear implants above, I claimed that the aim of the implant was to facilitate the entry of the hearing-impaired child into the hearing world. Two of the

necessary conditions of entry were sufficiently comptent speech production capabilities as well as the acquisition of an oral language. But as I claimed, intelligible speech production is virtually denied to many implant-using prelingually deaf children, and consequently, so too is *oral language* acquisition. Indeed, although intelligible *oral* language acquisition is only marginally possible, *language* acquisition need not be at all: "sign or speech can serve as the vehicle of language."[20]

As with other signed languages, ASL is not a manual version of English; it is, rather, a distinct language with a syntax and a grammar independent of English.[21] "Languages," as Harlan Lane has observed, "have evolved within communities in a way responsive to the needs of those communities. ASL is attuned to the needs of the deaf community in the United States; English is not."[22] This point has important consequences for the issue at hand. For the prelingually deaf child, signed languages are acquired with far greater facility than spoken languages are acquired by those using cochlear implants, and there is no evidence to indicate that the use of ASL will interfere with the child's ability to learn written English, or any other written languages.[23] On the contrary, the deaf children who perform the best on measures of educational and language achievement are the 10 percent who come from deaf parents and who learned ASL as a first language.[24] Thus, learning ASL as a primary language will enable the learning of written English as a second language, and this familiarity with written English leads to further successes in the educational and occupational disciplines to which the written word gives access, thereby increasing the Deaf person's links with the wider hearing community.

Placing prelingually deaf children in an environment where they can only learn oral language through an imperfect auditory system (even with cochlear implants) disadvantages many of them because not only do they fail to acquire an oral language, but perhaps more harmfully, their exposure to ASL is delayed, thus making their acquisition of ASL (and written English) far more difficult and incomplete.[25] The delay in the acquisition of ASL caused by the implant-using child's attempt to learn an oral language will delay the child's exposure to and engagement with the Deaf community, and is unlikely to help the child assimilate into the hearing community. Denying prelingually deaf children the opportunity to immerse themselves immediately in ASL puts them *between* two cultures and *within* neither of them, a situation we should strive to avoid.

THINKING CLEARLY ABOUT DEAFNESS AND DISABILITY

. . .

In my case for the legitimacy and importance of the Deaf community to the prelingually deaf child, I hope I have provided reasonable grounds upon which parents can refuse cochlear implants for their child. It is impossible, of course, to construct a convincing argument that will be applicable to all deaf children, given the different expressive capabilities (sign or oral) that such children will invariably possess. But I hope to have avoided some of the problematic elements that come with, on the one hand, the arguments of those who maintain that all cochlear implantation is a form of cultural genocide, and, on the other hand, the arguments of those who believe that cochlear implants are a panacea.

ACKNOWLEDGMENTS

I would like to thank the Fonds pour la Formation de Chercheurs et l'Aide à la Recherche (Quebec, Canada) for research funds while I was working on this project. I am thankful to the following people for their helpful comments and criticisms: Carl Elliott, Karen Lebacqz, Jamie MacDougall, Gilles Reid, Lainie Friedman Ross, Charles Weijer, Anna Zalewski, the editors of the Report, and three anonymous reviewers. I am also thankful to audiences at the 7th Annual Canadian Bioethics Society Conference in Vancouver (1995), at the McGill University Biomedical Ethics Unit in Montreal (1996), at the Montreal Children's Hospital (1996), at the Annual Meeting of the Society for Health and Human Values/Society for Bioethics Consultation in Cleveland (1996), and at the University of Virginia Health Sciences Center in Charlottesville (1997) who heard and commented upon earlier versions of the paper.

I would like to dedicate this paper to the memory of my first bioethics teacher, Benjamin Freedman.

REFERENCES

1 Thomas Balkany, "A Brief Perspective on Cochlear Implants," *NEJM* 328 (1993): 281–82, at p. 281.

2 National Institutes of Health, *Cochlear Implants in Adults and Children, NIH Consensus Statement* 13, no. 2 (1995): 1–30, at pp. 18–20.

3 Michael E. Glasscock, "Education of Hearing-Impaired Children in the United States," *The American Journal of Otology* 13, no. 1 (1992): 4–5, at p. 5.

4 Richard T. Miyamoto et al.," "Prelingually Deafened Children's Performance with the Nucleus Multichannel Cochlear Implant," *The American Journal of Otology* 14, no. 5 (1993): 437–45; John J. Shea III et al., "Speech Perception after Multichannel Cochlear Implantation in the Pediatric Patient." *The American Journal of Otology* 15, no. 1 (1994): 66–70; Harlan Lane, "Letters to the Editor," *The American Journal of Otology* 16, no. 3 (1995): 393–99.

5 Bruce J. Gantz et al., "Results of Multichannel Cochlear Implants in Congenital and Acquired Prelingual Deafness in Children: Five-year Follow-up," *American Journal of Otology* 15, Suppl. no. 2 (1994): 1–7.

6 Miyamoto et al., "Speech Perception and Speech Production Skills of Children with Multichannel Cochlear Implants."

7 Noel L. Cohen et al., "A Prospective, Randomized Study of Cochlear Implants," *NEJM* 328 (1993): 233–37.

8 The phrase "merely and wholly" disabled is inspired by Oliver Sacks (*The Man Who Mistook his Wife for a Hat*, p. 180), and is invoked to express the view that the deaf are disabled and nothing other than disabled people.

9 The convention in the literature is to put the word deaf in lower case when referring to the biological condition of not being able to hear, and upper case, Deaf, when referring to the cultural aspects of being deaf.

10 American Academy of Otolaryngology–Head and Neck Surgery Subcommittee on Cochlear Implants, "Status of Cochlear Implantation in Children," *The Journal of Pediatrics* 118, no. 1 (1991): 1–7; Balkany, "A Brief Perspective on Cochlear Implants."

11 The history of the education of deaf persons is indeed a tragic one, consisting of a series of ignorant and destructive decisions made by the hearing on behalf of the deaf. What runs through this history of the last two hundred years is a systematic suppression of the Deaf perspective. Of course, the great triumph for the Deaf is that despite the attempts of the hearing to do away with ASL, it survives to the present day largely unchanged from what it was, say, one hundred years ago. Two excellent accounts of this story are, Harlan Lane, *When the Mind Hears. A History of the Deaf* (New York: Vintage, 1984): Douglas C. Baynton, *Forbidden Signs: American Culture and the Campaign Against Sign Language* (Chicago: University of Chicago Press, 1996).

12 On this see, Sy Dubow, " 'Into the Turbulent Mainstream'— A Legal Perspective on the Weight to be Given to the Least Restrictive Environment in Placement Decisions for Deaf Children," *Journal of Law & Education* 18, no. 2 (1989): 215–28; Kathryn Ivers, "Towards a Bilingual Education

Policy in the Mainstreaming of Deaf Children," *Columbia Human Rights Law Review* 26 (1995): 439–82.

13 David A. Stewart, "Bi-Bi to MCE?" *American Annals of the Deaf* 138, no. 4 (1993): 331–37.

14 As quoted in Lane, *The Mask of Benevolence*, pp. 136–7.

15 Carol Padden and Tom Humphries, *Deaf in America: Voices from a Culture* (Cambridge, Mass.: Harvard University Press, 1988), p. 2.

16 Lane, *The Mask of Benevolence*, p. 45.

17 Helmer R. Myklebust, *The Psychology of Deafness: Sensory Deprivation, Learning and Adjustment* (New York: Grune and Stratton, 1960), pp. 241–42. This passage was quoted in Padden and Humphries, *Deaf in America*, p. 59.

18 Lane, *The Mask of Benevolence*, p. 172.

19 I am relying on the distinction between self-esteem and self-respect articulated by Michael Walzer in *Spheres of Justice*. According to Walzer, while self-esteem is a relational concept—one dependent upon the relative standing of citizens—self-respect is an external, normative concept—one dependent upon the "moral understanding of persons and positions" within the community. See, Michael Walzer, *Spheres of Justice: A Defense of Pluralism and Equality* (New York: Basic Books, 1983), pp. 272–80, at 274.

20 David M. Perlmutter, "The Language of the Deaf," *The New York Review of Books* 38, no. 7 (1991): 65–72, at p. 72.

21 Edward Klima and Ursula Bellugi, *The Signs of Language* (Cambridge, Mass.: Harvard University Press, 1979); Schein and Stewart, *Language in Motion;* Perlmutter, "The Language of the Deaf."

22 Lane, *The Mask of Benevolence*, p. 125.

23 Heather Mohay, "Letters to the Editor: Opposition from Deaf Groups to the Cochlear Implant," *The Medical Journal of Australia* 155, no. 10 (1991): 719–20.

24 As noted in Lane, *The Mask of Benevolence*, p. 138. See, Abraham Zweibel, "More on the Effects of Early Manual Communication on the Cognitive Development of Deaf Children," *American Annals of the Deaf* 132, no. 1 (1987): 16-20; Ann E. Geers and Brenda Schick, "Acquisition of Spoken and Signed English by Hearing-Impaired Children of Hearing-Impaired or Hearing Parents," *Journal of Speech and Hearing Disorders* 53, no. 2 (1988): 136–43; Stephen P. Quigley and Robert E. Kretschmer, *The Education of Deaf Children: Issues, Theory and Practice* (London: Edward Arnold, 1982).

25 Mohay, "Letters to the Editor: Opposition from Deaf Groups to the Cochlear Implant."

DEAF CULTURE, COCHLEAR IMPLANTS, AND ELECTIVE DISABILITY

Bonnie Poitras Tucker

In this excerpt from a longer article, Tucker addresses the claim that cochlear implants represent a threat to Deaf (with a capital D) culture by enabling partial hearing in deaf persons. Proponents of Deaf culture, she explains, understand deafness as a cultural identity rather than a disability, express pride in their shared use of American Sign Language (ASL), and reject efforts, such as the use of cochlear implants, to assimilate deaf persons into the hearing mainstream. In response to this position, Tucker, who is deaf, argues that inability to hear is genuinely disadvantageous, that learning English as well as ASL better overcomes these disadvantages than does learning ASL alone, and that cochlear implants expand the range of opportunities available to deaf children whereas hostility to mainstream hearing culture narrows those opportunities. She also criticizes those who reject cochlear implants yet demand costly accommodations for their deafness.

During the past decade, a growing concept of Deaf culture has taken root. Under this concept, people who cannot hear are viewed as either deaf (with a small d) or Deaf (with a capital D). Persons who view themselves as deaf are those who, although impaired in their ability to hear, have assimilated into hearing society and do not view themselves as members of a separate culture. People who call themselves "Deaf," however, view and define deafness as a cultural identity rather than as a disability for some purposes; they

Reprinted with permission of the author and the publisher from *Hastings Center Report*, vol. 28 (July–August 1998), pp. 6–9, 13–14, Copyright © 1998 by The Hastings Center.

insist that their culture and separate identity must be nourished and maintained.[1]

A cochlear implant is a surgically implanted device that is capable of restoring hearing and speech understanding to many individuals who are severely or profoundly deaf. Numerous studies show both the ability of profoundly deaf individuals to hear speech with cochlear implants and the ability of implanted deaf children to develop age-appropriate spoken and receptive language skills.[2] As reported in May 1998 to the Advisory Council of the National Institute on Deafness and Other Communication Disorders: "It has now been demonstrated that the long-term benefits of cochlear implants in children are not limited to speech recognition but extend into dramatically improved language learning and language skills."[3] In a recent survey, parents of 176 implanted children perceived that: (1) 44 percent of the children had greater than 70 percent open speech discrimination (using sound alone with no visual clues), (2) 61 percent of the children had greater than 50 percent open speech discrimination, and (3) 84 percent of the children had greater than 40 percent open speech discrimination.[4]

Because cochlear implants have the potential to ameliorate or eliminate ramifications of deafness, they are opposed by Deaf culturists, who view efforts to "cure" deafness or ameliorate its effects as an immoral means of killing Deaf culture.

The theory of Deaf culture is primarily premised on a shared language—American Sign Language (ASL). Individuals who communicate via ASL clearly *do* speak a different language. American Sign Language is visual rather than spoken, with its own syntax and grammar. ASL is quite different from signed English, which involves signing each English word as it is spoken, using English grammar and structure. In addition, some members of the Deaf cultural community claim to be part of a separate culture as a result of attending segregated (often residential) schools for Deaf children,[5] or as a result of their participation in Deaf clubs or wholly Deaf environments in which they socialize or work.

According to the leaders of the National Association of the Deaf (NAD), Deaf people like being Deaf, want to be Deaf, and are proud of their Deafness. Deaf culturists claim the right to their own "ethnicity, with [their] own language and culture, the same way that Native Americans or Italians [or blacks] bond together."[6] They claim the right to "personal diversity," which is "something to be cherished rather than fixed and erased." In short, they claim the right to their "birthright of silence."

Many individuals who are deaf, however, do not agree that these facts give rise to a true culture. The now deceased Larry G. Stewart, a leading member of the signing deaf community (a strong proponent and user of sign language), noted that "'[D]eaf culture' was not discovered; it was created for political purposes. The term has yet to be satisfactorily defined."[7] Dr. Stewart went on to say that "[i]n the larger sense of world cultures, the meaning of culture is so powerful and complex that to apply it so narrowly to a group of highly diverse deaf American citizens, whose members are as heterogeneous as the general population, simply makes no sense" (p. 129).

Although Deaf culturists equate being deaf to being a member of a racial or tribal minority, many deaf people find the analogy nonsensical. Deaf people lack one of the five critical senses. True deaf people such as this author are physically incapable of talking on the telephone alone. We have to use the phone with the aid of a third party—an interpreter or a relay service, both of which present extremely awkward situations. Most of us would *love* to be able to pick up the telephone and make a personal or business call when and how we feel like it without having to scramble to find an interpreter and without having to make the call with a third person privy to every word. We'd like to be able to go to a movie or a play regardless of whether captioning or interpreters are available. We'd like to be able to participate in group conversations, to hear the conversation at the dinner table. We'd like to be able to hear music; to hear our children and grandchildren laugh and cry; to listen to the radio when we are driving; to have a car phone; to be able to use the drive-up window at McDonald's; to hear the announcements at the airport, to be able to talk to the person in front of or behind us on a hiking trail; to be able to go to a professional meeting on the spur of the moment; to be able to get any job we want without having to consider how our deafness will interfere with the job duties. We'd particularly like to hear our own voices and to be able to control the tone and pitch and loudness of our voices. The list is endless. Why would any human being *want* to deny such pleasures to herself or her children?

Many members of the Deaf cultural community strongly desire to have Deaf children, who will be a part of their parents' Deaf culture. Some expectant Deaf parents visit geneticists for the purpose of determining whether their children are likely to be born deaf. As explained by Jamie Israel, a genetic counselor at Gallaudet University's genetic services center, "[m]any of our [Deaf] families are not interested in fixing or curing deaf genes . . . [m]any . . . couples come in and want . . . [D]eaf children."[8] If their children are *not* likely to be born deaf, Deaf parents may choose not to have children, or to abort children in gestation, just as hearing or deaf people who determine through genetic research that their children *are* likely to be born deaf may choose not to have children or to abort children in gestation.

The desire of parents to have children who will be like them and fit into their world is certainly understandable. But most parents want more for their children than they have. While this author's parents, for example, never went to college, they wanted all their children to have that opportunity. Similarly, although we cannot hear, most people who are deaf want our children and grandchildren to have that ability.

Dena S. Davis notes that "the primary argument against deliberately seeking to produce deaf children is that it violates the child's own autonomy and narrows the scope of her choices when she grows up; in other words, it violates her right to an 'open future.'"[9] Insisting that children who are deaf be raised in a Deaf cultural community denies these children the right to choose for themselves whether to accept or reject the larger hearing world.

Deaf culturists argue that parents should not make decisions about cochlear implants for their deaf children, that the children should be allowed to make such decisions for themselves when they are old enough to do so. However, experience has proven that early implantation is necessary for maximum efficacy of a cochlear implant. Thus, waiting ten or fifteen years to make the decision for a child

to have a cochlear implant is the same as deciding that the child will *not* have an implant. If a child who is deaf is going to learn to talk, he or she must begin learning at a *very* early age. A person who is deaf does not learn to speak at the age of twelve or older, the age at which the child is arguably old enough to decide for herself how she wants to live her life. But a child who is deaf who learns to speak and is part of the hearing world during childhood *can* learn to sign later in life and join the Deaf world.

Many of the leaders of the Deaf culture movement can speak, as a result of early oral training (or in a few cases because they became deaf later in life), and the majority of those leaders know perfect English—although they know ASL as well. Indeed, it is their oral skills that have enabled them to argue for Deaf isolationism so persuasively. Many of these leaders of Deaf culture, however, do not want today's deaf children to learn spoken English. Rather, they believe that spoken English should be rejected by Deaf people, and that Deaf people should use only ASL as their mode of "spoken" (actually signed) language. This is known as the "bi-bi," or "bilingual-bicultural" approach.[10] Under this approach, Deaf children are to learn ASL only, and not spoken *or* signed English. Bi-bi advocates believe that children who are deaf should be taught their "natural language" of ASL, which they consider to be the "birthright of all deaf children" (p. 60). Their rationale is expressed as follows:

> Natural sign not only serves deaf children as a means of communication between other sign language users but can support intellectual development and the acquisition of ideas in the same way that spoken language serves hearing people. It is, therefore, a folly, say bilingualists, to create an artificial sign system, such as SE [signed English] . . . when a bona fide sign language already exists. It is not only a folly but, say most supporters of bilingualism, a moral crime to attempt to force young deaf children to do something they cannot do, that is, learn spoken language as a first language. . . . (p. 63)

The contention on the part of the Deaf culture movement that children who are deaf are unable to "learn spoken language as a first language" is, of course, belied by the thousands of deaf children, including this author, who have learned spoken language as a first (and in many cases only) language. Nevertheless, advocates of biculturalism espouse the view that once a child who is deaf has acquired a strong "natural" language (ASL), the child can then be taught *written* (but not spoken) English as a second language. What biculturists do not explain, at least in any satisfactory manner, is why even if one accepts the proposition that sign language is more natural to deaf children than speech, learning ASL is more "natural" than learning signed English. Nor do biculturists explain why a child who is deaf should have to struggle with learning to read and write English as a second language, when even if the child is taught to sign only, it would be so much easier for the child to learn and sign English, and then apply those English signing skills when learning how to read and write.

The leaders of Deaf culture who espouse the most radical interpretation of the "bi-bi" movement and want to deny children who are deaf both spoken and signed English, would deny deaf children the very skills that allow many of the Deaf culture leaders to perform successfully in this hearing world. One oral deaf leader, Kevin Nolan, noted that "nearly all" the Deaf culture leaders he knows "have had the benefit of early oral education."[11] Mr. Nolan asks:

> Why should they deny children who are deaf the opportunity to realize the same oral successes that they themselves have experienced? . . . Having benefited from oral education in their own childhoods, why do they . . . deny their oral backgrounds—those very backgrounds that helped them to become the leaders that they are today? (p. T3)

When this author and many of the leaders of the Deaf culture movement were growing up, technology was very limited. Most people of our generation (born at least between 1940 and 1960) who are profoundly deaf were not able to obtain much, if any, benefit from hearing aids. (This author, for example, has never been able to wear a hearing aid.) The times have changed, drastically! Technology has *vastly* improved. Today's deaf children are able to wear

much-improved hearing aids or to have cochlear implants. And the technology is still improving rapidly. It is very likely that in ten to fifteen years, perhaps less, cochlear implants will have improved to the point where almost all children who are deaf could benefit very substantially from an implant.

Deaf culture advocates, however, are strongly opposed to research geared at "curing" deafness and are particularly opposed to placing cochlear implants in children. They assert that members of their minority group "are in no more need of a cure for their condition than are Haitians or Hispanics."[12] To many members of the Deaf cultural community, cochlear implants represent "the ultimate denial of deafness, the ultimate refusal to let deaf children be Deaf" (p. 40). As stated by Roz Rosen, former president of NAD, since "[h]earing is not a life or death matter . . . [it is] consequently not worth the medical, moral and ethical risk of altering a child."[13] In accord with this reasoning, Deaf culturists have strongly criticized the National Institute of Health's National Institute on Deafness and Other Communication Disorders, which gives federal grants for research geared at the prevention and treatment of deafness and other communication disorders.[14]

Gallaudet students and their families or friends have informed this author that cochlear implants are greatly frowned upon at Gallaudet, and that implanted individuals who attend Gallaudet are usually pressured (often by their peers rather than by staff or faculty members) to remove them or at least not to wear their processors. As one reporter succinctly stated:

> As anyone at Gallaudet knows, a student with a [cochlear implant] device . . . runs the risk of being shunned. "I have some friends with implants," says Scott Mohan, a sixth generation deaf senior at Gallaudet. "They just don't use them anymore."
>
> "You can understand why," says Keith Muller, Executive Director of the League for the Hard of Hearing in New York City. "Kids who try to speak in deaf schools are ridiculed. And the greater their oral success, the more they are criticized."[15]

The hatred with which Deaf culturists view cochlear implants is expressed in the ASL sign for a cochlear implant, which contains a two-fingered stab to the back of the neck, indicating a "vampire" in the cochlea.

One individual seeking information about cochlear implants sent a list of questions to selected cochlear implant recipients and parents of children with cochlear implants.[16] Questions asked included the following:

> (1) Do you think that having a cochlear implant takes away your Deaf pride?
> (2) Do you think that cochlear implants remove you as a member of Deaf culture?
> (3) Do you think that cochlear implants are a way for hearing people to break down Deaf society?
> (4) Do you think that a person should be allowed to choose whether or not to have a cochlear implant or should it be left up to the parents to decide? (Take into consideration that the longer you wait, the less likely it is that [the implant] will work).

At least several recipients of that questionnaire were angered by these questions. The responses of three individuals are illustrative.

To the question about whether cochlear implants take away "your Deaf pride," one respondent, Bill Boyle, noted, ". . . what the hell is deaf pride? Proud not to hear your child's voice, pianos, the birds in the trees? That's not pride, it's bull-headedness and selfishness. . . . I feel the implant enhances my pride. I am proud to be overcoming what was considered a severe handicap, proud to be part of the community as a whole, not to a 'club' of narrow minded people."[17]

To the question about whether cochlear implants "remove you as a member of Deaf culture," another recipient, Melissa Chaikof, responded:

> If the cochlear implant has removed my daughters from "[D]eaf culture," and it probably has, then that is fine by me. The [D]eaf culturists' opportunities in life are so limited, and my daughters' are not. Furthermore, it has been the choice of those in the "[D]eaf culture" to exclude those with implants from their group. . . .[18]

To the question about whether cochlear implants are a way for hearing people to break down Deaf so-

ciety, Ms. Chaikof stated: "In obtaining implants for our daughters, we did not have the ulterior motive of 'breaking down Deaf society. If that is an indirect result . . . [m]y concern for my daughters' futures is far greater than for the future of 'Deaf society.'"

The three respondents replied to the question about whether a person should be allowed to choose whether to have a cochlear implant or whether parents should make that decision as follows:

> (i) Mildred Oberkotter replied: "for young children, it is essential that parents choose what is best for their child's interest and [the child's ability to] function in his/her culture in which s/he is born. So much time and possible maximum value would be lost in language and auditory development if and when the child is cognitively ready to make such a decision for him/herself."[19]
> (ii) Melissa Chaikof replied: "I absolutely think that the decision as to whether or not to implant should be in the hands of the parents. . . and the implant team. Some children and some families make better candidates. For example, one implant team here will not implant children in total communication [sign and some speech] or manual [sign language only] programs . . . [T]he kids whose parents are committed to an auditory-verbal approach [learning to listen], as we are, stand a very high chance of success."
> (iii) Bill Boyle replied: "If this [question] is about children, it is an enormous responsibility for the parents to decide. *But*—it is a decision [for] the parents who truly believe that their decision will be in the best interest of their child, and not a decision [for] NAD or others to decide. Yes, the longer you wait, the less benefit, so leave the parents alone and let them decide. . . ."

. . . Cochlear implants do not, and likely will not, eliminate deafness altogether. An individual who has an implant is still deaf. The difference is, however, that the ramifications of deafness are significantly reduced. At the present time, it is known that most children, and people who become deaf later in life and have memory of normal hearing, do very well with cochlear implants, thus reducing (if not eliminating) the need for special schools, interpreters, and other costly accommodations. Such individuals who refuse today to have cochlear implants, yet demand costly accommodations, should, in this author's opinion, be viewed as acting unethically.

In spite of all that is said above, it is impossible not to recognize the source and validity of the anger, hostility, and solidarity expressed by the Deaf culturists who choose to reject hearing society and who do not wish to be "hearing" to any degree. Any individual with any compassion who knows anything of the history of people who are deaf must understand how the concept of Deaf culture came into existence. Many people who are deaf continue to live as second class citizens, as indicated not only by the rejection of deaf people by most hearing people but by the facts that:

> The average deaf person today reads at a fourth grade level. One in three drops out of high school. Only one in five who starts college gets a degree. Deaf adults make 30 percent less than the general population. Their unemployment rate is high, and when they are employed, it is usually in manual jobs such as kitchen workers, janitors, machine operators, tailors and carpenters, for which a strong command of English is not required . . .[20]

Rejecting hearing society, technology that will alleviate the ramifications of deafness, and the potential eradication of most deafness, however, is not the solution to the problems of deaf people. Rather, deaf people with cochlear implants, particularly children, have a wealth of opportunities and potential life experiences available to them. To deny such opportunities based on theories of segregation is indeed illogical.

REFERENCES

1 For an article explaining the viewpoint of Deaf culture, see Edward Dolnick, "Deafness as Culture," *Atlantic* 272, no. 3 (1993): 37–53.

2 See, for example, Susan B. Waltzman, Noel L. Cohen, Railey H. Gomolin, Janet E. Green, William H. Shapiro et al., "Open-Set Speech Perception in Congenitally Deaf Children Using Cochlear Implants," *American Journal of Otology* 18, no. 3 (1997): 342–49; "Progress Report, Outcomes for Paediatric Cochlear Implantation in Nottingham: Safe—Effective—Effecient," Nottingham Paediatric Cochlear Programme, University Hospital NHS Trust, Queens Medical Centre, Nottingham, England (May 1997); T.A. Zwolan, P. R. Kileny, S. A. Telian, "Self-Report

of Cochlear Implant Use and Satisfaction by Prelingually Deafened Adults," *Ear & Hearing* 17, no. 3 (1996): 198–210; Amy M. Robbins, "Implanted Children Can Speak, But Can They Communicate?" Paper Presented at the Sixth Symposium on Cochlear Implants in Children, University of Miami School of Medicine, Miami, Florida, February 1996; N. M. Young, J. C. Johnson, M. B. Mets, T. C. Hain, "Cochlear Implants in Young Children with Usher's Syndrome," *Annals of Otology, Rhinology & Laryngology* Suppl. 166, No. 9, Part 2 (1995): 342–45; Anne E. Geers and Jean S. Moog, eds., "Effectiveness of Cochlear Implants and Tactile Aids for Deaf Children: The Sensory Aids Study at Central Institute for the Deaf," *The Volta Review* 96, no. 5 (1994).

3 Report of Dr. Robert F. Naunton, Director, Division of Human Communications, National Institute of Deafness and Other Communication Disorders, 7 May 1998 (in the author's files).

4 Bonnie P. Tucker, *Cochlear Implants: A Handbook* (Jefferson, N.C.: McFarland & Co., 1998).

5 The vast majority of deaf children in the United States no longer attend such schools; the Individuals with Disabilities Education Act—enacted in 1973 for the purpose of providing children with disabilities with a free appropriate public education, primarily alongside children without disabilities—has resulted in sharp declines in special school enrollments. See, for example, Felicity Barringer, "Pride in a Soundless World: Deaf Oppose a Hearing Aid," *New York Times,* 16 May 1993.

6 Roslyn Rosen, "President Rosen on Cochlear Implants," *NAD Broadcaster,* December 1992, p. 6; see also, "The President Signs On," *NAD Broadcaster,* January 1991, p. 3.

7 Larry G. Stewart, "Debunking the Bilingual/Bicultural Snow Job in the American Deaf Community," *A Deaf American Monograph* 42 (1992): 129–42.

8 Abigail Trafford, "The Brave New World of Genetic Planning," *Washington Post,* 15 November 1994.

9 Dena S. Davis, "Genetic Dilemmas and the Child's Right to an Open Future," *Hastings Center Report* 27, no. 2 (1997): 7–15, at 9.

10 See, for example, Wendy Lynas, *Communication Options in the Education of Deaf Children* (London: Whurr Publishers, 1994).

11 Kevin Nolan, "Communication Chores: A Parent's Perspective," *Clarke Speaks* (Winter/Spring 1997): T3.

12 Dolnick, "Deafness as Culture," p. 37.

13 Rosen, "President Rosen on Cochlear Implants."

14 The author is a member of the National Advisory Council lto the National Institute on Deafness and Other Communication Disorders and has personal knowledge of such criticism.

15 M. Arana Ward, "As Technology Advances, A Bitter Debate Divides the Deaf," *Washington Post,* 11 May 1997.

16 E-mail by Kate T. Kubey of November 1996, submitted to the author by Mildred Oberkotter and Melissa K. Chaikof (in the author's files).

17 Response of Bill Boyle (in the author's files).

18 Response of Melissa K. Chaikof (in the author's files).

19 Response of Mildred Oberkotter (in the author's files).

20 Ward, "As Technology Advances."

THE HANUKKAH BUSH: ETHICAL IMPLICATIONS IN THE CLINICAL MANAGEMENT OF INTERSEX

Sherri A. Groveman (Morris)

Presenting her own experiences as an intersex individual—a person born with ambiguous genitalia—Groveman confronts the mainstream medical view that intersex is "a tragedy—a mistake of nature to be corrected, to the maximum possible extent, by medicine." She strongly criticizes physicians' (until recently standard) practice of pressuring parents of an intersex newborn to consent to surgery that will make the infant appear more normal (either male- or female-looking) and to hide the truth from the intersex individual for as long as possible. What parents need in these situations, Groveman contends, is emotional support, resources for education about intersex, and the freedom to make unpressured medical decisions for their child. What the intersex individual needs over the years, she argues, is the truth about his and/or her ambiguous sexuality, acceptance of his and/or her condition, and—before reaching the age of consent—no more surgery than is necessary for physical health. Groveman concludes by expressing the joy she felt upon discovering a support group for persons with her particular form of intersex, Androgen Insensitivity Syndrome, and her hope that other intersex individuals will find similar support.

As a young child of a conservative, but unobservant, Jewish household, I viewed Christmas as being about the large, aromatic firs and spruces adorning my friends' apartments, decorated with dazzling ornaments and surrounded by a profusion of foil-wrapped packages. Hanukkah, by contrast, was embodied in our home by only a small menorah on our window sill. Is it any wonder that I begged, pleaded, and cajoled my parents for a Christmas tree? Wisely, they would not relent.

Soon I discovered that the parents of some Jewish friends had instituted a custom of "Hanukkah bushes," which, to any honest observer, were clearly Christmas trees in drag. Seeing one for the first time it felt fake, hollow, half of something but all of nothing. My friends' parents, uncomfortable about their minority status, had been co-opted by the overwhelming pressure to make life "easier" for their children by diluting their heritage while assimilating to the dominant culture.

With the benefit of hindsigh, I am glad my parents did not yield to such pressure even as I regret they did not do more to educate me about my roots. Having now learned the history of my religion I have discovered all that is rich and precious about Hanukkah, dissipating any desire for a Christmas tree. My "Hanukkah bush" friends, by contrast, derive no such meaning from the Festival of Lights, but at the same time feel like frauds if they lay claim to actual Christmas trees. Did their parents' response to societal pressure, though well-intentioned to help these children "fit in," simply leave my friends incapable of functioning comfortably in either world? Can the same be said of doctors who importune parents to manage their intersex children with surgery and secrets?

I might mention, as a footnote to this parable, that the population of Jews in the world is no larger than the population of intersex persons. Thus, I suppose it is fortunate that pediatric endocrinologists are not the stewards of the world's religions, because with the same rationale they use to support surgery and secrecy in managing intersex—that is, that it is unfair to leave children's ambiguous genitals in their natural state, or even openly acknowledge to them that they are intersexed, because this will render them outcasts to the majority of society—these doctors might argue that it is unfair to obligate children to live with a religion shared by only a tiny fraction of the world's population. As a practical matter, of course, religious tolerance is an accepted norm in our society, whereas doctors perceive something inherently intolerable about intersex.

Intersex is a subject near and dear to my heart (and other parts of my anatomy). But it is also my personal history inflected by the burden of having lived almost all of my 40 years with the shame, secrecy, and isolation that are an inevitable byproduct of how my case was managed by the medical profession.

I have complete Androgen Insensitivity Syndrome (AIS), which is characterized by XY chromosomes and testes, but a complete inability, due to an androgen receptor defect, of the body to respond to the testosterone produced by the testes. Unable to virilize, my body, by preordination, simply developed along a female path. In my case, this was discovered 10 days after my birth, when my pediatrician noticed a swelling in my groin, suggesting a hernia. Exploratory surgery performed at two weeks revealed the presence of what seemed to be a testis. When the lab report confirmed this, my parents were told that it was medically necessary for them to consent to immediate gonadectomy. Lacking any better insight, they of course gave their consent.

In fact, there was no urgent medical necessity; my testes could have remained safely intact until puberty, at which time they should have been removed

to prevent any risk of cancer. But I strongly suspect that there were pressing "psychological" necessities for their removal in infancy: (1) my doctors' desire to rid me of any vestige of a male anatomy and render my body "congruent"; (2) the equal desire to avoid the need at puberty to explain the nature of the surgery that would have to be performed, raising questions the doctors did not want to have to answer; and (3) shards of a superstitious fear that, despite what medicine knew in 1958 about "testicular feminization" (as it was then called). I might somehow virilize if my troublesome gonads were left intact.

Unlike Hanukkah, where my parents were sufficiently inculcated with the traditions of their religion to inoculate them against the pressure to conform to the dominant messages surrounding them, my parents are not, alas, intersexed, and so to learn the "culture" of what this meant to their child they had to rely on doctors to translate the language and meaning of words such as "chromosomes" and "gonads" and "pseudohermaphrodite." Unfortunately, like most doctors even today, my doctors were steeped in a tradition that viewed intersexuality as a tragedy—a mistake of nature to be corrected, to the maximum extent possible, by medicine. This culture had been handed down to them without any concern for the long-term outcome of the recipients of such treatment protocols. Thus, they became self-appointed tour guides to a foreign country when they themselves had not bothered to ever communicate with the natives.

My experience over the past three years assisting families affected by AIS informs me that the most critical variable to achieving a better outcome for intersex patients is not surgical management followed up with platitudes and half-truths, but instead is the provision of resources for parents to be thoroughly educated about what intersex is, and to work through any anxiety or guilt they feel about having an intersex child. When parents are able to communicate their comfort and acceptance, the child's self-esteem can develop from a solid foundation. When parents are, by contrast, apprehensive, fearful, or ignorant about intersex, their child is left to flounder in a sea of confusion without support. Regrettably medicine has seen fit to "correct" what is between the child's legs while offering limited educational assistance and psychological support to either the child or her/his family.

Indeed, the sole instruction my parents received from my endocrinologists was one of "damage control," calculated to confirm a solid image that I was their daughter in the same breath that doctors enjoined them that they should not disclose my true diagnosis to anyone, least of all me. While informing my parents that I was "just like a normal female," my doctors offered no suggestions other than fabrication about how they should help me cope with the reality of having XY chromosomes and testes while lacking ovaries, a uterus, fallopian tubes, or fertility.

Fortuitously, my surgeon failed to diagnose that I have a vagina incapable of intromission; had he done so he likely would have suggested vaginoplasty, a procedure that continues to be recommended in childhood to this day, despite its nearly 80 percent failure rate when performed prior to adolescence. Had I had been born with more ambiguous looking genitals, the solution offered would have been more surgery, most likely to make my genitals appear "female," even at the expense of diminishing sexual sensation. Cultural imperative, masquerading as medical necessity, would have made such additional surgeries inevitable.

I spent my adolescence filled with shame, though I was never told the true details of my diagnosis. My trauma was needlessly compounded by my doctor's stony silence while examining me, and his asking me to lie naked on an examining table so that teams of interns and residents could inspect my genitals. Such experiences themselves, far more than the true facts I later learned about the nature of AIS, instilled a sense of freakishness that I have only recently shaken. It is, however, disheartening to hear that similar treatment of intersex adolescents continues to this day.

Ultimately, I unearthed the truth about having AIS in a medical school library when I was 20 by researching the possible causes for my primary amenorrhea and lack of pubic hair. It is disorienting when you have always considered yourself female to learn that you have XY chromosomes and once had testes. It is equally disorienting when you have always considered yourself loved and cared for to discover that your parents and doctors have lied and left you to your own devices to discover this truth.

I appreciate that because I am 40 years old my treatment protocol was a product of 1960s thinking. I am frightened, however, that as we approach the turn of the millennium conventional medical treatment continues to endorse a nearly identical protocol. Doctors continue to debate the patient's right to know the truth, seemingly oblivious to the idea that they do not "own" the patient's medical information. This conspiracy of silence stems from the same root as the continuing protocol to surgically alter intersex infants' anatomies—an inability to see intersex as anything other than shameful and pathologic. This, in turn, is communicated to the parents, whom I believe would be far less traumatized by the reality of intersex if they weren't receiving such negative cues from doctors.

Regrettably doctors fail to offer appropriate psychological support to parents or even communicate that the capacity to give and receive love is a function of the size of one's heart, not the size or appearance of one's genitals. Yet this capacity for healthy relationships is threatened at best, and more typically destroyed altogether, through the toxic mixture of silence and surgery which is offered up as the only "solution" to the child's intersex "problem."

In the aftermath of such surgery, doctors behave as though the "problem" has been cured ("you used to be intersexed but we fixed it")—as though being intersexed were an historic detail of the patient's life. Unfortunately, this too is communicated to the parents, who, in turn, assume that there is no need to offer their child a safe place to mourn and grieve what has occurred, or to help their child ascribe meaning to being intersexed. Often the parents are sufficiently uncomfortable and guilt-ridden about the whole affair that they are highly motivated to accept the doctor's revisionist history of the child's intersex state. Thus, the child has endured a personal holocaust while having to remain mute.

I believe, based upon my experiences overseeing the U.S. branch of the AIS Support Group, attending 10 AIS Support Group meetings in the U.S. and the U.K., and getting to know more than 100 intersex people, ranging in age from two months to 73 years, that under the best of circumstances learning the truth about being intersexed can be temporarily traumatic. But not knowing the truth culminates in experiences that are almost universally tragic. With limited inaccurate information, and in the face of an overarching sense of shame, the mind conjures a parade of horribles far worse than any truth. Indeed, of the more than 60 women with AIS whom I personally know, I have not heard of a single instance where someone has reported that it was worse to know the truth than to live with lies.

Fortunately, many pediatric endocrinologists are endorsing the approach of truthful disclosure at the same time that they are revisiting the wisdom of surgical management of intersex. Apart from the ethical implications of a protocol rooted in dissimulation, the paradigm of deceit is, quite simply, shortsighted. The reports of women affiliated with the AIS Support Group reveal that patients are driven to learn what it is about themselves that seems to cause a palpable silence whenever they are examined by doctors or broach the subject of their childhood/adolescent gonadectomies. To that end, some members of our support group became expert in reading their medical charts upside down, while others inspected their files when their doctors momentarily left the examining room.

But there are even more unusual, and often painful, ways this information is obtained. Some members report the "dreaded" information spilling out in the heat of arguments with stepparents or siblings. One woman in our U.K. group literally discovered she had AIS by buying a house. She applied for a mortgage which required that she provide proof of good health. To do so she had to sign a medical release. She had never been told she had AIS—just that she had an "ovarian" problem and couldn't have children, but that this had no bearing on her health. She innocently signed the release. A few weeks later her mortgage company called her and said "Every-

thing is fine but we need to know what this 'androgen insensitivity' thing is all about."

It is important to note that the significance of truth-telling has increased with the advent of intersex support groups, such as the AIS Support Group, the Intersex Society of North America, and the Coalition for Intersex Support Advocacy and Education. These support groups provide a culture for intersexuals as well as validation of feelings; they offer enormous psychological relief for parents of intersex children, as well as intersex adolescents and adults.

To illustrate, in the case of AIS, many parents are understandably concerned about how they will communicate to their daughters that they have XY chromosomes; these parents are typically uncomfortable about this fact themselves. However, at a recent meeting of the AIS Support Group our members decided to take a photograph with the adult women with AIS, and the fathers of children with AIS, forming "Y's" with their arms while the mothers of such children crossed their arms to form "X's." The ability to defuse tension about "the chromosome thing" quite visibly allowed these parents to feel more comfortable and accepting of the entire issue.

Perhaps it is fitting that I have used a holiday theme in this article. For it was the day after Christmas, in 1994 when I first discovered, while researching in a medical school library, that an AIS Support Group had recently been founded in the U.K. No gift I will receive in this lifetime will ever be as precious to me as discovering that information. My subsequent involvement with the support group has, remarkably, allowed me to view having AIS as a blessing—after all, if I didn't have AIS I would not have developed into the woman I believe God and nature intended me to be. This was certainly not the outcome my doctors would have predicted on a chilly September day when they removed my gonads and implored my parents never to tell me the truth. The miracle of life, however, is that we can evolve; I hope, in this holiday season, that this same miracle can touch those who will be privileged to care for the intersex children born while this article was being read.

THE SEDUCTION OF A SURGICAL FIX

Lisa Abelow Hedley

As the mother of a daughter born with dwarfism, Hedley presents her experiences in wrestling with the seductive allure of surgery that would increase her daughter's height. She begins by identifying two lessons one learns when one adjusts to the loss of the fantasy of raising an idealized child and begins to raise the child one actually has: (1) that flaws are an essential part of normal lives, and (2) that the pursuit of an imagined flawless life obstructs the true parental work of raising a well-adjusted child. Hedley then recounts what it was like for her and her husband to decide upon surgery for their daughter to prevent bowing of her legs—entailing a summer in bed wearing full leg casts and using bed pans—only to be informed of another option: extended limb-lengthening. This option would prolong the procedure by six months by attaching to their daughter's legs external fixators that would incrementally open day by day before the leg casts are put on, thereby increasing the girl's height by two to four inches. As Hedley explains, the parents strongly felt the seductive lure of moving their daughter toward normal height while also noticing the contradiction so often experienced by parents of disabled children: "We love you just the way you are . . . now change." In the end, they opted only for the surgery to prevent leg bowing, leaving until years later—and to their daughter—any decision about limb-lengthening. Hedley concludes by noting doctors' obligation to provide medically and psychologically appropriate guidance and parents' obligation to remain true to their child's best interests and to figure out when best to include them in decision-making.

As the mother of a child born with the form of dwarfism called achondroplasia, I struggle to let her be who she is and recognize that there are two children growing up: the one I perceive and the one she is—and ultimately all that matters is the one she is. That means not letting my fantasies get in the way, which is harder than it sounds.

When our LilyClaire was born ten years ago, everything was confusion: how to react, how to proceed, what to *do*. As the frantic first days unfolded, it seemed that all we could focus on was how to repair the flaws, and we would listen to anyone from a faith healer to a surgeon if we thought there was a "fix" for her in it. I remember thinking: we can put men in space, surely we can fix this.

In our case, there was no immediate fix on offer, because the flaws are molecular, embedded in

every cell of her body. So for us, the first order of business was to come to terms with a few central desires, not the least of which is that most troublesome one—the desire for normalcy. There are dangers both social and emotional in being different and a certain amount of safety in being normal. So as her guardian and protector, I am vulnerable to the enticing possibilities of a surgical fix that might bring her closer to that safety zone of normalcy.

When you are a parent busy adjusting to the loss of the idealized child and raising the one you do have, it takes time to come to terms with a couple of facts. First, flaws are an essential part of real, normal human lives. Second, the pursuit of some imagined, flawless life obscures the real parental work, which is to raise a resilient child who values herself. To do that you have to look closely at your own fantasies and balance them against the real medical and psychological needs of the child. This is the ongoing challenge and the best way to describe it is by example.

Parens, Erik, ed. *Surgically Shaping Children*, pp. 43–48. © 2006 The Johns Hopkins University Press. Reprinted with permission of The Johns Hopkins University Press.

It is April 2002. LilyClaire is 7 years old and my husband and I are sitting in the office of a pediatric orthopedic surgeon whom we respect immensely, who has monitored LilyClaire since she was born and who has carefully evaluated the latest X-rays of her very bowed legs.

"If I was a betting man, I would say we will need to operate by Christmas," he says.

"So, strictly speaking, we don't *need* to correct her bowing right now," I say, trying to understand why we would opt for breaking both of her legs in two places to straighten them when she walks perfectly well. "I mean, right now there is no medical proof that she is wearing down cartilage, or even the *certainty* that she will?"

I am very much attached to the notion of certainty even though I know there is no such thing in the world of medicine. I am also very susceptible to authority figures in white lab coats. So I am worrying about the goals we would reasonably hope to achieve by operating now: medical repair or fantasy-fix or something in between?

"So, all we are saying for sure," I continue, "is that she will have straighter legs and that might stave off future problems."

"That is correct, but I believe she *will* need it." Our doctor repeats his view that we will probably eventually have to make the correction to avoid damaging misalignment and wear and tear on LilyClaire's cartilage.

My husband sighs and shifts. He hates it when I engage in the "on the one hand, on the other hand" thing I was trained to do as a lawyer. But I am no longer a frantic mother in search of solutions. I am not a maniac for the fix. Nor am I the clear and precise thinker I can be on other issues in my life. I am a mother seesawing between the nagging desire to alleviate some of my daughter's difference, to feel we are doing something—and the strong belief that I have to protect my daughter against those marauding, seductive, and unattainable notions of normalcy. I am a mother who needs to be sure in my own mind that we are doing the right thing.

At that moment, I am enticed by the idea of straighter legs, thinking it really is one of those things that matters in the real everyday world of being LilyClaire on the playground, in the face of staring, curious strangers. It seems just then that straight legs really would make things easier. And LilyClaire herself hates the way her legs are shaped. She complains about them regularly, sometimes telling us her knees hurt. But it is generally a fleeting complaint, more like fatigue, I always think hopefully, than a clinical finding. Or not, I always worry at 3:00 a.m. when I can't sleep and vulnerabilities swirl.

There in that antiseptic outpatient cubicle, my mind is a blur of statistics and likelihoods of arthritis, breakdowns, and damage done by leaving this severe bowing untreated, not to mention thoughts of my daughter's anger with me when as an adult she asks why we didn't fix the bowing way back when we had the chance. But the more I question, the more I realize the futility of my questions. There are only so many facts and statistics available, and no matter how I twist and turn and combine them, they will never yield any definitive answers.

I don't feel our doctor's impatience, but I am pressured by the awareness that my ambivalence is taking up a lot of his time and the waiting area is teeming with kids in multiple casts and my husband is definitely antsy. He knows from years of life together that it is time to force the decision.

I have one last gasp of reticence. I know how wrenching it is to hold your child as she goes limp under anesthesia. What if it is for a nonessential medical procedure that you are relinquishing your precious child to possible surgical errors, uncertain outcomes, and God knows what other unknowns? It is clear to me that if I am being driven by the insatiable desire for normalcy, I am lost in my attempt to do the right thing.

I finally wear myself out and am persuaded that now is the time to operate to forestall potential permanent damage and not disturb school schedules. I am still reluctant, however, to abandon the notion that if we wait, we might find that six months from now she doesn't need the surgery yet. I also give one more glancing thought to her choice—the idea that at some point, now or in the future, she should be part of the decision. But right now she is whining and fidgety and I know she is still too young. I will be very clear with her about what we are doing, but I will not yet consult her.

So finally, *finally* we feel we have to have faith in the "betting man" whom we have decided to trust, and we convert that trust into the belief that we are doing the right thing. So we sign all of those scary papers, which commit LilyClaire to a summer of full leg casts and videos and bedpans. And we read the fine print about the hazards of surgery and tremble.

After we have signed and the tension is eased by the satisfaction of a decision made, we are told that this surgery is procedurally the same as extended limb-lengthening (known as ELL). It's like this: we could prolong the procedure by six months, put on external fixators that open incrementally day by day, then get the cast we will have anyway for eight weeks and thereby gain a little height. If we really want to.

"What is a *little* height?" we ask.

"Two to four inches."

I know this doctor, this "betting man," and know that he does not like the odds of ELL. We know about the infections and potential neurological and tendon damage, we know that he thinks it is risky and the outlook down the road unknown, and we know that he particularly does not approve of the procedure for young kids not yet able to decide for themselves.

All I can process for a few seconds is the 4 inches. Quick calculations bring me to the fact that for LilyClaire that could mean as much as 4 feet, 7 inches as an adult. More seduction toward the norm. But I respect our doctor for making sure to present all of the options in as unbiased a way as possible, and then I am confused all over again.

The concept of ELL surgery is so supremely seductive because on the surface it strikes you as a magic pill capable of stretching someone out of the musty air at the level of belt buckles and into the fine air of reasonably normal stature. This particular surgical fix has even more power than most to overshadow instinct, sense, facts, statistics, and clear thinking, because it directly addresses concerns that matter so much to a social little girl like LilyClaire. At age 7 she is already self-conscious about going into rooms full of strangers, worried about using public bathrooms and needing the stool at school when other girls can reach.

For details about what it's like to have the procedure, you have to turn to those who have done

ELL, and they are necessarily unreliable reporters. They have sublimated the awful, painful, frightening aspects and are confirmed in their belief, as they must be, that they did the right thing, the thing that has been their salvation. There is no going back from such a commitment, even, I find, for those who experienced complications and repeated surgeries to repair damage done by the ELL procedure itself.

So willing for a moment to suppress the risks, the question is: Can we take this shot and grab it before LilyClaire is old enough to have it affect her sense of self and psyche? I know fixing the bowing will do little to change the way people stare at her in airports, in supermarkets, on the street, and even that is appealing on some level, but height? Real height? That is something else again, even as I know it is no cure—just a measured amount of fix.

The lure of gaining a few inches on the sly, cloaked in medical necessity is achingly attractive. But then I know this is totally irrational—that is to say, it is a rationalization. It took years for my husband and me to know that we must never decide the ELL question for her, and here I am making room in my mind, preparing data space, for an elaborate rationale that will subvert all of my better judgment about the molecular reality, the *what is* reality, the identity building reality of LilyClaire. But the lines are so blurry, where cosmetic meets psychosocial meets medical necessity.

I know that an experience this profound would not go unnoticed by 7-year-old LilyClaire's rapier mind. When I was 7, I fell down a flight of stairs and split open my chin. I have vivid memories of straining to hear the doctors confabbing at the foot of my emergency room cot. They were discussing something about a little more pain now, but I would be happy later and I can remember wanting to scream at them, Include me here! This is my chin! My face! My pain! No. I know that this is already an age of awareness and she would bloody well get the very message I know we must never send: we love you, you're perfect the way you are . . . now change.

I have always believed every parent must choose her own course, and have always thought that I have been respectful of decisions either way. I am disappointed in myself because now I can actually observe the process by which it would be possible to come around to a position I have already decided is untenable for us.

But then the danger passes. The charm, attraction, and seduction of the fantasy fix fall away. We will stick with the first step to straighten the bowing so there will be no cartilage degeneration or progressive misalignment. Our doctor reassures me that we will, in fact, gain a little in height anyway. A centimeter or two. I glom onto that absurdly small increment as a little icing on the cake, but even that comes at a price. Even when the surgery ordeal is over and it is September and I am bored watching the fiftieth hour of rehab, I feel cheated that after all that we didn't get just a little more satisfaction, just a little more esthetic upside. And what's worse, I am disappointed in myself for being seduced by their promise.

It is March 2003. I never hear complaints of achy knees, and the long scars on the front of LilyClaire's shins have faded to pale pink, like most of the pain, the terrors of the hospital, the long boring summer, and the rehab. My daughter and I are reading a book on the couch on a rainy afternoon. I have to start up one of those conversations that neither of us likes: one where we have to explore the way LilyClaire has responded to a playmate's questions the day before about why she is so small, why her head is big, why she had to have casts on both legs and stay in bed all summer, even if she did have a super cool bed that went up and down and unlimited television time.

LilyClaire is furious that I told the other girl the party line we tell every one of her classmates, teachers, parents who ask: that it is because LilyClaire was born different and is just smaller because that's the way she is made, like some people are fatter and some skinny, some wear glasses, and so on. She was spitting mad when the girl left, but would only say that I had no right to explain her to people. Door slammed.

She forgave me by dinner and did not mention it again.

So now that a day has passed and we are reading together and discussing the way that her hair has gotten so beautifully long, I have decided to explore her reaction. Nothing like a little psycho babble in the afternoon.

"LilyClaire," I begin, "when people ask about the way you look, what would you like to tell them?"

"Nothing." And she trains her knowing and intense brown eyes on mine in a way that says do not mess with me on this one.

"Well, we have to say something." I am as determined as she is. I am very aware that people with dwarfism say they get tired of explaining themselves, of being seen first as a person with dwarfism second to everything else about them as people, and I wonder if she really does have to say something or not. But now that these questions crop up pretty regularly, it does seem that she ought to have some direct, proud, and reasonable response at the ready. "Why not just say 'because I have achondroplasia and this is the way dwarfs are supposed to look'?" I suggest.

"No. I will say that I fell out of a tree and broke my legs and shrank." And now those eyes are full of foreboding . . . they are saying loud and clear that the conversation is over.

"But honey, you know you have dwarfism, right?" Now I need to be sure she is not slipping into a fantasy and somehow undermining that all-important sense of self, rooted in reality but ever optimistic, that we have been nurturing.

"Of course. But I like the tree idea."

I imagine that LilyClaire would rather say she fell from a tree because she does not want to feel that heavy hand of fate upon her, which separates her so decisively from her peers. I imagine this fantasy is one of her first assertions as an individual about how she wants to be perceived, and who am I to argue with a bit of fiction about which she is so resolute? It is her way of trying to fit in, and part of her process of sorting out her reality. For the most part I am in awe of how deftly she already handles the paradox that it is both uniquely formative to have challenges and hard on a daily basis to manage the reality of being the one who is different.

As she matures, she will, I hope, be able to distinguish between wanting not to be different and wanting to be normal. I hope she will make peace with herself and her difference and focus less on how others perceive her. The struggle to be herself as an individual, flawed and yet perfect in her own way, is how she will embrace her own reality, just as it is one way any of us comes to terms with ourselves.

Even as I hope this kind of peace for her, it is the daily realities of staring and quizzical glances, outright questions, and the practical difficulties of doing some things for herself that drive me to feel I might do almost anything to alleviate her pain and self-consciousness if a palatable fix came along. Proving of course that, for parents like me, when it comes to surgical fixes, all you can be sure of is doubt. Nothing is clear or irrefutable. It is just that at some point you get exhausted by statistics, possibilities, and probabilities and decide just to act and that is when the internal arguments end . . . and you go for it . . . whatever it is you have decided on.

The seductive promise of surgery as repair mingles with the realities of surgery as medical solution by way of psychosocial rationale. Providing clear, medically and psychologically appropriate guidance and reasonable goals are the surgeon's and physician's challenges. Sorting through it all, while remaining true to the best interests of the child and, finally, figuring out when it is time for the child to participate in decision making about her care, are the grand parental challenges.

JUDGING OCTOMOM
Josephine Johnston

In this brief article, Johnston provides an ethical analysis of the "octomom" case. In this case, an unemployed single woman on public assistance, Nadya Suleman—who was already mother to six children—had eight more babies through the use of in vitro fertilization (IVF). Having conceived her first six children using IVF, Ms. Suleman apparently visited her fertility doctor in 2008 and demanded that he transfer her six remaining frozen embryos immediately; after warning her of the risks associated with multiple pregnancies, he complied. (Two of these embryos resulted in twins, hence the total of eight infants.) The American Society for Reproductive Medicine, Johnston notes, strongly advises against transferring more than two embryos in cases involving an apparently highly fertile woman such as Suleman. Judging that Suleman's fertility doctor acted irresponsibly in acceding to her request for all six embryos to be transferred, Johnston takes up the question of whether he should have refused to treat her at all—even if she had requested the transfer of only one or two embryos—in view of her existing parental obligations, her status as single and unemployed, and her dependence on public assistance. Should he have used something like the stringent social criteria typically employed by adoption agencies? Johnston ultimately argues in the negative, asserting that fertility clinics are not well positioned to make such judgments and therefore cannot be trusted to avoid unjust discrimination.

Just over a week after her eight babies were delivered by caesarean section in a California hospital, Nadya Suleman explained to an NBC reporter that her extraordinary pregnancy was the result of in

Reprinted with permission of the author and the publisher from *Hastings Center Report,* vol. 39 (May–June 2009), pp. 23–25. Copyright © 2009 by The Hastings Center.

vitro fertilization. Having conceived her first six children—four singletons and one set of twins—using IVF, Suleman said she visited her fertility doctor in 2008 and insisted that he transfer all of her six remaining frozen embryos at once. After warning her of the risks associated with a multiple birth, he'd done as she asked. All six embryos implanted, and two divided to create twins.

Awe at the successful delivery of her children quickly turned to ire when the press discovered that Suleman not only has six children already, but is an unemployed single mother on public assistance. Many feel she has irresponsibly created more mouths than she can possibly feed, and that the taxpayers of California are going to be left holding the babies, as it were.

Like many familiar with the ins and outs of fertility treatment, I initially assumed that the octuplets resulted from Suleman's body "overreacting" to fertility medications. I guessed that her physician had either failed to monitor her egg development adequately before inseminating her, or that she had intercourse around the time her body released a large number of eggs. The idea that IVF—the most controllable form of assisted reproductive technology—had been used in such clear contravention of current professional guidelines and practice was almost unthinkable.

In the early years of IVF, it was not unusual to transfer six embryos to a woman in the hope that just one would successfully implant. But as the technology has improved, multiple births have become more frequent. While high-order multiples were welcomed by some patients, a few sued their physicians for the costs and harms to mothers and infants associated with complicated premature births. In 1992, the Centers for Disease Control and Prevention began collecting statistics from fertility clinics and reporting clinic-specific success rates that highlighted not just the number of pregnancies achieved and infants born, but also the number and degree of multiple births. Among other goals, the CDC's reports aim to improve the safety of assisted reproduction technologies for women and their babies by pinpointing clinics that generate high numbers of multiples. As noted on the program's Web site, "Multiple birth is associated with poor infant and maternal health outcomes including pregnancy complications, preterm delivery, low birth weight, congenital malformations, and infant death."

The American Society for Reproductive Medicine also seeks to reduce the number of multiples born to its members' patients. To this end it recommends that when treating women of Nadya Suleman's age (under thirty five years) who have a favorable prognosis, physicians consider transferring only one and no more than two blastocysts (embryos at five or six days of development).[1] There is clearly some wiggle room here—for example, if Suleman's doctor was transferring embryos at day three of development (which are less likely to survive than embryos that have developed in the lab to the blastocyst stage), he might have argued for transferring two or three rather than one or two. But in a thirty-three-year-old woman who had successfully used IVF already, transferring six embryos is so far beyond the guidelines as to ignore them completely. And maybe Suleman's physician did simply ignore them: as John Robertson points out in his essay in this issue, the guidelines have few teeth.

When everyone else is reducing the number of embryo transfers, how might we understand the decision of Suleman's physician to transfer six? Maybe he is simply unskilled—his clinic does have very low success rates, even by the crudest measure, so perhaps, based on his past performance, he expected fewer embryos to implant (and he likely did not expect two of them to twin).

Or maybe he was listening not to ASRM guidelines or evolutions in clinical practice, but to his patient. Just exactly how much control fertility patients should have over the procedures they undergo is hotly debated, in bioethics and beyond. Patients have what is known as "dispositional authority" over their embryos—they can decide whether unused embryos should be frozen, whether either parent can use them in the event of death or divorce, and whether unused frozen embryos should eventually be discarded, donated to other would-be parents, or donated to research. Good clinics ask their patients to consider these issues even before embryos are made.

But dispositional authority does not require physicians to accede to any and all patient demands. Suleman's physician would have been well within his legal and moral rights if he refused a request that so flagrantly violated professional guidelines. Indeed, I believe he *should* have refused to transfer all six embryos at once because to do so was so very dangerous for both Suleman and her babies. The harder question, in my view, is whether he should have refused to treat her at all on account of her circumstances, even if she had come to him with a more reasonable request.

Many have noted that fertility clinics primarily treat the men and women having trouble conceiving, rather than the children they hope to bear. And many have contrasted the way fertility clinics frame their services and understand their goals with the way adoption agencies operate. Some in bioethics have argued that Suleman's fertility doctor should have turned her away on account of her existing obligations and her financial status; in essence, they contend that something like an adoption standard should have been applied to her.[2]

Fertility clinics aim to help people have babies, while adoption services aim to place parentless children in safe, loving homes. In the fertility clinic, doctors perform detailed assessments of both patient fertility and physical readiness to gestate a baby. They may learn something about the intended parent or parents' psychological well-being, but clinics do not require parent training or a home study, nor do social workers assess would-be parents' fitness, run criminal background checks, speak with references, or inquire into financial stability. While one can argue that the cost of fertility procedures can act as a de facto financial screen—most patients are probably financially stable enough to have adequate insurance or to be able to pay out-of-pocket—it's a very light and potentially uninformative substitute for the kind of detailed information adoption agencies gather.

Because adoption cases usually concern an existing child, state and private agencies may be legally—and, I would argue, morally—bound to investigate would-be parents. But while ASRM's ethics committee advises that physicians may decide to withhold services if they believe patients will be unable to provide adequate childrearing, it also makes clear that physicians are not morally obliged to do so except "when significant harm to future children is likely."[3] This seems a difficult standard to meet.

If the United States ever decided to regulate assisted reproduction, it could mandate that future children's welfare be taken into account, as is done in the United Kingdom. But as ASRM's ethics committee notes, clinics are not currently well-equipped to make such assessments, and when they do, their judgments may betray discrimination: in the past they have been held legally and morally blameworthy for denying services to single people and gay men and women.[4]

Fertility patients in the United States are treated more or less like anyone else trying to conceive: no preapproval is required. And this is probably the way it should stay. Fertility clinics are not suited to judge who will make a good parent. ASRM is right that clinics should refuse to provide treatment to individuals or couples it learns have "uncontrolled psychiatric illness, substance abuse, ongoing physical or emotional abuse, or a history of perpetuating physical or emotional abuse" (none of which seem to apply to Suleman).[5] But unless we have good evidence that the fertility industry is creating a child welfare problem, I see no reason to require clinics to probe deeper into their patients' circumstances than they currently do. While I agree that assisted reproduction invites a more careful approach to procreation than is taken "in the wild," I would be very suspicious of a new rule concerning parental fitness that stems from one highly unusual case. We know there are children in need of safer, healthier, and more supportive homes in this country, but we have little reason to think that asking fertility clinics to assess the fitness of would-be parents would do anything to address that problem.

NOTES

1   The Practice Committee of the Society for Assisted Reproductive Technology, The American Society for Reproductive Medicine, "Guidelines on the Number of Embryos Transferred," *Fertility and Sterility* 82, Suppl. 1 (2004): 1–2.

2   T. Murray, "Commentary: Are Eight Babies More Than Enough?" http://www.CNN.com, February 4, 2009; A. Caplan, "Ethics and Octuplets: Society Is Responsible," *Philadelphia Inquirer*, February 6, 2009, http://www.philly.com/inquirer/opinion/39190377.html.

3   The Ethics Committee of the American Society for Reproductive Medicine, "Child-Rearing Ability and the Provision of Fertility Services," *Fertility and Sterility* 82 (2004): 564.

4   B.E.S. Robinson, "Birds Do it. Bees Do It. So Why Not Single Women and Lesbians?" *Bioethics* 11 (1997): 217; *North Coast Women's Care Medical Group v. San Diego Country Superior Court* 189 P 3d 959 (Cal. 2008).

5   The Ethics Committee of the American Society for Reproductive Medicine, "Child-Rearing Ability and the Provision of Fertility Services."

AMPUTEES BY CHOICE

Carl Elliott

In this excerpt from a book chapter, Elliott discusses ethical, psychological, and cultural issues provoked by individuals who request the amputation of one or more of their healthy limbs and by physicians who comply with such requests. Should such a procedure, Elliott asks, be regarded as cosmetic surgery, as invasive psychological treatment, or as risky research? Individuals who request such amputations appear to suffer from a mismatch between the actual state of their body and their sense of how their body should be. Comparing this phenomenon with the self-image of presurgical transsexuals, with a variety of psychological disorders, and with relatively ordinary desires for changes in one's body or appearance, Elliott explores the way in which elective amputation and other psycho-medical phenomena that have become much more common in recent years might be fueled by such factors as psychiatry's expanding list of psychological disorders and the Internet's facilitation of a sense of group membership. Following this exploration, he adds the cautious note that new surgical procedures such as elective amputation are treated not as experimental procedures but as innovative therapies, "for which ethical oversight is much less uniform."

In January 2000 British newspapers began running articles about Robert Smith, a surgeon at Falkirk and District Royal Infirmary, in Scotland. Smith had amputated the legs of two patients at their request, and he was planning to carry out a third amputation when the trust that runs his hospital stopped him. These patients were not physically sick. Their legs did not need to be amputated for any medical reason. Nor were they incompetent, according to the psychiatrists who examined them. They simply wanted to have their legs cut off. In fact, both the men whose limbs Smith amputated have declared in public interviews how much happier they are, now that they have finally had their legs removed.[1]

Healthy people seeking amputations are not nearly as rare as one might think. In May 1998 a seventy-nine-year-old man from New York traveled to Mexico and paid $10,000 for a black-market leg amputation; he died of gangrene in a motel. In October 1999 a mentally competent man in Milwaukee severed his arm with a homemade guillotine, and then threatened to sever it again if surgeons reattached it. That same month a legal investigator for

From *Better Than Well: American Medicine Meets the American Dream* by Carl Elliott. Copyright © 2003 by Carl Elliott. Used by permission of W.W. Norton & Company, Inc.

the California state bar, after being refused a hospital amputation, tied off her legs with tourniquets and began to pack them in ice, hoping that gangrene would set in, necessitating an amputation. She passed out and ultimately gave up. Now she says she will probably have to lie under a train, or shoot her legs off with a shotgun.[2]

For the first time that I am aware of, we are seeing clusters of people seeking voluntary amputations of healthy limbs and performing amputations on themselves. The cases I have identified are merely those that have made the newspapers. On the Internet there are enough people interested in becoming amputees to support a minor industry. One discussion listserv has over 3,200 subscribers.

"It was the most satisfying operation I have ever performed," Smith told a news conference in February 2000. "I have no doubt that what I was doing was the correct thing for those patients."[3] Although it took him eighteen months to work up the courage to do the first amputation, Smith eventually decided that there was no humane alternative. Psychotherapy "doesn't make a scrap of difference in these people," psychiatrist Russell Reid, of Hillingdon Hospital in London, said in a BBC documentary on the subject, called "Complete Obsession."[4] "You can talk till the cows come home; it doesn't make any difference. They're still going to want their amputation, and I know that for a fact." Both Smith and Reid pointed out that these people may unintentionally harm or even kill themselves trying to amputate their own limbs. As retired psychiatrist Richard Fox observed in the BBC program, "Let's face it, this is a potentially fatal condition."

Yet the psychiatrists and the surgeon were all baffled by the desire for amputation. Why would anyone want an arm or a leg cut off? Where does this sort of desire come from? Smith has said that the request initially struck him as "absolutely, utterly weird." "It seemed very strange," Reid told the BBC interviewer. "To be honest, I couldn't quite understand it."

In 1977, mental health professionals published the first modern case histories of what Johns Hopkins University psychologist John Money termed "apotemnophilia"—an attraction to the idea of being an amputee.[5] Money distinguished apotemnophilia from "acrotomophilia," a sexual attraction to amputees. The suffix -philia is important here. It places these conditions in the group of psychosexual disorders called paraphilias, often referred to outside medicine as perversions. Fetishes are fairly common sorts of paraphilias. In the same way that some people are turned on by, say, shoes or animals, others are turned on by amputees. Not by blood or mutilation—pain is not usually what they are looking for. The apotemnophile's desire is to be an amputee, whereas the acrotomophile's desire is turned toward those who happen to be amputees. In the *Bulletin of the Menninger Clinic* that same year, another group of researchers described a patient who would have qualified as both an apotemnophile and an acrotomophile: a twenty-eight-year-old man who was sexually attracted to female amputees, and who intensely wished to be handicapped himself.[6] . . . I had never heard of apotemnophilia or acrotomophilia before the Falkirk story broke. I wondered: Was this a legitimate psychiatric disorder? Was there any chance that it might spread? Like Josephine Johnston, a lawyer from Dunedin who was writing a graduate thesis on the legality of these amputations (and who first brought the Falkirk case to my attention), I also wondered

about the ethical and legal status of surgery as a solution. Should amputation be treated like cosmetic surgery, or like invasive psychiatric treatment, or like a risky research procedure?

Reviewing the medical literature, it is easy to conclude that apotemnophilia and acrotomophilia are extremely rare. Fewer than half a dozen articles have been published on apotemnophilia, most of them in arcane journals.[7] Most psychiatrists and psychologists I have spoken with—even those who specialize in paraphilias—have never heard of apotemnophilia. On the Internet, however, it is an entirely different story. Acrotomophiles are known on the Web as "devotees," and apotemnophiles are known as "wannabes." "Pretenders" are people who are not disabled but use crutches, wheelchairs, or braces, often in public, in order to feel disabled. Various Web sites sell photographs and videos of amputees, display stories and memoirs, recommend books and movies, and provide chat rooms, meeting points, and electronic bulletin boards. Much of this material caters to devotees, who seem to be far greater in number than wannabes. It is unclear just how many people out there actually want to become amputees, but there exist numerous wannabe and devotee listservs and Web sites.

Like Robert Smith, I have been struck by the way wannabes use the language of identity and selfhood in describing their desire to lose a limb. "I have always felt I should be an amputee." "I felt, this is who I was." "It is a desire to see myself, be myself, as I 'know' or 'feel' myself to be." This kind of language has persuaded many clinicians that apotemnophilia has been misnamed—that it is not a problem of sexual desire, as the -philia suggests, but a problem of body image. What true apotemnophiles share, Smith said in the BBC documentary, is the feeling "that their body is incomplete with their normal complement of four limbs." Smith has elsewhere speculated that apotemnophilia is not a psychiatric disorder but a neuropsychological one, with biological roots.[8] Perhaps it has less to do with desire than with being stuck in the wrong body.

Yet what exactly does it mean to be stuck in the wrong body? Even people who use more conventional enhancement technologies often use the language of self and identity to explain why they want these interventions: a woman who says she is "not herself" unless she is on Prozac; a bodybuilder who says he took anabolic steroids because he wants to look on the outside the way he feels on the inside; a transsexual who describes her experience as "being trapped in the wrong body." The image is striking, and more than a little odd. In each case the true self is the one produced by medical science.

Some people are inclined to think of this language as a literal description. Maybe some people really do feel as if they have found their true selves on Prozac. Maybe they really did feel incomplete without cosmetic surgery. Yet it may be better to think of these descriptions not as literally true but as expressions of an ambivalent moral ideal—a struggle between the impulse toward self-improvement and the impulse to be true to oneself. Not that I can see no difference between a middle-aged man rubbing Rogaine on his head every morning and a man whose discomfort in his own body is so all-consuming that he begins to think of suicide. But we shouldn't be surprised when any of these people, healthy or sick, use phrases like "becoming myself" and "I was incomplete" and "the way I really am" to describe what they feel, because the language of identity and selfhood surrounds us. This is simply the language we use now to describe the way we live.

Perhaps the question to be answered is not only why people who want to be amputees use the language of identity to describe what they feel, but also what exactly they are using it to describe. One point of contention among clinicians is whether apotemnophilia is, as John Money thought, really a paraphilia. "I think that John Money confused the apotemnophiles and the acrotomophiles," Robert Smith wrote to me from Scotland. "The devotees I think are paraphilic, but not the apotemnophiles." The question here is whether we should view apotemnophilia as a problem of sexual desire—a variety of the same genre of conditions that includes pedophilia, voyeurism, and exhibitionism. Smith, in agreement with many of the wannabes I have spoken with, believes that apotemnophilia is closer to gender-identity disorder, the diagnosis given to people who wish to live as the opposite sex. Like these people, who are uncomfortable with their identities and want to change sex, apotemnophiles

are uncomfortable with their identities and want to be amputees. . . .

Many of the news reports about the case at the Falkirk and District Royal Infirmary identified Smith's patients as having extreme cases of body dysmorphic disorder. Like people with anorexia nervosa, who believe themselves to be overweight even as they become emaciated, people with body dysmorphic disorder are preoccupied with what they see as a physical defect: thinning hair, nose shape, facial asymmetry, the size of their breasts or buttocks. They are often anxious and obsessive, constantly checking themselves in mirrors and shop windows, or trying to disguise or hide the defect. They are often convinced that others find them ugly. Sometimes they seek out cosmetic surgery, but frequently they are unhappy with the results and ask for more surgery. Sometimes they redirect their obsession to another part of the body.[9] But none of this really describes most of the people who are looking for amputations—who, typically, are not convinced they are ugly, do not imagine that other people see them as defective, and are usually focused exclusively on amputation (rather than on, say, a receding hairline or bad skin). Amputee wannabes more often see their limbs as normal, but as a kind of surplus. Their desires frequently come with chillingly precise specifications: for instance, an above-the-knee amputation of the right leg. . . .

I am on the phone with Max Price, a graphic designer in Santa Fe, who has offered to talk to me about apotemnophilia. (He has asked me to change his name and the details of his life and history if I write about him, and I have.) Price is a charming man, articulate and well read, and despite my initial uneasiness about calling him, I am enjoying our conversation. I had corresponded by e-mail with a number of wannabes, but had not managed to talk to any of them until now. The conversation has taken on an easy intellectual tone, more like a discussion between colleagues than an interview. Price is telling me about his efforts to get doctors to adopt some guidelines for deciding when a person with apotemnophilia should have surgery. I am tossing out ideas, trying out some of my thoughts, and I wonder aloud about a relationship between apotemnophilia and obsessive-compulsive disorder.

I ask Price whether he feels that his desire is more like an obsession, a fantasy, or a wish. He says, "Well, it was definitely like an obsession. Until I cut my leg off, of course."

That brings me up short. I had been unaware that he had actually gone ahead with an amputation. "Ah," I say. I pause. Should I ask? I decide I should. "May I ask how you did it?" Price laughs. "It was kind of messy," he says. "I did it with a log splitter." He then explains, in a thoughtful, dispassionate manner, the details of his "accident" ten years ago—the research he had done on anesthesia and wound control, how he had driven himself to the emergency room after partially amputating his limb, the efforts of the hospital surgeons to reattach it. He lived with the reattached leg for six months, he said, until medical complications finally helped him persuade another surgeon to amputate it.

I met Price through an Internet discussion listserv called "amputee-by-choice," one of the larger lists. At first I had simply prowled through the archives and listened to the ongoing conversation. I found many of the archived messages very creepy. Here were people exchanging photographs of hands with missing fingers; speculating about black-market amputations in Russia; debating the merits of industrial accidents, gunshot wounds, self-inflicted gangrene, chain-saw slips, dry ice, and cigar cutters as means of getting rid of their limbs and digits. When I introduced myself to the active electronic group, however, the discussion abruptly stopped, like the conversation in a village pub when a stranger walks in. For several days only a handful of new messages were posted. But I had invited wannabes to get in touch with me individually, telling them that I was a university professor working on apotemnophilia, and over the next few days a dozen or so people responded. Some, like Price, were insightful and articulate. Some had become mental-health professionals, in part as a way of trying to understand their desires. The few who had managed an amputation seemed (somewhat to my surprise) to have made peace with their desires. But others obviously needed help: they were obsessive, driven, consumed. Many seemed to have other psychiatric problems: clinical depression, obsessive-compulsive disorder, eating disorders, transvestism of a type that sounded anything

but playful or transgressive. They did not trust psychiatrists. They did not want medication. They wanted to know if I could find them a surgeon. I felt like an ethnographer in a remote country, unfamiliar with the local customs, whom the natives believe can help them. I began to understand how Robert Smith must have felt. I also began to wonder at the strength of a desire that would take people to such lengths.

By all accounts, the Internet has been revolutionary for wannabes. I can see why. It took me months to track down even a handful of scientific articles on the desire for amputation. It took about ten seconds to find dozens of Web sites devoted to the topic. Every one of the wannabes and devotees I have talked with about the Internet says that it has changed everything for them. "My palms were actually sweating the first time I typed 'amputee' into a search engine," one wannabe wrote to me. But the results were gratifying. "It was an epiphany," she wrote. When Krafft-Ebing was writing *Psychopathia Sexualis,* people with unusual desires could live their entire lives without knowing that there was anyone else in the world like them. Today all it takes is a computer terminal. On the Internet you can find a community to which you can listen or reveal yourself, and instant validation for your condition, whatever it may be. This same wannabe told me that she has never spoken about her desire for amputation with a friend, a family member, or a mental-health professional, and that she never will. Yet she is a frequent anonymous participant on the wannabe discussion listserv. . . .

In his book *Stigma,* Erving Goffman writes about the way that most stigmatized groups, even as they are set apart from mainstream society, will find a group of people who share their particular standpoint in the world.[10] So that at the same time that the stigmatized person is cut off from the world of so-called normal people, who see the stigmatized person as deviant or subnormal, this group of sympathetic others reassure him that he is essentially human and normal despite his own self-doubts. We applaud this if the stigma comes from being part of a racial minority, or from being deaf, from having AIDS, but we worry if the stigma is something like dangerous drug use or pedophilia. Wannabes appear to be finding this kind of sympathetic group on the Internet. They thought they were alone, they thought they were crazy, and this group reassures them that they are not. From a therapeutic point of view, this kind of community-building may have mixed results. It gives the wannabes solidarity, but it also nourishes and shapes a desire that might otherwise wither away or take another form. . . .

Even if we assume that the obsessive desire for amputation is evidence of a psychiatric disorder, it is unclear why such a desire should be growing more common just now. Why do certain psychopathologies arise, seemingly out of nowhere, in certain societies and during certain historical periods, and then disappear just as suddenly? Why did young men in late-nineteenth-century France begin lapsing into fugue states, wandering the continent with no memory of their past, coming to themselves months later in Moscow or Algiers with no idea how they got there? What was it about America in the 1970s and 1980s that made it possible for thousands of Americans and their therapists to come to believe that two, ten, even dozens of personalities could be living in the same head? One does not have to imagine a cunning cult leader to envision alarming numbers of desperate people asking to have their limbs removed. One has only to imagine the right set of historical and cultural conditions.

So, at any rate, suggests the philosopher and historian of science Ian Hacking, who has attempted to explain just how "transient mental illnesses" such as the fugue state and multiple-personality disorder arise.[11] A transient mental illness is by no means an imaginary mental illness, though in what ways it is real (or "real," as the social constructionists would have it) is a matter for philosophical debate. A transient mental illness is a mental illness that is limited to a certain time and place. It finds an "ecological niche," as Hacking puts it. In the same way that the idea of an ecological niche helps to explain why the polar bear is adapted to the Arctic ecosystem, or the chigger to the South Carolina woods, Hacking's ecological niches help to explain the conditions that made it possible for multiple-personality disorder to flourish in late-twentieth-century America and the fugue state to flourish in nineteenth-century Bordeaux. If the niche disappears, the mental illness disappears along with it.

Hacking does not intend to rule out other kinds of causal mechanisms, such as traumatic events in childhood and neurobiological processes. His point is that a single causal mechanism isn't sufficient to explain psychiatric disorders, especially those contained within the boundaries of particular cultural contexts or historical periods. Even schizophrenia, which looks very much like a brain disease, has changed its form, outlines, and presentation from one culture or historical period to the next. The concept of a niche is a way to make sense of these changes. Hacking asks: What makes it possible, in a particular time and place, for this to be a way to be mad?

Hacking's books *Rewriting the Soul* and *Mad Travelers* are about "dissociative" disorders, or what used to be called hysteria. He has argued, I think very persuasively, that psychiatrists and other clinicians helped to create the epidemics of fugue in nineteenth-century Europe and multiple-personality disorder in late-twentieth-century America simply by the way they viewed the disorders—by the kinds of questions they asked patients, the treatments they used, the diagnostic categories available to them at the time, and the way these patients fit within those categories. He points out, for example, that the multiple-personality-disorder epidemic rode on the shoulders of a perceived epidemic of child abuse, which began to emerge in the 1960s and which was thought to be part of the cause of multiple-personality disorder. Multiple personalities were a result of childhood trauma; child abuse is a form of trauma. It seemed to make sense that if there were an epidemic of child abuse, we would see more and more multiples.

Sociologists have made us familiar with the idea of "medicalization," which refers to the way that a society manages deviant behavior by bringing it under the medical umbrella.[12] A stock example of medicalization is the way that homosexuality was classified by the American Psychiatric Association as a psychiatric disorder until the 1970s. Many enhancement technologies become popular only when they are conceptualized as treatments for medicalized conditions, such as Ritalin and Adderall for Attention Deficit Disorder (medicalized distractibility) or Paxil and Nardil for social phobia (medicalized shyness). Many technologies (including some of those used to treat medicalized conditions) are also used as "normalizing" procedures. Normalizing procedures bring a deviant behavior, characteristic, or personality type back within a range considered normal, or at least aesthetically acceptable. Cosmetic facial surgery for children with Down's syndrome is a normalizing procedure, in that it is performed not for medical reasons but to make the child look more like an ordinary child. Both "normalization" and "medicalization" are related to the processes that Hacking describes, but Hacking is onto something slightly different. By "transient mental illnesses" he does not have in mind new descriptions of old conditions so much as conditions that look new in themselves.[13]

Crucial to the way that transient mental illnesses arise is what Hacking calls "looping effects," by which he means the way a classification affects the thing being classified. Unlike objects, people are conscious of the way they are classified, and they alter their behavior and self-conceptions in response to their classification. Look at the concept of "genius," Hacking says, and the way it affected the behavior of people in the Romantic period who thought of themselves as geniuses. Look also at the way in which their behavior in turn affected the concept of genius. This is a looping effect: the concept changes the object, and the object changes the concept. To take a more contemporary example, think about the way that the concept of a "gay man" has changed in recent decades, and the way this concept has looped back to change the way that gay men behave. Looping effects apply to mental disorders too. In the 1970s, Hacking argues, therapists started asking patients they thought might be multiples if they had been abused as children, and patients in therapy began remembering episodes of abuse (some of which may not have actually occurred). These memories reinforced the diagnosis of multiple-personality disorder, and once they were categorized as multiples, some patients began behaving as multiples are expected to behave. Not intentionally, of course, but the category "multiple-personality disorder" gave them, as Hacking provocatively puts it, a new way to be mad.

I am simplifying a very complex and subtle argument, but the basic idea should be clear. By regarding a phenomenon as a psychiatric diagnosis—treating it, reifying it in psychiatric diagnostic manuals, developing instruments to measure it, inventing scales to rate its severity, establishing ways to reimburse the costs of its treatment, encouraging pharmaceutical companies to search for effective drugs, directing patients to support groups, writing about possible causes in journals—psychiatrists may be unwittingly colluding with broader cultural forces to contribute to the spread of a mental disorder.

Suppose doctors started amputating the limbs of wannabes. Would that contribute to the spread of the desire? Could we be faced with an epidemic of people wanting their limbs cut off? Most people would say, Clearly not. Most people do not want their limbs cut off. It is a horrible thought. The fact that others are getting their limbs cut off is no more likely to make these people want to lose their own limbs than state executions are to make people want to be executed. And if by some strange chance more people did ask to have their limbs amputated, that would be simply because more people with the desire were encouraged to "come out" rather than suffer in silence.

I'm not so sure. Clinicians and patients alike often suggest that apotemnophilia is like gender-identity disorder, and that amputation is like sex-reassignment surgery. Let us suppose they are right. Fifty years ago the suggestion that tens of thousands of people would someday want their genitals surgically altered so that they could change their sex would have been ludicrous. But it has happened. The question is, Why? One answer would have it that this is an ancient condition, that there have always been people who fall outside the traditional sex classifications, but that only during the past forty years or so have we developed the surgical and endocrinological tools to fix the problem.

But it is possible to imagine another story, that our cultural and historical conditions have not just revealed transsexuals but created them. That is, once "transsexual" and "gender-identity disorder" and "sex-reassignment surgery" became common linguistic currency, more people began conceptualizing and interpreting their experience in these terms. They began to make sense of their lives in a way that hadn't been available to them before, and to some degree they actually became the kinds of people described by these terms.

I don't want to take a stand on whether either of these accounts is right. It may be that neither is. It may be that there are elements of truth in both. But let us suppose that there is some truth to the idea that sex-reassignment surgery and diagnoses of gender-identity disorder have helped to create the growing number of cases we are seeing. Would this mean that there is no biological basis for gender-identity disorder? No. Would it mean that the term is a sham? No. Would it mean that these people are faking their dissatisfaction with their sex? Again, no. What it would mean is that certain social and structural conditions—diagnostic categories, medical clinics, reimbursement schedules, a common language to describe the experience, and, recently, a large body of academic work and transgender activism—have made this way of interpreting an experience not only possible but more likely.

Whether apotemnophilia (or, for that matter, gender-identity disorder) might be subject to the same kind of molding and shaping that Hacking describes is not clear. One therapist I spoke with, an amputee wannabe, believes that the desire for amputation, like multiple-personality disorder, is often related to childhood trauma. This is only one person's hypothesis, of course, and it may be wrong. But it is clear that sexual desire is malleable. It doesn't seem far-fetched to imagine that amputated limbs could come to be more widely seen as erotic, or that given the right set of social conditions, the desire for amputation could spread. For a thousand years Chinese mothers broke the bones in their daughters' feet and wrapped them in bandages, making the feet grow twisted and disfigured. To a modern Western eye, these feet look hideously deformed. But for centuries Chinese men found them erotic.

Hacking uses the term "semantic contagion" to describe the way in which publicly identifying and describing a condition creates the means by which that condition spreads. He says it is always possible for people to reinterpret their past in light of a new conceptual category. It is also possible for them to contemplate actions that they may not have contemplated before. When I was living in New Zealand, ten years ago, I had a conversation with Paul Mullen, who was then the chair of psychological medicine at the University of Otago, and who told me that he was a member of a government committee whose job it was to decide whether pornographic materials should be allowed into the country. I bristled at the idea of censorship, and asked him how he could justify being a part of something like that. He just laughed and said that if I could see what his committee was banning, I would change my mind. His position was that some sexual acts would never even occur to a person in an entire lifetime of thinking about sex if not for seeing them pictured in these books. He went on to describe to me various alarming acts that, it was true, had never occurred to me. Mullen was of the opinion that people were better off never having conceptualized such acts, and in retrospect, I think he may have been right.[14]

This is part of what Hacking is getting at, I think, when he talks about semantic contagion. The idea of having one's legs amputated might never even enter the minds of some people until it is suggested to them. Yet once it is suggested, and not just suggested but paired with imagery that a person's past may have primed him or her to appreciate, that act becomes possible. Give the wish for it a name and a treatment, link it to a set of related disorders, give it a medical explanation rooted in childhood memory, and you are on the way to setting up just the kind of conceptual category that makes it a treatable psychiatric disorder. An act has been redescribed to make it thinkable in a way it was not thinkable before. Elective amputation was once self-mutilation; now it is a treatment for a mental disorder. Toss this mixture into the vast fan of the Internet and it will be dispersed at speeds unimagined even a decade ago. . . .

I will confess that my opinions about amputation as a treatment have shifted since I began talking to wannabes. My initial thoughts were not unlike those of a magazine editor I approached about writing a piece on the topic, who replied, "Thanks. This is definitely the most revolting query I've seen for quite some time." Yet there is a simple, relentless logic to these people's requests for amputation. "I am suffering," they tell me. "I have nowhere else to turn." They realize that life as an amputee will not be easy. They understand the problems they will have with mobility, with work, with their social lives; they realize they will have to make countless adjustments just to get through the day. They are willing to pay their own way. Their bodies belong to them, they tell me. The choice should be theirs. What is worse: to live without a leg or to live with an obsession that controls your life? For at least some of them, the choice is clear—which is why they are talking about chain saws and shotguns and railroad tracks.

And to be honest, haven't surgeons made the human body fair game? You can pay a surgeon to suck fat from your thighs, lengthen your penis, augment your breasts, redesign your labia, even (if you are a performance artist) implant silicone horns in your forehead or split your tongue like a lizard's. Why not amputate a limb? At least Robert Smith's motivation was to relieve his patients' suffering.

It is exactly this history, however, that makes me worry about a surgical "cure" for apotemnophilia. Psychiatry and surgery have had an extraordinary and very often destructive collaboration over the past seventy-five years or so: clitoridectomy for excessive masturbation, cosmetic surgery as a treatment for an "inferiority complex," intersex surgery for infants born with ambiguous genitalia, and—most notorious—the frontal lobotomy. It is a collaboration with few unequivocal successes. Yet surgery continues to avoid the kind of ethical and regulatory oversight that has become routine for most areas of medicine. If the proposed cure for apotemnophilia were a new drug, it would have to go through a rigorous process of regulatory oversight. Investigators would be required to design controlled clinical trials, develop strict eligibility criteria, recruit subjects, get the trials approved by the Institutional Review Board, collect vast amounts of data showing that the drug was safe and effective, and then submit their findings to the U.S. Food and Drug Administration. But this kind of oversight is not required for new, unorthodox surgical procedures. (Nor, for that matter, is it required for new psychotherapies.) New surgical procedures are treated not like experimental procedures but like "innovative therapies," for which ethical oversight is much less uniform. . . .

NOTES

1 P. Taylor, "'My Left Foot Was Not Part of Me,'" *The Guardian,* February 6, 2000, 14; Tracey Lawson, "Therapist Praises Doctor's Bravery," *The Scotsman,* February 1, 2000; Clare Dyer "Surgeon Amputated Healthy Legs," *British Medical Journal* 320 (February 5, 2000): 332.

2 J. H. Burnett, "Southside Man Uses Homemade Guillotine to Sever Arm," *Milwaukee Journal Sentinel,* October 7, 1999; Stephen McGinty and Sue Leonard, "Secret World of Would-Be Amputees," *Sunday Times,* February 6, 2000; Michelle Williams, "Murder Trial Opens for Fetish M.D.," *Associated Press,* September 29, 1999.

3 Cherry Norton, "Disturbed Patients Have Healthy Limbs Amputated," *The Independent,* February 1, 2000.

4 BBC2 Horizon, "Complete Obsession," Transcript of television documentary, screened in United Kingdom Feb 17, 2000; downloaded November 27, 2000 at: www.bbc.co.uk/science/horizon/obsession.shtm. More recently, the Australian radio program "Soundprint" broadcast a documentary on amputee wannabes, available on-line at: http://soundprint.org/radio/display_show/ID/232/name/Wannabes.

5 J. Money, R. Jobaris, and G. Furth, "Apotemnophilia: Two Cases of Self-Demand Amputation as a Paraphilia," *Journal of Sex Research* 13:2 (May 1977): 114–25.

6 P. L. Wakefield, A. Frank, R. W. Meyers, "The Hobbyist: A Euphemism for Self-mutilation and Fetishism," *Bulletin of the Menninger Clinic* 41 (1977): 539–52.

7 W. Everaerd, "A Case of Apotemnophilia: a Handicap as a Sexual Preference," *American Journal of Psychotherapy* 37:2 (April 1983): 285–93; J. Money, "Paraphilia in Females: Fixation on Amputation and Lameness: Two Personal Accounts," *Journal of Psychology and Human Sexuality* 3:2 (1990): 165–72; R. L. Bruno, "Devotees, Pretenders and Wannabes: Two Cases of Factitious Disability Disorder," *Sexuality and Disability* 15:4 (Winter 1997): 243–60; Wakefield, Frank, and Meyers, "The Hobbyist." On acrotomophilia, see Grant Riddle, *Amputees and Devotees* (New York: Irvington Publishers, 1989).

8 Keren Fisher, Robert Smith, "More Work Is Needed to Explain Why Patients Ask for Amputation of Healthy Limbs," letter, *British Medical Journal* 320 (April 22, 2000): 1147. Smith and Gregg Furth also recently published a book titled *Amputee Identity Disorder: Information, Questions, Answers, and Recommendations About Self-Demand Amputation* (Portland, Ore.: 1stBooks Library, 2000).

9 Katherine A. Phillips, *The Broken Mirror: Understanding and Treating Body Dysmorphic Disorder* (New York: Oxford University Press, 1996). Phillips is a psychiatrist at Brown University who has also published extensively on body dysmorphic disorder in the medical literature. The patients she describes generally do not much resemble amputee wannabes, but she does briefly mention a man who asked a surgeon to remove his nose (p. 289).

10 Erving Goffman, *Stigma: Notes on the Management of a Spoiled Identity* (New York: Simon and Schuster, 1986; originally published in 1963).

11 See especially Ian Hacking, *Mad Travelers: Reflections on the Reality of Transient Mental Illness* (Charlottesville: University Press of Virginia, 1998) and Ian Hacking,

Rewriting the Soul: Multiple Personality and the Sciences of Memory (Princeton, N.J.: Princeton University Press, 1995).

12 Ivan Illich, *Limits to Medicine* (London: Marion Boyars, 2002); Peter Conrad and Joseph W. Schneider, *Deviance and Medicalization: From Badness to Sickness* (Philadelphia, Pa.: Temple University Press, 1992); Allan V. Horwitz, *Creating Mental Illness* (Chicago: University of Chicago Press, 2002).

13 What looks like an entirely new condition may on closer examination turn out to be a new variation on previously existing conditions. Hacking suggests, for instance, that some of the young men characterized as having fugue states would, in the terms of today, be characterized as having epilepsy or traumatic head injuries.

14 Mullen is also the coauthor of an interesting paper on the emergence of the idea of "stalking" in recent years. See P. E. Mullen, M. Pathe, and R. Purcell, "Stalking: New Constructions of Human Behaviour," *Australian and New Zealand Journal of Psychiatry* 35:1 (2001): 9–16.

COSMETIC SURGERY

COSMETIC SURGERY AND THE INTERNAL MORALITY OF MEDICINE

Franklin G. Miller, Howard Brody, and Kevin C. Chung

The authors confront the issue of whether cosmetic surgery is a legitimate medical practice. Medicine, they argue, is "governed by a moral framework consisting of goals proper to medicine, role-specific duties, and clinical virtues"; professional integrity requires adherence to this "internal morality of medicine." Underscoring the distinction between consumer sovereignty in the business world and patient autonomy in medicine, the authors argue that advertising for cosmetic surgery routinely violates the Code of Ethics for the American Society of Plastic and Reconstructive Surgeons. They conclude that, from the standpoint of the internal morality of medicine, cosmetic surgery is ethically questionable, located at best at the periphery of acceptable medical practice.

Cosmetic surgery is a fast-growing medical practice. In 1997 surgeons in the United States performed the four most common cosmetic procedures— liposuction, breast augmentation, eyelid surgery, and facelift—443,728 times, an increase of 150% over the comparable total for 1992.[1] Estimated total expenditures for cosmetic surgery range from $1 to $2 billion.[2] As managed care cuts into physicians' income and autonomy, cosmetic surgery, which is not covered by health insurance, offers a financially attractive medical specialty.

Although increasingly popular, cosmetic surgery is a most unusual medical practice. Invasive surgical operations performed on healthy bodies for the sake of improving appearance lie far outside the core domain of medicine as a profession dedicated to saving

lives, healing, and promoting health. These cosmetic procedures are not medically indicated for a diagnosable medical condition. Yet they pose risks, cause side effects, and are subject to complications, including pain, bruising, swelling, discoloration, infections, formation of scar tissue, nerve damage, hardening of implants, etc.[3] Moreover, cosmetic surgery is a consumer-oriented entrepreneurial practice, heavily promoted by advertising in newspapers, magazines, the yellow pages of the telephone directory, and by marketing on the World Wide Web. The remarkable nature of cosmetic surgery is reflected on in the following comments of a plastic surgeon: "But then on top of it all we actually operate on people who are normal. It's amazing that we're allowed to do that, the idea that we can get a permit to operate on someone who is totally normal is an unbelievable privilege."[4]

Is cosmetic surgery a medical privilege or an abuse of medical knowledge and skill? With the exception of feminist scholarship, which focuses on the personal and social meaning and value of cosmetic surgery for the lives of women, the bioethics literature has neglected to pay attention to moral issues posed by cosmetic surgery.[5] In this article we examine cosmetic surgery from the perspective of professional integrity and the internal morality of medicine—a perspective that we have explicated and defended in two previous essays.[6]

THE INTERNAL MORALITY OF MEDICINE

All members of our society are likely to become patients, vulnerable to life-threatening or disrupting conditions and in need of medical attention and treatment to cure, prevent, or ameliorate disease, injury, or bodily dysfunction. Owing to this vulnerability and need for professional care, medicine is not a morally neutral technique. Rather, it is a professional practice governed by a moral framework consisting of goals proper to medicine, role-specific duties, and clinical virtues. We call this framework "the internal morality of medicine." The professional integrity of physicians is constituted by loyalty and adherence to this internal morality.

A variety of formulations have been proposed for the goals of medicine. A recent report of an international group of scholars, convened by The Hastings Center, recommended a comprehensive list of four goals: (i) "the prevention of disease and injury and promotion and maintenance of health"; (ii) "the relief of pain and suffering caused by maladies"; (iii) "the care and cure of those with a malady, and the care of those who cannot be cured"; and (iv) "the avoidance of premature death and the pursuit of a peaceful death."[7] For our inquiry into the ethics of cosmetic surgery, this list is noteworthy in two respects. The designation of multiple goals signifies that medicine is too complex and diverse in its legitimate scope to be encompassed by any single, essential goal, such as healing or promoting health. If healing is the single essential goal of medicine, then it is obvious that cosmetic surgery does not belong within legitimate medical practice. But this essentialist perspective would also rule out a variety of medical practices, such as contraception and sterilization, which prima facie are not devoted to healing

or promoting health but are widely accepted as medically appropriate. The diversity of goals proper to medicine, and their openness to interpretation, makes mapping the moral domain of medicine complex and contested. Though broad in its scope, this list of goals is subject to limits. The central goal of relief of pain and suffering is confined to conditions that qualify as "maladies." What counts as a malady warranting medical attention may be subject to conflicting interpretations and may change over time. The important qualification, however, means that it is not within the purview of physicians to attempt to relieve any and all pain and suffering that may afflict human beings.

Specification of the goals of medicine is necessary but not sufficient for mapping the normative domain of medicine. In addition to being oriented to a set of proper goals, medicine is guided and constrained by a set of internal duties that pertain to the legitimacy of practices in pursuit of medical goals. We have identified four internal duties incumbent on physicians of integrity: (i) competence in the technical and humanistic skills required to practice medicine; (ii) avoiding disproportionate harms that are not balanced by the prospect of compensating medical benefits; (iii) refraining from the fraudulent misrepresentation of medicine as a scientific practice and clinical art; and (iv) fidelity to the therapeutic relationship with patients in need of care.[8] The internal morality of medicine also encompasses a set of clinical virtues—dispositions of character and conduct facilitating excellence in pursuit of the goals of medicine and the performance of professional duties. We hope to specify and explicate the medical virtues in a future undertaking, but this is not required for our purpose of critical examination of cosmetic surgery.

THE DISTINCTION BETWEEN BUSINESS AND MEDICINE

From the time of the ancient Greeks to the present, medicine as a professional practice has been distinguished from business.[9] Governance by an internal morality underlies this distinction. Business, to be sure, does not lie outside the domain of morality. But medicine is subject to specialized and more stringent ethical constraints than are characteristic of and appropriate to business enterprise. The distinction between consumers and patients and the use of advertising are two key aspects of the traditional contrast between business and professional medical practice; and both are relevant to the evaluation of cosmetic surgery in the light of the internal morality of medicine.

Central to business in a market economy is the doctrine of consumer sovereignty: that subjective preferences and money determine access to commodities in the marketplace. In medicine consumer sovereignty is attenuated, if not foreign to the domain. Medical care is provided by physicians who diagnose presenting problems and recommend medically indicated treatment or preventive interventions. Patients may demand specific medical interventions, particularly in the context of intense public attention to health and ready access to health information. But interventions that patients request or demand are medically appropriate only if they are consistent with diagnostic criteria, medical indications, and professional judgment.

Patient autonomy is not the same as consumer sovereignty. Ethical medical treatment depends on the informed consent of patients, who have a right to refuse treatment, including medically indicated lifesaving interventions. Patient autonomy, however, falls short of consumer sovereignty because patients do not have a right to receive whatever treatments they demand and are prepared to pay for. Preference and the ability to pay may be necessary for access to medical care in our society, but they are not sufficient. The extent to which cosmetic surgery is oriented toward and dependent on consumer demand is relevant to its moral assessment from the perspective of professional integrity.

In business, advertising functions as a standard means of linking sellers and buyers of products and services. Medical ethics, however, traditionally has prohibited advertising by physicians.[10] This traditional prohibition may have reflected, in part, a concern for status: marketing by advertising was considered beneath the dignity of learned professionals as distinct from tradesmen. The traditional prohibition eroded in the wake of the successful legal challenge by the Federal Trade Commission in 1978 of the American Medical Association's ban on

physician advertising. Nevertheless, the vulnerability of patients and the imbalance of knowledge and power between physicians and patients continue to make advertising by physicians ethically problematic. Here the truism applies that what is legal is not necessarily ethical.

Insofar as advertising by physicians is informational, it may alert individuals to unattended medical needs and appropriate treatments. But if it aims at stimulating demand for interventions that are not medically indicated, it potentially compromises professional integrity. Advertising cosmetic surgery puts physicians in the position of selling invasive procedures for which there is no medical need. Demand-stimulating advertising is especially problematic in medicine, since the willingness of physicians to provide treatments may operate as a legitimation in the mind of patients. That professionally qualified physicians are prepared to offer invasive procedures may encourage ambivalent patients to submit to medical intervention. Accordingly, advertising for interventions that are not medically needed to promote health is ethically suspect. What is acceptable business practice for selling consumer products and services is not necessarily appropriate for medical treatment. We argue below that the prevalence and unprofessional character of advertising contributes significantly to making the practice of cosmetic surgery ethically problematic.

MAPPING THE NORMATIVE DOMAIN OF MEDICINE

One of the major purposes of a conception of the internal morality of medicine is normative evaluation of practices by physicians to determine or question whether they belong within the proper domain of medicine. Violations of the internal morality of medicine consist of practices that are not supported by the goals of medicine and/or conflict with one or more of the internal duties of physicians. Examples include physician participation in capital punishment by lethal injection and prescribing anabolic steroids for athletes. Since these practices have nothing to do with treating or preventing a disease, injury, or malady, they do not serve the goals of medicine. Both involve causing or risking harms that are not compensated by medical benefits. Their performance by physicians fraudulently misrepresents medical practice by suggesting that it is proper for a physician to execute criminals or prescribe drugs to enhance athletic prowess. In addition, capital punishment is inconsistent with the context of a therapeutic relationship between physician and patient. Surgical procedures performed by a physician on close family members offer another example of a violation of the internal morality of medicine. Here the violation does not concern the goals of medicine, assuming that the procedure is medically indicated. However, the close family relationship has the potential to interfere substantially with competence (by impairing objectivity, clinical judgment, and thoroughness of medical inquiry) and with the therapeutic relationship between physician and patient.

In a previous essay we discussed a number of "borderline" medical practices, which belong within the legitimate domain of medicine but are not clearly supported by the goals of medicine and seem to conflict to some extent with one or more of the internal duties.[11] Examples include contraception and sterilization. On further reflection, we suggest that it is preferable to describe such procedures and practices as "peripheral" rather than borderline, since there are no precise, specifiable borders circumscribing unqualifiedly legitimate medical practices and defining violations. Among the definitions of "periphery" is "a zone constituting an imprecise boundary," which we think aptly characterizes the normative terrain. Thus we suggest a normative mapping of medicine that encompasses a core of legitimate medical practice, consistent with the goals and internal duties of medicine, a periphery of more or less acceptable procedures and practices outside the core, and a range of violations beyond the pale of medical legitimacy. Designating the zone within which a procedure or practice belongs is a matter of judgment based on coherence or fit with the internal morality of medicine.

Reasonable differences of opinion are likely with respect to mapping practices and procedures as within the core or the periphery. Consider the case of contraception and sterilization. Although not a disease or a malady, pregnancy is a condition that in our society brings women under medical attention. Unwanted pregnancy can be understood as a disability, which interferes with the ability of women to function normally in social life. This suggests the conclusion that contraception promotes the health of women. The health promotion rationale for contraception or sterilization is stronger in the case of women who are likely to experience serious health risks from becoming pregnant, which would support including these procedures within the core of medicine in these circumstances. Male sterilization via vasectomy, in contrast, would seem to lie more clearly in the periphery. If undertaken to prevent unwanted pregnancy, the pregnancy it prevents belongs to another person, not to the one sterilized. Unwanted paternity, unlike unwanted pregnancy, does not qualify as a medical condition to be prevented. Vasectomy, then, appears more like a "lifestyle" procedure than tubal ligation—a medical means of permitting sexual intercourse without risking pregnancy and paternity. This surgical procedure does pose some risks and complications not compensated by medical benefits. Yet we consider it an acceptable peripheral medical practice that does not threaten or violate professional integrity.

Is Cosmetic Surgery Compatible with the Internal Morality of Medicine? From the perspective of the ethics of the marketplace, governed by consumer sovereignty and honesty and fair play on the part of providers of commercial services, there appears to be nothing wrong with cosmetic surgery. It falls within the vast domain of commercial and consumer activity devoted to enhancing appearance. Cosmetic surgery involves certain risks and complications, but so does a range of other legitimate consumer activities, such as driving cars and engaging in recreational sports. In a "free society" what grounds are there for restricting the freedom of adults to purchase, and of medical practitioners to sell, cosmetic surgery? According to business ethics there are no ethical objections to cosmetic surgery as long as patients are adequately informed about risks and complications and are not subject to fraudulent marketing, and practitioners are technically competent. "Shaping up" by liposuction, for example, would seem to be an ethically acceptable, though less virtuous, alternative to jogging and working out, which are not without risks and potential complications.

Outside the minimalist ethics of the marketplace, a variety of value considerations are relevant to ethical appraisal of cosmetic surgery. The practice of cosmetic surgery may be criticized on the grounds that it is fueled by vanity and narcissistic fixation on bodily appearance. It reinforces intense concern with body image and culturally prescribed standards of beauty, especially among women, who are the major "consumers" of cosmetic surgery. It contributes to a youth culture that disdains and stigmatizes aging and the elderly. Cosmetic surgery upholds culturally specific standards of beauty— Caucasian, Anglo-Saxon, or Northern European— that stigmatize the appearance of ethnic groups that deviate from this standard. Finally, it promotes inequality between those who have and those who lack the resources to purchase the marketplace advantages of enhanced appearance via cosmetic surgery. None of these considerations, however, is relevant to the internal morality of medicine.

How, then, does cosmetic surgery stand with respect to the internal morality of medicine and professional integrity? It is difficult to find any solid support for cosmetic surgery within the goals of medicine. Those who seek to enhance their appearance by cosmetic surgery do not suffer from a diagnosable disease or injury. The qualifier "cosmetic" signifies that the surgery is not medically indicated or needed to promote health.

It might be objected that the description of cosmetic surgery as an appearance enhancement fails to do justice to the real, often prolonged, suffering from a negative body image that typically precedes the choice of cosmetic surgery.[12] The point is well taken, but it does not follow that the suffering involved belongs within the purview of medicine. As discussed above, the goals of medicine concern not all human suffering, but only that suffering connected with a malady. "Malady" in the medical context suggests an objectively diagnosable condition calling for medical treatment; and this is precisely what is lacking in the case of cosmetic surgery. The "need" for cosmetic surgery is a function entirely of subjective preference.

Kathy Davis conducted fieldwork in the Netherlands to study individuals who sought cosmetic surgery during a time in which it was covered by national health insurance. She observed 55 individuals who were examined by an official medical inspector to determine eligibility for cosmetic surgery. Davis observes,

> With one exception, a man with a cauliflower nose, I was never able to guess what the person had come in for. In some cases, I had a suspicion, as, for example, when a woman with a rather prominent nose appeared, only to have them dashed when she explained that she wanted an eyelid correction because her five-year-old son was always asking her 'why she had been crying.' My first impression confirmed that applicants for cosmetic surgery looked no different than the run-of-the-mill woman (or man) on the street and some were even decidedly attractive. Their appearance did not seem to warrant corrective measures as drastic as cosmetic surgery.[13]

Davis's inability to perceive the deficit in appearance prompting a request for cosmetic surgery was matched by a similar inability on the part of the responsible medical inspector. "Despite attempts to develop objective criteria for appearance, my observations of the Inspector's difficulties in actually making decisions about who should have cosmetic surgery presented a different picture. In practice, he routinely complained that he was unable to see why the applicant wanted cosmetic surgery."[14]

Whether all cosmetic surgery falls outside the core domain of medicine may be subject to conflicting interpretations. Reconstructive plastic surgery to correct ravages of disease and injuries as well as gross physical abnormalities constitutes a core medical practice. Reconstructive procedures. however, lie along a continuum, without any clear boundary between therapeutic reconstructive surgery for a diagnosable problem and purely cosmetic surgery. In addition, reconstructive surgery in response to deformity is guided by aesthetic considerations. Yet compare, for example, plastic surgery to remove a port-wine stain causing severe facial disfigurement, but without any functional impairment, with liposuction to produce a trimmer appearance or a facelift to "rejuvenate" facial features. The former appearance problem qualifies as a malady that is objectively discernable by all observers, and it is reasonable to describe corrective surgery as medically indicated.

In the latter cases the appearance problems giving rise to a request for cosmetic surgery are a matter entirely of subjective judgment. If surgery to remove a disfiguring port-wine stain is regarded as in part cosmetic, then at least some cosmetic procedures belong within the core of medical practice. This conclusion has no bearing, however, on the vast majority of purely cosmetic surgery procedures performed on normal bodies, which are not supported by the goals of medicine.

To give an aura of standard medical legitimacy to cosmetic surgery, cosmetic surgeons have concocted diagnostic categories warranting cosmetic surgical intervention, most notably, the "inferiority complex."[15] The extent to which this disposition to construct diagnostic categories can be taken is exemplified by Davis's account of a case conference by an eminent Dutch plastic surgeon, who described a rhinoplasty for a 15-year-old Moroccan girl. The rationale for surgery was explained in terms of a new syndrome: "inferiority complex due to racial characteristics."[16] Although on critical reflection such a medical diagnosis is apt to appear blatantly bogus, the felt need to invoke some diagnostic category to warrant cosmetic surgery testifies to the point that objective diagnosis underlies legitimate medical treatment.

Let us imagine for a moment what would be required of cosmetic surgery if we really believed that dissatisfaction with one's bodily appearance was a legitimate medical diagnosis. We have a model for such a state of affairs in the surgical treatment of transsexuals, who find their body appearance totally at odds with their perceived gender identity and suffer considerable anguish as a result. It is considered a legitimate surgical practice to operate on such persons to change their secondary sexual characteristics. But it is important to note how this is done in centers that can claim to be competent and comprehensive in their care. In particular, it is common to have sex change surgeons working very closely with teams of psychiatrists and other mental health workers, who do intensive screening of each applicant before the team decides that surgery should be performed. If the mental health assessment uncovers any evidence of psychological problems, so that managing those problems might relieve the gender dysphoria without doing surgery, then surgery is withheld and the appropriate psychotherapy is recommended instead.

This model suggests that if cosmetic surgeons truly believed that they were treating "real" psychiatric "maladies," then in order to provide minimally competent care, they ought to be working in tandem with mental health teams of this sort, and offering nonsurgical options to at least some of their patients. To our knowledge, very few if any cosmetic surgery offices and clinics are run in this fashion, which tends to suggest that cosmetic surgeons themselves do not take very seriously the claim that their practices are legitimated by the reality of psychiatric disease.

In addition to lacking support by the goals of medicine, cosmetic surgery is also ethically questionable with respect to the internal medical duties. These procedures pose risks of harm and have the potential for complications that are not compensated by any medical benefits. Furthermore, it is arguable that the willingness of physicians to perform cosmetic surgery on bodies that are not diseased, injured, or grossly abnormal fraudulently misrepresents medicine. This practice suggests a medical need and rationale for intervention, when in fact there is no diagnosable condition warranting medical treatment.

These considerations lead to the hardly surprising conclusion that cosmetic surgery lies outside the core of normative medical practice. But they leave open the question whether cosmetic surgery is a legitimate practice within the periphery of medicine or should be considered a violation of the internal morality of medicine. It is interesting to note that some of the early leaders of plastic surgery in the 1920s and 1930s expressed ethical concerns about cosmetic surgery.[17] They distinguished ethically appropriate reconstructive surgery in response to deformity and injury from purely cosmetic surgery, which they saw as the province of unprofessional "beauty doctors." For example, in an influential 1926 article published in *Annals of Surgery,* John Staige Davis wrote: "What is the ethical difference between doing an abdominal operation and removing wrinkles from a sagging face? The abdominal operation is necessary to the health of the patient, the operation for removal of wrinkles is unessential and is simply decorative surgery. True plastic surgery without question . . . is absolutely distinct and separate from what is known as cosmetic or decorative surgery."[18] Although a persuasive argument might be advanced that purely cosmetic surgery, not associated with any diagnosable deformity, violates the internal morality of medicine, we do not take this position. The continuum between reconstructive and cosmetic surgery, which makes it difficult to determine where the former ends and the latter begins, casts doubt on a blanket judgment that cosmetic surgery lies outside the domain of legitimate medical practice.

The Ethical Relevance of Advertising for Cosmetic Surgery Professional integrity concerns the fit between commitment to the norms of the internal morality of medicine and medical practice. All peripheral medical procedures and practices challenge professional integrity, since they are at best weakly supported by the goals of medicine, and they are apt to conflict with one or more of the internal duties. We submit that professional integrity is threatened, and potentially compromised, when peripheral procedures are not isolated or occasional occurrences within practice dedicated to core medical activities but are the predominant or exclusive focus of medical practice, as commonly characterizes cosmetic surgery. Moreover, the consumer-oriented, business context of cosmetic surgery risks compromising professional integrity, particularly insofar as it makes use of demand-stimulating marketing.

Advertisements for cosmetic surgery are prevalent in newspapers and the yellow pages of the telephone directory. Hundreds of sites on the World Wide Web are devoted to cosmetic surgery. For example, in the October 1997 yellow pages for suburban Washington, D.C., seven of the eight largest ads for physicians are for cosmetic surgery; and of those ads that take up one-quarter of a page or more, 18 of 31 are for cosmetic surgery. The weekly Health section of the *Washington Post* routinely contains ads placed by physicians for cosmetic surgery. These ads typically feature pictures of scantily clad, well-proportioned women and slogans such as "Bikini Time," "Let your mirror image be a masterpiece," "Reshape your future," "Spring into summer with a new look," "A New You for The New Millennium." In the *Washington Post Magazine* glossy ads have appeared recently for cosmetic surgery focusing on large-breasted women, with the slogans "Big and Believable," and "A Bustline for the Shoreline." These ads also feature the names, medical degrees, and board certification of plastic surgeons. Such advertisements juxtapose the lowest common denominator of marketing—sex sells—with markers of professional competence. The role of physician as salesman is displayed by the frequent offer in cosmetic surgery ads of free consultations, often with the aid of computer imaging. Targeted at women, these ads play on, and possibly contribute to, widespread dissatisfaction with body image and foster unrealistic expectations of what can be achieved by cosmetic surgery. Moreover, they give no indication of risks or complications from cosmetic surgery or the chance of less than fully satisfying outcomes.

The marketing of cosmetic surgery to consumers as a commercial service is particularly accentuated in a recent ad in the *Washington Post* health section. Under the bold headline, "Body Sculpting," it depicts the silhouette of a nude woman with an hourglass figure. Also in bold is the announcement of "100% Financing" followed by a list of cosmetic procedures offered and the following sales pitch: "Call today to arrange for a free consultation with one of our experienced plastic surgeons who'll use computer imaging to demonstrate how you could look after cosmetic surgery. You'll also learn about our finance plan with no down payment and low monthly payments."

It is revealing to evaluate the professional appropriateness of cosmetic surgery marketing by comparing samples of advertisements for cosmetic surgery, such as those described above, with statements from the Code of Ethics for the American Society of Plastic and Reconstructive Surgeons, approved in 1992.[19] Under the heading of Specific Principles, conditions are listed under which "Each member may be subject to disciplinary action, including expulsion." The category pertaining to advertising is the following: "The member . . . uses or participates in the use of any form of communication (including computer imaging and electronic communications) containing a false, fraudulent, deceptive, or misleading statement or claim." Included among unethical communication is a statement or claim that "[i]s intended or is likely to create false or unjustified expectations of favorable results"; "[a]ppeals primarily to layperson's fears, anxieties, or emotional vulnerabilities"; and "[i]s intended or likely to attract patients by use of puffery or exaggerated claims."

We contend that advertisements for cosmetic surgery routinely violate these professional ethical guidelines. They purvey misleading images and slogans, appeal to emotional vulnerabilities, and foster unrealistic expectations, rather than convey useful information about cosmetic surgery. These advertisements suggest that there is "a quick fix" for bodily improvement. They trade on glamour and dreams without drawing attention to risks and complications. Unprofessional advertising aimed at stimulating demand for invasive surgical procedures that are not medically indicated threatens, if not violates, professional integrity. Moreover, apart from the unprofessional character of much advertising for cosmetic surgery, the very use of advertising for cosmetic surgery is ethically problematic. Physicians should not be in the business of promoting medically unnecessary surgery on normal individuals.

It is a very basic component of the internal morality of medicine that physicians not be involved in the deliberate creation of disease just so that they can expand their practices and increase their earnings. For example, sprinkling resistant microorganisms into the town water supply would be the grossest possible violation of the internal morality of medicine. Yet if we imagine that an individual's dissatisfaction with his or her own bodily appearance is the (so-called) "disease" that cosmetic surgery is designed to treat, then it is arguable that the most extreme and misleading advertisements are analogous to this physician-as-Typhoid-Mary example. The ads are deliberately designed to convince people who might previously have thought that their appearance was acceptable that they are in fact seriously inadequate unless they seek a surgical correction for their newly discovered "problem."

An obvious rejoinder is that a medical "problem" can never be defined completely in isolation from the state of the art of medical therapy. On this view, advertising does not create a new perception of a problem that did not previously exist. Instead, people who all along had problems, but imagined that nothing practically could be done, are now being informed that a relatively safe and effective treatment exists so that they can be encouraged to come forward and seek relief. But this response seems disingenuous when we reflect how dependent body image is on the prevailing social norms of beauty. The more extreme ads for cosmetic surgery convey the message that the models shown in the ads represent the standard of beauty to which all sensible people should aspire, and that these models have achieved that standard of beauty precisely because they have themselves submitted to cosmetic surgery (perhaps numerous times). By promoting *dis-ease* and thus stimulating demand for cosmetic surgery, such advertisements clearly violate the internal morality of medicine.

IMPLICATIONS

Our argument suggests that cosmetic surgery is ethically questionable from the perspective of the internal morality of medicine, which makes it at best a peripheral medical practice. Ethical concern is heightened by the organization of cosmetic surgery as a consumer-oriented business supported by heavy use of marketing, much of which is misleading and unprofessional. Accordingly, we conclude that the current state of cosmetic surgery practice threatens professional integrity. Some might go further and conclude that cosmetic surgery does not belong within medicine.[20] This rigorist position may seem appealing theoretically but is unlikely to have any practical effect. More importantly, if cosmetic surgery should be ruled out of medicine because it does not serve the goals of medicine, then other widely endorsed procedures and practices that also are not supported by the goals of medicine, such as contraception and sterilization, may be ethically imperiled. We contend that the marketing of cosmetic surgery raises especially serious concern from the perspective of professional ethics—concern that ought to be addressed in practice. Cosmetic surgeons who engage in misleading or fraudulent advertising appear to want to have it both ways. In marketing cosmetic surgery, they use standard, but contextually objectionable, techniques of consumer advertising, coupled with drawing attention to their professional medical credentials. The incoherence between projection of professional competence and trust, and the reliance on sleazy advertising techniques, compromises professional integrity.

Those wishing to defend the ethics of cosmetic surgery as consistent with the internal morality of medicine may take comfort in our labeling of the practice as "peripheral" rather than as outside the boundaries. But the preceding discussion suggests that a price is paid when a practice is accepted as peripheral within medicine. The more a practice occupies a peripheral rather than a central position in relation to the goals and duties internal to medicine, the more physicians are obligated to free that practice from any association with potentially distracting or corrupting influences such as a profit motive. To see what this entails, recall how surgical sterilization was often handled by many physicians 20 or 30 years ago, when there tended to be more moral unease than there is today about the peripheral position of that practice. In a day when concern about informed consent had not yet been felt in most of medical practice, physicians went to great lengths to assure that patients were fully informed and had carefully thought about sterilization before being willing to do the procedure. It was as if these physicians were bending over backwards to demonstrate that it was not a desire to expand their practices and make more money that stimulated them to do those surgeries.

On this view, if cosmetic surgeons took the internal morality of medicine seriously, they would scrupulously refrain from ethically suspect advertising and minimize the profit-making orientation of their practice—even more so than physicians whose daily work was more safely nestled within the core of medicine. By contrast, in the practice of cosmetic surgery we find the coexistence of two factors: (i) a practice within medicine that is demonstrably quite peripheral; and (ii) heavy reliance on questionable advertising and other signs that an ethic of business rather than of medicine is operating. We conclude that a serious threat to the internal morality of medicine exists in the way this practice is conducted, even though we do not contend that the practice itself is totally outside the bounds of allowable medical activity.

Leaders of the medical profession, particularly those connected with the practice of plastic surgery, should take steps to curb unethical marketing of invasive procedures that are not medically indicated. In addition, they should promote attention to professional ethics in the context of specialty training of plastic surgeons. More broadly, teaching the internal morality of medicine, by precept and example, may discourage medical students and physicians in training from diverting their careers to a peripheral and ethically problematic practice, outside the core domain of medicine.

On the theoretical level we suggest that the critical evaluation of cosmetic surgery from the perspective of the internal morality of medicine demonstrates the significance of this ethical approach. Focus on the internal morality of medicine brings to light ethical considerations and concerns that lie beneath the surface of the mainstream of bioethics. As new interventions are developed that are aimed at enhancing human abilities and subjective well-being, in contrast to treating disease, injury, or dysfunction—e.g., growth hormone to combat the effects of aging, "cosmetic psychopharmacology," drugs to enhance sexual performance, and genetic engineering—attention to the internal morality of medicine and professional integrity is likely to grow more prominent, and this perspective is likely to achieve greater refinement and depth.

NOTES

1 American Society of Plastic and Reconstructive Surgeons (www.plasticsurgery.org).

2 Gillespie R. Women, the body and brand extension in medicine: Cosmetic surgery and the paradox of choice. *Women & Health* 1996:24:75.

3 Davis K. *Reshaping the Female Body: The Dilemma of Cosmetic Surgery.* New York: Routledge 1995:27–8.

4 Siebert C. The cuts that go deeper. *New York Times Magazine* 1996: July 7:24.

5 Sherwin S. Feminism and bioethics. In: Wolf S. M., ed. *Feminism & Bioethics.* New York: Oxford University Press, 1996:59.

6 Miller F. G., Brody H. Professional integrity and physician-assisted death. *Hastings Center Report* 1995;25(3):8–17; Brody H., Miller F. G. The internal morality of medicine: explication and application to managed care. *Journal of Medicine and Philosophy.* 1998; 23:384–410.

7 Callahan D. The goals of medicine: Setting new priorities [Special Supplement]. *Hastings Center Report* 1996; 25(6):S1–S26.

8 See note 6, Miller and Brody 1995.

9 Plato, *The Republic.* trans. HDP Lee. Harmondsworth, U.K.: Penguin, 1955:69–70.

10 Dyer A. R. Ethics, advertising and the definition of a profession. *Journal of Medical Ethics* 1985:11:72–8.

11 See note 6, Brody. Miller 1998:23:384–410.

12 See note 3, Davis 1995.

13 See note 3, Davis 1995:70.

14 See note 3, Davis 1995:72.

15 Haiken E. *Venus Envy: A History of Cosmetic Surgery.* Baltimore: Johns Hopkins University Press, 1997:90–130.

16 See note 3, Davis 1995:2.

17 See note 15, Haiken 1997:50–2, 93–103.

18 See note 15, Haiken 1997:93.

19 American Society of Plastic and Reconstructive Surgeons. *Code of Ethics,* rev. 1992.

20 Hyman D. A. Aesthetics and ethics: the implications of cosmetic surgery. *Perspectives in Biology and Medicine* 1990; 33:190–202.

COSMETIC SURGERY, SUSPECT NORMS, AND THE ETHICS OF COMPLICITY

Margaret Olivia Little

Cosmetic surgery, according to Little, is distinguished by the fact that the suffering medicine is asked to alleviate is a function of social norms—relating to appearance—rather than biological dysfunction. Little focuses on those cases of requested cosmetic surgery in which the content of the relevant norms "reflects, flows from, and reinforces a system of beliefs, attitudes, and practices that together involve deep injustice." Examples include breast augmentation to make women look like supermodels and surgeries designed to make African Americans look more white. Rejecting the view that doctors have responsibilities only to their patients, Little argues that medicine has to be accountable for its relationship to the suspect social norms and practices that often drive requests for cosmetic surgery. At the same time, the importance of physicians' avoiding complicity with unjust norms can conflict with the importance of relieving suffering, which may sometimes be accomplished by acceding to requests for the sorts of surgery in question. While some cosmetic surgeons apparently "side" with the suspect norms of appearance, exploiting their content and even adding to their force with manipulative advertising and the like (a concern addressed by Miller, Brody, and Chung), some cosmetic surgeons reject the norms in question while wanting to be responsive to the attendant suffering of individuals who request their services. Little addresses the moral tension experienced by the latter cosmetic surgeons by defending a holistic way of understanding the moral meaning of surgeons' actions. Accordingly, in addition to recommending a far more vigorous informed consent process than is typical today, she advises, "sometimes perform the surgery, and always fight the system."

Cosmetic surgery is often cited as a paradigm of "medical enhancement."[1] Most of the time, this classification is meant to signal the view that such surgery is not medically necessary—not needed, that is, for the maintenance or restoration of health. Under one publicly popular picture of what moves people to have cosmetic surgery (what we might call the "Beverly Hills" picture), such a conclusion follows from the view that the surgery isn't necessary in any sense: it is a luxury, motivated by pleasure—and pleasure born of vanity, to boot—rather than the need to avoid or end suffering. In reality, of course, the landscape is more mixed: while there are cultural enclaves in which the pursuit of "beauty by scalpel" is as excessive as any parody might imagine, requests for cosmetic surgery are often motivated by deep and genuine suffering, in which surgery is pursued, not from a desire for beauty, but from a desire to end a distressing sense of alienation from some body part or to escape incessant teasing. In these cases, classifying cosmetic surgery as beyond medical necessity is not meant to make light of the suffering, but to remind us that the suffering is not born of disease or physiological dysfunction: whatever necessity the surgeries might carry, it is not *medical* necessity.

Questions about cosmetic surgery's status as an enhancement in this sense of the term are clearly of importance when we are trying to decide whether its provision falls within the *duties* of medical practitioners and third-party payers. But there is another set of questions about cosmetic surgery's status as an enhancement that concerns a very different, and altogether more charged, issue—namely, whether it is *appropriate* for medicine to provide it. For enhancement is also sometimes used as a boundary concept, marking off the limits of what falls within medicine's purview; and questions recur about whether cosmetic surgeries fall on the far side of that boundary. This set of questions concerns, not whether medicine must provide cosmetic surgery, but whether it *ought* to.

The question is most familiarly raised about cosmetic surgery *tout court,* expressing concern about the very idea of medicine using its interventions to alter appearances. Raised in this way, the question is familiarly controversial. Those with a traditional conception of medicine's telos will be uneasy at the thought of using surgery to satisfy the dictates of fads and fashions, of incurring medical risk without providing medical benefit. Others will argue that the source of suffering is less important than the ability of medicine to alleviate it; indeed, some will extend the argument to ask why medicine shouldn't provide a little pleasure, and not just remove pain, as long as the risks aren't too high.

While this controversy is an interesting and important one, focusing our attention on the appropriateness of cosmetic surgery as such threatens to obscure a deeper and much graver issue about medicine's involvement with the cosmetic. Whatever we think about medicine being in the general business of altering appearances, I will argue that we should have special concerns about a specific class of cosmetic surgeries—namely, those whose moral status is complicated by their relationship to what I'll be calling "suspect norms of appearance." As I will explain, this moral issue is a nuanced one that won't be resolved simply by deciding how narrowly or broadly to draw medicine's telos or by weighing the risks and benefits of procedures to individual patients. In this essay, I want to isolate the nature of the concern I have in mind, to defend that it is important, and to suggest some of the implications it carries for the contours of medicine's moral responsibilities.

SURGERY AND SOCIAL NORMS

Cosmetic surgery, as a class, is distinctive in that the suffering medicine is asked to alleviate is in some sense due to social attitudes and norms rather than some disease or biological dysfunction. What distinguishes the distress suffered over some aspect of one's appearance from the pain, say, of a broken leg is that the former is parasitic on some value or aesthetic norm that society happens to hold. Perhaps the patient has internalized the norm and wants very much to meet it; perhaps she herself does not accept it but suffers because those who do accept the norm treat her differently. Concerns with appearance, then, reflect the influences of social attitudes, values, and preferences. I want to urge, though, that not all norms and pressures about appearance are on the same moral plane. Let me give three sets of cases to illustrate what I have in mind.

For the first case, imagine a society in which double chins are regarded as enormously attractive. While deeply held, the preference for voluptuous chins is understood to be a matter of aesthetic taste: those who possess only one chin are not vilified; they simply aren't anyone's idea of the dream Saturday-night date. In this society, as in ours, people differ in how much importance they place on being attractive, and some will be blithely carefree about the whole issue; but we can well imagine a person who has come to suffer deeply because he has just the one lonely chin. He has tried, we shall imagine, to shrug off this lack, to find compensating measures elsewhere in his life, even psychotherapy, all to no avail. He is self-conscious and miserable with his current chin, and requests a surgical implant.

The second case is all too real. Think of a young boy who has ears that stick straight out. Imagine further that he is one of the unfortunates who is teased mercilessly and constantly by his schoolmates and children of casual encounter. His parents have tried to comfort him and to offer him strategies for dealing with his tormentors, but to no avail. The taunting has begun to color his whole outlook on life: he becomes withdrawn, begins wetting the bed; his grades drop. His parents finally decide, with his enthusiastic support and relief, to request that a surgeon tuck his ears closer to his head.

The third case is also taken from our own society. Imagine a black person who, either because he has internalized certain messages or because he wishes to escape certain stigmas, requests procedures that will make him look more like a white European—narrowing the nose, thinning the lips, lightening the skin. Or again, imagine a woman who, increasingly distressed and dissatisfied with her size-eight body and the enormous gap she perceives between that body and the pictures of feminine physicality ubiquitous in popular culture, requests a series of surgeries that will bring her closer to the paradigm exemplified by super models—extensive liposuction, recontouring the cheekbones, perhaps a rib extraction or two, all finished off with breast augmentation.

Even if we stipulate that the levels of suffering are the same in these three cases, I want to urge that they are importantly different in terms of the moral considerations they raise. Start with the first case. Hopefully we can sympathize with the poor fellow who has but one chin: given his yearning to be attractive and the aesthetic tastes of his society, we can agree that he was dealt a bad hand in life's lottery. But in this sort of case, while the person suffers real pain that is indeed importantly parasitic on his society's attitudes and preferences, I don't think we would say that society is *culpable* for that pain. Society gets to have convergences of idiosyncratic preferences, tastes, fads, and fashions. Such conver-

gences will affect different people differently, but this difference alone does not mean that anything morally problematic is afoot. As the saying goes, not everything that is *unfortunate* is *unfair*. To give another example, in the United States more people are fanatical about basketball than about horse racing; very tall men therefore have a shot at becoming famous sports heroes in a way that very short men do not. A man whose sole desire in life is to reach megastardom in the sports world but who is only five feet tall has a dream that is very unlikely to come true. But again, while we may pity this person's distress and empathize with his misfortune, we should not regard it as pain that implicates society.

Turn now to the second case, to the boy whose ears stick out. Once again we find society expressing a certain preference, this time for a particular ear formation. In this case, though, something has gone wrong with society's reaction to those who deviate from the preferred appearance. Here the costs imposed for such deviation—the teasing, the ostracism—are grossly out of proportion to society's own reflective valuation of the norm. They are punitive, intolerant, in a word, *cruel*. In contrast to the first case, in which the society's aesthetic preference was strong but morally tolerant, in this case parts of society—children, say, and the parents, teachers, and other adults who are negligently permissive about the children's behavior—act immorally in the costs they mete out to those who fail to meet their preferences. We might call the attitude toward the boy a prejudice rather than a preference to mark the difference. Here society surely deserves blame for at least some of the boy's suffering—not because society has preferences or norms about appearance, but because it is immoral in its "enforcement" of those norms.

Now part of what is morally problematic about the third class of examples (illustrated by surgeries designed to make blacks look more white and women more like super models) is a similar inappropriateness in the enforcement of norms. Part of our unease about a black person being made to look more white results from the fact that the punishment inflicted on those with extremely black African features is often egregious, ranging from cruel teasing and ostracism to lessened opportunities in employment and housing. A similar story can be told for the norms of appearance that women face. While both men and women face pressures regarding their appearance, the pressures are neither symmetrical nor equal. Woman has tended historically to be *defined* by her appearance in a way man has not.[2] The virtue of beauty has been more central to female virtues than it has to male virtues, and woman has been more tightly associated or identified with body than with mind (a point that reappears historically as a premise undergirding the conclusion that woman is less rational than man).[3] Norms of appearance turn out to be, then, not norms of a *good-looking woman,* but norms of a *good woman,* full stop. Deviations from these norms of appearance are thus more highly punished than those applying to men (the pressure to "make the most of oneself" is for women a pressure that bespeaks an *obligation,* not a desideratum). After all, a man who fails in this category has failed in something that is only incidental to his nature; a woman has sinned against one of her deepest charges.

Part of what is morally problematic about the third class of cases, then, is that the cost imposed by society for failing to live up to its norms of appearance is here excessive, punitive, unfair, or cruel. But this problem isn't, I think, the full story about the third class of cases. I want to argue that there is another, very important source of moral unease in this third category. What is also problematic about these surgeries, I want to urge, is that the very *content* of the norms of appearance they involve is morally suspect. We feel a heightened moral unease about these cases, I want to urge, because the norms of appearance at issue are grounded in or get life from a broader system of attitudes and actions that is in fact *unjust.*

Consider the norm of attractiveness at issue in surgeries designed to make blacks look more white. We are not dealing here with some whimsical aesthetic preference. It is no *accident* that the standard of beauty prevalent in the West favors white European features over black African ones. It reflects a long-standing tradition in which being black is devalued and being white is valorized. Indeed, it reflects the remnants of a time-honored view—supported through history by major social institutions, especially science and religion—that the races are hierarchically arranged in nature, with

the white race standing as the exemplar of humanity, while the black race, quite literally subhuman, stands closer to the apes.[4] The racial and ethnic contours of our norms of attractiveness were shaped as part and parcel of this broader conception of humanity.

Our uneasiness at the example of the black trying to look more white, then, is not simply a result of the fact that it involves racial features. There is something more presumptively problematic about incentives and pressures for blacks to look white than there is about incentives and pressures for whites to play with the exoticism of looking black. The former takes place against a broad context of devaluing blackness and a pressure to assimilate to an unjust paradigm of humanness.

Once again the point continues with the norms of appearance that are applied to women. Throughout history, woman and the "feminine" has been cast in roles of contamination, infection, and danger.[5] The resulting alienation toward features regarded as distinctly or especially feminine gets reflected in the norms of appearance applying to the feminine: in some cultures, it appears as a hatred of female fat, in others, as a hatred of female body hair. In virtually all cultures, it shows up in the fact that women's norms of appearance tend to be farther from the natural, the average, or the usual than are men's (e.g. fewer decades of a woman's life than a man's count as candidates for beauty)—a point that helps explain why women's standards of appearance are usually much harder to meet than are men's. Further, as several historians have noted, the idea of beauty has been defined as the object of the male, not female, gaze.[6] Given that the nature and worth of woman are seen as residing so largely in her appearance, subliminally we begin to believe that the nature and worth of woman reside largely, if not exhaustively, in her existence as an object of male gaze. Consequently, the content of women's norms of appearance have a much greater tendency to objectify women than do men's norms of appearance—a theoretical point that is borne out all too vividly when we look at images of women in "entertainment" and advertising.[7] At heart, the norms of women's appearance reflect, not aesthetic whim, but distorted, unjust conceptions of woman herself.

In the third classification, then, the content of the standards is part and parcel of an unjust social ideology. The examples so far adduced have involved race and gender, but I don't mean to suggest that the problem is limited to these categories. Put generally, it seems to me that norms of appearance occupy a morally suspect status when their content reflects, flows from, and reinforces a system of beliefs, attitudes, and practices that together involve deep injustice. If any one central theme is common to such oppressive systems, as we might call them, it is perhaps the view that some group occupies less than full human status; and certainly categories other than race and gender have been the target of such ideological exclusions. Take for instance the case of children with Down's syndrome. Such children have distinctive facial features that publicly "mark" them; as such they often encounter hurtful teasing and distorted expectations. At the very least such cases belong in our second category, as instances in which society is culpably cruel in the costs it imposes for failing to meet some norm. But such cases may also fit the third category, for the *content* of the norms invoked may well be morally suspect. That is, while it may be that we have a merely aesthetic dislike of the facial features typical of those with Down's syndrome, it may be that the reason we have such an aesthetic reaction is because of some historical association these features have with a certain conception of "idiocy," namely, one in which "idiots" were regarded as occupying something less than full human status. The extent to which such a conception continues subterraneously to inform those norms, and for the norms to reinforce a broader system of unfairly constraining practices, is the extent to which the content of the norms themselves inherit a status that is morally suspect.

The cases of cosmetic surgery that raise special moral concern, then, are cases in which the dissatisfaction or distress that people ask medicine to alleviate results, not from morally innocuous preferences, but from practices or ideologies that are morally troubling—for instance, suffering that stems from cruel teasing, or distress that arises from trying to meet the pressures of a norm whose content is steeped in injustice. The question now at issue is whether this concern is one that is relevant to the moral responsibilities of *medicine*. Does the fact that the demand for such surgeries arises in problematic contexts count as a morally salient consideration for medicine's practices; does it carry any ethical implications for medicine as an institution or for surgeons as individual professionals?

One mainstream view of medicine's responsibilities contends that it does not. According to this view, much as we may abhor the attitudes and pressures that lie behind such surgeries, it is not and cannot be within medicine's purview to pass judgment on them or to use them as factors in determining what surgeries should be performed. After all, it is urged, to perform a surgery is not to agree with the values underwriting the request—physicians often disagree with patients' values or preferences, but respect for patient autonomy requires that they not automatically substitute their own values for the patient's. In short, while the moral unease we feel at surgeries designed to make blacks look more white or women look more like super models may point to an important agenda for general society, medicine's role-specific duty must be to bracket these concerns, to take the situation as it is found, and to focus on its primary charge: having compassion for patients' suffering and alleviating it where possible.

However appealing such a view is on first glance, it fails to do justice to the moral contours of the situation. Whatever we might decide about the all-things-considered moral permissibility of performing such surgeries, we must surely agree that they call for *some* sort of moral hesitancy. That is, a surgeon who finds herself in a community of Stepford women trying to look pneumatic, or in a racist state whose government pays for blacks to look more white, must surely feel some moral unease at using her role to such purposes. To put it somewhat differently, even if the surgeon decides to go ahead with the surgeries—to alleviate, say, the extreme censure the patients would otherwise face—there will be a moral *residue* to doing so. But the model of medical responsibility that underwrites this response provides no means for explaining or grounding this modest, and thoroughly intuitive, notion. Even if the suspect nature of the norms leaves the surgeries permissible, it is far too strong to say that it is of no moral salience to the surgeon at all.

I think that the mainstream model gets the wrong answer because it's looking in the wrong place. It assumes that the moral covenant at issue in these worrisome surgeries is the surgeon's covenant to the individual patients who stand before her. It casts the moral question, that is, in terms of the physician-patient relationship, an approach which, not surprisingly, delivers the familiar advice to alleviate the patient's suffering and respect his autonomy wherever possible. But the moral complication such surgeries present to medicine concerns another relationship altogether—the relation between the surgeon, or indeed medicine as an institution, and the suspect norms and practices themselves. We focus the moral issue too tightly if we focus only on the duty to relieve suffering, for as real as this duty is, there is a further issue about the physician's relationship to the system that causes that suffering. The deeper moral issue these cosmetic surgeries raise is, in short, the issue of *complicity*.

ACTING WITH INTEGRITY

What is it permissible to do in the face of cruel bullying or of pressures backed by suspect norms? When is it acceptable to accommodate these pressures, and when does doing so count as "selling out" or "giving in"? What paths from suffering can one take without a loss of integrity? When is one to be cheered for taking measures to escape the unfairly punitive system, and when is one to be judged an "Uncle Tom" or a "recruit of the patriarchy"? These questions hopefully give some indication of the complexity of the moral terrain here. Concerns about complicity are *nuanced* concerns. They are not reducible to moral concerns about the aggregate net utility of one's actions, or to concerns about the wrongs one might do to some specified individuals. To be complicitous is to bear some improper relation *to the evil* of some practice or set of attitudes. Just what relation is it?

Put in broadest brushstrokes, let me suggest that one is complicitous when one endorses, promotes, or unduly benefits from norms and practices that are morally suspect. How we unpack this schematic answer depends on the context, of course. Certainly, the worst cases are those that involve explicit (if sometimes subtle) endorsement and exploitation of

the norms and practices themselves. In the practice of cosmetic surgery, we find this sort of crass complicity represented all too well. The widespread practices of advertising to create demand, of under-emphasizing risks and overclaiming results, of suggesting procedures over and above the ones initially requested by the patient, are bad enough; the point here is that the promotions often exploit the suspect norms themselves. When the surgeries suggested to blacks are predictably for narrower noses rather than broader ones, when advertisement rhetoric plays to women's anxieties that anything over size four is fat, when patients report that surgeons suggest breast augmentations more often than they suggest breast reduction, we have patterns that reflect and endorse the content of the suspect norms. Matters are worse when such exploitation is done for the purpose of personal gain. Whether or not medicine in general should be pursued simply to make money (an issue I'm bracketing here), performing surgeries involving suspect norms solely for personal gain deserves heightened scrutiny—think of acting the Uncle Tom to make one's *second* million. Indeed, whatever the motive, there is something presumptively troubling about a practice that reaps profit from making society more white and women more like Barbie Dolls, if only because those who profit from the system run a tremendous danger of becoming invested in seeing it continue.

There are, then, cases in which practitioners of medicine have, in essence, "sided" with the suspect norms of appearance, exploiting their content and counterfactually sustaining their force. These cases deserve our ethical scrutiny and our ethical censure. But the theoretically more challenging, because more subtle, aspect of complicity remains yet to be addressed. Obviously, the picture presented here, while depressingly common, does not describe all cosmetic surgeons. Just as patients have a variety of motives for requesting cosmetic surgery, not all of which fit stereotypes of shallow vanity, surgeons have a variety of motives for performing such surgeries, not all of which fit stereotypes of cynical exploitation. Many surgeons are morally decent folk—a few even morally heroic—whose intentions betray no endorsement of the norms that underwrite many patients' requests. They decry the pressures that lead to patients' suffering, much as they would decry the prevalence of a virus, and would change that aspect of society if they could; in the meantime, though, they are motivated by the genuinely noble goal of relieving the distress they find. (Indeed, the now-classic moral defense for performing frivolous or worrisome cosmetic surgeries is that it funds *pro bono* work doing reconstructive surgery on those with severe disfigurements.)

Certainly, we want to mark off these activities as different from the crass ones. But the deeper question is whether the difference is sufficient to free them from all dangers of complicity. The question is whether purity of motive suffices to insulate actions. Take, for instance, first-person worries about one's own possible complicity. Such questions only arise when one abhors a system—one wouldn't *worry* about participating in an activity one endorsed. The surgeon who is asked to make blacks look more like whites under a system of apartheid feels tension at the prospect of performing such surgeries precisely *because* she regards apartheid as evil. Questions about complicity often start, not end, with the judgment that one disapproves of a system or practice. Reflecting on these points presses us to question whether an approach that grants us absolution from complicity as long as we don't want to support a suspect system might be drawing the moral lines too cleanly.

The residual concern is that complicity might arise, not just when one subjectively endorses the suspect system, but when one's actions in fact end up reinforcing it. Clearly, one's actions can de facto serve to promote a system one does not intentionally set out to bolster, and the danger is particularly deep for the actions of medicine. For one thing, medicine enjoys an extraordinarily high institutional status in society; its participation in such surgeries can easily be regarded as sanctioning the importance and appropriateness of those norms. When the institution of medicine helps turn society white or women into Barbie Dolls, those maneuvers can seem to be backed by one of the central institutional authorities of our society. Further danger arises from the fact that the institution of medicine, in addition to occupying high status, is primarily concerned with health and healing. Its participation can unwittingly bring

suspect surgeries under that umbrella, so that the norms of appearance get blurred with norms of "health" and "normalcy," reinforcing sexist and racist conceptions of what the paradigm human is like. And the mere fact that medical interventions, which in general are associated with risk and invasiveness, are used to achieve some end tends to elevate the importance of that end: the tacit inference is that it must be *worth* doing, and not simply idiosyncratically desired, if it justifies taking such risks. (This outcome is especially true when surgeries are designed merely to gratify a patient's desire to meet the norm. When the deployment of medicine's social role is not the alleviation of suffering, but the satisfaction of the desire to meet a norm of appearance, the norm itself becomes elevated in stature—the opposite of what we want to see happen when the norms are suspect.)

But what are the contours of moral responsibility here? Are we now to conclude that duty demands us to avoid anything that will causally reinforce a suspect system? Do our own conceptions of our actions count for nothing? If we are tempted by the view that intention is the sole arbiter of complicity, it is surely in part because we recoil at the thought that the morality of our actions should be held hostage in this way to the existence of the suspect system, which would end up not only causing harm but grounding a startling extensive prohibition against measures that might help alleviate that harm.

The question here is what counts as "participating in" a suspect system one does not endorse; and it misses the nuance of complicity simply to equate that notion with causal reinforcement of a system. For the nuance of complicity (and the reason I think it is such a useful concept) is located precisely in the fact that responsibility for such causal effect should sometimes be laid at our doorstep and sometimes at the doorstep of the suspect system.

Let me suggest a different approach to the issue. When even well-intentioned actions unwittingly play a large role in legitimizing and reinforcing the suspect norms under discussion, they do so because of the *meaning* that those surgeries carry for others—they do so because others see in them a legitimization of or pressure to meet norms. This approach gives us better direction for understanding the terrain of responsibilities here. Clearly, one should not be held hostage to all possible interpretations of our actions, to all the meanings others might attach to our behavior. But it is negligence to ignore the interpretations that others may naturally be expected to place on our actions given the broad context in which they take place. That is, while one is not responsible, for instance, when others willfully or negligently misinterpret one's actions, one cannot simply turn a blind eye to all but the meanings one *wishes* others would see in our actions: we have a duty to forestall those interpretations that, while unintended, would be completely natural given the larger background context in which the action takes place.

If something like this notion is right, then the key to analyzing complicity is found when we remember that the meaning carried by actions, just as the meaning carried by words, is determined *holistically*. It is not found in individual features of an action—it is not equivalent to its effects, and it is certainly not solipsistically determined by our intention. Meaning emerges, rather, as a function of a broad context, including, significantly, the backdrop of other actions one performs. This idea suggests that we refocus our moral attention. Instead of examining the morality of an individual piece of surgery, we must examine the context in which that individual act of surgery takes place. The broad implication is, in essence, a conditional form of the motto, "If you're not part of the solution, you're part of the problem." If one must perform surgeries to help people meet suspect norms of appearance (out of concern for their suffering, say), then one must maintain an overall stance of fighting the norms. The only way to participate in the surgeries without de facto promoting the evil whose effects one decries is to locate the surgery in a broader context of naming and rejecting the evil norms. One's purpose and meaning—that of alleviating the extreme burdens the system places on some—can be expressed only if one's broader actions stand squarely against the norms.

Even in pursuing surgery from motives that are distant from the suspect norms, then, one must be cognizant of, and take into account, the possible side effects of one's actions. One has a responsibility to maintain and make clear the meaning of the action,

and to factor in the increased pressure others may in fact feel as a result of having surgically "improved" appearance. At the very least, this responsibility would require those who perform the surgeries to speak out publicly against the suspect content of the norms—to be a general voice against, rather than promoter of, the norms and practices in question. But it will also issue in more specific recommendations driven by the specific contours of the suspect system's content. Let me give an example drawing from the case of women's appearance.

A true appreciation of the special injustices underlying norms of women's appearance would influence and enrich our idea of what constitutes proper informed consent for such surgeries. Take for instance the matter of informing patients of the options they face. It may seem needless to recount the option of not pursuing surgery, but in fact doing so is not at all unimportant. One of the insidious ways sexism works is by gradually constricting the options that women imaginatively conceive for themselves. Such constriction happens, of course, with women's norms of appearance: the presumption for certain appearances is so heavy that our models of acceptable appearance occupy a narrow range. Medicine can take proactive steps to counteract this constriction by responsibly underscoring the option not to pursue surgery.

I don't mean that medicine should issue some vague admonition for women to rest content with their current appearance: to do so would be naive if not condescending. But far more use could be made of women's own differing experiences with cosmetic surgery and appearance. Some prospective patients arrive at medicine's doorstep less decided on the procedures than others. It would help stretch their imaginative options if one gave these women access (through videos, conversations, or written narratives) to a wide variety of women's experience: experiences from women who decided to go through with the surgery and are happy, from those who did so and have regrets, and from women who decided in the end not to have the surgery at all. And, again, it is important for women to have access to studies and narratives that bring to life the various real-life experiences women have of their bodies and society's reaction to them, not only that benefits are portrayed more realistically, but that the dangers and risks—social as well as medical—are understood. To give just one example, some defend breast augmentation as empowering, for large breasts enable one to "rivet men's gaze."[8] But it is not the power to rivet men's gaze when and only when one desires that gaze, and there are many circumstances in which having a man's gaze riveted at one's breasts is anything but what one desires, as when one is trying to be taken seriously as a job candidate.

CONCLUSION

Whatever we think of the general idea of medicine altering appearance, we should have special, and deep, concerns about medicine participating in practices that reflect and reinforce certain suspect norms of appearance. Medicine and surgeons must beware the extent to which their participation in cosmetic surgeries involving such norms ends up contributing to a broad and unjust system of constraining pressures and forces. For while we want to alleviate what can be very real pain, the danger arises that, in doing so, we will be acting in a way that is complicitous with the very evils that give rise to it.

Yet there is surely some role for medicine to perform surgeries even in cases involving suspect norms. There is a limit to the suffering we require victims of the norm to bear before taking measures to escape that suffering, and health-care professionals are sometimes the only ones who can alleviate that distress. Determining medicine's proper role in helping people meet suspect norms of appearance, then, is a complicated task, for there are two relations a physician must properly juggle—her relation to the individual patient, and her relation to the system of norms.

The tension between the duties grounded in these respective relations, I have argued, can be somewhat lessened when we remember that the relation one must maintain to the norms is *holistically* defined: one must, if one participates in such surgeries at all, maintain an overall stance of fighting against the system. Such a general stance can leave room for occasions of helping a distressed patient by performing surgery that admittedly involves the suspect norms. There is all the difference in the world, that is, between, on the

one hand, a surgeon who promotes, suggests, and aggressively advertises these surgeries, who performs them whether the patient requests it out of self-abnegation, desire for power, or anguish, who is glad when, for instance, trends in women's figures and faces change because shifting fads mean repeat business, and who is vaguely pleased that there is so much pressure on women to meet the norms because it means increased profits, and, on the other hand, a surgeon who does not suggest or promote the suspect surgeries, who helps her patients explore other options, who speaks out against the pressures women face, but who occasionally uses her surgical skills in cases where there seems no other path out of true suffering. Medicine does indeed have two duties to attend to when thinking about whether to perform the troubling surgeries, but I think they can be somewhat reconciled: sometimes perform the surgery, and always fight the system.

NOTES

1 This article is a companion piece to my article, "Suspect Norms of Appearance and the Ethics of Complicity," in *In the Eye of the Beholder: Ethics and Medical Change of Appearance,* ed. Inez de Beaufort, Medard Hilhorst, and Soren Holm (Scandinavian University Press, 1997), pp. 151–67; some paragraphs in this essay are taken from that article.

2 See Sandra Lee Bartky, *Femininity and Domination: Studies in the Phenomenology of Oppression.* (New York and London: Routledge, 1990), especially chapters 3 and 5; Susan Bordo, *Unbearable Weight: Feminism, Western Culture, and the Body* (Berkeley: University of California Press, 1993).

3 Sherry Ortner, "Is Female to Nature as Male Is to Culture?" in *Women, Culture and Society,* ed. Michelle Zimbalist and Louise Lamphere (Stanford: Stanford University Press, 1974); Carolyn Merchant, *The Death of Nature* (San Francisco: Harper and Row, 1980); Genevieve Lloyd, "Reason, Gender, and Morality in the History of Philosophy," *Social Research* 50, no. 3 (Autumn 1983): 490–513.

4 For examples and discussion, see Stephen Jay Gould, *The Mismeasure of Man* (New York and London: W. W. Norton & Co., 1981).

5 See Merchant, *The Death of Nature,* and Lloyd, "Reason, Gender, and Morality."

6 Arthur Marwick, *Beauty in History* (London: Thames and Hudson, 1988); Reena N. Glazer, "Women's Body Image and the Law," *Duke Law Journal* 43 (1993): 113–47.

7 See Susan Bordo, *Unbearable Weight.*

8 I am indebted to my colleague Alisa Carse for the example and skeptical analysis.

MAKEOVER
Peter D. Kramer

In this excerpt from Chapter 1 of his landmark book, *Listening to Prozac*, Kramer, a psychiatrist, reflects upon his experience with several patients who took the anti-depressant Prozac in the first few years after it entered the market. He gives special emphasis to the case of a remarkable, resilient woman, Tess, who originally sought help for depression but got far more from the drug than she or Kramer anticipated. As Kramer explains, individuals on Prozac sometimes not only overcome depression (or some other psychiatric condition such as obsessive-compulsive disorder or anxiety), but also transform into different sorts of people. These patients are not only restored to normal health and functioning; the effect of the medication extends to transforming their personalities—in the case of Tess, enhancing her "social popularity, business acumen, self-image, energy, flexibility, sexual appeal." In view of such transformations of personality, Kramer coins the now popular term "cosmetic psychopharmacology." While transformations such as these may seem obviously welcome, Kramer contends, they also raise a panoply of difficult professional, social, and philosophical issues. These issues include the proper role of the doctor, the continuity of human selves, the meaning of mental illness, the plasticity of diagnostic categories, the components of personal identity, the relationship between biochemistry and achievement, and the role of drugs—both legal and illegal—in a stressful, competitive culture. Prozac, Kramer concludes, forces us to question conventional thinking about all of these issues.

My first experience with Prozac involved a woman I worked with only around issues of medication. A psychologist with whom I collaborate had called to say she was treating a patient who had accomplished remarkable things in adult life despite an especially grim childhood; now, in her early thirties, the patient had become clinically depressed. Would I see her in consultation? My colleague summarized the woman's history, and I learned more when Tess arrived at my office.

Tess was the eldest of ten children born to a passive mother and an alcoholic father in the poorest public-housing project in our city. She was abused in childhood in the concrete physical and sexual senses which everyone understands as abuse. When Tess was twelve, her father died, and her mother entered a clinical depression from which she had never recovered. Tess—one of those inexplicably resilient children who flourish without any apparent source of sustenance—took over the family. She managed to remain in school herself and in time to steer all nine siblings into stable jobs and marriages.

Her own marriage was less successful. At seventeen, she married an older man, in part to provide a base outside the projects for her younger brothers and sisters, whom she immediately took in. She never went to the movies alone with her husband; the children came along. The weight of the family was always on her shoulders. The husband was alcoholic, and abusive when drunk. Tess struggled to help him stop drinking, but to no avail. The marriage soon became loveless. It collapsed once the children—Tess's siblings—were grown and one of its central purposes had disappeared.

Meanwhile, Tess had made a business career out of her skills at driving, inspiring, and nurturing others. She achieved a reputation as an administrator capable of turning around struggling companies by addressing issues of organization and employee morale, and she rose to a high level in a large corporation. She still cared for her mother, and she kept one foot in the projects, sitting on the school committee, working with the health clinics, investing personal effort in the lives of individuals who mostly would disappoint her.

It is hard to overstate how remarkable I found the story of Tess's success. I had an image of her beginnings. The concrete apartment in which she cared for her younger brothers and sisters was recently destroyed with great fanfare on local television. Years earlier, my work as head of a hospital clinic had led me to visit that building. From the start, it must have been a vertical prison, a place where to survive at all could be counted as high ambition. To succeed as Tess had—and without a stable family to guide or support her—was almost beyond imagining.

That her personal life was unhappy should not have been surprising. Tess stumbled from one prolonged affair with an abusive married man to another. As these degrading relationships ended, she would suffer severe demoralization. The current episode had lasted months, and, despite a psychotherapy in which Tess willingly faced the difficult aspects of her life, she was now becoming progressively less energetic and more unhappy. It was this condition I hoped to treat, in order to spare. Tess the chronic and unremitting depression that had taken hold in her mother when she was Tess's age.

Though I had learned some of this story before my consultation with Tess, the woman, when I met her, surprised me. She was utterly charming.

I have so far recounted Tess's history as if it were extraordinary, and it is. At the same time, people like Tess are familiar figures in a psychiatrist's practice. Often it will be the most competent child in a chaotic family who will come for help—the field even has a name for people in Tess's role, "parental children," and a good deal is written about them. Nor is it uncommon for psychiatric patients to report having had a depressed mother and an absent father.

What I found unusual on meeting Tess was that the scars were so well hidden. Patients who have struggled, even successfully, through neglect and abuse can have an angry edge or a tone of aggressive sweetness. They may be seductive or provocative, rigid or overly compliant. A veneer of independence may belie a swamp of neediness. Not so with Tess.

She was a pleasure to be with, even depressed. I ran down the list of signs and symptoms, and she had them all: tears and sadness, absence of hope, inability to experience pleasure, feelings of worthlessness, loss of sleep and appetite, guilty ruminations, poor memory and concentration. Were it not for her many obligations, she would have preferred to end her life. And yet I felt comfortable in her presence. Though she looked infinitely weary, something about Tess reassured me. She maintained a hard-to-place hint of vitality—a glimmer of energy in the eyes, a sense of humor that was measured and not self-deprecating, a gracious mix of expectation of care and concern for the comfort of her listener.

It is said that depressed mothers' children, since they have to spend their formative years gauging mood states, develop a special sensitivity to small cues for emotion. In adult life, some maintain a compulsive need to please and are thought to have a knack for behaving just as friends (or therapists) prefer, at whatever cost to themselves. Perhaps it was this hypertrophied awareness of others that I saw in Tess. But I did not think so, not entirely. I thought what I was seeing was a remarkable and engaging survivor, suffering from a particular scourge, depression.

I had expected to ask how Tess had managed to do so well. But I found myself wondering how she had done so poorly.

Tess had indeed done poorly in her personal life. She considered herself unattractive to men and perhaps not even as interesting to women as she would have liked. For the past four years, her principal social contact had been with a married man—Jim—who came and went as he pleased and finally rejected Tess in favor of his wife. Tess had stuck with Jim in part, she told me, because no other men approached her. She believed she lacked whatever spark excited men; worse, she gave off signals that kept men at a distance.

Had I been working with Tess in psychotherapy, we might have begun to explore hypotheses regarding the source of her social failure: masochism grounded in low self-worth, the compulsion of those abused early in life to seek out further abuse. Instead, I was relegated to the surface, to what psychiatrists call the phenomena. I stored away for further consideration the contrast between Tess's charm and her social unhappiness. For the moment, my function was to treat my patient's depression with medication.

I began with imipramine, the oldest of the available antidepressants and still the standard by which others are judged. Imipramine takes about a month to work, and at the end of a month Tess said she was substantially more comfortable. She was sleeping and eating normally—in fact, she was gaining weight, probably as a side effect of the drug. "I am better," she told me. "I am myself again."

She did look less weary. And as we continued to meet, generally for fifteen minutes every month or two, all her overt symptoms remitted. Her memory and concentration improved. She regained the vital force and the willpower to go on with life. In short, Tess no longer met a doctor's criteria for depression. She even spread the good word to one of her brothers, also depressed, and the brother began taking imipramine.

But I was not satisfied.

It was the mother's illness that drove me forward. Tess had struggled too long for me to allow her, through any laxness of my own, to slide into the chronic depression that had engulfed her mother.

Depression is a relapsing and recurring illness. The key to treatment is thoroughness. If a patient can put together a substantial period of doing perfectly well—five months, some experts say; six or even twelve, say others—the odds are good for sustained remission. But to limp along just somewhat improved, "better but not well," is dangerous. The partly recovered patient will likely relapse as soon as you stop the therapy, as soon as you taper the drug. And the longer someone remains depressed, the more likely it is that depression will continue or return.

Tess said she was well, and she was free of the signs and symptoms of depression. But doctors are trained to doubt the report of the too-stoical patient, the patient so willing to bear pain she may unwittingly conceal illness. And, beyond signs and symptoms, the recognized abnormalities associated with a given syndrome, doctors occasionally consider what the neurologists call "soft signs," normal findings that, in the right context, make the clinical nose twitch.

I thought Tess might have a soft sign or two of depression.

She had begun to experience trouble at work—not major trouble, but something to pay attention to. The conglomerate she worked for had asked Tess to take over a company beset with labor problems. Tess always had some difficulty in situations that required meeting firmness with firmness, but she reported being more upset by negotiations with this union than by any in the past. She felt the union leaders were unreasonable, and she had begun to take their attacks on her personally. She understood conflict was inevitable; past mistakes had left labor-management relations too strained for either side to trust the other, and the coaxing and cajoling that characterized Tess's management style would need some time to work their magic. But, despite her understanding, Tess was rattled.

As a psychotherapist, I might have wondered whether Tess's difficulties had a symbolic meaning. Perhaps the hectoring union chief and his foot-dragging members resembled parents—the aggressive father, the passive mother—too much for Tess to be effective with them. In simpler terms, a new job, and this sort especially, constitutes a stressor. These viewpoints may be correct. But what level of stress was it appropriate for Tess to experience? To be rattled even by tough negotiations was unlike her.

And I found Tess vulnerable on another front. Toward the end of one of our fifteen-minute reviews of Tess's sleep, appetite, and energy level, I asked about Jim, and she burst into uncontrollable sobs. Thereafter, our meetings took on a predictable form. Tess would report that she was substantially better. Then I would ask her about Jim, and her eyes would brim over with tears, her shoulders shake. People do cry about failed romances, but sobbing seemed out of character for Tess.

These are weak reeds on which to support a therapy. Here was a highly competent, fully functional woman who no longer considered herself depressed and who had none of the standard overt indicators of depression. Had I found her less remarkable, considered her less capable as a businesswoman, been less surprised by her fragility in the face of romantic disappointment, I might have declared Tess cured. My conclusion that we should try for a better medication response may seem to be based on highly subjective data—and I think this perception is correct. Pharmacotherapy, when looked at closely, will appear to be as arbitrary—as much an art, not least in the derogatory sense of being impressionistic where ideally it should be objective—as psychotherapy. Like any other serious assessment of human emotional life, pharmacotherapy properly rests on fallible attempts at intimate understanding of another person.

When I laid out my reasoning, Tess agreed to press ahead. I tried raising the dose of imipramine, but Tess began to experience side effects—dry mouth, daytime tiredness, further weight gain—so we switched to similar medications in hopes of finding one that would allow her to tolerate a higher dose. Tess changed little.

And then Prozac was released by the Food and Drug Administration. I prescribed it for Tess, for entirely conventional reasons—to terminate her depression more thoroughly, to return her to her "premorbid self." My goal was not to transform Tess but to restore her.

But medications do not always behave as we expect them to.

Two weeks after starting Prozac, Tess appeared at the office to say she was no longer feeling weary. In retrospect, she said, she had been depleted of energy for as long as she could remember, had almost not known what it was to feel rested and hopeful. She had been depressed, it now seemed to her, her whole life. She was astonished at the sensation of being free of depression.

She looked different, at once more relaxed and energetic—more available—than I had seen her, as if the person hinted at in her eyes had taken over. She laughed more frequently, and the quality of her laughter was different, no longer measured but lively, even teasing.

With this new demeanor came a new social life, one that did not unfold slowly, as a result of a struggle to integrate disparate parts of the self, but seemed, rather, to appear instantly and full-blown.

"Three dates a weekend," Tess told me. "I must be wearing a sign on my forehead!"

Within weeks of starting Prozac, Tess settled into a satisfying dating routine with men. She had missed out on dating in her teens and twenties. Now she reveled in the attention she received. She seemed even to enjoy the trial-and-error process of learning contemporary courtship rituals, gauging norms for sexual involvement, weighing the import of men's professed infatuation with her.

I had never seen a patient's social life reshaped so rapidly and dramatically. Low self-worth, competitiveness, jealousy, poor interpersonal skills, shyness, fear of intimacy—the usual causes of social awkwardness—are so deeply ingrained and so difficult to influence that ordinarily change comes gradually if at all. But Tess blossomed all at once.

"People on the sidewalk ask me for directions!" she said. They never had before.

The circle of Tess's women friends changed. Some friends left, she said, because they had been able to relate to her only through her depression. Besides, she now had less tolerance for them. "Have you ever been to a party where other people are drunk or high and you are stone-sober? Their behavior annoys you, you can't understand it. It seems juvenile and self-centered. That's how I feel around some of my old friends. It is as if they are under the influence of a harmful chemical and I am all right—as if I had been in a drugged state all those years and now I am clearheaded."

The change went further: "I can no longer understand how they tolerate the men they are with." She could scarcely acknowledge that she had once thrown herself into the same sorts of self-destructive relationships. "I never think about Jim," she said. And in the consulting room his name no longer had the power to elicit tears.

This last change struck me as most remarkable of all. When a patient displays any sign of masochism, and I think it is fair to call Tess's relationship with Jim masochistic, psychiatrists anticipate a protracted psychotherapy. It is rarely easy to help a socially self-destructive patient abandon humiliating relationships and take on new ones that accord with a healthy sense of self-worth. But once Tess felt better, once the weariness lifted and optimism became possible, the masochism just withered away, and she seemed to have every social skill she needed.

Tess's work, too, became more satisfying. She responded without defensiveness in the face of adamant union leaders, felt stable enough inside herself to evaluate their complaints critically. She said the medication had lent her surety of judgment; she no longer tortured herself over whether she was being too demanding or too lenient. I found this remark noteworthy, because I had so recently entertained the possibility that unconscious inner conflicts were hampering Tess in her dealings with the labor union. Whether the conflicts were real or illusory, the problem disappeared when the medication took effect. "It makes me confident," Tess said, a claim I since have heard from dozens of patients, none of whom had been given a hint that this medication, or any medication, could do any such thing.

Tess's management style changed. She was less conciliatory, firmer, unafraid of confrontation. As the troubled company settled down, Tess was given a substantial pay raise, a sign that others noticed her new effectiveness.

Tess's relations to those she watched over also changed. She was no longer drawn to tragedy, nor did she feel heightened responsibility for the injured. Most tellingly, she moved to another nearby town, the farthest she had ever lived from her mother.

Whether these last changes are to be applauded depends on one's social values. Tess's guilty vigilance over a mother about whom she had strong ambivalent feelings can be seen as a virtue, one that medication helped to erode. Tess experienced her "loss of seriousness," as she put it, as a relief. She had been too devoted in the past, at too great a cost to her own enjoyment of life. . . .

There is no unhappy ending to this story. It is like one of those Elizabethan dramas—Marlowe's *Tamburlaine*—so foreign to modern audiences because the Wheel of Fortune takes only half a turn: the patient recovers and pays no price for the recovery. Tess did go off medication, after about nine months, and she continued to do well. She was, she reported, not quite so sharp of thought, so energetic, so free of care as she had been on the medication, but neither was she driven by guilt and obligation. She

was altogether cooler, better controlled, less sensible of the weight of the world than she had been.

After about eight months off medication, Tess told me she was slipping. "I'm not myself," she said. New union negotiations were under way, and she felt she could use the sense of stability, the invulnerability to attack, that Prozac gave her. Here was a dilemma for me. Ought I to provide medication to someone who was not depressed? I could give myself reason enough—construe it that Tess was sliding into relapse, which perhaps she was. In truth, I assumed I would be medicating Tess's chronic condition, call it what you will: heightened awareness of the needs of others, sensitivity to conflict, residual damage to self-esteem—all odd indications for medication. I discussed the dilemma with her, but then I did not hesitate to write the prescription. Who was I to withhold from her the bounties of science? Tess responded again as she had hoped she would, with renewed confidence, self-assurance, and social comfort.

I believe Tess's story contains an unchronicled reason for Prozac's enormous popularity: its ability to alter personality. Here was a patient whose usual method of functioning changed dramatically. She became socially capable, no longer a wallflower but a social butterfly. Where once she had focused on obligations to others, now she was vivacious and fun-loving. Before, she had pined after men; now she dated them, enjoyed them, weighed their faults and virtues. Newly confident, Tess had no need to romanticize or indulge men's shortcomings.

Not all patients on Prozac respond this way. Some are unaffected by the medicine; some merely recover from depression, as they might on any antidepressant. But a few, a substantial minority, are transformed. Like Garrison Keillor's marvelous Powdermilk biscuits, Prozac gives these patients the courage to do what needs to be done. . . .

No doubt doctors should be unreservedly pleased when their patients get better quickly. But I confess I was unsettled by [another patient's] enthusiasm, and by Tess's as well. I was suspicious of Prozac, as if I had just taken on a cotherapist whose charismatic style left me wondering whether her magic was wholly trustworthy.

The more rational component to my discomfort had to do with Tess. It makes a psychiatrist uneasy to watch a medicated patient change her circle of friends, her demeanor at work, her relationship to her family. All psychiatrists have seen depressed patients turn manic and make decisions they later regret. But Tess never showed signs of mania. She did not manifest rapid speech or thought, her judgment remained sound, and, though she enjoyed life more than she had before, she was never euphoric or Pollyannaish. In mood and level of energy, she was "normal," but her place on the normal spectrum had changed, and that change, from "serious," as she put it, to vivacious, had profound consequences for her relationships to those around her.

As the stability of Tess's improvement became clear, my concern diminished, but it did not disappear. Just what did not sit right was hard to say. Might a severe critic find the new Tess a bit blander than the old? Perhaps her tortured intensity implied a complexity of personality that was now harder to locate. I wondered whether the medication had not ironed out too many character-giving wrinkles, like overly aggressive plastic surgery. I even asked myself whether Tess would now give up her work in the projects, as if I had administered her a pill to cure warmheartedness and progressive social beliefs. But in entertaining this thought I wondered whether I was clinging to an arbitrary valuation of temperament, as if the melancholy or saturnine humor were in some way morally superior to the sanguine. In the event, Tess did not forsake the projects, though she did make more time for herself.

Tess, too, found her transformation, marvelous though it was, somewhat unsettling. What was she to make of herself? Her past devotion to Jim, for instance—had it been a matter of biology, an addiction to which she was prone as her father had been to alcoholism? Was she, who defined herself in contrast to her father's fecklessness, in some uncomfortable way like him? What responsibility had she for those years of thralldom to degrading love? After a prolonged struggle to understand the self, to find the Gordian knot dissolved by medication is a mixed pleasure: we want some internal responsibility for our lives, want to find meaning in our errors. Tess was happy, but she talked of a mild, persistent sense of wonder and dislocation.

My discomfort with Tess's makeover had another component. It is all very well for drugs to do small things: to induce sleep, to allay anxiety, to ameliorate a well-recognized syndrome. But for a drug's effect to be so global—to extend to social popularity, business acumen, self-image, energy, flexibility, sexual appeal—touches too closely on fantasies about medication for the mind. Patients often have extreme fears about drugs, stemming from their apprehension that medication will take over in a way that cannot be reversed, that drugs will obliterate the self. For years, psychiatrists have reassured patients that medication merely combats illness: "If the pills work," I and others have said, "they will restore you to your former self. I expect you to walk in here in a few weeks and say, 'I'm myself again.'" Medication does not transform, it heals.

When faced with a medication that does transform, even in this friendly way, I became aware of my own irrational discomfort, my sense that for a drug to have such a pronounced effect is inherently unnatural, unsafe, uncanny.

I might have come to terms with this discomfort—the unexpected soon becomes routine in the world of pharmacology. But Tess's sense of dislocation did not disappear immediately, and her surprise at her altered self helped me to understand the more profound sources of my own concern. The changes in Tess, which I saw replicated in other patients given Prozac, raised unsettling issues.

Many of these were medical issues. How, for example, would Prozac affect the doctor's role? To ameliorate depression is all very well, but it was less clear how psychiatrists were to use a medication that could lend social ease, command, even brilliance. Nor was it entirely clear how the use of antidepressants for this purpose could be distinguished from, say, the street use of amphetamine as a way of overcoming inhibitions and inspiring zest.

Other questions seemed to transcend any profession, to bear directly on the way members of our culture see themselves and one another. How were we to reconcile what Prozac did for Tess with our notion of the continuous, autobiographical human self? And always there was the question of how society would be affected by our access to drugs that alter personality in desirable ways.

I wondered what I would have made of Tess had she been referred to me just before Jim broke up with her, before she had experienced acute depression. I might have recognized her as a woman with skills in many areas, one who had managed to make friends and sustain a career, and who had never suffered a mental illness; I might have seen her as a person who had examined her life with some thoroughness and made progress on many fronts but who remained frustrated socially. She and I might suspect the trouble stemmed from "who she is"—temperamentally serious or timid or cautious or pessimistic or emotionally unexpressive. If only she were a little livelier, a bit more carefree, we might conclude, everything else would fall into place. . . .

Confronted with a patient who had never met criteria for any illness, what would I be free to do? If I did prescribe medication, how would we characterize this act?

For years, psychoanalysts were criticized for treating the "worried well," or for "enhancing growth" rather than curing illness. Who is not neurotic? Who is not a fit candidate for psychotherapy? This issue has been answered through an uneasy social consensus. We tolerate breadth in the scope of psychoanalysis, and of psychotherapy in general; few people today would remark on a patient's consulting a therapist over persistent problems with personality or social interactions, though some might object to seeing such treatments covered by insurance under the rubric of illness.

But I wondered whether we were ready for "cosmetic psychopharmacology." It was my musings about whether it would be kosher to medicate a patient like Tess in the absence of depression that led me to coin the phrase. Some people might prefer pharmacologic to psychologic self-actualization. Psychic steroids for mental gymnastics, medicinal attacks on the humors, antiwallflower compound—these might be hard to resist. Since you only live once, why not do it as a blonde? Why not as a peppy blonde? Now that questions of personality and social stance have entered the arena of medication, we as a society will have to decide how comfortable we are with using chemicals to modify personality in useful, attractive ways. We may mask the issue by defining less and less severe mood states as pathol-

ogy, in effect saying, "If it responds to an antidepressant, it's depression." Already, it seems to me, psychiatric diagnosis had been subject to a sort of "diagnostic bracket creep"—the expansion of categories to match the scope of relevant medications.

How large a sphere of human problems we choose to define as medical is an important social decision. But words like "choose" and "decision" perhaps misstate the process. It is easy to imagine that our role will be passive, that as a society we will in effect permit the material technology, medications, to define what is health and what is illness.

Tess's progress also seemed to blur the boundary between licit and illicit drug use. How does Prozac, in Tess's life, differ from amphetamine or cocaine or even alcohol? People take street drugs all the time in order to "feel normal." Certainly people use cocaine to enhance their energy and confidence. "I felt large. I mean, I felt huge," is how socially insecure people commonly explain why they abuse cocaine or amphetamine. Uppers make people socially attractive, obviously available. And when a gin drinker takes a risk, we are tempted to ask whether the newfound confidence is not mere "Dutch courage."

In fact, it is people from Tess's background—born poor to addicted and dependent parents, and then abused and neglected—who are most at risk to use street drugs. A cynic may wonder whether in Tess's case drug abuse has sneaked in through the back door, whether entering the middle class carries the privilege of access to socially sanctioned drugs that are safer and more specific in their effects than street drugs, but are morally indistinguishable in terms of the reasons they are taken and the results they produce. I do not think it is possible to see transformations like Tess's without asking ourselves both whether street-drug abusers are self-medicating unrecognized illness and whether prescribed-drug users are, with their doctors' permission, stimulating and calming themselves in quite similar ways.

More unsettling to me than questions of definition—licit versus illicit—was an issue raised by Tess's renewed professional success: how might a substance like Prozac enter into the competitive world of American business? Psychiatrists have begun to recognize a normal or near-normal mental condition called "hyperthymia," which corresponds loosely to what the Greeks called the sanguine temperament. Hyperthymia is distinct from mania and hypomania, the disorders in which people are grandiose, frenetic, distractible, and flawed in their judgment. Hyperthymics are merely optimistic, decisive, quick of thought, charismatic, energetic, and confident.

Hyperthymia can be an asset in business. Many top organizational and political leaders require little sleep, see crises as opportunities, let criticism roll off their backs, make decisions easily, exude confidence, and hurry through the day with energy to spare. These qualities help people succeed in complex social and work situations. They may be considered desirable or advantageous even by those who have quite normal levels of drive and optimism. How shall we respond to the complaint that a particular executive lacks decisiveness and vigor? By prescribing Prozac? In Tess's work, should the negotiators on the union side be offered Prozac, too? The effect of Prozac on Tess's style in her corporate work—and [another patient's] in his architectural practice—raises questions about how a drug that alters personality might be used in a competitive society.

Nor is it possible to witness Tess's transformation without fearing that a drug like Prozac might bolster other unfortunate tendencies in contemporary culture. Even Prozac's main effect in Tess's treatment—the relief it provided from social vulnerability—might, in societal terms, prove a mixed blessing. Tess had come for medication treatment only after a prolonged effort at self-understanding through psychotherapy. But I could imagine a less comfortable scenario: A woman much like Tess, abused and neglected in childhood, though not fully aware to what extent and to what effect, seeks treatment in a society that prefers to ignore victimization and that values economy over thoroughness in health care; the woman seems subdued and angry, is discontented for reasons she cannot easily put into words. By what means will her doctor attempt to help her? Would Prozac, alone, be enough?

But my central concern, as I watched Tess's story unfold, involved her personhood. Tess had every right, on the basis of both childhood experience and unhappiness in adult life, to be socially vulnerable in adulthood. But once she had taken Prozac, she—and those who knew her—had to explain her newfound social success on medication. If her self-destructiveness with men and her fragility at work disappeared in response to a biological treatment, they must have been biologically encoded. Her biological constitution seems to have determined her social failures. But how does the belief that a woman who was abused as a child and later remains stuck in abusive relationships largely because of her biologically encoded temperament affect our notions of responsibility, of free will, of unique and socially determinative individual development? Are we willing to allow medications to tell us how we are constituted?

When one pill at breakfast makes you a new person, or makes your patient, or relative, or neighbor a new person, it is difficult to resist the suggestion, the visceral certainty, that who people are is largely biologically determined. I don't mean that it is impossible to escape simplistic biological materialism, but the drama, the rapidity, the thoroughness of drug-induced transformation make simplicity tempting. Drug responses provide hard-to-ignore evidence for certain beliefs—concerning the influence of biology on personality, intellectual performance, and social success—that heretofore we as a society have resisted. When I saw the impact of medication on patients' self-concept, I came to believe that even if we tried to understand these matters complexly, new medications would redraw our map of those parts of the self that are biologically responsive, so that we would arrive, as a culture, at a new consensus about the human condition.

An indication of the power of medication to reshape a person's identity is contained in the sentence Tess used when, eight months after first stopping Prozac, she telephoned me to ask whether she might resume the medication. She said, "I am not myself."

I found this statement remarkable. After all, Tess had existed in one mental state for twenty or thirty years; she then briefly felt different on medication. Now that the old mental state was threatening to re-emerge—the one she had experienced almost all her adult life—her response was "I am not myself." But who had she been all those years if not herself? Had medication somehow removed a false self and replaced it with a true one? Might Tess, absent the invention of the modern antidepressant, have lived her whole life—a successful life, perhaps, by external standards—and never been herself?

When I asked her to expand on what she meant, Tess said she no longer felt like herself when certain aspects of her ailment—lack of confidence, feelings of vulnerability—returned, even to a small degree. Ordinarily, if we ask a person why she holds back socially, she may say, "That's just who I am," meaning shy or hesitant or melancholy or overly cautious. These characteristics often persist throughout life, and they have a strong influence on career, friendships, marriage, self-image.

Suddenly those intimate and consistent traits are not-me, they are alien, they are defect, they are illness—so that a certain habit of mind and body that links a person to his relatives and ancestors from generation to generation is now "other." Tess had come to understand herself—the person she had been for so many years—to be mildly ill. She understood this newfound illness, as it were, in her marrow. She did not feel herself when the medicine wore off and she was rechallenged by an external stress.

On imipramine, no longer depressed but still inhibited and subdued, Tess felt "myself again." But while on Prozac, she underwent a redefinition of self. Off Prozac, when she again became inhibited and subdued—perhaps the identical sensations she had experienced while on imipramine—she now felt "not myself." Prozac redefined Tess's understanding of what was essential to her and what was intrusive and pathological. . . .

Beyond the effect on individual patients, Tess's redefinition of self led me to fantasize about a culture in which this biologically driven sort of self-understanding becomes widespread. Certain dispositions now considered awkward or endearing, depending on taste, might be seen as ailments to be pitied and, where possible, corrected. Tastes and judgments regarding personality styles do change. The romantic, decadent stance of Goethe's young Werther and Chateaubriand's René we now see as merely immature, overly depressive, perhaps in need of treatment. Might we not, in a culture where overseriousness is a medically correctable flaw, lose our taste for the melancholic or brooding artists—Schubert, or even Mozart in many of his moods?

These were my concerns on witnessing Tess's recovery. I was torn simultaneously by a sense that the medication was too far-reaching in its effects and a sense that my discomfort was arbitrary and aesthetic rather than doctorly. I wondered how the drug might influence my profession's definition of illness and its understanding of ordinary suffering. I wondered how Prozac's success would interact with certain unfortunate tendencies of the broader culture. And I asked just how far we—doctors, patients, the society at large—were likely to go in the direction of permitting drug responses to shape our understanding of the authentic self. . . .

By the time Tess's story had played itself out, I had seen perhaps a dozen people respond with comparable success to Prozac. Hers was not an isolated case, and the issues it raised would not go away. Charisma, courage, character, social competency—Prozac seemed to say that these and other concepts would need to be re-examined, that our sense of what is constant in the self and what is mutable, what is necessary and what contingent, would need, like our sense of the fable of transformation, to be revised.

ASPIRIN FOR THE MIND? SOME ETHICAL WORRIES ABOUT PSYCHOPHARMACOLOGY

Carol Freedman

Contrary to the common view that regards emotions as types of pleasure or pain, a view (which she attributes to Kramer) that likens emotional problems to headaches, Freedman argues that emotions—unlike headaches—are ways of interpreting the world and one's situation in it. If, accordingly, we regard emotional problems as related to reasons, and not just to causes, we should maintain a commitment to address these problems with insight and understanding; failure to do so, Freedman contends, involves a failure to respect what it is to be a self. The growing success of biological psychiatry, as understood by Kramer, encourages us to think of emotional problems as similar to headaches. Kramer's approach, she concludes, "jeopardizes our dignity as responsible persons who owe it to ourselves to struggle toward insight through dialogue."

In describing the extreme sensitivity to rejection of his patient Lucy, Peter Kramer recounts the following disagreement he had with Sophie Lowenstein Freud.

> Sophie Freud suggested that all people are rejection-sensitive, in the sense that rejection hurts them, but that Lucy might be more skilled than most at *perceiving* rejection. . . .
>
> . . . Sophie Freud's comment . . . is grounded in the belief that all people—if they perceive themselves to be rejected—feel the same pain internally. They differ only according to how small a cue they need to recognize rejection. . . . If all people are similar in how they translate loss into pain, then the instrument we are adjusting is not the internal amplifier but the external receiver—we are asking the person to create an artificial attentional deficit, to ignore loss. . . .
>
> The alternative view—one that seems more likely—is that sensitive people, when they perceive rejection, feel it more keenly. . . . The *primary* deficit is increased amplification. . . .
>
> For the most part, I do not believe that either medicine or psychotherapy makes people less perceptive. But . . . [o]nce we turn down the amplification, small slights, even if they are noticed for a moment, may pass without being registered into memory. . . . In this sense, a *secondary* effect of reduced amplification is reduced perception (emphasis added).[1]

Kramer's disagreement with Sophie Freud might seem to be only an academic quarrel. Kramer argues that when people feel rejected they *first* ex-

perience the *pain* of loss, and then the heightened *perception* of loss. Sophie Freud argues, conversely, that what comes first is the heightened *perception* of loss and then the *pain* of loss. They are not disagreeing about the ultimate effect of treatment: for either way the aim is to alter people's perception. They are disagreeing about whether such alteration comes about as a direct or indirect result of treatment. What difference could such a distinction really make?

I want to argue that such a distinction *does* matter. It isn't just a coincidence that Kramer describes his treatment of patients like Lucy as a process of reducing their internal amplifier as opposed to adjusting their external receiver. Analogies in this case have ethical significance. When Kramer discusses the psychological problems he treats with Prozac they are often made to sound like headaches: pains or deficiencies that give rise to particular modes of perception or cognition without being particular modes of perception or cognition themselves. Psychopharmaceuticals, to follow the analogy, are like aspirin.

I want to argue, against the tenor of Kramer's *Listening to Prozac,* that emotional disturbances are often not like headaches, and that once we see this it becomes ethically problematic to treat such disturbances with drugs. Even if we grant, then, that drugs and understanding can realize the same ends of psychic health, the means often make an ethical difference. For what is at stake is a conception of ourselves as responsible agents, not machines.

Central to *Listening to Prozac* is Kramer's claim that Prozac allows us to see a whole spectrum of psychological problems as physical disorders. People who are particularly sensitive to rejection, for example, have problems with their serotonin levels. For the sake of argument, I'll grant Kramer this finding. But I want to challenge some assumptions he makes about what it's like to *experience* emotional problems. In particular, he implies that psychological disturbances are best understood merely as kinds of pain, as is shown in the analogy he makes between rejection-sensitivity and panic disorder.

Panic attacks, he writes, are now understood by psychiatrists as "'heightened pain in response to loss.'"[2] And this means that the agoraphobia or agrophobia that tend to characterize those who suffer from panic attacks are not *meaningful*. It is not as if one's fear of going over a bridge expressed a terror of being unsupported and insignificant, the way one felt as a small child. For Kramer, "there [is] no special symbolic significance to the bridge, no meaning traceable to childhood trauma or current ambivalence; the only significance of the bridge [is] as an unpleasant place in which to suffer spontaneous panic."[3] Rejection-sensitivity, to follow the analogy, is just a tendency to feel heightened pain in response to loss. And the situations that occasion such pain aren't meaningful.[4]

That Kramer is prone to think of rejection-sensitivity in this way has, I think, less to do with scientific evidence, than with fairly old and unreflective judgments we make at the level of ordinary practice. If Kramer's description of rejection-sensitivity sounds convincing it is more because he is appealing to some common ways we think about the emotions or emotional states,[5] rather than that he is appealing to new developments made possible by ever more sophisticated advances in biological psychiatry.

One common way of thinking about the emotions involves viewing them as noncognitive. What distinguishes an emotion from a cognition, on this view, is a kind of pleasure or pain. These pleasures or pains are influenced by, and influence, cognitions—for example, anger may be caused by the belief that I have been insulted, and it can cause the belief that the offender deserves a piece of my mind. According to this view, emotions are separate from the beliefs that cause them and that they cause. They are not *essentially* connected. It is this sense in which they are like headaches. I do not intend to defend a particular cognitive view

of the emotions at length here, but only to raise some questions about the coherence of Kramer's noncognitive account and to examine its ethical implications.[6]

A key question for Kramer's account of emotion is whether it can do justice to the way we *experience* emotion, and in particular to the way in which we see emotion as connected in a *meaningful* way to the situations that cause it. Consider Kramer's case of Lucy. When Lucy was ten her mother was violently murdered. At the time, Lucy showed no immediate reaction. She was productive and responsible, despite the fact that her father focused primarily on his work and not on her. When Lucy first saw Kramer she was a young adult who tended either to become interested in men who were dismissive of her and wild, or to experience heightened feelings of rejection with men who seemed to treat her well. Lucy suffered from deep and protracted moods: "disorganized, paralyzed, hopelessly sad, overtaken by unfocused feelings of urgency."[7] Kramer doesn't deny that we should think of Lucy's current sensitivity to rejection as caused by her past. Even if he thinks of feelings of rejection as nothing more than kinds of pain, he might still think of the places and people Lucy seeks to avoid as meaningful in the sense that they bear a resemblance to the people and places that gave rise to her early experiences of painful rejection. But they are no more meaningful on this view than is my wanting to avoid eating too many hot dogs because eating five once made my stomach upset. Lucy's earliest feelings of rejection on this view were nothing but severe pains occasioned by the murder of her mother. And such early experiences changed Lucy biologically so that she became more prone to feel the pain of rejection. Kramer could argue, then, that because she *associates* such pain with the early experiences that caused it, she seeks to avoid situations that she thinks resemble those early ones.

There are, I think, many problems with understanding the genesis and nature of rejection-sensitivity in this way. But the problem I want to highlight concerns the understanding of emotional states as akin to pleasures or pains that we merely *associate* with types of situations—as if it makes sense to say that Lucy associates the pain of rejection with losing her mother in the way that one might associate a kind of stomach pain with hot dogs. If we reflect carefully about emotional pain, we will realize that the relationship between it and the way we see the situation that we believe causes emotional pain is not like the relationship between physical pain and the way we see the situation that we believe causes physical pain.[8] One notable difference is the fact that emotions are intentional: what I take to be the source of my anger is not separable from the anger itself. There is not my anger, on the one hand, and what I'm angry about on the other. If I am angry about the fact that you are late, then if as I see it you are no longer late, there is no anger. There could be anger about something else. But anger cannot exist without an object in the way that a physical pain can exist without its cause.[9] It is in this sense that emotions are not merely caused by what we take them to be about. And this is why we don't merely *associate* them with what we take them to be about in the way that we might associate hot dogs with stomach pain.

But there is another significant difference between emotions and physical pleasures and pains: the way I see the situation that I believe causes my emotional pain seems from my point of view to *justify* my pain. This notion is revealed by the kinds of reasons we offer for our emotions in contrast to our stomach aches or other physical pains. When we ask someone why their stomach hurts we are in effect asking, "how did it happen that your stomach got upset, what is the *explanation?*" But when we ask Lucy why she feels rejected by her boyfriend, or father, or mother we are not in effect asking, "how did it happen that you came to feel rejected?" We want more than an *explanation*; we want to hear her *justification*. We want to know why Lucy takes feeling rejected to be *merited* by her situation. What sort of evidence does she think there is for believing that certain others don't really care for her? What as she sees it justifies her level of feeling rejected: what as she sees it merits the view that she is alone in the world, and that no one will ever love her.

Sometimes when we justify our emotions, our reasons terminate in nothing but our own likes and dislikes. When asked, for instance, why I hope there will be vanilla rather than chocolate ice cream at the party, I might respond by saying merely, "because I like vanilla better." But often our reasons for emotions don't terminate in what could be called such "subjectivist" reasons.[10] Why do I feel rejected by the death of my mother? Because it is the worst thing in the world to have no one who sees you standing out in a crowd, who is primarily interested in *your* feelings, achievements, opinions, actions; because I am like an orphan now; I am not whole; there is no one holding me up and watching out for me. And as I feel it, this rejection is not just a matter of how I see things: I am not alone just because I see it that way, and being alone is not bad merely because I don't like it. Being a young girl who feels rejected by the death of her mother is feeling like *the most terrible* thing in the world has happened.

Imagine, then, that when Lucy was a little girl she failed to feel rejected by the murder of her mother. Her failure would be a very different kind of failure from the person who failed to feel a pin prick his finger, or whose knee didn't jump when his reflexes were tested. Both cases reveal problems. The person who doesn't feel the pin prick is not working the way humans usually work; some mechanism is not in normal order. But this explanation does not capture Lucy's problem. For hers is a failure of *insight*—a failure to *see* how really devastating it is to lose the person who has been the center of her world. In this way, emotions are like beliefs. When one feels an inappropriate emotion, it is often like "missing something"—more like a false belief than like failing to feel the prick of the pin or the thump of the hammer. There is a problem, then, with the fact that Kramer thinks of rejection as nothing but a kind of pain, and with rejection-sensitivity as a tendency to feel that pain. Such a view might appeal to our unreflective judgments about the emotions. But such judgments are confirmed neither by scientific evidence, nor by philosophical reflection.[11]

Kramer's account of rejection-sensitivity is unclear because he seems to assume that much of his view follows once we regard a psychological problem as a "quasi-biological quasi-entity."[12] But the fact that a psychological problem is physical does not tell us what it is like for the person having it.[13] We cannot assume that it is merely a kind of pain, that it is like a headache. That this distinction matters ethically when it comes to psychopharmacology is what I want to argue now.

INSIGHTFUL FEELINGS

Psychotherapy in its most basic form carries with it a certain conception of who we are: namely, rational creatures of insight. We can have severely distorted views of the world, and do extremely destructive and inappropriate things. But the psychotherapeutic assumption is that (1) we, often unconsciously, take our distorted and destructive attitudes to be justified; and (2) our justifications, however wrong, are sourced in insight. One of the central goals of psychotherapy is to get the patient to see that she really does take herself to have good reasons for her feelings, and that those reasons originate with insight. This is a deeply respectful and humane aspect of the psychotherapeutic view: our distorted and misguided attitudes are the outgrowth of insightful ones, our craziness the outgrowth of sanity. In Lucy's case, for example, the goal is to get her to see the reasons she takes for her sensitivity to rejection—that is, to get her to see how her conception of herself as deserving rejection is confirmed as she sees it by the fact that her mother abandoned her and her father spent so much time away from home. And this goal is a very small part of the complicated story of justification. The final goal is to get her to see the insight at the heart of her distorted and disturbed view of herself and others: a little girl who really did lose the *central support* of her life, who saw how *utterly irreplacable* such support was.

At the heart of the psychotherapeutic approach is, I think, a view that is indispensible to maintaining the idea of a *self*. To lose a conception of our attitudes as grounded in reasons is to lose a self. If mechanistic causality is the only kind of causality at work in our explanations of why we do and feel what we do, then we are not describing the feelings and behaviors of a self. For central to the idea of a self is the idea of a creature who may legitimately be held responsible. Without a view of ourselves as acting on reasons, we cease to be creatures who may legitimately be held responsible.[14] We become machines. And this means that it is not legitimate for us to ask whether the self may be explainable in mere mechanistic terms, whether it is in fact a machine. For a machine is not a self, and whether there are selves in the world is not a question *for us*. A world without selves is not *our* world. And so, the following sorts of questions must sometimes be answerable in nonmechanistic terms. Why do you think that? Why do you feel that? Why did you do that? The answers, in other words, do not always refer to some physical process: for example, "because my serotonin is too high," "because I'm feeling sick," "because my C-fibers fired in a certain way." Rather, for example: I think abortion is morally permissible *because* I think the fetus is not a person; I feel angry at my friend *because* I think she insulted me; and I came home early *because* I wanted to watch the baseball game on television.[15]

It is important to make one clarification. In what I have said, and will say, I emphasize the essential connection between being a self and acting on reasons, and ultimately rational agency. When many hear this claim, it pushes a button: there is something "off" about seeing ourselves as rational. Surely that's not the right way to describe our emotions. It makes us sound too cool, too calculating. Perhaps I could say instead, "creatures who act on interpretations, self-interpreting animals."[16] But this formulation misses something important, as I see it, that is captured by the idea of acting on reasons. An interpretation is something I don't have to believe is justified, or true. It is not something I have to be committed to. But emotions, for the most part, are our way of being oriented toward what we take to be the true and the good. We might be deeply misguided. But emotions define our characters precisely because they express our deepest beliefs, not just our interpretations. I talk of reasons and rationality, then, with ambivalence. It seems to me that we either lack the language to capture a certain reality, or our conception of reason is so wedded to logic and calculation, as some feminists would argue, that we can only associate the word with certain images.

So being a self means that we will sometimes act, feel, and think for *reasons*. It is important, then, to understand the difference between two types of causality: mechanistic and rational. The therapeutic story about Lucy is an example of rational causality. We take her current way of seeing the world to be one she believes is *justified* by her life and experiences.

Her boyfriend turns away every now and then to change the channel on the television, and she feels painfully rejected. As she sees it, when someone's attention to her is distracted she is being *ignored*. Being ignored is not being cared for; it is not a far cry away from being abandoned. Such a way of interpreting things is justified as Lucy sees it because that is what experience has shown her—for example, her father's constant turning away from her at a time in her life when she already felt lost and alone. Her conception of herself as ignored and not cared for is rationally caused in the sense that it is something she believes to be grounded in good reasons.

A headache, on the other hand, is an example of mechanistic causation. I might have a headache that is caused by psychological stress—my bank account is running low, I'm late on the rent, or my child has the flu. In this sense my headache is caused by my interpretations: I believe I am not succeeding in supporting and caring for my child properly, and am, therefore, a bad parent. These are interpretations I take myself to be justified in having. We could say, then, that the beliefs that give rise to my headache are rationally caused. But this doesn't mean the headache is so caused. For the relationship between the headache and my interpretations is mechanistic: I don't take my headache to be *justified* by the way I see the world. My headache is not something I take to be grounded in good reason. Rather it is the *result* of a way of seeing the world that I take myself to have good reasons for.[17]

In making a distinction between two kinds of causality the point is not to deny the intimate connection between our interpretations and our embodiment. The point is not to be a dualist: as if there were pure mind and pure body. The point is that we are dehumanized if we are reduced to mere mechanism. And that means that we must distinguish between those actions and attitudes that we are going to regard as interpretative and those that we are going to regard as physical.

For Kramer, feeling rejected is like having a bad headache, and suffering from rejection-sensitivity is like being prone to suffer from a bad headache. To see Lucy's problem as unconnected to her self-interpretations, as a problem of "internal amplification," is to see it as mechanistically caused. It is like

a headache in the sense that it might be caused by self-interpretations that are themselves rationally caused. So a by-product of Lucy's view of herself as undeserving of love may be the feeling of, and proneness to feeling, rejection. And her feeling of rejection might cause a change in her self-interpretations. But the relationship between the self-interpretations that both cause, and are caused by, the feeling of rejection is mechanistic. The feeling of rejection is, like a headache, just a kind of pain. And in this sense, it is typically not something one takes oneself to have *reason* to feel.

I would like to propose that seeing our psychological problems as like headaches has the following ethical implications. Crudely put, you could think of psychological problems as existing on a spectrum. At one extreme are problems that are clearly untreatable by insight and understanding. At the other end of the spectrum are problems whose prospects for being treatable by insight and understanding are not so clear. When it comes to the ethical appropriateness of treating psychological problems with drugs there is, in one sense, only one relevant question: *can* the problem be treated with insight or understanding? If we judge the problem to be one that only responds to physical intervention, then that seems to be sufficient for determining that drug use is ethically appropriate. But it doesn't mean that if we judge that the problem *can* be treated with drugs, then it is ethically appropriate to do so. It is here the headache analogy becomes relevant. If you are suffering from a headache, then whether it is ethically appropriate for you to take aspirin doesn't seem to hang on whether drugs are the only way to remove your discomfort. We might believe that thinking good thoughts while sitting in the bathtub could relieve your pain, but that seems to have no bearing on whether it is ethically appropriate for you to take an aspirin. You have a headache. It is painful. Aspirin will help. That is all there is to it.

That we have this ethical judgment about headaches is grounded, I think, in the fact that they are mechanistically caused. Emotional problems, I've suggested, can be like suffering from false beliefs.[18] Lucy, for example, is *wrong* to see herself as ignored and abandoned by her boyfriend just because he changes the channel on the television. And her false beliefs, we can imagine, are grounded in something like a *mistake in reasoning*. So Lucy might be right to see her father's treatment of her as a case of being ignored and abandoned. But she is mistaken to believe further that when others fail to pay her undivided attention *they* don't care for her, and that she is undeserving of the love of a good person. When we see someone's problem as a mistake in reasoning, there is an imperative to help them understand their error. For that is the way we value our capacity as creatures who act on reasons. Valuing the fact that we act on reasons means trying to correct mistakes in reasoning with other reasons.[19] To think it is appropriate to "cure" mistakes of reasons mechanistically is to regard our rational capacity as of little significance or importance. That—insofar as we live in a world of selves—is something we are in no position to do. It is in this sense that it matters what means we use to 'cure' our psychological problems.[20]

To know that a psychological problem responds to drugs, then, is not sufficient for determining that such treatment is ethically appropriate. We will want to know how the problem is caused—mechanistically or rationally. And that is not answered for us merely by knowing that the problem is physical and that it responds to drugs. There will certainly be considerable variation among those psychological problems that might be resolvable with insight and understanding: there will be those problems that are better addressed with psychotherapy and those that are not; those problems that require long-term psychotherapy and those that do not. These will be tough cases ethically. Even if we judge our problems to be rationally caused by our self-interpretations, they might still respond to drugs. Then we will have to consider our reservations about taking drugs in light of the following questions. How long in therapy is too long? Does treating the problem with drugs facilitate therapy, and in that sense is it in the service of insight and understanding? With cases at this end of the spectrum, however, it will be clear that once we see our problem as rationally caused, our objective should be insight and understanding. So drug use in these cases ought always to be in the service of insight and understanding, and there should always be a healthy resistance to drugs.[21] For many emotional problems are precisely not like headaches. They are not *just* painful. And so, even if drugs work, that's not all there is to it.[22]

The headache analogy reveals how important it is for us to describe the problems we treat with drugs as problems *of the body*—problems that can no doubt *affect* the mind without themselves being "of the mind." We aren't troubled by the way vitamins affect our minds, for example, because we think of ourselves as attending to the body so that the mind can "do its thing." Treating our emotional problems with drugs might sometimes be like taking vitamins or fixing low blood sugar. But if we think of all emotional problems as mechanical problems, we lose our personhood. It is too easy, and dangerous to think of all psychopharmacological drugs as like aspirin, or vitamins.

What is particularly interesting about the headache analogy is the extent to which it appeals to ordinary experience. Scientists can tell you that your problem is "of the body," and mean that it is your hormones, or your serotonin, or something similar. But a headache is "of the body" at the level of felt experience; it is a pain. We define it as bodily, as mechanistically caused, in our *own* understanding of it. The task of determining causation is infinitely complicated. Whether biological psychiatry can definitively show that a psychological problem is caused by a physical problem, as opposed to merely being physically realized, is questionable.[23] It is no wonder, then, that Kramer appeals to something like the headache analogy. It seems to make his way of describing emotional problems more persuasive. For we as ordinary people can appreciate the extent to which emotional problems are bodily. They seem to be like pains. I'm afraid that this is how our culture is being encouraged to think about emotional problems by the current revolution in biological psychiatry. What I have argued, however, is that our unreflective understanding of emotion is mistaken. Much of the appeal of Kramer's analogy, then, is in the end ungrounded.

CONCLUSION

My argument can be summarized as follows.

(1) The familiar view that emotions are merely kinds of pleasures and pains is not something science

can show. To describe the physiology of a psychological state doesn't tell us what it is like to experience such a state and, in this respect, doesn't inform us as to what an emotion is.

(2) On my view, emotions are not merely like pains that are caused by and cause beliefs, interpretations, and perceptions. Emotions, unlike headaches, are themselves ways of believing and interpreting, even though they are physically realized and viscerally felt.

(3) When an emotional problem is sourced in our interpretations or reasons, then we should have a basic commitment to addressing it with insight and understanding. Otherwise, we are not respecting what it is to be a self. For central to maintaining the idea of a self is the commitment to regard some of our actions and attitudes as justified by our reasons, not explained in mechanistic terms. My view concedes that the treatment of some emotional problems that are sourced in our reasons may be facilitated by medication. But even in such cases there should be a healthy resistance to drugs.[24]

(4) The current revolution in biological psychiatry—as interpreted in Peter Kramer's *Listening to Prozac*—encourages us to think of emotional problems as like headaches. This is a convenient view, for if we can say that what someone is *experiencing* is just pain, then there is little doubt that her problem should be regarded in mechanistic terms. We don't need a scientist to tell us the physiology of headaches to believe that it is appropriate to treat headaches with aspirin.

(5) Kramer's view is troubling, then, because it makes it too easy for us to see ourselves in mechanistic terms. In this sense it jeopardizes our dignity as responsible persons who owe it to ourselves to struggle toward insight through dialogue.[25]

NOTES

1 Peter Kramer, *Listening to Prozac* (New York: Penguin Books, 1993), pp. 103–04.

2 Kramer, *Listening to Prozac*, p. 77.

3 Kramer, *Listening to Prozac*, p. 82.

4 Kramer's general tendency to see emotional problems as meaningless is evident in the way he contrasts his view with psychoanalysis. See, especially, *Listening to Prozac*, chapter 4.

5 Though Kramer describes rejection-sensitivity as a disorder of *mood,* it is still appropriate to talk here of his view of

emotion. For while rejection-sensitivity is not described as an emotion per se, it is described as an affective, as distinct from a cognitive, problem. It seems in this sense to be essentially emotional in nature.

In the chapter on self-esteem, for example, Kramer says explicitly that medication treats affective, as distinct from cognitive, problems. He emphasizes a number of times throughout the chapter that self-esteem, insofar as it is an affective condition, is not primarily a matter of self-understanding. Self-esteem can *influence* self-understanding, but not the other way around. See, especially, pp. 208–12, 221.

6 The contemporary philosophical literature on the emotions is dominated by attempts of one form or another to defend a cognitive view of the emotions. See, for example: Robert Roberts, "What an Emotion Is: A Sketch," *Philosophical Review*, Vol. 97, n. 2 (1988); Cheshire Calhoun, "Cognitive Emotions?" in *What is an Emotion?* ed. Cheshire Calhoun and Robert Solomon (New York: Oxford University Press, 1984), pp. 327–42; Amelie Oksenberg Rorty, "Explaining Emotions," in *Explaining Emotions*, ed. Amelie Oksenberg Rorty (Berkeley: University of California Press, 1980), pp. 103–26; Ronald de Sousa, *The Rationality of Emotion* (Cambridge: MIT Press, 1987); Patricia Greenspan, *Emotions and Reasons* (New York: Routledge, 1988); Anthony Kenny, *Action, Emotion and Will* (New York: Humanities Press, 1964); and Irving Thalberg, *Perception, Emotion and Action* (New Haven: Yale University Press, 1977).

7 Kramer, *Listening to Prozac*, p. 69.

8 One could argue that emotions are pains or pleasures that we associate with cognitions in an *essential,* rather than contingent, way. We could call such a view a "causal cognitive" account. For according to such a view emotion would not be a pain or pleasure that is associated with cognition *in the way* that physical pains are associated with cognitions. And so, emotions would not be, to make a familiar philosophical argument, like *sensations*. Kramer, however, views emotions as akin to sensations. In criticizing his view, then, I am not criticizing a "causal cognitive" view, but a view of emotion as akin to sensation.

The "causal cognitive" view, for the most part, captures the basic structure of Hume's account of the "indirect passions"—even though Hume himself is not always Humean. See, in particular, his discussion of pride in *The Treatise*, ed. L.A. Selby-Bigge and P.H. Niditch (New York: Oxford University Press, 1990), pp. 275–89. Others who often sound like endorsers of the causal cognitive view include Robert Gordon, *The Structure of Emotions* (Cambridge: Cambridge University Press, 1987). For a reading of Gordon that makes his view look causal, see Robert Roberts's review in *Philosophical Review,* Vol. 99, No. 2 (1990). Freud explicitly endorses what could be called a weak version of the "causal cognitive" view—where emotion tends to be associated with beliefs of a certain sort, though the two can be separated. But Freud misdescribes his own insights here. That his explicit theory of emotion often fails to do justice to the practice of psychoanalysis is argued quite persuasively by Jonathan Lear in *Love and Its Place in Nature* (New York: Farrar, Straus and Giroux, 1990), pp. 91–93.

9 For some classic discussions of the nature of emotional causes and objects, see Irving Thalberg, *Perception, Emotion and Action,* excerpted in Calhoun and Solomon, *What is an Emotion?* pp. 291–304; Anthony Kenny, *Action, Emotion and Will,* excerpted in Calhoun and Solomon, *What is an Emotion?* pp. 279–90; and Robert Solomon, "Emotions and Choice," also excerpted in Calhoun and Solomon, *What is an Emotion?*

10 The distinction between "subjectivist" and "objectivist" reasons is one way of capturing Charles Taylor's distinction between "weak" and "strong" evaluation. See his, "What is Human Agency?" in *Philosophical Papers I,* (Cambridge: Cambridge University Press, 1985), pp. 15–44.

11 I am not denying that *some* psychological disturbances might be nothing but kinds of pain. The main problem with Kramer's account is that he wants to entertain the possibility that all emotional disorders should be conceived on the model of rejection-sensitivity—this is what we are led to believe, he suggests, when we "listen to Prozac." What I am challenging, then, is the view that Kramer is accurately giving us anything like the model of emotional disturbance.

12 Kramer, *Listening to Prozac,* p. 105.

13 To talk about what a mental state "is like" is, for many, another way of talking about the subjective irreducibility of mental states. See, for example, Thomas Nagel's "What Is It Like to Be a Bat?" in *Mortal Questions* (Cambridge: Cambridge University Press, 1979), pp. 165–80. When I use the phrase, "what it is like . . .," however, I am not making any claims about the subjective irreducibility of mental states. I am just questioning whether the activity of describing the biological nature of mental states can adequately determine whether such states are, for example, pains, desires, or beliefs.

14 That we cannot deny the truth of the perspective from which we are responsible agents is argued by, among others, Thomas Nagel in "Moral Luck," in *Mortal Questions,* pp. 24–38, and Peter Strawson in "Freedom and Resentment," *Proceedings of the British Academy,* vol. 48 (1962), pp. 1–25.

That responsible agency requires acting on reasons is essentially uncontroversial in the contemporary philosophical literature on the topic. *What* counts as acting on a reason, however, and *why* responsible agency requires acting on a reason are questions that motivate much disagreement. For some well-known discussions, see Donald Davidson, "Actions, Reasons and Causes," in *Actions and Events* (New York: Oxford University Press, 1989), pp. 3–20; Harry Frankfurt, "Freedom of the Will and the Concept of a Person," in *The Importance of What We Care About* (New York: Cambridge University Press, 1988), pp. 11–25; Charles Taylor, "What Is Human Agency?" and Susan Wolf, "Sanity and the Metaphysics of Responsibility," in *Responsibility, Character, and the Emotions,* ed. Ferdinand Schoeman (New York: Cambridge University Press, 1987),

pp. 46–62. For a nice summary of different stories of how human action originates, see David Velleman, "The Guise of the Good," *Nous* 26:1 (1992), pp. 3–5.

15 To describe a case of causation as rational is compatible with "the body's" playing a role in two senses. First, insofar as we are embodied creatures, it will always be the case that we depend upon the body's functioning in order for our rational processes to operate. It is assumed, then, that when a rational explanation holds, certain mechanistic processes are required as well. We all need sleep and proper nutrition, for example. But insofar as the self requires a domain of rational explanation, there must be some legitimate distinction between the kind of minimal role the body plays in cases of rational causation, as compared to the significant role it plays in cases of mechanistic causation.

Second, to say that the self requires cases of rational causation does not preclude there also being mechanistic explanations for the same cases. So for any instance when an explanation in terms of an agent's reasons holds, there might *also* be a physical explanation that holds as well. I can accurately describe my walking in the house and turning on the television both as, "I came home because I wanted to watch the ballgame," and "my C-fibers caused my muscles to move." There might be two levels of explanation in this sense. That is why understanding mental phenomena in physical terms does not settle whether there is also a rational account to be told. All that the self requires is that a rational explanation sometimes be true.

16 The expression, "self-interpreting animals" comes from Charles Taylor's essay "Self-interpreting Animals," in *Philosophical Papers I,* pp. 45–76.

17 This is not to say that one's headache could not be rationally caused. I could make it my objective to have a headache. I might unconsciously see having physical pain as something there is good reason to have—perhaps to get my husband's sympathy, or because I believe I am a bad parent and I deserve to suffer discomfort. But this is not the typical case. In the typical case my headache is the by-product of attitudes that I take myself to be justified in having. Usually the attitudes are rationally caused; the headache is not.

18 One of the complicated implications of thinking of emotions as like beliefs is that it is not clear how we are to treat someone who is experiencing painful, but *justified* emotion. If it were always, and simply, the case that seeing the truth helped an agent—by perhaps motivating action in the long run that protects her from harm—then feeling justified emotion should always be encouraged. But since it is not clear that the truth always benefits an agent, we will sometimes have to weigh our commitment to reducing suffering against our commitment to grasping the truth.

19 It might be objected that even if we grant that understanding matters, it doesn't follow that such understanding must be achieved through insight. As a compatibilist might argue, all that matters is that we are creatures who act on reasons; it doesn't matter how we got to be such creatures. Suffice it to say, however, that I am assuming a compatibilism of a

Strawsonian sort. On the one hand, whether determinism is true doesn't matter when it comes to our status as responsible agents. On the other hand, from within the practical standpoint, it is as if determinism is false. I am interested in showing what follows from within the practical standpoint. And that means that if it matters that I get from point *a* to point *b* by rational means, than it also matters that I get to point *a* by rational means.

20 There are at least two other important arguments for why the means matter when it comes to treating psychological problems: one has to do with the kind of good that character is, and the other has to do with the importance of suffering. While I don't have the space here to look at such arguments in depth, it is worth mentioning how my argument supplements and corrects these arguments in important ways.

So, for example, when articulating why character is the kind of thing that ought to be achieved in certain ways, it is not enough merely to say it is valued as the product of our will. For there are many things that we may be responsible for—like a stress headache—that we don't think it is wrong to treat with drugs. It is because character is the product of our will in the sense that it is sourced in *our reasons,* then, that explains why it should not be achieved primarily in mechanistic ways. And it is not enough to say that character is the kind of good that is valued as the product of effort and discipline. For what matters is that character be changed as a result of a certain *kind* of effort and discipline: the kind that follows, among other things, from the fact that character is sourced in reasons.

The argument that there is intrinsic value in suffering, that it has value apart from the ends it promotes, is also supplemented by my argument. For it is difficult to imagine how suffering could have such intrinsic value if it were *just pain*; that is, if it involved no insight, if it were not cognitive. And so, my argument is a way of explaining why insight as a means to psychic health matters.

21 But what are we to say about someone who has important commitments—like finishing his novel—who doesn't want to spend the time it would take to change himself through understanding? I would argue that while someone like this

has good reason to take drugs for his emotional problems, there is always a kind of *loss* involved in not choosing to pursue understanding as the preferable way of correcting problems that are sourced in our reasons. Ethical life is not just about seeking to minimize pain. It involves evaluating a variety of goods, and making tough choices. Sometimes the goods we choose between are incommensurable, and we are left "missing out" on something valuable even when our choices are justified. But the basic commitment to correct problems that are sourced in our reasons through understanding is a good of such fundamental value to us as rational agents, that to fail to make it a priority involves a fundamental loss. It might sometimes be justified. But doing the right thing in such a case should still leave us with some reluctance and ambivalence.

22 Once we recognize that many emotional problems are not just painful, it follows that the purpose of psychotherapy is not just to relieve suffering. It will often be a *primary* goal of psychotherapy to change perception. And this raises difficult questions about the conception of therapy as *health care.* Suffice it to say that I don't think it is in the interest of psychotherapy to misdescribe what it does in the attempt to gain credibility and funding.

23 For an excellent discussion of the limits of biological psychiatry's ability to mark out the causes of mental illness, see Colin A. Ross and Alvin Pam, *Pseudoscience in Biological Psychiatry* (New York: John Wiley and Sons, 1995).

24 Having a healthy resistance to psychopharmacology does not mean believing that anyone should be coerced into having therapy or denied access to safe medication. It does mean, however, believing that psychotherapy should be treated as a legitimate form of treatment, and that people should be provided with a real opportunity to get it—something that is beginning to sound radical in our present age of managed-care.

25 I am indebted for criticism to Michael Della Rocca, Jodi Halpern, Carol Rovane, Lawrence Vogel, members of the "enhancement technologies" project at the Hastings Center, and audiences at Connecticut College and Worcester Polytechnic Institute.

PROZAC, ENHANCEMENT, AND SELF-CREATION
David DeGrazia

Opening with a case about a woman brooding over her sense of self and life direction, DeGrazia asks two questions about her request for a prescription to Prozac in the absence of any diagnosable psychiatric condition. First, is her request itself morally problematic? Second, should a psychiatrist refuse to prescribe Prozac in a case like this one? Stressing that the use of Prozac in these circumstances would be an instance of biomedical *enhancement* rather than treatment—since the patient is not ill and is already functioning normally—DeGrazia focuses on issues related to personal identity. He responds to concerns voiced by some commentators that the use of psychotropic medications for enhancement purposes and self-transformation are inauthentic, claiming instead that such "self-creation projects" can be perfectly authentic. After addressing a range of distinct concerns about "cosmetic psychopharmacology"—including the concern raised by Freedman about trivializing emotional problems—DeGrazia suggests that often the wisest path includes the more arduous road of psychotherapy. He concludes, however, that in general such decisions ought to be left to competent adults like the woman featured in the case, and that it can often be a responsible choice for psychiatrists to accede to such requests for Prozac.

Marina's history is notable for significant childhood neglect. After her parents split up when she was four, her father became distant and mostly uninvolved and her mother suffered from depression and a borderline case of alcoholism. Although involved in Marina's day-to-day life, she was inconsistently available on an emotional level. Because Marina was the oldest child and apparently "had her shit together," she was often called on to help out with her younger sister and two brothers, who had a variety of problems ranging from depression to juvenile delinquency to significant obsessive-compulsiveness. Due to the distraction of other family members' more dramatic struggles, many of Marina's own needs were never met. However nurturing this "parentified" child was, she never felt nurtured.

Although by her own account she had a troubled adolescence—doing less well than she wanted in school, flirting with drug use and reckless sexual encounters—she managed to get accepted to a good university. Settling down considerably, she excelled in college and got into a top business school, where she continued her academic success. Throughout this period, her primary source of emotional sustenance came from several close friendships. Although these relationships were generally strong, Marina sometimes bristled from perceived putdowns and betrayals by those she held dear. Her family's demands for advice and assistance persisted, but coming to un-

derstand how her overreaching family oppressed her, she established some reasonable boundaries with her mother and siblings, an achievement made easier by living in a different city. Her romantic life she considered a failure. Her intense work ethic afforded little time for dating, and the men she wound up with tended to be distant, rejecting, and sometimes emotionally abusive.

Marina has also always been somewhat obsessional. She has been disturbed by thoughts about death since adolescence and overly concerned with the possibility of tragedy befalling her or her family, although these thoughts occur fleetingly and do not disrupt her functioning. For many years, her recurring sexual fantasies have featured powerful older men. She is troubled and disgusted with herself when these fantasies drive her to consume late-night hours pursuing the half-hearted titillation of sex-oriented internet chat rooms.

As she approaches age thirty, Marina is rather successful in nearly everyone's estimation: She is a wellpaid manager for a large computer company, she has close friends, and she has several pastimes that she genuinely enjoys (especially bicycling and guitar). Yet Marina finds herself brooding and pensive, wondering about her life and its direction. She seeks out a psychiatric consultation, which takes place over four sessions, and accepts the psychiatrist's conclusion that she has no diagnosable disorder. When he suggests that psychotherapy might nevertheless be of help to her, she is inhibited by the prospect of paying for many sessions out of pocket (since her HMO will not cover them). Still, she

Reprinted with permission of the publisher from *Hastings Center Report*, vol. 30 (March–April 2000), pp. 34–40. Copyright © 2000 by The Hastings Center.

wants changes. At work, she feels overly tentative, unsure, too prone to worry about possible errors. In her social life, she hates how she endlessly interprets the latest transactions with friends and the way she is attracted to men who are bad for her. She feels alienated by her obsessional thoughts, considering them ridiculous and bothersome even if not harmful.

After extended periods of introspection, fueled by her impending birthday and the discussions that took place in the psychiatric consultation, Marina decides that she wants to become more outgoing, confident, and decisive professionally; less prone to feelings of being socially excluded, slighted, or unworthy of a good partner; and less obsessional generally. She calls the psychiatrist who provided the consultation, whom she likes, and explains that she has heard that Prozac sometimes produces transformations like the ones she seeks—and more quickly and less expensively than could be expected from therapy. Marina requests a prescription for Prozac.

Is Marina's request morally problematic? Should a psychiatrist refuse to prescribe Prozac in a situation like this one? What may give us greatest pause about her request is that she wants to use a medication to change her personality and become a different sort of person. Is either the goal of major self-transformation or the means of using a prescription drug morally problematic? If so, why?

In a highly insightful set of reflections on Prozac, Carl Elliott makes the provocative claim that deliberately changing one's personality through use of Prozac is *inauthentic* because it results in a personality and life that are not really one's own. Thus he states that it "would be worrying if Prozac altered my personality, even if it gave me a better personality, simply because it isn't *my* personality"; and he asks, "What could seem less authentic, at least on the surface, than changing your personality with an antidepressant?"[1] Elliott's thesis suggests that it would be inauthentic, and therefore morally problematic, for Marina to use Prozac for the purpose of changing her personality; indeed, if the drug had its intended effect, the resulting personality would not really be hers.

But however intuitively appealing this reasoning may be, it is undermined by its misleading image of the self as "given," static, something there to be discovered. One can be true to oneself even as one deliberately transforms and to some extent creates oneself. In fact, a transformation such as Marina proposes can be a perfectly authentic piece of what I will call *self-creation.*

What is at issue here is clearest in cases of personality change that, like Marina's, are uncontroversially cases of enhancement, that is, of "interventions designed to improve human form or functioning beyond what is necessary to sustain or restore good health."[2] Often, enhancements are understood as interventions to produce improvements in human form or function that do not respond to genuine medical needs, where the latter are defined in terms of disease, normal functioning, or prevailing medical ideology, but sometimes enhancements are picked out by the nature of their *means* rather than their goals. Some means of self-improvement, such as exercise or education, are considered natural, virtuous, or otherwise admirable. By contrast, means that are perceived as artificial, as involving corrosive shortcuts, or as perverting medicine are often thought to render the intended self-improvement morally suspect (as with steroid use to improve athletic performance).

Marina's intended use of Prozac implicates the concept of enhancement both because she is not mentally ill and because many would see her use of Prozac as an artificial shortcut that perverts the medical enterprise. Her case, and those at issue in this paper, are cases of what Peter Kramer calls "cosmetic psychopharmacology" in his landmark book, *Listening to Prozac.*[3] Kramer uses the term to describe Prozac's effect on patients who are not really ill and who become "better than well": more energetic, confident, and socially attractive. It is worth noting that to varying degrees, certain other drugs—such as Ritalin and other "smart drugs," Propranolol for reducing normal anxiety and enhancing musical performance, and the "happy pill" ginseng—raise at least some of the issues associated with cosmetic psychopharmacology.[4] But this paper will concentrate on Prozac, which apparently produces the most extensive transformations of personality and therefore presents the issues of enhancement and self-creation in the clearest light.

PROJECTS OF SELF-CREATION

Elliott's remarks about Prozac and authenticity occur within a broader discussion of the values pervading contemporary American culture. I do not dispute Elliott's claim that having a sense of spiritual emptiness (reflecting our culture's hollowness) can be preferable to Prozac-induced complacency.[5] What interests me here is his description of the ethics of authenticity, to which he ascribes two leading ideas, and the possible implications of this approach for people like Marina (pp. 181–82).

The first idea Elliott identifies is that life is a project whose meaning depends on how we live and for which we are largely responsible. I agree with this claim. The second idea may be broken into two parts. First, figuring out how one should live requires introspection, because there is no unique external standard for living meaningfully. Here again I agree (while noting the role introspection plays in Marina's growth). Second, one has to discover and be true to oneself in order to live an authentic life. To the extent that this assertion suggests that the self is "given," a pre-existing reality that might be discovered and to which one's actions should conform or "be true," it strikes me as highly problematic. And it seems fair to read this assertion as depending on the image of a static self, since Elliott uses the assertion to argue that Prozac-driven changes of personality are inauthentic and lead to a personality that isn't really one's own. (I don't mean to suggest that he *fully* embraces the image of a static self, just that his remarks on Prozac appear to promote this image to a degree that I consider distorting.)

The ideas of authenticity, of being true to oneself, and of self-creation provoke issues pertaining to personal identity. But what sense of identity is at issue? One sense of the term, analyzed by Locke, Parfit, and kindred philosophers, is that of numerical identity over time: a thing at one time is numerically identical with something at another time if and only if they are one and the same object, even if that object undergoes qualitative change. In this sense of identity, the problem of personal identity is to specify the conditions that must be satisfied for a person to continue to exist through time. While this sense of personal identity raises interesting practical issues

concerning, for example, the definition of death and the authority of advance directives, it is not central to this discussion.

The sense of personal identity at the heart of the concepts of authenticity and self-creation is connected with our self-conceptions—with what we consider most important to who we are, our self-told narratives about our own lives. Your inner story allows you to get your bearings when you act, especially when confronting difficult or momentous decisions.[6] It is what comes apart when a person has an identity crisis, when she is left wondering, in an important sense, who she is.[7] In this sense of identity, one could become a different person by undergoing a major change of outlook and values. And this is the notion Kramer has in mind when he describes the transforming effects of Prozac: Someone on Prozac might acquire a new sense of self—or identity—and strike others as having become "a new person."

All of this suggests that the self, in the second sense of identity, can change over time. Indeed, the feeling that a self might undergo *too much* change may underlie some of the common discomfort with cosmetic psychopharmacology. But how malleable is the self, and to what extent can one actively change oneself? It is important to have a tenable view on these issues before considering whether self-creation via Prozac can be authentic.

One possible view envisions the self as completely "given," although to discover its shape and true colors one may have to dig (with reflection, therapy, or the like). One can find the self but not change it; any change is due to forces outside one's agency. One version of this view takes a person's "inner core," the values that define the individual, to be entirely constructed by society.[8]

In another possible position, essentially the opposite of the first, the self is as amorphous and malleable as Silly Putty. In Sartre's view, we human beings are thrown into the world without any determinate nature. What we choose determines what we are, so we are completely responsible for what we become. With nothing except ourselves determining our actions and identity, we shoulder the burden of "radical freedom." Thus we may shape ourselves into one form one day without limiting what we can shape ourselves into the next day. In this view, we are entirely self-creating, leaving no room for discovering anything about oneself except perhaps what one freely chooses to be.[9]

These two extreme views about self-malleability strike me as highly implausible. A little reflection suggests that we can reshape ourselves *to some extent.* We may try with some success to become more disciplined—or less disciplined, for the workaholics and perfectionists among us. We may work at being more generous or more patient or more willing to stand up to authority, and sometimes we may succeed. We may aspire to orient ourselves more toward a relationship—or less. And when we accomplish change in ourselves, it does not seem that this change is entirely independent of our agency (as it would be if the impetus were simply social forces, human nature, or one's genetic makeup).

But if human phenomenology suggests a capacity for self-change through our agency, it does not suggest an unlimited capacity. Persons with addictions and obsessive-compulsive disorders, for example, know that their will is not the only force driving their actions. And all of us are frequently reminded that there are limits to what we can accomplish in changing our characters and behavior just as there are limits to what our bodies can achieve in sports.

If such self-shaping is possible, it is only one crucial process that determines what we and our lives become. The possibilities for self-creation are limited by its enmeshment with other crucial processes and factors (p. 138). One of these is the genetically determined cycle of life, which we are not free to escape: the neediness of infancy and childhood, the relative turbulence of adolescence, the gradual loss of physical powers in advanced age, and so on. Other crucial factors concern the tools we are given to work with, especially our particular genetic endowment and the quality of our early environment. A final crucial influence derives from the unexpected, random, yet momentous consequences of the things we choose. I once decided somewhat reluctantly to attend a Halloween party where I happened to meet the woman who later became my wife and the mother of my child. While self-creation is possible, the range of possibilities available to an individual is at once opened up and limited by other major processes and factors that shape our lives.

In this moderate view, self-creation is conceived of in the way suggested by Jonathan Glover, for whom it is a process in which we are "consciously shaping our own characteristics."[10] I understand Glover to mean specifically the conscious and deliberate shaping of one's own personality, character, or life direction. Glover captures the interplay of self-directed shaping as well as its limits by comparing the self to wood that can be sculpted, "respecting the constraints of natural shape and grain" (p. 136).

People who are engaged in self-creation seek to change themselves. Marina, for example, wants to change her personality. While she has been tentative, socially a bit mistrustful, and somewhat obsessive for as long as she can remember, she would like to be free of these personality traits. But this raises a conceptual issue: If Marina loses these characteristics, will the resulting person really be Marina?[11]

Elliott's remarks about Prozac suggest not, but I think a negative answer here is profoundly mistaken—and not just because of the associated image of a static self. For, again, what is identity in the relevant sense all about? It is about one's self-conception, what a person considers most important to who she is, her self-told inner story. That means that it is ultimately up to Marina to determine what counts as Marina and what counts as not-Marina; the story is hers to write (within the constraints set by the various factors beyond her control). And she wants to get rid of the traits in question, if she can. In general, whether certain personality traits are definitive of someone depends on whether she identifies with them—that is, whether she owns them (pun intended) autonomously. An example will help make the point.

Imagine two people, Nina and Xena, both of whom are inveterate, addicted cigarette smokers. Both spend a lot of money on the habit, both find it very inconvenient at times, and both are unsure they could muster the willpower to quit if they tried. Is being a smoker part of their respective identities? In my view, that depends on further detail.

Suppose that they have different attitudes toward their addiction. Nina finds it alien and out-of-character and wishes she never smoked that first cigarette. Xena, meanwhile, delights in being contrarian and knows that smoking and addiction generally are contrary to what most people consider good sense. While in a way her addiction deprives her of the freedom not to smoke—she just has to light up periodically—Xena is autonomously a smoker, precisely because she identifies with smoking along with its delightfully contrarian associations. So while both women are smokers, being a smoker is part of Xena's identity but not part of Nina's, and the difference lies in their distinct value systems.

This consequence should not be surprising, since who we are has everything to do with what we value. Further, what we value largely determines our projects of self-creation. Thus if Marina is able to rid herself of traits with which she doesn't identify, and decides that the "real Marina" does not have those traits, no one is in a position to correct her.

What legitimate basis might there be, then, for the idea that it would be inauthentic for Marina to change her personality? Do the means of making a personality change—in this case, using Prozac—matter here? Some would answer affirmatively, contending that these means represent an unnatural or artificial shortcut to self-improvement. But consider a path to desired self-change that would be regarded as natural, admirably laborious, and clearly within the bounds of accepted psychiatric practice: psychotherapy. Successful psychotherapy sometimes produces a shift in personality that the patient considers an improvement.[12] Now suppose Marina wanted to change her personality through the long, hard work of therapy. If she were willing to pay for it, I can imagine no reasonable objection to her enhancement project ("cosmetic psychotherapy," we might call it, keeping in mind that she is not genuinely ill). So I take it that therapy is an authentic and otherwise legitimate way of facilitating self-creation, even where enhancement is the goal.

The question is, why should the supposedly unnatural shortcut of Prozac use make any significant difference to the authenticity of Marina's self-creation project? That it is "unnatural"—that it works directly on her biochemistry rather than indirectly, as therapy does—simply seems irrelevant; the shortcut would still be authentic because Marina's values and self-conception are the basis for the chosen means. That it involves a shortcut might even, in some ways, make it admirable from a prudential standpoint. After all, it is her time and money that will be consumed here. While therapy may offer a patient some advantages that Prozac does not, if Marina believes those advantages do not offset the efficiency she hopes to find in Prozac, it is hard to see the justification for paternalistically judging that her values and self-conception are not authoritative for her own life. If they are admitted to be authoritative for judging what is good in her life (her best interests), then they should be authoritative for determining what constitutes her life, thus what is authentic for her. If this is right, then Prozac, no less than psychotherapy, can be an authentic part of a project of self-creation.

SOME REMAINING WORRIES

If the preceding arguments have been sound, they show that using Prozac can be an authentic part of a self-creation project, even in cases that involve enhancement. This conclusion of possible authenticity seems generalizable to other cases of cosmetic psychopharmacology—at least assuming that an adult with decisionmaking capacity is deciding only for herself, since decisions for children and incapacitated adults raise special issues.[13] But even if the charge of inauthenticity is wrong-headed, it does not follow that cosmetic psychopharmacology is ethically justified or wise. There remain some substantial ethical concerns about cosmetic psychopharmacology for capable adults like Marina. In the end, I do not think these concerns demonstrate that Marina's psychiatrist should refrain from prescribing Prozac for her, or that Marina should exclude Prozac from her project of self-creation. But I will only gesture in the direction of an adequate reply to each concern.

One concern is that Prozac, and other pharmaceuticals that could be used for enhancement purposes, are not available to all who might want and stand to benefit from them.[14] Forty million or so Americans lack health insurance, and many others are insured by plans that do not cover prescriptions for psychiatric medications or that provide coverage only when one has a diagnosible illness. Of course, the relatively wealthy can still opt to pay out of pocket. But the overall picture is one in which cosmetic psychopharmacology is likely to benefit mainly those who are relatively well off and otherwise advantaged. Thus by exacerbating existing gaps between the haves and have-nots in our society, cosmetic psychopharmacology raises issues of social and economic fairness.

These concerns about unfairness are legitimate. But the unfairness derives from our economic system—including our system of health care finance, which promotes the interests of the private insurance industry at nearly everyone's expense—rather than from Marina's or her psychiatrist's choices. In my view, they and everyone else should fight for greater justice in the distribution of income, wealth, and health care access, but doing so is compatible with Marina's use of Prozac. In fact, if Marina is right that taking Prozac would cost less than psychotherapy, her project raises a milder problem about justice than does therapy, since the more expensive approach would be available to even fewer people.

Another worry is that cosmetic psychopharmacology tends to promote some very troubling cultural values. Part of what drives Marina's interest, for example, is her desire to be more efficient at work and her longing for a more attractive personality. Since she is already professionally successful and has good friendships, one might think her desire for self-improvement reflects our culture's disturbing tendency to valorize hyper-competitiveness and "designer" personalities. Thus her plan and her psychiatrist's involvement (if he goes along) raise the issue of complicity with suspect social norms.[15]

I agree that our society overvalues competitiveness and other yuppie qualities. But it seems to me that reasonable people could disagree with this judgment, and that in any case, responsibility for this problem too should be located in our broader culture, not placed in the laps of Marina and her psychiatrist. If there is a responsibility to change the culture, it is everyone's, and it should not be arbitrarily imposed on particular individuals in ways that interfere with their self-regarding projects.

Some critics also feel that widespread use of Prozac and similar drugs, unlike psychotherapy, promotes biopsychiatry's agenda of reducing emotional and personal struggles to mechanistic terms—as if these struggles were just another form of pain to be treated with a new pill.[16] According to critics, this agenda threatens our self-conceptions as reasonable agents. But people might not be equally troubled by the possibility that using Prozac supports biopsychiatry's agendas. In any event, Marina and her psychiatrist have no obligation to promote the image of human beings as reasonable agents. We are such agents, but we are also feeling creatures; self-esteem problems, suspiciousness, and compulsiveness are connected with our agency, but they are also closely connected to unpleasant feelings, which Prozac may help to alleviate. Besides, even if Prozac lends itself to a mechanistic view of the self in some ways, Marina's plan for changing herself and her life direction is a powerful expression of her own agency.

Another concern is that cosmetic psychopharmacology can encourage social quietism because patients may favor drug-induced complacency over active struggle to change the social conditions that contribute to their discontent, with the result that these social problems are left untouched.[17] But while there may be some risk of social quietism, the risk attaches to all uses of mood-improving drugs, not just to cases of cosmetic psychopharmacology, as well as to mainstream religions and many other clearly acceptable practices and institutions that can brighten our outlooks.

Critics have also pointed to problems that may arise if people pursue cosmetic psychopharmacology for competitive reasons, such as Marina's desire to become a more confident businessperson. If nearly everyone in a particular competitive environment makes the same choice, the result will be self-defeating: there will be the expense and other personal costs of taking the drug but no advantage acquired over others (just as most law school applicants take an LSAT prep course without gaining a competitive advantage).[18] Meanwhile, those who would prefer not to take the drug may feel social pressure and possibly coercion to do so; they may fear falling too far behind.[19] At least with respect to Prozac, however, concerns about self-defeating drug enhancements and excessive social pressure to take it are rather speculative. We are still far from such a scenario.[20] What to do if and when it arrives is not at all obvious (just as there is no obvious solution to the problem concerning the LSAT prep course), but the mere possibility of such a scenario does not cast significant moral doubt on Marina's enhancement project.

Finally, we should not ignore whatever risks are associated with the drug in question, especially since some risks may remain unknown while others may be hard to discern accurately amid the glitter of the drug's celebrated benefits. This concern highlights the importance of an informed consent process that includes a responsible, balanced, and thorough discussion of risks; it does not justify paternalistically preventing use of the drugs in question.

PERMISSIBILITY AND PRUDENCE

As the tone of this essay may have revealed, I believe the kind of self-transformation Marina proposes can be quite admirable. At the very least, transformation via cosmetic psychopharmacology can be a perfectly authentic piece of self-creation, in that the resulting personality and life are very much one's own. One can identify with certain traits, authentically pursue them, and change oneself—while maintaining one's identity—within a project of self-creation.

At the same time, the *wisest* path toward desired self-creation may often include the slow, arduous road of psychotherapy, despite its considerable costs. For those who are willing to work and confront some unpleasantness about themselves or their lives, and who possess at least ordinary introspective capacities, psychotherapy offers insights that are generally not available from other sources or activities. Moreover, the changes in personality, character, or life plans that result from this vigorous work stand a decent chance of enduring, while people who go the route of cosmetic psychopharmacology may need to take the drugs indefinitely to maintain the desired changes. In effect, it may turn out that therapy is the less expensive option after all, at least in the long run.

If Marina were my friend or family member, I would urge her to consider extended therapy very seriously. I might even try to make the case that its likely benefits more than offset its added costs. But the values that ultimately count here, the ones that must be translated into benefits and costs of various weights, are Marina's. If she assesses her options with her eyes wide open, she should be allowed to select that which she believes is best for her. It is, after all, her identity.

NOTES

1 C. Elliott, "The Tyranny of Happiness: Ethics and Cosmetic Psychopharmacology," in *Enhancing Human Traits: Ethical and Social Implications,* ed. E. Parens (Washington, D.C.: Georgetown University Press, 1998), pp. 177–188, at 182, 186. Erik Parens, who edited the excellent anthology that contains Elliott's article, seems to concur with him. Thus Parens speaks of "appreciating that drugs like Prozac are good at promoting self-fulfillment as opposed to authenticity" (E. Parens, "Is Better Always Good? The Enhancement Project," in *Enhancing Human Traits,* pp. 1–28, at 23).

2 E. T. Juengst, "What Does *Enhancement* Mean?" in *Enhancing Human Traits,* pp. 29–47, at 29.

3 P. D. Kramer, *Listening to Prozac* (New York: Viking Press, 1993).

4 See L. H. Diller, "The Run on Ritalin: Attention Deficit Disorder and Stimulant Treatment in the 1990s," *Hastings Center Report* 26, no. 2 (1996): 12–18; C. Mills, "One Pill Makes You Smarter: An Ethical Appraisal of the Rise of Ritalin," *Report from the Institute for Philosophy and Public Policy* 18, no. 4 (1998): 13–17; P. J. White-house et al., "Enhancing Cognition in the Intellectually Intact," *Hastings Center Report* 27, no. 3 (1997): 14–22; J. Slomka, "Playing with Propranolol," *Hastings Center Report* 22, no. 4 (1992): 13–17; and J. Glover, *What Sort of People Should There Be?* (London: Penguin, 1984), pp. 71–72 (on ginseng).

5 See ref. 1, Elliott, "The Tyranny of Happiness," pp. 178, 186.

6 J. Glover, *I: The Philosophy and Psychology of Personal Identity* (London: Penguin, 1988), p. 152.

7 Marya Schechtman emphasizes this point in what may be the strongest theoretical exploration of this sense of personal identity *(The Constitution of Selves* [Ithaca, N.Y.: Cornell University Press, 1996], esp. Part II).

8 This position is helpfully explored and criticized in ref. 6, Glover, *I,* ch. 17.

9 J. P. Sartre, *Being and Nothingness,* tr. H. E. Barnes (New York: Philosophical Library, 1943).

10 See ref. 6, Glover, *I,* p. 131.

11 Kramer raises this conceptual issue in the case of his own patients (ref. 3, *Listening to Prozac,* pp. 18–19).

12 Sometimes a personality change may result from the patient's rewriting her inner story, since this story is about who she is. Cf. ref. 6, Glover, *I,* p. 153. For a classic background work, see Sigmund Freud, *Introductory Lectures on Psychoanalysis* (New York: Norton, 1960 [1920]).

13 Much of the concern about Ritalin, for example, focuses on parental consent on behalf of children, sometimes in apparent conflict with their best interests. See ref. 4, Diller, "The Run on Ritalin" and Mills, "One Pill Makes You Smarter."

14 D. W. Brock, "Enhancements of Human Function: Some Distinctions for Policymakers," in ref. 1, *Enhancing Human Traits,* pp. 48–69, at p. 59.

15 Cf. ref. 1, Elliott, "The Tyranny of Happiness." Regarding this problem in connection with Ritalin, see ref. 4, Diller, "The Run on Ritalin," p. 17; and regarding the more frightening case of prescribing for children, see ref. 4, Mills, "One Pill Makes You Smarter," pp. 16–17. For an insightful discussion of complicity with suspect cultural norms, see Margaret Olivia Little, "Cosmetic Surgery, Suspect Norms, and the Ethics of Complicity," in ref. 1, *Enhancing Human Traits,* pp. 162–76.

16 This viewpoint is powerfully developed in Carol Freedman, "Aspirin for the Mind? Some Ethical Worries about Psychopharmacology," in ref. 1, *Enhancing Human Traits,* pp. 135–50.

17 See ref. 1, Elliott, "The Tyranny of Happiness," p. 180; ref. 4, Glover, *What Sort of People Should There Be?,* pp. 72–73 and ref. 4, Diller, "The Run on Ritalin," pp. 14–15.

18 See ref. 14, Brock, "Enhancements of Human Function," p. 60.

19 See ref. 4, Diller, "The Run on Ritalin," p. 16 and Slomka, "Playing with Propranolol," p. 15.

20 We are probably closer in the cases of Ritalin for school-children and Propranolol for professional musicians (see cites in previous note). My sense is that the associated difficulties are so closely tied to the features of a particular drug and the social context in which it is used, that we cannot profitably generalize from a viable solution for one drug to cosmetic psychopharmacology in general.

OTHER TYPES OF NEUROENHANCEMENT

ONE PILL MAKES YOU SMARTER: AN ETHICAL APPRAISAL OF THE RISE OF RITALIN
Claudia Mills

Responding to the explosive growth in American children's use of the stimulant Ritalin since the early 1990s, Mills notes that the drug is now often prescribed for children who exhibit fairly normal childlike behaviors such as making careless errors in schoolwork, failing to pay attention, and squirming in their seats. The thought that we are increasingly drugging our children in order to get them to conform to adult expectations tends to disturb us, she argues, although it is difficult to say exactly what about this trend is genuinely disturbing. In the end, what is most troubling about the rise of Ritalin use in children, according to Mills, is neither the means of improving performance—a pill—nor the inequitable distribution of this means, but the goal of hyper-achievement. Our society's relentless pursuit of this goal, she concludes, may rob our children of their opportunity to be children.

The statistics at least *seem* alarming. The production of Ritalin, an amphetamine derivative used for the treatment of attention deficit disorder in children (and, lately, in adults as well), has risen a whopping 700 percent since 1990. According to figures given by Lawrence Diller in *Running on Ritalin,* over the decade, the number of Americans using Ritalin has soared from 900,000 to almost 5 million—the vast majority children from the ages of 5 to 12, though there is a significant rise in Ritalin use among teens and adults as well. No comparable rise is reported in other countries, though a much smaller surge has taken place in Canada and Australia. In Virginia

Report from the Institute for Philosophy & Public Policy, vol. 18, no. 4 (1988). pp. 13–17. Also in Verna Gehring and William Galston, eds., *Philosophical Dimensions in Public Policy* (Transaction, 2002). Copyright © 2002 by Transaction Publishers. Reprinted by permission of Transaction Publishers.

Beach, Va. (perhaps the most egregious example), 17 percent of fifth-grade boys were taking Ritalin in 1996 to control behavior problems and improve school performance. (Boys on Ritalin outnumber girls in a ratio of 3.5 to 1; when I was recently complaining to another mother about my own son's academic difficulties, she said simply, "Welcome to the world of boys.")

Stimulants have been used to treat behavior problems in children since 1937; Ritalin itself appeared on the market in the 1960s to treat what was then called "hyperactivity"—impulsive, disruptive behavior by children who just "couldn't sit still." In recent years, however, the root problem has been identified as "attention deficit disorder" (ADD), either with or without attendant hyperactivity.

Symptoms of ADD, according to the standard survey used in its diagnosis, include: "often fails to give close attention to details or makes careless mistakes in schoolwork," "often has difficulty organizing tasks and activities," and "often avoids, dislikes, or is reluctant to engage in tasks that require mental effort (such as schoolwork or homework)." Symptoms of ADD-H (the variant with hyperactivity) include: "often fidgets with hands or feet or squirms in seat" and "often has difficulty playing or engaging in leisure activities quietly." Ritalin, by most accounts, is remarkably effective in getting such children to settle down and pay attention, with resultant (at least short-term) gains in parental sanity and academic achievement.

The fear, stated quite baldly, is that as a society we are drugging our children in ever-larger numbers to get them to conform to adult expectations. Dislikes homework? Makes careless mistakes? Squirms in seat? To many it seems that we are drugging our children to get them to stop being *children*. I myself feel profoundly troubled by the rise of Ritalin—and by my own temptation to use it for my child, who, yes, makes careless mistakes and has been known to fidget. But, I will argue, it is surprisingly difficult to pinpoint any justifiable sources of discomfort here—both harder than one might think, and more illuminating. The effort to do so will lead us into an exploration of a range of issues about how we view our children and ourselves.

Here, then, are some possible responses to our concerns about the rise of Ritalin, followed by some speculations about the deeper—and legitimate—fears that fuel these concerns.

RATIONALES FOR TREATMENT

On some accounts, the rise in Ritalin simply reflects our commendably growing willingness to treat a serious and common disorder that has too long been left untreated. That there is soaring use of any drug is not itself a problem, if the drug is treating a genuine medical condition that responds favorably to treatment. If there is some real disorder in the area of children's brains that controls their ability to pay attention (current research is focusing on the prefrontal cortex), and this disorder is causing problems in school and home, and it can be easily treated, *shouldn't* it be treated? Why should children have to struggle with their schoolwork, and parents struggle with discipline, if the root cause of disappointing academic performance and poor behavior is a medical one that can be easily treated? On one expert's estimate attention deficient disorder is even now underdiagnosed, and so we should expect—and welcome—a further doubling of Ritalin use in response.

However, it is unclear that there really is any one, clearly identified "thing" that "is" attention deficit disorder. Diller argues persuasively that when parents or doctors speak of a child as "having" ADD, this tends to mean only that the child in fact scored positively on a certain number of questions on the kind of survey described earlier. Certainly diagnosis of ADD is inexact, to say the least—often based largely on reported frustration by parents and teachers sometimes made (as admitted by some teachers I've spoken to in my own local schools) by prescribing Ritalin on a trial basis and seeing if it works.

The trouble with the latter approach is that Ritalin almost always "works," in that it almost always enhances performance, at least in the short term (Diller reports that there is no evidence of long-term improvement in children taking Ritalin). According to one study cited by Diller, "stimulants had essentially the same effects on normal children as on children with attention or behavior problems." Diller notes an increasing amount of what has been called "diagnostic bracket creep," as the criteria for diagnosis become ever more loose and generous, allowing more borderline ADD children to benefit from drug treatment.

Now, it can be argued that it shouldn't matter whether children receiving Ritalin have some underlying "brain disorder" that causes inattention, or whether they are inattentive for other, less physiologically based reasons. Why is the *cause* of a condition relevant to whether or not we have reason to try to treat it? For example, if parents are debating whether or not to treat an abnormally short child with growth hormone, David B. Allen and Norman Fost have argued that it shouldn't matter whether the child's height is caused by a hormone deficiency or by his genetic endowment: What should matter is whether this is causing a problem for him, and whether it can be successfully treated.

With the diagnosis of attention deficit disorder so elastic, however, one begins to wonder whether the "disorder" in question is simply that the child places at the lower end of the spectrum for behavior or achievement—that is, that parents, clinging stubbornly to Lake Wobegon fantasies, insist that all children generally and their own children in particular should be "above average," or certainly not below average. (I have discovered from my own experience that teachers are also quick to suggest an ADD evaluation for a child with any academic difficulties.) If attention or behavior problems interfere with a child's achieving his or her "full potential," parents and teachers may be increasingly tempted to turn to medication, even where this can mean not just allowing their children to perform "normally," but raising them significantly above the norm. Diller mentions one student whose use of Ritalin allowed him to become his high school's valedictorian: Off the drug, he still performed well, but his grades slipped, from straight A's to A's intermingled with B's.

Some of us will be troubled by using Ritalin in such cases. But why shouldn't every child be able to use whatever means are available to improve his or her performance, whatever his starting point? If we were to raise poor performers to the mean, but refuse to raise average performers above the mean, this could seem unfair to the superior performers. Why shouldn't they have a chance at enhancement, too?

RITALIN AS A MEANS OF ENHANCEMENT

As Ronald Cole-Turner points out, in his article in this issue, most of us are already "enhancement enthusiasts." We not only strive to improve our children all the time, but would criticize parents who neglected to do so. If we give children Ritalin to enhance their academic performance—well, don't we send them to school in the first place for the same reason? It doesn't seem all that problematic to want our children to be more attentive, more responsive, better behaved, better able to learn: Isn't better, by definition, *better*? Cole-Turner argues, however, that while the goal of enhancement may be a legitimate one (I will raise doubts about this below), we need also to look at the means. Means *do* matter.

First, some means may be problematic in themselves, including the use of drugs. A friend with whom I was discussing the rise in Ritalin use voiced the reactions of many in saying, "Putting kids on drugs? Uh-uh." Now, drugs of any kind are often attended with a myriad of negative (and perhaps not yet discovered) side effects. But stimulants like Ritalin have been used to treat behavior problems in children for six decades with few observed ill effects. Ritalin causes insomnia, which can be avoided by not taking it in the evening; some children experience suppressed appetite. But the vast majority experience no distressing side effects at all.

The term "drugs" generally carries with it a stigma: When we think of "children on drugs," we think first of illegal drug use; when we talk about "drugging our children," we visualize children wandering through the day in a dopey, feel-good haze. It is important to free Ritalin from such unwarranted associations. Its use is legal, although controlled, and, far from inducing a fuzzy "drugged" state, it works to increase the ability to pay attention. With Ritalin, children don't "tune out," but "tune in." Or so we might claim.

Second, as Cole-Turner argues, some means to an end may be valued for their own sake and in their own right—either because they also represent ends that we value, or because we value reaching the end only after an experience of striving and struggle. If we choose a "quick fix" to solve our problems and achieve our goals, we may end up achieving different goals altogether, or, at the least, give up the long and ultimately more rewarding journey to our destination. In the case of Ritalin, the fear is that we will be content to give "problem children" a couple of little pills every day, rather than put in the extra effort as parents and teachers to reach them and teach them, to help them learn and grow in a more messy and non-medicalized way. Specifically, the fear is that we will see Ritalin as a means of bypassing tough and loving parental discipline or real (and expensive) commitments to shouldering the rising costs of effective public education.

Now, clearly we value parental love and discipline and the long journey of education as ends in themselves, not just as means to producing more successful children. Focusing for the moment on education, we don't send children to school simply to get them to acquire a certain body of knowledge and master a certain body of skills, but because the process of learning is itself valuable. I still remember the thrill the first time I really "got" long division. Or the shock of joy with which I first learned, from my high school American history teacher, that there really are two sides to every question. We may worry that Ritalin provides an easy way out of facing the challenge—and reward—of truly educating our children. For teachers who can teach and classroom environments in which children can learn cost vastly more than daily doses of Ritalin.

To this concern about Ritalin, I have two responses. First, Ritalin could be defended as a means, not of bypassing the journey of education, but of permitting certain children to engage in the journey more fully, to pay attention to the journey in all its richness. Ritalin doesn't substitute for learning; it at best assists in providing one of the preconditions for learning—the ability to pay attention to what is being taught. Ritalin or no Ritalin, we will still need to teach our children, both how to behave and how to learn, in the most creative ways possible.

This suggests, second, that when it comes to parents and to teaching, we do not need to fear that we will take the easy way out, because, quite simply, there *is* no easy way out. Cole-Turner points out correctly that while new means "may relocate our human struggle, they do not eliminate it." Even if we are what Gerald Klerman has called "pharmacological calvinists," who reject drug-based solutions as too easy, who value the hard way just because it's hard, this gives us no reason to resist Ritalin. Anyone who is a parent or teacher knows that there will be no shortage of hard work in raising and educating children. If hard is what we want, we're home free: however hard we want parenting and teaching to be, it will be hard enough.

EQUALITY AND COMPETITIVENESS

As I approach what I take to be the most serious worry about Ritalin, let me mention one other objection that is sometimes raised to it and other programs of medical enhancement. This objection concedes that Ritalin can provide genuine and legitimate advantages for those who use it, but charges that these advantages are not distributed fairly. Responsible diagnoses of attention deficit disorder are expensive and beyond the budget of many families, who are already poorly served by an inadequate health care system. With the rise of Ritalin, whose use is concentrated among white, upper-middle-class families, the children of the rich get cognitively richer, and the children of the poor fall ever further behind.

This objection, if it stands on its merits, could be met by efforts to equalize provision of Ritalin (as well as access to medical care generally). If racial or class disparities in Ritalin use were our chief concern, the solution would be obvious. But in my view, the biggest problem with Ritalin lies not with the kids who don't get it, but with (at least some of) those who do.

The real reason that I remain uncomfortable with the rise of Ritalin concerns not the means of enhancement, but the goal itself—what our motives are for seeking enhancement so diligently and desperately, and, even more, what we as a society are currently counting as enhancement. What, in the end, are we trying to gain?

Now, there are clear advantages to being able to pay attention, clear advantages to being able to learn. Dan Brock notes that often our efforts at enhancement are meant to provide us with "intrinsic goods" that we value for their own sake. If these are what we are seeking in putting our children on

Ritalin, this doesn't seem particularly troubling. But it seems to me, chiefly as an observer of my own life in one white, upper-middle-class American neighborhood, that many of us want more than this. We don't want to be better than our own imperfect selves; we want to be better than somebody else. We don't want Garrison Keillor's vision of a world where all the children are above average—we want a world where our own children are more above average than anybody else's. A friend of mine who is a principal in an affluent suburban elementary school says that in his school there are only three kinds of children: gifted, very gifted, and extremely gifted. We have grade inflation because so many students and parents insist on getting top grades that now teachers give top grades to almost everybody. And we give our children Ritalin in part because we cannot bear that they be below average; indeed, we cannot bear that they not be above average. This goal itself is troubling to me independent of any questions about the means to achieve it.

Of course, as Brock observes, such a goal is ultimately self-defeating: once everyone achieves the same relative enhancement, the competitive benefit of the enhancement disappears. But it may be a long time before we figure this out. And in the meantime we have to live in the world that we have been creating.

The concerns that I am raising now are targeted not only against Ritalin use, but against other, more familiar and widely accepted means of enhancement as well. For I don't think that our non-pharmaceutical strategies to produce better, brighter children are themselves beyond reproach. When I compare my own childhood experiences with those of my children, I feel a sorrow that I think runs deeper than mere nostalgia for a sentimentalized version of one's own past.

When I was a child, competitive sports didn't begin until fairly late in elementary school; now they begin for some children in kindergarten or even preschool. Children who wait until third or fourth grade to join a soccer or basketball team find themselves at an insuperable competitive disadvantage. In fact, in my neighborhood, a number of the children have already burned out on a sport and decided to drop it by the age at which children a generation ago were just beginning. I began piano lessons in third grade; my own children began in kindergarten. How else can they keep up with everyone else's children who have also been studying music from the cradle—indeed, with children who listened to tapes of Mozart in utero?

And so middle-class children have childhoods in which they are chauffeured by their ever-more-frantic parents from one enrichment activity to another: two sports, two musical instruments, Scouts, Odyssey of the Mind, after-school language programs, science discovery programs, theater workshops. Parents who have a different vision of what childhood might be are reluctant to pursue it, for fear that their children will be left too far behind. One parenting magazine recently published an article about a family that actually chose not to participate in any after-school activities, where this was considered sufficiently unusual to merit a feature article in a national magazine.

The irony in all this is that Ritalin is prescribed for attention deficit disorder. Yet as we struggle to enhance our children faster than our neighbors manage to enhance theirs, we fill our lives with an even greater level of distractions. Diller speculates that if Huck Finn and Tom Sawyer walked out of Twain's pages and into a suburban American school today, they might well find themselves on Ritalin. He worries about our inability to tolerate and appreciate a range of temperaments and personality styles. I worry about this, too, but more about whether we are losing the ability to let children be children—or at least to let them be average children, not gifted, very gifted, or extremely gifted, savoring childhood as it slips by all too quickly.

If we want our kids to pay attention, maybe we have to begin paying attention to what it is that's worth paying attention *to*.

SOURCES

Lawrence H. Diller, *Running on Ritalin: A Physician Reflects on Children, Society, and Performance in a Pill* (Bantam Books, 1998), and "The Run on Ritalin: Attention Deficit Disorder and Stimulant Treatment in the 1990s," *Hastings Center Report*, vol. 26, no. 2 (1996); Erik Parens, "Is Better Always Good? The Enhancement Project," *Hastings Center Report*, vol. 28, no. 1 (1998) (Parens quotes Dan

Brock and David B. Allen and Norman Fost, and Peter J. Whitehouse, Eric Juengst, Maxwell Mehlman, and Thomas H. Murray, "Enhancing Cognition in the

Intellectually Intact," *Hastings Center Report,* vol. 27, no. 3 (1997) (this article cites Gerald Klerman on "pharmacological calvinism").

MONITORING AND MANIPULATING BRAIN FUNCTION: NEW NEUROSCIENCE TECHNOLOGIES AND THEIR ETHICAL IMPLICATIONS

Martha J. Farah and Paul Root Wolpe

In this excerpt from a much longer article, Farah and Wolpe begin by explaining that the recent explosion of interest in the ethics of neuroscience has resulted from two main factors: (1) advances in technologies that permit us to monitor brain function in significant ways and (2) our bourgeoning capacity to manipulate brain function with precision and control. (The present excerpt concerns the second factor.) Regarding brain enhancement, the authors describe such technologies as selective serotonin reuptake inhibitors (SSRIs) including Prozac, psychotropic drugs that enhance cognitive function, transcranial magnetic stimulation, and brain-machine interfaces. They then examine in detail the use of medications to enhance cognition and memory in particular. Following this descriptive overview, Farah and Wolpe identify and discuss the ethical issues provoked by the manipulation of brain function for enhancement purposes. They conclude with the thesis that these technological advances reinforce the scientific image of human beings as part of the natural world while threatening some traditional notions of selfhood and soul.

Congress christened the 1990s "the decade of the brain," and this was apt from the vantage point of the early 21st Century. Great strides were made in both basic and clinical neuroscience. What the current decade may, in retrospect, be remembered for is the growth of neuroscience beyond those two categories, "basic" and "clinical," into a host of new applications. From the measurement of mental processes with functional neuroimaging to their manipulation with ever more selective drugs, the new capabilities of neuroscience raise unprecedented ethical and social issues. These issues must be identified and addressed if society is to benefit from the neuroscience revolution now in progress.

Reprinted with permission of the authors and publisher from *Hastings Center Report,* vol. 34 (May–June 2004), pp. 35–36, 40–44. Copyright © 2004 by The Hastings Center.

Like the field of genetics, cognitive neuroscience raises questions about the biological foundations of who we are. Indeed, the relation of self and personal identity to the brain is, if anything, more direct than that of self to the genome. In addition, the ethical questions of neuroscience are more urgent, as neural interventions are currently more easily accomplished than genetic interventions. Yet compared to the field of molecular genetics, in which ethical issues have been at the forefront since the days of the 1975 Asilomar meeting on recombinant DNA, relatively little attention has been paid to the ethics of neuroscience.

This situation is changing, as bioethicists and neuroscientists are beginning to explore the emerging social and ethical issues raised by progress in neuroscience. In the Society for Neuroscience's recently formulated mission statement, bioethical issues figure prominently.[1] Numerous articles, meetings, and symposia have appeared on the subject.[2] The term "neuroethics," which originally referred to bioethical issues in clinical neurology, has now been adopted to refer to ethical issues in the technological advances of neuroscience more generally.[3] (Unfortunately, the term is also used to refer to the neural bases of ethical thinking, a different topic.[4])

Neuroethics encompasses a broad and varied set of bioethical issues. Some are similar to those that have arisen previously in biomedicine, such as the safety of new research and treatment methods, the rationing of promising new therapies, and predictive testing for future illnesses when no cure is available (as with Alzheimer's or Huntington's disease). Other neuroethical issues, however, are unique to neuroscience because of the particular subject matter of that field. The brain is the organ of the mind and consciousness, the locus of our sense of selfhood. Interventions in the brain, therefore, have different ethical implications than interventions in other organs. In addition, our growing knowledge of mind-brain relations is likely to affect our definitions of competence, mental health and illness, and death. Our moral and legal conceptions of responsibility are likewise susceptible to change as our understanding of the physical mechanisms of behavior evolves. Our sense of the privacy and confidentiality of our own thought processes may also be threatened by technologies that can reveal the neural correlates of our innermost thoughts.

Many of the new social and ethical issues in neuroscience result from one of two developments. The first is the ability to monitor brain function in living humans with a spatial and temporal resolution sufficient to capture psychologically meaningful fluctuations of activity. The second is the ability to alter the brain with chemical or anatomical selectivity that is sufficient to induce specific functional changes. . . .

BRAIN ENHANCEMENT

The psychopharmacology of the mid-twentieth century depended entirely on serendipity. The antihistamine chlorpromazine was accidentally found to calm agitated schizophrenic patients and reduce their psychosis. Another early drug investigated for its antipsychotic properties, imipramine, turned out to be ineffective for that purpose, but was observed to lift the mood of some of the patients taking it. When a small number of patients with major depression tried it, the therapeutic effect was dramatic, and imipramine continues to be used as an antidepressant today. The second antidepressant to be discovered, iproniazid, was hither-to used as an antibiotic for treating patients with tuberculosis when its mood-elevating properties were observed. Similar accidental discoveries led to the identification of amphetamine as a stimulant in the course of refining a treatment for asthma, and meprobamate as an anti-anxiety treatment in the course of testing an antibiotic.[5]

Such lucky accidents were then augmented by trial and error tests with other molecules of similar structure. Parallel to this development, researchers began to understand the effects of these drugs on brain function, identifying the specific neurotransmitter systems affected by the drugs and the mechanisms by which the drugs interacted with these systems. The advent of direct-binding assays in the 1960s provided the first direct approach to testing and comparing the affinity of a drug for different neurotransmitter receptors, and the tools of the molecular biology revolution, including the cloning of rare subtypes of receptors, allowed for the design of highly selective agonists, antagonists, and other molecules to influence selectively the process of neurotransmission.

The continual improvement in side-effect profile of modern psychotropic medications is due to the increasing selectivity of drug action made possible by the methods of molecular neuroscience. "Selective" is the first S in SSRI, the class of drugs to which fluoxetine (Prozac) belongs. New drugs with ever more selective actions on the neurochemistry of mood, anxiety, attention, and memory are under development. Although intended for therapy, many of these drugs affect brain function in healthy people, raising the possibility of their use for enhancement of normal function rather than remediation of dysfuntion.

The enhancement potential of some medications is, in itself, nothing new, and the attempts of human beings to use chemical substances to alter normal affective and cognitive traits is as old as the drinking of alcohol. Until recently, however, psychotropic drugs had significant risks and side effects that limited their attractiveness. This situation is changing as side-effect profiles become more tolerable. In addition, therapy in conjunction with other drugs is an increasingly common strategy for counteracting the remaining side effects. For example, the most trouble-some side effect for users of SSRIs is sexual dysfunction, which responds well to the drug sildenafil (Viagra). Other drugs specifically developed to counteract the sexual side effects of SSRIs are in development and clinical trials. The result of both new designer drugs and adjuvant drugs is the same: increasingly selective alteration of our mental states and abilities through neurochemical intervention, with correspondingly less downside to their use by anyone, sick or well.

Technical advances in non-pharmaceutical methods for altering brain function are also creating potential enhancement tools. Transcranial magnetic stimulation (TMS) and, more rarely, vagus nerve stimulation and deep-brain stimulation have already been used to improve mental function or mood in patients with medically intractable neuropsychiatric illnesses.[6] Research on the effects of non-pharmaceutical methods on brain function in normal individuals has been limited to the relatively less invasive TMS. Mood effects on normal healthy subjects have been investigated in the context of basic research on mood and brain function,[7] and at least one laboratory is devoted to the development of TMS methods for enhancing normal cognition.[8] Finally, there is growing research interest in computer augmentation of brains. Most research on brain-machine interfaces currently focuses on capturing and using movement command signals from the brain and carrying sensory inputs to the brain, for example from a video camera.[9] One research program is tackling memory augmentation by developing a prosthetic hippocampus that can be interfaced with a rodent brain.[10] The motivation for this research is partly scientific, to better understand neural coding of sensory, motor, and memory information, and partly clinical, to help patients with paralysis and peripheral sensory impairments.

Nevertheless, the military's substantial support for this research suggests that some think normal healthy individuals might someday be enhanced by neural prostheses.[11] . . .

ENHANCEMENT OF COGNITION

Our current ability to enhance cognition through the direct alteration of brain function involves two types of cognitive function: attention and memory. "Attention" is used here in its broadest sense, including active use of working memory, executive function, and other forms of cognitive self-control. These are the cognitive abilities most obviously deficient in the syndrome of Attention Deficit Hyperactivity Disorder (ADHD). These same abilities vary in their strength within the normal population. Indeed it seems likely that ADHD represents the lower tail of the whole population distribution rather than a qualitatively different state of functioning, discontinuous with the normal population.[12]

Drugs targeting the neurotransmitter systems dopamine and norephinephrine are effective in treating ADHD, and have been shown to improve normal attentional function as well. Methyphenidate (Ritalin) and amphetamine (Adderal), as well as modafinil (Provigil, a newer drug approved for regulating sleep) have been shown to enhance attention across a variety of different tests in healthy young volunteers.[13]

Do these laboratory-measured improvements translate into a noticeable improvement of real world cognitive performance? No experimental evidence is available, but the growing illicit use of ADHD medications on college campuses suggests that many young adults believe their cognition is enhanced by the drugs.[14] Parents also appear to find real world benefits for their normal children with ADHD medication: In certain school districts the proportion of boys taking methylphenidate exceeds the most generous estimates of ADHD prevalence.[15]

Memory is the other cognitive ability that can, at present, be manipulated to some degree by drugs. Interest in memory enhancement has so far been confined to the middle-aged and elderly, whose memory ability undergoes a gradual decline even in the absence of dementia. The most commonly used method involves manipulation not of memory circuits per se but of cerebrovascular function. Herbal supplements such as Gingko Biloba affect memory mainly by increasing blood flow within the brain. However, the effectiveness of this treatment is questionable.[16] How close are we to more specific and effective memory enhancement for healthy older adults?

As the molecular biology of memory progresses, it presents drug designers with a variety of entry points through which to influence the specific processes of memory formation. A huge research effort is now being directed to the development of memory-boosting drugs.[17] The candidate drugs target various stages in the molecular cascade that underlies memory formation, including the initial induction of long-term potentiation (LTP) and the later stages of memory consolidation. There is reason to believe that some of the products under development would work for enhancement as well as therapy. For example, treatment of healthy human subjects with an ampakine, which enhances LTP, improved performance in a dose-dependent manner.[18]

Few consider memory enhancement for the young to be a goal. Although some specialized pursuits such as certain competitive card games could conceivably benefit from super-memory, evidence suggests that the forgetting rates of normal young humans are optimal for most purposes.[19] Empirically, prodigious memory has been linked to difficulties with thinking and problem solving,[20] and computationally, the effect of boosting the durability of individual memories is to decrease the ability to generalize.[21]

Indeed, in some circumstances reduced learning would confer benefit. Memories of traumatic events can cause lifelong suffering in the form of post traumatic stress disorder (PTSD), and methods are being sought to prevent the consolidation of such memories by intervening pharmacologically immediately following the trauma.[22] Drugs that interfere with the consolidation of memories in general, such as benzodiazepines, are well known.[23] Extending these methods beyond the victims of trauma, to anyone wishing to avoid remembering an unpleasant event, is yet another way in which the neural bases of memory could be altered to enhance normal function.

ETHICAL ISSUES IN ENHANCEMENT

Although the promise of enhancement is easy to identify—smarter, more cheerful, and more capable

people—the risk is harder to articulate. Most people feel at least some ambivalence about neuropsychological enhancement, but distinguishing realistic or compelling arguments from generalized fear is often difficult.

Many of the ethical issues raised by neuropsychological enhancement also arise with other types of enhancement.[24] Cosmetic surgery and the use of human growth hormone for healthy children who are naturally short, for example, are medical enhancements that do not affect brain function, and though both are controversial, both are generally accepted. Enhancement techniques that affect brain function through more familiar and non-neuroscience-based interventions such as biofeedback, meditation, tutoring, or psychotherapy are not seen as objectionable, and, in fact, are often seen as laudable. What, then, are the objections to using pharmaceutical or other neurotechnological means to achieve the same ends as behavioral techniques? Much recent discussion has focused on this question.[25] Although few if any ethical concerns arise uniquely in connection with neuroscience-based methods, two concerns seem particularly salient in the context of neural interventions for enhancement compared with other biomedical interventions whose targets are not psychological, on the one hand, and behavioral interventions for psychological enhancement, on the other.[26]

The first of these concerns is safety. Safety is a concern with all medications and procedures, but in comparison to other comparably elective treatments such as cosmetic surgery or growth hormone treatment, neuroscience-based enhancement involves intervening in a far more complex system. We are therefore at greater risk of unanticipated problems when we tinker. Would endowing learners with super-memory interfere with their ability to understand what they have learned and relate it to other knowledge? Might today's Ritalin users face an old age of premature cognitive decline? These are empirical questions, of course, which can only be answered in time. So far, medications such as SSRIs and stimulants have good safety records, and their long-term effects may even be positive. For example, SSRIs have been shown to be neuroprotective over the long term.[27] A recent study of the effects of Ritalin on rat brain development showed both desirable and undesirable effects on later adult behavior.[28] Nevertheless, drug safety testing does not routinely address long-term use, and relatively little evidence is available on long-term use by healthy subjects. It remains an open empirical issue whether the net effects of these or other yet-to-be developed drugs are positive or negative.

The second concern about neuroscience-based enhancement is more complex and difficult to state succinctly. This is actually a group of related concerns resulting from the many ways in which neuroscience-based enhancement intersects with our understanding of what it means to be a person, to be healthy and whole, to do meaningful work, and to value human life in all its imperfection. The recent report of the President's Council on Bioethics emphasized these issues in its discussion of enhancement. At the heart of this group of concerns is the problem of reconciling our understanding of persons and brains.[29]

Among the widely shared intuitions about persons are the following: Persons have a kind of value that is independent of any commodity or capability they bring to the world. Persons are responsible for their actions and deserve blame or respect depending on those actions. Persons lead lives that have meaning, and although it is difficult to say exactly what is meant by "meaning" in this context, most of us would agree that accomplishments in life are made meaningful partly by the effort they require. Finally, persons endure over time; although some of their characteristics may change, there is a self that remains constant for as long as the person can be said to exist.

Brains are physical systems and as such do not share any of the foregoing qualities. Of course, neuroscience-based enhancements work because changes to the brain result in changes to the person. To use such enhancements, without infringing on our personhood, can seem a contradiction, or at least perplexing, and raises a number of concerns. Maximizing the performance capabilities of an already healthy, functional person can be viewed as commodifying human abilities. Improving behavior pharmacologically seems to detract from the responsibility of the person for his or her own actions. Reducing the effort needed for personal accomplishments by neurochemical means may reduce their meaning as well. And the changing of abilities, memories, and moods at will by swallowing a pill may undermine the idea of a constant "self."

PENDING CHALLENGES

Technologies for monitoring and manipulating the brain have developed rapidly over the last few decades and are poised for continued growth. Some of the ethical problems posed by these developments have immediate practical consequences. Examples of such problems include the illusory accuracy of brain images in forensic contexts and the unknown safety of long-term stimulant use by healthy adults and children. Other ethical problems are on the horizon, pending further technological progress. For example, brain imaging will not pose a serious threat to privacy until scanning methods can reliably deliver useful information about individual subjects. Although this is not the case at present, the development is foreseeable and could have enormous practical consequences.

Another way in which developments in neuroscience will influence society is less tangible than those just mentioned, but no less consequential. Both brain imaging and brain-based enhancement are forcing us to confront the fact that we are physical systems. If specific abilities, personality traits, and dispositions are manifest in characteristic patterns of brain activation and can be manipulated by specific neurochemical interventions, then they must be part of the physical world. Our intuitions about personhood do not mesh easily with this realization. At the very least, the realization calls for a considerably more nuanced idea of personal responsibility in law and morality.[30] More generally, it will prove challenging to traditional ideas regarding the soul, or the non-material component of the human mind.

ACKNOWLEDGEMENTS

The authors thank the editor and reviewers for extremely helpful comments on an earlier draft of this article, and Arthur Caplan for discussion and encouragement. The writing of this article was supported by NSF grants 0226060 and 0342108, NIH grants R21-DA01586, R01-DA14129 and R01-HD043078.

NOTES

1 Available at www.sfn.org.

2 M.J. Farah, "Emerging ethical issues in neuroscience," *Nature Neuroscience* 5 (2002): 1123–29; J. Illes, M.P Kirschen, and J. Gabrieli, "From Neuroimaging to Neuroethics," *Nature Neuroscience* 6 (2003): 205; D. Marcus, ed., *Neuroethics Mapping the Field Conference,* Proceedings of The Dana Foundation, 2002; A. Roskies, "Neuroethics for the New Millenium," *Neuron* 35 (2002): 21–23.

3 P.R. Wolpe, "Neuroethics," *Encyclopedia of Bioethics,* 3rd edition (Farmington Hills, Mich.: Macmillan Reference, 2004).

4 See Roskies, "Neuroethics for the New Millenium," 2002.

5 S.H. Barondes, *Better than Prozac: Creating the Next Generation of Psychiatric Drugs* (London, Oxford University Press, 2003).

6 G.S. Mahli and P. Sachdev, "Novel Physical Treatments for the Management of Neuropsychiatric Disorders," *Journal of Psychosomatic Research* 53 (2002): 709–19.

7 M. George, E. Wasserman, and R. Post, "Transcranial Magnetic Stimulation: A Neuropsychiatric Tool for the 21st century," *Journal of Neuropsychiatry Clinical Neuroscience* 8 (1996): 373–82.

8 A.W. Snyder et al., "Savant-like Skills Exposed in Normal People by Suppressing the Left Fronto-temporal Lobe," *Journal of Integrative Neuroscience* 2 (2003): 149–58.

9 J. Donoghue, "Connecting Cortex to Machines: Recent Advances in Brain Interfaces,"*Nature Neuroscience Supplement* 5 (2002): 1085–88.

10 Available at www.usc.edu/programs/pibbs/site/faculty/berger_t.

11 H. Hoag, "Neuroengineering: Remote control," *Nature* 423 (2003): 796–798.

12 NIH, *Diagnosis and Treatment of Attention Deficit Hyperactivity Disorder,* NIH Consensus Statement 16, no. 2 (1998): 1–37.

13 R. Elliott et al., "Effects of Methylphenidate on Spatial Working Memory and Planning in Healthy Young Adults," *Psychopharmacology* 131 (1997): 196-206; M.A. Mehta et al., "Methylphenidate Enhances Working Memory by Modulating Discrete Frontal and Parietal Lobe Regions in the Human Brain," *Journal of Neuroscience* 20 (2000): RC65; D.C. Turner et al., "Cognitive Enhancing Effects of Modafinil in Healthy Volunteers," *Psychopharmacology* 165 (2003): 260–69.

14 Q. Babcock and T. Byrne, "Student Perceptions of Methylphenidate Abuse at a Public Liberal Arts College," *Journal of American College Health* 49 (2000): 143–45.

15 L.H. Diller, "Running on Ritalin: Attention deficit disorder and stimulant treatment in the 1990s," *Hastings Center Report* 26 (1996): 12–14.

16 P.E. Gold, L. Cahill, and G.L. Wenk, "Ginkgo Biloba: a cognitive enhancer?," *Psychological Science in the Public Interest* 3 (2002): 2–11.

17 G. Lynch, "Memory enhancement: the search for mechanism-based drugs," *Nature Neuroscience* 5 (2002): 1035–1038.

18 M. Ingvar et al., "Enhancement by an Ampakine of Memory Encoding in Humans," *Experimental Neurology* 146 (1997): 553–59.

19 J. Anderson, *The adaptive characteristics of thought* (Hillsdale, NJ: Erlbaum, 1990).

20 A.R. Luria, *The Mind of a Mnemonist* (Cambridge, Mass.: Harvard University Press, 1968).

21 J.L. McClelland, B.L. McNaughton, and R.C. O'Reilly, "Why there are complementary learning systems in the hippocampus and neocortex: Insights from the successes and failures of connectionist models of learning and memory," *Psychology Review* 102 (1995): 419–457.

22 R.K. Pittman, K.M. Sanders, R.M. Zusman, A.R. Healy, F. Cheema, and N.B. Lasko, "Pilot study of secondary prevention of posttraumatic stress disorder with propranolol," *Biological Psychiatry* 15 (2002): 189–192.

23 S.E. Buffett-Jerrott and S.H. Stewart, "Cognitive and sedative effects of benzodiazepine use," *Current Pharmaceutical Design* 8 (2002): 45–58.

24 See C. Elliot, *Better than Well: American Medicine Meets the American Dream* (New York: Norton, 2003); E. Parens, (Ed.) *Enhancing Human Traits: Social and Ethical Implications* (Washington: Georgetown University Press, 2000).

25 M.J. Farah et al., "Neurocognitive Enhancement: What Can We Do? What Should We Do?" *Nature Reviews Neuroscience* 5 (2004): 421–25; P.R. Wolpe, "Treatment, enhancement, and the ethics of neurotherapeutics," *Brain and Cognition* 50 (2003): 387–395.

26 J.D. Moreno, "Neuroethics: An Agenda for Neuroscience and Society," *Nature Reviews Neuroscience* 4 (2003): 149–53.

27 V. Sanchez, J. Camarero, B. Esteban, M.J. Peter, A.R. Green and M.I. Colado, The mechanisms involved in the longlasting neuroprotective effect of fluoxetine against MDMA ('ecstasy')-induced degeneration of 5-HT nerve endings in rat brain," *British Journal of Pharmacology* 134 (2001): 46–57.

28 W.A. Carlezon Jr., S.D. Mague, and S.L. Andersen, "Enduring Behavioral Effects of Early Exposure to Methylphendate in Rats," *Biological Psychiatry* (2003): 1330–37.

29 L. Kass, *Beyond Therapy: Biotechnology and the Pursuit of Happiness* (New York: Harper Collins 2003).

30 S. Morse, "Brain and Blame,"*Georgetown Law Journal* 84 (1996).

ANNOTATED BIBLIOGRAPHY

Buchanan, Allen: "Moral Status and Human Enhancement," *Philosophy and Public Affairs* 37 (Fall 2009), pp. 346–381. In this imaginative article, Buchanan explores what human enhancements might mean for the moral status of people like present-day human beings. Buchanan argues that moral status is best understood as a threshold concept rather than a matter of degree, and that understanding moral status in this way is likely to protect the status of unenhanced human beings even in a world in which some human beings are enhanced to a point of dramatic cognitive superiority.

Caplan, Arthur L.: "Death as an Unnatural Process," *EMBO Reports* 6 (2005), pp. S72–S75. In this very readable discussion, Caplan argues that aging can be understood as more disease-like than as natural and inevitable.

Dees, Richard H.: "Better Brains, Better Selves? The Ethics of Neuroenhancements," *Kennedy Institute of Ethics Journal* 17 (December 2007), pp. 371-395. Responding to a wide range of concerns about neuroenhancements, Dees argues that few proposed uses of these technologies would be wrong in principle.

DeGrazia, David: "Enhancement Technologies and Human Identity," *Journal of Medicine and Philosophy* 30 (June 2005), pp. 261–283. Responding in part to the work of the President's Council on Bioethics, DeGrazia examines the relationship between enhancement and human identity. His thesis is that a lucid, plausible conception of identity largely neutralizes the charges that use of biotechnologies for enhancement purposes is inauthentic and threatens core human characteristics.

Dreger, Alice D.: "'Ambiguous Sex'—or Ambivalent Medicine? Ethical Issues in the Treatment of Intersexuality," *Hastings Center Report* 28 (May–June 1998), pp. 24–36. Examining the history and cultural meaning of the treatment of intersexuality, Dreger criticizes standard medical approaches to these conditions on ethical grounds and offers several suggestions toward a better approach.

Elliott, Carl: *Better Than Well: American Medicine Meets the American Dream* (New York: Norton, 2003). Elliott explores the cultural, psychological, and ethical ramifications of medical enhancement and a variety of controversial medical treatments in American society, with special emphasis on the value Americans place on individuality and self-improvement.

———, and Tod Chambers, eds.: *Prozac as a Way of Life* (Chapel Hill, NC: University of North Carolina Press, 2004). The eleven essays in this volume offer groundwork for a philosophical discussion of the ethical and cultural dimensions of selective serotonin reuptake inhibitors. Focusing on the growing use of medication as a means of enhancement, authors from the fields of bioethics, psychiatry, and psychology address issues connected with personal identity, the elasticity of psychiatric diagnosis, and aggressive marketing by drug companies.

Farah, Martha J.: "Neuroethics: The Practical and the Philosophical," *Trends in Cognitive Science* 9 (January 2005), pp. 34–40. This article provides an overview of ethical concerns, both practical and philosophical, that surround the emergence of new technologies in cognitive neuroscience.

Fenton, Elizabeth: "Liberal Eugenics and Human Nature: Against Habermas," *Hastings Center Report* 36 (November–December 2006), pp. 35–42. Replying to Jürgen Habermas's case against making genetic enhancements to one's children, Fenton challenges his assumption that a clear line can be drawn between what is natural and what is manufactured.

Kramer, Peter D.: *Listening to Prozac* (New York: Viking, 1993). In this classic and exceptionally well-written discussion, Kramer introduces the concept of cosmetic psychopharmacology in sharing his experiences with patients who have used the antidepressant Prozac. The book addresses a variety of ethical and philosophical issues including the appropriate boundaries of medical practice, the meaning of mental illness, and personal identity.

Levy, Neil: *Neuroethics: Challenges for the Twenty-First Century* (Cambridge: Cambridge University Press, 2007). This volume offers an outstanding introduction to the issues of neuroethics. In connection with the use of new brain imaging technologies and various types of brain manipulation, Levy addresses ethical issues as well as such philosophical topics as free will, selfhood, and the nature of the mind.

Parens, Erik: "Authenticity and Ambivalence: Toward Understanding the Enhancement Debate," *Hastings Center Report* 35 (May–June 2005), pp. 34–41. Parens argues that the differences between critics and proponents of enhancement technologies tend to be exaggerated, and that both groups share the moral ideal of authenticity while understanding this ideal in different terms.

————, ed.: *Enhancing Human Traits: Ethical and Social Implications* (Washington, DC: Georgetown University Press, 1998). This anthology serves as an excellent introduction to such biomedical enhancements as cosmetic surgery, antidepressants for "the worried well," and genetic enhancements. The thirteen essays explore conceptual, ethical, policy-related, and cultural issues provoked by efforts to enhance human traits with biomedical means.

President's Council on Bioethics, *Beyond Therapy: Biotechnology and the Pursuit of Happiness* (Washington, DC: President's Council on Bioethics, 2003). This report investigates the potential implications of using biotechnology "beyond therapy" in seeking better children, superior individual performance, avoidance of the usual effects of aging, and happiness. The PCB intends with this report "to advance the nation's awareness and understanding of a critical set of bioethical issues and to bring them beyond the narrow circle of bioethics professionals into the larger public arena."

Wilson, Bruce E., and William G. Reiner: "Management of Intersex: A Shifting Paradigm," *Journal of Clinical Ethics* 9 (Winter 1998), pp. 360–369. After introducing the clinical phenomenon of intersex and the multiple meanings of the terms *male* and *female*, the authors criticize the old treatment paradigm for intersex, which paternalistically promoted early surgical intervention, and recommend an approach that affords parents and the intersex individual, as he or she matures, a greater role in decision making.

CHAPTER 4

HUMAN AND ANIMAL RESEARCH

INTRODUCTION

This chapter focuses primarily on ethical issues in biomedical research using human subjects. Investigations of these issues employ some of the same ethical concepts and principles discussed in the previous two chapters. Here, too, one finds an emphasis on the value of individual autonomy and on the requirements of informed consent or, in the case of incompetent patients, proxy consent consistent with either the substituted-judgment standard or the best-interests standard. At the same time, a concern unique to research is its potential benefits to society as a whole. In addition to confronting issues related to the requirements of informed consent and (to a lesser extent) proxy consent, this chapter features a discussion of randomized clinical trials in general and a closely related discussion of specific problems associated with research in developing countries.

In addition to examining these topics pertaining to human research, this chapter includes an extensive discussion of the ethics of biomedical research involving animal subjects. Animals lack the decision-making capacity required for informed consent and never have had such capacity (precluding meaningful substituted judgments); nor can it be plausibly argued, in most cases, that serving as a research subject promotes an animal's best interests. Is the use of animals as research subjects morally justified? If so, what is the justification for animal research, under what conditions can it be ethically conducted, and can the answers to these questions be integrated into a coherent overall account of research ethics that addresses human research subjects as well?

CONCEPTUAL ISSUES

Before examining some of the ethical issues raised by human research, we should clarify the meaning of *human research* (or *human experimentation*) and the distinction often drawn between therapeutic and nontherapeutic research. In the biomedical context, *therapy* ordinarily refers to a set of activities whose primary purpose is to relieve suffering, restore or maintain health, or prolong life. Therapy takes many forms. Medical treatment, diagnosis, and even some preventive measures (e.g., vaccine injections) are typically classified as forms of therapy. It is important to notice that the primary aim of therapy is to benefit the recipient. In contrast, *research* or *experimentation* refers to a set of scientific activities whose primary purpose is to contribute to generalizable knowledge about the chemical, physiological, or psychological processes involved in human (or sometimes animal) functioning. In human research, human beings serve as subjects.

A distinction has often been drawn between therapeutic and nontherapeutic research. As with all research, *therapeutic research* is concerned with the acquisition of generalizable knowledge. However, in therapeutic research the patient-subjects are themselves expected (or at least hoped) to benefit medically from the new drug, vaccine, treatment, or diagnostic procedure under investigation. For example, the first patients on kidney dialysis machines and the first recipients of coronary bypass surgery were participants in medical experiments. The techniques in question had never been tried on human subjects, so the use of these techniques on the patient-subjects was experimental. Furthermore, medical professionals gained information that furthered their research and contributed to generalizable knowledge. At the same time, the new techniques provided a form of therapy designed to alleviate the patient-subjects' own medical problems. They hoped to benefit from procedures that were thought to offer promise of proving more effective than any other therapy available. By contrast, *nontherapeutic research* is often characterized as research whose sole aim is to furnish data that contributes to generalizable knowledge. Providing therapy for the research subjects is not regarded as an aim of nontherapeutic research.

In practice, however, it is difficult to draw a clear line between therapeutic and nontherapeutic research. Therapeutic research is not conducted solely to benefit patient-subjects since the purpose of all research is to contribute to generalizable knowledge. Moreover, the therapeutic project may require patient-subjects to undergo additional procedures unrelated to their own therapy. They may have to give blood samples or undergo catheterization, for example. Such additional procedures are nontherapeutic for the patients and may carry risks unrelated to their own therapy. Nontherapeutic research, in turn, may indirectly provide medical benefits (such as a thorough medical checkup) for subjects.

Despite these complications, which somewhat obscure the distinction between therapeutic and nontherapeutic research, many commentators find the distinction helpful in exploring ethical issues pertaining to research. For example, it is commonly believed that in therapeutic research it is morally acceptable to impose somewhat higher risk to patient-subjects than would be acceptable in nontherapeutic research. The acceptance of the therapeutic/nontherapeutic distinction is reflected in codes of research ethics that continue to employ it. For example, the Declaration of Helsinki, reprinted in this chapter, implies the distinction by announcing, in addition to basic principles for all medical research, several principles for medical research combined with medical care. (Earlier versions of this ethical code more explicitly distinguished what it called *clinical research* and *nonclinical research*.) Some commentators today find it clearer and more helpful to articulate a distinction between research that "offers the prospect of direct medical benefit" to subjects and research that does not.[1]

THE JUSTIFICATION OF RESEARCH USING HUMAN SUBJECTS

Many biomedical research projects entail some risk to subjects. New drugs may prove toxic, for example. Some studies involve deliberately exposing subjects to a disease such as malaria before they can be used to test the efficacy of a new treatment. What moral justification is available for research that puts human subjects at risk?

The most commonly offered justification for human research is utilitarian in character and features two main claims. First, human experimentation enhances the discovery of new diagnostic and therapeutic techniques. For example, past research has enabled the development of cardiovascular surgery, renal transplantation, and the control of poliomyelitis. Second, controlled experiments are necessary for sound medical practice. Iatrogenic illnesses (illnesses caused by medical interventions) are preventable only if clinical research provides necessary data about human reactions to specific therapies. In the past, physicians employed many techniques that were of no benefit and sometimes even harmed patients. For example, neither the blood-letting common in the eighteenth century nor the practice of freezing the stomachs of patients with ulcers in the twentieth century proved to have any therapeutic value. Yet both practices were believed to be therapeutic. Well-designed, controlled research projects, it is argued, will help to minimize the use of worthless or harmful procedures. The utilitarian conclusion is that human experimentation is not just morally permissible, but morally required, because its future benefits and prevention of harm to many will far outweigh its harmful consequences to some research subjects.

Sometimes a different sort of argument, based on considerations of fairness—or perhaps gratitude—is advanced to justify human research and to defend the view that individuals have a duty to participate as research subjects. The argument can be stated simply. We are the beneficiaries of advances that past biomedical research made possible. Without the use of human subjects, these advances would not have occurred. Having benefited from the sacrifices made by past research subjects, we have a fairness-based (or gratitude-based) obligation to reciprocate by serving as subjects ourselves. One possible reply to this argument is that current participation in research will primarily benefit individuals in the future; few persons who made sacrifices in the past will be alive to benefit from the so-called "reciprocity" of people today serving as research subjects. A proponent of the fairness-based argument might respond that what is important is not that particular subjects be "paid back" for their past services; the idea is rather that humanity has made sacrifices for presently living individuals, who should in turn be willing to make sacrifices for humanity. Another reply to the fairness-based argument claims that medical progress, while extremely important, is a moral goal. As such, it cannot compete with rights of an individual, including the right to decline to serve as a subject. Moral goals, no matter how important, may be pursued only within the constraints of respecting people's rights. Thus no one has a duty to participate in research.[2]

Discussions of whether or not individuals have a duty to serve as research subjects sometimes reflect what may be called *the protection model* of participation in research. This model emphasizes that research participation typically involves risks to subjects, highlighting the importance of adequate subject protection. The protection model is at least partly inspired by historical examples, such as the Tuskegee syphilis study (which is discussed below), in which subjects were not adequately protected. In recent years, however, what may be called *the access model* of participation in research has emerged into prominence. This model stresses that participation in research can, in the absence of effective therapies for some illnesses, benefit subjects. AIDS activists argued in the 1980s and early 1990s—before there were effective treatments for HIV (human immunodeficiency virus) infection—that participation in clinical trials testing the efficacy of various treatments could benefit HIV-positive individuals. Activists often asserted that these patients have a right to participate in promising studies. Similar access-based claims have also been made on behalf of women, African Americans, children, and other groups who have been in some way underrepresented in research. Whether one views the ethics of research participation mainly in terms of the protection model or in terms of the access model, the requirements of informed consent and proxy consent remain matters of paramount concern.

THE INFORMED-CONSENT REQUIREMENT

Most of the literature on the ethics of human research is concerned with specifying the conditions under which research involving human subjects is ethically acceptable. Since World War II, more than thirty different guidelines and codes of ethics identifying these conditions have been formalized. Foremost among these are two codes included in this chapter, the Nuremberg Code and the Declaration of Helsinki. Common to all these documents is the principle that research may not be conducted on human subjects without their informed consent (or, as some codes allow, the consent—where appropriate—of a proxy). Discussions of this requirement are commonplace in the literature on human research, and some of the major topics connected with informed consent are treated in this chapter.

One major topic is the justification of the informed-consent requirement. Arguments in favor of requiring that human beings not be used as research subjects without their informed consent are similar to those favoring the requirement in the context of the physician-patient relationship. The primary argument, advanced from a deontological perspective, rests on the principle of respect for autonomy or the value of individual self-determination. Respect for human beings as persons requires protection and promotion of their autonomy. Research that uses human subjects without their consent violates that autonomy and is therefore morally unacceptable. One major proponent of this position, Paul Ramsey, holds that informed consent is the "chief canon of loyalty" between the biomedical researcher and the patient-subject. It serves as a deontological check on any attempt to justify the use of human subjects solely on utilitarian grounds, insofar as it affirms that human beings are not objects to be used, without their consent, for others' benefit. In Ramsey's view, only individuals who are (1) capable of knowingly involving themselves in a common cause with the researcher and (2) willing to participate as research subjects may serve in that capacity.[3]

Some of the literature on informed consent in research focuses on special causes for concern where individuals from certain "vulnerable" groups serve as subjects. These causes for concern often involve one or more of the following factors: (1) the fact of vulnerability itself, (2) egregious historical failures on the part of researchers to comply with the informed-consent requirement, and (3) cultural complexities in implementing this requirement.

Some groups of individuals are inherently vulnerable due to their incapacity to make informed decisions regarding their medical care and their dependence on others to protect their interests. Examples include children, incompetent elderly patients, and individuals who suffer from psychiatric or other mental disorders that may affect decision-making capacity. Members of the latter group are vulnerable on account of both the social stigma associated with these disorders and their significant potential for reducing or eliminating decision-making capacity.

Perhaps the most notorious historical example of ethical noncompliance with the informed-consent requirement is that of Nazi researchers who performed many gruesome experiments on nonconsenting adults without any regard for their interests. The Nuremberg Code was written in the wake of these atrocities. Somewhat less well-known are what have come to be called "the radiation experiments." During the Cold War with the Soviet Union, federal agencies in the United States funded and in some cases conducted research projects in which hundreds of Americans were exposed to high doses of radiation. Often the subjects were from such vulnerable groups as newborns, the terminally ill, prisoners, mentally retarded persons, racial minorities, or the indigent. Frequently, subjects had no opportunity to provide consent of any kind, much less informed consent.[4]

Another notorious episode in American research history involved a federally funded, longitudinal study in Tuskegee, Alabama, of the consequences of untreated syphilis in which all of the subjects were black men. Among the shocking facts about this research is that, after penicillin was discovered, subjects were not informed of its availability, although it was known to be effective in treating syphilis. Because the violation of the subjects' right to self-determination was apparently related to racism, this episode also suggests cultural reasons for concern about the implementation of the informed-consent requirement. In fact, some commentators use the Tuskegee experience as a backdrop to a broader cultural concern regarding the use of minority research subjects: an uncomfortable tension between avoiding the perpetuation of negative stereotyping while being prepared to note racially correlated differences that may be medically significant.[5]

Psychiatric research presents in subtler ways both historical and cultural causes for concern. Available evidence suggests that for decades well-intentioned psychiatric researchers have frequently violated the rights of subjects.[6] One recurring problem is the regular absence of procedures that could ensure that supposedly competent patients have, in fact, provided voluntary and informed consent. While such ethical problems in psychiatric research may be viewed as a historical cause for concern, the reasons for concern are also cultural. For one thing, persisting societal prejudice against persons with mental illness probably makes it easier, in practice, for researchers and the public to overlook their rights. Furthermore, the culture of the biomedical research community is so strongly pro-research that it has proved unreliable in protecting subjects' rights against the tide of utilitarian efforts to use them as means to the end of biomedical progress.[7]

PROXY CONSENT FOR RESEARCH SUBJECTS INCAPABLE OF INFORMED CONSENT

Since children, especially young children, cannot give informed consent due to their lack of decision-making capacity, any research that involves them as subjects may seem to violate the informed-consent requirement. The same may be said of adult patients who are incompetent due to mental illness, severe retardation, or dementia. Concerns are alleviated somewhat in the case of research that is reasonably expected to benefit the subject. In this case, as with validated therapies, it is usually agreed that proxies, such as parents or other legal guardians, can legitimately consent on the incompetent individual's behalf. However, when the procedure is not intended to benefit the subject directly but solely to acquire knowledge that will benefit future patients, the participation of the child or incompetent adult is more problematic. Is it ever right for proxies to permit incompetent subjects to participate in nontherapeutic research?

It is widely accepted today that promising research offering no prospect of direct benefits for incompetent subjects may be acceptable if it entails no more than "minimal risk" for the subjects. Proponents of research using children cite its benefits to children as a group; results of studies on adults cannot be simply extrapolated to children because the bodies of children and adults are significantly different. In addition, some diseases, like infantile autism, are unique to children. Not to involve them in research would therefore greatly impoverish pediatric medicine, making children as a class "therapeutic orphans." (This argument assumes that what can be learned from therapeutic research is insufficient to solve this practical problem.) To some extent, similar arguments apply to mentally ill individuals and to elderly patients with Alzheimer's disease or other conditions that compromise mental functioning. Many of these individuals lack decision-making capacity occasionally, intermittently, or even permanently. Some research on their illnesses (e.g., studies of severe psychosis or late-stage Alzheimer's disease) would appear to require the use of incompetent subjects. If only persons who are capable of providing informed consent were used in research, we might never achieve sufficient understanding of some mentally compromising conditions to develop effective treatments for them. For these and other reasons, the use of certain classes of incompetent individuals as research subjects seems necessary for progress in pediatrics and in particular areas of psychiatry, geriatrics, and other subfields of medicine. In view of these potential gains, most commentators accept the validity of proxy consent under some circumstances. Their acceptance of proxy consent follows the lead of the Declaration of Helsinki, the first major code of research ethics to address the participation of incompetent subjects.

EXPERIMENTAL DESIGN AND RESEARCH IN DEVELOPING NATIONS

Questions about informed and proxy consent also arise in discussions of randomized clinical trials (RCTs). Considered the "gold standard" of clinical research, the RCT is a comparison of two or more treatment arms—scientifically controlled with random assignment of subjects—to study the efficacy of new therapies. In one of this chapter's readings, Samuel Hellman and Deborah S. Hellman argue that RCTs present an ethical dilemma admitting of no comfortable solution. Typically, at the beginning of a study or at some point during the study, they maintain, researchers have an opinion about which treatment arm is preferable in terms of the patient-subjects' best interests. But while sharing that opinion seems required out of fidelity to the patient—that is, promotion of his or her best interests—doing so would ruin the study, according to the authors.

Although today it is widely appreciated that RCTs can place researchers in conflicting roles, not all commentators consider the problem intractable. In a reading reprinted in this chapter, Don Marquis attempts to resolve this problem. For purposes of discussion, he focuses on decisions about inviting patients to enroll in a trial, not decisions connected with their best interests during a trial; and he focuses on studies that compare two treatments as opposed to studies that compare one or more treatments and a placebo. Marquis argues that the solution rests in a full appreciation of informed consent. On his proposal, a physician may be fully justified in (1) recommending the treatment he or she considers superior and (2) asking whether the patient would like to enroll in an RCT in which subjects may or may not receive the recommended treatment. Recommending a treatment permits the physician to fulfill the duty of fidelity while providing crucial information to the patient, who can then make an informed decision in response to the offer of enrolling in the study.

A distinct solution is offered by Paul Litton and Franklin Miller in an article reprinted here. Stressing the different aims of clinical medicine and clinical research, Litton and Miller deny an assumption made by the Hellmans and Marquis: that physicians, even when acting as researchers, have the same duty of fidelity to subjects as they do to their patients. Recognizing that this assumption is unjustified, the authors argue, permits the research enterprise to avoid undue restrictions while assuring appropriate respect and protections for research subjects.

In recent years, issues about proper study design have been provoked with special urgency by a series of placebo-controlled studies, conducted in developing countries, to assess the efficacy of a particular regimen involving zidovudine (AZT). Some background information will help to clarify the issues. While AIDS is a major problem in "first-world" or developed countries, it is far more devastating in certain developing countries in which a frighteningly high percentage of the population is infected with HIV. Years ago an American clinical trial showed that the rate of transmission of HIV from pregnant women to fetuses is cut by two thirds through a specific regimen involving AZT. These experimental results sparked an interest in helping women and infants in developing countries. But the regimen that had already been proven effective was extremely expensive. Moreover, it required that women receive counseling and undergo HIV testing early in pregnancy, comply with an extensive oral regimen and with intravenous administration of AZT during labor and delivery, and refrain from breastfeeding. Such requirements struck many officials as virtually impossible to implement in developing countries; researchers, public health experts, and officials from Ivory Coast, Uganda, several other African countries, and Thailand agreed that a briefer course of oral AZT treatment for pregnant women, if it proved effective, would be a more realistic regimen in their nations. Trials were designed to study the efficacy of an oral regimen of AZT administered in the late stages of pregnancy, and all but one of these trials included a placebo arm.

A crucial ethical question emerged and remains with us retrospectively now that these studies have been completed: Considering what was known about the effectiveness of AZT in reducing transmission, was it ethically permissible to commence a trial including a placebo arm in which subjects did not receive AZT? According to one school of thought, such studies treated some subjects unjustly. Because researchers had good reason to believe that even a short course of oral AZT would be more effective than no treatment, willingness to include a placebo arm entailed a willingness to impose a serious disadvantage on subjects in that arm. (Some commentators called for an alternative study design that would have compared the effectiveness of the rigorous regimen validated by the American trial against the effectiveness of a short course of oral AZT; one study did in fact employ such a design.) Proponents of this school of thought have cited the Declaration of Helsinki, which asserts that in biomedical research, "considerations related to the well-being of the human subject should take precedence over the interests of science and society." Prior to a substantial revision of the code in 2000, these critics also cited another statement that no longer appears: "In any medical study, every patient—including those of a control group, if any— should be assured of the best proven diagnostic and therapeutic method."

An opposing school of thought maintains that placebo controls were necessary to ensure that short-course AZT was better than no treatment at all. From this perspective, it is irrelevant that effective preventive treatment for mother-fetus transmission of AZT was available elsewhere in the world, because it was not available in the developing countries in question. In a reading reprinted in this chapter, Baruch Brody defends a standard that he believes appropriate (and preferable to the statement from the Declaration of Helsinki just quoted): "All participants in the study, including those in the control group, should not be denied any treatment *that should otherwise be available to [them] in light of the practical realities of health care resources available in the country in question.*" In Brody's view, the AZT trials in question probably satisfied this standard.

These trials have provoked other ethical concerns in addition to those related to study design and the inclusion of a placebo arm. Another issue concerns the possibility of coercion. Some commentators have argued that subjects were unable to make a genuinely voluntary choice about enrollment. Living in extreme poverty and lacking access even to basic health care, pregnant women who were offered the choice of joining a study that provided some chance of receiving AZT treatment were in no position to decline. In response to this concern, Brody agrees that it was reasonable for the women, in their circumstances, to enroll in the study to gain possible benefit for themselves and their fetuses, but he denies that any coercion was involved. A coercive offer, he maintains, involves a threat to make someone worse off than he or she would have been without the offer—and this was not the case in these studies.

A third concern about the AZT trials in developing countries is that the citizens of these countries were exploited insofar as the short course of AZT, even if it proved effective, would not be available to them following the study. In a reading reprinted in this chapter, Leonard H. Glantz, George J. Annas, Michael A. Grodin, and Wendy K. Mariner argue that in order for such trials to be justified, the risks or burdens imposed on trial participants must be offset by the prospect of actual benefit to the citizens of the developing country. Thus, if the trial yields beneficial knowledge, benefits must actually reach individuals in the country in which the trial took place; otherwise, the subjects will have been exploited. A practical upshot of this approach is that those who plan trials in developing nations must identify, in advance of commencing a trial, the source and amount of funding for providing any benefits of the research to the local populace—a moral requirement that was not satisfied in the case of the African maternal-fetal HIV transmission studies. Although the short-course regimen did prove effective, and some efforts have been made to expand access to it in the countries in question, Glantz et al. are correct that the feasibility of providing access to local citizens was not established in advance. Moreover, access to the beneficial treatment has only been partial.

According to Brody, however, legitimate concerns about exploitation will be met if the subjects themselves—not necessarily the broader local community—are provided access to effective treatment following the study. The subjects, not other citizens in the same countries, bear any risks and burdens associated with participation in the trials. Brody's reasoning is consonant with another statement from the Helsinki code: "At the conclusion of the study, patients entered into the study are entitled to be informed about the outcome of the study and to share any benefits that result from it, for example, access to interventions identified as beneficial in the study or to other appropriate care or benefits." Moreover, as recently amended, the Declaration of Helsinki states that "[t]he protocol should describe arrangements for post-study access by study subjects to interventions identified as beneficial in the study or access to other appropriate care or benefits." This requirement addresses the concern of Glantz et al. regarding the prospective identification of means for providing post-trial access to any benefits identified in the study—or to "other appropriate care or benefits"—but it applies only to study participants rather than to the broader local community.

In another reading reprinted here, the participants in a 2001 Conference on Ethical Aspects of Research in Developing Countries suggest a somewhat different direction for ensuring that study subjects and communities are not exploited in research conducted in developing countries. Contrary to Brody and Glantz et al., the conference participants argue that there are many benefits—not only interventions identified as beneficial during a study—that should be considered in fairly compensating study participants and/or the broader community. The authors distinguish benefits to participants during the research (e.g., health services unrelated to the study), benefits to the population during the research (e.g., public health measures, employment), and benefits to the population after the research (only one example of which is the reasonable availability of an intervention identified as effective). Thus, they argue that a "fair benefits" framework is more defensible than a "reasonable availability" requirement.

ANIMAL RESEARCH

The use of animals in biomedical research intended to benefit humans raises its own set of troubling questions. Some questions concern the moral status of animals while others concern the importance of the research. Regarding the first set of issues, should animals be regarded as having any significant moral status? If so, is their moral status the same as that of humans, so that whatever is morally impermissible in the case of humans is also impermissible in the case of animals? If that is the case, then it would seem that animals, like humans, could be ethically used in very little nontherapeutic research that entails substantial risks or harm to the subjects. If, on the other hand, animals have moral status but less than that possessed by human beings, how is this judgment to be justified? In general, what characteristics must a being possess to be entitled to moral consideration? What is required for full moral status? Note that if one contends that humans have exclusive, or radically superior, moral status on the basis of certain characteristics—such as autonomy, moral agency, or some degree of rationality—one provokes the *problem of nonparadigm humans*. The problem is that any criterion that apparently excludes animals from the domain of moral status (or full moral status) will apparently also exclude certain human beings who lack the characteristic in question.

Regarding the importance of the research, is there a genuine need to use animals in experiments intended to benefit humans? More precisely, if animals' moral status does not preclude their use in nontherapeutic research that poses significant risks to the animal subjects, how valuable must the sought knowledge be to justify a particular experiment? Is the use of animals necessary to obtain that knowledge? Or could alternatives to animal research yield equally useful information?

In its "International Guiding Principles for Biomedical Research Involving Animals," reprinted in this chapter, the Council for International Organizations of Medical Sciences (CIOMS) apparently assumes that the moral status of animals does not preclude their use in research, including nontherapeutic research posing significant risks. At the same time, CIOMS asserts that researchers have a responsibility to minimize animal subjects' pain, distress, and discomfort and must use alternatives to animal research wherever feasible. One might consider CIOMS's position a moderate view on animals' moral status and the ethics of animal research.

Representing a different view, Peter Singer has influentially argued that animals' interests must be given *equal consideration* to comparable human interests—so that, for example, a human's and an animal's interest in avoiding suffering should be considered equally morally important.[8] Failure to meet this standard, Singer contends, is *speciesism*, which is morally analogous to racism and sexism. Applying the principle of equal consideration, Singer condemns the vast bulk of animal experimentation for causing great harm to sentient animals while rarely achieving important research goals. He argues that the use of animals in research is justified only in those rare instances when using a human of comparable mental capacities would also be justified.

Responding to Singer's arguments and to what he calls "the animal rights view," Carl Cohen, in a reading reprinted in this chapter, argues against extending the principle of equal consideration to animals and in favor of speciesism. Because only members of the human community have moral rights, he contends, animals are appropriately used to advance biomedical research. Indeed, according to Cohen, we have an obligation to increase the total amount of animal research to protect human subjects and benefit future human patients. Edwin Converse Hettinger, also in this chapter, responds directly and in detail to each of Cohen's major arguments. He argues, among other things, that Cohen has not responded adequately to the problem of nonparadigm humans, that utilitarianism (which assumes equal consideration for humans and animals) supports relatively little animal research, and that the promise of alternative methods is much greater than Cohen allows. In the chapter's final reading, David DeGrazia sketches what he takes to be four reasonable views regarding animals' moral status and then traces the implications of these views for the ethics of animal research in light of what is known—and what is uncertain—about the associated benefits, costs, and harms. After exploring the issue of possible alternatives to animal research, he concludes with several policy suggestions that are presented as "points of overlapping consensus or palatable compromises where consensus is unavailable."

NOTES

1 See, e.g., National Bioethics Advisory Commission (NBAC), *Research Involving Persons with Mental Disorders That May Affect Decisionmaking Capacity,* Vol. I: *Report and Recommendations of the National Bioethics Advisory Commission* (Rockville, MD: NBAC, 1998), pp. 44–46.

2 For an argument more or less along these lines, see Hans Jonas, "Philosophical Reflections on Experimenting with Human Subjects," in Paul Freund, ed., *Experimentation with Human Subjects* (New York: Braziller, 1970), pp. 1–31.

A less frequently advanced but interesting line of argument in support of the claim that people sometimes have a duty to serve as research subjects runs as follows. Sometimes threats to the community are so grave that some people's interests must be sacrificed or, to put it another way, some people have to make sacrifices. In times of war, according to the argument, conscription into the military is justified if volunteers are not forthcoming in sufficient numbers. In times of famine, when not everyone can eat, those who have more than enough to eat may be required to relinquish some of their food, and some individuals (say, those who are extremely feeble and likely to die anyway) may have to suffer the consequences of not receiving food. In research, the argument continues, there may be times when individuals must be "conscripted" for research—say, to test a promising vaccine during an epidemic. (Note that this argument might be advanced from a utilitarian standpoint or from a deontological perspective.) Whatever its merits, it differs from the two more prominent sorts of argument just presented in that it applies only in rare circumstances (e.g., epidemics) and not generally.

3 Paul Ramsey, *The Patient as Person* (New Haven, CT: Yale University Press, 1970).

4 Advisory Committee on Human Radiation Experiments, *Final Report* (Washington, DC: U.S. Government Printing Office, 1995).

5 See, e.g., Patricia King, "The Dangers of Difference," *Hastings Center Report* 22 (November-December 1992), pp. 35–38.

6 See, e.g., Alexander Morgan Capron, "Ethical and Human-Rights Issues in Research on Mental Disorders That May Affect Decision–Making Capacity," *New England Journal of Medicine* 340 (May 6, 1999), pp. 1430–1434.

7 *Ibid.*

8 Peter Singer, *Animal Liberation* (New York: Avon Publishers, 1975; 2nd edition 1990).

THE NUREMBERG CODE

The Nuremberg Code of Ethics in Medical Research was developed by the Allies after the Second World War. During the war crimes trials in Germany, this code provided the standards against which the practices of Nazis involved in human experimentation were judged. The Nuremberg Code emphasizes the centrality of voluntary consent. Its first and longest article discusses consent in great detail. The code also sets forth other criteria that must be met before any experiment using human beings as subjects can be judged morally acceptable.

(1) The voluntary consent of the human subject is absolutely essential. This means that the person involved should have legal capacity to give consent; should be so situated as to be able to exercise free power of choice, without the intervention of any element of force, fraud, deceit, duress, overreaching, or other ulterior form of constraint or coercion; and should have sufficient knowledge and comprehension of the elements of the subject matter involved as to enable him to make an understanding and enlightened decision. This latter element requires that before the acceptance of an affirmative decision by the experimental subject there should be made known to him the nature, duration, and purpose of the experiment; the method and means by which it is to be conducted; all inconveniences and hazards reasonably to be expected; and the effects upon his health or person which may possibly come from his participation in the experiments.

The duty and responsibility for ascertaining the quality of the consent rests upon each individual who initiates, directs or engages in the experiment. It is a personal duty and responsibility which may not be delegated to another with impunity.

(2) The experiment should be such as to yield fruitful results for the good of society, unprocurable by other methods or means of study, and not random and unnecessary in nature.

(3) The experiment should be so designed and based on the results of animal experimentation

Reprinted from *Trials of War Criminals Before the Nuremberg Military Tribunals* (Washington, DC: U.S. Government Printing Office, 1948).

and a knowledge of the natural history of the disease or other problem under study that the anticipated results [will] justify the performance of the experiment.

(4) The experiment should be so conducted as to avoid all unnecessary physical and mental suffering and injury.

(5) No experiment should be conducted where there is an a priori reason to believe that death or disabling injury will occur; except, perhaps, in those experiments where the experimental physicians also serve as subjects.

(6) The degree of risk to be taken should never exceed that determined by the humanitarian importance of the problem to be solved by the experiment.

(7) Proper preparations should be made and adequate facilities provided to protect the experimental subject against even remote possibilities of injury, disability, or death.

(8) The experiment should be conducted only by scientifically qualified persons. The highest degree of skill and care should be required through all stages of the experiment of those who conduct or engage in the experiment.

(9) During the course of the experiment the human subject should be at liberty to bring the experiment to an end if he has reached the physical or mental state where continuation of the experiment seems to him to be impossible.

(10) During the course of the experiment the scientist in charge must be prepared to terminate the experiment at any stage, if he has probable cause to believe, in the exercise of good faith,

superior skill and careful judgment required of him that a continuation of the experiment is likely to result in injury, disability, or death to the experimental subject.

DECLARATION OF HELSINKI
World Medical Association

In 1964 the Eighteenth World Medical Assembly, meeting in Helsinki, Finland, adopted an ethical code to guide physicians and other investigators who conduct medical research involving human subjects. This code has been amended eight times; the version reprinted here is the most recent (2008) version. The Declaration of Helsinki has much in common with the Nuremberg Code, most fundamentally the requirement of informed consent. Two differences, however, are especially noteworthy. First, the Declaration of Helsinki notes that some, but not all, medical research is combined with medical care. Accordingly, it articulates, in addition to basic principles for all medical research, a set of principles for medical research combined with medical care (also known as *clinical research* or *therapeutic research*). Second, while the Nuremberg Code does not address research on subjects who are unable to provide informed consent, the Helsinki code addresses such research, asserting the ethical acceptability under certain conditions of what is usually called "proxy consent." Recent amendments include clarifications regarding (1) the circumstances in which use of placebo controls is justified, and (2) subjects' post-trial access to procedures identified as beneficial during the course of the trial or to alternative medical care.

A. INTRODUCTION

1. The World Medical Association (WMA) has developed the Declaration of Helsinki as a statement of ethical principles for medical research involving human subjects, including research on identifiable human material and data.

   The Declaration is intended to be read as a whole and each of its constituent paragraphs should not be applied without consideration of all other relevant paragraphs.

2. Although the Declaration is addressed primarily to physicians, the WMA encourages other participants in medical research involving human subjects to adopt these principles.

3. It is the duty of the physician to promote and safeguard the health of patients, including those who are involved in medical research. The physician's knowledge and conscience are dedicated to the fulfilment of this duty.

4. The Declaration of Geneva of the WMA binds the physician with the words, "The health of my patient will be my first consideration," and the International Code of Medical Ethics declares that, "A physician shall act in the patient's best interest when providing medical care."

5. Medical progress is based on research that ultimately must include studies involving human subjects. Populations that are underrepresented in medical research should be provided appropriate access to participation in research.

6. In medical research involving human subjects, the well-being of the individual research subject must take precedence over all other interests.

7. The primary purpose of medical research involving human subjects is to understand the causes, development and effects of diseases and improve preventive, diagnostic and therapeutic interventions (methods, procedures and treatments). Even the best current interventions must be evaluated continually through research for their safety, effectiveness, efficiency, accessibility and quality.

8. In medical practice and in medical research, most interventions involve risks and burdens.

9. Medical research is subject to ethical standards that promote respect for all human subjects and protect their health and rights. Some research populations are particularly vulnerable and need special protection. These include those who cannot give or refuse consent for themselves and those who may be vulnerable to coercion or undue influence.

10. Physicians should consider the ethical, legal and regulatory norms and standards for research involving human subjects in their own countries as well as applicable international norms and standards. No national or international ethical, legal or regulatory requirement should reduce or eliminate any of the protections for research subjects set forth in this Declaration.

B. PRINCIPLES FOR ALL MEDICAL RESEARCH

11. It is duty of physicians who participate in medical research to protect the life, health, dignity, integrity, right to self-determination, privacy, and confidentiality of personal information of research subjects.

12. Medical research involving human subjects must conform to generally accepted scientific principles, be based on a thorough knowledge of the scientific literature, other relevant sources of information, and adequate laboratory and, as appropriate, animal experimentation. The welfare of animals used for research must be respected.

13. Appropriate caution must be exercised in the conduct of medical research that may harm the environment.

14. The design and performance of each research study involving human subjects must be clearly described in a research protocol. The protocol should contain a statement of the ethical considerations involved and should indicate how the principles in this Declaration have been addressed. The protocol should include information regarding funding, sponsors, institutional affiliations, other potential conflicts of interest, incentives for subjects and provisions for treating and/or compensating subjects who are harmed as a consequence of participation in the research study. The protocol should describe arrangements for post-study access by study subjects to interventions identified as beneficial in the study or access to other appropriate care or benefits.

15. The research protocol must be submitted for consideration, comment, guidance and approval to a research ethics committee before the study begins. This committee must be independent of the researcher, the sponsor and any other undue influence. It must take into consideration the laws and regulations of the country or countries in which the research is to be performed as well as applicable international norms and standards but these must not be allowed to reduce or eliminate any of the protections for research subjects set forth in this Declaration. The committee must have the right to monitor ongoing studies. The researcher must provide monitoring information to the committee, especially information about any serious adverse events. No change to the protocol may be made without consideration and approval by the committee.

16. Medical research involving human subjects must be conducted only by individuals with the appropriate scientific training and qualifications. Research on patients or healthy volunteers requires the supervision of a competent and appropriately qualified physician or other health care professional. The responsibility for the protection of research subjects must always rest with the physician or other health care professional and never the research subjects, even though they have given consent.

17. Medical research involving a disadvantaged or vulnerable population or community is only justified if the research is responsive to the health needs and priorities of this population or community and if there is a reasonable likelihood that this population or community stands to benefit from the results of the research.

18. Every medical research study involving human subjects must be preceded by careful assessment of predictable risks and burdens to the individuals and communities involved in the research in comparison with foreseeable benefits to them and to other individuals or communities affected by the condition under investigation.

19. Every clinical trial must be registered in a publicly accessible database before recruitment of the first subject.

20. Physicians may not participate in a research study involving human subjects unless they are confident that the risks involved have been adequately assessed and can be satisfactorily managed. Physicians must immediately stop a study when the risks are found to outweigh the potential benefits or when there is conclusive proof of positive and beneficial results.

21. Medical research involving human subjects may only be conducted if the importance of the objective outweighs the inherent risks and burdens to the research subjects.

22. Participation by competent individuals as subjects in medical research must be voluntary. Although it may be appropriate to consult family members or community leaders, no competent individual may be enrolled in a research study unless he or she freely agrees.

23. Every precaution must be taken to protect the privacy of research subjects and the confidentiality of their personal information and to minimize the impact of the study on their physical, mental and social integrity.

24. In medical research involving competent human subjects, each potential subject must be adequately informed of the aims, methods, sources of funding, any possible conflicts of interest, institutional affiliations of the researcher, the anticipated benefits and potential risks of the study and the discomfort it may entail, and any other relevant aspects of the study. The potential subject must be informed of the right to refuse to participate in the study or to withdraw consent to participate at any time without reprisal. Special attention should be given to the specific information needs of individual potential subjects as well as to the methods used to deliver the information. After ensuring that the potential subject has understood the information, the physician or another appropriately qualified individual must then seek the potential subject's freely-given informed consent, preferably in writing. If the consent cannot be expressed in writing, the non-written consent must be formally documented and witnessed.

25. For medical research using identifiable human material or data, physicians must normally seek consent for the collection, analysis, storage and/or reuse. There may be situations where consent would be impossible or impractical to obtain for such research or would pose a threat to the validity of the research. In such situations the research may be done only after consideration and approval of a research ethics committee.

26. When seeking informed consent for participation in a research study the physician

should be particularly cautious if the potential subject is in a dependent relationship with the physician or may consent under duress. In such situations the informed consent should be sought by an appropriately qualified individual who is completely independent of this relationship.

27. For a potential research subject who is incompetent, the physician must seek informed consent from the legally authorized representative. These individuals must not be included in a research study that has no likelihood of benefit for them unless it is intended to promote the health of the population represented by the potential subject, the research cannot instead be performed with competent persons, and the research entails only minimal risk and minimal burden.

28. When a potential research subject who is deemed incompetent is able to give assent to decisions about participation in research, the physician must seek that assent in addition to the consent of the legally authorized representative. The potential subject's dissent should be respected.

29. Research involving subjects who are physically or mentally incapable of giving consent, for example, unconscious patients, may be done only if the physical or mental condition that prevents giving informed consent is a necessary characteristic of the research population. In such circumstances the physician should seek informed consent from the legally authorized representative. If no such representative is available and if the research cannot be delayed, the study may proceed without informed consent provided that the specific reasons for involving subjects with a condition that renders them unable to give informed consent have been stated in the research protocol and the study has been approved by a research ethics committee. Consent to remain in the research should be obtained as soon as possible from the subject or a legally authorized representative.

30. Authors, editors and publishers all have ethical obligations with regard to the publication of the results of research. Authors have a duty to make publicly available the results of their research on human subjects and are accountable for the completeness and accuracy of their reports. They should adhere to accepted guidelines for ethical reporting. Negative and inconclusive as well as positive results should be published or otherwise made publicly available. Sources of funding, institutional affiliations and conflicts of interest should be declared in the publication. Reports of research not in accordance with the principles of this Declaration should not be accepted for publication.

C. ADDITIONAL PRINCIPLES FOR MEDICAL RESEARCH COMBINED WITH MEDICAL CARE

31. The physician may combine medical research with medical care only to the extent that the research is justified by its potential preventive, diagnostic or therapeutic value and if the physician has good reason to believe that participation in the research study will not adversely affect the health of the patients who serve as research subjects.

32. The benefits, risks, burdens and effectiveness of a new intervention must be tested against those of the best current proven intervention, except in the following circumstances:

- The use of placebo, or no treatment, is acceptable in studies where no current proven intervention exists; or

- Where for compelling and scientifically sound methodological reasons the use of placebo is necessary to determine the efficacy or safety of an intervention and the patients who receive placebo or no treatment will not be subject to any risk of serious or irreversible harm. Extreme care must be taken to avoid abuse of this option.

33. At the conclusion of the study, patients entered into the study are entitled to be informed about the outcome of the study and to share any benefits that result from it, for example, access to interventions identified as beneficial in the study or to other appropriate care or benefits.

34. The physician must fully inform the patient which aspects of the care are related to the research. The refusal of a patient to participate in a study or the patient's decision to withdraw from the study must never interfere with the patient-physician relationship.

35. In the treatment of a patient, where proven interventions do not exist or have been ineffective, the physician, after seeking expert advice, with informed consent from the patient or a legally authorized representative, may use an unproven intervention if in the physician's judgment it offers hope of saving life, re-establishing health or alleviating suffering. Where possible, this intervention should be made the object of research, designed to evaluate its safety and efficacy. In all cases, new information should be recorded and, where appropriate, made publicly available.

INTERNATIONAL GUIDING PRINCIPLES FOR BIOMEDICAL RESEARCH INVOLVING ANIMALS

Council for International Organizations of Medical Sciences

The Council for International Organizations of Medical Sciences (CIOMS) is an international organization that was established by the World Health Organization and Unesco in 1949. In this 1985 statement, CIOMS assumes both (1) that the use of animals in biomedical research is morally appropriate and (2) that such use of animals entails responsibility for their welfare. Reflecting these assumptions, CIOMS presents 11 principles that are intended to provide a framework for more specific policies in individual nations. These principles include an endorsement of the use of alternatives to animal research whenever feasible and the injunction to regard the minimization of animal subjects' pain, distress, and discomfort "as ethical imperatives."

BASIC PRINCIPLES

I. The advancement of biological knowledge and the development of improved means for the protection of the health and well-being both of [humans] and of animals require recourse to experimentation on intact live animals of a wide variety of species.

II. Methods such as mathematical models, computer simulation and in vitro biological systems should be used wherever appropriate.

III. Animal experiments should be undertaken only after due consideration of their relevance for human or animal health and the advancement of biological knowledge.

IV. The animals selected for an experiment should be of an appropriate species and quality, and the minimum number required to obtain scientifically valid results.

V. Investigators and other personnel should never fail to treat animals as sentient, and should regard their proper care and use and the avoidance or minimization of discomfort, distress, or pain as ethical imperatives.

VI. Investigators should assume that procedures that would cause pain in human beings cause pain in other vertebrate species, although more needs to be known about the perception of pain in animals.

VII. Procedures with animals that may cause more than momentary or minimal pain or distress should be performed with appropriate sedation, analgesia, or anesthesia in accordance with accepted veterinary practice. Surgical or other painful procedures should not be performed on unanesthetized animals paralysed by chemical agents.

VIII. Where waivers are required in relation to the provisions of article VII, the decisions should not rest solely with the investigators directly concerned but should be made, with due regard to the provisions of articles IV, V, and VI, by a suitably constituted review body. Such waivers should not be made solely for the purposes of teaching or demonstration.

IX. At the end of, or, when appropriate, during an experiment, animals that would otherwise suffer severe or chronic pain, distress, discomfort, or disablement that cannot be relieved should be painlessly killed.

X. The best possible living conditions should be maintained for animals kept for biomedical purposes. Normally the care of animals should be under the supervision of veterinarians having experience in laboratory animal science. In any case, veterinary care should be available as required.

XI. It is the responsibility of the director of an institute or department using animals to ensure that investigators and personnel have appropriate qualifications or experience for conducting procedures on animals. Adequate opportunities shall be provided for in-service training, including the proper and humane concern for the animals under their care. . . .

EXPERIMENTAL DESIGN AND RANDOMIZED CLINICAL TRIALS

OF MICE BUT NOT MEN: PROBLEMS OF THE RANDOMIZED CLINICAL TRIAL

Samuel Hellman and Deborah S. Hellman

Hellman and Hellman argue that an ethical dilemma confronts the use of randomized clinical trials, that is, controlled comparisons of two or more treatment arms (one of which may involve a placebo) in which subjects are randomly assigned to the different groups. According to the authors, such studies require researchers to enter into two largely incompatible roles. (1) As *physicians,* they are ethically required to act in their patients' best interests. (2) As *scientists,* they are expected to address rigorously the question of whether a particular therapy is effective, or how effective it is compared with others, in the hope of offering a genuine benefit to future patients. At some point in a study, the authors contend, researchers usually have an opinion about which treatment arm is more advantageous—but disclosing that judgment would ruin the study, while nondisclosure would mean failing to act in their patients' best interests. Hellman and Hellman conclude by suggesting that several research techniques might be sufficiently rigorous to offer viable alternatives to randomized clinical trials.

As medicine has become increasingly scientific and less accepting of unsupported opinion or proof by anecdote, the randomized controlled clinical trial has become the standard technique for changing diagnostic or therapeutic methods. The use of this technique creates an ethical dilemma.[1,2] Researchers participating in such studies are required to modify their ethical commitments to individual patients and do serious damage to the concept of the physician as a practicing, empathetic professional who is primarily concerned with each patient as an individual. Researchers using a randomized clinical trial can be described as physician-scientists, a term that expresses the tension between the two roles. The physician, by entering into a relationship with an individual patient, assumes certain obligations, including the commitment always to act in the patient's best interests. As Leon Kass has rightly maintained, "the physician must produce unswervingly the virtues of loyalty and fidelity to his patient."[3] Though the ethical requirements of this relationship have been modified by legal obligations to report wounds of a suspicious nature and certain infectious diseases, these obligations in no way conflict with the central ethical obligation to act in the best interests of the patient medically. Instead, certain nonmedical interests of the patient are preempted by other social concerns.

The role of the scientist is quite different. The clinical scientist is concerned with answering questions—i.e., determining the validity of formally constructed hypotheses. Such scientific information, it is presumed, will benefit humanity in general. The clinical scientist's role has been well described by Dr. Anthony Fauci, director of the National Institute of Allergy and Infectious Diseases, who states the goals of the randomized clinical trial in these words: "It's not to deliver therapy. It's to answer a scientific question so that the drug can be available for everybody once you've established safety and efficacy."[4] The demands of such a study can conflict in a number of ways with the physician's duty to minister to patients. The study may create a false dichotomy in

the physician's opinions: according to the premise of the randomized clinical trial, the physician may only know or not know whether a proposed course of treatment represents an improvement; no middle position is permitted. What the physician thinks, suspects, believes, or has a hunch about is assigned to the "not knowing" category, because knowing is defined on the basis of an arbitrary but accepted statistical test performed in a randomized clinical trial. Thus, little credence is given to information gained beforehand in other ways or to information accrued during the trial but without the required statistical degree of assurance that a difference is not due to chance. The randomized clinical trial also prevents the treatment technique from being modified on the basis of the growing knowledge of the physicians during their participation in the trial. Moreover, it limits access to the data as they are collected until specific milestones are achieved. This prevents physicians from profiting not only from their individual experience, but also from the collective experience of the other participants.

The randomized clinical trial requires doctors to act simultaneously as physicians and as scientists. This puts them in a difficult and sometimes untenable ethical position. The conflicting moral demands arising from the use of the randomized clinical trial reflect the classic conflict between rights-based moral theories and utilitarian ones. The first of these, which depend on the moral theory of Immanuel Kant (and seen more recently in neo-Kantian philosophers, such as John Rawls[5]), asserts that human beings, by virtue of their unique capacity for rational thought, are bearers of dignity. As such, they ought not to be treated merely as means to an end; rather, they must always be treated as ends in themselves. Utilitarianism, by contrast, defines what is right as the greatest good for the greatest number—that is, as social utility. This view, articulated by Jeremy Bentham and John Stuart Mill, requires that pleasures (understood broadly, to include such pleasures as health and well-being) and pains be added together. The morally correct act is the act that produces the most pleasure and the least pain overall.

A classic objection to the utilitarian position is that according to that theory, the distribution of pleasures and pains is of no moral consequence. This element of the theory severely restricts physicians from being utilitarians, or at least from following the theory's dictates. Physicians must care very deeply about the distribution of pain and pleasure, for they have entered into a relationship with one or a number of individual patients. They cannot be indifferent to whether it is these patients or others that suffer for the general benefit of society. Even though society might gain from the suffering of a few, and even though the doctor might believe that such a benefit is worth a given patient's suffering (i.e., that utilitarianism is right in the particular case), the ethical obligation created by the covenant between doctor and patient requires the doctor to see the interests of the individual patient as primary and compelling. In essence, the doctor-patient relationship requires doctors to see their patients as bearers of rights who cannot be merely used for the greater good of humanity.

As Fauci has suggested,[4] the randomized clinical trial routinely asks physicians to sacrifice the interests of their particular patients for the sake of the study and that of the information that it will make available for the benefit of society. This practice is ethically problematic. Consider first the initial formulation of a trial. In particular, consider the case of a disease for which there is no satisfactory therapy—for example, advanced cancer or the acquired immunodeficiency syndrome (AIDS). A new agent that promises more effectiveness is the subject of the study. The control group must be given either an unsatisfactory treatment or a placebo. Even though the therapeutic value of the new agent is unproved, if physicians think that it has promise, are they acting in the best interests of their patients in allowing them to be randomly assigned to the control group? Is persisting in such an assignment consistent with the specific commitments taken on in the doctor-patient relationship? As a result of interactions with patients with AIDS and their advocates, Merigan[6] recently suggested modifications in the design of clinical trials that attempt to deal with the unsatisfactory treatment given to the control group. The view of such activists has been expressed by Rebecca Pringle Smith of Community Research Initiative in New York: "Even if you have a supply of compliant martyrs, trials must have some ethical validity."[4]

If the physician has no opinion about whether the new treatment is acceptable, then random assignment is ethically acceptable, but such lack of enthusiasm for the new treatment does not augur well for either the patient or the study. Alternatively, the treatment may show promise of beneficial results but also present a risk of undesirable complications. When the physician believes that the severity and likelihood of harm and good are evenly balanced, randomization may be ethically acceptable. If the physician has no preference for either treatment (is in a state of equipoise[7,8]), then randomization is acceptable. If, however, he or she believes that the new treatment may be either more or less successful or more or less toxic, the use of randomization is not consistent with fidelity to the patient.

The argument usually used to justify randomization is that it provides, in essence, a critique of the usefulness of the physician's beliefs and opinions, those that have not yet been validated by a randomized clinical trial. As the argument goes, these not-yet-validated beliefs are as likely to be wrong as right. Although physicians are ethically required to provide their patients with the best available treatment, there simply is no best treatment yet known.

The reply to this argument takes two forms. First, and most important, even if this view of the reliability of a physician's opinion is accurate, the ethical constraints of an individual doctor's relationship with a particular patient require the doctor to provide individual care. Although physicians must take pains to make clear the speculative nature of their views, they cannot withhold these views from the patient. The patient asks from the doctor both knowledge and judgment. The relationship established between them rightfully allows patients to ask for the judgment of their particular physicians, not merely that of the medical profession in general. Second, it may not be true, in fact, that the not-yet-validated beliefs of physicians are as likely to be wrong as right. The greater certainty obtained with a randomized clinical trial is beneficial, but that does not mean that a lesser degree of certainty is without value. Physicians can acquire knowledge through methods other than the randomized clinical trial. Such knowledge, acquired over time and less formally than is required in a randomized clinical trial, may be of great value to a patient.

Even if it is ethically acceptable to begin a study, one often forms an opinion during its course—especially in studies that are impossible to conduct in a truly double-blinded fashion—that makes it ethically problematic to continue. The inability to remain blinded usually occurs in studies of cancer or AIDS, for example, because the therapy is associated by nature with serious side effects. Trials attempt to restrict the physician's access to the data in order to prevent such unblinding. Such restrictions should make physicians eschew the trial, since their ability to act in the patient's best interests will be limited. Even supporters of randomized clinical trials, such as Merigan, agree that interim findings should be presented to patients to ensure that no one receives what seems an inferior treatment.[6] Once physicians have formed a view about the new treatment, can they continue randomization? If random assignment is stopped, the study may be lost and the participation of the previous patients wasted. However, if physicians continue the randomization when they have a definite opinion about the efficacy of the experimental drug, they are not acting in accordance with the requirements of the doctor-patient relationship. Furthermore, as their opinion becomes more firm, stopping the randomization may not be enough. Physicians may be ethically required to treat the patients formerly placed in the control group with the therapy that now seems probably effective. To do so would be faithful to the obligations created by the doctor-patient relationship, but it would destroy the study.

To resolve this dilemma, one might suggest that the patient has abrogated the rights implicit in a doctor-patient relationship by signing an informed-consent form. We argue that such rights cannot be waived or abrogated. They are inalienable. The right to be treated as an individual deserving the physician's best judgment and care, rather than to be used as a means to determine the best treatment for others, is inherent in every person. This right, based on the concept of dignity, cannot be waived. What of altruism, then? Is it not the patient's right to make a sacrifice for the general good? This question must be considered from both positions—that of the patient and that of the physician. Although patients may decide to waive this right, it is not consistent with the

role of a physician to ask that they do so. In asking, the doctor acts as a scientist instead. The physician's role here is to propose what he or she believes is best medically for the specific patient, not to suggest participation in a study from which the patient cannot gain. Because the opportunity to help future patients is of potential value to a patient, some would say physicians should not deny it. Although this point has merit, it offers so many opportunities for abuse that we are extremely uncomfortable about accepting it. The responsibilities of physicians are much clearer; they are to minister to the current patient.

Moreover, even if patients could waive this right, it is questionable whether those with terminal illness would be truly able to give voluntary informed consent. Such patients are extremely dependent on both their physicians and the health care system. Aware of this dependence, physicians must not ask for consent, for in such cases the very asking breaches the doctor-patient relationship. Anxious to please their physicians, patients may have difficulty refusing to participate in the trial the physicians describe. The patients may perceive their refusal as damaging to the relationship, whether or not it is so. Such perceptions of coercion affect the decision. Informed-consent forms are difficult to understand, especially for patients under the stress of serious illness for which there is no satisfactory treatment. The forms are usually lengthy, somewhat legalistic, complicated, and confusing, and they hardly bespeak the compassion expected of the medical profession. It is important to remember that those who have studied the doctor-patient relationship have emphasized its empathetic nature.

> [The] relationship between doctor and patient partakes of a peculiar intimacy. It presupposes on the part of the physician not only knowledge of his fellow men but sympathy. . . . This aspect of the practice of medicine has been designated as the art; yet I wonder whether it should not, most properly, be called the essence.[9]

How is such a view of the relationship consonant with random assignment and informed consent? The Physician's Oath of the World Medical Association affirms the primacy of the deontologic view of patients' rights: "Concern for the interests of the subject must always prevail over the interests of science and society."[10]

Furthermore, a single study is often not considered sufficient. Before a new form of therapy is generally accepted, confirmatory trials must be conducted. How can one conduct such trials ethically unless one is convinced that the first trial was in error? The ethical problems we have discussed are only exacerbated when a completed randomized clinical trial indicates that a given treatment is preferable. Even if the physician believes the initial trial was in error, the physician must indicate to the patient the full results of that trial.

The most common reply to the ethical arguments has been that the alternative is to return to the physician's intuition, to anecdotes, or to both as the basis of medical opinion. We all accept the dangers of such a practice. The argument states that we must therefore accept randomized, controlled clinical trials regardless of their ethical problems because of the great social benefit they make possible, and we salve our conscience with the knowledge that informed consent has been given. This returns us to the conflict between patients' rights and social utility. Some would argue that this tension can be resolved by placing a relative value on each. If the patient's right that is being compromised is not a fundamental right and the social gain is very great, then the study might be justified. When the right is fundamental, however, no amount of social gain, or almost none, will justify its sacrifice. Consider, for example, the experiments on humans done by physicians under the Nazi regime. All would agree that these are unacceptable regardless of the value of the scientific information gained. Some people go so far as to say that no use should be made of the results of those experiments because of the clearly unethical manner in which the data were collected. This extreme example may not seem relevant, but we believe that in its hyperbole it clarifies the fallacy of a utilitarian approach to the physician's relationship with the patient. To consider the utilitarian gain is consistent neither with the physician's role nor with the patient's rights.

It is fallacious to suggest that only the randomized clinical trial can provide valid information or that all information acquired by this technique is valid. Such experimental methods are intended to reduce error and bias and therefore reduce the uncertainty of the result. Uncertainty cannot be eliminated, however. The scientific method is based on increasing probabilities and increasingly refined approximations of truth.[11] Although the randomized clinical trial contributes to these ends, it is neither unique nor perfect. Other techniques may also be useful.[12]

Randomized trials often place physicians in the ethically intolerable position of choosing between the good of the patient and that of society. We urge that such situations be avoided and that other techniques of acquiring clinical information be adopted. For example, concerning trials of treatments for AIDS, Byar et al.[13] have said that "some traditional approaches to the clinical-trials process may be unnecessarily rigid and unsuitable for this disease." In this case, AIDS is not what is so different; rather, the difference is in the presence of AIDS activists, articulate spokespersons for the ethical problems created by the application of the randomized clinical trial to terminal illnesses. Such arguments are equally applicable to advanced cancer and other serious illnesses. Byar et al. agree that there are even circumstances in which uncontrolled clinical trials may be justified: when there is no effective treatment to use as a control, when the prognosis is uniformly poor, and when there is a reasonable expectation of benefit without excessive toxicity. These conditions are usually found in clinical trials of advanced cancer.

The purpose of the randomized clinical trial is to avoid the problems of observer bias and patient selection. It seems to us that techniques might be developed to deal with these issues in other ways. Randomized clinical trials deal with them in a cumbersome and heavy-handed manner, by requiring large numbers of patients in the hope that random assignment will balance the heterogeneous distribution of patients into the different groups. By observing known characteristics of patients, such as age and sex, and distributing them equally between groups, it is thought that unknown factors important in determining outcomes will also be distributed equally. Surely, other techniques can be developed to deal with both observer bias and patient selection.

Propective studies without randomization, but with the evaluation of patients by uninvolved third parties, should remove observer bias. Similar methods have been suggested by Royall.[12] Prospective matched-pair analysis, in which patients are treated in a manner consistent with their physician's views, ought to help ensure equivalence between the groups and thus mitigate the effect of patient selection, at least with regard to known covariates. With regard to unknown covariates, the security would rest, as in randomized trials, in the enrollment of large numbers of patients and in confirmatory studies. This method would not pose ethical difficulties, since patients would receive the treatment recommended by their physician. They would be included in the study by independent observers matching patients with respect to known characteristics, a process that would not affect patient care and that could be performed independently any number of times.

This brief discussion of alternatives to randomized clinical trials is sketchy and incomplete. We wish only to point out that there may be satisfactory alternatives, not to describe and evaluate them completely. Even if randomized clinical trials were much better than any alternative, however, the ethical dilemmas they present may put their use at variance with the primary obligations of the physician. In this regard, Angell cautions, "If this commitment to the patient is attenuated, even for so good a cause as benefits to future patients, the implicit assumptions of the doctor-patient relationship are violated."[14] The risk of such attenuation by the randomized trial is great. The AIDS activists have brought this dramatically to the attention of the academic medical community. Techniques appropriate to the laboratory may not be applicable to humans. We must develop and use alternative methods for acquiring clinical knowledge.

REFERENCES

1 Hellman S. Randomized clinical trials and the doctor-patient relationship: an ethical dilemma. Cancer Clin Trials 1979; 2:189–93.

2 *Idem.* A doctor's dilemma: the doctor-patient relationship in clinical investigation. In: Proceedings of the Fourth National Conference on Human Values and Cancer, New York, March 15–17, 1984. New York: American Cancer Society, 1984:144–6.

3 Kass L. R. Toward a more natural science: biology and human affairs. New York: Free Press, 1985:196.

4 Palca J. AIDS drug trials enter new age. Science 1989; 246:19–21.

5 Rawls J. A theory of justice. Cambridge, Mass.: Belknap Press of Harvard University Press, 1971:183–92, 446–52.

6 Merigan T. C. You *can* teach an old dog new tricks—how AIDS trials are pioneering new strategies. N Engl J Med 1990; 323:1341–3.

7 Freedman B. Equipoise and the ethics of clinical research. N Engl J Med 1987; 317:141–5.

8 Singer P. A, Lantos J. D, Whitington P. F., Broelsch C. E, Siegler M. Equipoise and the ethics of segmental liver transplantation. Clin Res 1988; 36:539–45.

9 Longcope W. T. Methods and medicine. Bull Johns Hopkins Hosp 1932; 50:4–20.

10 Report on medical ethics. World Med Assoc Bull 1949; 1:109, 111.

11 Popper K. The problem of induction. In: Miller D, ed. Popper selections. Princeton, N.J.: Princeton University Press, 1985:101–17.

12 Royall R. M. Ethics and statistics in randomized clinical trials. Stat Sci 1991; 6(1):52–62.

13 Byar D. P, Schoenfeld D. A, Green S. B, et al. Design considerations for AIDS trials. N Engl J Med 1990; 323:1343–8.

14 Angell M. Patients' preferences in randomized clinical trials. N Engl J Med 1984; 310:1385–7.

HOW TO RESOLVE AN ETHICAL DILEMMA CONCERNING RANDOMIZED CLINICAL TRIALS

Don Marquis

Marquis addresses an apparent dilemma that arises when a physician considers enrolling patients in a randomized clinical trial and when the physician has an opinion about which treatment arm is preferable. (For the purpose of discussion, he focuses on trials that compare two treatments as opposed to one or more treatments and a placebo). On the one hand, the physician has a duty to promote the patient's best interests and so seemingly may not recommend enrollment in a study in which the patient might not receive the treatment the physician considers preferable. On the other hand, recognition of this duty and its apparent implication creates an obstacle to achieving sufficient enrollment for the study to generate significant results. After arguing against two popular strategies for resolving this problem, Marquis contends that "[t]aking informed consent seriously resolves the dilemma." On his proposal, a physician can both (1) recommend the treatment that he or she considers superior and (2) ask whether the patient would like to enroll in a randomized clinical trial in which he or she may or may not receive that treatment.

An apparent ethical dilemma arises when physicians consider enrolling their patients in randomized clinical trials. Suppose that a randomized clinical trial comparing two treatments is in progress, and a physician has an opinion about which treatment is better. The physician has a duty to promote the patient's best medical interests and therefore seems to be obliged to advise the patient to receive the treatment that the physician prefers. This duty creates a barrier to the enrollment of patients in randomized clinical trials.[1–10] Two strategies are often used to resolve the dilemma in favor of enrolling patients in clinical trials.

THE "EITHER YOU KNOW WHICH IS BETTER OR YOU DON'T" STRATEGY

According to one strategy, physicians should not recommend one treatment over another if they do not really know which one is better, and they do not really know which treatment is better in the absence of data from randomized clinical trials.[11] Data from uncontrolled studies are often influenced by the desire on both the investigator's part and the patient's part to obtain positive results.[12] Journal editors are more likely to publish reports of studies with positive results than reports of studies with negative results.[13] A treatment recommendation based on weaker evidence than that obtained from a randomized clinical trial is like a recommendation based on a mere hunch or an idiosyncratic preference.[14] Thus, according to this argument, in the absence of data from a randomized clinical trial, evidence that

provides an adequate basis for recommending a treatment rarely exists, and the enrollment dilemma is based on a mistake.

This strategy for resolving the dilemma is simplistic. It assumes that evidence available to physicians can be only one of two kinds: gold standard evidence or worthless prejudice. But clinical judgments may be based on evidence of intermediate quality, including physicians' experience with their own patients, their conversations with colleagues concerning their colleagues' experience, their evaluation of the results of nonrandomized studies reported in the literature, their judgment about the mechanism of action of one or both treatments, or their view of the natural history of a given disease. Evidence need not be conclusive to be valuable; it need not be definitive to be suggestive. Because all good physicians allow evidence of intermediate quality to influence their professional judgment when a relevant randomized clinical trial is not being conducted, it is unreasonable to claim that such evidence has no worth when a relevant randomized clinical trial is being conducted. Therefore, the "either you know which is better or you don't" strategy for dealing with the enrollment dilemma is not persuasive.

ADOPTING A LESS STRICT THERAPEUTIC OBLIGATION

The dilemma about enrolling patients in randomized clinical trials is generated by the claim that a physician has a strict therapeutic obligation to inform the patients of the physician's treatment preference, even when the preference is based on evidence that is not of the highest quality. The dilemma could be resolved if the physician's therapeutic obligation were less strict. This strategy was developed by Freedman.[14,15] He argued that the standard for determining whether a physician has engaged in medical malpractice or committed some other violation punishable by a professional disciplinary body is the standard of good practice as determined by a consensus of the medical community. There is no consensus about which of two treatments being compared in a randomized clinical trial is superior. (Otherwise, why conduct the trial?) Therefore, enrolling a patient in the trial does not violate the physician's therapeutic obligation to the patient, regardless of the physician's treatment preference. In addition, a patient who consults a physician with a preference for treatment A could have consulted a physician who preferred treatment B. Therefore, enrolling a patient in a randomized clinical trial in order to be randomly assigned (perhaps) to treatment B does not make such a patient worse off than he or she would otherwise have been.

Despite these points, compelling arguments for the stricter interpretation of therapeutic obligation remain. In the first place, consider what physicians expect when they seek professional advice from their malpractice attorneys, their tax advisors, or for that matter, their own physicians. Surely they expect—and believe they have a right to expect—not merely minimally competent advice, but the best professional judgments of the professionals they have chosen to consult. In the second place, patients choose physicians in order to obtain medical advice that is, in the judgment of those physicians, the best available. If physicians do not provide such advice, then they tacitly deceive their patients, unless they disclose to their patients that they are not bound by this strict therapeutic obligation. Physicians should adopt the strict therapeutic obligation.

A RESOLUTION

The clash between a strict therapeutic obligation and a less strict one is only apparent. On the one hand, the less strict therapeutic obligation is supported by the argument that it is morally permissible to offer to enroll a patient in a randomized clinical trial. On the other hand, the strict therapeutic obligation is supported by the arguments concerning treatment recommendations. Recommending is different from

offering to enroll. A recognition of this difference provides the basis for a solution to the dilemma.

Suppose that a randomized clinical trial is being conducted to compare treatments A and B and that a physician prefers A and informs the patient of this preference. All physicians have an obligation to obtain their patients' informed consent to treatment. A physician has respected this right only if he or she explains to the patient the risks and benefits of reasonable alternatives to the recommended treatment and offers the patient an opportunity to choose an alternative, if that is feasible. Either treatment B or enrollment in the trial comparing A and B is a reasonable alternative to treatment A, because presumably, A is not known to be superior to B: Indeed, there is some evidence that enrollment in a randomized clinical trial is a superior therapeutic alternative when a trial is available.[16] Respect for a patient's values is a central purpose of informed consent. A particular patient may place a greater value on participation in a study that will contribute to medical progress and to the well-being of patients in the future than on the unproved advantages of following the physician's recommendation. Therefore, a physician can both recommend a treatment and ask whether the patient is willing to enroll in the randomized clinical trial.

This resolution is based on the recognition that there can be evidence of the superiority of a treatment that falls short of the gold standard for evidence but is better than worthless. It also takes into account the good arguments for the view that physicians have a strict obligation to recommend the best treatment on the basis of their professional judgment, even when the recommendation is based on evidence that falls short of the gold standard. Nevertheless, because all physicians have an obligation to take informed consent seriously, because respect for informed consent entails offering a patient the reasonable alternatives to the recommended treatment, and because enrollment in an appropriate randomized clinical trial is often a reasonable therapeutic option, one could argue that offering a patient the opportunity to be enrolled in a clinical trial is not only morally permissible but, in many cases, also morally obligatory, if a relevant trial is being conducted and if enrollment in it is feasible. Taking informed consent seriously resolves the dilemma about whether to enroll patients in randomized clinical trials.

Is this analysis clinically realistic? Some may argue that if clinicians inform their patients that they prefer treatment A, then few of their patients will consent to participate in a trial comparing A with B. Furthermore, many clinicians may be unwilling to invest the time necessary to explain the option of enrollment in a trial, particularly if it seems unlikely that a patient, knowing the physician's preference for one of the treatments, will choose to participate in the trial.

On the other hand, in recent years the public has been exposed to a barrage of medical information and misinformation. Explaining to patients the difference between solid scientific evidence of the merits of a treatment and weaker evidence of its merits is worthwhile, whether or not a relevant randomized clinical trial is being conducted. When a relevant trial is being conducted, offering the patient enrollment in the trial should not impose on the physician a large, additional burden of explanation. Physicians can promote enrollment by explaining that their preference is based only on limited evidence, which may or may not be reliable. They can also explain that data from randomized clinical trials have often shown that the initial studies of new treatments were overly optimistic.[17]

In addition, using this informed-consent strategy to resolve the enrollment dilemma may not be morally optional. My analysis is based on two important obligations of physicians. The first is the strict obligation to recommend the treatment that is, in the physician's professional judgment, the best choice for the patient. The second is the obligation to obtain the patient's informed consent to the recommended treatment. The duty of obtaining informed consent implies that the physician is obligated to offer the patient the opportunity to enroll in a clinical trial when one is available, even if the physician has a treatment preference. The physician owes this duty to the individual patient, not simply to future patients who may benefit from advances in medical knowledge. Thus, the informed-consent strategy for resolving the dilemma about enrolling patients in randomized clinical trials leads to the conclusion that physicians have a greater duty to offer their patients enrollment in trials than has previously been realized. A strict, thoroughly defensible, therapeutic obligation need not interfere with the conduct of randomized clinical trials.

I am indebted to Erin Fitz-Gerald, Nina Ainslie, Stephen Williamson, Sarah Taylor, Jerry Menikoff, Don Hatton, and Ron Stephens for their criticisms.

REFERENCES

1 Chalmers T. C. The ethics of randomization as a decision-making technique and the problem of informed consent. Report of the 14th conference of cardiovascular training grant program directors, June 3–4, 1967. Bethesda, Md.: National Heart Institute, 1967:87–93.

2 Shaw L. W, Chalmers T. C. Ethics in cooperative clinical trials. Ann N Y Acad Sci 1970; 169:487–95.

3 Kolata G. B. Clinical trials: methods and ethics are debated. Science 1977;198:1127–31.

4 Wikler D. Ethical considerations in randomized clinical trials. Semin Oncol 1981; 8:437–41.

5 Schafer A. The ethics of the randomized clinical trial. N Engl J Med 1982;307:719–24.

6 Marquis D. Leaving therapy to chance. Hastings Cent Rep 1983;13:40–7.

7 Gifford R. The conflict between randomized clinical trials and the therapeutic obligation. J Med Philos 1986; 11:347–66.

8 Hellman S, Hellman D. S. Of mice but not men: problems of the randomized clinical trial. N Engl J Med 1991; 324:1585–9.

9 Gifford R. Community equipoise and the ethics of randomized clinical trials. Bioethics 1995; 9:127–48.

10 Markman M. Ethical difficulties with randomized clinical trials involving cancer patients: examples from the field of gynecologic oncology. J Clin Ethics 1992; 3:193–5.

11 Spodick D. H. Ethics of the randomized clinical trial. N Engl J Med 1983; 308:343.

12 Passamani E. Clinical trials — are they ethical? N Engl J Med 1991; 324:1589–92.

13 Altman L. Negative results: a positive viewpoint. New York Times. April 29, 1986:B6.

14 Freedman B. Equipoise and the ethics of clinical research. N Engl J Med 1987; 317:141–5.

15 *Idem.* A response to a purported ethical difficulty with randomized clinical trials involving cancer patients. J Clin Ethics 1992; 3:231–4.

16 Davis S, Wright P. W., Schulman S. F, et al. Participants in prospective, randomized clinical trials for resected non-small cell lung cancer have improved survival compared with nonparticipants in such trials. Cancer 1985; 56:1710–8.

17 Sacks H, Chalmers T. C, Smith H. Jr. Randomized versus historical controls for clinical trials. Am J Med 1982; 72:233–40.

A NORMATIVE JUSTIFICATION FOR DISTINGUISHING THE ETHICS OF CLINICAL RESEARCH FROM THE ETHICS OF MEDICAL CARE

Paul Litton and Franklin G. Miller

Litton and Miller address an assumption made by many research ethics documents and commentators: "that physicians, whether acting as care givers or researchers, have the same duty of beneficence toward their patients and subjects: . . . optimal medical care." Underscoring the different aims of clinical medicine and research, while restricting their analysis to competent adults, the authors reject this therapeutic orientation to research ethics in favor of an alternative approach. Citing the moral philosophy of T. M. Scanlon as a theoretical foundation, Litton and Miller embrace a framework of seven ethical requirements for clinical research. While noting that this framework entails very significant obligations on the part of investigators to their subjects, the authors deny that it entails a requirement of clinical equipoise (a requirement embraced by "The Declaration of Helsinki" and the authors of the two preceding articles), which Litton and Miller regard as ethically unnecessary. They go on to argue that the therapeutic orientation to research ethics and the equipoise requirement underlying it are excessively paternalistic before illustrating their own approach with several cases. Litton and Miller conclude that their approach is properly respectful of patient-subjects as persons while permitting clinical research to advance without undue restrictions.

In the research ethics literature, there is strong disagreement about the ethical acceptability of placebo-controlled trials, particularly when a tested therapy aims to alleviate a condition for which standard treatment exists.[1] Recently, this disagreement has given rise to debate over the moral appropriateness of the principle of clinical equipoise for medical research.[2] Underlying these debates are two fundamentally different visions of the moral obligations that investigators owe their subjects.

Some commentators and ethics documents claim that physicians, whether acting as care givers or researchers, have the same duty of beneficence toward their patients and subjects: namely, that they must provide optimal medical care. In discussing placebo surgery in research on refractory Parkinson's disease, Peter Clark succinctly states this view: "The researcher has an ethical responsibility to act in the best interest of subjects."[3] The Declaration of Helsinki,

From *Journal of Law, Medicine & Ethics*, vol. 33 (2005), pp. 566–574.
Copyright © 2005 by Blackwell Publishing Ltd. Reproduced with permission of Blackwell Publishing Ltd.

a leading code of ethics for clinical research, also appears to accept this ethical view when it embraces the physician's oath, "The health of my patient will be my first consideration."[4]

We, however, argue that researchers owe significant moral obligations to patient-subjects, but do not have the same duty of therapeutic beneficence that binds physicians treating patients. Thus far, while both sides have provided reasons for their respective views and critiques of contrary perspectives, neither side has shown how its view is rooted in and justified by a more general account of what we morally owe to each other. This paper provides that needed, theoretical moral justification for distinguishing the ethical guidelines governing medical care and research, respectively. We examine whether there are legitimate reasons for patient-subjects to demand the ethical orientation of therapeutic beneficence in the research setting, and whether there are otherwise good reasons from the physician-researchers' perspective to conclude that they owe their subjects the same duties owed to patients under medical care. Our inquiry is limited to normal competent adults as the set of potential research subjects, recognizing that the ethics of conducting research on children and mentally incompetent persons requires separate treatment.

CONTRASTING ETHICAL PERSPECTIVES ON THE RELATIONSHIP BETWEEN PHYSICIAN-INVESTIGATORS AND RESEARCH SUBJECTS

The distinctive goals of medical care and clinical research are central to the debates regarding the proper ethical standards for these practices. Clinical medicine aims to promote the well-being of individual patients. Ethically, the potential benefits of diagnostic and therapeutic measures prescribed to patients must outweigh the risks posed to them, precisely because physicians must practice medicine with primary loyalty to caring for their patients. The essential purpose of clinical research, however, is to produce generalizable medical knowledge that will improve medical care for future patients. Physician-investigators conduct experiments to test the safety and effectiveness of therapies and diagnostic tools on groups of research subjects. In clinical trials a subject receives treatment or a diagnostic measure based on the scientific design of the research protocol and not on an individualized medical assessment. Assessing the ethical justification of a protocol involves considering the risks and possible benefits to the participating subjects, as well as the potential benefits to *society*.

In a recent paper, Trudo Lemmens and Paul Miller acknowledge that clinical care and research have different aims and practices, but argue that those differences do not have any *normative significance* that could *justify* allowing the investigator to deviate from the physician's preeminent duty to act in the best interest of her patient.[5] In their view, resting a distinct set of ethical standards for research on its distinctive goal represents, without argument, an arbitrary "sheer re-definition" of research ethics.[6]

Lurking behind their criticism is the belief that there is a convincing argument for binding clinical researchers to the medical care ethic. Paul Miller and Charles Weijer explicate such an argument in defending the principle of clinical equipoise for medical research. They contend:

> Patients come to their physicians for expert advice and treatment. By virtue of illness and the power of physicians to aid and assist them in coping with it, patients are in a vulnerable position vis-á-vis physicians. Given the pervasive understanding of the overriding mission of medicine as providing care for the ill, patients enter relationships with physicians with the *reasonable expectation* that their physicians' recommendations always will be consistent with, and indeed intended to promote, their best interests.[7]

On this view, because patients are "sufficiently troubled to seek medical attention" from physicians, who have superior knowledge and the ability to help, they, as patient-subjects, may reasonably expect their physician-investigators to use their discretion only in a manner consistent with their patient-subjects' best interests. We call this position, "the therapeutic orientation to the ethics of clinical research."

MORAL APPROACH OUTLINED

In arguing that physician-investigators do not owe patient-subjects the duty of therapeutic beneficence within the research context, we examine systematically the question raised by Miller and Weijer: is it reasonable for persons (ill or healthy) to expect or demand physicians to treat them according to the medical care ethic when enrolled in, or invited to enroll in, research? In other words, would patient-subjects have reasonable grounds to complain that they were not treated according to the medical care ethic even though their physician-researchers fulfilled a set of ethical requirements formulated distinctly for medical research?

The structure of the argument presented is based on the account of moral reasoning offered by T. M. Scanlon.[8] In Scanlon's account, our reasoning about right and wrong is structured by our shared motivation to find "principles for the general regulation of behavior that others, similarly motivated, could not reasonably reject."[9] These principles imply permissions and restrictions on action that are reasonable to impose on one another within different contexts, given that we are seeking to find principles to serve as the terms of mutual respect among persons. Stated differently, principles that no one could reasonably reject entail the legitimate expectations and moral duties for which we are accountable within interpersonal relationships.

This account of moral reasoning assumes a normative idea of persons as creatures distinguished by their capacities "to assess reasons and to govern their lives according to this assessment."[10] It is also informed by the idea that we are committed to relating to each other on terms that mutually respect each individual's value as a reasons-assessing, self-directed person in pursuit of a meaningful life.[11] These normative commitments embodied in ordinary moral reasoning explain why, in assessing a proposed principle of morality, we have reason to take seriously any consideration "that virtually anyone capable of living a rationally self-directed worthwhile life has at least prima facie reason to care about."[12] For example, any person capable of governing her own life has reason to care about avoiding pain, being healthy, having sufficient material resources, having what happens to them depend on the choices they make, and so on.[13] These are the kinds of considerations that plausibly may provide a reason to reject a proposed principle for how we may relate to one another.

At issue, in assessing a proposed ethical principle, is whether the principle, if generally acted upon, expresses an attitude respectful of the value of the persons potentially affected by the principle's adoption. It is important to note that this framework is not meant to offer an algorithm for settling the ethical issue at hand. Rather, explicating this account of moral reasoning is meant to expose the deeper normative assumptions behind the forthcoming arguments. The moral question examined here is whether principles that no one can reasonably reject dictate that patient-subjects enrolled in clinical research may reasonably expect or demand from physician-researchers treatment in accordance with the medical care ethic.

THE NORMATIVE SIGNIFICANCE OF THE GOAL OF CLINICAL RESEARCH

Are there ethical standards for clinical research that depart from the ethics of medical care? The major reason to find a separate research ethic concerns the significant social value underlying the distinctive goal of research to develop generalizable knowledge for the improvement of medical care. If a proposed set of ethical guidelines for research is more conducive to producing valid and medically useful knowledge than adopting the therapeutic orientation for research, then there is a prima facie reason to endorse the proposed set.

We need not belabor the point that we have strong reason to value medical research. It "has increased the well-being of humans in much of the world. And it has done so in all its many guises, from early epidemiological research, such as John Snow's investigations of the cholera outbreaks in London in the mid-nineteenth century, to current studies of treatments administered in controlled settings."[14] "Thanks to the efforts of researchers in both the public and private sectors, diseases that had struck fear and dread into the lives of our parents and grandparents—yellow fever, polio, rheumatic fever—no longer haunt our consciousness."[15] In short, the extensive benefits that we have come to expect from medical care undoubtedly depend upon the discoveries of medical research. The best way to achieve the goal of medical research—generalizable medical knowledge—is by designing research protocols that aim precisely at testing hypotheses by means of rigorous scientific methods. In contrast to medical care, the purpose of these research methods is not to promote the best interests of the research subjects involved. Understanding the pathophysiology of diseases and evaluating novel potential treatments and diagnostic tools require controlled experimentation involving groups of individuals, including patients with the diseases under investigation. Observations produced in the course of medical care of individual patients have limited scientific value and validity, owing to biases in the selection of patients and the assessment of outcomes. Validating medical hypotheses, therefore, requires researchers to compare results achieved from controlled experimentation on groups of patients. Treatments typically must be limited to the protocolized care prescribed, and not based on individual needs, to reach valid results. Finally, as noted, producing generalizable medical knowledge requires the use of purely research interventions to measure study outcomes—such as blood draws taken over time and biopsies—that are not administered for the purposes of medical care.

It follows that the distinctive goal of research *is* normatively significant: there are good reasons to design research protocols for the purpose of producing socially important, generalizable medical knowledge. The goal of research and the most effective and scientifically rigorous means of achieving it provide reasons to posit research ethical requirements that do not include a duty on physician-investigators to maintain primary loyalty to their subjects' best medical interests.[16] Importantly, a rule requiring the medical care ethic for research, if strictly applied, would make clinical research largely impossible to conduct because it would prohibit any research interventions posing risks to subjects without sufficiently compensating benefits to them, individually. Indeed, there is an unacknowledged tension in the view that the medical care ethic must govern clinical research: it exalts the value of medical care for persons who are afflicted with a treatable condition yet simultaneously advocates guidelines for research which, if strictly followed, would severely hinder the efforts that under-gird and increase its value by developing relevant medical knowledge.

Nevertheless, the good reasons not to bind research to the medical care ethic, by themselves, are not sufficient to justify a different set of duties for physicians conducting medical research. We must ask whether these prima facie reasons to expose patient-subjects to risk without compensating benefit to them are trumped by other considerations, including the respect owed to them as persons. Even though the goal of research is eminently worthwhile, it would still be wrong for researchers to depart from the ethics of medical care if, all things considered, they do owe subjects the same duties owed to patients.

We argue that the good reasons to conduct research without the therapeutic orientation of medical care are *not* trumped by what physician-investigators owe patient-subjects. Of course, rejecting the medical care ethic for research does not imply that investigators owe only weak or no duties to subjects. Physician-researchers must respect the value of patient-subjects as persons. Accordingly, investigators *do* have very significant obligations to them,

corresponding with the legitimate demands to which patient-subjects may hold them.

A DISTINCT SET OF ETHICAL STANDARDS FOR RESEARCH

The recent work of Emanuel, Wendler, and Grady provides a valuable starting point for discussing ethical principles that are sufficient for respecting patient-subjects participating in the discovery of medical knowledge.[17] The authors put forth seven ethical requirements on clinical research as an elucidation of protections embedded in several widely-recognized documents and codes.[18] These requirements "aim to minimize the possibility of exploitation [of subjects] by ensuring that [they] are not merely used but are treated with respect while they contribute to the social good."[19] According to this framework, a research protocol must (1) have "social, scientific, or clinical value," that justifies exposing subjects to potential harm; (2) be scientifically rigorous; (3) select subjects fairly on the basis of scientific objectives and not, for example, because of vulnerability or privilege; (4) minimize the risks to individual subjects, and have potential benefits to those subjects and/or society that outweigh or are proportionate to the risks; (5) be reviewed and approved prospectively by a committee of independent and qualified evaluators; (6) be conditioned, to the extent possible, on the voluntary and informed consent of its participating subjects; and (7) ensure that enrolled subjects are shown respect, which includes protecting their privacy, monitoring their well-being, and providing opportunities to withdraw. The moral duties implied by these requirements are quite substantial, even if they do not include the duty of therapeutic beneficence.

Emanuel and colleagues assert that clinical equipoise is implied by their ethical framework. This widely endorsed principle prohibits assigning treatments in clinical trials known to be inferior to established therapy. It has been argued elsewhere that clinical equipoise confuses the ethics of clinical research with the ethics of medical care.[20] We do not repeat the argument here but affirm the conclusion that clinical equipoise is not a necessary component of an ethical framework appropriate to clinical research. Therefore, it is important to recognize that our version of the ethical requirements on clinical research does not presuppose or imply clinical equipoise or any other version of equipoise.

As characterized by Emanuel and colleagues, the seven ethical principles of clinical research reflect the way "reasonable people would want to be treated"[21] when invited to participate and when enrolled in research. Indeed, "these requirements are precisely the types of considerations that would be invoked to justify clinical research if it were challenged."[22] Correlatively, these requirements reflect the considerations on which someone could base an ethical challenge to a research protocol or the way in which a physician-investigator engages with a patient-subject.

Each of the seven principles expresses a respectful attitude toward the worth of each patient-subject. For example, with respect to requiring research to have social or scientific value, an investigator who asked persons to dedicate their time and expose themselves to some level of risk for a trivial or useless hypothesis would thereby express disregard for their time and health. Similarly, employing scientifically invalid principles and methods shows disrespect for the time and health of research participants, as well as disrespects their decision to help discover scientifically valid knowledge. The standard for a favorable risk-benefit ratio also recognizes the value of research participants as persons. It requires that risks to patient-subjects be minimized, acknowledging the interest every person has to avoid harm. Potential benefits to patient-subjects and society must outweigh the risks to the participants precisely because all participants have reason to reject being exposed to harms without some compensating reason.

Respecting the value of a patient-subject as a person does not require that the reasonable and minimized risks of research to which she is exposed be outweighed solely by the potential medical benefits *to her* from the research interventions. Competent adults generally do not need protection from their ability to choose to take on reasonable risks when there are important and meaningful reasons, from an individual's point of view, even if those reasons are unrelated to one's best medical interests. For example, by enrolling in research, some persons understandably

derive meaning from their illness by seeing it as an opportunity to help alleviate the suffering of people afflicted with the same condition in the future. Others who have benefited from medical care and, therefore, from the participation of research subjects in the past, enroll in research as a symbolic act of gratitude. Some research participants choose to join the fight against a particular disease to honor the memory of a family member who succumbed to it. The respect due to these research participants does not provide reason to prohibit them, even if ill, from assuming reasonable and minimized risks that are not outweighed by the medical benefits to them, individually.

BEING ILL AND SEEKING MEDICAL CARE: A REASON TO REQUIRE THE MEDICAL CARE ETHIC?

In order to justify the therapeutic orientation to the ethics of clinical research, one must articulate the legitimate reason subjects have to demand therapeutic beneficence from a researcher even when the researcher meets the ethical requirements specified by Emanuel and colleagues. Put differently, an objection to our view must put forth a reasonable ground to reject the thesis that physician-researchers do not have an obligation to maintain primary loyalty to the best medical interests of their patient-subjects as long as they invite patients to enroll in research that satisfies the seven ethical requirements.

Miller and Weijer propose a basis for patient-subjects to legitimately demand therapeutic beneficence from a researcher, at least with regard to clinical trials testing a new therapy. Recall that they start with the premise that research subjects are initially ill patients seeking expert care and advice from physicians. Their vulnerability due to illness, in conjunction with the superior knowledge of their physicians, makes it reasonable for them to expect protection from being used by physicians in any way contrary to their best interests. Kathleen Cranley Glass presumably appeals to similar reasoning when she emphasizes that "in most randomized clinical trials are persons seeking medical care."[23]

This ground for supporting the therapeutic orientation, and rejecting our position, is unconvincing.

First, this line of argument conflates the questions of when it is ethically permissible for a physician personally treating a patient to invite her into research, and the separate question regarding what ethical standards should govern the investigator-subject relationship in the course of a research protocol. Even if we assumed that it is ethical for a physician treating a patient to invite her into research only when it is in her best medical interests, we still must consider what standards should guide the activity of performing general research on persons. Many research subjects are recruited into research by physician-investigators who have no prior treating relationships with them as patients. Furthermore, even if a clinical trial is considered to be the best medical option for a given patient, it will likely include research procedures that are not intended for, or justified by, the medical benefit to subjects.

Second, the proposed ground for the therapeutic orientation to research overstates the vulnerability of ill persons as a class. Clearly, there are very seriously ill people who are in an especially vulnerable state because of their anxiety, pain, desperate need to find a cure, and so on. A physician-investigator must not exploit such vulnerabilities. Moreover, under the seven principles for research, it would be unethical to withhold effective treatment to such ill persons for research purposes if withholding treatment exposes a person to grave risk. But for the vast majority of patients, it would, in fact, be *disrespectful* for physicians to relate to them merely as the vulnerable sick. There is an important distinction between being ill and being viewed by others as occupying only a passive role due to illness. Having a medical condition does not imply that one is *merely* sick. Most ill persons can assess reasons and live according to those assessments. As such, physicians and researchers must respect those capacities. If competent, an ill person can understand that participation in a research protocol is not for therapeutic purposes. Of course, some patients will not be able to grasp that idea and, perhaps, on that basis, may not be eligible to participate in research; however, it is implausible to suggest that having any medical condition implies an inability to engage rationally with a physician except for one's own best medical interests.

PATERNALISM AND REASONS TO REJECT THE MEDICAL CARE ETHIC FOR RESEARCH

Insisting on the medical care ethic for research conveys the message that individuals should never be allowed to give up their "right" to optimal treatment from physicians, regardless of the significant safeguards against exploitation that are required and regardless of the circumstances under which informed consent is obtained. Indeed, Benjamin Freedman and his colleagues, in explicating the normative grounds for the principle of clinical equipoise, suggest that patients have an inalienable right to the medical care ethic: "As a normative matter, [the principle of clinical equipoise] defines ethical trial design as prohibiting any compromise of a patient's right to medical treatment by enrolling in a study."[24] David Steinberg echoes that position: "People who agree to participate in clinical investigations do not relinquish the right to optimal medical care."[25] However, patient-subjects have good reason to reject that view as unjustifiably paternalistic.

The therapeutic orientation to the ethics of clinical research is unduly paternalistic not simply because it forbids a physician-investigator from honoring a person's choice to opt out of the role as patient. It implies that even when the threat of exploitation has been safeguarded against, and even when the conditions under which someone could choose to opt out of the role of patient are fair, patients are forbidden from doing so. It treats potential subjects merely as the vulnerably ill and ignores the good reasons they have to be able to participate in research that aims to help others and is not necessarily in their best medical interests.

The therapeutic orientation ignores that persons have reason to want the ways in which they are treated [to] depend on the choices they make, especially when placed in a sufficiently good position to make an informed decision.[26] First, persons have reason to want their informed decisions respected because they express what is meaningful to them through their choices.[27] In the present context, a rule requiring the therapeutic orientation to clinical trials would deny individuals the opportunity to express altruism and gratitude to prior research subjects and investigators who have made possible important medical advances. It would prevent some individuals from finding meaning in their illnesses by contributing to the discovery of interventions that will alleviate the suffering of persons in the future. One might maintain that the medical care ethic would not preclude research participants from expressing altruism, gratitude, or related attitudes. However, requiring that research be governed by therapeutic beneficence would unduly restrict the ability of patient-subjects to express gratitude and altruism because it limits the potential value of research (by making much of research impossible) and eliminates the possibility of reasonable sacrifice (by requiring research to be consistent with one's best medical interests). Because those implications are rooted in an unacceptable view of patient-subjects as merely passively ill, it is unacceptably paternalistic.

Second, persons have reason to want others to treat them in accordance with their informed choices out of respect for their ability to govern their own lives. In the present context, it is demeaning to competent adult persons who understand the risks and benefits of enrolling in a protocol, and who comprehend what they might be forgoing by leaving the therapeutic setting, to be forbidden from contributing to research that involves withholding treatment but nonetheless is safeguarded by the substantial moral protections of the investigator-subject relationship.[28] Those who support the medical care ethic for research perhaps might contend that it would always be irrational for a person to leave the protected role of being a patient to become "merely" a research subject.[29] But such a claim would be demeaning to individuals, given the extensive ethical protections provided by the articulated requirements for research, including the limits on acceptable risk, careful monitoring of enrolled subjects, and the duties on investigators to clarify for potential subjects the differences between research participation and medical care and their alternatives to research before obtaining informed consent. The ethical requirements on research, as outlined, make it reasonable for persons, including many persons

with medical conditions, to accept the role of subject, not patient.

REFLECTION ON SPECIFIC EXAMPLES

To assess our argument that patient-subjects do not have reasonable grounds to expect investigators to be bound by the medical care ethic, it will be helpful to examine specific practical examples. Consider the following hypothetical scenario. A patient-subject, enrolled in a clinical trial that satisfies the seven ethical requirements for clinical research, develops intermittent headaches for one week following a lumbar puncture (LP) to measure study outcomes. The subject complains to the investigator and the IRB that he has been wronged because the LP was not administered for his medical care but solely to serve the purposes of research. Is this a valid complaint?

The subject has no reasonable grounds for complaint as long as the following conditions obtain: (1) the clinical trial offered a reasonable prospect of generating clinically valuable knowledge; (2) the LP was necessary to produce scientifically valid data; (3) the subject was properly screened, and no medical conditions were detected that would make an LP contraindicated; (4) the LP was performed according to optimal practice aimed at minimizing risks of post-LP headache; (5) the protocol was reviewed and approved by a competent IRB; (6) the subject gave informed consent, which included a clear disclosure in conversation with the investigator and in the consent document that the LP was administered for research purposes and not for medical care, and that it carried a risk of headache; and (7) the subject was carefully monitored during the course of research participation and received standard treatment for post-LP headache. In sum, the subject was not exposed to any degree of harm that was uncompensated by the worth of the study; the investigator provided him with a fair opportunity not to enroll; and, presumably, this competent subject had reasons for choosing to enroll.

As a second example, consider the following non-therapeutic research protocol. To test hypotheses concerning the pathophysiology of depression, investigators recruit persons diagnosed with major depression who are not currently receiving treatment for a study lasting four weeks, which employs brain scans and other non-invasive investigative procedures. The primary risk to these subjects is the potential worsening of symptoms or lack of improvement due to a delay in receiving standard medically-indicated treatment. A protocol of this sort can meet the seven ethical requirements on clinical research. These subjects were not receiving any medical [treatment] for depression, thus they were not exposed to the harm of being taken off a regimen that was working for them. Furthermore, the potential harm they faced could be minimized by close monitoring, and if delay in medical treatment began to pose serious risks to a subject, investigators could remove him from the study and recommend standard treatment. Moreover, despite being diagnosed with depression, there is no sound reason to assume that these subjects are not competent to understand fully that they are participating in research, which aims to understand brain physiology and not to provide medical care.[30] Such subjects are able to give informed consent after understanding the risks of non-treatment and that medical care was an alternative.

Again, it appears that their investigators are not disregarding their value as persons. On the stipulation that these patient-subjects were competent and had intelligible reasons to enroll, the researcher has better reason to accept gratefully their decision to enroll rather than to "protect" them by prohibiting any risk-taking unrelated to their individual best medical interests. In fact, we should understand investigators as expressing respect for their value as persons by trying to find more effective treatment for their illness. Under these conditions, it is incumbent on someone who insists upon the medical care ethic for research with patient-subjects to illuminate the reason why their value as persons is not respected, which would ground a legitimate demand for therapeutic beneficence in this context.

With respect to a third example, we contend, perhaps more controversially, that a subject who enrolls in a randomized placebo-controlled trial that meets the ethical requirements on research, despite the existence of standard treatment for his condition, could not reasonably expect to be treated according to the medical care ethic. Again, if the seven ethical requirements were met, as stipulated, the subject

understood that he would be given, for research purposes, either the experimental agent or placebo, and, that he would be bypassing standard treatment available to him. We acknowledge that it is disputed whether placebo controls, where proven effective therapy is available, satisfy the second requirement of scientific necessity.[31] But notice that even if the use of a placebo control is unethical in a given clinical trial because it would be scientifically unnecessary, our key point should not be lost: namely, that if the requirements on clinical research have been satisfied, then the departure from the ethics of medical care does not count as wronging research subjects.

Putting aside disputes about the scientific need for placebos, there is no relevant moral distinction between allowing a subject to undergo a non-therapeutic intervention that poses some risks without any compensating medical benefit to her (as in our first example), and permitting a person with a treatable medical condition to forgo standard therapy temporarily when she knowingly bypasses such treatment without assuming any serious risk. Morally, the scenarios are the same: a person, informed that she is under no obligation to assume the risks posed by a research protocol, agrees to expose herself to a reasonable, limited degree of risk, without compensating medical benefit to her, for the sake of generating medical knowledge. Indeed, subjects in the non-therapeutic psychiatric study that enrolled subjects with untreated depression and in a placebo-controlled trial might be taking on precisely the same risk: temporarily forgoing standard or experimental treatment. If investigators would not express any disrespectful attitude toward the value of subjects in the former study, there is no reason to think that the subjects randomized to placebo would be wronged.

AN OBJECTION BASED ON THE THERAPEUTIC MISCONCEPTION

A recent study by Appelbaum and colleagues, encompassing a wide range of clinical trials, indicates that a substantial proportion of participants confuse the provision of treatment within randomized trials with the patient-centered therapy of standard medical care.[32] It might be objected to our position that the prevalence of the "therapeutic misconception" provides a reason to reject principles of research ethics that permit placebo-controlled trials when proven effective treatment exists. Patients harboring a therapeutic misconception will not understand or appreciate that they may receive suboptimal treatment, thus invalidating their informed consent.

However, by itself, the empirical fact that many subjects misconceive their investigators' intentions as therapeutic does not provide a reason to require the medical care ethic for research. That some subjects participate under the therapeutic misconception might indicate that investigators are not making acceptable efforts to clarify for research subjects the purpose of their studies and the basis on which interventions are assigned. The data from the study by Appelbaum and colleagues, however, do not show that subjects are incapable of understanding the distinction between the goals of research and medical care. Moreover, the cause of many instances of the therapeutic misconception may, in fact, be due to physician-investigators who primarily see their clinical trials from a therapeutic perspective.[33] If that were the case, the data provide good reason for investigators to acquire a better understanding of the distinctive ethical standards that bind them, as opposed to providing a reason to endorse the therapeutic orientation to the ethics of research.

ANOTHER OBJECTION: THE PERSPECTIVE OF THE PHYSICIAN-INVESTIGATOR

Thus far, by asking what patient-subjects reasonably may demand from physician-investigators, our approach has focused exclusively on the perspective of the research subject. However, an objector to our position might argue that the perspective of the reasonable research subject is morally irrelevant. The objection would maintain that physicians always have a duty to act in the best interests of persons to whom they attend. After all, physicians have been trained for this very purpose. This line of objection even finds support in the Declaration of Helsinki, referred to earlier, which without distinguishing subjects from patients, endorses the physician's oath in expounding ethical principles for medical research: "The health of my patient will be my first consideration."[34]

The proposed objection fails, however. First, despite the position of the Helsinki Declaration, the objection is incongruous with moral principles implicit in our accepted societal practices in other contexts. Specifically, for example, forensic psychiatrists who fulfill a necessary role in our criminal justice system are not governed by the ethical principles of the medical care setting when examining potential or actual criminal defendants. "As numerous commentators have recognized, were forensic psychiatrists to be charged with pursuing subjects' best interests and avoiding harm—as are their clinical colleagues—their evaluations would be worthless to the courts."[35] The practices of military and occupational medicine also represent contexts in which we accept a deviation from the undivided loyalty that we expect from medical care physicians. These practices reflect the principle that the duties binding physicians should change depending upon the societal role they fulfill in a particular context, and thereby reject the principle that physicians are always governed by the medical care ethic. Similar to the forensic psychiatrist, the physician-investigator cannot conduct research competently without departing from the ethics of medical care.

Second, the proposed rejoinder, which takes as irrelevant the reasonable expectations of subjects, embraces an odd and unacceptable understanding of interpersonal moral obligations. The objection incoherently implies that an investigator can violate a duty owed to a research subject, and thereby wrong the subject, even though the subject would not have reasonable grounds to claim that his investigator breached any legitimate expectation to which he could hold her. Under the objector's view, the alleged duty of investigators to provide optimal medical care bears no connection to the nature of the research enterprise and the interpersonal nature of the investigator-subject relationship; rather, it appears to be an absolute prohibition lacking any cogent rationale. We maintain that if physician-investigators have a duty to treat subjects in the same way they would treat patients, then that duty must correspond with the expectations of subjects that are justified by legitimate reasons, taking into consideration the good reasons to conduct research outside the framework of the medical care ethic.

CONCLUSION

The reasons to value generalizable medical knowledge and the most effective and rigorous means to produce it present a prima facie rationale to endorse ethical standards for research that depart from the medical care ethic. Strict adherence to the medical care ethic in the research setting would render impossible much of the clinical research we value because it would prohibit interventions posing risks to subjects that are not outweighed by benefits to them individually. The ethical principles for research articulated by Emanuel and colleagues sufficiently recognize the worth of patient-subjects as persons, capable of assessing reasons and directing their lives according to those assessments. Indeed, it is disrespectful to confine a person with a medical condition to the passive role of the vulnerably ill. Likewise, it is unacceptably paternalistic to prevent persons from acting on very good reasons to enroll in research when there is a significant and respectful ethical framework available, formulated in light of the valuable goal of research.

ACKNOWLEDGEMENTS

The authors thank Zeke Emanuel and Dave Wendler for very helpful comments on previous drafts of this article.

REFERENCES

1 See e.g., J. Sugarman, "Using Empirical Data to Inform the Ethical Evaluation of Placebo Controlled Trials," *Science and Engineering Ethics* 10 (2004): 29–35; F. G. Miller and H. Brody, "What Makes Placebo-Controlled Trials Unethical?" *American Journal of Bioethics* 2, no. 2 (2002): 3–9; R. M. Veatch, "Subject Indifference and the Justification of Placebo-Controlled Trials," *American Journal of Bioethics* 2, no. 2 (2002): 12–13; T. Lemmens and P. B. Miller, "Avoiding a Jekyll-And-Hyde Approach to the Ethics of Clinical Research and Practice," *American Journal of Bioethics* 2, no. 2 (2002): 14–17; E. J. Emanuel and F. G. Miller, "The Ethics of Placebo-Controlled Trials— A Middle Ground," *N. Engl. J. Med.* 345 (2001): 915–19; B. Freedman, K. C. Glass, C. Weijer, "Placebo Orthodoxy in Clinical Research II: Ethical, Legal, and Regulatory Myths," *Journal of Law, Medicine & Ethics* 24 (1996): 252–59.

2 See e.g., F. G. Miller and H. Brody, "A Critique of Clinical Equipoise: Therapeutic Misconception in the Ethics of Clinical Trials," *Hastings Center Report* 33, no. 3 (2003): 19–28; C. Weijer and P. B. Miller, "Therapeutic Obligation in Clinical Research," *Hastings Center Report* 33, no. 3 (2003): 3.

3 P. Clark, "Placebo Surgery For Parkinson's Disease: Do the Benefits Outweigh the Risks?" *Journal of Law, Medicine & Ethics* 30 (2002): 58–68, at 62.

4 World Medical Association, "Declaration of Helsinki: Ethical Principles for Medical Research Involving Human Subjects," adopted in 1964 and amended in 1975, 1983, 1989, 1996, and 2000, reprinted in *JAMA* 284 (2000): 3043–45.

5 T. Lemmens and P. B. Miller, *supra* note 1.

6 *Id.* at 14, 15. David Steinberg similarly questions the ethical relevance of the divergent goals of research and care: "The dominant goals of clinical research and clinical care may differ; however, the existence of a goal does not suffice as its moral justification." D. Steinberg, "Clinical Research should not be Permitted to Escape the Ethical Orbit of Clinical Care," *American Journal of Bioethics* 2, no. 2 (2002): 27–28, at 27.

7 P. B. Miller and C. Weijer, "Rehabilitating Equipoise," *Kennedy Institute of Ethics Journal* 13 (2003): 93–118, at 110–11.

8 T. M. Scanlon, *What We Owe To Each Other* (Cambridge, MA: Harvard University Press, 1998).

9 *Id.* at 4.

10 *Id.* at 106.

11 R. Kumar, "Reasonable Reasons in Contractualist Moral Argument," *Ethics* 114, no. 1 (2003): 6–37, at 14.

12 *Id.* at 14.

13 *Id.* at 14; Scanlon, *supra* note 8, at 204, 251.

14 E. J. Emanuel et al., "Scandals and Tragedies of Research with Human Participants (Introduction to Part I)," in E. J. Emanuel et. al., eds., *Ethical and Regulatory Aspects of Clinical Research* (Baltimore: The Johns Hopkins University Press, 2003): 1–5, at 1.

15 E. J. Emanuel et al., "Preface," in E. J. Emanuel et. al. eds., *Ethical and Regulatory Aspects of Clinical Research* (Baltimore: The Johns Hopkins University Press, 2003): xv–xviii, at xv.

16 For a discussion of the different *legal* duties that should guide clinical research and practice, respectively, based on the different ethical duties supported by the distinctive goals of those enterprises, see E. H. Morreim, "Litigation in Clinical Research: Malpractice Doctrines Versus Research Realities," *Journal of Law, Medicine & Ethics* 32 (2004): 474–484.

17 E. J. Emanuel, D. Wendler, and C. Grady, "What Makes Clinical Research Ethical?" *JAMA* 283 (2000): 2701–2711.

18 *Id.* at 2701–2702. These documents include the Nuremberg Code, the Declaration of Helsinki, the Belmont Report, International Guidelines for Biomedical Research Involving Human Subjects, as well as others.

19 *Id.* at 2701, citing R. J. Levine, *Ethics and Regulation in Clinical Research,* 2nd ed. (New Haven: Yale University Press, 1988).

20 F. G. Miller and H. Brody, *supra* note 1.

21 E. J. Emanuel, D. Wendler, and C. Grady, *supra* note 17, at 2708.

22 *Ibid.*

23 K. C. Glass, Letter to the Editor, "Clinical Equipoise and the Therapeutic Misconception," *Hastings Center Report* 33, no. 5 (2003): 5–6, at 5.

24 B. Freedman, K. C. Glass, C, Weijer, *supra* note 1, at 253.

25 Steinberg, *supra* note 6, at 27.

26 Scanlon, *supra* note 8, at 248–56.

27 *Id.* at 252.

28 *Id.* at 253.

29 So, for example, Rousseau argues that a choice to become a slave should not be respected precisely because it is irrational or unacceptably foolish:

> Now, since, in the relations between men, the worst that can happen to someone is for him to see himself at the discretion of someone else, would it not have been contrary to good sense to begin by surrendering into the hands of a leader the only things for whose preservation they needed his help? What equivalent could he have offered them for the concession of so fine a right?

J. J. Rousseau, "Discourse on the Origin of Inequality," in D. A. Cress, trans., *Basic Political Writings* (Indianapolis: Hackett Publishing, 1987): at 72.

Steinberg, in fact, makes this argument, stating that "no rational person would sign" a consent form that informed a potential subject that the ethics governing the protocol deviated from the ethics of medical care. Steinberg, *supra* note 6, at 27.

30 P. S. Appelbaum, T. Grisso, E. Frank, et al., "Competence of Depressed Patients for Consent to Research," *American Journal of Psychiatry* 156 (1999): 1380–84.

31 E. J. Emanuel and F. G. Miller, *supra* note 1; B. Freedman, K. C. Glass, C. Weijer, *supra* note 1.

32 P. S. Appelbaum, C. W. Lidz, T. Grisso, "Therapeutic Misconception in Clinical Research: Frequency and Risk Factors," *IRB* 26, no. 2 (2004): 1–8.

33 F. G. Miller and D. L. Rosenstein, "The Therapeutic Orientation to Clinical Trials," *N. Engl. J. Med.* 348 (2003): 1383–86.

34 World Medical Association, *supra* note 4.

35 P. S. Appelbaum, "A Theory of Ethics for Forensic Psychiatry," *The Journal of the American Academy of Psychiatry and the Law* 25 (1997): 233–247, at 239.

CLINICAL TRIALS IN DEVELOPING COUNTRIES

RESEARCH IN DEVELOPING COUNTRIES: TAKING BENEFIT SERIOUSLY

Leonard H. Glantz, George J. Annas, Michael A. Grodin, and Wendy K. Mariner

The authors confront the issue of whether it can be acceptable for researchers in wealthy countries to enroll citizens of developing countries in clinical trials. Citing guidelines published by the Council for International Organizations of Medical Sciences, the authors argue that to justify such trials, the risks or burdens imposed on trial participants must be offset by the prospect of actual benefit to the inhabitants of the developing country. Thus, if the trial yields beneficial knowledge, benefits must actually reach individuals in the country in which the trial took place; otherwise, the subjects will have been exploited. A practical implication of this approach is that "an essential prerequisite to designing ethical research in underdeveloped countries is identifying the source and amount of funding for providing the fruits of the research to the people of the developing country"—a moral requirement that was not satisfied in recent African AZT studies. The authors then consider and reply to a wide range of objections to the ethical standard they propose.

An April 1998 *New York Times Magazine* article described Ronald Munger's efforts to obtain blood samples from a group of extremely impoverished

Reprinted with permission of Leonard H. Glantz and the publisher from *Hastings Center Report*, vol. 28 (November–December 1998), pp. 38–42. Copyright © 1998 by The Hastings Center.

people in the Philippine Island of Cebu.[1] Munger sought the blood to study whether there was a genetic cause for this group's unusually high incidence of cleft lip and palate. One of many obstacles to the research project was the need to obtain the cooperation of the local health officer. It was not clear to

Munger, or the reader, whether the health officer had a bona fide interest in protecting the populace or was looking for a bribe. The health officer asked Munger a few perfunctory questions about informed consent and the study's ethical review in the United States, which Munger answered. Munger also explained the benefits that mothers and children would derive from participating in the research. The mothers would learn their blood types (which they apparently desired) and whether they were anemic. If they were anemic, they would be given iron pills. Lunch would be served, and raffles arranged so that families could win simple toys and other small items.

Munger told the health officer that if his hypotheses were correct, the research would benefit the population of Cebu: if the research shows that increased folate and vitamin B6 reduces the risk of cleft lip and palate, families could reduce the risk of facial deformities in their future offspring. The reporter noted that the health officer "laughs aloud at the suggestion that much of what is being discovered in American laboratories will make it back to Cebu any time soon." Reflecting on his experience with another simple intervention, iodized salt, the health officer said that when salt was iodized, the price rose threefold "so those who need it couldn't afford it and those who didn't need it are the only ones who could afford it."

The simple blood collecting mission to Cebu illustrates almost all the issues presented by research in developing countries. First is the threshold question of the goal of the research and its importance to the population represented by the research subjects. Next is the quality of informed consent, including whether the potential subjects thought that participation in the research was related to free surgical care that was offered in the same facility (although it clearly was not) and whether one could adequately explain genetic hypotheses to an uneducated populace. Finally, there is the question whether the population from which subjects were drawn could benefit from the research. This research intervention is very low risk—the collection of 10 drops of blood from affected people and their family members. The risk of job or insurance discrimination that genetic research poses in this country did not exist for the Cebu population; ironically, they were protected from the risk of economic discrimination by the profound poverty in which they lived.

Even this simple study raises the most fundamental question: "Why is it acceptable for researchers in developed countries to use citizens of developing countries as research subjects?" A cautionary approach to permitting research with human subjects in underdeveloped countries has been recommended because of the risk of their inadvertent or deliberate exploitation by researchers from developed countries. This cautionary approach generally is invoked when researchers propose to use what are considered "vulnerable populations," such as prisoners and children, as research subjects.[2] Vulnerable populations are those that are less able to protect themselves, either because they are not capable of making their own decisions or because they are particularly susceptible to mistreatment.[3] For example, children may be incapable of giving informed consent or of standing up to adult authority, while prisoners are especially vulnerable to being coerced into becoming subjects. Citizens of developing countries are often in vulnerable situations because of their lack of political power, lack of education, unfamiliarity with medical interventions, extreme poverty, or dire need for health care and nutrition. It is the dire need of these populations that may make them both appropriate subjects of research and especially vulnerable to exploitation. This combination of need and vulnerability has led to the development of guidelines for the use of citizens of developing countries as research subjects.

CIOMS GUIDELINES

In 1992, the Council for International Organizations of Medical Sciences (CIOMS), in collaboration with the World Health Organization, published guidelines for the appropriate use of research subjects from "underdeveloped communities."[4]

Like other human research codes, the CIOMS guidelines combine the protection of subjects' rights with protection of their welfare; as subjects become less able to protect their own rights (and therefore become more vulnerable), researchers and reviewers must increase their efforts to protect the welfare of subjects.[5] Perhaps the most important statement in these guidelines is what appears to be the injunction against using subjects in developing countries if the research could be carried out reasonably well in developed countries. Commentary to guideline 8 notes, for example, that there are diseases that rarely or never occur in economically developed countries, and that prevention and treatment research therefore needs to be conducted in the countries at risk for those diseases. The conclusion to be drawn from the substance of these guidelines is that in order for research to be ethically conducted, it must offer the potential of actual benefit to the inhabitants of that developing country.

In order for underdeveloped communities to derive potential benefit from research, they must have access to the fruits of such research. The CIOMS commentary to guideline 8 states that, "as a general rule, the sponsoring agency should ensure that, at the completion of successful testing, any product developed *will* be made reasonably available to inhabitants of the underdeveloped community in which the research was carried out: exceptions to this general requirement should be justified, and agreed to by all concerned parties before the research is begun."[6] This statement is directed at minimizing exploitation of the underdeveloped community that provides the research subjects. If developed countries use inhabitants of underdeveloped countries to create new products that would be beneficial to both the developed and the underdeveloped country, but the underdeveloped country cannot gain access to the product because of expense, then the subjects in the underdeveloped countries have been grossly exploited. As written, however, this CIOMS guideline is not strong or specific enough to prevent exploitation. Exemplifying this problem are recent short course zidovudine (AZT) studies in Africa that were approved and conducted despite the existence of the CIOMS guidelines.[7]

THE AFRICAN MATERNAL-FETAL HIV TRANSMISSION STUDIES

The goal of the short course AZT studies was to see if lower doses of the drug AZT than those used in the United States could reduce the rate of maternal-child transmission of HIV. It was well established that doses of AZT that cost $800 (not taking into account screening and other related costs) reduced maternal-fetal transmission of HIV by as much as two-thirds in the United States.[8, 9] If the developed countries had been willing to subsidize the cost of this regimen in Africa, no additional research would have been needed. But because many African countries could not afford this expense, the decision was made to attempt to see if lower (and therefore cheaper) doses would prevent maternal-fetal HIV transmission. Several impoverished countries were chosen as research sites. The justification for conducting research in those countries was not that they suffered from a disease that did not afflict people in developed countries, and not because no treatment existed, but because their impoverishment made an existing therapy unavailable to them (as long as developed countries refused to subsidize the costs).[10]

The issue, as always, is to determine the ethical acceptability of the proposed research *before* it is conducted. In a case like this, where the researchable problem exists *solely* because of economic reasons, the research hypothesis must contain an economic component. The research question should be formulated as follows:

(1) We know that a given regimen of AZT will reduce the rate of maternal-child transmission of HIV.

(2) Maternal-child transmission of HIV in many African countries is a serious problem but the effective AZT regimen is not available because it is too expensive.

(3) If an effective AZT regimen costs $X, then it will be made available in the country in which it is to be studied.

(4) Therefore, we will conduct trials in certain African countries to see if $X worth of AZT will effectively reduce maternal-child transmission of HIV in those countries.

The most important part of the development of this research question is number 3. Without knowing what dollar amount X actually represents, it is impossible to formulate a research question that can lead to any benefit to the citizens of the country in which the research is to be conducted. There is no way to determine what $X represents in the absence of committed funding. Therefore, an essential prerequisite to designing ethical research in underdeveloped countries is identifying the source and amount of funding for providing the fruits of the research to the people of the developing country in which it is to be studied as a condition of the research being approved.

If a study found, for example, that $50 worth of AZT has the same effect as $800 worth of AZT, it would greatly benefit the developed world. Developed countries, which currently spend $800 per case on drugs alone, could pay substantially less for this preventive measure, and, because the research was conducted elsewhere, none of their citizens would have been put at any risk. At the same time, if the underdeveloped country could not afford to spend $50 any more than it could spend $800, then it could not possibly derive information that would be of any benefit to its population. This is the definition of exploitation.[11]

It is only now that an effort is being made to determine how to raise the money to actually provide AZT to prevent maternal-child HIV transmission (as well as the other costly services that go with the appropriate administration of the drug) to the impoverished African countries that provided the human subjects.[12] These efforts began after parallel studies conducted in Thailand reported that lower doses of AZT reduced maternal-fetal transmission of HIV.[13] The Thai government had committed to providing the AZT before its trials began. In the African trials, however, no one "ensured" that at the completion of successful testing the product would be made reasonably available, thereby violating the CIOMS guidelines.[14] The guidelines say that there can be exceptions to this general requirement, but that exceptions must be "justified" and "agreed to by all concerned parties." It is not clear to whom the exception must be "justified" or on what grounds. Moreover, if the "concerned parties" are the sponsor and/or the investigator and the host country, they may not adequately represent the interests of the research subjects. The fact that representatives of the research community and officials of the host countries agree to exploit the population does not make the research any less exploitive.[15]

RULES FOR ETHICAL RESEARCH IN DEVELOPING COUNTRIES

We believe the standards for research in developing countries should include the following.

There should be a rebuttable presumption that researchers from developed countries will not conduct research in developing countries unless it can be shown that a direct benefit *will* be bestowed upon the residents of that country if the research proves to be successful. The person or entities proposing to conduct the study must demonstrate that there is a realistic plan, which includes identified funding, to provide the newly proven intervention to the population from which the potential pool of research subjects is to be recruited. In the absence of a realistic plan and identified funding, the population from which the research subjects will be drawn cannot derive benefit from the research. Therefore, the benefits cannot outweigh the risks, because there are, and will be, no benefits. Only by having committed funding and a plan to make a successful intervention available can it be determined that there will be sufficient benefit to justify conducting research on the target population. The distribution plan must be realistic. Where the health care infrastructure is so undeveloped that it would be impossible to deliver the intervention even if it were free, research would be unjustified in the absence of a plan to improve that country's health care delivery capabilities.

Some might argue that this standard is too strict and that it would reduce the amount of research that could be conducted in certain countries. The answer, of course, is that if the benefits of the research are not made available to the inhabitants of that country, they have lost nothing by the lack of such research. Others might argue that research in underdeveloped countries is justified if it might benefit the individual research subjects, even if it will not benefit anyone else in the population. However, research is, by definition, designed to create generalizable knowledge, and is legitimate in a developing country only if its purpose is to create generalizable knowledge that will benefit the citizens of that country. If the research only has the potential to benefit the limited number of individuals who participate in the study, it cannot offer the benefit to the underdeveloped country that legitimizes the use of its citizens as research subjects. It should be emphasized that research whose goal is to prevent or treat large populations is fundamentally public health research, and public health research makes no sense (and thus should not be done) if its benefits are limited to the small population of research subjects.

It might be argued that there is no requirement that such a plan be devised prior to conducting research in the United States, and, therefore, that by adopting such a requirement we would be imposing a higher standard for research conducted in developing countries than we do for research conducted in the United States.

This argument only further demonstrates the differences between wealthy and poor countries. The reality in the United States is that regardless of the very significant gaps in insurance and Medicaid coverage and the health care discrepancies between the rich and poor, medical interventions are relatively widely available, especially when compared to developing countries. Upon the successful completion of the research that demonstrated the effectiveness of the 076 regimen in reducing maternal-child transmission, the primary beneficiaries of this new preventive intervention in the United States were poor women and their newborns. Unlike the United States, absent a plan to pay for a new intervention and lacking the infrastructure to deliver an intervention, it is virtually guaranteed that the intervention will not be generally available in a developing country.

The more accurate analogy to the African AIDS trials would be if investigators proposed the 076 protocol in the United States knowing that only poor women would be recruited as research subjects and that, if successful, the intervention would not be made generally available to poor women. Such research would be clearly unethical. Not only would this be a gross violation of the ethical principle of distributive justice, it would be a violation of the regulatory obligation of the equitable selection of subjects.[16]

A further objection is that one cannot always trust what a government or another potential funder promises. What is to prevent the promisor from reneging? The answer is, nothing. One can try to expose the funder to embarrassment and other pressures that might cause it to live up to the promise upon which researchers and subjects relied. However, the potential unethical behavior in the future by the funder is no excuse for not having a realistic plan at the outset. Furthermore, if we take this obligation

seriously, this should only occur once per funder. After reneging once, they cannot be relied upon again to justify research in the future.

An additional objection to our position is that it will restrict access to new interventions because once a new intervention is developed, the price will come down and therefore the intervention will become available to the people of the impoverished country. The answer is to ask those who control the pricing of interventions if this will be the case in any particular instance. One could have asked Glaxo if it would reduce its price once it was shown that lower doses of AZT were effective. If the answer is yes, one can proceed. If the answer is no, or "we have not decided," there seems to be no justification to proceed if the current price would significantly restrict availability. There is nothing magical about pricing. Pricing is in the absolute control of manufacturers and there is no need to guess or speculate about what will happen to price. Indeed, this objection to our argument would justify conducting the full 076 trial itself in developing countries. The price *might* come down enough so that determining the efficacy of short course AZT regimens might not be needed at all. Such speculation should not be sufficient to put subjects at risk.

Finally, it might be argued that there are diseases that only affect people in developing countries for which there are no effective treatments, but that the treatments that might be discovered could be expensive. The argument continues that it is not right to fail to develop treatments that could benefit some affected people because it will not be available to most affected people. This objection raises quite a different issue from the one addressed in this article. The impetus for such research is the absence of effective treatment and not the absence of economic resources. We have discussed research intended to determine whether effective but unaffordable interventions would work if used in lower, less expensive dosages. The researchable issue arises from an economic circumstance. The only way such research could offer any benefit is by "curing" the economic problem by establishing that the less expensive form of the intervention will be affordable and available. Absent knowledge of financial resources, one might well be creating a new unaffordable, and therefore useless, intervention. In contrast, in the case in which one is developing a new intervention, not because of poverty, but because no known effective intervention exists, and the disease is prevalent in a particular geographic area, the issue is quite different. In such a case one is not conducting research to try to "cure" the effects of poverty but rather because of the need to create new knowledge to treat a currently untreatable disease. However, even this case may raise problems similar to the ones addressed here. If one were to try to develop an intervention for such a condition and chose research subjects from impoverished segments of a society, knowing that only the richest segment of that society could benefit from that intervention, such subject selection would be unethical for many of the reasons we have discussed.

Our proposal to require researchers and their funders to develop realistic plans to make their interventions available to the relevant population of the developing country in which the research is proposed should not be controversial. It is well accepted in principle not only by groups like CIOMS, but by the funders of many of the African HIV trials, including the Centers for Disease Control and Prevention and the National Institutes of Health.[17] The principle is often honored in the breach, however. Research funders who hope that their studies will yield beneficial knowledge may neglect the steps necessary to ensure that the benefits will be made available. Ethical codes have not been sufficiently specific or enforceable to protect research subjects from exploitation. It is essential to replace vague promises with realistic plans that must be reviewed and approved before the research commences.

In at least one other instance it has been suggested that economic issues be addressed in the review of proposed research projects. The U.S. National Research Council's Committee on Human Genome Diversity recommended that "Arrangements regarding financial interests in the products or outcomes of the research should be negotiated as *part of the original project review* and informed-consent process."[18]

It is essential that the wealthier countries of the world use their resources, both financial and technological, to help resolve the health problems that afflict the poor of the world. Doing so will undoubtedly require research. But research is a means to solving health problems, not an end in itself. The goal must be to create interventions that will benefit the people of the countries in which the research is conducted. They will benefit only if the knowledge gained produces interventions that are affordable and accessible. This needs to be determined as a condition of approval before research is conducted so that limited research funds are not wasted, and research subjects are not drawn from populations that will not be able to benefit from the research.

REFERENCES

1 Lisa Belkin, "The Clues Are in the Blood," *New York Times Magazine,* 26 April 1998.

2 Michael Grodin and Leonard Glantz, eds., *Children as Research Subjects: Science, Ethics, and Law* (New York: Oxford University Press, 1994).

3 Wendy K. Mariner, "Distinguishing 'Exploitable' from 'Vulnerable' Populations: When Consent Is Not the Issue," in *Ethics and Research on Human Subjects: Proceedings,* ed. Zbigniew Bankowski and Robert J. Levine (Geneva: CIOMS, 1993), pp. 44–55.

4 Zbigniew Bankowski and Robert J. Levine. eds., *Ethics and Research on Human Subjects: International Guidelines* (Geneva: CIOMS. 1993), pp. 25–32. 43–46.

5 Sharon Perley, Sev S. Fluss, Zbigniew Bankowski, and Francoise Simon. "The Nuremberg Code: An International Overview," in *The Nazi Doctors and the Nuremberg Code,* ed. George J. Annas and Michael A. Grodin (New York: Oxford University Press, 1992), pp. 149–73.

6 Bankowski and Levine, *Ethics and Research,* p. 26. Emphasis added.

7 George Annas and Michael Grodin, "Human Rights and Maternal-Fetal HIV Transmission Prevention Trials in Africa," *American Journal of Public Health,* 88, no. 4 (1998): 560–63.

8 Edward Connor, Rhoda Sperling, Richard Gelber et al., "Reduction of Maternal-Infant Transmission of Human Immunodeficiency Virus Type 1 with Zidovudine Treatment," *NEJM* 331 (1994): 1173–80.

9 "Recommendation of the U.S. Public Health Service Task Force on the Use of Zidovudine to Reduce Prenatal Transmission of Human Immunodeficiency Virus," *MMWR Morbidity and Mortality Weekly Reports* 43 (1994): 1–20.

10 Harold Varmus and David Satcher, "Ethical Complexities of Conducting Research in Developing Countries," *NEJM* 337 (1997): 1003–1005.

11 The per capita health care expenditures of most of the African countries involved in mother-to-child HIV transmission prevention trials range from $5 to $22 U.S. *World Bank Sector Strategy Health Nutrition and Population,* 1997.

12 M. Bunce, "Chirac Seeks Worldwide Relief for AIDS in Africa," *Boston Globe,* 8 December 1997.

13 "Administration of Zidovudine During Late Pregnancy and Delivery to Prevent Perinatal HIV Transmission—Thailand 1996–1998," *MMWR Morbidity and Mortality Weekly Reports* 47, no. 8 (1998): 151–54. The editorial note states that "to implement these findings, ministries of health, donor agencies, and other interested agents *should* develop policies and practices to strengthen access to prenatal care, testing and counseling for HIV infections, and provision of ZDV for HIV-infected pregnant women."

14 Bankowski and Levine, *Ethics and Research,* p. 45.

15 As the National Research Council's Committee on Human Genome Diversity properly put it, in the context of research on human subjects, "[s]ensitivity to the special practices and beliefs of a community cannot be used as a justification for violating universal human rights." Committee on Human Genetic Diversity, *Evaluating Human Genetic Diversity* (Washington, D.C.: National Academy Press, 1997), p. 65.

16 45 CFR 46.111(a)(3).

17 Varmus and Satcher, "Ethical Complexities of Conducting Research in Developing Countries."

18 *Evaluating Human Genetic Diversity,* at pp. 55–68. Emphasis added.

ETHICAL ISSUES IN CLINICAL TRIALS IN DEVELOPING COUNTRIES
Baruch Brody

Brody addresses three moral criticisms of recent clinical trials in developing countries that tested the efficacy of short-course AZT regimens in reducing maternal-fetal transmission of HIV: (1) that subjects who received placebos were treated unjustly; (2) that subjects' dire circumstances coerced them into agreeing to participate in the trials; and (3) that the developing countries in question were exploited insofar as they would not have access to the AZT regimens under study even if they proved effective (as argued by Glantz et al.). In response to the first criticism, Brody argues that the trials probably met the following appropriate standard of justice: "all participants in the study, including those in the control group, should not be denied any treatment *that should otherwise be available to [them] in light of the practical realities of health care resources available in the country in question*." He responds to the second criticism by analyzing the concept of coercion and arguing that subjects were not coerced on any reasonable construal of this concept. Regarding the third criticism, Brody suggests that legitimate concerns about exploitation will be met if the subjects themselves—not necessarily the broader local community—are provided access to effective treatment following the study.

Since the publication of the results of AIDS Clinical Trials Group (ACTG) 076, it has been known that an extensive regimen of Zidovudine provided to the mother and to the newborn can drastically reduce (25.5 to 8.3%) the vertical transmission of HIV.[1] Unfortunately, the regimen in question is quite expensive and beyond the means of most developing countries, some of which are the countries most in

need of effective techniques for reducing vertical transmission. This realization led to a series of important clinical trials designed to test the effectiveness of less extensive and less expensive regimens of antiretroviral drugs. These trials were conducted by researchers from developed countries in the developing countries which were in need of these less expensive regimens.

These new trials have been very successful. The Thai CDC trial showed a 50% reduction (18.9 to 9.4%) in transmission from a much shorter antepartum regimen of Zidovudine combined with a more modest intrapartum regimen.[2] The PETRA trial showed that Zidovudine and Lamivudine provided in modest intrapartum and postpartum regimens also significantly reduced transmission, whether or not they were provided antepartum.[3] There was a trend to more reduction of transmission if they were provided in a short antepartum regimen (16.5 to 7.8%) than if they were not (16.5 to 10.8%). Most crucially, there was no reduction (16.5 to 15.7%) if they were not provided postpartum. Finally, a single dose of nevirapine provided intrapartum and postpartum was shown in HIVNET 012 to significantly reduce transmission (21.3 to 11.9%).[4] In all cases except HIVNET 012, the control group received only a placebo. In HIVNET 012, the control group received a modest regimen of intrapartum and postpartum Zidovudine.

As a result of these trials, developing countries with some financial capabilities have the opportunity to drastically reduce vertical transmission by proven less expensive regimens. This constitutes an important contribution of these trials. Unfortunately, the poorest developing countries (including some in which these trials have been run) may not be able to afford even these shorter regimens unless the drugs in question are priced far less expensively for those countries. Efforts have begun to make that possible.[5]

There have been many critics of these trials who have argued that they were unethical. Some have gone on to attempt to explain how the information might have been obtained in other more ethical trials while others have not. My focus in this paper is not on that question. Instead, *I want to focus on the arguments offered in support of the claim that these trials were unethical.* I see the critics as advancing three very different criticisms, although the critics often do not carefully distinguish them. We will do so to enable each criticism to be analyzed. The *first criticism* is that an *injustice was done to the control group* in each of these trials (with perhaps the exception of HIVNET 012) since they were denied proven effective therapy as they only received a placebo. The *second criticism* is that the *participants in the trial were coerced* into participating, and did not give voluntary consent, because they had no real choice about participating since antiretroviral

therapy was otherwise unavailable to them. The *third criticism* is that the *countries in question were exploited* by the investigators from the developed countries since they were testing the effectiveness of regimens that would not be available after the trial to the citizens of the countries in which the trials were conducted.

THE JUSTICE OF THE USE OF THE PLACEBO CONTROL GROUP

The scientific importance of the use of concurrent placebo control groups is well illustrated by the PETRA trial. If there had been no such control group, and the various regimens had been compared to the historical control group in ACTG 076, then the intrapartum only arm would have been judged a success, since its transmission rate was only 15.7% as compared to the 25.5% transmission rate in the control group in ACTG 076. But it actually was no better than the placebo control group in PETRA (16.5%). When the rate of transmission varies from one setting to another, you really cannot use historical control groups. Despite this scientific value, the critics have argued that it was wrong to use a placebo control arm because the patients in that arm were being denied a proven therapy (the 076 regimen) and were being offered nothing in its place.[6] The critics claim that this did not meet the standard found in *earlier versions* of the Declaration of Helsinki: "In any medical study, every patient, including those of a control group, if any, should be assured of the best proven diagnostic and therapeutic method."[7]

Defenders of these trials quite properly note that none of the participants in these trials would otherwise have received any antiretroviral therapy, so nothing was being denied to them that they would otherwise have received. How then, ask the defenders, can the members of the control group have been treated unjustly? This led to a proposed, very controversial and eventually rejected, revision of the Declaration of Helsinki which read: "In any biomedical research protocol every patient-subject, including those of a control group, if any, should be assured that he or she will not be denied access to the best proven diagnostic, prophylactic, or therapeutic method that would otherwise be available to him or her."[8] The point is then that the justice or injustice of what is done to the control group depends on what the members of that group *would* have received if the trial had not been conducted.

While the reality of what the members of the control group would have received is obviously relevant, I am not satisfied that this proposed revision would have properly taken that into account. Would it be just, for example, to use such a placebo control group in a trial in a developed country where the antiretroviral therapy is widely available except to members of some persecuted minority, from whom the control group is drawn? They *would* not have received the treatment if the trial had not been conducted, although they *should* have, given the resources available in the developed country. Their use in a placebo control group is not therefore justified. The proposed revision made too much reference to what would have occurred and not enough to what should have occurred.

A recent workshop proposed instead that "study participants should be assured the highest standard of care practically attainable in the country in which the trial is being carried out."[9] This seems better, although it may suggest too much. Suppose that the treatment is practically attainable but only by inappropriately cutting corners on other forms of health care which may have a higher priority. I would suggest, therefore, that the normative nature of the standard be made explicit. It would then read that all participants in the study, including those in the control group, should not be denied any treatment *that should otherwise be available to him or her in light of the practical realities of health care resources available in the country in question.* The question for IRBs reviewing proposals for such research is then precisely the question of justice.

On that standard, the trials in question were probably not unjust, although there is some debate about the Thai CDC trial in light of donated resources that became available in Thailand between its being planned and its being implemented.[10] Such trials will be harder to justify in the future given the current availability of proven much less expensive therapies which should be available even in some of the poorest countries. It is of interest to note that HIVNET 012 was not a placebo-controlled trial, but it was a superiority trial, and active controlled trials are less problematic scientifically when they are superiority trials. That may well be the way future transmission trials will be run.

COERCIVE OFFERS

It has been suggested by other critics that the participants in these trials were coerced into participating because of their desperation. "The very desperation of women with no alternatives to protect their children from HIV infection can be extremely coercive," argue one set of critics.[11] One of the requirements of an ethical trial is that the participants voluntarily agree to participate, and how can their agreement to participate be voluntary if it was coerced?

This line of thinking is analogous to the qualms that many have about paying research subjects substantial sums of money for their participation in research. Such inducements are often rejected on the grounds that they are coercive, because they are too good to refuse. The ICH [International Conference on Harmonization] Guidelines for Good Clinical Practice is one of many standards which incorporate this approach when it stipulates that the "IRB/IEC should review both the amount and method of payment to subjects to assure that neither present problems of coercion or undue influences on the research subject."[12]

Normally, coercion involves a threat to put someone below their baseline unless they cooperate with the demands of the person issuing the threat.[13] As the researchers were not going to do anything to those who chose not to participate, they were clearly not threatening them. Further evidence of this comes from the reflection that threats are unwelcome to the parties being threatened, and there is no reason to suppose that the potential subjects saw the request to participate as something unwelcome. Even the critics recognize this. The potential subjects were being offered an opportunity that might improve their situation. This was an offer "too good to refuse," not a threat.

Should we expand the concept of coercion to include these very favorable offers? There are several reasons for thinking that we should not. First, it is widely believed that offering people valuable new opportunities is desirable. Moreover, the individuals in question want to receive these offers, and denying them the opportunity to receive them seems paternalistic or moralistic.[14] It is important that participants understand that what they are being offered is a chance to receive a treatment that may reduce transmission (since this is a randomized placebo-controlled trial of a new regimen), and ensuring that is essential for the consent to be informed. As long as care is taken to ensure that this information is conveyed in a culturally sensitive fashion, and is understood, then there seems to be little reason to be concerned about coercion simply because a good opportunity is being offered to those with few opportunities.

A colleague and I are currently working on one residual concern in this area. It has to do with studies in which there is a potential for long-term harms to subjects which they inappropriately discount because the very substantial short-term benefits cloud their judgment. This may be a ground for concern in some cases, but it is difficult to see how it would apply to the vertical transmission trials. For those trials, it is appropriate to conclude that concerns about coercion were unfounded.

EXPLOITATION OF SUBJECTS

The final criticism of the trials is that they are exploitative of developing countries and their citizens because the interventions in question, even if proven successful, will not be available in these countries. To quote one of the critics: "To use a population as research subjects because of its poverty and its inability to obtain care, and then to not use that knowledge for the direct benefit of that population, is the very definition of exploitation. This exploitation is made worse by the fact that richer nations will unquestionably benefit from this research . . . [they] will begin to use these lower doses, thereby receiving economic benefit."[15]

There are really two claims being advanced in that quotation. The second, that the developed countries ran these trials to discover cheaper ways of treating their own citizens, is very implausible since pregnant women in developed countries are receiving even more expensive cocktails of drugs both to treat the woman and to reduce transmission. The crucial issue is whether the trials are exploitative of the developing countries.

There seems to be a growing consensus that they are exploitative unless certain conditions about future availability in the country in question are met. The Council for International Organizations of Medical Sciences (CIOMS) is the source of this movement, as it declared in its 1992 guidelines that "as a general rule, the initiating agency should insure that, at the completion of successful testing, any products developed will be made reasonably available to residents of the host community or country."[16] A slightly weaker version of this requirement was adopted by a recent workshop which concluded that "studies are only appropriate if there is a reasonable likelihood that the populations in which they are carried out stand to benefit from successful results."[17]

This growing consensus is part of what lies behind the effort to secure these benefits by negotiating more favorable prices for the use of the tested drugs in developing countries. It seems highly desirable that this goal be achieved. But I want to suggest that it should be viewed as an aspiration, rather than a requirement, and that a different, more modest requirement must be met to avoid charges of exploitation.

A good analysis of exploitation is that it is a wrong done to individuals who do not receive a fair share of the benefits produced by an activity in which they take part, even if they receive some benefit.[18] This is why a mutually beneficial activity, one from which both parties will be better off, can still be exploitative if one of the parties uses their greater bargaining power to harvest most of the benefits and the other party agrees because they need whatever modest benefit is being left for them.

As we apply this concept to the trials in question, we need to ask who needs to be protected from being exploited by the trials in question. It would seem that it is the participants. Are they getting a fair share of the benefits from the trial if it proves successful? This is a particularly troubling question when we consider those in the control group, whose major benefit from participation may have been an unrealized possibility of getting treated. If we judge that the participants have not received enough, then it is they who must receive more. An obvious suggestion is that they be guaranteed access to any regimen proved efficacious in any future pregnancies (or perhaps even that they be granted access to antiretroviral therapy for their own benefit). This would be analogous to familiar concepts of subjects receiving continued access to treatment after their participation in a trial is completed.

I certainly support every reasonable effort to increase access to treatments which will reduce vertical transmission. But imposing the types of community-wide requirements that have been suggested, but not necessarily justified if the above analysis is correct, may prevent important trials from being run because of the potential expense. Such proposals should be treated as moral aspirations, and exploitation should be avoided by focusing on what is owed to the subjects who have participated in the trials. It is they, after all, who are primarily at risk for being exploited.

These observations are about research in developing countries in general, and not just about research on vertical transmission. Three lessons have emerged. The standard for when a placebo control group is justified is a normative standard (what they should have received if they were not in the trial) rather than a descriptive standard (what they would have received if they were not in the trial). Coercion is not a serious concern in trials simply because attractive offers are made to the subjects. Legitimate concerns about exploiting subjects should be addressed by ensuring their future treatment, rather than by asking what will happen in their community at large.

NOTES

1 E. M. Connor, R. S. Sperling, R. Gelber, et al., "Reduction of Maternal-Infant Transmission of Human Immunodeficiency Virus Type I with Zidovudine Treatment," *New England Journal of Medicine,* 331 (1984): 1173–80.

2 N. Shaffer, R. Chuachoowong, P. A. Mock, et al., "Short-Course Zidovudine for Perinatal HIV Transmission in Bangkok, Thailand: A Randomised Controlled Trial," *Lancet,* 353 (1999): 773–80.

3 Conference data cited in K. DeCock, M. Fowler, E. Mercier, et al., "Prevention of Mother-to-Child HIV Transmission in Resource Poor Countries," *JAMA,* 283 (2000): 1175–82.

4 L. A. Guay, P. Musoke, T. Fleming, et al., "Intrapartum and Neonatal Single-Dose Nevirapine Compared with Zidovudine for Prevention of Mother-to-Child Transmission of HIV-1 in Kampala, Uganda," *Lancet,* 354 (2000): 795–802.

5 P. Brown, "Cheaper AIDS Drugs Due for Third World," *Nature,* 405 (2000): 263.

6 P. Lurie and S. M. Wolfe, "Unethical Trials of Interventions to Reduce Perinatal Transmission of the Human Immunodeficiency Virus in Developing Countries," *New England Journal of Medicine,* 337 (1997): 853–56.

7 World Medical Association, Declaration of Helsinki, Principle 11.3.

8 "Proposed Revision of the Declaration of Helsinki," *Bulletin of Medical Ethics,* 18–21 (1999).

9 Perinatal HIV Intervention Research in Developing Countries Workshop Participants, "Science Ethics and the Future of Research into Maternal Infant Transmission of HIV-1," *Lancet,* 353 (1999): 832–35.

10 P. Phanuphak, "Ethical Issues in Studies in Thailand of the Vertical Transmission of HIV," *New England Journal of Medicine,* 338 (1998): 834–35.

11 E. Tafesse and T. Murphy, Letter, *New England Journal of Medicine,* 338 (1998): 838.

12 ICH, *Guideline for Good Clinical Practice* (Geneva: IFPMA, 1996), guideline 3.1.8.

13 R. Nozick, "Coercion." In Morgenbesser S., ed. *Philosophy, Science, and Method* (New York: St. Martin's, 1969).

14 M. Wilkinson and A. Moore, "Inducement in Research," *Bioethics,* 11 (1997): 373–89.

15 I. Glantz and M. Grodin, Letter, *New England Journal of Medicine,* 338 (1998): 839.

16 CIOMS, *International Ethical Guidelines for Biomedical Research Involving Subjects* (Geneva: CIOMS, 1992), 68.

17 Perinatal HIV Intervention Research in Developing Countries Workshop Participants, "Science Ethics and the Future of Research into Maternal Infant Transmission of HIV-1," *Lancet,* 353 (1999): 832–35.

18 A. Wertheimer, *Exploitation* (Princeton, N.J.: Princeton University Press, 1996).

FAIR BENEFITS FOR RESEARCH IN DEVELOPING COUNTRIES
Participants in the 2001 Conference on Ethical Aspects of Research in Developing Countries

This joint statement by participants in a 2001 conference challenges the thesis (embraced by Glantz et al.) that, in order to avoid exploitation, interventions proven safe and effective through research in developing countries must be made "reasonably available" in those countries. After analyzing the concept of exploitation for the sake of explicitness, the authors argue that the reasonable availability requirement fails to avoid exploitation in many cases and wrongly regards interventions under investigation as the only relevant sort of benefits. In place of the reasonable availability requirement, the authors offer a Fair Benefits framework, which incorporates principles of collaborative partnership (between investigators and the local population), transparency (regarding agreements reached and community consultation), and fair benefits. The fair benefits principle distinguishes benefits to trial participants and benefits to the local population both during and following research. Extending well beyond the benefits of medical interventions validated in a trial, the benefits identified as appropriate to consider in avoiding exploitation include health services unrelated to the trial, public health measures, employment, and development of a community's research or medical care capacity.

Collaborative, multinational clinical research, especially between developed and developing countries, has been the subject of controversy. Much of this attention has focused on the standard of care used in randomized trials. Much less discussed, but probably more important in terms of its impact on health, is the claim that, in order to avoid exploitation, interventions proven safe and effective through research in developing countries should be made "reasonably available" in those countries.[1,2]

This claim was first emphasized by the Council for International Organizations of Medical Sciences: "As a general rule, the sponsoring agency should agree in advance of the research that any product developed through such research will be made reasonably available to the inhabitants of the host community or country at the completion of successful testing."[1] The reasonable availability requirement has received broad support, with disagreement focusing on two elements. First, how strong or explicit should the commitment to provide the drug or vaccine be at the initiation of the research study? Some suggest that advanced discussions without assurances are sufficient, while others require advance guarantees that include identifiable funding and distribution networks.[2–6] Second, to whom must the drugs and vaccines be made available? Should the commitment extend only to the participants in the study, the community from which

From *Science* 298 (2002), pp. 2133–2134. Reprinted with permission from AAAS.

participants have been recruited, the entire country, or the region of the world? Although these disagreements have ethical and practical implications, there is a deeper question about whether reasonable availability is necessary, or the best way, to avoid exploitation in developing countries.[7]

What constitutes exploitation? A exploits B when B receives an unfair level of benefits as a result of B's interactions with A.[8] The fairness of the benefits B receives depends on the burdens that B bears as a result of the interaction, and the benefits that A and others receive as a result of B's participation. Fairness is the crucial aspect, not equality of benefits. Although being vulnerable may increase the chances for exploitation, it is neither necessary nor sufficient for exploitation.

The potential for clinical research to exploit populations is not a major concern in developed countries since there are processes, albeit haphazard and imperfect, for ensuring that interventions proven effective are introduced into the healthcare system and benefit the general population.[9] In contrast, target populations in developing countries often lack access to regular health care, political power, and an understanding of research. They may be exposed to the risks of research, while access to the benefits of new, effective drugs and vaccines goes predominantly to people in developed countries and the profits go to the biopharmaceutical industry. This situation fails to provide fair benefits and thus constitutes the paradigm of exploitation.[1,2,5,6,10,11]

By focusing on a particular type of benefit, the reasonable availability requirement fails to avoid exploitation in many cases. First, and most importantly, the ethical concern embedded in exploitation is about the amount or level of benefits received and not the type of benefits.[8] Reasonable availability fails to ensure a fair share of benefits; for instance, it may provide for too little benefit when risks are high or benefits to the sponsors great. Moreover, it applies only to phase III research that leads to an effective intervention; it is inapplicable to phase I and II and unsuccessful phase III studies.[12] Consequently, reasonable availability fails to protect against the potential of exploitation in a great deal of research conducted in developing countries. Furthermore, reasonable availability embodies a narrow concept of benefits. It does not consider other potential benefits of research in developing countries, including training of health-care or research personnel, construction of health-care facilities and other physical infrastructure, and provision of public health measures and health services beyond those required as part of the research trial. Finally, insisting on reasonable availability precludes the community's deciding which benefits it prefers.

Reasonable availability should not be imposed as an absolute ethical requirement for research in developing countries without affirmation by the countries themselves. The authors,[13] who are from developed countries and African developing countries, have proposed an alternative to reasonable availability to avoid exploitation in developing countries: Fair Benefits. This framework would supplement the usual conditions for ethical conduct of research trials, such as independent review by an institutional review board or research ethics committee and individual informed consent. In particular, Fair Benefits relies on three widely accepted ethical conditions. First, the research must address a health problem of the developing country population, although, as with HIV/AIDS, it could also be relevant to other populations.[7] Second, the research objectives, not vulnerability of the population, must provide a strong justification for conducting the research in this population. For instance, the population may have a high incidence of the disease being studied or high transmission rates

of infection necessary to evaluate a vaccine. Third, the research must pose few risks to the participants, or the benefits to them clearly must outweigh the risks.[7]

The Fair Benefits framework requires satisfaction of the following three additional fundamental principles to protect developing communities from exploitation.

Fair benefits. In assessing whether studies offer a fair level of benefits, the population could consider benefits from both the conduct and results of research. Among potential benefits to research participants are additional diagnostic tests, distribution of medications and vaccinations, and emergency evacuation services. Research might also provide collateral health services to members of the population not enrolled in the research, such as determining disease prevalence and drug resistance patterns, or providing interventions such as antibiotics for respiratory infections or the digging of boreholes for clean water. Conducting research usually entails the benefits of employment and enhanced economic activity for the population as well.

Reasonable availability of a safe and effective intervention may provide an important benefit for the population after the completion of some research trials. Alternatively, other postresearch benefits might include capacity development, such as enhancing health-care or research facilities, providing critical equipment, other physical infrastructure such as roads or vehicles, training of health-care and research staff, and training of individuals in research ethics. Furthermore, any single research trial could be an isolated endeavor or form part of a long-term collaboration between the population and the researchers. Long-term collaboration embodies engagement with and a commitment to the population; it can also provide the population with long-term training, employment, investment, and additional research on other health issues. Finally, profits from direct sales of proven interventions or from intellectual property rights can be shared with the developing country. It is not necessary to provide each of these benefits; the ethical imperative is for a fair level of benefits overall—not an equal level.

Collaborative partnership. Collaborative partnership means that researchers must engage the population in developing, evaluating, and benefiting from the research. Currently, there is no shared, international standard of fairness. In part this is because of conflicting conceptions of international distributive justice.[14,15] Ultimately, the determination of whether the benefits are fair and worth the risks cannot be entrusted to people outside the population, no matter how well intentioned. They may be ill-informed about the health, social, and economic context and are unlikely to appreciate the importance of the proposed benefits to the host community. The relevant population for the Fair Benefits framework is the community that is involved with the researchers, bears the burdens of the research, and would be the potential victims of exploitation. There is no justification for including an entire region or every citizen of a country in the distribution of benefits and decision-making, unless the whole region or country is involved in the research study. To avoid exploitation, it is the village, tribe, neighborhood, or province whose members are approached for enrollment, whose health-care personnel are recruited to staff the research teams, whose physical facilities and social networks are utilized to conduct the study who must receive the benefits from research and determine what constitutes a fair level of benefits.

The population's decision about whether research is worthwhile and fair must be free and uncoerced.[16] Practically, this means that a decision not to participate in the proposed research is a realistic alternative. Deciding if a population can really refuse will not be easy. Nonetheless, proceeding with a research trial requires that the population in which it is to be conducted genuinely supports it.

Transparency. The lack of an international standard for fairness and the disparity in bargaining power between populations and researchers in developing countries and sponsors and researchers from developed countries means that even in the presence of collaborative partnership, the community might agree to an unfair level of benefits. The Fair Benefits framework can be used to catalog the array of benefits that are provided in different research studies (see Table, this page). An independent

body, such as the World Health Organization, could establish a central and publicly accessible repository of all the formal and informal benefit agreements of previous studies. This repository would allow populations, researchers, and others to make independent and transparent comparisons of the level of the benefits provided in particular studies to ensure their fairness.

To further facilitate transparency, this body should develop a program of community consultations that actively informs the communities, researchers, and others in developing countries likely to participate in research about previously negotiated agreements. These consultations would also provide forums in

---

The Fair Benefits Framework*

Fair Benefits

Benefits to Participants During the Research

Improvements to health and health care
Collateral health services unnecessary for research study

Benefits to Population During the Research

Collateral health services unnecessary for research study
Public health measures
Employment and economic activity

Benefits to Population After the Research

Reasonable availability of effective intervention
Research and medical care capacity development
Public health measures
Long-term research collaboration
Sharing of financial rewards from reseach results

Collaborative Partnership

Community involvement at all stages
Free, uncoerced decision-making by population bearing the burdens of the research

Transparency

Central, publicly accessible repository of benefits agreements
Process of community consultations

*It is not necessary to provide each benefit.

which all interested parties could deliberate on the fairness of the agreements. Over time, such a central repository and the community consultations would generate a collection of critically evaluated benefits agreements that would become a kind of "case law" generating shared standards of fair benefits.

REFERENCES AND NOTES

1 *International Ethical Guidelines for Biomedical Research Involving Human Subjects* [Council for International Organizations of Medical Science (CIOMS), Geneva, 1993], guidelines 8 and 15.

2 P. Wilmshurst, *B.M.J.* **314**, 840 (1997).

3 Joint United National Program on HIV/AIDS (UNAIDS), *Ethical Considerations in HIV Preventive Vaccine Research* (UNAIDS, Geneva, 2000).

4 National Bioethics Advisory Commission, *Ethical and Policy Issues in International Research: Clinical Trials in Developing Countries* (Government Printing Office, Washington, DC, April 2001).

5 L. H. Glantz *et al.*, *Hastings Center Rep.* **28**, 38 (1998).

6 G. J. Annas, M. A. Grodin, *Am. J. Public Health* **88**, 560 (1998).

7 E. J. Emanuel, D. Wendler, C. Grady, *JAMA* **283**, 2701 (2000).

8 A. Wertheimer, *Exploitation* (Princeton Univ. Press, Princeton, NJ, 1999), chap. 1.

9 N. Black, *B.M.J.* **323**, 275 (2001).

10 M. Angell, *N. Engl. J. Med.* **337**, 847 (1997).

11 H. T. Shapiro, E. M. Meslin, *N. Engl. J. Med.* **345**, 139 (2001).

12 http://clinicaltrials.gov/ct/gui/info/

13 Meeting held 26 to 28 March 2001 in Blantyre, Malawi. It was cosponsored by the Department of Clinical Bioethics and NIAID of the NIH (USA) and the University of Malawi College of Medicine. Author affiliations at www.sciencemag.org/cgi/content/full/298/5601/2133/DC1

14 J. Rawls, *The Law of Peoples* (Harvard Univ. Press, Cambridge, MA, 1999).

15 T. Pogge, *World Poverty and Human Rights* (Polity Press, Cambridge, UK, 2002), chap. 1 and 4.

16 A. Wertheimer, *Coercion* (Princeton Univ. Press, Princeton, NJ, 1987), chap. 1, 11, and 12.

17 We thank D. R. Broadhead, D. Brock, and J. Killen for support and comments.

ANIMAL RESEARCH

THE CASE FOR THE USE OF ANIMALS IN BIOMEDICAL RESEARCH
Carl Cohen

Identifying himself as a speciesist, Cohen defends the extensive use of animals in biomedical research. Against the "animal rights" view, he contends that animals are incapable of moral agency and therefore lack moral rights. Against Peter Singer's view, which extends to animals the principle of equal consideration of interests, he maintains that animals' interests are not due equal consideration because animals lack the moral standing of humans; speciesism is therefore not analogous to racism and sexism. Indeed, Cohen argues, we have an obligation to expand animal research both to protect potential human subjects and to benefit future patients with advances in biomedicine. In his view, our obligations toward animals (e.g., not to be cruel to them) are minimal and do not compare in importance with our obligations to beings who have rights—namely, human beings.

Using animals as research subjects in medical investigations is widely condemned on two grounds:

first, because it wrongly violates the *rights* of animals,[1] and second, because it wrongly imposes on sentient creatures much avoidable *suffering*.[2] Neither of these arguments is sound. The first relies on a mistaken understanding of rights; the second relies on a mistaken calculation of consequences. Both deserve definitive dismissal.

WHY ANIMALS HAVE NO RIGHTS

A right, properly understood, is a claim, or potential claim, that one party may exercise against another. The target against whom such a claim may be registered can be a single person, a group, a community, or (perhaps) all humankind. The content of rights claims also varies greatly: repayment of loans, nondiscrimination by employers, noninterference by the state, and so on. To comprehend any genuine right fully, therefore, we must know *who* holds the right, *against whom* it is held, and *to what* it is a right.

Alternative sources of rights add complexity. Some rights are grounded in constitutional law (e.g., the right of an accused to trial by jury); some rights are moral but give no legal claims (e.g., my right to your keeping the promise you gave me); and some rights (e.g., against theft or assault) are rooted both in morals and in law.

The differing targets, contents, and sources of rights, and their inevitable conflict, together weave a tangled web. Notwithstanding all such complications, this much is clear about rights in general: they are in every case claims, or potential claims, within a community of moral agents. Rights arise, and can be intelligibly defended, only among beings who actually do, or can, make moral claims against one another. Whatever else rights may be, therefore, they are necessarily human; their possessors are persons, human beings.

The attributes of human beings from which this moral capability arises have been described variously by philosophers, both ancient and modern: the inner consciousness of a free will (Saint Augustine[3]); the grasp, by human reason, of the binding character of moral law (Saint Thomas[4]); the self-conscious participation of human beings in an objective ethical order (Hegel[5]); human membership in an organic moral community (Bradley[6]); the development of the human self through the consciousness of other moral selves (Mead[7]); and the underivative, intuitive cognition of the rightness of an action (Prichard[8]). Most influential has been Immanuel Kant's emphasis on the universal human possession of a uniquely moral will and the autonomy its use entails.[9] Humans confront choices that are purely moral; humans—but certainly not dogs or mice—lay down moral laws, for others and for themselves. Human beings are self-legislative, morally *autonomous.*

Animals (that is, nonhuman animals, the ordinary sense of that word) lack this capacity for free moral judgment. They are not beings of a kind capable of exercising or responding to moral claims. Animals therefore have no rights, and they can have none. This is the core of the argument about the alleged rights of animals. The holders of rights must have the capacity to comprehend rules of duty, governing all including themselves. In applying such rules, the holders of rights must recognize possible conflicts between what is in their own interest and what is just. Only in a community of beings capable of self-restricting moral judgments can the concept of a right be correctly invoked.

Humans have such moral capacities. They are in this sense self-legislative, are members of communities governed by moral rules, and do possess rights. Animals do not have such moral capacities. They are not morally self-legislative, cannot possibly be members of a truly moral community, and therefore cannot possess rights. In conducting research on animal subjects, therefore, we do not violate their rights, because they have none to violate.

To animate life, even in its simplest forms, we give a certain natural reverence. But the possession of rights presupposes a moral status not attained by the vast majority of living things. We must not infer, therefore, that a live being has, simply in being alive, a "right" to its life. The assertion that all animals, only because they are alive and have interests, also possess the "right to life"[10] is an abuse of that phrase, and wholly without warrant.

It does not follow from this, however, that we are morally free to do anything we please to animals. Certainly not. In our dealings with animals, as in our dealings with other human beings, we have obligations that do not arise from claims against us based on rights. Rights entail obligations, but many of the things one ought to do are in no way tied to another's entitlement. Rights and obligations are not reciprocals of one another, and it is a serious mistake to suppose that they are.

Illustrations are helpful. Obligations may arise from internal commitments made: physicians have obligations to their patients not grounded merely in their patients' rights. Teachers have such obligations to their students, shepherds to their dogs, and cowboys to their horses. Obligations may arise from differences of status: adults owe special care when playing with young children, and children owe special care when playing with young pets. Obligations may arise from special relationships: the payment of my son's college tuition is something to which he may have no right, although it may be my obligation to bear the burden if I reasonably can; my dog has no right to daily exercise and veterinary care, but I do have the obligation to provide these things for her. Obligations may arise from particular acts or circumstances: one may be obliged to another for a special kindness done, or obliged to put an animal out of its misery in view of its condition—although neither the human benefactor nor the dying animal may have had a claim of right.

Plainly, the grounds of our obligations to humans and to animals are manifold and cannot be formulated simply. Some hold that there is a general obligation to do no gratuitous harm to sentient creatures (the principle of nonmaleficence); some hold that there is a general obligation to do good to sentient creatures when that is reasonably within one's power (the principle of beneficence). In our dealings with animals, few will deny that we are at least obliged to act humanely—that is, to treat them with the decency and concern that we owe, as sensitive human beings, to other sentient creatures. To treat animals humanely, however, is not to treat them as humans or as the holders of rights.

A common objection, which deserves a response, may be paraphrased as follows:

> If having rights requires being able to make moral claims, to grasp and apply moral laws, then many humans—the brain-damaged, the comatose, the senile—who plainly lack those capacities must be without rights. But that is absurd. This proves [the critic concludes] that rights do not depend on the presence of moral capacities.[1, 10]

This objection fails; it mistakenly treats an essential feature of humanity as though it were a screen for sorting humans. The capacity for moral judgment that distinguishes humans from animals is not a test to be administered to human beings one by one. Persons who are unable, because of some disability, to perform the full moral functions natural to human beings are certainly not for that reason ejected from the moral community. The issue is one of kind. Humans are of such a kind that they may be the subject of experiments only with their voluntary consent. The choices they make freely must be respected. Animals are of such a kind that it is impossible for them, in principle, to give or withhold voluntary consent or to make a moral choice. What humans retain when disabled, animals have never had.

A second objection, also often made, may be paraphrased as follows:

> Capacities will not succeed in distinguishing humans from the other animals. Animals also reason; animals also communicate with one another; animals also care passionately for their young; animals also exhibit desires and preferences.[11, 12] Features of moral relevance—rationality, interdependence, and love—are not exhibited uniquely by human beings. Therefore [this critic concludes], there can be no solid moral distinction between humans and other animals.[10]

This criticism misses the central point. It is not the ability to communicate or to reason, or dependence on one another, or care for the young, or the exhibition of preference, or any such behavior that marks the critical divide. Analogies between human families and those of monkeys, or between human communities and those of wolves, and the like, are entirely beside the point. Patterns of conduct are not at issue. Animals do indeed exhibit remarkable behavior at times. Conditioning, fear, instinct, and intelligence all contribute to species survival. Membership in a community of moral agents nevertheless remains impossible for them. Actors subject to moral judgment must be capable of grasping the generality of an ethical premise in a practical syllogism. Humans act immorally often enough, but only they—never wolves or monkeys—can discern, by applying some moral rule to the facts of a case, that a given act ought or ought not to be performed. The moral restraints imposed by humans on themselves are thus highly abstract and are often in conflict with the self-interest of the agent. Communal behavior among animals, even when most intelligent and most endearing, does not approach autonomous morality in this fundamental sense.

Genuinely moral acts have an internal as well as an external dimension. Thus, in law, an act can be criminal only when the guilty deed, the *actus reus,* is done with a guilty mind, *mens rea.* No animal can ever commit a crime; bringing animals to criminal trial is the mark of primitive ignorance. The claims of moral right are similarly inapplicable to them. Does a lion have a right to eat a baby zebra? Does a baby zebra have a right not to be eaten? Such questions, mistakenly invoking the concept of right where it does not belong, do not make good sense. Those who condemn biomedical research because it violates "animal rights" commit the same blunder.

IN DEFENSE OF "SPECIESISM"

Abandoning reliance on animal rights, some critics resort instead to animal sentience—their feelings of pain and distress. We ought to desist from the imposition of pain insofar as we can. Since all or nearly all experimentation on animals does impose pain and could be readily forgone, say these critics, it should be stopped. The ends sought may be worthy, but those ends do not justify imposing agonies on humans, and by animals the agonies are felt no less. The laboratory use of animals (these critics conclude) must therefore be ended—or at least very sharply curtailed.

Argument of this variety is essentially utilitarian, often expressly so[13]; it is based on the calculation of the net product, in pains and pleasures, resulting from experiments on animals. Jeremy Bentham, comparing horses and dogs with other sentient creatures, is thus commonly quoted: "The question is not, Can they reason? nor Can they talk? but, Can they suffer?"[14]

Animals certainly can suffer and surely ought not to be made to suffer needlessly. But in inferring, from these uncontroversial premises, that biomedical research causing animal distress is largely (or wholly) wrong, the critic commits two serious errors.

The first error is the assumption, often explicitly defended, that all sentient animals have equal moral standing. Between a dog and a human being,

according to this view, there is no moral difference; hence the pains suffered by dogs must be weighed no differently from the pains suffered by humans. To deny such equality, according to this critic, is to give unjust preference to one species over another; it is "speciesism." The most influential statement of this moral equality of species was made by Peter Singer:

> The racist violates the principle of equality by giving greater weight to the interests of members of his own race when there is a clash between their interests and the interests of those of another race. The sexist violates the principle of equality by favoring the interests of his own sex. Similarly the speciesist allows the interests of his own species to override the greater interests of members of other species. The pattern is identical in each case.[2]

This argument is worse than unsound; it is atrocious. It draws an offensive moral conclusion from a deliberately devised verbal parallelism that is utterly specious. Racism has no rational ground whatever. Differing degrees of respect or concern for humans for no other reason than that they are members of different races is an injustice totally without foundation in the nature of the races themselves. Racists, even if acting on the basis of mistaken factual beliefs, do grave moral wrong precisely because there is no morally relevant distinction among the races. The supposition of such differences has led to outright horror. The same is true of the sexes, neither sex being entitled by right to greater respect or concern than the other. No dispute here.

Between species of animate life, however—between (for example) humans on the one hand and cats or rats on the other—the morally relevant differences are enormous, and almost universally appreciated. Humans engage in moral reflection; humans are morally autonomous; humans are members of moral communities, recognizing just claims against their own interest. Human beings do have rights; theirs is a moral status very different from that of cats or rats.

I am a speciesist. Speciesism is not merely plausible; it is essential for right conduct, because those who will not make the morally relevant distinctions among species are almost certain, in consequence, to misapprehend their true obligations. The analogy between speciesism and racism is insidious. Every sensitive moral judgment requires that the differing natures of the beings to whom obligations are owed be considered. If all forms of animate life—or vertebrate animal life?—must be treated equally, and if therefore in evaluating a research program the pains of a rodent count equally with the pains of a human, we are forced to conclude (1) that neither humans nor rodents possess rights, or (2) that rodents possess all the rights that humans possess. Both alternatives are absurd. Yet one or the other must be swallowed if the moral equality of all species is to be defended.

Humans owe to other humans a degree of moral regard that cannot be owed to animals. Some humans take on the obligation to support and heal others, both humans and animals, as a principal duty in their lives; the fulfillment of that duty may require the sacrifice of many animals. If biomedical investigators abandon the effective pursuit of their professional objectives because they are convinced that they may not do to animals what the service of humans requires, they will fail, objectively, to do their duty. Refusing to recognize the moral differences among species is a sure path to calamity. (The largest animal rights group in the country is People for the Ethical Treatment of Animals; its codirector, Ingrid Newkirk, calls research using animal subjects "fascism" and "supremacism." "Animal liberationists do not separate out the *human* animal," she says, "so there is no rational basis for saying that a human being has special rights. A rat is a pig is a dog is a boy. They're all mammals."[15])

Those who claim to base their objection to the use of animals in biomedical research on their reckoning of the net pleasures and pains produced make a second error, equally grave. Even if it were true—as it is surely not—that the pains of all animate beings must be counted equally, a cogent utilitarian calculation requires that we weigh all the consequences of the use, and of the nonuse, of animals in laboratory research. Critics relying (however mistakenly) on animal rights may claim to ignore the beneficial results of such research, rights being trump cards to which interest and advantage must give way. But an argument that is explicitly framed in terms of interest and benefit for all over the long run must attend also to the disadvantageous consequences of not using animals in research, and to

all the achievements attained and attainable only through their use. The sum of the benefits of their use is utterly beyond quantification. The elimination of horrible disease, the increase of longevity, the avoidance of great pain, the saving of lives, and the improvement of the quality of lives (for humans and for animals) achieved through research using animals is so incalculably great that the argument of these critics, systematically pursued, establishes not their conclusion but its reverse: to refrain from using animals in biomedical research is, on utilitarian grounds, morally wrong.

When balancing the pleasures and pains resulting from the use of animals in research, we must not fail to place on the scales the terrible pains that would have resulted, would be suffered now, and would long continue had animals not been used. Every disease eliminated, every vaccine developed, every method of pain relief devised, every surgical procedure invented, every prosthetic device implanted—indeed, virtually every modern medical therapy is due, in part or in whole, to experimentation using animals. Nor may we ignore, in the balancing process, the predictable gains in human (and animal) well-being that are probably achievable in the future but that will not be achieved if the decision is made now to desist from such research or to curtail it.

Medical investigators are seldom insensitive to the distress their work may cause animal subjects. Opponents of research using animals are frequently insensitive to the cruelty of the results of the restrictions they would impose.[2] Untold numbers of human beings—real persons, although not now identifiable—would suffer grievously as the consequence of this well-meaning but shortsighted tenderness. If the morally relevant differences between humans and animals are borne in mind, and if all relevant considerations are weighed, the calculation of long-term consequences must give overwhelming support for biomedical research using animals.

CONCLUDING REMARKS

Substitution The humane treatment of animals requires that we desist from experimenting on them if we can accomplish the same result using alternative methods—in vitro experimentation, computer simulation, or others. Critics of some experiments using animals rightly make this point.

It would be a serious error to suppose, however, that alternative techniques could soon be used in most research now using live animal subjects. No other methods now on the horizon—or perhaps ever to be available—can fully replace the testing of a drug, a procedure, or a vaccine, in live organisms. The flood of new medical possibilities being opened by the successes of recombinant DNA technology will turn to a trickle if testing on live animals is forbidden. When initial trials entail great risks, there may be no forward movement whatever without the use of live animal subjects. In seeking knowledge that may prove critical in later clinical applications, the unavailability of animals for inquiry may spell complete stymie. In the United States, federal regulations require the testing of new drugs and other products on animals, for efficacy and safety, before human beings are exposed to them.[16, 17] We would not want it otherwise.

Every advance in medicine—every new drug, new operation, new therapy of any kind—must sooner or later be tried on a living being for the first time. That trial, controlled or uncontrolled, will be an experiment. The subject of that experiment, if it is not an animal, will be a human being. Prohibiting the use of live animals in biomedical research, therefore, or sharply restricting it, must result either in the blockage of much valuable research or in the replacement of animal subjects with human subjects. These are the consequences—unacceptable to most reasonable persons—of not using animals in research.

Reduction Should we not at least reduce the use of animals in biomedical research? No, we should increase it, to avoid when feasible the use of humans as experimental subjects. Medical investigations putting human subjects at some risk are numerous and greatly varied. The risks run in such experiments are usually unavoidable, and (thanks to earlier experiments on animals) most such risks are minimal or moderate. But some experimental risks are substantial.

When an experimental protocol that entails substantial risk to humans comes before an institutional review board, what response is appropriate? The investigation, we may suppose, is promising and deserves support, so long as its human subjects are protected against unnecessary dangers. May not the investigators be fairly asked, Have you done all that you can to eliminate risk to humans by the extensive testing of that drug, that procedure, or that device on animals? To achieve maximal safety for humans we are right to require thorough experimentation on animal subjects before humans are involved.

Opportunities to increase human safety in this way are commonly missed; trials in which risks may be shifted from humans to animals are often not devised, sometimes not even considered. Why? For the investigator, the use of animals as subjects is often more expensive, in money and time, than the use of human subjects. Access to suitable human subjects is often quick and convenient, whereas access to appropriate animal subjects may be awkward, costly, and burdened with red tape. Physician-investigators have often had more experience working with human beings and know precisely where the needed pool of subjects is to be found and how they may be enlisted. Animals, and the procedures for their use, are often less familiar to these investigators. Moreover, the use of animals in place of humans is now more likely to be the target of zealous protests from without. The upshot is that humans are sometimes subjected to risks that animals could have borne, and should have borne, in their place. To maximize the protection of human subjects, I conclude, the wide and imaginative use of live animal subjects should be encouraged rather than discouraged. This enlargement in the use of animals is our obligation.

Consistency Finally, inconsistency between the profession and the practice of many who oppose research using animals deserves comment. This frankly ad hominem observation aims chiefly to show that a coherent position rejecting the use of animals in medical research imposes costs so high as to be intolerable even to the critics themselves.

One cannot coherently object to the killing of animals in biomedical investigations while continuing to eat them. Anesthetics and thoughtful animal husbandry render the level of actual animal distress in the laboratory generally lower than that in the abattoir. So long as death and discomfort do not substantially differ in the two contexts, the consistent objector must not only refrain from all eating of animals, but also protest as vehemently against others eating them as against others experimenting on them. No less vigorously must the critic object to the wearing of animal hides in coats and shoes, to employment in any industrial enterprise that uses animal parts, and to any commercial development that will cause death or distress to animals.

Killing animals to meet human needs for food, clothing, and shelter is judged entirely reasonable by most persons. The ubiquity of these uses and the virtual universality of moral support for them confront the opponent of research using animals with an inescapable difficulty. How can the many common uses of animals be judged morally worthy, while their use in scientific investigation is judged unworthy?

The number of animals used in research is but the tiniest fraction of the total used to satisfy assorted human appetites. That these appetites, often base and satisfiable in other ways, morally justify the far larger consumption of animals, whereas the quest for improved human health and understanding cannot justify the far smaller, is wholly implausible. Aside from the numbers of animals involved, the distinction in terms of worthiness of use, drawn with regard to any single animal, is not defensible. A given sheep is surely not more justifiably used to put lamb chops on the supermarket counter than to serve in testing a new contraceptive or a new prosthetic device. The needless killing of animals is wrong; if the common killing of them for our food or convenience is right, the less common but more humane uses of animals in the service of medical science are certainly not less right.

Scrupulous vegetarianism, in matters of food, clothing, shelter, commerce, and recreation, and in all other spheres, is the only fully coherent position the critic may adopt. At great human cost, the lives of fish and crustaceans must also be protected, with equal vigor, if speciesism has been forsworn. A very few consistent critics adopt this position. It is the reductio ad absurdum of the rejection of moral distinctions between animals and human beings.

Opposition to the use of animals in research is based on arguments of two different kinds—those relying on the alleged rights of animals and those relying on the consequences for animals. I have argued that arguments of both kinds must fail. We surely do have obligations to animals, but they have, and can have, no rights against us on which research can infringe. In calculating the consequences of animal research, we must weigh all the long-term benefits of the results achieved—to animals and to humans—and in that calculation we must not assume the moral equality of all animate species.

REFERENCES

1 Regan T. The case for animal rights. Berkeley, Calif.: University of California Press, 1983.

2 Singer P. Animal liberation. New York: Avon Books, 1977.

3 St. Augustine. Confessions. Book Seven. 397 A.D. New York: Pocketbooks, 1957:104–26.

4 St. Thomas Aquinas. Summa theologica. 1273 A.D. Philosophic texts. New York: Oxford University Press, 1960:353–66.

5 Hegel GWF. Philosophy of right. 1821. London: Oxford University Press, 1952:105–10.

6 Bradley F. H. Why should I be moral? 1876. In: Melden AI, ed. Ethical theories. New York: Prentice-Hall, 1950:345–59.

7 Mead G. H. The genesis of the self and social control. 1925. In: Reck A. J, ed. Selected writings. Indianapolis: Bobbs-Merrill, 1964:264–93.

8 Prichard H. A. Does moral philosophy rest on a mistake? 1912. In: Cellars W, Hospers J, eds. Readings in ethical theory. New York: Appleton-Century-Crofts, 1952:149–63.

9 Kant I. Fundamental principles of the metaphysic of morals. 1785. New York: Liberal Arts Press, 1949.

10 Rollin B. E. Animal rights and human morality. New York: Prometheus Books, 1981.

11 Hoff C. Immoral and moral uses of animals. N Engl J Med 1980; 302:115–8.

12 Jamieson D. Killing persons and other beings. In: Miller H. B, Williams WH, eds. Ethics and animals. Clifton, N.J.: Humana Press, 1983:135–46.

13 Singer P. Ten years of animal liberation. New York Review of Books. 1985; 31:46–52.

14 Bentham J. Introduction to the principles of morals and legislation. London: Athlone Press, 1970.

15 McCabe K. Who will live, who will die? Washingtonian Magazine. August 1986:115.

16 U.S. Code of Federal Regulations, Title 21, Sect. 505(i). Food, drug, and cosmetic regulations.

17 U.S. Code of Federal Regulations, Title 16, Sect. 1500.40-2. Consumer product regulations.

THE RESPONSIBLE USE OF ANIMALS IN BIOMEDICAL RESEARCH
Edwin Converse Hettinger

> Hettinger responds directly to Cohen's defense of animal research. Against Cohen's thesis that only human beings can have rights, Hettinger argues that one need not be a moral agent to possess rights, as suggested by the examples of human infants and severely retarded humans. Regarding Cohen's embrace of speciesism, Hettinger advances several arguments in an effort to demonstrate the incoherence of attributing moral status to a being on the basis of species membership rather than on the basis of the individual's characteristics. He goes on to argue that utilitarianism—which incorporates a principle of equal consideration of interests—supports animal research only in those cases where it also supports research on human beings whose mental capacities are comparable to those of animals. Hettinger next contends that the promise of alternatives to animal research is much greater than Cohen allows, before sketching an equal-consideration approach to the human use of animals.

Carl Cohen's defense of the use of animals for biomedical research in *The New England Journal of Medicine*[1] raises most of the major issues in the moral controversy concerning human treatment of nonhuman animals. It exhibits the major lines of attack against both animal rights advocates (such as Tom Regan)[2] and utilitarian animal-liberationists (such as Peter Singer).[3] It is also a showcase of the most common mistakes made by those who seek to defend the current human use of animals. . . .

DO ALL HUMANS BUT NO ANIMALS HAVE RIGHTS?

Cohen argues that only human beings can have rights.

> Rights arise, and can be intelligibly defended, only among beings who actually do, or can, make moral claims against one another. Whatever else rights may be, therefore, they are necessarily human; their possessors are persons, human beings. (p. 104)

Cohen is correct in maintaining that rights cannot arise unless there exist moral agents for whom these rights claims make sense. To say that some being has a right is to say (at least in part) that some other being has obligations to treat the right holder

in certain ways specified by that right. So if there were no beings more cognitively and morally capable than pigs or dogs, there would be no rights.

However, the fact that rights claims require the existence of duty bearers does not imply that only those duty bearers can have rights. Even Cohen would grant that human infants have rights, yet they are not duty bearers. Thus, some creatures possess rights despite being unable to invoke them against others or to recognize and respect others' rights.

Cohen attempts to avoid this objection by shifting his criterion of rights possession to the *capacity* for being a moral agent, rather than actually being a moral agent.

> Animals. . . are not beings of a kind capable of exercising or responding to moral claims. Animals therefore have no rights, and they can have none. . . . The holders of rights must have the capacity to comprehend rules of duty. . . . (p. 104)

However, most people would grant that severely retarded humans have rights (Cohen does), and yet they do not have "the capacity to comprehend rules of duty." Thus if having the capacity to be a duty bearer is necessary for the possession of rights, then severely retarded humans cannot have rights.

Cohen responds to this point with his talk of "kinds."

Reprinted with permission of the author and the publisher from *Between the Species*, vol. 5, no. 3 (Summer 1989), pp. 123–31.

The capacity for moral judgment that distinguishes humans from animals is not a test to be administered to human beings one by one. Persons who are unable, because of some disability, to perform the full moral functions natural to human beings are certainly not for that reason ejected from the moral community. The issue is one of kind. Humans are of such a kind that they may be the subject of experiments only with their voluntary consent. The choices they make freely must be respected. Animals are of such a kind that it is impossible for them, in principle, to give or withhold voluntary consent or to make a moral choice. What humans retain when disabled, animals have never had. (p. 106)

Cohen seems to be claiming that the capacity for moral agency is essential to human beings and is necessarily lacking in other animals. Thus, severely retarded humans, because they are human, retain the capacity for moral agency even in their retarded state. Animals by their very nature lack this capacity. Since the capacity for moral agency confers rights, severely retarded humans have rights, whereas animals do not.

But many severely retarded humans could never carry out even the quasi-moral functions that some animals can perform. Dogs, for example, can be obedient, protective, and solicitous, while there are severely retarded humans who could not achieve these minimal moral abilities despite our best efforts. Given this fact, it just is not plausible to claim that severely retarded humans have the capacity for moral agency, while claiming that psychologically sophisticated animals do not. Cohen certainly has not given us any reason to accept this claim. He simply assumes that being a member of a biological species guarantees that one has certain capacities, despite overwhelming evidence that marginal members of species often lack capacities normal for that kind of creature. We need a strong argument before we should reject the obvious point that some animals have a greater capacity for moral behavior (however minimal) than do some severely retarded human beings.

Cohen might argue that severely retarded humans have the capacity for moral agency despite lacking the ability to realize that capacity. But why should we accept such an attenuated notion of capacity? Certainly capacities can be left unrealized,

but if there is no possibility that they could ever be developed, what sense is there in claiming that the capacity is present? I see no reason to accept the notion that there can be unrealizable capacities.

IS SPECIESISM DEFENSIBLE?

Perhaps Cohen would agree that severely retarded humans lack the capacity for moral agency but thinks this is unimportant. He may be arguing that we should treat the severely retarded as human beings and that since human beings have rights (presumably because many of them are moral agents), severely retarded humans have rights as well. On this reading, Cohen is suggesting that we treat individuals according to their biological kind and ignore their individual characteristics. Moral status is to be determined by species membership, not individual qualities. This is "speciesism": the view that species membership is by itself a morally legitimate reason for treating individuals differently.

Peter Singer and others have argued that speciesism is "a form of prejudice no less objectionable than racism or sexism."[4] Cohen's speciesist perspective concerning the moral status of animals vis-à-vis humans does coincide uncomfortably with the outlook of racists and sexists toward blacks and women. Both judge according to class membership while ignoring individual qualities.

Cohen responds to this charge of speciesism by embracing it:

I am a speciesist. Speciesism is not merely plausible; it is essential for right conduct, because those who will not make the morally relevant distinctions among species are almost certain, in consequence, to misapprehend their true obligations. The analogy between speciesism and racism is insidious. Every sensitive moral judgment requires that the differing natures of the beings to whom obligations are owed be considered. (p. 109)

This passage defends the truism that there often are differences between members of distinct species which are morally relevant in determining how we should treat them. But this is not what is at issue in the debate over speciesism. Singer, Regan, and other opponents of speciesism are not suggesting that we ignore morally relevant differences between members of different species and treat them all identically. (They are not suggesting, for example, that dogs be allowed at the dinner table or be allowed to vote.) What rejecting speciesism commits one to is being unwilling to use difference in species by itself as a reason for treating individuals differently. Similarly, rejecting racism and sexism commits one to not using race or sex by itself as a reason for differential treatment. Cohen's truism does not support speciesism in this problematic sense.

The analogy between speciesism and racism or sexism is deficient in one respect. Species classification marks broader differences between beings than does racial or sexual classification. Thus attempting to justify differential treatment on the basis of species membership alone (as Cohen does) is not *just* as morally objectionable as doing so on the basis of race or sex, since members of different species are more likely to require differential treatment than are members of different races or sexes (within a species). For example, in determining what sort of food or shelter to provide, it would be much more important to know a creature's species than it would be to know a person's race or sex.

But this does not imply that difference in species by itself is a morally legitimate reason for treating individuals differently, while difference in race or sex considered by itself is not. Arguing that a woman should be prohibited from combat because of her sex fails to provide a morally relevant reason for the recommendation. Arguing for this on the grounds that this woman lacks the required physical capacities is to provide a morally relevant reason. Similarly, arguing that a chimpanzee should be experimentally sacrificed rather than a human, simply because it is a chimpanzee, gives no morally relevant reason for the recommendation. However, arguing that the chimpanzee does not value or plan for its future life to the extent that the human does is to provide such a reason.

Thus even though considerations of species are frequently more closely correlated with morally relevant features than are considerations of race or sex, species membership by itself (like racial or sexual class membership) is not a morally legitimate reason for differential treatment. Speciesism is thus a moral mistake of the same sort as racism and sexism: it advocates differential treatment on morally illegitimate grounds.

The illegitimacy of judgments based on species membership alone becomes especially clear when comparing the moral status of a severely retarded human with that of psychologically sophisticated animals, since here the individual does not have what most members of the species have. The morally relevant differences which *usually* exist between individuals of two different biological kinds (and hence which would frequently justify treating them differently) are lacking when comparing severely retarded humans with psychologically sophisticated animals. Any plausible morally relevant characteristic—whether it be rationality, self-sufficiency, ability to communicate, free choice, moral agency, psychological sophistication, fullness of life, and so on—is possessed by some animals to a greater extent than by some severely retarded humans. In this case, to classify by biological kind and to argue for differential treatment on that basis alone obscures and ignores morally relevant features rather than relying on them. We should not treat individuals on the basis of group or kind membership when their individual characteristics are readily apparent and relevant.

Thus, Cohen's argument fails on this second interpretation, as well. His appeal to biological kind to justify differential moral status of severely retarded humans and psychologically sophisticated animals is an unjustified form of speciesism. Unless Cohen can show us that there is some morally relevant difference between severely retarded humans and psychologically sophisticated animals, his position is open to the following objection: if experimenting on severely retarded humans is a violation of their rights, then experimenting on psychologically sophisticated animals violates their rights, as well.

DOES UTILITARIANISM JUSTIFY ANIMAL EXPERIMENTATION?

Utilitarians hold that the right policy is the one whose consequences maximize the satisfaction of interests. In this calculation the interests of all affected parties are fairly taken into account. Utilitarians who oppose animal experimentation do so not on the grounds that animal rights are violated but because they think that the overall good resulting from these experiments is not sufficient to justify their negative consequences. The benefits which result from animal experimentation (such as an increase in scientific and medical knowledge) either do not outweigh the costs (e.g., animal pain and death) or could be achieved in a less costly fashion.

Cohen rejects the utilitarian critic's position that the like interests of humans and animals should be given equal moral weight. He denies that similar amounts of human and animal pain are equally morally significant.

> The first error is the assumption, often explicitly defended, that all sentient animals have equal moral standing. Between a dog and a human being, according to this view, there is no moral difference; hence the pains suffered by dogs must be weighed no differently from the pains suffered by humans. . . . If all forms of animate life . . . must be treated equally, and if therefore in evaluating a research program the pains of a rodent count equally with the pains of a human, we are forced to conclude (1) that neither humans nor rodents possess rights, or (2) that rodents possess all the rights that humans possess. . . . One or the other must be swallowed if the moral equality of all species is to be defended. (pp. 108–9)

This argument misses the mark. To claim that animals "have equal moral standing" and should have their like interests treated equally implies neither that there are no moral differences between humans and animals nor that we should treat animals in the same manner that we do humans.

From the utilitarian position that the right act is the one which maximizes the net satisfaction of interests it follows that it is morally preferable to give a human a slightly less amount of pain than to give an animal a slightly greater amount of pain (or *vice versa*). If the pains are of equal intensity and consequence, then one should be morally indifferent. The fact that one is the pain of a human and the other is the pain of an animal is not by itself morally relevant.

This is not to say that the same type of experiment on a human and an animal would cause each the same amount of pain and suffering and that we should be indifferent to which being we use. Giving

a typical chimpanzee a deadly virus in order to test a vaccine is likely to cause less pain and suffering than giving a typical human the deadly virus for the same purpose. The greater psychological sophistication of the human, its greater intelligence and self-consciousness, makes possible a greater degree of pain and suffering. (Sometimes the reverse is true, however.)[5]

Even though pain and suffering would often be minimized by experimenting on an animal instead of a typical human, that does not show that we may morally discount the pain and suffering of animals. We must still count the pain and suffering of animals equally with the like pain and suffering of humans. But in cases where a human will suffer more, we should prefer the use of animals (and *vice versa*).

Cohen is thus mistaken in thinking that giving equal consideration to the like interests of animals and humans makes moral discriminations between the two impossible. For a utilitarian, equal consideration (or equal moral standing) does not imply identical treatment. Cohen has given us no cogent reason for rejecting the view that the like pains of humans and animals must be given equal moral weight. Since the pain of the animals on whom we experiment cannot be discounted, Cohen's utilitarian justification for the biomedical use of animals becomes far more difficult to achieve.

Cohen argues that even if "the pains of all animate beings must be counted equally" (p. 109), a utilitarian calculus would still come out in support of the biomedical use of animals:

> The sum of the benefits of their use is utterly beyond quantification. The elimination of horrible disease, the increase of longevity, the avoidance of great pain, the saving of lives, and the improvement of the quality of lives (for humans and for animals) achieved through research using animals is so incalculably great that the argument of these critics, systematically pursued, establishes not their conclusion but its reverse: to refrain from using animals in biomedical research is, on utilitarian grounds, morally wrong. (p. 110)

Substantial benefits have resulted (and continue to result) from biomedical experimentation, much of which involves the use of animals. And although a utilitarian benefit/cost analysis would reach the conclusion that it would be wrong to stop the use of animals entirely, it would not justify Cohen's call for an increase in the biomedical use of animals. Cohen can reach this conclusion only by abandoning utilitarianism (and its principle of equal consideration of like interests), by adopting the speciesist position which treats animal pain and distress as insignificant when it is a means to human benefit, and by being overly pessimistic about the possibility of alternatives to animal use.

THE POSSIBILITY OF SUBSTITUTION

Whether research using living creatures is justified on utilitarian grounds depends in large part on the availability of substitute procedures. A utilitarian benefit/cost analysis (which must consider alternative, less costly ways to achieve these benefits) would find that some, perhaps many, but certainly not all experiments using animals are morally justifiable. *Some* use of living beings continues to be necessary and justifiable. Even developing alternatives to the biomedical use of animals often requires the use of animals. At present substitute techniques are not sufficiently developed to eliminate this use entirely (and they may never be).[6]

Nevertheless, Cohen is overly pessimistic about the possibility of alternatives to the current biomedical use of animals. His speciesism prevents him from appreciating or even acknowledging the numerous substitute procedures that are being developed. A recent report by the U.S. Congress' Office of Technology Assessment (OTA) on alternatives to animal use in research, testing, and education is much more encouraging about the potential for alternatives.[7] This study presents numerous suggestions involving the replacement, reduction, and refinement of the use of animals. In addition to the promising techniques of in vitro experimentation and computer simulation (which Cohen mentions), the OTA report suggests:

1. Coordinating investigations and sharing information (to reduce duplicative experiments when necessary for validating the original research);

2. Replacing the use of higher animals with lower animals (invertebrates for vertebrates and cold-blooded for warm-blooded animals);

3. Using plants instead of animals;

4. Sharing animals (e.g., getting several tissues from one animal);

5. Designing experiments which use statistical inferences and whose design provides reliable information despite the use of fewer animals;

6. Decreasing the pain and distress in animal experimentation by altering the experimental design and by using anesthetics and tranquilizers;

7. Using non-living chemical and physical systems that mimic biological functions;

8. Using human and animal cadavers; and

9. Teaching by demonstration instead of by individual student use of animals.

Recent amendments to the Animal Welfare Act[8] and the Public Health Service Act,[9] as well as legislation concerning the education of health professionals,[10] all encourage alternatives to the current methods of animal use.[11] Cohen's pessimistic assessment of these alternatives flies in the face of a growing trend of using already existing alternatives and of developing new substitute procedures. Experiments which cause animals pain, distress, or death are clearly not justifiable when such substitute procedures are available.

SHOULD WE INCREASE BIOMEDICAL ANIMAL USE?

Cohen argues that in order to achieve maximum safety for humans "the wide and imaginative use of live animal subjects should be encouraged rather than discouraged" (p. 112). Cohen is right that some experiments which subject humans to risk could be conducted using animals without loss in the significance of the results. Furthermore, risky experiments which are necessary *should* be performed on psychologically less sophisticated creatures. An increase in psychological sophistication brings with it a wider range of interests, a greater ability to experience satisfaction (and dissatisfaction), and the possibility of leading a fuller life. Inflicting suffering or death on these creatures causes greater harm.

In advocating an increase in the biomedical use of animals Cohen not only ignores the available alternatives but disregards the widespread experimental misuse of animals, as well. Numerous books and articles have persuasively documented that many experiments using animals have been unprofessional, of dubious scientific merit, repetitive, or cruel.[12] Two video tapes are especially persuasive; "Unnecessary Fuss," about head injury research involving baboons at the University of Pennsylvania,[13] and "Tools for Research," a general review of research using animals over the last twenty years.[14] The flurry of recent legislation concerning animal welfare cited above shows a growing public recognition of the misuse of laboratory animals. Government regulations for the care of laboratory animals have been developed to prevent these sorts of experiments, as well.[15] Cohen's suggestion that we encourage the wide and imaginative use of live animal subjects, instead of limiting this use and working to find substitute techniques, shows blatant disregard for this widely acknowledged problem.

CAN A CONSISTENT POSITION CONCERNING ANIMAL USE BE DEVELOPED?

Cohen charges his anti-speciesist opponents with inconsistency or absurdity: "Scrupulous vegetarianism, in matters of food, clothing, shelter, commerce, and recreation, and in all other spheres, is the only fully coherent position the critic may adopt" (p. 113). The person who eats veal and then strenuously objects to the killing of cats in relatively painless medical experiments *is* inconsistent. We do not *need* to eat animals for food (certainly not mammals); carefully chosen vegetarian diets are perfectly healthy. We do need the ongoing results of biomedical research and for some of this research the use of living creatures continues to be required.

Cohen is right that the use of animals in biomedical research is less difficult to defend than are other uses of animals. (Only one out of every hundred animals used is for this purpose.)[16] But the anti-speciesist critic of current biomedical uses of animals need not be committed to prohibiting all uses of animals. Since anti-speciesism allows for discriminating between animals, critics can consistently object to the raising, slaughtering, and consumption of veal calves while not objecting to commercial shrimp farming and shrimp consumption. A critic might also object to repeated surgery on healthy animals in the training of veterinarians and not object to the use of chick embryos for toxicity testing. The recommendation that experimenters substitute cold-blooded animals for warm-blooded ones or invertebrates for vertebrates is also perfectly consistent. These suggestions are not speciesist, since species membership *per se* is not the justification offered for differential treatment. Differences in the fullness of life, in psychological sophistication, and in the capacity for suffering are what motivates these suggestions.

Thus, one can argue for limiting animal use in biomedical research without embracing the extreme position prohibiting all uses of any animals for whatever reason. Cohen can successfully saddle only his most extreme opponents with this consequence. A more circumspect skepticism about the legitimacy of a significant portion of laboratory animal use is possible. Advocates of limiting the use of animals in biomedical research can consistently advocate the limited use of animals in other areas, as well. Both extremes—the absolute prohibition of all animal use, as well as Cohen's speciesist encouragement of such use—should be avoided. . . . [17]

NOTES

1 Carl Cohen, "The Case for the Use of Animals in Biomedical Research," *New England Journal of Medicine* 315 (1986): 865–70. [All page references are to section 10 of this volume]

2 Tom Regan, *The Case for Animal Rights* (Berkeley, Calif.: University of California Press, 1983).

3 Peter Singer, *Animal Liberation* (New York: Avon Books, 1975).

4 Peter Singer, "Animal Liberation" in *People, Penguins, and Plastics*, ed. Donald VanDeVeer and Christine Pierce (Belmont, Calif.: Wadsworth, 1986), p. 31.

5 Peter Singer, *Practical Ethics* (Cambridge: Cambridge University Press, 1979), p. 53.

6 Office of Technology Assessment (OTA), *Alternatives to Animal Use in Research, Testing, and Education,* publication

no. OTA-BA-273 (Washington, D.C.: U.S. Government Printing Office, 1986), p. 138.

7 Ibid.

8 The Food Security Act of 1985 (Public Law 99–198).

9 The Health Research Extension Act of 1985 (Public Law 99–158).

10 The Health Professions Educational Assistance Amendments of 1985 (Public Law 99–129).

11 See OTA, *Alternatives to Animal Use in Research, Testing, and Education,* chap. 13.

12 See Singer, *Animal Liberation,* chap. 2; Richard Ryder, "Speciesism in the Laboratory" in *In Defense of Animals,* ed. Peter Singer (New York: Basil Blackwell, 1985) pp. 77–88; Dale Jamieson and Tom Regan, "On the Ethics of the Use of Animals in Science," in *And Justice for All*

(Totowa, N.J.: Rowman and Littlefield, 1982), pp. 169–96; Bernard Rollin, *Animal Rights and Human Morality* (Buffalo, N.Y.: Prometheus Books, 1981), chap. 3.

13 Available from People for the Ethical Treatment of Animals, P.O. Box 42516, Washington, D.C. 20015.

14 Available from Bullfrog Films, Inc., Olney, Penn.

15 See National Institutes of Health, *Guidelines for the Care and Use of Laboratory Animals,* NIH publication no. 85-23 (Bethesda, Md.: National Institutes of Health, 1985).

16 See OTA, *Alternatives to Animal Use in Research, Testing, and Education,* p. 43.

17 I would like to thank Beverly Diamond, John Dickerson, Martin Perlmutter, and Hugh Wilder for helpful suggestions on earlier drafts of this paper.

ON THE ETHICS OF ANIMAL RESEARCH
David DeGrazia

DeGrazia begins his discussion by arguing, contrary to the Nuffield Council of Bioethics, that the issue of animals' moral status is unavoidable in any serious investigation of the ethics of animal research. After providing conceptual, historical, and legislative background, he contends that animals clearly have some moral status and distinguishes four reasonable views regarding their moral status. DeGrazia next explores the uncertainty involved in evaluating the benefits of animal research before cataloguing its major costs and harms to research subjects. With benefits, costs, and harms in view, he draws out the implications of the aforementioned positions on animals' moral status for the ethics of animal research before raising the issue of alternatives to animal research. DeGrazia concludes the essay by advancing several suggestions for public policy.

INTRODUCTION

Few moral issues are as polarizing as the use of non-human animals in biomedical research. Contrary to some at the poles, this issue is also enormously complex. Moreover, the stakes are high. From 50 to 100 million animals are involved in such experiments annually (Orlans, 1998, p. 400). And, according to many proponents of animal research, biomedical progress requires the continuation of experiments upon live animals. The purpose of this chapter is to

convey some of the complexity of this important issue, sketch and evaluate leading positions, and offer several ethical and policy recommendations.

Reflection on the ethics of animal research inclines most people toward neither absolute abolitionism nor a pure *laissez-faire* approach, but to something (perhaps not well defined) in between. From such a moderate standpoint, it may seem obvious that some animal research is justified. Imagine an experiment that would cause mild pain or distress to 100 rats before they are painlessly killed, and is very likely to succeed, thereby validating a cure for a disease that currently kills tens of thousands of children every year: no scientifically promising

From R. E. Ashcroft et al., editors, *Principles of Health Care Ethics,* 2nd edition (Wiley, 2007). Reproduced with permission of the author and Blackwell Publishing Ltd.

alternative to this experiment is known. Although it may seem perfectly obvious that this experiment passes moral muster, this judgment is not self-justifying. After all, most of us would condemn an experiment that caused pain or distress—not to mention death—to human subjects *who neither consented to participate nor stood to benefit from their participation.* Yet, the rats in the imagined study neither consent nor stand to benefit. They are sacrificed for the benefit of others. The judgment that the experiment is justified while similar coercive use of humans would not be justified implies that the *moral status* of rats is, in some sense, less than that of humans.

More generally, any justification of animal research requires assumptions about moral status. Naturally, the same is true of principled opposition to animal research, because such opposition assumes that animals' moral status is too substantial to permit their sacrifice for others' (humans' or animals') benefit. My first thesis, then, is that consideration of animals' moral status is inescapable in any responsible investigation of the ethics of animal research.

In its admirable, well-researched report, the Nuffield Council on Bioethics (NCB) disagrees:

> 'The debate is not best characterized in terms of the relative moral status of humans and animals but in terms of what features of humans and animals are of moral concern . . . Once those features are identified, the question [is] how they should be taken into account in moral reasoning. Are they factors to be weighed against others, or do they function as absolute prohibitions?' (NCB, 2005, p. 57; cf. Rachels 2004).

The NCB identifies *sentience, higher cognitive capacities, the capacity to flourish, sociability, and possession of a life* as morally relevant features (NCB, 2005, p. 41).

However, this proposal is deeply problematic. First, deciding which features are morally relevant can be as controversial as debates about moral status. For example, contrary to the NCB's list, I do not believe that an amoeba's being alive is morally relevant—just as I doubt that life *per se* confers moral status. Second, even if we confidently endorsed a list of morally relevant features, as the NCB notes, we must decide how to take these features into

account. If sentience is morally relevant, we must ask whether, say, rats' sentience justifies (1) an absolute prohibition against causing rats pain, (2) a presumption against causing them pain *equal* to the presumption against causing humans (unconsented) pain, or (3) a presumption against causing pain that is *weaker* than that against causing humans pain. The NCB notes that we must decide between absolute constraints and balancing considerations. But on what basis? Note that any endorsement of balancing will be unhelpful without a specification of *how* to balance different factors. Should a rat's pain count as much as a human's pain, or less? And, if less, how much less? Answers to the questions raised in this paragraph, I suggest, are intelligible only on the basis of assumptions about animals' moral status.

Before we take up the issue of moral status, some background should be helpful.

BACKGROUND

In this chapter, 'animal research' will refer to two broad endeavours. First is animal usage in the *pursuit of original scientific knowledge.* This category divides into *basic research,* which pursues new knowledge of biological processes and functions, and *applied research,* which seeks new biological, medical or veterinary knowledge in order to promote human, animal or environmental health. Second, *testing* on animals evaluates chemicals and other products for safety.

Animal research dates back to classical Greece and Rome and, further east, to early Arabic medicine after the fall of Rome (NCB, 2005, pp. 15-29). Although little animal research was conducted in medieval Europe, animal experiments led to several important discoveries—for example, about blood circulation and the function of lungs—in the seventeenth and eighteenth centuries. The volume of animal research greatly increased in the nineteenth century. Partly in response to the pioneering experiments of François Magendie and Claude Bernard in that century, a notable antivivisection movement emerged in Britain. The 1876 (British) Cruelty to Animals Act, the world's first legislation regulating animal research, established a system requiring licences for experimentation on animals.

Despite continuing protests, animal research grew steadily for most of the twentieth century. Responding to both society's interest in animal research and its ethical concerns, British scientists William Russell and Rex Burch published in 1959 a landmark work that established the 'three Rs'— *Refinement* of techniques to reduce suffering, *Reduction* of numbers of animal subjects and *Replacement* of live animals wherever possible—as central concerns for conscientious members of the profession (Russell and Burch, 1959). Public pressure for increased regulation in Great Britain led to the 1986 Animals (Scientific Procedures) Act, which regulates the research use of all vertebrates and, by a subsequent modification, octopi. Prominent in this legislation is a requirement of harm/benefit assessments of proposed experiments.

In the United States, the (Laboratory) Animal Welfare Act became law in 1966, following widespread outrage that pet dogs were being stolen and sold to research laboratories. At first, it was primarily a pet protection bill. Subsequent amendments significantly increased the requirements for the care and use of research animals. Although this legislation has never covered farm animals, or even rats and mice— the animals most commonly used in research—Public Health Service (PHS) policy covers all vertebrate animals in PHS-funded research. But PHS policy leaves rats and mice unprotected in privately funded research—a major gap in American regulation.

Today, member states of the European Union are legally bound by the 1986 EU Directive EEC 86/609. Among its provisions are a requirement for special authorization to conduct experiments likely to cause severe, prolonged pain in animals; requirements for breeders and suppliers; and the prohibition of animal use where a valid alternative exists. A more recent ban on the use of animals in cosmetics testing took effect in 2009.

Is the policy status quo morally defensible? That depends, in significant measure, on how we should understand animals' moral status.

MORAL STATUS

A being has *moral status* if he or she is morally important in his or her own right, and not merely because how he or she is treated may affect others' interests. All *moral agents*—that is, all beings who have moral responsibilities—have moral status. Rocks do not. They have no conscious or sentient life (even potentially), so nothing we do to them can possibly matter to them. We cannot harm or benefit rocks. Similarly with cars (although what one does to a car can matter to its owner), because our treatment of a car does not matter to it and therefore does not harm or benefit it in any morally significant sense. Common sense suggests that only beings who have interests—or a welfare—have moral status. So having interests is necessary for moral status. If having interests is also sufficient for moral status, then many animals have moral status. Do they?

One historically prominent view answers negatively. According to this *no-status view,* animals' interests have no moral importance except where our treatment of animals affects human interests. That kicking a dog may upset some people, or damage an owner's property, is morally important on this view; that it hurts the dog does not directly matter. The no-status view is enormously implausible in the case of sentient animals, who have interests, and its historical prominence seems to have more to do with humans' self-interested bias and power over animals than with moral insight. Here, I quickly suggest two reasons to reject the no-status view. First, it does not adequately account for our considered judgment that cruelty to animals is wrong; an adequate account must acknowledge the moral status of cruelty's victims. Second, it has trouble explaining why it is wrong to mistreat those human beings who are sentient yet, due to injury or genetic anomaly, lack (even potentially) advanced capacities such as moral agency and linguistic competence—capacities commonly believed to confer special moral status on human persons (DeGrazia, 1996, pp. 40–3, 54–6). Hereafter in this chapter, I will assume that (sentient) animals have at least some moral status, that how we treat them has non-derivative moral importance and that they are beings to whom moral agents can have obligations.

Among the theories ascribing moral status to animals, significant differences appear. Let us first distinguish *equal-consideration views* and *unequal-(less-than-equal-) consideration views.*

The language of 'consideration' focuses on how important, morally, animals' interests are in comparison with prudentially comparable human interests. Take for example, one's interest in not suffering (to some degree, however measured), an interest humans and animals share. How important is animal suffering (in its own right)? Equal-consideration (EC) views maintain that comparable interests have equal moral weight, regardless of the interest bearer's species. This implies that sentient beings have *equal moral status at the level of basic consideration,* but perhaps not with respect to certain interests that do not seem prudentially comparable across species. For example, most commentators agree that death typically harms a person more than it harms, say, a mouse, so that their interests in staying alive are not prudentially comparable (not presumptively equal)—in which case equal consideration is consistent with the judgment that killing persons is generally worse than killing mice. (For a fuller discussion of noncomparable interests, see DeGrazia, 1996, ch. 8). Unequal-consideration (UC) views hold that animals' interests have some (non-derivative) moral importance but less than what persons' comparable interests have—implying that animals have moral status, but less than persons.

The major representatives of EC views are *utilitarianism* and *animal rights theories.* Utilitarianism grants sentient beings equal consideration by counting everyone's comparable interests equally in its directive to maximize utility or net welfare (Singer, 1990, although here he stresses equal consideration more than utilitarianism). Animal rights theories afford stronger protection for the vital interests of humans and certain animals (those claimed to have rights), generally resisting appeals to utility as a justification for sacrificing those interests. In this chapter I use the term *animal rights views* somewhat narrowly to refer to views in which rights generally trump appeals to utility (Regan, 1983; Pluhar, 1995). Some use the term more broadly to refer to all equal-consideration views or even all views granting moral status to animals.

UC theories have received less attention in the literature than EC views and the no-status view. One UC theory is the *two-tier theory,* according to which persons or humans deserve full, equal consideration whereas other sentient beings deserve some non-trivial, but less-than-equal, consideration (Warren, 1997; McMahan, ch. 3). Another UC theory is a *sliding-scale model* of moral status, according to which sentient beings deserve consideration in proportion to their level of cognitive, emotional and social complexity. (I describe this model, without endorsing it, in DeGrazia 1996, ch. 3) This model is likely to stipulate that beyond some threshold of complexity such as personhood, one deserves full consideration—consistent with two-tier theories and the considered judgment that all persons deserve equal consideration.

Each theory of moral status just sketched is, unlike the no-status view, a serious contender. Each is supported by substantial arguments and each faces important challenges. In this chapter, I assume that both EC and UC theories are fairly reasonable and will not attempt to adjudicate between them. Before exploring the implications of these theories, let us examine the possible benefits and harms associated with animal research.

THE ISSUE OF BENEFITS

Proponents of animal research stress its benefits, which accrue mostly to humans but also to animals. The claim of benefits extends to the use of animals in basic research, in modelling diseases and developing therapeutic interventions, in pharmaceutical research and development, and in toxicity testing. Now, in the case of many advances in biomedicine and veterinary science, animal research has certainly been part of the pathway to progress. But it does not logically follow that animal research was necessary for such progress. There may be multiple paths to a particular goal. In justifying animal research, we tend to focus on the path actually taken; relatively little attention (and even less funding) has been given to other possible paths. This raises the issue of alternatives to animal research.

Some critics of animal research hold that it impedes biomedical progress. They doubt that nonhuman animals are reliable models for human beings. Obviously, mice, rats and dogs are not the same as humans. And surely the methodological difficulties of extrapolating data from non-human subjects to the human situation are substantial. It is probably fair to assert that animal models can be misleading, with serious consequences. Some critics argue, for example, that reliance on animal models delayed the development of an effective polio vaccine for many years (LaFollette and Shanks, 1996, ch. 8). And critics often cite the disaster involving thalidomide, which was licensed following animal research for use by pregnant women (a group on which the drug was not tested) as a treatment for morning sickness, leading to the birth of thousands of children with major limb deformities.

Nevertheless, it seems reasonable to assume that, due to many continuities and similarities across species, well-chosen animal models often furnish valuable data on the road to bio-medical advances. But what if there are other, non-animal roads to progress? It would greatly vitiate the moral case for animal research if the latter were unnecessary. So how extensive are the benefits that *only* animal research can provide?

Confronting this complex issue requires comparing (1) progress that results, or has resulted, from use of animal subjects with (2) progress that could result, or could have resulted, from optimal non-animal methods. But progress of type (2) is hypothetical because investments in the study of alternatives pale in comparison with investments in animal research. So, we must speculate to estimate the value of (2). Yet, unless proponents of animal research can compare the values of (1) and (2) rather persuasively—as seems doubtful—then, although they can assert that animal research has yielded benefits, they are in no position to say that it was *necessary* for those benefits.

We must also remember that particular benefits from animal studies are only *possible and hoped for*, whereas the harms to animals are typically immediate and certain. (Countless animal studies harm animals without producing benefits.) Any honest cost/benefit analysis must multiply the value of hoped-for benefits *by the (<1) probability of achieving them*, before considering the predictable costs and harms. This often overlooked fact is critical not only to utilitarianism but also to all positions that regard costs and benefits as relevant to the justification of animal research. In light of both (1) the need to factor in likelihood of success in any honest cost/benefit analysis and (2) the issue of non-animal al-

ternatives, the value of animal research would seem to be less than what proponents typically claim.

Yet its value may sometimes be sufficient to justify the associated costs and harms. Perhaps an animal experiment is the only possible way to achieve some important benefit—such as knowledge about a new veterinary technique's viability. Or perhaps non-animal means to some human benefit would be so costly or harmful to humans as to be unacceptable. (In principle, we *could* always use human subjects to learn about human biology, effective therapies and toxicity, but doing so might require coercion of human subjects or unacceptable risks to them.) Suppose we assume that animals can be useful models in pursuit of some substantial benefit *and* that no non-animal alternative is both scientifically viable and morally acceptable. Does this justify animal research? Not necessarily, for we must also consider harms and costs.

HARMS AND COSTS

In addressing harms and costs associated with animal research, we are likely to think first of harms caused in experimental procedures. These harms range from none (e.g., in simply observing animals) to severe (e.g., in prolonged deprivation of food, water or sleep; force-feeding a substance until subjects die; induction of cancer tumours; brain damage). Intermediate cases include the taking of frequent blood samples, holding an animal in restraints in an inhalation chamber and performing a caesarean section on a pregnant animal.

Additional sources of harm for animal subjects include the following:

- *Acquisition*—usually through breeding but sometimes through the capture of wild animals;

- *Transportation to the research facility*;

- *Housing conditions,* which typically confine animals to small spaces, often without enrichment or access to conspecifics;

- *Handling* of animal subjects, sometimes including the use of restraints; and

- *Death*—if continued life for the animal subject would be worth living.

In cost/benefit assessments, harms count as 'costs'. Of course, so do costs in the ordinary sense. Government-funded research uses taxpayers' money. Research funded by for-profit companies—say, in product testing—uses stockholders' money.

Where non-animal research methods are employed, harms to animal subjects are avoided whereas financial costs are not. Wherever animal methods are not replaced, the other two Rs, reduction and refinement, loom large. Harms and costs are minimized by using the smallest possible number of animals consistent with scientific objectives. Refinements, meanwhile, involve fine-tuning experimental conditions and procedures in light of a sensitive appreciation of animal subjects' needs. Providing an instructive illustration of the latter, the NCB offers this list of rats' and mice's husbandry needs: housing in stable, compatible groups; enough space for exercise and normal social behaviour; a solid floor with a wood-shaving substrate; sufficient height for rearing; nesting material; material to gnaw; and refuges (NCB, 2005, p. 211).

With the benefits, harms and costs associated with animal research in view, let us return to theories of moral status and explore their ethical implications.

SOME DIFFERING IMPLICATIONS

The animal rights approach has almost no interest in cost/benefit considerations because it opposes harming some individuals (without their valid consent) for others' benefit. Although this approach might seem to preclude animal research, it does not. For it can consistently permit (1) research that does not harm its subjects at all and (2) research that promotes animal subjects' best interests—therapeutic veterinary research. Moreover, insofar as current policy permits *minimal-risk* research on human children, who cannot consent in the relevant sense, an animal rights theory might permit this third category as well. But it would preclude the vast majority of animal experiments currently conducted. It would also reject the hypothetical experiment described earlier in this chapter despite its extraordinarily favourable benefit/cost ratio.

The other EC view, utilitarianism, would embrace the hypothetical experiment because its expected utility is higher than that of any known alternative. Utilitarianism would also justify some

animal research conducted today. Even more-than-minimal-risk, non-therapeutic research is acceptable on this view so long as the expected benefits—factoring in the likelihood of achieving them and giving animals' interests equal weight to humans' comparable interests—outweigh the total costs, and no alternative offers a better benefit/cost ratio. Then again, utilitarianism's commitment to equal consideration entails that rather little animal research is justified. Meanwhile, utilitarians must grapple with the fact that their theory seems open, in principle, to the coercive use of human subjects in some circumstances.

Compared with utilitarianism, UC theories will be considerably more welcoming of animal research because they grant animals' interests (e.g., avoiding suffering) less weight than comparable human interests. The main difference between the two-tier theory and the sliding-scale model, both UC views, is this: the former would give all sentient nonhuman animals' interests the same weight, whereas the latter would give their interests more weight if the animals in question are more complex. But, more importantly, no UC theory will be *laissez-faire* about animal research. Recognizing that animals have moral status and that they are not mere tools for research, UC views would likely reject a great deal of current research. Examples include frivolous experiments lacking real benefits (e.g., the infamous cat sex experiments (Wade, 1976)), research offering non-essential benefits (e.g., testing new cosmetics), research causing excessive harm (e.g., Harry Harlow's maternal deprivation studies on monkeys (Harlow and Zimmerman, 1959)) and experiments that are clearly replaceable (cosmetics testing in general). UC views would also seek to minimize the harms associated with acquisition, transport, handling, housing and experimental procedures. The challenges of accommodating the needs of animal subjects' might lead such views to ban or severely limit the use of certain 'higher' mammals, such as primates, whose social and psychological needs are especially hard to meet.

These implications of EC and UC theories motivate another thesis: no reasonable view of animals' moral status can justify the full extent of animal research conducted today. Moreover, all reasonable views would permit some animal research, though animal rights theories would permit precious little. But our discussion of the theories' implications has tacitly assumed that there are no viable alternatives to animal research. Is that so?

WHAT ABOUT ALTERNATIVES?

Although the term 'alternatives' is often used to refer to the *replacement* of live animal use with non-animal techniques, the term is sometimes used more broadly to refer to the other Rs as well: *reduction* in the number of animals used to that needed for scientific validity and *refinement* of techniques to minimize suffering. It is difficult to imagine morally serious opposition to reduction and refinement, so let's focus on replacement.

Replacement alternatives can be either 'complete' or 'incomplete'. Complete replacements use no animal-derived materials. Examples include mathematical and computer modelling studies of biological processes, predictions based on chemical properties of molecules, analyses of epidemiological data, research on human cell or tissue cultures, and studies directly involving human volunteers. Incomplete replacements use some biological materials derived from living or humanely killed animals—for example, cell or tissue cultures from a small number of sacrificed animals—or use animals thought to be insentient such as horseshoe crabs or insects.

The alternatives movement has made considerable progress in recent years (Stephens, Goldberg and Rowan, 2001). With respect to replacements, the most progress has been made in the area of testing. Since the late 1990s several alternatives have achieved regulatory acceptance and widespread adoption. Examples include an in vitro test for phototoxicity and Corrositex, a kind of synthetic skin, to test skin corrosivity. Providing an indication of progress, the Netherlands and Great Britain have stopped using animals for testing cosmetics—and the European Union has banned cosmetics testing with effect from 2009 (NCB, 2005, p. 235).

Although alternatives, including replacements, have made significant inroads in testing, one might doubt the feasibility of replacing animals in original

biological research. Nevertheless, there have been advances in this area as well. For example, an in vitro method has proven to be a viable substitute for mouse-based methods of producing monoclonal antibodies. Sometimes computer modelling is effective in simulating biological systems. Meanwhile, some progress has involved and will continue to involve the use of human beings. Volunteers sometimes participate in physiological studies or in testing diagnostic techniques. Epidemiological studies can help identity factors contributing to particular diseases. Human tissue and cell cultures (e.g., tumour cell lines, neuronal cell culture lines) represent an important growth area. Though often overlooked, the use of new imaging technology—such as PET scans and magnetic resonance imaging—permits study of the live human brain without invasive procedures on people or animals. Finally, the use of stem cells derived from embryos or, less controversially, from adults has enormous research promise.

Inasmuch as regulatory and financial support for alternatives to animal research is in its infancy, it is very difficult to predict how far, scientifically, alternatives can lead. What is clear is that heavy investment in and development of alternatives should be a very high priority on any reasonable view of animals' moral status.

SOME SUGGESTIONS

The ethics of animal research is enormously complex. Even if we settled the hard factual issues (e.g., the validity of animal models, the prospects for alternatives, the sentience or insentience of particular animals) and conceptual issues (e.g., how to evaluate the harm of death in the case of animals), the issue of moral status would remain. I have discussed representatives of both EC and UC views not out of politeness to representatives of different views; I honestly find all of these views reasonable. Even if one theory is the most reasonable, several others are within reason and none is an obvious winner.

Although this plurality of reasonable views impedes the quest for a detailed ethics of animal research, it does not prevent us from identifying points of overlapping consensus or palatable compromises where consensus is unavailable. In this spirit, I close with several policy suggestions:

1. *There should be a massive public investment in alternatives research.* Inasmuch as animals have moral status, they cannot be regarded—merely or even primarily—as tools for human use. On any reasonable view, there must be a presumption against animal research. And, at this time, we know relatively little about the full promise of alternatives. (Apparently, the NCB shares the spirit of my suggestion: 'The Working Party therefore agrees that there is a moral imperative to develop as a priority scientifically rigorous and validated alternative methods for those areas in which Replacements do not currently exist' (NCB, 2005, p. XIX).)

2. *Animal experiments should not be permitted where viable replacement alternatives are known to exist.*

3. *Where animal research is permitted, housing conditions must meet the basic needs—physical, psychological and social—of animal subjects.* Barren housing is a source of major harm to research animals. Although meeting the basic needs of animal subjects is costly, nothing less is appropriate for beings with moral status. Presumably, this requirement will be considerably easier to satisfy in the case of rodents, the animals most commonly used in research, than in the case of 'higher' mammals, especially primates.

4. *Wild animals should never be captured for laboratory research.* Breeding avoids the harms associated with forcing an animal to transition from one form of life to a radically different sort of existence.

5. *Great apes should not be used in research unless their participation is voluntary and/or compatible with the best interests of individual research subjects.* Some great apes currently live in captivity. If all their basic needs are met—which is far from easy to ensure—they may be appropriately used in two circumstances: (1) where they freely choose to participate (e.g., by accepting an 'invitation' to take part in language-learning exercises and not resisting continued participation) and (2) where there is no other known means to help them (therapeutic veterinary research). As I have argued elsewhere, the cognitive, emotional and social complexity of great apes suggests that they are 'borderline persons' who deserve protections comparable with those afforded to humans of uncertain personhood (DeGrazia, 2005). (The same is true for dolphins. But as it appears impossible to meet their basic needs while they are held captive, I reject any research on dolphins that maintains them in captivity longer than necessary to benefit the dolphin subjects themselves.)

6. *Toxicity testing on live animals should be banned.* We have made much progress in developing alternatives to animal testing. With a massive public investment in alternatives, progress should accelerate. Although some representatives of business may chafe at this suggested ban, their priority—maximizing profits—is less important than minimizing harm to beings with moral status.

7. *Public funding for animal research that aims at original scientific knowledge, both basic and applied, should be reduced to some relatively small fraction—say, 10%—of current levels.* That seems a reasonable compromise between EC views, which would justify little animal research, and UC views, which would preserve considerably more of the status quo. This requirement would strongly encourage consideration of alternatives and greatly reduce harm to animal subjects while protecting the very best, most important animal research. The money saved here could more than pay for the massive increase in public funding for alternatives research recommended above.

REFERENCES

DeGrazia D. *Taking Animals Seriously: Mental Life and Moral Status.* Cambridge: Cambridge University Press, 1996.

DeGrazia D. On the question of personhood beyond *Homo sapiens.* In: Singer P, ed. *In Defense of Animals,* 2nd edition. Oxford: Blackwell, 2005; pp. 40–53.

Harlow H, Zimmerman R. Affectional responses in the infant monkey *Science* 1959; **130**: 421–432.

LaFollette H, Shanks N. *Brute Science.* London: Routledge, 1996. McMahan J. *The Ethics of Killing.* Oxford: Oxford University press, 2002.

NCB. *The Ethics of Research Involving Animals.* London: 2005.

Orlans B. History and ethical regulation of animal experimentation: an international perspective. In: Kuhse H. Singer P, eds. *A Companion to Bioethics.* Oxford: Blackwell, 1998; pp. 399–410.

Pluhar E. *Beyond Prejudice.* Durham, NC: Duke University Press, 1995.

Rachels J. Drawing lines. In: Sunstein C. Nussbaum M, eds. *Animal Rights.* Oxford: Oxford University Press, 2004; pp. 162–74.

Regan T. *The Case for Animal Rights.* Berkeley CA: University of California Press, 1983.

Russel W, Burch R. *The Principles of Humane Experimental Technique.* London: Methuen, 1959.

Singer P. *Animal Liberation,* 2nd edition. New York: New York Review. 1990.

Stephens M, Goldberg A, Rowan A. The first forty years of the alternatives approach. In: Salem D, Rowan A, eds. *The State of the Animals 2001.* Washington, DC: Humane Society Press, 2001: pp.121–135.

Wade N. Animal rights: NIH cat sex study brings grief to New York museum. *Science* 1976; **194**: 162–167.

Warren MA. *Moral Status.* Oxford: Oxford University Press, 1997.

ANNOTATED BIBLIOGRAPHY

Appelbaum, Paul S., et al.: "False Hopes and Best Data: Consent to Research and the Therapeutic Misconception," *Hastings Center Report* 17 (April 1987), pp. 20–24. The authors focus on the potential conflict in randomized clinical trials between seeking generalizable knowledge and serving patients' best interests. After arguing that patient-subjects commonly labor under the "therapeutic misconception"—the denial of the possibility that one's participation in RCTs can be seriously disadvantageous to oneself—the authors maintain that proper educational efforts can dispel this misconception for many subjects.

Brody, Baruch A.: *The Ethics of Biomedical Research: An International Perspective* (New York: Oxford University Press, 1998). This book analyzes major issues of research ethics through a review of differing policies throughout the world (especially North America, Western Europe, and the Pacific Rim). Topics covered include genetic research, reproductive research, research on vulnerable subjects, drug approval and the research process, and research on animals.

Buchanan, Allen: "Judging the Past: The Case of the Human Radiation Experiments," *Hastings Center Report* 26 (May–June 1996), pp. 25–30. Using the human radiation experiments as a case study, Buchanan argues for the legitimacy of retrospective moral judgments and traces implications of this thesis for how present practices and institutions should be judged.

DeGrazia, David: *Animal Rights: A Very Short Introduction* (Oxford: Oxford University Press, 2002). In this short volume, DeGrazia explores the mental life, interests, and moral status of animals before addressing the issues of meat-eating, the keeping of pets and zoo animals, and animal research.

Emanuel, Ezekiel J., et al. (ed.): *Ethical and Regulatory Aspects of Clinical Research* (Baltimore: Johns Hopkins University Press, 2003). This volume is intended as a reference guide for the ethical issues confronted by professionals who conduct biomedical research. Divided into ten parts and followed by a helpful set of appendices, the book is especially thorough in addressing leading topics within human research ethics.

Hawkins, Jennifer S., and Ezekiel J. Emanuel (eds.): *Exploitation and Developing Countries: The Ethics of Clinical Research* (Princeton: Princeton University Press, 2008). This book represents an effort by philosophers and bioethicists to explore the meaning of exploitation, to address the issue of when research in developing countries should count as exploitative, and to consider what can be done practically to minimize the chances for exploitation in this context. Within the literature on human research ethics, this book is exceptional for its philosophical depth.

Hellman, Deborah: "Trials on Trial," *Report from the Institute for Philosophy & Public Policy* 18 (Winter/Spring 1998), pp. 13–18. Hellman explores the ethical issues associated with placebo-controlled trials of the effectiveness of anti-retroviral drugs in reducing mother-to-infant transmission of HIV. In an exceptionally balanced and in-depth discussion, she examines the issues from the perspectives of the patient, the researcher, and the public health official, before concluding that in the context under discussion "the usual interpretations of both the equipoise principle and the standard of care principle are inapt."

Holmes, Helen Bequaert: "Can Clinical Research Be Both Ethical and Scientific?" *Hypatia* 4 (Summer 1989), pp. 154–165. Holmes argues that conflicts between physicians' therapeutic and research obligations in clinical research may result, in part, from excessive faith in the objectivity of science and in statistics. She contends that feminist approaches to clinical research hold promise for more satisfactorily dealing with the ethical and scientific issues involved.

Jonas, Hans: "Philosophical Reflections on Experimenting with Human Subjects," in Paul Freund, ed., *Experimentation with Human Subjects* (New York: Braziller, 1970), pp. 1–31. In this classic essay, Jonas challenges common arguments for the view that the use of human subjects in medical experimentation is morally justified. While Jonas does not argue that all such research is unjustified, he maintains that researchers and other scientists should be the first volunteers in justifiable research.

Kahn, Jeffrey, Anna C. Mastroianni, and Jeremy Sugarman, eds.: *Beyond Consent: Seeking Justice in Research* (New York: Oxford University Press, 1998). This edited volume examines the concept of justice and its application to human subjects research through the different lenses of important research populations: children, the vulnerable sick, captive and convenient populations, women, people of color, and subjects in international settings.

Kopelman, Loretta M.: "Group Benefit and Protection of Pediatric Research Subjects: *Grimes v. Kennedy Krieger* and the Lead Abatement Study," *Accountability in Research* 9 (Summer 2002), pp. 177–192. Kopelman examines a legal case concerning a lead abatement study, drawing implications for the ethics of pediatric research.

London, Alex John: "Justice and the Human Development Approach to International Research," *Hastings Center Report* 35 (January–February 2005), pp. 24–37. Noting that the debate about the ethics of clinical research in developing countries has generally avoided issues of global justice, London addresses these issues in a way that highlights the connections between medical research, the social determinants of health, and justice.

Lurie, Peter, and Sidney M. Wolfe: "Unethical Trials of Interventions to Reduce Perinatal Transmission of the Human Immunodeficiency Virus in Developing Countries," *New England Journal of Medicine* 337 (September 18, 1997), pp. 853–856. The authors contend that because zidovudine has already been shown effective in reducing perinatal transmission of HIV, placebo-based trials in developing countries are unethical for failing to provide subjects in the placebo arm with the standard of care. In order to prevent the exploitation of vulnerable individuals, they argue, research ethics must embrace and maintain universal standards for the treatment of human subjects.

Macklin, Ruth: "International Research: Ethical Imperialism or Ethical Pluralism?" *Accountability in Research* 7 (Spring 1999), pp. 59–83. Against ethical relativism Macklin defends universal moral principles along with a pluralistic view about what specific research practices are appropriate in different cultural contexts. Employing this framework, she engages the ethics of placebo-controlled AZT trials in developing countries and ethical issues provoked by HIV vaccine trials.

National Bioethics Advisory Commission (NBAC): *Research Involving Persons with Mental Disorders That May Affect Decisionmaking Capacity,* vol. I: *Report and Recommendations of the National Bioethics Advisory Committee* (Bethesda, MD: NBAC, 1998). This report provides an overview of ethical issues in research involving subjects whose psychiatric conditions may affect their decision-making capacity. Attempting to reconcile the importance of progress in psychiatric research with the ethical imperative of protecting subjects' rights, the report includes numerous recommendations, including a call for a highly visible, independent panel that would review the most controversial research protocols in this area.

National Commission for the Protection of Human Subjects of Biomedical and Behavioral Research: *The Belmont Report: Ethical Principles and Guidelines for the Protection of Human Subjects of Research.* DHEW (OS) 78-0012. *The Belmont Report. Appendix,* vols. 1, 2. DHEW (OS) 78-0013, 78-0014. (Bethesda, MD, 1978). This report was produced by a commission established under the National Research Act (P.L. 93–348). The commission's purpose was to develop ethical guidelines for the conduct of research involving human subjects and to make recommendations for the application of these guidelines to research conducted or supported by the Department of Health, Education, and Welfare. *The Belmont Report* is the commission's final and most general report. Other reports, listed below, concern narrower topics. The appendices to this report and to the ones listed below contain many useful papers and other materials that were reviewed by the commission prior to formulating its recommendations.

____: *Report and Recommendations: Research Involving Children.* DHEW (OS) 77-0004. *Appendix: Research Involving Children.* DHEW (OS) 77-0005. (Bethesda, MD: 1977).

____: *Report and Recommendations: Research Involving Prisoners.* DHEW (OS) 76-131. *Appendix: Research Involving Prisoners.* DHEW (OS) 76-132. (Bethesda, MD: 1976).

____: *Report and Recommendations: Research Involving Those Institutionalized as Mentally Infirm.* DHEW (OS) 78-0006. *Appendix: Research Involving Those Institutionalized as Mentally Infirm.* DHEW (OS) 78-0007. (Bethesda, MD, 1978).

Nuffield Council on Bioethics: *The Ethics of Research Involving Animals* (London: Nuffield Council on Bioethics, 2005). This report, published by the leading bioethics council in Great Britain, provides an in-depth discussion of the ethics of animal research. The topics addressed include the history of animal research, the moral status of animals, their cognitive lives, the use of animals in various categories of research, and alternatives to animal research. The final section addresses issues of public policy and law.

Smith, Jane A., and Kenneth M. Boyd: *Lives in the Balance: The Ethics of Using Animals in Biomedical Research* (Oxford: Oxford University Press, 1991). This book is a report of a working party of the Institute of Medical Ethics (Great Britain) that met eighteen times to examine ethical issues related to animal research. Notable for both thoroughness and moderation, the book is especially helpful in addressing scientific aspects of the study of animals' mental states.

CHAPTER 5

DEATH AND DECISIONS REGARDING LIFE-SUSTAINING TREATMENT

INTRODUCTION

Decisions regarding life-sustaining treatment frequently emerge from a complex dynamic involving physicians, patients, and families. A wide range of ethical questions and concerns can be raised about such decisions. This chapter begins by engaging some conceptual questions about death itself. Attention is then focused on the refusal of life-sustaining treatment by competent adults. A further concern is the ethics of do-not-resuscitate (DNR) orders, and discussion on this score leads to a consideration of more general questions related to the concept of medical futility. Next, in conjunction with a consideration of treatment decisions for incompetent adults, substantial attention is given to the topic of advance directives.

THE DEFINITION AND DETERMINATION OF DEATH

Two groups of patients are at the center of controversy in recent discussions of the definition and determination of death. In the first group are patients whose *entire* brain has irreversibly ceased functioning. They are irreversibly unconscious, but cardiopulmonary function (heartbeat and respiration) is successfully maintained by a respirator and allied technology. These patients are usually identified either as "brain-dead" or "whole-brain-dead." Here they will be referred to as "brain-dead." In a second group of patients, brain-stem function is sufficient to sustain respiration and heartbeat, but brain damage—typically involving the cerebrum—is so severe that consciousness has been *irreversibly* lost. This group of patients includes those who are in a permanent coma and those whose "persistent vegetative state" (PVS) is permanent.[1] Are the patients in each of these groups alive or dead? In any case, what is the morally appropriate treatment for patients in each group?

The traditional standard for the determination of death is the permanent loss of respiration and heartbeat. According to this standard, brain-dead patients are alive so long as technological support systems sustain cardiopulmonary functioning. In 1968 an ad hoc committee of the Harvard Medical School issued an influential report. In this report, the ad hoc committee specified a set of tests for the identification of a permanently nonfunctioning (whole) brain—that is, the condition of brain death. In the view of the ad hoc committee, when this condition has been diagnosed, "death is to be declared and *then* the respirator turned off."[2] In essence, then, the ad hoc committee advanced a new standard for the determination of death. A brain-dead patient is a dead patient, even if cardiopulmonary function is being maintained by artificial means.

It is a matter of substantial importance whether brain-dead patients are alive or dead. For example, taking the vital organs of these patients for transplantation purposes is morally unproblematic if they are dead—presuming, of course, that appropriate consent procedures have been followed. If they are alive, however, taking their vital organs would presumably be the cause of their death. There are other important implications for the way we think and the way we talk. When a respirator is withdrawn from a brain-dead patient, how are we to conceptualize this action? If the patient is still alive, then it is appropriate to describe the removal of the respirator as the withdrawal of life-sustaining treatment, and it makes sense to say that we are allowing the patient to die. However, if the patient is already dead when we remove the respirator, it does not make sense to say that we are allowing the patient to die.

The substance of the Harvard proposal is reflected in the approach taken by the President's Commission for the Study of Ethical Problems in Medicine and Biomedical and Behavioral Research. In its 1981 report, *Defining Death,* the commission recommended that all states adopt the Uniform Determination of Death Act:

> An individual who has sustained either (1) irreversible cessation of circulatory and respiratory functions, or (2) irreversible cessation of all functions of the entire brain, including the brain stem, is dead. A determination of death must be made in accordance with accepted medical standards.

The whole-brain standard of death that is built into the Uniform Determination of Death Act has achieved widespread public acceptance in the United States, and yet the adequacy of the whole-brain standard continues to be challenged both on theoretical and clinical grounds.[3] Some of those who reject the whole-brain approach argue for a higher-brain approach (as explained below).

In one of this chapter's selections, James L. Bernat, an early proponent of the whole-brain approach, defends the view against some criticisms that have been raised against it, mostly by academics. He argues that the view captures our ordinary concept of death reasonably well and, more importantly, has proven a workable basis for public policy across the globe. Bernat also argues that other approaches compare unfavorably to the whole-brain approach on these measures. The alternatives that he considers include the higher-brain approach and approaches that characterize death in terms of brain-stem function or the circulatory-respiratory system. Bernat acknowledges that critics of the whole-brain approach have made some sound philosophical points, but he denies that any of the proposed alternatives makes more sense as a foundation for policy and practice.

Responding directly to Bernat and others, Jeff McMahan defends a higher-brain approach, distinguishing between the human organism and the person to whom the organism belongs at a given time. According to the higher-brain approach, a person dies upon irreversibly losing the capacity for consciousness. The organism can continue to live, McMahan argues, even after the associated person has died, because irreversible loss of consciousness entails the person's death but not that of the associated organism. A patient in a permanent vegetative state is, on this view, already dead. Inducing cardiac arrest in such a patient cannot, therefore, constitute a killing of the person. Likewise, if the patient is already dead, then the removal of his or her organs for transplantation cannot count as killing him or her, either.

Others find fault with any approach that seems to redefine "death." As Robert D. Truog and Franklin G. Miller point out in their paper, there are patients who are classified as brain dead whom many observers would consider to be still alive: these patients are warm to the touch, digest and metabolize food, mature sexually, and can even reproduce. Truog and Miller argue that, even if a brain-death approach otherwise makes medical and philosophical sense, the medical profession invites distrust and suspicion on the part of the general public when it denies that these patients are still alive. Instead, the authors suggest relaxing the dead donor rule, which currently requires that prospective organ donors be dead before their organs may be removed. As an alternative to the dead donor rule, Truog and Miller propose a strict ethical requirement of prior informed consent and a condition of irreversible unconsciousness. Their approach would avoid invoking what they see as the dubious concept of brain death, while protecting the rights of prospective donors and maintaining at least the current supply of donor organs for transplant.

COMPETENT ADULTS AND THE REFUSAL OF LIFE-SUSTAINING TREATMENT

Regarding the refusal of life-sustaining treatment by competent adults, there seem to be noteworthy differences among the following: (1) cases in which a patient, by accepting life-sustaining treatment, would return to a state of health; (2) cases in which a patient, by accepting life-sustaining treatment, would simply continue a severely compromised existence; and (3) cases in which a terminally ill patient, by accepting life-sustaining treatment, would merely *prolong the dying process.*

Refusal of treatment in cases of the first type is relatively uncommon but typically dramatic. The most discussed example involves a Jehovah's Witness who refuses to accept a blood transfusion for religious reasons. It is widely acknowledged, at least in theory, that respect for individual autonomy requires recognition of the right of a competent adult Jehovah's Witness to refuse a life-sustaining blood transfusion.[4]

In conjunction with ongoing developments in the courts, refusal of treatment in cases of the second type is probably becoming increasingly common. By and large, the law now recognizes the right of a competent adult—and not just one who is terminally ill or in the process of dying—to refuse life-sustaining treatment. Consider in this regard the example of a patient whose life is severely compromised by the presence of a painful and debilitating form of arthritis. This patient is coincidentally being treated for pneumonia and is temporarily dependent upon a respirator until the antibiotics have a chance to take effect. The pneumonia is entirely curable and the patient, however much compromised from a quality-of-life standpoint, is not in the process of dying. If the patient now decides to forgo the respirator, we cannot simply say that the patient has chosen not to prolong the dying process. Accordingly, although considerations of individual autonomy provide a strong moral warrant for the right to refuse life-sustaining treatment in general, some commentators would take issue with the right to refuse treatment in this kind of case because they are concerned about the implications of accepting quality-of-life considerations. It can also be argued that the refusal of life-sustaining treatment in this kind of case is tantamount to suicide,[5] an approach taken by Vicki Michel in one of this chapter's readings. Michel's discussion is also notable for its presentation of a disability-rights perspective on the issues at stake.

In another reading in this chapter, Tia Powell and Bruce Lowenstein focus attention on the case of a chronically disabled woman who chose to refuse life-sustaining treatment. The patient, who suffered a brain-stem stroke at the age of 37, remained mentally alert but was rendered quadriplegic and unable to speak. As described by Powell and Lowenstein, much of the ethical tension in the case can be traced to the fact that staff members working with the patient in a rehabilitation facility felt that she had decided too rapidly that she could not adjust to a life with serious disability.

Refusal of treatment in cases of the third type has a strong foundation in both morality and law and is certainly common. In many cases of terminal illness, "aggressive" treatment is capable of warding off death—for a time. However, it is often questionable whether such treatment is in a patient's best interest, and a competent adult is generally considered to have both a moral and a legal right to refuse treatment that would merely prolong the dying process.

Depending upon a patient's circumstances, life-sustaining treatment can take a variety of forms—for example, mechanical respiration, cardiopulmonary resuscitation, kidney dialysis, surgery, antiobiotics, and artificial nutrition and hydration. It is sometimes claimed that the provision of food and water is so fundamentally different from other forms of life-sustaining treatment that it may never be omitted. Those who systematically oppose withholding nutrition and hydration often call attention to the symbolic significance of food and water—their intimate connection with notions of care and concern. However, most commentators insist that there is no reason to apply a different standard to artificial nutrition and hydration. In their view, artificial nutrition and hydration—just like other life-sustaining treatments—will sometimes fail to offer a patient a net benefit, and the decision of a competent patient to refuse them must be respected.

In one of the selections in this chapter, the AMA Council on Ethical and Judicial Affairs acknowledges and endorses the right of competent patients to forgo life-sustaining treatment. The council explicitly argues against the view that it is never permissible to forgo artificial nutrition and hydration. One other issue discussed by the council is noteworthy. Although it is clear that medical decision making is sometimes influenced by the fact that many physicians are more comfortable with withholding a life-sustaining treatment to begin with rather than withdrawing it once it has been initiated, the council insists that there is no ethically significant distinction between withholding and withdrawing life-sustaining treatment.

DNR ORDERS AND MEDICAL FUTILITY

When a patient undergoes cardiac arrest, resuscitation techniques can sometimes restore heartbeat and thereby prolong life, yet in many cases a dying patient would not welcome attempts at cardiopulmonary resuscitation (CPR), and in some cases there is virtually no likelihood of success. In one of this chapter's readings, Tom Tomlinson and Howard Brody identify three distinct rationales for do-not-resuscitate (DNR) orders. Two of the identified rationales involve quality-of-life judgments. Insisting that quality-of-life judgments must ultimately be made by the patient or the patient's family (if the patient is incompetent), Tomlinson and Brody argue that it is inappropriate in such cases for a physician to write a DNR order without the permission of the patient or family. With regard to a third rationale, however, they contend that there is no need for the physician to secure the permission of the patient or family before writing a DNR order. They rely at this point on the concept of futility. In their view, sometimes "resuscitation would almost certainly not be successful," and the "decision that CPR is unjustified because it is futile is a judgment that falls entirely within the physician's expertise."

Although many patients and their families feel there is an ongoing need to assert a patient's right to refuse life-sustaining treatment against a perceived tendency among physicians to overtreat, it is also true that many physicians increasingly feel the need to assert a professional prerogative to limit treatment in the face of requests from patients and (more commonly) from families that "everything be done." If patients or their families desire treatments considered futile by physicians, are physicians justified in refusing to provide them? Clearly, Tomlinson and Brody would respond in the affirmative. However, the meaning of "futility" is presently the source of intense controversy in biomedical ethics, as is the ethical significance of the concept. Mark R. Wicclair, in this chapter, distinguishes various senses of futility and ultimately recommends that physicians avoid the language of futility in expressing their opposition to a given treatment.

ADVANCE DIRECTIVES AND TREATMENT DECISIONS FOR INCOMPETENT ADULTS

The rigors of incurable illness and the dying process frequently deprive previously competent patients of their decision-making capacity. How can a person best ensure that his or her personal wishes with regard to life-sustaining treatment (in various possible circumstances) will be honored even if decision-making capacity is lost? Although communication of one's attitudes and preferences to one's physician, family, and friends surely provides some measure of protection, it is frequently asserted that the most effective protection comes through the formation of advance directives.

There are two basic types of advance directives, and each has legal status in almost all, if not all, of the states. In executing an *instructional* directive, a person specifies instructions about his or her care in the event that decision-making capacity is lost. Such a directive, especially when it deals specifically with a person's wishes regarding life-sustaining treatment in various possible circumstances, is commonly called a *living will.* In executing a *proxy* directive, a person specifies a substitute decision maker to make health-care decisions for him or her in the event that decision-making capacity is lost. The legal mechanism for executing a proxy directive is often called a *durable power of attorney for health care.* Since purging ambiguities from even the most explicit written directives is difficult, as is foreseeing all the contingencies that might give rise to a need for treatment decisions, many commentators recommend the execution of a durable power of attorney for health care even if a person has already executed a living will.[6]

If a patient lacks decision-making capacity and has not executed a proxy directive, a surrogate decision maker must be identified; ordinarily this is a member of the family or a close personal friend. If the patient has provided an instructional directive, the surrogate is, of course, expected to follow the stated instructions. However, sometimes an instructional directive provides insufficient guidance for the treatment decision at hand, and frequently a surrogate decision maker must function in the absence of any instructional directive. In applying the *substituted-judgment* standard, the surrogate decision maker is expected to consider the patient's preferences and values and make the decision that the patient would have made if he or she had been able to choose. If no reliable basis exists to infer what the patient would have chosen, then the surrogate decision maker is expected to retreat to the *best-interests* standard. In applying the best-interests standard, the surrogate decision maker is expected to choose in accordance with the patient's best interests, which may reduce to choosing what a reasonable person in the patient's circumstances would choose.[7]

The Patient Self-Determination Act, passed by Congress in October 1990, requires all health-care institutions (e.g., hospitals and nursing homes) receiving federal funds to inform patients of their right to formulate advance directives. Nevertheless, advance directives remain problematic in many ways. Especially worrisome are concerns that can be raised about the construction, implementation, and force of instructional directives. For one thing, many of the standard-form living wills that have emerged in conjunction with state statutes can be activated only upon the diagnosis of a "terminal illness," a category that has usually been interpreted to exclude both a patient in a permanent vegetative state and one who is existing in a severely compromised state as a result of a progressively debilitating disease (e.g., Alzheimer's). Other phrases commonly found in living wills are also problematic. For example, suppose a patient signs a form that authorizes withholding or withdrawing life-sustaining treatment if there is "no reasonable expectation that I will regain a meaningful quality of life." Unless a person provides a further specification of what counts for him or her as "a meaningful quality of life," numerous problems of interpretation can arise. Another important question is whether physicians can ever be justified in refusing to honor the provisions of a patient's instructional directive.

In one of this chapter's selections, Thomas A. Mappes considers some of the many problems that can be raised about the construction and implementation of advance directives, especially instructional directives. In the final selection of this chapter, Rebecca Dresser focuses attention on patients who are incompetent, severely compromised, yet conscious and not terminally ill. The point of departure for her discussion is the *Wendland* case, in which the California Supreme Court refused to authorize the cessation of nutrition and hydration for Robert Wendland, a man who was left severely brain damaged as a result of an automobile accident. Dresser writes that "*Wendland* may signal a developing legal consensus," and she explores some of the implications of this consensus, especially in reference to advance directives.

NOTES

1 The phrase *persistent vegetative state* (PVS) continues to be the source of confusion. When a patient's vegetative state is identified as "persistent," it is certainly implied that the vegetative state has endured for a significant period of time. (In fact, according to a reigning clinical standard, a vegetative state must last at least a month before it can be diagnosed as persistent.) Is it also implied in calling a vegetative state "persistent" that it is irreversible, that is, permanent? Some writers in biomedical ethics speak of a patient's vegetative state as "persistent" only when it is believed that the condition is permanent. In this sense, a persistent vegetative state entails that the condition is permanent. More commonly, however, the

phrase "persistent vegetative state" is used in a contrasting way. In this sense, a persistent vegetative state does not entail that the condition is permanent. When PVS is understood in this way, there is no contradiction in saying that a patient has recovered from PVS. Of course, whenever a patient has been in a vegetative state for a significant period of time, a medical determination of irreversibility is of central practical importance. For further clarification of PVS and the difference between permanent vegetative state and permanent coma, see Ronald E. Cranford, "Definition and Determination of Death: Criteria for Death," in Warren R. Reich, ed., *Encyclopedia of Bioethics*, rev. ed. (New York: Macmillan, 1995), pp. 531–533.

2 The Ad Hoc Committee of the Harvard Medical School to Examine the Definition of Brain Death, "A Definition of Irreversible Coma," *JAMA* 205 (August 6, 1968), p. 338.

3 See, for example, *Journal of Medicine and Philosophy* 26 (October 2001). The articles in this issue are grouped under the title "Revisiting Brain Death." Some critics of the whole-brain approach are opposed to the higher-brain approach as well. See, for example, Michael Potts et al., eds., *Beyond Brain Death: The Case Against Brain Based Criteria for Human Death* (Dordrecht: Kluwer, 2000).

4 See, for example, Ruth Macklin, "Consent, Coercion, and Conflicts of Rights," *Perspectives in Biology and Medicine* 20 (Spring 1977), pp. 360–371. For a discussion of added complexities, see Dena S. Davis, "Does 'No' Mean 'Yes'? The Continuing Problem of Jehovah's Witnesses and Refusal of Blood Products," *Second Opinion* 19 (January 1994), pp. 35–43.

5 The morality of suicide is discussed in Chapter 6.

6 Some commentators also recommend that patients complete a "values history," a document that is designed to provide background information on patient values and attitudes. A values history might function as a supplement to an instructional directive, intended to guide any necessary interpretation, or it could be intended as a resource for one's designated proxy or surrogate.

7 For one articulation of the "standard wisdom" regarding surrogate decision making for incompetent adults, see Dan W. Brock, "Surrogate Decision Making for Incompetent Adults: An Ethical Framework," *Mount Sinai Journal of Medicine* 58 (October 1991), pp. 388–392. In contrast, John Hardwig calls for a fundamental revision in the theory of surrogate (proxy) decision making. He challenges the appropriateness of exclusively patient-centered standards of surrogate decision making, and he argues that it is morally unsound to expect proxy decision makers to disregard their own interests and those of other family members. See John Hardwig, "The Problem of Proxies with Interests of Their Own: Toward a Better Theory of Proxy Decisions," *Journal of Clinical Ethics* 4 (Spring 1993), pp. 20–27.

THE DEFINITION AND DETERMINATION OF DEATH

THE WHOLE-BRAIN CONCEPT OF DEATH
REMAINS OPTIMUM PUBLIC POLICY

James L. Bernat

After briefly tracing the origins of the concept of whole-brain death, Bernat defends this approach as capturing more effectively than other approaches the standard concept of death. He criticizes the higher-brain approach, favored by some scholars but not reflected in public policy anywhere in the world, as failing to reflect what ordinary people mean by "death," namely the irreversible loss of the critical functions of the organism as a whole. In Bernat's view the whole-brain concept also provides a more clinically reliable criterion for death than does the higher-brain criterion, and is superior in other respects to the brain-stem and circulatory-respiratory criteria proposed by others. While conceding to critics that the whole-brain criterion suffers from some conceptual and practical weaknesses, Bernat emphasizes that it has proven a workable basis for public policy in many countries around the world. Any competitor, he believes, must show that it, too, translates into policies that would be intuitively acceptable and would maintain public confidence in the medical profession. Bernat admits, however, that flaws may exist in the procedures by which determinations of brain death are presently made. If such flaws exist, then these procedures should be supplemented by clinical tests for cessation of all intracranial blood flow, so as to avoid false determinations that death has occurred.

The definition of death is one of the oldest and most enduring problems in biophilosophy and bioethics. Serious controversies over formally defining death began with the invention of the positive-pressure mechanical ventilator in the 1950s. For the first time, physicians could maintain ventilation and, hence, circulation on patients who had sustained what had been previously lethal brain damage. Prior to the development of mechanical ventilators, brain injuries severe enough to induce apnea quickly progressed to cardiac arrest from hypoxemia. Before the 1950s, the loss of spontaneous breathing and heartbeat ("vital functions") were perfect predictors of death because the functioning of the brain and of all other organs ceased rapidly and nearly simultaneously thereafter, producing a unitary death phenomenon. In the pre-technological era, physicians and philosophers did not have to consider whether a human being who had lost certain "vital functions" but had retained others was alive, because such cases were technically impossible.

With the advent of mechanical support of ventilation, (permitting maintenance of circulation) the previous unitary determination of death became ambiguous. Now patients were encountered in whom some vital organ functions (brain) had ceased totally and irreversibly, while other vital organ functions (such as ventilation and circulation) could be maintained, albeit mechanically. Their life status was ambiguous and debatable because they had features of both dead and living patients. They resembled dead patients in that they could not move or breathe, were utterly unresponsive to any stimuli, and had lost brain stem reflex activity. But they also resembled living patients in that they had main-

tained heartbeat, circulation and intact visceral organ functioning. Were these unfortunate patients in fact alive or dead?

In a series of scientific articles addressing this unprecedented state, several authors made the bold claim that patients who had totally and irreversibly lost brain functions were dead, despite their continued heartbeat and circulation.[1] In the 1960s, they popularized the concept they called "brain death" to acknowledge this idea.[2] The intuitive attractiveness of the concept of "brain death" led to its rapid acceptance by the medical and scientific community, and to legislators expeditiously drafting public laws permitting physicians to determine death on the basis of loss of brain functioning.[3] Interestingly, largely by virtue of its intuitive appeal, the academy, medical practitioners, governments, and the public accepted the validity of brain death prior to the development of a rigorous biophilosophical proof that brain dead patients were truly dead. Medical historians have emphasized utilitarian factors in this rapid acceptance, because a determination of brain death permitted the desired societal goals of cessation of medical treatment and organ procurement.[4]

The practice of determining human death using brain death tests has become worldwide over the past several decades. The practice is enshrined in law in all 50 states in the United States and in approximately 80 other countries, including nearly all of the developed world and much of the undeveloped world.[5] A 1995 conference on the definition of death sponsored by the Institute of Medicine concluded that, despite certain theoretical and practical shortcomings, the practice of diagnosing brain death was so successful and so well accepted by the medical profession and the public that no major public policy changes seemed desirable.[6]

Yet despite this consensus, from its beginning, a persistent group of critics have attacked the concept

From *Journal of Law, Medicine & Ethics*, vol. 34, no. 1 (2006), pp. 35–43. Copyright © 2006 by Blackwell Publishing, Ltd. Reproduced with permission of Blackwell Publishing, Ltd.

and practice of brain death as being conceptually invalid or a violation of religious beliefs.[7] Recently, through the intellectual leadership of Alan Shewmon, additional critics have concluded that the concept of brain death is incoherent, anachronistic, unnecessary, a legal fiction, and should be abandoned.[8] In this essay I show that, despite admitted shortcomings, the classical formulation of whole-brain death remains both conceptually coherent and forms a solid foundation for public policy surrounding human death determination and organ transplantation.

AN ANALYSIS OF DEATH

Defining death is a formidable task.[9] In their rigorous, thoughtful, and highly influential book *Defining Death*,[10] the President's Commission for the Study of Ethical Problems in Medicine and Biomedical and Behavioral Research chose as their conceptual foundation the analysis of death that I published with my Dartmouth colleagues Charles Culver and Bernard Gert.[11] Our analysis was conducted in three sequential phases: (1) the philosophical task of determining the definition of death by making explicit the consensual concept of death that has been confounded by technology; (2) the philosophical and medical task of determining the best criterion of death, a measurable condition that shows that the definition has been fulfilled by being both necessary and sufficient for death; and (3) the medical-scientific task of determining the tests of death for physicians to employ at the patient's bedside to demonstrate that the criterion of death has been fulfilled with no false positive and minimal false negative determinations. Most subsequent scholars have accepted this method of analysis, if not our conclusions, with two recent exceptions.[12]

Following a series of published critiques and rebuttals of our position over the past two decades, I concluded that much of the disagreement over our account of death resulted from the lack of acceptance by dissenting scholars of the "paradigm of death." By "paradigm of death" I refer specifically to a set of conditions and assumptions that frame the discussion of the topic of death by identifying the nature of the topic, the class of phenomena to which it belongs, how it should be discussed, and its con-

ceptual boundaries.[13] Accepting a paradigm of death permits scholars to rationally analyze and discuss death without falling victim to the fallacy of category noncongruence and consequently talking past each other. But the paradigm remains useful even if scholars do not agree on all its elements, because it can help clarify the root of their disagreement.

My paradigm of death comprises seven sequential elements. First, the word "death" is a common, nontechnical word that we all use correctly to refer to the cessation of a human being's life. The philosophical task of defining death seeks not to redefine it by contriving a new meaning, but rather to divine and make explicit the implicit meaning of death that we all accept but that has been made ambiguous by technological advances. Some scholars have gone astray by not attempting to capture our consensual concept of death and instead redefining death for ideological purposes or by overanalyzing death to a metaphysical level of abstraction—thereby rendering it devoid of its ordinary meaning.[14]

Second, death is fundamentally a biological phenomenon. We all agree that life is a biological entity; thus also should be its cessation. Accepting that death is a biological phenomenon neither denigrates the richness and beauty of various cultural and religious practices surrounding death and dying, nor denies societies their proper authority to govern practices and establish laws regulating the determination and time of death. But death is an immutable and objective biological fact and not fundamentally a social contrivance.[15] For the definition and criterion of death, the paradigm thus exclusively considers the ontology of death and ignores its normative aspects.

Third, we restrict our analysis to the death of higher vertebrate species for which death is univocal. That is, we mean the same phenomenon of "death" when we say our cousin died as we do when we say our dog died. Although individual cells within organisms and single-celled organisms also die, our analysis of defining human death is simplified by restricting our purview to the death of related higher vertebrate species. Determining the death of cells, organs, protozoa, or bacteria are valid biophilosophical tasks but are not the task at hand here.

Fourth, the term "death" can be applied directly and categorically only to organisms. All living organisms must die and only living organisms can die. Our use of language may seem to confuse this point, for example, when we say "a person died." But by this usage we are referring directly to the death of the living organism that embodied the person, not to a living organism ceasing to be a person. Personhood is a psychosocial construct that can be lost but cannot die, except metaphorically. Similarly, other uses of the term "death" such as "the death of a culture" clearly are metaphorical and fall outside the paradigm.[16]

Fifth, a higher vertebrate organism can reside in only one of two states, alive or dead: no organism can be in both states or in neither. Based on the theory of fuzzy sets, the concept that the world does not easily divide itself into sets and their complements, Amir Halevy and Baruch Brody proposed that an organism may reside in a transitional state between alive and dead that shares features of both states.[17] This claim appears plausible when considering cases of gradual, protracted dying, in which it may be difficult and even appear arbitrary to identify the precise moment of death. But this claim ignores the important distinction between our ability to identify an organism's biological state and the nature of that state. Simply because we currently lack the technical ability to always accurately identify an organism's state does not necessitate postulating an in-between state. Using the terminology of fuzzy set theory as a guide, the paradigm requires us to view alive and dead as mutually exclusive (non-overlapping) and jointly exhaustive (no other) sets.

Sixth, and inevitably following from the preceding premise, death must be an event and not a process. If there are only two exclusive underlying states of an organism, the transition from one state to the other, at least in theory, must be sudden and instantaneous, because of the absence of an intervening state. Disagreement on this point, highlighted since the original debate over 30 years ago in *Science* by Robert Morison and Leon Kass,[18] centers on the difference between our ability to accurately measure the presence of a biological state and the nature of that biological state. To an observer, it may appear that death is an ineluctable process within which it is arbitrary to stipulate the moment of death, but such an observation simply underscores our cur-

rent technical limitations. For technical reasons, the event of death may be determinable with confidence only in retrospect. As my colleagues and I first observed in 1981, death is best conceptualized not as a process but as the event separating the biological processes of dying and bodily disintegration.[19]

Seventh and finally, death is irreversible. By its nature, if the event of death were reversible it would not be death but rather part of the process of dying that was interrupted and reversed. Advances in technology permit physicians to interrupt the dying process in some cases and postpone the event of death. So-called "near-death experiences," reported by some critically ill patients who subsequently recovered, do not indicate returning from the dead but are rather recalled experiences that result from alterations in brain physiology during incipient dying that was reversed in a timely manner.[20]

THE DEFINITION OF DEATH

Given the set of assumptions and conditions comprising the paradigm of death, we can now explore the definition, criterion, and tests of death. Defining death is the conceptual task of making explicit our understanding of it. It poses an essential question: what does it mean for an organism to die, particularly in our contemporary circumstance in which technology can compensate for the failure of certain vital organs?

We all agree that by "death" we do not require the cessation of functioning of every cell in the body, because some integument cells that require little oxygen or blood flow continue to function temporarily after death is customarily declared. We also do not simply mean the cessation of heartbeat and respiration, though this circumstance will lead to death if untreated. Although some religious believers assert that the soul departs the body at the moment of death, this is not an adequate definition of death because it is not what religious believers fundamentally mean by "death."

Beginning early in the brain-death debate, Robert Veatch advocated a position that became known as the "higher-brain formulation of death."[21] He claimed that death should be defined formally as "the irreversible loss of that which is considered to be essentially significant to the nature of man." He expressly rejected the idea that death should be related to an organism's "loss of the capacity to integrate bodily function" asserting that "man is, after all, something more than a sophisticated computer."[22] His project attempted not to reject brain death, but to refine the intuitive thinking underlying the brain death concept by emphasizing that it was the cerebral cortex that counted in a brain death concept and not the more primitive integrating brain structures.

Irrespective of the attractiveness of this idea, (it has spawned a loyal following[23]) the higher-brain formulation contains a fatal flaw as a candidate for a definition of death: it is not what we mean when we say "death." Its logical criterion of death would be the irreversible loss of consciousness and cognition, such as that which occurs in patients in an irreversible persistent vegetative state (PVS). Thus a higher-brain formulation of death would count PVS patients as dead. However, despite their profound and tragic disability, all societies, cultures, and laws consider PVS patients as alive. Thus, despite its potential merits, the higher-brain formulation fails the first condition of the paradigm: to make explicit our underlying consensual concept of death and not to contrive a new definition of death.

In 1981, my colleagues and I strove to capture the essence of the concept of human death that formed the intuitive foundation of the brain-based criterion of death. We defined death as "the cessation of functioning of the organism as a whole."[24] This definition utilized a biological concept proposed by Jacques Loeb in 1916.[25] Loeb explained that organisms are not simply composites of cells, tissues, and organs, but possess overarching functions that regulate and integrate all systems to maintain the unity and interrelatedness of the organism to promote its optimal functioning and health. The organism as a whole comprises that set of functions that are greater than the mere sum of the organism's parts.

More recently, biophilosophers have advanced the concept of "emergent functions" to explain this type of phenomenon with greater conceptual clarity.[26] An emergent function is a property of a whole that is not possessed by any of its component parts, and that cannot be reduced to one or more of its component parts. The physiological correlate of the organism as a whole is the set of emergent functions of the organism. The irretrievable loss of the organism's emergent functions produces loss of the critical functioning of the organism as a whole and therefore is the death of the organism.

In early writings on brain death, a few scholars proposed similar ideas. Most noteworthy was Julius Korein who asserted that the brain was the "critical system" of the organism whose loss indicated the organism's death.[27] Using thermodynamics theory, Korein argued that once the critical system was irretrievably lost (death), an irreversible and unstoppable process ensued of increasing entropy that constituted the process of bodily disintegration. The concept of the demise of the organism's critical system relies on concepts analogous to the cessation of functions of the organism as a whole.

Examples of critical functions of the organism as a whole include: (1) consciousness, which is necessary for the organism to respond to requirements for hydration and nutrition; (2) control of circulation, respiration, and temperature control, which are necessary for all cellular metabolism; and (3) integrating and control systems involving chemoreceptors, baroreceptors, and neuroendocrine feedback loops to maintain homeostasis. Death is the irreversible and permanent loss of the critical functions of the organism as a whole.

THE CRITERION OF DEATH

The next task is to identify the criterion of death, the general measurable condition that satisfies the definition of death by being both necessary and sufficient for death. There are several plausible candidates for a criterion of death. Among brain death advocates, three separate criteria have been proposed: (1) the whole-brain formulation, the criterion recommended by the Harvard Committee and the President's Commission, and accepted throughout the United States and in most parts of the world; (2) the higher-brain formulation, popular in the academy but accepted in no jurisdictions anywhere; and (3) the brain stem formulation accepted in the United Kingdom.[28]

The whole-brain criterion requires cessation of all brain clinical functions including those of the cerebral hemispheres, diencephalon (thalamus and hypothalamus), and brain stem. Whole-brain theorists require widespread cessation of neuronal functions because each part of the brain serves the critical functions of the organism as a whole. The brain stem initiates and controls breathing, regulates circulation, and serves as the generator of conscious awareness through the ascending reticular activating system. The diencephalon provides the center for bodily homeostasis, regulating and coordinating numerous neuroendocrine control systems such as those regulating body temperature, salt and water regulation, feeding behavior, and memory. The cerebral hemispheres have an indispensable role in awareness that provides the conditions for all conscious behavior that serves the health and survival of the organism.

Clinical functions are those that are measurable at the bedside. The distinction between the brain's clinical functions and brain activities, recordable electrically or through other laboratory means, was made by the President's Commission in *Defining Death* though, for the sake of brevity, it did not appear in the Uniform Determination of Death Act proposed by the Commission.[29] All clinical brain functions measurable at the bedside must be lost and the absence must be shown to be irreversible. But the whole-brain criterion does not require the loss of all neuronal activities. Some neurons may survive and contribute to recordable brain activities (by an electroencephalogram, for example) but not to clinical functions.[30] The precise number, location, and configuration of the minimum number of critical neuron arrays remain unknown.

Despite the fact that the whole-brain criterion does not require the cessation of functioning of every brain neuron, it does rely on a pathophysiological process known as brain herniation to assure widespread destruction of the neuron systems responsible for the brain's clinical functions.[31] When the brain is injured diffusely by trauma, hypoxicischemic damage during cardiorespiratory arrest or asphyxia, meningoencephalitis, or enlarging intracranial mass lesions such as neoplasms,[32] brain edema causes intracranial pressure to rise to levels exceeding mean arterial blood pressure. At this point, intracranial circulation ceases and nearly all brain neurons that were not destroyed by the initial brain injury are secondarily destroyed by lack of

intracranial circulation. Thus the whole-brain formulation provides a fail-safe mechanism to eliminate false-positive brain death determinations and assure the loss of the critical functions of the organism as a whole. Showing the absence of all intracranial circulation is sufficient to prove widespread destruction of all critical neuronal systems. Similarly, it satisfies Korein's requirement for the loss of the irreplaceable critical system of the organism.

The higher-brain formulation fails to provide an adequate criterion of death because its conditions are insufficient for the loss of the critical functions of the organism as a whole. Its criterion is the irreversible loss of consciousness and cognition. The most common clinical manifestation of this condition is the PVS, caused by diffuse damage to the cerebral hemispheres, thalami, or disconnections between those structures.[33] In most cases of PVS, brain-stem neurons and their functions remain intact, so PVS patients, although unaware, have retained wakefulness and sleep-wake cycles (through the function of the intact ascending reticular activating system), have continued control of respiration and circulation by the intact medulla, and retain other brain-stem mediated regulatory functions.[34] The higher-brain formulation, thus, serves as neither an adequate definition nor criterion of death.

The criterion of the brain-stem formulation is the loss of consciousness and the capacity for breathing.[35] Diffuse damage to the brain stem that is sufficient to destroy the ascending reticular activating system and the medullary breathing center satisfies this criterion. But the brain-stem formulation does not require commensurate damage to the diencephalon or cerebral hemispheres. It therefore leaves open the possibility of misdiagnosis of death because of a pathological process that appears to destroy brain-stem activities but that permits some form of residual conscious awareness that cannot be easily detected. It thus lacks the fail-safe feature of whole-brain death to test for and guarantee the irreversible loss of these critical systems.

As a criterion of death, the circulation formulation fails for precisely the opposite reason of the higher-brain and brain-stem formulations. Whereas the higher-brain and brain-stem criteria both fail because they are necessary but not sufficient for death, the circulation criterion fails because it is sufficient but not necessary for death. The loss of all systemic circulation produces the destruction of all bodily organs and tissues so it is clearly a sufficient condition for death. But it is unnecessary to require the cessation of functions of organs that do not serve the critical functions of the organism as a whole.[36]

THE TESTS OF DEATH

Brain death tests must be used to determine death only in the unusual case in which a patient's ventilation is being supported. If positive-pressure ventilation is neither employed nor entertained, the traditional tests of death—prolonged absence of breathing and heartbeat—can be used successfully. These traditional tests are absolutely predictive that the brain will be rapidly destroyed by lack of blood flow and oxygen, at which time death will have occurred. Traditional examinations for death, in addition to testing for heartbeat and breathing, always included tests for responsiveness and pupillary reflexes that directly measure brain function.

The bedside tests satisfying the whole-brain criterion of death have been designed with a sufficiently high degree of concordance to permit the drafting of widely accepted clinical practice guidelines on the determination of brain death.[37] The tests require demonstrating the loss of all clinical brain functions, irreversibility, and a known structural process sufficient to produce the clinical findings. Laboratory tests showing the absence of intracranial blood flow or the absence of electrical activity in the hemispheres and brain stem can be used to confirm the clinical diagnosis to expedite the determination.[38]

Irreversibility is an indispensable requirement for brain death. There is general belief that irreversibility can be adequately demonstrated by conducting serial neurological examinations, excluding potentially reversible factors, and demonstrating a structural cause that is sufficient to account for the clinical signs. But, while highly plausible, these conditions have never been proved to assure irreversibility. Two recent factors prompted me to reassess my previous position that irreversibility could be proved solely by clinical factors and to suggest that a laboratory test showing cessation of all in-

tracranial blood flow should become mandatory in brain death determination.

There are several published studies documenting the alarming frequency of physician variations and errors in performing brain death tests,[39] despite clear guidelines for performing and recording the tests. Patients with "chronic brain death" have been reported who were diagnosed as brain dead but whose circulation and visceral organ functioning were successfully physiologically maintained for months or longer.[40] Eelco Wijdicks and I questioned whether all of the reported patients were correctly diagnosed, and if some brain-damaged but not brain dead patients were included because of inadequate examinations and resultant incorrect brain death determinations.[41] Reacting to both these findings, I proposed that the mere assertion of irreversibility may no longer be sufficient to diagnose brain death and that a test showing cessation of all intracranial blood flow, such as transcranial Doppler ultrasonography, radionuclide angiography, or computed tomographic angiography, should become mandatory, at least if there is any question about the diagnosis or if the examiner is inexperienced.[42]

PUBLIC POLICY ON DEATH

Brain death is widely regarded as the prime example of a formerly contentious bioethical and biophilosophical issue that has been resolved to the point of widespread public consensus.[43] Evidence for this consensus is the enactment of effective and well-accepted brain death laws and policies throughout the world.[44] In the United States, the Uniform Determination of Death Act, recommended by the President's Commission and the National Conference of Commissioners on Uniform State Laws,[45] has been enacted in most states, and others have enacted statutes with similar language. Contemporaneously, the Law Reform Commission of Canada produced a similar statute.[46]

But an observer unaware of this consensus and public acceptance, who relied solely on reading the output of scholarly articles and university conferences on brain death, would reach a far different conclusion. The publication of anti-brain death articles has never been greater than during the past decade.

Yet, despite those arguments, the 1995 Institute of Medicine conference on brain death recommended no changes in public laws in the United States,[47] no jurisdiction has abandoned its brain death statute, and there is evidence that many additional countries have embraced the practice of determining brain death during the past decade of scholarly dissention.[48] What accounts for the mismatch between public acceptance and scholarly agitation?

Higher-brain proponents continue to accept brain death but argue that the criterion of death should be changed to the higher-brain formulation. Brain stem death proponents also accept the conceptual validity of brain death but hold that the criterion of death should be the brain stem formulation. Religious authorities continue a debate that has raged for 40 years about whether brain death is compatible with the doctrines of the world's principal religious traditions.[49] Protestantism, including fundamentalism, has accepted brain death.[50] The debate in Roman Catholicism was largely settled by Pope John Paul's 2000 pronouncement embracing brain death as consistent with Catholic teachings.[51] In Judaism, brain death is accepted by Reform and Conservative authorities, but an Orthodox rabbinic debate continues between those who declare brain death compatible with Jewish law and those who do not.[52] Brain death determination is also practiced in several Islamic societies,[53] Hindi societies,[54] and in Confucian-Shinto Japan.[55]

The principal active opponents within the academy are those who reject the concept of brain death outright and promote the concept that a human being is not dead until the systemic circulation ceases and all organs are destroyed. The circulation proponents see no special role for brain functions in a determination of death. Alan Shewmon, the intellectual leader of the circulationists, has written eloquently on the conceptual problems inherent within the whole-brain (or any brain criterion) formulation.[56] He cites evidence that the brain performs no qualitatively different forms of integration than the spinal cord and argues that therefore it should enjoy no special status above other organs in death determination. He claims further that his cases of "chronic brain death" show that the concept of brain death is inherently counterintuitive, for how could a dead body gestate infants or grow?[57]

Another critic, Robert Taylor, has called the brain death concept a "legal fiction" that is accepted by society in a manner analogous to the concept of legal blindness. Taylor explains that legal blindness is a concept invented by society to permit people who are functionally blind from severe visual impairment to receive the same social benefits as those enjoyed by people who are totally blind. We all know that most people who are declared legally blind are not truly blind. But we employ a legal fiction and use the term "blindness" in a biologically incorrect way for its socially beneficial purpose. Taylor argues that, by analogy, we know that people we declare "brain dead" are not truly dead, but we consider them dead for the socially beneficial goal of organ procurement.[58]

As a longstanding proponent of whole-brain death, I acknowledge that the whole-brain formulation, although coherent, is imperfect, and that my attempts to defend it have not adequately addressed all valid criticisms. But my inadequacies must be viewed within the larger context of the relationship of biology to public policy. Our attempts to conceptualize, understand, and define the complex and subtle natural concepts of life and death remain far from perfect. Perhaps we will never be able to achieve uniform definitions of life and death that everyone accepts and that no one criticizes for conceptual or practical shortcomings.

In the real world of public policy on biological issues, we must frequently make compromises or approximations to achieve acceptable practices and laws. For these compromises to be tolerable, generally they should be minor and not affect outcomes. For example, in the current practice of organ donation after cardiac death (formerly known as non-heart-beating organ donation), I and others raised the question of whether the organ donor patients were truly dead after only five minutes of asystole. The five-minute rule was accepted by the Institute of Medicine as the point at which death could be declared and the organs procured.[59] Ours was a biologically valid criticism because, at least in theory, some such patients could be resuscitated after five minutes of asystole and still retain measurable brain function. If that was true, they were not yet dead at that point so their death declaration was premature.

But thereafter I changed my position to support programs of organ donation after cardiac death. I decided that it was justified to accept a compromise on this biological point when I realized that donor patients, if not already dead at five minutes of asystole, were incipiently and irreversibly dying because they could not auto-resuscitate and no one would attempt their resuscitation. Because their loss of circulatory and respiratory functions was permanent if not yet irreversible, there would be no difference whatsoever in their outcomes if their death were declared after five minutes of asystole or after 60 minutes of asystole. I concluded that, from a public policy perspective, accepting the permanent loss of circulatory and respiratory functions rather than requiring their irreversible loss was justified. The good accruing to the organ recipient, the donor patient, and the donor family resulting from organ donation justified overlooking the biological shortcoming because, although the difference in the death criteria was real, it was inconsequential.

Of course Alan Shewmon is correct that not all bodily system integration and functions of the organism as a whole are conducted by the brain (though most are) and that the spinal cord and other structures serve relevant roles. And Robert Taylor is correct that many people view brain death as a legal fiction and regard such patients "as good as dead" but not biologically dead. But despite its shortcomings, the whole-brain formulation remains coherent on the grounds of the critical functions of the organism as a whole and on the additional grounds of Korein's critical system theory. The whole-brain death formulation comprises a concept and public policy that make intuitive and practical sense and have been well accepted by the public throughout many societies. Therefore, while I am willing to acknowledge that whole-brain death formulation remains imperfect, I continue to support it because on the public policy level its shortcomings are relatively inconsequential.

Those scholars attacking the established whole-brain death formulation have a duty to show that their proposed alternative formulations not only more accurately represent biological reality, but also can be translated into successful public policy that is intuitively acceptable and maintains public confidence in physicians' accuracy in death determination and in the integrity of the organ procurement enterprise. Although I acknowledge certain weakness of the whole-brain death formulation, I hold that it most accurately maps our consensual implicit concept of death in a technological age and, as a consequence, it has been accepted by societies throughout the world.

REFERENCES

1 The early history of "brain death" is discussed in M. S. Pernick, "Brain Death in a Cultural Context: The Reconstruction of Death 1967–1981," in S. J. Youngner, R. M. Arnold, and R. Schapiro, eds., *The Definition of Death: Contemporary Controversies* (Baltimore: Johns Hopkins University Press, 1999): 13–33; and M. N. Diringer and E. F. M. Wijdicks, "Brain Death in Historical Perspective," in E. F. M. Wijdicks, ed., *Brain Death* (Philadelphia: Lippincott Williams & Wilkins, 2001): 5–27. Early reports from France described *coma dépassé* (a state beyond coma). See P. Mollaret and M. Goulon, "Le Coma Dépassé (Mémoire Préliminaire)" *Revue Neurologique* 101 (1959): 3–15. The Harvard Medical School report was the earliest widely publicized article to claim that such patients were dead. See "A Definition of Irreversible Coma: Report of the Ad Hoc Committee of the Harvard Medical School to Examine the Definition of Brain Death," *JAMA* 205 (1968): 337–340.

2 "Brain death" is the colloquial term for human death determination using tests of absent brain functions. But it is an unfortunate term because it is inherently misleading. It falsely implies that there are two types of death: brain death and ordinary death, instead of unitary death tested using two sets of tests. It also wrongly suggests that only the brain is dead in such patients. Robert Veatch stated that because of these shortcomings he uses the term only in quotation marks (personal communication November 4, 1995).

3 In 1970, Kansas became the first state to enact a death statute incorporating the new concept of brain death, a mere two years after the Harvard Medical School report. See I. M. Kennedy, "The Kansas Statute on Death – An Appraisal," *New England Journal of Medicine* 285 (1971): 946–950, at 946.

4 See G. S. Belkin, "Brain Death and the Historical Understanding of Bioethics," *Bulletin of the History of Medical Allied Sciences* 58 (2003): 325–361; E. F. M. Wijdicks, "The Neurologist and Harvard Criteria for Brain Death," *Neurology* 61 (2003): 970–976; M. Giacomini, "A Change of Heart and a Change of Mind? Technology and the Redefinition of Death in 1968," *Social Science & Medicine* 44 (1997): 1465–1482; and M. S. Pernick, *supra* note 1.

5 In nearly all states, brain death is incorporated into the statute of death. In a few jurisdictions, brain death is permitted in administrative regulations. See H. R. Beresford, "Brain Death," *Neurologic Clinics* 17 (1999): 295–306. For international practices of brain death, see E. F. M. Wijdicks,

"Brain Death Worldwide: Accepted Fact but No Global Consensus in Diagnostic Criteria," *Neurology* 58 (2002): 20–25.

6   S. J. Youngner, R. M. Arnold, and R. Schapiro, eds., *The Definition of Death: Contemporary Controversies* (Baltimore: Johns Hopkins University Press, 1999).

7   See, for example, R. D. Truog, "Is it Time to Abandon Brain Death?" *Hastings Center Report* 27, no. 1 (1997): 29–37; R. M. Taylor, "Re-examining the Definition and Criterion of Death," *Seminars in Neurology* 17 (1997): 265–270; P. A. Byrne, S. O'Reilly, and P. M. Quay, "Brain Death—An Opposing Viewpoint," *JAMA* 242 (1979): 1985–1990; and J. Seifert, "Is Brain Death Actually Death? A Critique of Redefinition of Man's Death in Terms of 'Brain Death,'" *The Monist* 76 (1993): 175–202.

8   Alan Shewmon's recent works on this topic include D. A. Shewmon, "The Brain and Somatic Integration: Insights into the Standard Biological Rationale for Equating 'Brain Death' with Death," *Journal of Medicine and Philosophy* 26 (2001): 457–478; and D. A. Shewmon, "The 'Critical Organ' for the Organism as a Whole: Lessons from the Lowly Spinal Cord," *Advances in Experimental Medicine and Biology* 550 (2004): 23–42. Other scholars agreeing with him also published works following his article in the *Journal of Medicine and Philosophy.*

9   H. K. Beecher, chairman of the landmark 1968 Harvard Medical School Committee report (see note 1), later warned: "Only a very bold man, I think, would attempt to define death." See H. K. Beecher, "Definitions of 'Life' and 'Death' for Medical Science and Practice," *Annals of the New York Academy of Sciences* 169 (1970): 471–474.

10 President's Commission for the Study of Ethical Problems in Medicine and Biomedical and Behavioral Research, *Defining Death: Medical, Legal and Ethical Issues in the Determination of Death* (Washington, DC: U.S. Government Printing Office, 1981): at 31–43.

11 J. L. Bernat, C. M. Culver and B. Gert, "On the Definition and Criterion of Death," *Annals of Internal Medicine* 94 (1981): 389–394.

12 Alan and Elisabeth Shewmon recently claimed that my approach is futile because language constrains our capacity to conceptualize life and death. They regard death as an "ur-phenomenon" that is "…conceptually fundamental in its class; no more basic concepts exist to which it can be reduced. It can only be intuited from our experience of it…" See D. A. Shewmon and E. S. Shewmon, "The Semiotics of Death and its Medical Implications," *Advances in Experimental Medicine and Biology* 550 (2004): 89–114. Winston Chiong also rejected my analytic approach claiming that there can be no unified definition of death. Yet, he agreed that the whole-brain criterion of death is the most coherent concept of death. See W. Chiong, "Brain Death Without Definitions," *Hastings Center Report* 35 (2005): 20–30.

13 I have discussed these conditions in greater detail in J. L. Bernat, "The Biophilosophical Basis of Whole-Brain Death," *Social Philosophy & Policy* 19, no. 2 (2002): 324–342.

14 Robert Veatch exemplifies a scholar who has attempted to redefine death for the purpose of considering patients in persistent vegetative states as dead, despite the fact that all societies consider them alive. See, for example, R. M. Veatch, "The Impending Collapse of the Whole-Brain Definition of Death," *Hastings Center Report* 23, no. 4 (1993): 18–24. Linda Emanuel abstracted death to a clinically unhelpful metaphysical level: "there is no state of death…to say 'she is dead' is meaningless because 'she' is not compatible with 'dead.'" See L. L. Emanuel, "Reexamining Death: The Asymptotic Model and a Bounded Zone Definition," *Hastings Center Report* 25, no. 4 (1995): 27–35.

15 For a scholar who argues that the definition of death is largely a normative social matter, see R. M. Veatch, "The Conscience Clause: How Much Individual Choice in Defining Death Can Our Society Tolerate?" in S. J. Youngner, R. M. Arnold, and R. Schapiro, eds., *The Definition of Death: Contemporary Controversies* (Baltimore: Johns Hopkins University Press, 1999): 137–160.

16 In this regard, I disagree with Jeff McMahan that there are two types of death: death of the organism and death of the person. See J. McMahan, "The Metaphysics of Brain Death," *Bioethics* 9 (1995): 91–126.

17 A. Halevy and B. Brody, "Brain Death: Reconciling Definitions, Criteria, and Tests," *Annals of Internal Medicine* 119 (1993): 519–525.

18 R. S. Morison, "Death: Process or Event?" *Science* 173 (1971): 694–698 and L. Kass, "Death as an Event: A Commentary on Robert Morison," *Science* 173 (1971): 698–702. The Shewmons (see note 12) recently described the process vs. event argument as "tiresome" because, as a consequence of linguistic constraints, death can be understood only as an event.

19 J. L. Bernat, C. M. Culver, and B. Gert, "On the Definition and Criterion of Death," *Annals of Internal Medicine* 94 (1981): 389–394.

20 S. Parnia, D. G. Waller, R. Yeates, and P. Fenwick, "A Qualitative and Quantitative Study of the Incidence, Features, and Etiology of Near Death Experiences in Cardiac Arrest Survivors," *Resuscitation* 48 (2001): 149–156.

21 R. M. Veatch, "The Whole Brain-Oriented Concept of Death: An Outmoded Philosophical Formulation," *Journal of Thanatology* 3 (1975): 13–30; R. M. Veatch, "Brain Death and Slippery Slopes," *Journal of Clinical Ethics* 3 (1992): 181–187; and R. M. Veatch, "The Impending Collapse of the Whole-Brain Definition of Death," *Hastings Center Report* 23, no. 4 (1993): 18–24.

22 R. M. Veatch, *supra* note 21, at 23.

23 See, for example, M. B. Green and D. Wikler, "Brain Death and Personal Identity," *Philosophy and Public Affairs* 9 (1980): 105–133; S. J. Youngner and E. T. Bartlett, "Human Death and High Technology: The Failure of the Whole Brain Formulation," *Annals of Internal Medicine* 99 (1983): 252–258; and K. G. Gervais, *Redefining Death* (New Haven: Yale University Press, 1986).

24 J. L. Bernat, C. M. Culver, and B. Gert, "On the Definition and Criterion of Death," *Annals of Internal Medicine* 94 (1981): 389–394. I later refined the definition to require only the permanent loss of the *critical* functions of the organism as a whole, in response to exceptional cases raised, but this is mostly quibbling. See J. L. Bernat, "Refinements in the Definition and Criterion of Death," in S. J. Youngner, R. M. Arnold, and R. Schapiro, eds., *The Definition of Death: Contemporary Controversies* (Baltimore: Johns Hopkins University Press, 1999): 83–92.

25 J. Loeb, *The Organism as a Whole* (New York: G. P. Putnam's Sons, 1916).

26 See, for example, the explanation of emergent functions in M. Mahner and M. Bunge, *Foundations of Biophilosophy* (Berlin: Springer-Verlag, 1997): at 29–30.

27 J. Korein, "The Problem of Brain Death: Development and History," *Annals of the New York Academy of Sciences* 315 (1978): 19–38. For the most recent refinement of Korein's argument, see J. Korein and C. Machado, "Brain Death: Updating a Valid Concept for 2004," *Advances in Experimental Medicine and Biology* 550 (2004): 1–14.

28 I have discussed these three formulations in greater detail in J. L. Bernat, "How Much of the Brain Must Die in Brain Death?" *Journal of Clinical Ethics* 3 (1992): 21–26.

29 The text of *Defining Death* makes clear that the President's Commission found an important distinction between brain clinical functions and brain activities. See President's Commission for the Study of Ethical Problems in Medicine and Biomedical and Behavioral Research, *Defining Death: Medical, Legal and Ethical Issues in the Determination of Death* (Washington, DC: U.S. Government Printing Office, 1981): at 28–29.

30 Residual EEG activity seen on unequivocally brain dead patients has been described by M. M. Grigg, M. A. Kelly, G. G. Celesia, M. W. Ghobrial, and E. R. Ross, "Electroencephalographic Activity after Brain Death," *Archives of Neurology* 44 (1987): 948–954.

31 F. Plum and J. B. Posner, *The Diagnosis of Stupor and Coma,* 3rd ed., (Philadelphia: F. A. Davis, 1980): at 88–101.

32 These are the most common causes of brain death. See D. Staworn, L. Lewison, J. Marks, G. Turner, and D. Levin, "Brain Death in Pediatric Intensive Care Unit Patients: Incidence, Primary Diagnosis, and the Clinical Occurrence of Turner's Triad," *Critical Care Medicine* 22 (1994): 1301–1305.

33 H. C. Kinney and M. A. Samuels, "Neuropathology of the Persistent Vegetative State: A Review," *Journal of Neuropathology and Experimental Neurology* 53 (1994): 548–558.

34 Multi-Society Task Force on PVS, "Medical Aspects of the Persistent Vegetative State. Parts I and II," *New England Journal of Medicine* 330 (1994): 1499–1508, 1572–1579.

35 Conference of Medical Royal Colleges and their Faculties in the United Kingdom, "Diagnosis of Brain Death," *British Medical Journal* 2 (1976): 1187–1188; and C. Pallis, *ABC of Brainstem Death* (London: British Medical Journal Publishers, 1983).

36 I have provided more extensive arguments with examples to support this claim in J. L. Bernat, "A Defense of the Whole-Brain Concept of Death," *Hastings Center Report* 28, no. 2 (1998): 14–23 at 18–19.

37 The Quality Standards Subcommittee of the American Academy of Neurology, "Practice Parameters for Determining Brain Death in Adults [Summary Statement]," *Neurology* 45 (1995): 1012–1014. The tests accepted in various European countries are described and compared in W. F. Haupt and J. Rudolf, "European Brain Death Codes: A Comparison of National Guidelines," *Journal of Neurology* 246 (1999): 432–437.

38 The clinical and confirmatory tests for brain death are described in detail in E. F. M. Wijdicks, "The Diagnosis of Brain Death," *New England Journal of Medicine* 344 (2001): 1215–1221.

39 See, for example, R. E. Mejia and M. M. Pollack, "Variability in Brain Death Determination Practices in Children," *JAMA* 274 (1995): 550–553; and M. Y. Wang, P. Wallace, and J. B. Gruen, "Brain Death Documentation: Analysis and Issues," *Neurosurgery* 51 (2002): 731–735.

40 D. A. Shewmon, "Chronic 'Brain Death': Meta-analysis and Conceptual Consequences," *Neurology* 51 (1998): 1538–1545.

41 E. F. M. Wijdicks and J. L. Bernat, "Chronic 'Brain Death': Meta-analysis and Conceptual Consequences," (letter to the editor) *Neurology* 53 (1999): 1639–1640.

42 I defend this claim in J. L. Bernat, "On Irreversibility as a Prerequisite for Brain Death Determination," *Advances in Experimental Medicine and Biology* 550 (2004): 161–167.

43 This conclusion was reached by Alexander Capron, the former Executive Director of the President's Commission (see note 10), in A. M. Capron, "Brain Death—Well Settled Yet Still Unresolved," *New England Journal of Medicine* 344 (2001): 1244–1246.

44 E. F. M. Wijdicks, "Brain Death Worldwide: Accepted Fact but No Global Consensus in Diagnostic Criteria," *Neurology* 58 (2002): 20–25.

45 President's Commission for the Study of Ethical Problems in Medicine and Biomedical and Behavioral Research, *Defining Death: Medical, Legal and Ethical Issues in the Determination of Death* (Washington, DC: U.S. Government Printing Office, 1981): at 72–84.

46 Law Reform Commission of Canada, *Criteria for the Determination of Death* (Ottawa: Law Reform Commission of Canada, 1981).

47 R. A. Burt, "Where Do We Go from Here?" in S. J. Youngner, R. M. Arnold, and R. Schapiro, eds., *The Definition of Death: Contemporary Controversies* (Baltimore: Johns Hopkins University Press, 1999): 332–339.

48 See E. F. M. Wijdicks, *supra* note 5, at 22–23.

49 In the early brain death era, commentators asserted that brain death was compatible with the world's principal religions. See F. J. Veith, J. M. Fein, M. D. Tendler, R. M. Veatch, M. A. Kleiman, and G. Kalkines, "Brain Death: I. A Status Report of Medical and Ethical Considerations," *JAMA* 238 (1977): 1651–1655.

50 C. S. Campbell, "Fundamentals of Life and Death: Christian Fundamentalism and Medical Science," in S. J. Youngner, R. M. Arnold, and R. Schapiro, eds., *The Definition of Death: Contemporary Controversies* (Baltimore: Johns Hopkins University Press, 1999): 194–209.

51 Some Catholic commentators had long claimed that brain death violated Catholic teachings. See P. A. Byrne, et al., *supra* note 7. But in August, 2000, in an address to the 18th Congress of the International Transplantation Society meeting in Rome, the Pope asserted that brain death was fully consistent with Catholic doctrine. For a detailed historical discussion of earlier statements on brain death from Vatican academies, an account of the process of Vatican decision making, and an explanation of the Pope's recent statement, see E. J. Furton, "Brain Death, the Soul, and Organic Life," *The National Catholic Bioethics Quarterly* 2 (2002): 455–470.

52 The rabbinic debate is explained in F. Rosner, "The Definition of Death in Jewish Law," in S. J. Youngner, R. M. Arnold, and R. Schapiro, eds., *The Definition of Death: Contemporary Controversies* (Baltimore: Johns Hopkins University Press, 1999): 210–221.

53 Saudi Arabia represents a conservative interpretation of Islam and brain death is accepted there. See B. A. Yaqub and

S. M. Al-Deeb, "Brain Death: Current Status in Saudi Arabia," *Saudi Medical Journal* 17 (1996): 5–10.

54 S. Jain and M. C. Maheshawari, "Brain Death–The Indian Perspective," in C. Machado, ed., *Brain Death* (Amsterdam: Elsevier, 1995): 261–263.

55 M. Lock, "Contesting the Natural in Japan: Moral Dilemmas and Technologies of Dying," *Culture, Medicine and Psychiatry* 19 (1995): 1–38.

56 See Shewmon, *supra* note 8.

57 See Shewmon, *supra* note 40.

58 R. M. Taylor, "Re-examining the Definition and Criterion of Death," *Seminars in Neurology* 17 (1997): 265–270.

59 I made this point in a review of a pre-publication draft of the Institute of Medicine report. See, Institute of Medicine, *Non-Heart-Beating Organ Transplantation: Practice and Protocols* (Washington DC: National Academy Press, 2000): at 22–24. The same point was made in reference to an earlier publication of the Institute of Medicine in J. Menikoff, "Doubts about Death: The Silence of the Institute of Medicine," *Journal of Law, Medicine & Ethics* 26 (1998): 157–165.

AN ALTERNATIVE TO BRAIN DEATH

Jeff McMahan

In this response to Bernat and other defenders of the whole-brain criterion of death, McMahan defends a higher-brain or cerebral-death criterion. McMahan's position requires drawing a metaphysical distinction between the human *organism* and the *person* to whom that organism belongs. He supports his conclusion by appealing to two scenarios. The first is a hypothetical case of cerebrum transplantation, in which we intuitively believe that the person travels with his brain from one organism to another. The second involves actual cases of dicephalic twins, in which a single human organism appears to support two distinct persons. Although he agrees with Bernat that a human *organism* dies when it irreversibly loses its capacity for integrated functioning of its major organs and systems, McMahan denies that loss of the brain's critical regulatory functions is part of our concept of death. He argues that the difference between a *person's* life and death cannot depend on whether the brain, rather than artificial life support, performs these critical functions. Whole-brain death, he concludes, is sufficient for the death of a person, but not necessary. The only necessary condition is irreversible loss of consciousness.

SOME COMMON BUT MISTAKEN ASSUMPTIONS ABOUT DEATH

Most contributors to the debate about brain death, including Dr. James Bernat, share certain assumptions. They believe that the concept of death is uni-

From *Journal of Law, Medicine & Ethics*, vol. 34, no. 1 (2006), pp. 44–48. Copyright © 2006 by Blackwell Publishing, Ltd. Reproduced with permission of Blackwell Publishing, Ltd.

vocal, that death is a biological phenomenon, that it is necessarily irreversible, that it is paradigmatically something that happens to *organisms,* that we are human organisms, and therefore that our deaths will be deaths of organisms. These claims are supposed to have moral significance. It is, for example, only when a person dies that it is permissible to extract her organs for transplantation.

It is also commonly held that our univocal notion of death is the permanent cessation of integrated functioning in an organism and that the criterion for determining when this has occurred in animals with brains is the death of the brain as a whole—that is, brain death. The reason most commonly given for this is that the brain is the irreplaceable master control of the organism's integration.

Before presenting my own view, let me say something about a couple of these assumptions and about the case for brain death. It is, perhaps, a measure of the heretical cast of my mind that I reject *all* of these widely shared assumptions.

I do not think the concept of death is univocal. When Jesus says that "whosoever liveth and believeth in me shall never die," he does not mean that some human organisms will remain functionally integrated forever. He means that believers will never cease to exist. (Admittedly, Jesus did not use the English word "die." But this seemed an intelligible use of the word to the translators.)

But "death" also has a biological meaning. It makes sense to say that when a unicellular organism, such as an amoeba, undergoes binary fission, it ceases to exist; but in the biological sense it does not *die*. There is no cessation of functioning that turns this once-living organism into a corpse. So death as a biological phenomenon is different from the ceasing to exist of a living being and may or may not involve an entity's ceasing to exist. It is intelligible, for example, to say that when an animal organism dies, it does not cease to exist. Rather, it simply becomes a corpse. The living animal becomes a dead animal—but nothing ceases to exist until the animal organism disintegrates.

I also do not think our concept of death makes it a necessary truth that death is irreversible. If that were true, the claim that Lazarus was raised from the dead, or that Jesus was resurrected, would be incoherent. I think these claims are false; but if it were a conceptual truth that death is irreversible, they would not be false, but nonsensical.

I do think, however, that there is something true and important in the idea that death as a biological phenomenon is irreversible. It may well be a conceptual truth that an organism can be revived from death only by a violation of the laws of nature—that

is, only by a literal miracle of the sort that Jesus is thought by some to have performed. For in cases not involving miracles, if an organism that was thought to be dead is restored to integrated functioning, our tendency is to conclude that we were mistaken in assuming that it was dead. (Subsequent references to irreversibility should be understood as having the implicit qualification "except by miracle.")

Some people, of course, will say that the organism was dead but was non-miraculously restored to life. To make this claim acceptable, they will need to offer good reasons for thinking the organism was dead, given that it is now alive. For reasons that I will give later, I think that nothing of importance depends on this. It is just a question of how we use certain words. But for those who believe that we are organisms and that we always have special value or sanctity while we are alive, this is a very important issue indeed.

While we are considering whether death is necessarily irreversible, I should mention that I am puzzled that Bernat and others define death as the permanent cessation of functioning—or of the critical functions—of an organism as a whole.[1] Surely what they should say is that it is the irreversible cessation of functioning. (By "irreversible" I mean irreversible in principle, not in practice.) If an organism stops functioning but its functioning could be recovered by means of a device that we do not in fact possess, it is not dead. There are, however, metaphysically determined constraints on what kind of device this could be. It would, for example, have to restore the same life, not create a new one.

Let me explain why the notion of irreversibility is preferable to that of permanence. Suppose there is an organism in which integrated functioning has ceased but could be revived. If it is up to you whether to revive the functioning, your decision now will determine whether the organism was dead a moment ago. For if you decide to revive the functioning, the cessation will not have been permanent and the organism will have been alive a moment ago. But if you decide not to revive it, you thereby make permanent the cessation of functioning that occurred in the past. But whether the organism was dead a moment ago is a matter of its intrinsic state at the time; it cannot be determined retroactively by what you do now. (Bernat, I should note, urges a similar point in his cogent objections to the proposal for non-heart-beating organ donation.[2])

BRAIN DEATH AND THE CESSATION OF INTEGRATED FUNCTIONING

Turn now to the central contention of the defenders of brain death, which is that at least certain critical functions of the brain are necessary for integrated functioning in the organism. (I put aside the interesting question whether they are also sufficient.) This claim raises two related questions. First, what counts as the right sort of integration? Second, is the claim empirical or conceptual?

There are several ways in which the functions of the various organs and subsystems of an organism might be integrated so as to maintain homeostasis and resist entropy. It might be, for example, that integration occurs via a central integrator, a master control that receives signals from the various organs and subsystems, processes them, and then sends return signals that coordinate the functions of the organism's many parts. The defenders of brain death typically claim that the only possible central integrator is the brain. They say that the brain is irreplaceable, that nothing else could possibly carry out its regulative functions.

Critics of brain death, by contrast, often speculate that a mechanical brain—or to be more precise, a mechanical substitute for the brain stem—could adequately replicate the regulative functions of the brain and hence could be the central integrator of a living human organism. Some, indeed, have claimed that the resources of the modern intensive care unit (ICU) already constitute an external and multifaceted substitute for the regulatory functions of the brain stem.[3]

In defending the irreplaceability of the brain, Bernat writes that, "although some of the brain's regulatory functions may be replaced mechanically, the brain's functions of awareness, sentience, sapience, and its capacities to experience and communicate cannot be reproduced or simulated by any machine."[4] Let us grant that this is true. The problem is that these are not somatic regulatory functions.[5]

A second way in which the functions of an organism's various organs and subsystems might be

integrated is through decentralized interaction, in which these parts achieve coordination by sending, receiving, and processing signals among themselves. In a series of papers, Alan Shewmon has argued that this sort of decentralized integration of functioning can and sometimes does occur among the parts of an organism without any input from the brain at all.[6] He cites numerous actual cases involving high cervical transection, functional isolation of the brain in Guillain-Barré Syndrome, or even brain death with artificially induced respiration in which there is a high degree of functional integration in the absence of regulation by the brain—and, indeed, without any central integrator at all. He notes, for example, that some brain dead organisms have the same range of functions as certain uncontroversially living patients in an ICU, and yet maintain these functions with *fewer* sources of external support.

If the familiar claims about the necessary role of the brain in integrating the functions of an organism are empirical claims, I think that Shewmon's cases and arguments force the defender of brain death to admit defeat. But it is possible for the defender of brain death to respond to Shewmon's challenge by interpreting the claim that the brain is necessary for integrated functioning as a conceptual rather than empirical claim.

The defender of brain death can, in other words, retreat to the claim that while certain forms of integrated functioning can be sustained via an artificial central regulator or via decentralized interaction, these forms of integration are not the kind of integration that is necessary for life in a human organism. Only the brain as central regulator can provide that.

This may be a reasonable interpretation of Bernat's claim that "the brain is the critical system of the organism without which the remaining organs may continue to function independently but cannot together comprise an organism as a whole."[7] He might be saying that, even if all the organs are alive and doing their job, they cannot together constitute a living organism without the mediation of the brain.

There are various responses to such a view. One is to ask how much the brain must contribute to the integration of functioning among the parts of the organism in order for the organism to be alive. Clearly it need not regulate *every* aspect of functioning. Indeed, it seems that those who would defend the idea that somatic regulation by the brain is a conceptually necessary condition for life in a human organism must accept something like the following. First we have to identify a range of "critical" regulatory functions. As long as the brain continues to carry out any single one of these functions, that is sufficient for life in the organism. For if we were to insist on the necessity of the brain's carrying out more than one, then an organism in which the brain carried out only one critical regulatory function would be dead—but it would not be brain dead.

But now imagine a case in which only one critical regulatory function is being carried out by the brain. All others are being carried out by external life support. Suppose that right at the moment the brain is about to lose the capacity to carry out this one remaining critical function, a mechanical replacement takes over for it with perfect efficiency. Could *this* be the difference between life and death? Note that, because the mechanical replacement would carry out the regulatory functions in exactly the same way the brain did, the state of the organism would be unchanged apart from this one small change in the brain itself. It is very hard to believe that such a change could make the difference between life and death in an organism, either as a matter of fact or, especially, as a matter of conceptual necessity.

If presented only with information about the loss of supposed critical functions in the brain and information about the unchanged but externally supported functioning of the various organs and subsystems within the organism, most people, I suspect, would not know what to say about whether such an organism was alive or dead. Our concept of death simply fails to deliver an immediately intuitive verdict that the organism is dead. This strongly suggests that the loss by the brain of critical regulatory functions is no part of our *concept* of death.

Another response is simply to point to the case of human embryos, which seem to be living human organisms whose somatic functions are not regulated or integrated by the brain. If this is a correct description, it cannot be a necessary truth that the kind of integrated functioning necessary for life must be regulated to some degree by the brain.

There are a great many other problems with the notion of brain death but I will not rehearse them here.[8] Instead I will conclude by sketching an alternative view.

AN ALTERNATIVE UNDERSTANDING OF DEATH

I accept that it is largely correct to say that a human organism dies when it irreversibly loses the capacity for integrated functioning among its various major organs and subsystems. But the death of a human organism will necessarily be *my* death only if I am an organism. The view that we are organisms is the most important of the widely shared assumptions that I noted at the outset. But, as I mentioned, I think it is mistaken.

The question whether we are organisms is not a biological question, or even a scientific question—just as it is not a scientific question whether a statue and the lump of bronze of which it is composed are one and the same thing or distinct substances. Whether we are organisms is also, and more obviously, not an ethical question. It is a metaphysical question.

There are two arguments that convince me that the answer to this question is "no." One appeals to the hypothetical case of brain transplantation—or, better yet, cerebrum transplantation. If my cerebrum were successfully grafted onto the brain stem of my identical twin brother (whose own cerebrum had been excised), I would then exist in association with what was once his organism. What was formerly my organism would have an intact brain stem and might, therefore, be idling nicely in a persistent vegetative state without even mechanical ventilation. Since I can thus in principle exist separately from the organism that is now mine, I cannot be identical with it.

The second argument appeals not to a science fiction scenario but to an actual phenomenon: dicephalus. Certain instances of dicephalic twinning, in which two heads spout from a single torso, seem to be clear cases in which a single organism supports the existence of two distinct people. The transitivity of identity prevents us from saying that *both* these people *are* that organism; for that implies that the people are identical, that is, that there are not really two people but only one. And because each twin's relation to the organism is the same as the other's, it cannot be that one twin but not the other is the organism. The best thing to say, therefore, is that neither of them is identical to the organism. Since we are essentially the same kind of thing they are, we cannot be organisms either.

If I am right that we are not organisms, what are we? The most widely held alternative view is that each of us is essentially a cartesian soul—that is, a nonmaterial conscious entity that in life is linked with a particular brain and body but at death continues to exist and indeed remains conscious and is psychologically continuous with the person prior to death. Because the soul, so conceived, is nonphysical, it can be individuated only by reference to a single field of consciousness. Thus, any conscious state that is not accessible in my field of consciousness must belong to a different person, or soul. This conception of the soul is, however, undermined by what we know about the results of hemispheric commissurotomy—a procedure in which the tissues connecting a patient's cerebral hemispheres are surgically severed. This procedure gives rise, at least in certain experimental settings, to two separate centers of consciousness in a single human organism. If persons were cartesian souls, we would have to conclude that the procedure creates two persons where formerly there was only one. Since this is clearly not what happens, we cannot be cartesian souls.[9]

How should we think about the problem of determining what kind of thing we essentially are? Here is a quick thought-experiment. Imagine that you were facing the prospect of progressive dementia. At what point would you cease to exist? To most of us it seems clear that you would persist at least as long as the brain in your body retained the capacity for consciousness. For there would be somebody there, and who might it be, if not you? But would you still survive if your brain irreversibly lost the capacity for consciousness? It seems that the only thing there that might qualify as you would be a living human organism. But if I am right that you are not a human organism and there would be nothing else there for you to be, it seems that you must have ceased to exist when your brain lost the capacity for consciousness. I infer from this that you are in fact a mind, a mind that is necessarily embodied.

Recall now my earlier claim that the concept of death is not univocal. The term "death" can refer to our ceasing to exist (as in the earlier quotation from Jesus) or it can refer to a biological event in the history of an organism. This makes things easy; for we already have the two concepts of death that we require if I am right that we are not organisms.

An organism dies in the biological sense when it loses the capacity for integrated functioning. The best criterion for when this happens is probably a circulatory-respiratory criterion. There is bound to be considerable indeterminacy about how much functional integration is required for life in an organism. But if we are not organisms, this is of little consequence.

What it is important to be able to determine is when we die in the nonbiological sense—that is, when we cease to exist. If we are embodied minds, we die or cease to exist when we irreversibly lose the capacity for consciousness—or, to be more precise, when there is irreversible loss of function in those areas of the brain in which consciousness is realized. The best criterion for when this happens is a higher-brain criterion—for example, what is called "cerebral death." But I do not pretend to any expertise here.

Note that when I say the right criterion of our death is a higher-brain criterion, I am not claiming that a human organism in a persistent vegetative state is dead. If persistent vegetative state involves the loss of the capacity for consciousness, then neither you nor I could ever exist in a persistent vegetative state. But you could be survived by your organism, which could remain biologically alive in a persistent vegetative state even though you were dead (that is, had ceased to exist). My view thus avoids the embarrassing implication of most proposals for a higher-brain criterion of death that an organism with spontaneous respiration and heartbeat might be dead.

From an ethical point of view, what matters is not whether an organism remains alive, but whether one of us continues to exist. Of course, we cannot survive unless our organisms remain alive (though this might change if brain transplantation were to become possible). Indeed, although brain death is not sufficient for the biological death of a human organism, it is sufficient for the death or ceasing to exist of a person.

The problematic cases are those in which a person has ceased to exist but her organism remains alive. Might it be permissible to remove the organs from such an organism for transplantation? I believe that it would be, provided that this would not be against the expressed will of the person whose organism it was. But if the person had consented in advance, there would be no moral objection to killing the unoccupied organism in order to use its organs to save the lives of others.

The organism itself cannot be harmed in the relevant sense, it has no rights, and it is not an appropriate object of respect in the Kantian sense. I believe that the treatment of a living but unoccupied human organism is governed morally by principles similar to those that govern the treatment of a corpse. The latter also cannot be harmed or possess rights. But respect for the person who once animated a corpse dictates that there are certain things that must not be done to it. Taking its organs for transplantation with the person's prior consent is not one of these.

REFERENCES

1 J. L. Bernat, "A Defense of the Whole-Brain Concept of Death," *Hastings Center Report* 28, no. 2 (1998): 14–23, at 17.

2 See J. L. Bernat, "Defending Challenges to the Concept of 'Brain Death,'" *at* <http://www.lahey.org/NewsPubs/ Publications/Ethics/JournalFall1998/Journal_Fall1998_ Feature.asp> (last visited December 5, 2005); and M. A. DeVita and R. M. Arnold, "The Concept of Brain Death," *at* <http://www.lahey.org/NewsPubs/ Publications/Ethics/ JournalWinter1999/Journal_Winter1999_ Dialogue.asp> (last visited December 5, 2005).

3 For an early suggestion of this sort, see M. B. Green and D. Wikler, "Brain Death and Personal Identity," *Philosophy and Public Affairs* 9 (1980): 105–33, at 113.

4 Bernat, *supra* note 1, at 19.

5 Bernat also claims that "consciousness, which is required for the organism to respond to requirements for hydration, nutrition, and protection, among other needs," is therefore among the "critical functions of the organism as a whole." *Ibid.,* at 17. But this still does not make it a somatic regulatory function of the brain.

6 See, for example, A. Shewmon, "Recovery from 'Brain Death': A Neurologist's Apologia," *Linacre Quarterly* 64 (1997): 30–96; A. Shewmon, "Chronic 'Brain Death,'" *Neurology* 51 (1998): 1538–45; and A. Shewmon, "The Disintegration of Somatic Integrative Unity: Demise of the Orthodox but Physiologically Untenable Physiological Rationale for 'Brain Death,'" manuscript on file with the author.

7 Bernat, *supra* note 2.

8 See J. McMahan, *The Ethics of Killing: Problems at the Margins of Life* (New York: Oxford University Press: 2002): chapter 5, section 1.2.

9 For further argument, see McMahan, *supra* note 8, at 7–24.

THE DEAD DONOR RULE AND ORGAN TRANSPLANTATION

Robert D. Truog and Franklin G. Miller

The dead donor rule states that patients must be declared dead before their vital organs can be removed for transplantation. Truog and Miller criticize the rule for three reasons. First, the dead donor rule has motivated the redefinition of death as "brain death," which leads physicians to classify certain individuals as dead whom many laypeople consider to be still alive. The second concern, related to the first, is that the redefinition of death has undermined trust in the transplantation enterprise by suggesting that doctors are altering the definition of death just in order to increase the organ supply. Third, the dead donor rule limits the supply of transplantable organs more than the authors believe to be ethically required: some organs are unusable, or less likely to thrive after transplantation, if not harvested before brain death occurs. For these reasons, the authors advocate replacing the dead donor rule with a rule requiring that prospective donors or their surrogates give informed consent and specify conditions under which vital organs may be removed. The authors suggest that, with proper safeguards, including a condition of irreversible unconsciousness, the only patients who would die under such a rule would be those who otherwise would have died from the withdrawal of life support.

Since its inception, organ transplantation has been guided by the overarching ethical requirement known as the dead donor rule, which simply states that patients must be declared dead before the removal of any vital organs for transplantation. Before the development of modern critical care, the diagnosis of death was relatively straightforward: patients were dead when they were cold, blue, and stiff. Unfortunately, organs from these traditional cadavers cannot be used for transplantation. Forty years ago, an ad hoc committee at Harvard Medical School, chaired by Henry Beecher, suggested revising the definition of death in a way that would make some patients with devastating neurologic injury suitable for organ transplantation under the dead donor rule.[1]

The concept of brain death has served us well and has been the ethical and legal justification for thousands of lifesaving donations and transplantations. Even so, there have been persistent questions about whether patients with massive brain injury, apnea, and loss of brain-stem reflexes are really dead. After all, when the injury is entirely intracranial, these patients look very much alive: they are warm and pink; they digest and metabolize food, excrete waste, undergo sexual maturation, and can even reproduce. To a casual observer, they look just like patients who are receiving long-term artificial ventilation and are asleep.

The arguments about why these patients should be considered dead have never been fully convincing. The definition of brain death requires the complete absence of all functions of the entire brain, yet many of these patients retain essential neurologic function, such as the regulated secretion of hypothalamic hormones.[2] Some have argued that these patients are dead because they are permanently unconscious (which is true), but if this is the justifica-

From *New England Journal of Medicine*, vol. 359, no. 7 (August 14, 2008), pp. 674–675. Copyright © 2008 Massachusetts Medical Society. All rights reserved.

tion, then patients in a permanent vegetative state, who breathe spontaneously, should also be diagnosed as dead, a characterization that most regard as implausible. Others have claimed that "brain-dead" patients are dead because their brain damage has led to the "permanent cessation of functioning of the organism as a whole."[3] Yet evidence shows that if these patients are supported beyond the acute phase of their illness (which is rarely done), they can survive for many years.[4] The uncomfortable conclusion to be drawn from this literature is that although it may be perfectly ethical to remove vital organs for transplantation from patients who satisfy the diagnostic criteria of brain death, the reason it is ethical cannot be that we are convinced they are really dead.

Over the past few years, our reliance on the dead donor rule has again been challenged, this time by the emergence of donation after cardiac death as a pathway for organ donation. Under protocols for this type of donation, patients who are not brain-dead but who are undergoing an orchestrated withdrawal of life support are monitored for the onset of cardiac arrest. In typical protocols, patients are pronounced dead 2 to 5 minutes after the onset of asystole (on the basis of cardiac criteria), and their organs are expeditiously removed for transplantation. Although everyone agrees that many patients could be resuscitated after an interval of 2 to 5 minutes, advocates of this approach to donation say that these patients can be regarded as dead because a decision has been made not to attempt resuscitation.

This understanding of death is problematic at several levels. The cardiac definition of death requires the irreversible cessation of cardiac function. Whereas the common understanding of "irreversible" is "impossible to reverse," in this context irreversibility is interpreted as the result of a choice not to reverse. This interpretation creates the paradox that the hearts of patients who have been declared dead on the basis of the irreversible loss of cardiac function have in fact been transplanted and have successfully functioned in the chest of another. Again, although it may be ethical to remove vital organs from these patients, we believe that the reason it is ethical cannot convincingly be that the donors are dead.

At the dawn of organ transplantation, the dead donor rule was accepted as an ethical premise that did not require reflection or justification, presumably because it appeared to be necessary as a safeguard against the unethical removal of vital organs from vulnerable patients. In retrospect, however, it appears that reliance on the dead donor rule has greater potential to undermine trust in the transplantation enterprise than to preserve it. At worst, this ongoing reliance suggests that the medical profession has been gerrymandering the definition of death to carefully conform with conditions that are most favorable for transplantation. At best, the rule has provided misleading ethical cover that cannot withstand careful scrutiny. A better approach to procuring vital organs while protecting vulnerable patients against abuse would be to emphasize the importance of obtaining valid informed consent for organ donation from patients or surrogates before the withdrawal of life-sustaining treatment in situations of devastating and irreversible neurologic injury.[5]

What has been the cost of our continued dependence on the dead donor rule? In addition to fostering conceptual confusion about the ethical requirements of organ donation, it has compromised the goals of transplantation for donors and recipients alike. By requiring organ donors to meet flawed definitions of death before organ procurement, we deny patients and their families the opportunity to donate organs if the patients have devastating, irreversible neurologic injuries that do not meet the technical requirements of brain death. In the case of donation after cardiac death, the ischemia time inherent in the donation process necessarily diminishes the value of the transplants by reducing both the quantity and the quality of the organs that can be procured.

Many will object that transplantation surgeons cannot legally or ethically remove vital organs from patients before death, since doing so will cause their death. However, if the critiques of the current methods of diagnosing death are correct, then such actions are already taking place on a routine basis. Moreover, in modern intensive care units, ethically justified decisions and actions of physicians are already the proximate cause of death for many patients—for instance, when mechanical ventilation is withdrawn. Whether death occurs as the result of ventilator withdrawal or organ procurement, the ethically relevant precondition is valid consent by the patient or surrogate. With such consent, there is no harm or wrong done in retrieving vital organs before death, provided that anesthesia is administered. With proper safeguards, no patient will die from vital organ donation who would not otherwise die as a result of the withdrawal of life support. Finally, surveys suggest that issues related to respect for valid consent and the degree of neurologic injury may be more important to the public than concerns about whether the patient is already dead at the time the organs are removed.

In sum, as an ethical requirement for organ donation, the dead donor rule has required unnecessary and unsupportable revisions of the definition of death. Characterizing the ethical requirements of organ donation in terms of valid informed consent under the limited conditions of devastating neurologic injury is ethically sound, optimally respects the desires of those who wish to donate organs, and has the potential to maximize the number and quality of organs available to those in need.

NOTES

1 A definition of irreversible coma: report of the ad hoc committee of the Harvard Medical School to examine the definition of brain death. *JAMA* 1968;205:337–40.

2 Truog RD. Is it time to abandon brain death? *Hastings Cent Rep* 1997;27:29–37.

3 Bernat JL, Culver CM, Gert B. On the definition and criterion of death. *Ann Intern Med* 1981;94:389–94.

4 Shewmon DA. Chronic "brain death": meta-analysis and conceptual consequences. *Neurology* 1998;51:1538–45.

5 Miller FG, Truog RD. Rethinking the ethics of vital organ donation. *Hastings Cent Rep* (in press).

COMPETENT ADULTS AND THE REFUSAL OF LIFE-SUSTAINING TREATMENT

WITHHOLDING AND WITHDRAWING LIFE-SUSTAINING TREATMENT
Council on Ethical and Judicial Affairs, American Medical Association

In this brief excerpt from a much longer report, the AMA Council on Ethical and Judicial Affairs presents a series of clarifications related to the right of a competent patient to forgo life-sustaining treatment. In conjunction with a consideration of the traditional distinction between ordinary and extraordinary treatments, the council rejects the idea that it is never permissible to forgo artificial nutrition and hydration. Also rejected is the view that there is an ethically significant distinction between *withholding* and *withdrawing* life-sustaining treatment.

The principle of patient autonomy requires that physicians respect a competent patient's decision to forgo any medical treatment. This principle is not altered when the likely result of withholding or withdrawing a treatment is the patient's death.[1] The right of competent patients to forgo life-sustaining treatment has been upheld in the courts (for example, *In re Brooks Estate,* 32 Ill2d 361, 205 NE2d 435 [1965]; *In re Osborne,* 294 A2d 372 [1972]) and is generally accepted by medical ethicists.[1]

Decisions that so profoundly affect a patient's well-being cannot be made independent of a patient's subjective preferences and values.[2] Many types of life-sustaining treatments are burdensome and invasive, so that the choice for the patient is not simply a choice between life and death.[3] When a patient is dying of cancer, for example, a decision may have to be made whether to use a regimen of chemotherapy that might prolong life for several additional months but also would likely be painful, nauseating, and debilitating. Similarly, when a patient is dying, there may be a choice between returning home to a natural death, or remaining in the hospital, attached to machinery, where the patient's life might be prolonged a few more days or weeks. In both cases, individuals might weigh differently the value of additional life vs the burden of additional treatment.

The withdrawing or withholding of life-sustaining treatment is not inherently contrary to the principles of beneficence and nonmaleficence. The physician is

obligated only to offer sound medical treatment and to refrain from providing treatments that are detrimental, on balance, to the patient's well-being. When a physician withholds or withdraws a treatment on the request of a patient, he or she has fulfilled the obligation to offer sound treatment to the patient. The obligation to offer treatment does not include an obligation to impose treatment on an unwilling patient. In addition, the physician is not providing a harmful treatment. Withdrawing or withholding is not a treatment, but the forgoing of a treatment.

Some commentators argue that if a physician has a strong moral objection to withdrawing or withholding life-sustaining treatment, the physician may transfer the patient to another physician who is willing to comply with the patient's wishes.[1] It is true that a physician does not have to provide a treatment, such as an abortion, that is contrary to his or her moral values. However, if a physician objects to withholding or withdrawing the treatment and forces unwanted treatment on a patient, the patient's autonomy will be inappropriately violated even if it will take only a short time for the patient to be transferred to another physician.

Withdrawing or withholding some life-sustaining treatments may seem less acceptable than others. The distinction between "ordinary" vs "extraordinary" treatments has been used to differentiate ethically obligatory vs ethically optional treatments.[4] In other words, ordinary treatments must be provided, while extraordinary treatment may be withheld or withdrawn. Varying criteria have been proposed to distinguish ordinary from extraordinary treatment.

Reprinted with permission of the AMA from "Decisions Near the End of Life," *JAMA*, vol. 267, no. 16 (April 22/29, 1992), pp. 2229–2233.

Such criteria include customariness, naturalness, complexity, expense, invasiveness, and balance of likely benefits vs burdens of the particular treatment.[4,5] The ethical significance of all these criteria essentially are subsumed by the last criterion—the balance of likely benefits vs the burdens of the treatment.[4]

When a patient is competent, this balancing must ultimately be made by the patient. As stated earlier, the evaluation of whether life-sustaining treatment should be initiated, maintained, or forgone depends on the values and preferences of the patient. Therefore, treatments are not objectively ordinary or extraordinary. For example, artificial nutrition and hydration have frequently been cited as an objectively ordinary treatment which, therefore, must never be forgone. However, artificial nutrition and hydration can be very burdensome to patients. Artificial nutrition and hydration immobilize the patient to a large degree, can be extremely uncomfortable (restraints are sometimes used to prevent patients from removing nasogastric tubes), and can entail serious risks (for example, surgical risks from insertion of a gastrostomy tube and the risk of aspiration pneumonia with a nasogastric tube).

Aside from the ordinary vs extraordinary argument, the right to refuse artificial nutrition and hydration has also been contested by some because the provision of food and water has a symbolic significance as an expression of care and compassion.[6] These commentators argue that withdrawing or withholding food and water is a form of abandonment and will cause the patient to die of starvation and/or thirst. However, it is far from evident that providing nutrients through a nasogastric tube to a patient for whom it is unwanted is comparable to the typical human ways of feeding those who are hungry.[5] In addition, discomforting symptoms can be palliated so that a death that occurs after forgoing artificial nutrition and/or hydration is not marked by substantial suffering.[7,8] Such care requires constant attention to the patient's needs. Therefore, when comfort care is maintained, respecting a patient's decision to forgo artificial nutrition and hydration will not constitute an abandonment of the patient, symbolic or otherwise.

There is also no ethical distinction between withdrawing and withholding life-sustaining treatment.[1,4,9] Withdrawing life support may be emotionally more difficult than withholding life support because the physician performs an action that hastens death. When life-sustaining treatment is withheld, on the other hand, death occurs because of an omission rather than an action. However, as most bioethicists now recognize, such a distinction lacks ethical significance.[1,4,9] First, the distinction is often meaningless. For example, if a physician fails to provide a tube feeding at the scheduled time, would it be a withholding or a withdrawing of treatment? Second, ethical relevance does not lie with the distinction between acts and omissions, but with other factors such as the motivation and professional obligations of the physician. For example, refusing to initiate ventilator support despite the patient's need and request because the physician has been promised a share of the patient's inheritance is clearly ethically more objectionable than stopping a ventilator for a patient who has competently decided to forgo it. Third, prohibiting the withdrawal of life support would inappropriately affect a patient's decision to initiate such treatment. If treatment cannot be stopped once it is initiated, patients and physicians may be more reluctant to begin treatment when there is a possibility that the patient may later want the treatment withdrawn.[1]

While the principle of autonomy requires that physicians respect competent patients' requests to forgo life-sustaining treatments, there are potential negative consequences of such a policy. First, deaths may occur as a result of uninformed decisions or from pain and suffering that could be relieved with measures that will not cause the patient's death. Further, subtle or overt pressures from family, physicians, or society to forgo life-sustaining treatment may render the patient's choice less than free. These pressures could revolve around beliefs that such patients' lives no longer possess social worth and are an unjustifiable drain of limited health resources.

The physician must ensure that the patient has the capacity to make medical decisions before carrying out the patient's decision to forgo (or receive) life-sustaining treatment. In particular, physicians must be aware that the patient's decision-making capacity can be diminished by a misunderstanding of the medical prognosis and options or by a treatable state of depression. It is also essential that all efforts be made to maximize the comfort and dignity of patients who are dependent on life-sustaining treatment and that patients be assured of these efforts. With such assurances, patients will be less likely to forgo life support because of suffering or anticipated suffering that could be palliated.

The potential pressures on patients to forgo life-sustaining treatments are an important concern. The Council believes that the medical profession must be vigilant against such tendencies, but that the greater policy risk is of undermining patient autonomy.

REFERENCES

1 *Deciding to Forego Life-Sustaining Treatment: A Report on the Ethical, Medical, and Legal Issues in Treatment Decisions.* Washington, DC: President's Commission for the Study of Ethical Problems in Medicine and Biomedical and Behavioral Research; 1987.

2 Brock D. W. Death and dying. In: Veatch R. M, ed. *Medical Ethics.* Boston, Mass: Jones & Bartlett Publishing Inc; 1989.

3 Office of Technology Assessment Task Force. *Life-Sustaining Technologies and the Elderly.* Philadelphia, Pa: Science Information Resource Center; 1988.

4 Beauchamp T. L, Childress J. F. *Principles of Biomedical Ethics.* 3rd ed. New York, NY: Oxford University Press; 1989.

5 Lynn J., Childress J. F. Must patients always be given food and water? *Hastings Cent Rep.* October 1983: 17–21.

6 Ramsey P. *The Patient as Person.* New Haven, Conn: Yale University Press; 1970: 113–129.

7 Schmitz P., O'Brien M. Observations on nutrition and hydration in dying patients. In: Lynn J., ed. *By No Extraordinary Means: The Choice to Forgo Life-Sustaining Food and Water.* Bloomington, Ind: Indiana University Press; 1986.

8 Billings J. A. Comfort measures for the terminally ill: is dehydration painful? *J Am Geriatr Soc.* 1985; 33:808–810.

9 *Guidelines on the Termination of Life-Sustaining Treatment and the Care of the Dying: A Report by the Hastings Center.* Briarcliff Manor, NY: Hastings Center; 1987.

REFUSING LIFE-SUSTAINING TREATMENT AFTER CATASTROPHIC INJURY: ETHICAL IMPLICATIONS

Tia Powell and Bruce Lowenstein

Powell and Lowenstein present and discuss a case in which a severely disabled patient decided to refuse life-sustaining treatment (nutrition and hydration) in order to bring about her death. The authors compare and contrast this case with the more widely known case of Elizabeth Bouvia. They then express reservations about the suggestion that patient autonomy should be suspended for an extensive period of time as a patient undergoes rehabilitation in response to catastrophic injury. Powell and Lowenstein ultimately endorse the right of a competent disabled patient to refuse life-sustaining treatment, "no matter how much we may lament such a choice."

In theory, a competent patient may refuse any and all treatments, even those that sustain life. The problem with this theory, confidently and frequently asserted, is that the circumstances of real patients may so confound us with their complexity as to shake our confident assumptions to their core.

Journal of Law, Medicine & Ethics, vol. 24 (Spring 1996), pp. 54–61. Copyright © 1996 by Blackwell Publishing, Ltd. Reproduced with permission of Blackwell Publishing, Ltd.

For instance, it is not the case that one may always and easily know which patients are competent. Indeed, evaluation of decision-making capacity is notoriously difficult. Not only may reasonable and experienced evaluators, say a judge and a psychiatrist, disagree, but also a person's capacity may change from hour to hour and may extend to some decisions yet not to others. And yet it is on this subtle art of capacity evaluation that life and death decisions often turn, especially when patients decline life-sustaining treatment.

An evaluation of capacity may consider the impact of serious medical or psychiatric illness, as well as the patient's life circumstances. A number of authors have addressed decision-making capacity in the setting of depression, fatal illness, and end-of-life treatment decisions.[1] Less commonly, these factors have been examined in the context of competent patients with chronic disability, rather than terminal illness.[2] In the world of rehabilitation medicine and disability, which is so strikingly different from acute medicine in other ways, assumptions about decision-making capacity may also differ. These different assumptions may lead to a crisis when chronically disabled (but not dying) patients refuse life-sustaining treatments. This crisis, in turn, forces a reexamination of the concept of decisional capacity in the rehabilitation context. In particular, the impact of catastrophic trauma on decisional capacity is judged differently in acute intensive care settings than in rehabilitation settings.

We review a complex case that highlights the difficulty in evaluating capacity to refuse life-sustaining treatments in the rehabilitation setting. As we shall see, the determination of this patient's capacity hinges on diverse factors, including depression, physician countertransference, and the ethos of disability and rehabilitation medicine. Although factors specific to the context of disability deserve careful examination in evaluations of capacity, we do not think, in this case or in general, that disabled patients should be held to a different standard of capacity than other patients.

CASE PRESENTATION: BB

BB was a thirty-seven-year-old woman, in good health, employed, and pursuing a marital separation. Without warning, she suffered a brain-stem stroke in November 1993, resulting in the diagnosis of locked-in syndrome. She was left fully alert mentally, although quadriplegic and unable to speak; she preserved limited voluntary head movement, vertical gaze, blinking, and minimal voluntary movement of her left arm.

Before her stroke, BB had a history of major depression with psychotic features, with one previous psychiatric hospitalization ten years earlier. Over the past decade, her symptoms were well controlled with weekly psychotherapy and medications. She

was an effective and skilled professional in a competitive technical field.

Roughly ten weeks after her injury, BB was transferred to a rehabilitation facility for possible weaning from a ventilator and for assistance with communication and mobility devices. She began to learn to communicate by means of an elaborate state-of-the-art computer system; she also had an appropriately modified power wheelchair.

BB expressed great eagerness to proceed with ventilatory weaning. After some difficulty, she succeeded in breathing without the ventilator. However, her success disappointed her, to the surprise of the staff. In this fashion, the medical team learned of BB's wish to die.

Although engaged in psychotherapy since her admission to the rehabilitation facility, BB had not confided in her therapists her desire to die. Indeed, although she exuded feelings of tension, anger, and anguish, she had kept psychotherapeutic contacts generally superficial. Now, the focus of psychotherapy shifted toward exploring the reasons why BB wanted to die. She described great suffering, which was primarily psychological rather than physical. She did not believe that she could ever accept life with her extreme physical limitations.

BB's treatment team encouraged her to reconsider. They informed BB that many persons who suffer catastrophic injury have suicidal ideas early in their rehabilitation, yet, after two or more years, may regain their desire to live. Thus, a decision to forgo life-sustaining treatment should wait until then.[3] On the basis of this information, BB promised to postpone for at least six months her wish to die.

However, three weeks later, BB changed her mind. She took three days to write a letter, using her specially adapted computer communication system. She cogently and forcefully described her reasons for wanting to die, and to do so by stopping all nutrition, hydration, and medications, except for morphine as needed to control pain. She further stated that she wished to die at the rehabilitation hospital.

This new stance prompted formal evaluation of BB's capacity to make medical decisions, and specifically to forgo life-sustaining treatment. BB's attending psychologist and psychiatrist carefully reviewed the issue of her capacity to make this irrevocable medical decision. Her cognition clearly allowed her to understand her prognosis and to participate in everyday decisions. She had no formal thought disorder and no current evidence of disabling depression. However, BB had manifested significant fluctuations of mood since admission, as well as waxing and waning of her interest in her care, in a fashion consistent with early reaction to catastrophic injury. Because of these symptoms, the staff feared BB might indeed lack capacity, and engaged a forensic psychiatrist to evaluate her. This evaluation confirmed BB's capacity, as judged from the standpoint of an expert who was not involved in her daily care.

BB's family participated in discussions about her prognosis and wishes. They appreciated the enormity of BB's suffering, but fervently hoped that she would postpone her decision to die. They also supported her right to make her own decision.

Distress was great for many members of the staff who had worked with BB. In particular, members of her team felt extreme discomfort with the timing of BB's request. Were she to wait two years, a number of staff members said that they would still regret her decision to die, but that they would feel that her choice would be more truly the product of informed consent.

Meanwhile, BB's attending physician felt he could not continue to act as her doctor if she wanted to terminate food and fluid. The physician himself had recently been given a potentially fatal diagnosis. His determination to fight his own illness by every possible means stood in direct contrast to BB's choice. Physician and patient, both facing life and death decisions, chose opposite courses. Perhaps, for this reason, or others, the physician described to BB his idea of the suffering she would endure as she died of starvation and dehydration. He would not offer her pain medication, for to do so, in his opinion, would hasten her death, in violation of his ethical and personal beliefs.

At this point, BB and her doctor parted ways. After intense discussions among the staff, another physician—reluctantly and courageously—accepted BB as a patient.

The staff investigated various alternative discharge plans for BB. Of note, local hospices refused to accept BB, arguing that her request constituted assisted suicide. They would only accept a patient whose *illness,* and not whose choice, was leading to

an imminent death. BB's disability made the option of dying at home an impossibility, as she would need significant assistance to manage pain, possible seizures, and routine care.

The staff requested an ethics consultation, but BB refused to meet with the ethicist, noting correctly that she had already been examined by an extraordinary number of health professionals. In addition, communication for her was physically arduous and time-consuming. The ethicist, however, did meet with the staff and the administration several times. These meetings focused on the process by which BB's decisions had evolved, rather than on the outcome. Initially, many staff members objected to carrying out a plan that they could not condone, just because the law permitted, indeed required, that they do so. The ethicist presented a different point of view. Staff members who believed that they could not ethically carry out BB's wishes could withdraw from her care. However, the ethicist urged them not to view their obligation as first and foremost a legal one, but rather as an ethical response to their competent yet suffering patient, who stated so movingly that caring for her as she died was the only way to care for her at all. In the ethicist's opinion, it is not always up to the health professional to determine how or when a patient dies, either because of medical limitations or because of legal power; yet this fact does not relieve caregivers from their obligation to care for the dying patient to the best of their ability.

The staff continued to work closely with BB, acknowledging her right to cease food and fluid, but encouraging her to wait or reconsider. BB wrote letters of thanks and farewell to many who had cared for her. Then, on August 15, 1994, she stopped receiving food and fluid. Over a period of about two weeks, she became gradually unresponsive, and ultimately fell into a coma. She denied significant amounts of pain, and required only minimal analgesics. During the first week of September, BB died.

RELEVANT CASES: DISABILITY AND REFUSAL OF LIFE-SUSTAINING TREATMENT

The most widely known—and quite controversial—case of a conscious patient who wished to die by refusing food and fluid while hospitalized is that of Elizabeth Bouvia.[4] Ms. Bouvia was a twenty-eight-year-old woman with cerebral palsy, a life-long, progressively degenerative neuromuscular disorder. Ms. Bouvia was quadriplegic, had significant chronic pain, and depended on a gastrostomy tube for nutrition. She had, disability notwithstanding, graduated from college, attended graduate school in social work, married, and suffered a miscarriage. Bouvia gained notoriety through a protracted and ultimately successful legal battle to secure the right to be cared for in a hospital while she died from starvation and dehydration. (Ms. Bouvia has not yet exercised that right.)

Bouvia's case is similar to BB's in a number of ways. First, both cases call into question the traditional distinction between refusing treatment, which may inadvertently lead to death, and actively seeking death. For instance, when a patient refuses a treatment like chemotherapy because the procedure itself is invasive, painful, or otherwise burdensome, that refusal may result in death. However, we accept this refusal more readily because we can say that the illness kills the patient, who has merely let nature take its course. The point for both Bouvia and BB was not simply to avoid an onerous or invasive treatment that *might* prolong life. They explicitly wanted to die. In order to die, they rejected a treatment—food and fluid—that had nothing in particular to do with illness, but is necessary to sustain life in all persons. Thus, Bouvia and BB did not first object to a treatment, and then reluctantly accept that their refusal might lead to death. They first and primarily objected to life with their disability, and then seized on treatment refusal as a means to end life.

For both Bouvia and BB, the overt wish to die led to evaluations of their capacity to make medical decisions. In both cases, the notion that a desire to die was in itself proof of incapacity was raised and rejected. Further, the Bouvia case helped establish, along with the case of Nancy Cruzan,[5] that nutrition and hydration are medical treatments, and are not inherently different from other life-sustaining measures, such as ventilatory support.

But Bouvia and BB are not alike in all respects. When Bouvia attempted to die by starvation, she had lived with cerebral palsy for her entire twenty-eight years. The duration of her disability sets her radically apart from individuals who have recently suf-

fered catastrophic illness or injury, such as stroke, traumatic quadriplegia, or severe Guillain-Barre syndrome. In these persons, the onset of impairment is sudden and unexpected; the symptoms and inabilities are foreign and frightening. The dependency that ensues is often complete, following fast on a life with no knowledge of physical limitation. The sense of loss may be overwhelming.

Recently, a number of competent patients with severe permanent paralysis have fought for and won the right to stop life-sustaining treatments. These cases are more similar to BB's case than to Bouvia's in the onset and timing of their disability. Included in this group are patients with amyotrophic lateral sclerosis, locked in syndrome,[6] and spinal cord injury (SCI).[7]

Two of these cases bear closer examination. First, an eighteen-year-old male athlete suffered a C1 lesion with quadriplegia and ventilatory dependence after a diving accident.[8] He developed severe, painful spasticity of the head and face, which was unresponsive to medication. Two months post-injury, he told his parents that he wanted to die. They urged him to postpone his decision until he could complete rehabilitation efforts. He acquired a motorized wheelchair and advanced communication technology, and returned home to live with his family. This young man persisted in his wish to die. He requested legal proceedings to document his competency and to protect his parents. A judge acceded to his request that his parents remove him from the ventilator. He died twenty-five months after sustaining his injury.

Second, Ridley[9] presents the case of a twenty-three-year-old man with a high cervical injury sustained in a diving accident while he was intoxicated. This patient had a complex history of psychiatric disturbance, including substance abuse and multiple hospitalizations. After asking to die, he was evaluated by a psychiatrist, found competent and removed from the respirator.

Thus, in a number of cases, patients with catastrophic injuries have proved competent and exercised the right to refuse life-sustaining treatment. However, these cases are controversial, and not all ethicists or health-care professionals support such decisions.[10]

CHALLENGES TO AUTONOMY

Because of legal precedents and their own ethical principles, the Ethics Committee of the American Academy of Neurology has published a position statement strongly defending the right of competent but profoundly paralyzed patients to cease all treatments.[11]

However, professionals who focus on rehabilitation medicine may not endorse such a position. Indeed, these professionals, at least in the initial phase of patients' recovery from traumatic injury, suggest that in some cases physicians override patient autonomy, particularly in regard to refusing life-sustaining treatment. For instance, Caplan, Callahan, and Haas suggest that because newly disabled patients have limited experience with disability and lack information about their options and outcomes, some level of paternalism may be justified in their early care and rehabilitation.[12] Caplan, Callahan, and Haas offer three reasons why the competence of patients with recent traumatic injuries may be questioned. They suggest that, first, such patients may not be able adequately to evaluate the risks and benefits of rehabilitation, the results of which may take months or years to appreciate. Second, they argue that it takes time—of an unspecified amount—to cope with the threat to self-identity posed by catastrophic injury. Third, they believe that surrogates may also have impaired judgment because they suffer, as do the patients, from the first two problems. Thus, Caplan, Callahan, and Haas opt for a kind of temporary suspension of patient autonomy, during which significant decision-making authority will accrue to the health-care team, which may "initially ignore or override patient and family choice." However, Caplan, Callahan, and Haas also impose on rehabilitation providers a duty to maximize autonomy and to return decision-making authority to patients once they have had an "opportunity to accommodate to the realities of their functional impairments."[13]

Some aspects of this model closely resemble ordinary standards for decision making in emergency care. In the immediate aftermath of significant trauma, patients often cannot make informed refusals of treatment, either because the patient's mental status is unclear or because physicians may not yet have made a reliable estimate of damage and prognosis. The difficulty with Caplan, Callahan, and Haas's proposal does not arise, therefore, from the idea of a temporary abridgment of autonomy, but from the related questions of how long to accept such an infringement on patients' rights, and how to determine what constitutes a sufficient opportunity to appreciate disability. Caplan, Callahan, and Haas do not offer specific answers to either of these questions, and this reticence leaves severely disabled patients in jeopardy. Are they suggesting that we suspend patients' rights to refuse treatment for the six months to two years that clinical lore suggests are necessary to reintegrate identity after catastrophic trauma? We would not support such a lengthy extension of emergency decision-making power for health-care providers. We do favor extremely careful evaluations of capacity, along with maximal efforts to teach patients about options for rehabilitation, and to offer the best possible treatments. However, we would reserve for competent disabled patients the right to refuse life-saving care, no matter how much we may lament such a choice. . . .

REFERENCES

1 T. E. Quill, "Death and Dignity—A Case of Individualized Decision Making," *N. Engl. J. Med.,* 324 (1991): 691–94; S. Block and A. Billings, "Patient Requests for Euthanasia and Assisted Suicide in Terminal Illness," *Psychosomatics,* 36 (1995): 445–57; H. M. Chochinov et al., "Desire for Death in the Terminally Ill," *American Journal of Psychiatry,* 152 (1995): 1185–91; and M. Sullivan and S. Youngner, "Depression, Competence, and the Right to Refuse Lifesaving Treatment," *American Journal of Psychiatry,* 151 (1994): 971–78.

2 J. Shapiro, "No Less Worthy a Life," in J. Shapiro, *No Pity: People with Disabilities Forging a New Civil Rights Movement* (New York: Times Books, 1993): ch. 9; V. Michel, "Suicide by Persons with Disabilities Disguised as the Refusal of Life-Sustaining Treatment," *HEC Forum,* 7 (1995): 122–31; and B. Ridley, "Tom's Story: A Quadriplegic Who Refused Rehabilitation," *Rehabilitation Nursing,* 14 (1989): 250–53.

3 D. Patterson et al., "When Life Support Is Questioned Early in the Care of Patients with Cervical-Level Quadriplegia," *N. Engl. J. Med.,* 238 (1993): 506–09.

4 For further discussion of Bouvia, see: G. Annas, "When Suicide Prevention Becomes Brutality: The Case of Elizabeth Bouvia," *Hastings Center Report,* 14, no. 2 (1984): 20–21; G. Annas, "Elizabeth Bouvia: Whose Space

Is This Anyway?," *Hastings Center Report,* 16, no. 2 (1986): 24–25; and F. Kane, "Keeping Elizabeth Bouvia Alive for the Public Good," *Hastings Center Report,* 15, no. 6 (1985): 5–8.

5 *Cruzan v. Director, Missouri Dep't of Health,* 497 U.S. 261 (1990).

6 *Satz v. Perlmutter,* 362 So. 2d 160 (Fla. App. Ct. 1978), *aff'd,* 379 So. 2d 359 (Fla. 1980); and *In re Requena,* No. P-326-86E (N.J. Super. Ct. Ch. Div. Sept. 24. 1986), *aff'd per curiam,* No. A-442-86T5 (N.J. Super. Ct. App. Div. Oct. 6, 1986). For amyotrophic lateral sclerosis, see *In re Farrell,* 108 N.J. 335, 529 A.2d 404 (N.J. 1987). For locked in syndrome, see *In re Rodas,* No. 86PR139 (Colo. Dist. Ct. Jan. 22, 1987), *modified,* (Colo. Dist. Ct. Apr. 3. 1987). All above cases are cited in J. Bernat et al., "Competent Patients with Advanced States of Permanent Paralysis Have the Right to Forgo Life-Sustaining Therapy," *Neurology,* 43 (1993): 224–25.

7 F. Maynard and A. Muth, "The Choice to End Life as a Ventilator-Dependent Quadriplegic," *Archives of Physical Medicine and Rehabilitation,* 68 (1987): 862–64.

8 *Id.* A C1 lesion is an injury sustained to the upper part of the spinal cord. The injury results in quadriplegia and ventilatory dependence.

9 Ridley, *supra* note 2.

10 J. R. Thobaben, "The Case of Mr. Sims," *HEC Forum,* 7 (1995): 94–109.

11 Report of the Ethics and Humanities Subcommittee of the American Academy of Neurology, "Position Statement: Certain Aspects of the Care and Management of Profoundly and Irreversibly Paralyzed Patients with Retained Consciousness and Cognition," *Neurology,* 43 (1993): 222–23.

12 A. Caplan, D. Callahan, and J. Haas, "Ethical and Policy Issues in Rehabilitation Medicine," *Hastings Center Report,* 17, no. 4 (1987): S1–S20.

13 *Id.* at 12.

SUICIDE BY PERSONS WITH DISABILITIES DISGUISED AS THE REFUSAL OF LIFE-SUSTAINING TREATMENT

Vicki Michel

Michel focuses attention on a series of court cases in which a disabled person who is not terminally ill has sought to refuse life-sustaining treatment in order to end his or her life. She believes that such cases are most accurately described as cases in which a person with disabilities has chosen suicide. Courts typically hold in these cases that a competent adult cannot be forced to accept life-sustaining treatment, but Michel—giving voice to a disability-rights perspective—is critical of the attitude toward disability often found in the thinking of the courts. In her view, the courts are far too ready to conclude that life as a dependent person is meaningless; thus, she charges them with discrimination on the basis of disability. She insists that courts have a responsibility to consider the context of a person's life and, in particular, to remember how the eradication of social barriers to a meaningful life can create life possibilities for a person with disabilities.

Cases involving the refusal of life-sustaining treatment by competent persons arise in three basic forms. First, there are those involving a terminally ill person who refuses the burden of continued treatment with the result that death comes somewhat

sooner (by weeks or months) than it would have if treatment had been continued. These situations can be fairly described as involving "the process of dying" and courts and ethicists have agreed that no other interests should override the patient's choice about treatment during that process.

Second are those cases involving religious objections to treatment. These usually involve refusals of blood transfusions by Jehovah's Witnesses, and

From HEC Forum, vol. 7, nos. 2–3 (1995), pp. 122–131. © 1995 Kluwer Academic Publishers. Reprinted with kind permission from Springer Science and Business Media.

physicians find them particularly difficult because the medical prognosis is often one of return to health and normal functioning if the blood transfusion is given and death if it is not. Because Jehovah's Witnesses generally accept other medical treatment it is not reasonable to argue that this particular treatment refusal constitutes a suicide attempt; from a legal perspective the general right to make treatment decisions is strengthened by the First Amendment right to free exercise of religion. As a result, the dominant view has been to uphold the right to refuse treatment in this context.

The third group of cases is the one I am going to address in this article. The cases in this group have been analyzed by the courts as cases about refusal of life-sustaining treatment. They involve nonterminally ill people with disabilities who ask to stop eating or to have ventilator support withdrawn in order that they may end their lives. It is clear from the facts of these cases that the person both intends and wants to die, unlike the situations in the first two categories of cases. Despite the clarity of the intention courts uniformly have refused to analyze these situations as involving suicide. This was demonstrated most recently in the case of *Thor v. Superior Court*[1], a decision by the California Supreme Court involving a quadriplegic prisoner who was refusing food and medical treatment. Like the *Bergstedt, Rodas, Rivlin, McAfee* and *Bouvia* cases before it, this case would be more accurately described as a case about a person with disabilities choosing suicide rather than simply another case about a competent patient refusing life-sustaining treatment.

Descriptively naming these cases matters because calling them treatment refusal cases masks the courts' judgments about the quality of life of persons with disabilities. By focusing on a person's right to make choices about life and death, courts act and speak as if disability is not an issue and in particular ignore the social conditions that may cause persons with disabilities to want to be dead rather than continue to struggle against social prejudice and discrimination. To the extent that this occurs, the respect for persons that is supposed to underlie the priority given to the value of personal autonomy is undermined in these court decisions. At the same time, to insist that a disability perspective is essen-

tial to understanding these cases creates the danger that in attempting to advocate for people with disabilities we risk imposing our view of their lives on them—that is, we may find ourselves telling people they *should* want to continue the struggle rather than give in to the social barriers to a meaningful life that they experience.

The tension between these concerns has been evident since Elizabeth Bouvia first asked Riverside County Hospital psychiatric ward, over ten year ago, to care for her while she starved herself to death. The February–March 1984 issue of *The Disability Rag* (an advocacy publication for the community of people with disabilities) was primarily devoted to articles about the case of Elizabeth Bouvia. In 1983, Elizabeth Bouvia was a 26-year-old woman with cerebral palsy who used a wheelchair, was married, and was in graduate school in social work. That year Ms. Bouvia suffered a series of losses that included a miscarriage, the breakup of her marriage, and being told that she would never be employable. Before long, Ms. Bouvia, whose life was of course much more complex than this description captures, became the focal point of a vehement dispute between civil libertarians and disability activists, a dispute which has not yet really cooled down and which has had a series of subsequent cases to fuel it over the years. The dispute is about whether a person with disabilities has a "right to die" that encompasses a right to refuse to eat and drink and then to refuse any medical means of nutrition and hydration necessitated by the refusal to take food and fluids by mouth. The physicians at Riverside said no—they were not willing to participate in a suicide, which is how they defined what Ms. Bouvia was up to. Ms. Bouvia's lawyer on the other hand tried to define it as a refusal of medical treatment, and although Elizabeth Bouvia failed to get the agreement of the Riverside trial court, she was eventually able to establish through a California Second District Court of Appeal decision in 1986 that physicians could not legally administer nutrition and hydration over her objection even if her refusal to eat hastened her death.

Some members of the disability community objected. Paul Longmore, Ph.D., at that time a program specialist with the Program on the Study of Disability and Society at the University of Southern

California, said the courts have appropriated disability rights to support the right to suicide. "It isn't a right to die case at all. It's a disability case. When society has given us the right to live with dignity, then we will talk about the right to die. Not before"[2] (p. 5).

Subsequent cases have adopted the analytic structure established in *Bouvia*. A competent person cannot be forced to accept life-sustaining treatment over his or her objection. My argument is not with this statement as a general matter but rather with the attitude toward disability revealed in the decisions, an attitude which suggests that the court would have treated the case differently if the central character had not had a severe disability. The court in *Bouvia* said, "All decisions permitting cessation of. . .life-support procedures to some degree hastened the arrival of death. In part, at least, this was permitted because the quality of life during the time remaining in those cases had been terribly diminished. In Elizabeth Bouvia's view the quality of her life has been diminished to the point of hopelessness, uselessness, unenjoyability and frustration. She, as the patient, lying helplessly in bed, unable to care for herself, may consider her existence meaningless. She cannot be faulted for so concluding"[3] (p. 304).

Would a court ever make such a statement about a person without disabilities? Judicial comments like this simply reflect the societal view that not only is dependency the worse thing that can befall a person, but that life as a dependent person is a meaningless existence. Thus, it should have come as no surprise that the four mental health experts who spoke with Elizabeth Bouvia during her stay in Riverside concluded that her decision to end her life was reasonable. This despite the fact that when a person without disabilities voices a desire to die, he or she is first assumed to be clinically depressed and an appropriate candidate for psychiatric treatment.

Kenneth Bergstedt became a quadriplegic as the result of a swimming accident at age ten. His father cared for him and he lived what seemed to be a satisfactory life until he was thirty-one and his father was terminally ill. At that point Mr. Bergstedt asked the court to affirm that he had a right to die by refusing further ventilator support. The Nevada Supreme Court did so, denying that what Mr. Bergstedt wanted was to commit suicide. "If a competent adult is beset with an irreversible condition such as quadriplegia, where life must be sustained artificially and under circumstances of total dependence, the adult's attitude or motive may be presumed not to be suicidal"[4] (p. 627). The court also said that "the State has no overriding interest in interfering with the natural process of dying among citizens whose lives are irreparably devastated by injury or illness to the point where life may be sustained only by contrivance or radical intervention"[4] (p. 626). But does this make sense as a description of Kenneth Bergstedt's twenty-one years of life using ventilator support after his accident? Interestingly the court elsewhere in its opinion acknowledged that Kenneth led a meaningful life and noted that "it appeared to us that Kenneth needed some type of assurance that society would not cast him adrift in a sea of indifference after his father's passing"[4] (p. 628). To the point, the court said, "It is beyond cavil in one sense, that Kenneth was taking affirmative measures to hasten his own death. It is equally clear that *if Kenneth had enjoyed sound physical health but had viewed life as unbearably miserable because of his mental state, his liberty interest would provide no basis for asserting a right to terminate his life with or without the assistance of other persons. Our societal regard for the value of an individual life . . . would never countenance an assertion of liberty over life under such circumstances*"[4] (p. 625). (emphasis added)

In other words, only if a person has serious disability does his or her liberty interest in being able to choose to die take precedence over the social interest in preserving individual lives! This is a shocking statement, but it and statements like it in other similar cases go unaddressed in the literature except in journals like *The Disability Rag* and *Issues in Law and Medicine* which tend to be dismissed as publications committed to advocacy.

Concerns about attitudes toward disability sometimes get tangled up with the concerns that arise from a right-to-life perspective. The right-to-life perspective makes life itself the ultimate value, leading to a view that killing, suicide, and letting die are all moral wrongs whether the person involved is competent, senile, or permanently unconscious. Personal autonomy in this view will generally be trumped by the value of life itself. The mainstream bioethics literature, on the other hand, has made autonomy the value that generally trumps anything else. Consistent with this view, the ACLU as counsel for Elizabeth Bouvia took the position that persons with disabilities have the same right to choose death by refusal of life-sustaining treatment as persons without disabilities. As a statement of a general principle this may not be objectionable, but such a statement does not take account of the context of people's lives and in each of the cases that have reached the courts context has been both critical and unaccounted for in the legal proceedings. Kenneth Bergstedt was facing the impending loss of his care taker, his father. Elizabeth Bouvia had been told she would never be employable and was dealing with a miscarriage and a failing marriage as mentioned earlier.

The case of Larry McAfee in Georgia demonstrates the dramatic change in intention which can occur when the context changes through the opening up of life opportunities for a person with disabilities. McAfee was a quadriplegic, as a result of a motorcycle accident, who seemed likely to do well at rehabilitation in the years following the accident despite the devastating loss of his relationship with grandparents who were very important to him. But when insurance money ran out he had only Medicaid funding which was not sufficient to support living at home with attendants. McAfee went to court to get permission to end his ventilator support and die, but his case got the attention of disability activists who eventually energized both him and his parents; this led to opportunities to use his engineering talents and to get home care rather than state institutional care. McAfee no longer wanted to die although he made clear he would kill himself if forced to return to an institution[5] (ch. 9).

The point made by the disability community is that it is not the disability itself that makes life so unbearable that suicide seems a reasonable solution, but rather the conditions that people with disabilities have to contend with, including both social attitudes and the lack of accommodation and opportunity. When a person with disabilities says he or she wants to die it is outrageously discriminatory to *assume* this is a reasonable choice, whereas someone without those disabilities would be referred for suicide prevention services. It should be shocking to hear a person's lawyer say, as Elizabeth Bouvia's lawyer did, that people with disabilities can't work and that "For Elizabeth Bouvia a natural death is the sanctuary from an existence so painful and degrading that its intentional infliction would be shunned as cruel, inhumane and repugnant."[6]

In 1983, disability activists wanted to talk to Elizabeth Bouvia. They hoped to convince her that she had other options. She rejected their efforts. In December 1983 she made a public statement including the following: "I appreciate the concern of disabled persons and the disabled community but would ask them to express their support for me by agreeing that my choice, as a competent individual, is mine to make, however much any other person disagrees with that choice"[2] (p. 5). Here is the tension between the civil libertarian and disability advocacy positions.

But the court opinions don't reflect the tension or the complexity. Instead they deny the reality of suicide by calling it treatment refusal and they say explicitly that they would treat the case differently if it involved someone who was not disabled. These sentiments merit critical analysis regardless of whether one agrees with the courts' ultimate holdings because they amount to discrimination on the basis of disability. These cases say that if you are not disabled and you are suicidal the state has an interest in making sure your decision is not due to mental disorder, and to promote that interest can insist on psychiatric evaluation and involuntary hospitalization for diagnosis and sometimes treatment. But if you are a person with disabilities your desire to end your life is presumed reasonable. In addition, if you want to accomplish your demise by refusing to eat, even if you are capable of taking food by mouth, your refusal will be considered a refusal of medical treatment despite the fact that you didn't need medical treatment to get nourishment until you refused to eat.

The most recent decision of this kind, the California Supreme Court decision in the *Thor* case mentioned earlier, illustrates this analytic structure perfectly.[1,7]

Howard Andrews was an inmate serving a life sentence. In 1991, he jumped off a wall in prison and sustained injuries causing him to become quadriplegic. There seems to be agreement that Andrews was depressed both prior to and after this incident. Subsequently, he refused spoon feeding, which was an effective way for him to receive nutrition as long as he cooperated. He also refused treatment for medical problems. Dr. Thor, the prison physician, went to court for permission to place a gastrostomy tube to feed Andrews over his objection. The trial and appellate courts held that Andrews had a right to refuse life-sustaining treatment and the California Supreme Court affirmed their decision.

In one sense the decision is unremarkable. It can be viewed as simply consistent with other California opinions (*Bartling, Bouvia,* etc.) which have said that competent, non-terminally ill persons' rights to refuse life-sustaining treatment outweigh any asserted state interests in keeping them alive. But it is worth looking at Andrews' situation more closely. When we do, the case looks more like a *real* "right to die" case than like a treatment refusal case. Andrews, after all, apparently attempted suicide by jumping off a wall prior to his becoming quadriplegic. He is refusing spoon feeding, not artificial nutrition and hydration, and no one has yet asserted that spoon feeding is medical treatment. In this case, the need for feeding as medical treatment arises only from the refusal of spoon feeding, not from the patient's inability to tolerate spoon feeding, as is typical in most other artificial feeding cases.

Thus this case seems to be about a suicide attempt, not a treatment refusal. The amicus brief from the California Medical Association (CMA) is the only brief in the case that acknowledges this. The brief asserts that it doesn't matter whether Andrews is attempting suicide; he has a right to refuse an unwanted medical intervention no matter what caused his underlying medical condition. This is a defensible position. It does not pretend that refusing life-sustaining treatment is never attempted suicide and it suggests that the state interest in preventing suicide is not very compelling.

What is disturbing about the court's opinion? The court notes that "with respect to the prevention of suicide, the state has expressed a limited interest at best," and goes on to say, "a necessary distinction

exists between a person suffering from a serious life-threatening disease or debilitating injury who rejects medical intervention that only prolongs but never cures the affliction and an individual who deliberately sets in motion a course of events aimed at his or her own demise and attempts to enlist the assistance of others."[1] Howard Andrews seems to be in the latter category, but the court inexplicably places him in the former.

Noting that Andrews has a "profoundly disabling" condition that causes him to be totally dependent on others, the court accepts the Nevada Supreme Court's view in *Bergstedt* that, "as the quality of life diminishes because of physical deterioration, the State's interest in preserving life may correspondingly decrease." In other words, the court believes it is Andrews' disability that causes the state to have little interest in preserving his life. This analysis is reinforced by footnote 16 of the opinion which says, "Under the facts of this case we have no occasion to address and therefore do not decide any related issues that might arise in the event an otherwise healthy inmate with no underlying affliction engages in a course of conduct for nonmedical reasons, such as a hunger strike, that subsequently necessitates therapeutic intervention to prevent death."[1] Howard Andrews was such a healthy inmate who jumped off a wall presumably for "non-medical" reasons and then refused spoon feeding, also for nonmedical reasons, thus "necessitat[ing] therapeutic intervention."

This is not to suggest that the state should force feed quadriplegic inmates who have decided that death is a better alternative than life in prison in that condition. But it is disturbing to find that the court treats an inmate with disabilities differently from one without disabilities, who similarly decides to choose death over life in prison and to accomplish this refuses to eat. The court gives every indication that the state's interest in preserving the life of a person without disabilities would be viewed as more substantial.

The fact that Andrews was in prison added a factor that should have helped the court see the relevance of context in considering an "autonomous" decision to die. The CMA in its amicus brief was again the only participant to raise ethical concerns stemming from the inherently coercive character of incarceration. The CMA brief suggested that, because the prison environment puts the voluntariness of inmate decisions into question, there should be judicial involvement before accepting a decision to refuse life-sustaining treatment. CMA raises the question of whether a disabled prisoner has had access to rehabilitative services that meet the community care standards, to a physician of his choosing, to visitors, to a social support system, and so on. The ironic thing about this very valid point is that it is the very lack of access to these things *outside* of prisons that can lead to despair and the desire to die on the part of people with disabilities.

The difficult question is how courts are to take context into account. The Nevada Supreme Court in the *Bergstedt* decision made an attempt in this direction despite also buying into the questionable analytic structure discussed above. The court created a new state interest that must be considered in cases where a competent person who is not terminally ill wants to reject life-sustaining treatment. This is the "state's interest in encouraging the charitable and humane care of afflicted persons"[4] (p. 628). The court noted that efforts to improve the lives of people with disabilities "are indicative of the highest social character—a society attuned to the worth of an individual irrespective of physical or mental handicap"[4] (p. 628).

Although the tone here sounds somewhat patronizing of people with disabilities and also seems to view opportunities for them as a matter of charity rather than entitlement, the court is still moving in the right direction. At least a court with a case like Larry McAfee's would have to explore his life circumstances and consider whether he was aware of all his options. And under the Nevada decision each of these cases would *have* to be reviewed by a judge.

The cases described here are certainly just the tip of the iceberg. They are not likely to have had major impact on the lives of people with disabilities generally compared to the years of activist struggle that led to both local victories and ultimately to the passage of the Americans with Disabilities Act. But it is worth wondering why the bioethics literature includes so little from a disability rights perspective and why in both these "right to die" cases and in the cases about treatment decisions for newborns with disabilities so little weight is given to that perspective. Perhaps it is unrealistic to expect this literature to reflect a more constructive and contextual understanding of difference than others. I hope not. Martha Minow has given the question of difference thoughtful consideration in her book, *Making All the Difference.*[8] In a chapter titled "Dying and Living" she makes a point that will serve well as my conclusion and as something ethics committees and courts would do well to keep in mind. "Preserving life in a doubtful case may be the only way to guard against underestimations of the potential life experience of the disabled person. Once we recognize the extent to which social attitudes construct the meaning of disabilities—that disabilities are critically relational in their social meaning and their actual impact on people's lives—we may work for changes in institutional arrangements to benefit those who have been labeled handicapped. The historical record cautions against underestimating and stigmatizing those whose prospects may well change with medical advances and changes in social attitudes. Hence, the fact of life alone—and the possibilities for change that it implies—may supply the core meaning to its quality"[8] (p. 321).

REFERENCES

1 *Thor v. Superior Court* 21 Cal Rptr. 2d.357 (1993).

2 *The Disability Rag.* Feb/Mar; 1984.

3 *Bouvia v. Superior Court* 225 Cal Rpt. 297 (Cal. App 2d Dist 1986).

4 *McKay v. Bergstedt* 801 P2d 617 (Nev. 1990).

5 Shapiro P. *No Pity.* New York, N.Y.: New York Times Books; 1993.

6 Memorandum of Points and Authorities in Support of Application for TRO and injunctions in the Bouvia case, Nov. 1, 1983.

7 The following discussion of the *Thor* case is adapted from *Ethical Currents* #35; September 1993.

8 Minow M. *Making All the Difference.* Ithaca, N.Y.: Cornell University Press; 1993.

ETHICS AND COMMUNICATION IN DO-NOT-RESUSCITATE ORDERS
Tom Tomlinson and Howard Brody

Tomlinson and Brody emphasize the importance of distinguishing among three distinct rationales for DNR orders: (1) CPR would be futile and thus offer no medical benefit; (2) there would be an unacceptable quality of life *after* CPR; (3) there is presently—*before* CPR—an unacceptable quality of life. In their view, whereas the first rationale involves a purely medical judgment, the second and third involve judgments that are properly made by the patient or the patient's family. Also, whereas the first and second do not imply that other forms of life-prolonging treatment are inappropriate, the third does have such an implication. The authors analyze the proper purposes of physician communication with patients and families by reference to the underlying rationale of a DNR order. They also argue that failure to make clear the underlying rationale of a DNR order is a potent source of confusion among professional staff.

Despite the extensive literature devoted to do-not-resuscitate (DNR) orders, they continue to raise vexing problems for physicians, house staff, nurses, and policy makers. The difficulties include physicians' ambivalence about who should be consulted before a DNR order is written, the frustration of house officers and nurses who are asked to continue complicated or invasive treatments of a patient for whom a DNR order has been written, and hospital administrators' uncertainty and confusion over what their DNR policies should be.

Many of these problems arise from the failure to distinguish among three distinct rationales for DNR orders and to appreciate their differing implications. Although some commentators, notably Annas,[1] have insisted that different justifications for a DNR order should be explicitly distinguished, the majority view has lumped them all together uncritically:

> A decision not to resuscitate is considered for a variety of reasons: a request by a patient or family; advanced age of the patient; poor prognosis; severe brain damage; extreme suffering or disability in a chronically or terminally ill patient; and in some instances, the enormous cost and personnel commitment as opposed to the low probability of patient recovery.[2]

Each of the reasons listed may be good in one circumstance or another. But this shopping-list approach hides important differences among three distinct rationales that need to be better articulated and understood.

THREE RATIONALES FOR DNR

No Medical Benefit A commonly accepted ethical principle is that physicians have no obligation to provide, and patients and families have no right to demand, medical treatment that is of no demonstrable benefit.[3] Patients or families may wrongly imagine that a futile treatment would be beneficial, but this imagined benefit does not generate a right to receive treatment; otherwise, patients would be entitled to demand and receive laetrile and other quack therapies from their physicians.[4]

Although published data on survival after cardiopulmonary resuscitation (CPR) will not always be decisive in individual cases,[5,6] we believe there are circumstances when a DNR order is justified because resuscitation would almost certainly not be successful, and so would be of no benefit to the patient. This rationale for DNR orders has been discussed by Blackhall.[7]

Poor Quality of Life After CPR A second reason for withholding CPR is that the quality of life that would result after the cardiac arrest and the subsequent CPR effort is unacceptable, even though survival might be prolonged. The life that would remain might be of little or no benefit to the patient (as with permanent loss of consciousness), or the benefits might be far outweighed by likely burdens. For example, a patient who is physically disabled after a previous arrest may still have a life whose quality is acceptable to him or his family; but it can be predicted that if he should have another arrest, he would almost certainly deteriorate further into a condition he would consider unacceptable. The crucial feature of this rationale is that the arrest, the resuscitation effort, or both threaten a change in the patient's quality of life, from one that is at least minimally acceptable to one that is unacceptable.

Poor Quality of Life Before CPR The third rationale also involves a judgment about the quality of life, but here the judgment concerns the patient's current quality of life—before any anticipated arrest and resuscitation. Although the patient may survive the resuscitation, his current quality of life is judged to be unacceptable, either to him or to his family if he is incompetent. This rationale might be applied to a patient who was severely incapacitated, mentally or physically, or who suffered intolerably from a terminal or chronic disease. The crucial difference between this and the second rationale is that the judgment here concerns the patient's current quality of life, not merely the quality of life after an arrest.

With these distinctions in hand, it becomes apparent how vague many previous recommendations have been concerning the proper use of resuscitation. An example is the maxim advocated by the National Council on Cardiopulmonary Resuscitation and Emergency Cardiac Care, and often quoted with approval: "The purpose of CPR is the prevention of sudden, unexpected death. CPR is not indicated in certain situations, such as in cases of terminal irreversible illness where death is not unexpected."[1,8] "Cases of terminal irreversible illness" do not unequivocally exemplify just one kind of rationale for DNR orders, as this principle would suggest. A terminally ill patient may reasonably be given a DNR order for any of the three reasons just described, depending on the facts of the case. There could even be

cases of terminal irreversible illness in which a DNR order would *not* be justified, because the resuscitation would not be futile and the patient would judge the quality of life both before and after the arrest to be acceptable.

This last possibility suggests the ethical danger of applying a single rule for the use of CPR unambiguously to all terminally ill patients, and also the ethical importance of the distinctions we have made. In what follows, we will substantiate the claim that these are distinctions that make a difference—for the ethics of DNR decisions, for communication with patients and families, for communication among health professionals, and for hospital policies. In these discussions, we will refer to two important contrasts among the three rationales.

CONTRASTS AMONG THE THREE RATIONALES

Relevance of Patient's Values The first important difference among the rationales concerns the relevance of the patient's or family's values to the justification for the DNR decision. When the decision is based on there being no medical benefit in resuscitation, then the value that the patient or the patient's family might place on the patient's life after an arrest is irrelevant: resuscitation would not provide any meaningful prolongation of the patient's life and so could not provide anything that the patient or his family could reasonably value. Consequently, when resuscitation offers no medical benefit, the physician can make a reasoned determination that a DNR order should be written without any knowledge of the patient's values in the matter. The decision that CPR is unjustified because it is futile is a judgment that falls entirely within the physician's technical expertise.

By contrast, when the rationale depends on an assessment of the patient's quality of life, either before or after CPR, it requires the application of a set of values that determine whether the benefit of continued life outweighs any associated harm such as pain or disability. Since the physician's values may well differ from those of the patient or the patient's family acting as proxy, and since the patient has both a legal and a moral right to accept or refuse treatment in accordance with his or her values, the values

TABLE 1   Contrasts Among Rationales for DNR Orders

Rationale	Patient's values relevant?	Implications for other treatments?
No medical benefit	No	No
Poor quality of life after CPR	Yes	No
Poor quality of life before CPR	Yes	Yes

used to make these quality-of-life determinations are properly the patient's. Therefore, the justification of a DNR order on the basis of either one of the quality-of-life rationales described above is not purely a matter for expert judgment: it requires that the decision be based on the values of the individual patient.

Generalizability to Other Treatments The other important area of contrast among the three rationales concerns their specificity to the event of an arrest and subsequent resuscitation, and the generalizations they allow about the appropriateness of treatment options besides CPR.

Both "no medical benefit" and "poor quality of life after CPR" are rationales that limit the scope of their judgments to resuscitation. A decision that resuscitation will be futile concerns that treatment alone and does not imply futility for other life-prolonging treatments. So too, the judgment that an arrest and subsequent resuscitation would result in an unacceptable quality of life for the patient pertains to the undesirable consequences of those specific events; it implies nothing about the consequences of other life-threatening events and their related treatments.

On the other hand, a DNR order based on the unacceptable quality of a patient's current life, before an anticipated or possible arrest, does not involve a judgment tied exclusively to the arrest and to CPR. Instead, it is a judgment that death would be preferable to continued survival, because of the burdens imposed either by disease or by necessary life-prolonging treatment. Therefore, the same logic that supports the DNR order also supports the withholding or withdrawing of other life-prolonging measures, other things being equal.

These contrasts are summarized in Table 1.

COMMUNICATION WITH PATIENTS AND FAMILIES

The differences we have described among the three rationales have implications for the proper purposes of communicating with patients and families about DNR decisions. They also provide a basis for evaluating some of the published research in this area.

When the absence of medical benefit is the rationale for a DNR order, communication with the patient or family should aim at securing an understanding of the decision the physician has already made. Eliciting the patient's values or involving the family in the decision is not required because the decision is based on medical expertise. Rather, the discussion should inform them of the medical realities and attempt to persuade them of the reasonableness of the DNR order. (This is not to say that the physician should callously override or ignore the wishes of a patient or family that insists on resuscitation.)

When one of the quality-of-life rationales is involved, discussions with the patient or family have a different objective. Contemplating a DNR order justified by a quality-of-life rationale, a physician needs the patient's or family's permission (as an exercise of their rights), not merely their understanding (out of concern for their welfare). In such cases, it is inappropriate for the physician to begin by trying to persuade the patient or family to agree to the DNR order. It is presumptuous for the physician to believe that a DNR order is justified before he or she has knowledge of the only set of values—the patient's—that is relevant to a quality-of-life decision.

If we are correct on these points, then the President's Commission is wrong in claiming, with regard to all resuscitation decisions, that "the great weight accorded to competent patients' self-determination means that attending physicians have a duty to ascertain patients' preferences."[8] The right of self-determination, as well as the patient's preferences, is irrelevant to the determination that resuscitation would be of no medical benefit. When this is the rationale for a DNR decision, the physician has no duty to ascertain the patient's preferences.

Charlson et al. err on the other side by suggesting that DNR decisions should be discussed only with "patients whose hospital course is characterized by a slow, progressive deterioration," because statistically such patients account for the lowest post-CPR success and survival rates.[6] But these facts support their recommendation only on the false assumption that the sole valid reason for giving a DNR order is that CPR would be of no medical benefit.

Several recent studies of doctor-patient communication in DNR decisions are unhelpful when they do not distinguish among rationales. What, for example, should be made of the study[9] that indicated that one third of the DNR orders documented no discussion with either patient or family? We don't know how many of these cases involved DNR decisions based on the lack of medical benefit. In such cases, there would be no need for discussion, since the justification for the order would not rest on information about the patient's values or preferences. Other data showing a higher rate of communication[10] cannot be applauded until we know whether the communication had the proper objectives, pursuing understanding or permission only when each was appropriate. Future empirical studies in this area need to account explicitly for the ethical differences among the three rationales.

COMMUNICATION AMONG PHYSICIANS AND STAFF

In our experience, DNR orders can be potent sources of misunderstanding, dissension, and anger among the professional staff. These problems arise at least partly from uncertainty about which of the three rationales is being applied in a particular case.

An example is the case, described by Stuart Youngner,[11] of an elderly woman who had had a series of strokes but remained mentally alert. Both she and her family requested that if she should have a cardiac arrest, no resuscitative efforts should be made. Accordingly, she was given a DNR order. When she had a cardiac arrhythmia, however, she was successfully defibrillated. Both the patient and

the family were very upset at what they considered a violation of their directive. Some physicians agreed; others did not consider the arrhythmia an arrest and so disagreed that the patient's wishes had been violated.

Youngner uses this case simply to illustrate that there can be disagreement over what constitutes a cardiac arrest. But this way of framing the problem makes the dispute seem semantic and legalistic, when it is more than that. The question of whether defibrillation fell under the scope of the DNR order is better answered by looking to the rationale behind the request of the patient and family and their physician's agreement. Was the order made because resuscitation was thought to be of no medical benefit? If so, defibrillation might not be covered under that rationale, if it were the physician's judgment that a fibrillation could be treated more successfully than another arrest mechanism, such as a complete heart block. Was the issue worry about the quality of life after an arrest? Again, it might be thought that damage after a successful resuscitation from fibrillation would be less severe than that after other forms of arrest. Only if the original order were grounded in concern for the patient's quality of life before CPR would its interpretation be unambiguous. In that case, no life-prolonging treatment for any form of cardiac arrest would be acceptable, because the life to be prolonged had been judged as unacceptable by the patient, independently of any further facts about the mechanism of the arrest or the characteristics of the resuscitation.

As this example illustrates, proper understanding or interpretation of a DNR order is impossible without knowing the rationale behind it. Unfortunately, one study reports that for almost half of DNR orders there is no written explanation or justification to serve as a guide.[9] Another study revealed that physicians writing DNR orders invariably intended the order to include other interventions besides CPR—antibiotics, blood transfusions, antiarrhythmic drugs. Nevertheless, 43 percent of the patients' charts failed to mention these other interventions.[12] Lipton found that in "60 percent of the cases physicians did not specify the intent or philosophy of the overall treatment plan subsequent to DNR designation" and that in only 35 percent of the cases was there any mention of other specific types of care to be either continued or withdrawn.[13]

In practice, clearly, the terms "DNR" or "no code" are left both ambiguous and vague. The ambiguity arises from the existence of two meanings—the explicit "no CPR" and the often inferred "no extraordinary measures." The vagueness arises under both meanings because the other treatments to be withheld, if any, can only be guessed at when the rationale for the order is missing. It is therefore not surprising that if three staff members hear that a patient has been assigned a "no code," they will each construct an idea of what the patient's true management plan is, and the three imagined plans may be radically different.

HOSPITAL POLICY

Some proposed DNR policies have tried to avoid both ambiguity and vagueness by insisting that a DNR order should have no implication for the continuation of other treatments besides CPR.[2,8] As the data show, this has simply not worked, for an obvious reason. One of the three rationales for DNR—indeed, the one that may be used most frequently—does have implications for other modes of treatment. If it does not, the DNR order is illogical or unfounded. Thus, hospital staff members who continue to believe that at least some DNR orders imply conclusions about other management options are correct, formal hospital policies notwithstanding. We therefore reject this principle as invalid for guiding hospital DNR policies.

DNR forms that simply include options for withholding other types of treatment besides CPR[12] are also inadequate. When they offer options independently of the overall rationale for the DNR order, the forms invite the automatic withholding of other treatments whenever a DNR decision is made, even when the rationale for that decision may not readily generalize to other life-prolonging treatments.

Finally, our analysis also suggests difficulties with DNR policies that combine categories of patient care with resuscitation status. A typical scheme divides patients into groups assigned to receive "full support, including CPR," "full support, excluding

CPR," or "modified support, excluding CPR."[14] The trouble with such schemes is that they do not connect the use of the no-CPR categories to the rationale for the decision not to use CPR, which leads to incoherent treatment plans or unjustified generalization from the patient's no-CPR status. Thus, a patient whose no-CPR order was based on an unacceptable quality of life before CPR could be placed in the category requiring full support, excluding CPR. This would require nursing and medical staff to continue other treatments that were also unjustified, leading to the miscommunication and anger we have mentioned. Also, a patient could be assigned to the "modified support, excluding CPR" category merely on the basis of his or her no-CPR status, when such a generalization was unjustified by the rationale for the resuscitation decision.

REFERENCES

1 Annas G. J. CPR: when the beat should stop. Hastings Cent Rep 1982; 12(5):30–1.
2 Miles S. H., Cranford R., Schultz A. L. The do-not-resuscitate order in a teaching hospital: considerations and a suggested policy. Ann Intern Med 1982; 96:660–4.
3 President's Commission for the Study of Ethical Problems in Medicine and Biomedical and Behavioral Research. Making health care decisions: a report on the ethical and legal implications of informed consent in the patient-practitioner relationship. Vol. 1. Washington, D.C.: Government Printing Office, 1982:43–4. (Publication no. 0-383-515/8673.)
4 Brett A. S., McCullough L. B. When patients request specific interventions: defining the limits of the physician's obligation. N Engl J Med 1986; 315:1347–51.
5 Bedell S. E., Delbanco T. L., Cook E. F., Epstein F. H. Survival after cardiopulmonary resuscitation in the hospital. N Engl J Med 1983; 309:569–76.
6 Charlson M. E., Sax F. L, MacKenzie C. R., Fields S. D., Braham R. L., Douglas R. G. Jr. Resuscitation: How do we decide? A prospective study of physicians' preferences and the clinical course of hospitalized patients. JAMA 1986; 255:1316–22.
7 Blackhall L. J. Must we always use CPR? N Engl J Med 1987; 317:1281–5.
8 President's Commission for the Study of Ethical Problems in Medicine and Biomedical and Behavioral Research. Deciding to forego life-sustaining treatment. Washington, D.C.: Government Printing Office, 1983. (Publication no. 0-402-884.)
9 Youngner S. J., Lewandowski W., McClish D. K., Juknialis B. W., Coulton C., Bartlett E. T. 'Do not resuscitate' orders:

incidence and implications in a medical intensive care unit. JAMA 1985; 253:54–7.

10 Bedell S. E., Pelle D., Maher P. L., Cleary P. D. Do-not-resuscitate orders for critically ill patients in the hospital: How are they used and what is their impact? JAMA 1986; 256:233–7.

11 Youngner S. J. Do-not-resuscitate orders: no longer secret, but still a problem. Hastings Cent Rep 1987; 17(1):24–33.

12 Uhlmann R. E., Cassel C. K., McDonald W. J. Some treatment-withholding implications of no-code orders in an academic hospital. Crit Care Med 1984; 12:879–81.

13 Lipton H. L. Do-not-resuscitate decisions in a community hospital: incidence, implications, and outcomes. JAMA 1986; 256:1164–9.

14 Daila F., Boisaubin E. V., Sears D. A. Patient care categories: an approach to do-not-resuscitate decisions in a public teaching hospital. Crit Care Med 1986; 14:1066–7.

MEDICAL FUTILITY: A CONCEPTUAL AND ETHICAL ANALYSIS

Mark R. Wicclair

Wicclair explores some of the difficulties associated with the view that judgments of futility can provide a justification for the refusal of physicians to make certain treatments available to patients. His analysis is developed by reference to three senses of futility: (1) physiological futility; (2) futility in relation to the patient's goals; and (3) futility in relation to standards of professional integrity. In Wicclair's view, judgments of futility almost always involve a reference to evaluative standards. Thus, since he believes that the language of futility tends to communicate a false sense of scientific objectivity, he ultimately recommends that physicians not use such language in expressing their opposition to providing certain treatments.

There is a growing consensus that patients who possess decision-making capacity have an ethical and legal right to accept or refuse medical interventions, including life-sustaining treatment.[1] Advance directives enable persons to express their wishes before losing decision-making capacity, and when patients who lack decision-making capacity have not executed advance directives with unambiguous instructions, surrogates can accept or refuse medical interventions on their behalf. However, a right to accept or refuse treatments *if they are offered* by physicians does not entail a right to demand or receive treatments that physicians are unwilling to offer. In fact, there is increasing support for the position that physicians are not obligated to give patients or their surrogates an opportunity to accept or refuse *medically futile* treatments.[2]

It might be thought that physicians are uniquely qualified to make determinations of medical futility because such judgments are based on knowledge and expertise that physicians possess and patients and surrogates lack. But is this belief correct? To answer this question, it is necessary to distinguish three senses of "futility": (1) Physiological futility: A medical intervention is futile if there is no reasonable chance that it will achieve its direct physiological (medical) objective.[3] For example, CPR is futile in this sense if there is no reasonable chance that it will succeed in restoring cardiopulmonary function; dialysis is futile if there is no reasonable chance that it will succeed in cleansing the patient's blood of toxins; and tube feeding is futile if there is no reasonable chance that it will succeed in providing the patient with life-sustaining nutrition. (2) Futility in relation to the patient's goals: A medical intervention is futile if there is no reasonable chance that it will achieve the patient's goals. For example, if the patient's goal is to survive to leave the hospital, CPR is futile in this sense if there is no reasonable chance that it will enable the patient to do so. (3) Futility in relation to standards of professional integrity: A medical intervention is futile if there is no reasonable chance that it will achieve any goals that are compatible with norms of professional integrity.[4]

1. PHYSIOLOGICAL FUTILITY

Judgments of futility in the first sense (i.e., physiological futility) appear to be based on expertise that physicians possess and patients and surrogates typically lack. Physicians have scientific and clinical expertise that enables them to ascertain the likely physiological effects of medical interventions, and most patients and surrogates lack this ability. Consequently, if anyone is capable of determining that a medical intervention (e.g., CPR, chemotherapy, or dialysis) is unlikely to have a specified physiological effect in a particular case, it is the physician and not the patient or the patient's surrogate. However, there are still two reasons for doubting that the scientific and clinical expertise of physicians uniquely qualifies them to make futility judgments in this sense.

First, although their scientific and clinical expertise enables physicians to determine whether, in relation to a particular standard of reasonableness, there is a reasonable chance that a specified physiological outcome will occur, setting the standard of reasonableness involves a value judgment that goes beyond such expertise. Suppose a 79-year-old severely demented man is hospitalized with pneumonia. He appears to be responding to intravenous antibiotics. His physician believes that it is important to decide whether CPR should be initiated in the event of a cardiopulmonary arrest. The physician's scientific and clinical expertise uniquely qualifies her to determine whether the chance of restoring cardiopulmonary function is greater than X percent. However, unless X equals zero, that expertise does not uniquely qualify her to determine whether the chance of restoring cardiopulmonary function is reasonable or worthwhile only if it is greater than X percent.

Second, although the scientific and clinical expertise of physicians enables them to determine whether a medical intervention is likely to achieve a specified outcome, determining whether a particular outcome is an appropriate objective for a medical intervention involves value judgments that go beyond that expertise. Suppose a physician concludes that it would be futile to amputate the leg of a terminally ill cancer patient because an amputation would neither prevent the spread of the cancer nor significantly reduce pain. But the patient wants an amputation because he is disgusted by the thought of having a cancerous leg. Insofar as an amputation would achieve the patient's objective of removing a source of disgust and extreme displeasure, it would not be futile to the patient. The scientific and clinical expertise of the physician uniquely qualifies her to determine whether an amputation is likely to prevent the spread of the cancer or significantly reduce pain. However, that expertise does not uniquely qualify her to evaluate the patient's goal and to determine that the amputation is futile (inappropriate) even if there is a reasonable chance of achieving the patient's goal.

If a patient or surrogate wants a medical intervention that the physician deems to be futile because she concludes that there is no reasonable chance that the intervention will achieve its direct physiological (medical) objective, the physician can attempt to justify not offering it by citing standards of professional integrity. For example, the physician can claim that it is incompatible with those norms either (1) to attempt resuscitation when there is less than an X percent chance that it will restore cardiopulmonary function or (2) to amputate a limb because it disgusts a patient. However, the physician's decision not to offer a treatment would then involve a judgment of futility in the third sense (which will be considered later).

2. FUTILITY IN RELATION TO THE PATIENT'S GOALS

A medical intervention is futile in the second sense if there is no reasonable chance that it will achieve the patient's goals. Patients and surrogates may require assistance in identifying and clarifying goals, and physicians can sometimes provide such assistance. However, ordinarily physicians are not uniquely qualified to identify a patient's goals.

Even when patients or their surrogates and physicians agree on goals, there are two possible sources of disagreement about whether a treatment is futile in relation to those goals. First, the patient or surrogate and the physician might disagree about the *probability* of achieving the patient's goals by means of the treatment. Suppose that the patient's primary goal is to survive to leave the hospital. The physician concludes that the chance of achieving this goal by means of CPR if the patient were to experience cardiac arrest is close to nil. The patient agrees that CPR would be futile if the physician were right, but the patient refuses to accept the physician's conclusion. Instead, he insists that there is a very good chance that he would survive to leave the hospital if he were to receive CPR after experiencing cardiac arrest. In such cases, the disputed judgments call for scientific and clinical expertise that physicians have and patients and surrogates typically lack. Consequently, in situations of this kind, the expertise of physicians appears to uniquely qualify them to make futility determinations.

Second, even if a patient or surrogate and the physician agree on the probability of achieving the patient's goals, they might disagree about whether the probability is high enough to warrant treatment. Whereas a physician might conclude that treatment is futile because of the low probability of achieving the patient's goals, the patient or surrogate might believe that despite the poor odds, it is still worth a try. As it is sometimes put, "there is always a chance for a miracle," and the patient or surrogate may not want to foreclose whatever slim chance there is. This disagreement between the physician and the patient or surrogate concerns the standard for determining whether the probability of achieving a specified outcome is "reasonable." To recall what was said in relation to the first sense of futility, although the scientific and clinical expertise of physicians enables them to determine whether, in relation to a particular standard of reasonableness, a chance of producing a specified outcome is reasonable, setting that standard involves a value judgment that goes beyond such expertise. Again, the physician can attempt to justify a particular standard of reasonableness by citing standards of professional integrity. However, the physician's decision to not offer treatment would then involve a judgment of futility in the third sense.

3. FUTILITY IN RELATION TO STANDARDS OF PROFESSIONAL INTEGRITY

The reasoning underlying the claim that physicians are uniquely qualified to make determinations of futility in the third sense is as follows. Since the best treatment choice for patients is a function of their individual preferences and values, the scientific and clinical expertise of physicians ordinarily does not uniquely qualify them to make treatment decisions for patients. However, as practitioners of medicine, physicians have a special responsibility to uphold standards of professional integrity. These are standards for the medical profession, and not merely personal standards of individual physicians. For example, performing abortions or withdrawing life support might be contrary to the personal standards of a particular physician, but she might not hold that it is improper for *any* physician to perform an abortion or withdraw life support. That is, she need not believe that it is wrong to perform such actions *as a physician*.

Among other things, standards of professional integrity identify the proper goals of medicine and the appropriate objectives and uses of medical interventions. These standards provide a basis for claiming, say, that whereas certain surgical procedures (e.g., surgically altering the size and shape of a person's nose) are properly used for cosmetic purposes, others (e.g., an amputation of a healthy leg or arm) are not.

Of more relevance to futility determinations, standards of professional integrity might provide a basis for a principle such as the following: A medical intervention is futile if the probability of achieving any appropriate treatment goal by means of that intervention is too low. Suppose a physician recommends a Do Not Resuscitate (DNR) order to a patient with widely metastasized liver cancer. The patient responds that she *wants* CPR if she suffers cardiopulmonary arrest. The physician carefully explains the burdens of CPR and states that it is futile because the patient is within a group that has less than a 1 percent chance of surviving to leave the hospital. The patient responds that any chance of extending her life, even if it will be spent in the hospital, is worthwhile to her, and clearly outweighs the burdens of CPR. The physician can still maintain that CPR is futile because resuscitative efforts would be incompatible with norms of professional integrity. In effect, the physician would be claiming that the use of CPR in this case would constitute a *misuse* of that medical procedure.

It is important to recognize that this account of futility decisions is not based on the presumed special scientific and clinical expertise of physicians. Rather, it is based on norms associated with standards of professional integrity and the alleged special responsibility of physicians to uphold those norms. The term "standards of professional integrity" is ambiguous. It can be used descriptively or prescriptively (in an evaluative sense). Descriptively, "standards of professional integrity" can refer to: (1) an individual physician's standards (i.e., the physician's conception of the proper goals of medicine, the appropriate objectives and uses of medical interventions, and so forth), or (2) customary or currently accepted standards relating to the proper goals of medicine, the appropriate objectives and uses of medical interventions, and so forth. On some questions (e.g., whether Laetrile is an appropriate treatment for cancer) there may be enough agreement among members of the medical profession to warrant referring to "customary or currently accepted standards." However, on other questions (e.g., whether tube feeding is appropriate for patients who have been in a persistent vegetative state for over a month), there may be insufficient agreement. Prescriptively, "standards of professional integrity" refers to *valid* or *legitimate* standards. Such standards are valid if and only if their content is *worthy* of being adopted and maintained by members of the medical profession.[5]

If determinations that medical interventions are futile in the third sense can justify decisions to deny patients or their surrogates an opportunity to accept or refuse treatments, it can only be when futility judgments are based on *valid* standards of professional integrity.[6] Suppose Ms. P is a 76-year-old patient with lung cancer who suffers renal failure. Her physician is Dr. Q, and dialyzing patients under these circumstances is contrary to Dr. Q's conception of the appropriate objectives and uses of dialysis. Suppose it is not contrary to valid standards of professional integrity to dialyze Ms. P. If Dr. Q of-

fers to refer Ms. P or her surrogate to a nephrologist who would be willing to dialyze Ms. P, then Dr. Q might justifiably assert that *he* is not obligated to dialyze her. However, Dr. Q cannot justifiably claim that Ms. P or her surrogate should be denied an opportunity to accept or refuse dialysis because dialyzing Ms. P would violate *his* and/or *customary* standards of professional integrity.

CONCLUSION

It is beyond the scope of this essay to provide criteria for identifying valid standards of professional integrity. By way of a modest conclusion about determinations of medical futility, however, I will suggest the following. The statement that a medical intervention is futile communicates a sense of scientific objectivity and finality and tends to suggest that clinical data alone can decisively demonstrate that it is justified to deny patients or surrogates an opportunity to accept or refuse the treatment. However, standards of professional integrity almost always are an essential component of judgments of futility in every sense, and these standards are *evaluative*. Whereas a medical intervention may be futile in relation to one conception of the proper goals of medicine and the appropriate objectives and uses of that intervention, it may not be futile in relation to another conception. For example, according to one conception of the proper objectives and uses of mechanical ventilation, it may be futile for patients with advanced Alzheimer's disease; and according to another conception, ventilatory support may not be futile for such patients. Similarly, according to one conception of the proper objectives and uses of CPR, resuscitative efforts can be futile if the probability of survival until discharge is less than 2 percent; and according to another conception, resuscitative efforts may not be futile in the same circumstances. A key issue, then, is whether or not the medical intervention is *appropriate* from the perspective of valid standards of professional integrity.

Since the term "futility" tends to communicate a false sense of scientific objectivity and finality and to obscure the evaluative nature of the corresponding judgments, it is recommended that physicians avoid using the term to justify not offering medical interventions. Instead of saying, "life-extending treatment is not an option because it is futile," it is recommended that physicians explain the specific grounds for concluding that life-support generally, or a particular life-sustaining measure, is inappropriate in the circumstances. Whereas the statement that life-sustaining treatment is futile tends to discourage discussion, explaining the grounds for concluding that (some or all) life-extending interventions are inappropriate in the circumstances tends to invite discussion and point it in the right direction.

NOTES

1 See Alan Meisel, "The Legal Consensus About Forgoing Life-Sustaining Treatment: Its Status and Prospects," *Kennedy Institute of Ethics Journal,* Vol. 2, No. 4 (December 1992), pp. 309–45.

2 See, for example, Tom Tomlinson and Howard Brody, "Futility and the Ethics of Resuscitation," *Journal of the American Medical Association,* Vol. 264, No. 10 (Sept. 12, 1990), pp. 1276–1280; Lawrence J. Schneiderman, Nancy S. Jecker, and Albert R. Jonsen, "Medical Futility: Its Meaning and Ethical Implications," *Annals of Internal Medicine,* Vol. 112, No. 12 (June 15, 1990), pp. 949–954; and Steven

H. Miles, "Medical Futility," *Law, Medicine & Health Care,* Vol. 20, No. 4 (Winter 1992), pp. 310–15.

3 This sense of futility might be further identified as "*specific* physiological futility" to distinguish it from "*general* physiological futility." A medical intervention is futile in the latter sense if there is no reasonable chance that it will have *any* physiological effect. However, it is rarely, if ever, the case that a medical intervention is unlikely to have *any* physiological effect. For example, although a blood transfusion or chemotherapy may not extend a patient's life, each is likely to produce some physiological changes (e.g., an alteration in blood count).

4 See Tomlinson and Brody, "Futility and the Ethics of Resuscitation."

5 Alternatively, validity can be understood as a *procedural* concept. For example, it might be said standards are valid if: (1) they were adopted through a fair democratic process open to physicians and the general public, or (2) they would be adopted if such a process were followed.

6 Even if physicians are not obligated to *offer* medically futile treatments to patients or their surrogates, it may still be appropriate to *discuss* treatment goals and plans with patients or their surrogates before implementing a decision to forgo such treatments. As Youngner puts it, "Don't offer, perhaps, but please discuss." Stuart J. Youngner, "Futility in Context," *Journal of the American Medical Association,* Vol. 264, No. 10 (Sept. 12, 1990), p. 1296.

ADVANCE DIRECTIVES AND TREATMENT DECISIONS FOR INCOMPETENT ADULTS

SOME REFLECTIONS ON ADVANCE DIRECTIVES
Thomas A. Mappes

Mappes discusses some of the problems associated with the construction and implementation of advance directives. He argues that standard-form living wills typically fail to address adequately the problem posed by the prospect of existence in a severely debilitated but nonterminal condition, and he further argues that this problem is not easily solved, even if a person resolves to craft a more customized instructional directive. Mappes also provides a discussion of the relative importance of proxy and instructional directives. Next, he argues that although advance directives have a very weighty moral authority, physicians are sometimes justified in refusing to honor the instructional directives of patients. Finally, he briefly considers both "the past wishes versus present interests problem" and the "problem of incompetent revocation."

Reprinted with permission of the American Philosophical Association from *Newsletter on Philosophy and Medicine,* in *APA Newsletters,* vol. 98, no. 1, Fall 1998, pp. 106–111.

There is no doubt in my mind that advance directives can be a valuable and important tool for many of us, but it has become increasingly clear that these instruments (especially living wills) are more problematic than originally anticipated.[1] In calling attention to some of the problems associated with the construction and implementation of advance directives, I do not really mean to suggest that advance directives are unworthy of enthusiasm, but I do want to insist that our enthusiasm needs to be somewhat tempered by an awareness of various limitations and problems.

There are two basic types of advance directives. In executing an *instructional* directive, a competent person specifies instructions about his or her care in the event that decision-making capacity is lost. An instructional directive, especially when it deals specifically with a person's wishes regarding life-sustaining treatment in various possible circumstances, is commonly called "a living will." In executing a *proxy* directive, a competent person specifies a substitute decision maker (i.e., a health-care agent) to make health-care decisions for him or her in the event that decision-making capacity is lost. The legal mechanism for executing a proxy directive is often called a "durable power of attorney for health care."

It is helpful at this point to remind ourselves of the sense behind a living will. Most of us can easily imagine medical circumstances in which the continuation of our lives would be of no value to us. I would certainly say, in the event that I should fall into a persistent vegetative state (PVS), that the continuation of my life would have no value for me. [All references to PVS in this paper assume that the vegetative state is reasonably believed to be irreversible (i.e., permanent).] Moreover, in some cases, I—and I think many others—would want to say something even stronger—not just that the continuation of my life has *no* value for me, but that it has *negative* value. If I were terminally ill and undermined by pain, constraint, and/or indignity, with no reasonable prospect of relief, I would be inclined to say that I am better off dead; that is, it is in my best interests for my life not to continue. Now, if I am competent (i.e., if I retain decision-making capacity) at this point, I can refuse life-sustaining treatment. But, as we all know, the rigors of incurable illness and the dying process frequently deprive previously competent agents of their decision-making capacity. A living will is a device that allows me to exercise some measure of control over the circumstances of my death. In a living will, I express my personal wishes with regard to life-sustaining treatment in various possible circumstances. At its core, then, the living will is an expression of patient autonomy; the principal value that is being expressed is the value of self-determination. I am presently incompetent and cannot make decisions about life-sustaining treatment, but the living will has allowed me to make such decisions *prospectively.* I make decisions—while I am still competent—about how I want to be treated if I become incompetent, and the living will is the instrument that confers authority on these decisions and renders them efficacious.

A COMMON SHORTCOMING IN STANDARD-FORM LIVING WILLS: THE CIRCUMSTANCES TYPICALLY REQUIRED FOR ACTIVATION OF A LIVING WILL ARE TOO RESTRICTIVE

In speaking now of standard-form living wills, I have in mind principally the various forms that have emerged in conjunction with state statutes. In my judgment, most of these standard forms share a central shortcoming, to this effect, the circumstances typically required for activation of a living will are *too restrictive.* The problem I have in mind here was more extreme in the first generation of living wills but is still cause for concern in many states, including my own (Maryland).

The core of the problem is the way in which activation of a living will is so frequently tied to the presence of "terminal illness" or a "terminal condition"—categories that have usually been interpreted to exclude both a patient in a persistent vegetative state and one who is mired in a severely compromised state, for example, as a result of stroke or Alzheimer's disease. Although the definition of a "terminal condition" is itself a notoriously problematic issue, a terminal condition is often understood as a condition that is incurable and irreversible and, regardless of medical intervention, will lead to death in some suitably short period of time. Thus, a PVS patient is not necessarily terminally ill. Although irreversibly unconscious and hopelessly compromised, the patient might be sustained in this state for

10, 20, 30, 40 or more years. Similarly, a desparately compromised stroke victim might be in a relatively stable state and thus not qualify as terminally ill. And the Alzheimer's patient, despite the fact that he or she is significantly debilitated and on a progressively worsening trajectory, also fails to qualify as terminally ill.

Many states (including my own) have by now effectively acted to deal with the first aspect of the problem that I am worried about; they have simply revised their standard-form living wills to ensure that the existence of PVS is an independent basis upon which to activate a living will. Although I find this development with regard to PVS an entirely welcome one, I am convinced that the other aspect of the overall problem remains largely unsolved. Even if the PVS issue has been effectively resolved in second generation standard-form living wills, it still remains the case that the circumstances typically required for activation of a living will are too restrictive.

Many of us, I believe, are deeply concerned about the prospect of existence in a *severely debilitated but nonterminal condition,* and we would like our living will to somehow address this concern. Would I, for example, want to be sustained as an Alzheimer's patient if I no longer had any idea who my friends and family were? Would I want antibiotics for my pneumonia in such a state? Would I even want nutrition and hydration in such a state? But with the emergence of such questions things get much more complicated. In fact, we are now faced with a whole new layer of complexity.

ANOTHER LAYER OF COMPLEXITY: DESIGNING AN INSTRUCTIONAL DIRECTIVE RESPONSIVE TO THE PROSPECT OF EXISTENCE IN A SEVERELY DEBILITATED BUT NONTERMINAL CONDITION

I am ruminating for a moment in terms of my own value system, recognizing of course that diverse personal and cultural values will lead different individuals to very different points of view on the issues at stake in this new layer of complexity. For one thing, I am not a religious person, so my attitudes and beliefs do not take account of any doctrinal authority

or tradition. Obviously, many others will want to ensure that anything they say at this point would be in accord with the religious tradition they have embraced.

Certain general phrases come to my mind. I would not want life-sustaining treatment for myself in the event that I no longer have, and there is no reasonable possibility that I will regain, a "meaningful quality of life." That phrase certainly captures part of what I want to say, but were I to put it (or something like it) in an instructional directive, what would I really accomplish? Unless I go on to specify in some detail what counts *for me* as a *meaningful* quality of life, my instructional directive will be hopelessly vague. Other ideas are floating around in my mind. I certainly do not want to be condemned to an existence that I (as a presently competent person) would consider—here are the words— "demeaning" or "degrading" or "undignified." Perhaps I should add something like the following to my instructional directive: I do not want life-sustaining treatment if there is no reasonable prospect that I will recover from an *undignified* state of existence. Once again, we encounter the problem of vagueness. Unless I go on to specify in some detail what counts *for me* as an *undignified* state of existence, I will have provided very little effective guidance in my instructional directive.

Here is one other concern that I would consider very central to any instructional directive that I might want to prepare. I do not wish for my continued existence in a severely compromised state to be a burden—either an emotional or a financial burden—on those with whom I have shared my life—that is, my family and friends. I'm not at all sure exactly how to phrase what I want to say on this score; I only know that I am very strongly invested in this consideration, and I think many other people are as well. Perhaps I want to say something like this: Even if my life in a severely compromised state seems on balance to provide more benefits than burdens *for me,* I would not want my life to be sustained if the *collective burdens* to me, my family and friends are significant enough to outweigh the *collective benefits* to me, my family, and friends. At any rate, I think I have the prerogative as a presently competent person to stipulate that I do not want decisions about the continuation of my life in a severely compromised state to be made without regard for the impact of these decisions on my family and friends.

In focusing attention on some phrases that I resonate with, here is where I wind up. I don't want my life in a severely compromised state to be sustained if I no longer have a "meaningful" quality of life or if I am mired in an "undignified" state or if my continued existence constitutes a "significant burden" for those who love me. Now, on the one hand, I am interested in incorporating such phrases into an instructional directive that is more comprehensive than standard-form living wills. But, on the other hand, I recognize that numerous problems of interpretation are likely to arise unless I more effectively specify the meaning of these various phrases. Although this task is not an insurmountable one, I believe it is a very difficult one, even for those of us who have already thought a good bit about the issues at stake. One natural alternative is simply to include such phrases in an instructional directive and concurrently execute a proxy directive with the intention of having one's health-care agent resolve any problems of interpretation. If this strategy is chosen, of course, it would certainly be important for a person to discuss these matters in some detail with one's health-care agent.

THE RELATIVE VALUE OF ADVANCE DIRECTIVES

Should everyone have advance directives? It is very doubtful that an affirmative answer to this question could be sustained, but it does seem to me that there are very good reasons for many people to have at least some type of advance directive. Perhaps the best way to think about this is simply to say that, depending on individual circumstances, and depending on the type of advance directive we have in mind, there are more powerful reasons for some people to have advance directives than for other people to have them.

Let's focus attention first on the relative importance of a proxy directive. In many states, there is now established an explicit hierarchy for the identification of a surrogate decision maker for an incompetent person who has not executed a proxy

directive. In Maryland, for example, the hierarchy looks like this:

- court-appointed guardian
- spouse
- adult child
- parent
- adult sibling
- close friend or other relative

I am reflecting, once again, in terms of the circumstances of my own life. There is no doubt in my mind that were I to lose decision-making capacity, I would want my spouse to make health-care decisions for me. But in Maryland, she will be empowered to do so even if I never execute a proxy directive appointing her as my health-care agent. So, in a way, it seems like I don't have a very compelling incentive to execute a proxy directive. But now I reflect further: What would happen if, for whatever reason, my spouse could not function as my surrogate? According to the established Maryland hierarchy, my parents are next in line, but they are approaching 80 and I would not want this responsibility to fall on them. So I reach this point in my deliberations: It makes sense for me to have a proxy directive in which I appoint my spouse as my health-care agent and, taking account of the possibility that she might ultimately be unable to function as my health-care agent, I name one of my three sisters as my backup health-care agent. And yet, since my first choice for a health-care decision maker is in accord with the state hierarchy, it may not seem like I have a really powerful incentive to have a proxy directive in place.

Suppose on the other hand that I were a gay male in a long-term relationship with my male partner. I would certainly execute a proxy directive naming my male partner as my health-care agent, because the more traditional logic of the state hierarchy is not about to lead to the identification of my partner as my surrogate decision maker. And similarly, anyone whose first choice for a surrogate decision maker does not accord with the reigning hierarchy has a very powerful motive for establishing a proxy directive. Suppose a person looks at the relevant state hierarchy and says: "You mean it's my brother who would make health-care decisions for me? My brother's a space cadet! I wouldn't trust him to take out the garbage." The person who says that is a person who has a very powerful incentive to execute a proxy directive.

Now, there is another consideration in all of this and, for me, it turns out to be a consideration of decisive importance. In Maryland, the health-care agent—that is, the person formally named in a proxy directive—has broader powers with regard to end-of-life decision making than does a surrogate identified in terms of the state hierarchy. A surrogate is authorized to reject life-sustaining treatment *only if* the patient is in a terminal condition, is in a so-called end-stage condition, or is in a persistent vegetative state; a health-care agent is not restricted to these three circumstances. Thus, for me, taking account of the fact that I would very much like to guard against the possibility of a prolonged existence in a severely compromised state, it would be very imprudent not to execute a proxy directive.

A more remote possibility also enters my mind. What if I were tragically injured and hospitalized in a state such as New York, where at present a surrogate (as contrasted with a designated health-care agent or proxy) essentially has no legal right to refuse life-sustaining treatment for a patient who has lost decision-making capacity? As a resident of Maryland, I already have a very strong reason to establish a proxy directive. When I consider that I am also a potential visitor to a state such as New York, I realize that the overall case for my having a proxy directive is at least slightly stronger. Of course, if I were a resident of New York, I would conclude that my need for a proxy directive (especially in the absence of a very explicit living will) was truly compelling.

Let's shift our focus now to the relative importance of instructional directives. I think I want to say, other things being equal, that the older a person is, the more compelling is the reason to think seriously about executing a living will. Do we really want to suggest that it is important for (healthy) young adults to have a living will? In teaching biomedical ethics to undergraduate students, I find that I do not so much want to encourage young adults to execute a living will at this point in their life as to educate

them so that they will have the understanding necessary to think seriously about the possibility of doing so in due time.

A related consideration seems more or less obvious to me. Other things being equal, the more endangered a person's health, the more compelling is the reason to think seriously about the possibility of executing a living will. Further, in this vein, once a person is identified as a "heart" patient, or a "kidney" patient, or an ALS patient, it becomes possible to forsee with greater concreteness what sort of decline and dying process might lie ahead. And then, with appropriate education and support from both health-care professionals and family, it becomes more realistic to think through exactly what one might want in terms of life-sustaining treatment. Thus it becomes more feasible to craft a customized instructional directive, and I think there is often very good sense in doing so.

Instructional directives might well be of special value for individuals whose treatment preferences are unusual or at odds with what family members might be expected to favor. Instructional directives might also be of special value for those who would like to insulate their loved ones from the perceived burdens of end-of-life decision making, those who do not consider any likely surrogate or possible health-care agent sufficiently trustworthy or otherwise adequate to the task, and those who are essentially devoid of close personal ties. Of course, living wills originally evolved as a form of protection against overtreatment, and for most of us, that concern—despite a competing concern that cost controls now operative in the health-care system create a significant risk of undertreatment—may still provide a fairly strong incentive for establishing a living will, regardless of our age, degree of health, or special circumstances.

Let's ask then why so few people do in fact have living wills. One reason is obvious. On any given day, if I have a choice between working on my living will and working in the garden (or some such thing), I will probably decide to work in the garden. Thinking about my death is a rather unpleasant task; designing a new garden plot is a much more engaging activity. Moreover, the cultural and religious attitudes of many people are in various ways at odds with the whole idea of planning for death.[2] Closely related is the fact that some people are simply repelled by the thought that their choices could actually be implicated in the moment and manner of their death. However, I also want to suggest that the issues and concerns that can arise in drafting a living will can be very intimidating. I do not say that I am typical in the following regard, but I also do not think I am alone in saying that I have never seen a standard-form living will that did not make me nervous in some way, and often nervous in four or five different ways at once. On the other hand, how many of us are prepared to strike out on our own and craft our own document?[3] Better perhaps to share our thoughts and concerns with our health-care agent and trust his or her judgment.

Joanne Lynn develops a related line of thought in an article entitled, "Why I Don't Have a Living Will." Lynn registers a host of complaints against standard-form living wills but, in the end, simply prefers a model of family decision making. She writes:

> I believe I have a trustworthy family and a supportive circle of friends. I would prefer to endure the outcome if they "err" in predicting my preferences, or even if they choose to ignore my preferences other than the preference for family decision-making, rather than to remove from them the opportunity and the burden of making the choices. I do not want anyone else presuming to impose what are taken to be my desires as expressed elsewhere upon that family.[4]

Many people, I believe, do not have living wills essentially because they feel secure within the fabric of family life. If difficult end-of-life decisions must be made for a family member who has lost decision-making capacity, then so be it; the decision-making resources of the family will be adequate to the task. Thus, from this point of view, there is simply no compelling need for living wills.

JUSTIFIED VERSUS UNJUSTIFIED REFUSALS TO HONOR ADVANCE DIRECTIVES

When patients have in fact gone to the trouble of establishing advance directives—and here I am thinking primarily of instructional directives—do physicians typically pay sufficient attention to them? There is perhaps good reason to believe the answer to this question is no, but rather than directly exploring worries that might arise on this score, I will briefly consider a closely related and more fundamental question: Is it ever justified for physicians to refuse to honor the advance directives of patients?[5]

Surely the value of patient autonomy is sufficient to ground a very strong moral presumption that advance directives should be followed, but a moral presumption is one thing and an unconditional moral requirement is something else. Advance directives must be accorded a very weighty moral authority, but I believe it is just wrongheaded to say that refusals to honor them can never be justified.

Suppose a person has explicitly written the following into an instructional directive: "Never put me on a ventilator." At face value, this instruction is as plain as anything could possibly be. It says, "*never* put me on a ventilator." But suppose further that this person, otherwise in good health, has been injured, is presently incompetent, and needs the temporary assistance of a ventilator in order to recover. The family of the patient insists that this instruction should be disregarded. The patient's daughter speaks for the family: "Look, Mom didn't really mean she wouldn't want a ventilator in this instance. She wrote that instruction after watching granddad's tortured existence on a ventilator in his last days. Mom only meant that she did not want her dying process to be prolonged on a ventilator." In this sort of case I think it would be morally perverse to "honor" a patient's advance directive. Surely we do not show respect for patient autonomy by slavishly following a written instruction when there is compelling reason to believe the written instruction does not convey what the patient really meant to say.

Here is a similar case that once arose at a hospital in my community. An ALS patient essentially decided that he would not want his life to be prolonged past the point at which he had lost all awareness, and he wanted to write an instructional directive to this effect. He explained what he wanted to say to a lawyer, who responded, very wrongly, "oh, you mean brain death." So the patient wound up with an instructional directive saying that he wanted life-prolonging treatment until he was brain dead, but this instruction was clearly not the one he meant to give. Now, I would say, in such a case, to the extent that there is clear evidence—based on the testimony of family and friends—that a written instruction does not in fact represent the actual wishes of a formerly competent patient, that a refusal to follow this instruction is morally permissible and perhaps even morally required.

I will briefly mention one other consideration relevant to the claim that the refusal to honor the provisions of an instructional directive might sometimes be justified. There is certainly an important difference in an instructional directive between a patient's *refusing* and *requesting* certain forms of treatment. If a patient's instructional directive requests an experimental and very expensive form of treatment, and there is no mechanism in terms of which the treatment can be funded, there is certainly no obligation to provide it. Similarly, if a patient's instructional directive requests a so-called "medically ineffective" or "futile" treatment, there may well be no obligation to provide it.

TWO REMAINING PROBLEMS

Two final problems are sufficiently important to warrant explicit mention. The first can be identified as the "past wishes versus present interests problem." The second can be identified as the "problem of incompetent revocation."

The past-wishes-versus-present-interests problem is associated with the following kind of case. Someone has unambiguously stipulated in an advance directive that life-sustaining treatment should not be provided if she becomes seriously mentally debilitated; this patient is now severely mentally debilitated but is "pleasantly senile" and does not appear to be suffering. The problem is that life-sustaining treatment, although clearly incompatible with her *past wishes,* appears to be in her *present interests.* And there is a body of opinion that insists that the patient's present interests should take priority over the patient's past wishes.[6] A related issue involves the concept of personal identity. If mental deterioration is so severe that there is good reason to doubt that the present patient is essentially the "same person" as the one who executed the instructional directive, then what is the

moral authority of the one to determine what happens to the other?[7]

My own view on the past-wishes-versus-present-interests problem is that the patient's past wishes should ultimately take priority over the patient's present interests, but I think this is a very difficult problem and I have constructed a more developed case to help us feel its force.

Albert H is a 77-year-old man who lives in a nursing home. His wife is deceased but their only child, a son, visits his father at least three times a week. Albert H began to exhibit the first signs of senility in his late sixties and his condition rapidly deteriorated. At this point he is categorized as severely but "pleasantly" demented. Albert H needs constant supervision and assistance with basic tasks but seems undisturbed by his situation. He loves to watch TV and smoke cigars. He seldom recognizes his son but talks enthusiastically with him and anyone else who will listen. He tells the same stories over and over again; in fact, he often tells the same story to a person 4 or 5 times in a row, forgetting that he has just told the story. Almost all of his stories derive from memories of childhood; he seems to have virtually no memories of his adult life. Apart from his mental deterioration, Albert H has no notable health problems.

When Albert H was in his early sixties, he had executed a formal advance directive. Among other things, he had clearly specified that, were he to become seriously mentally impaired, he should not be given life-sustaining treatments, including antibiotics. The problem now is that Albert H has contracted pneumonia, and this disease will probably be fatal unless it is countered with an antibiotic. Although Albert H's son is aware of his father's advance directive, he nevertheless believes that an antiobiotic should be provided. He argues that his father presently has no conception of the "indignity" of his existence. Since his life, however compromised, clearly has value to him (i.e., to Albert H), his son contends, it is in his best interest that the antiobiotic be provided.

Should Albert H's advance directive be overridden in this case? Is Albert H presently the same person as the person who wrote the advance directive? If not, does that former person have the right to dictate what happens to Albert H?[8]

Our final problem—a closely related one—is the problem of incompetent revocation.[9] A previously competent patient has unambiguously rejected some form of life-sustaining treatment in his or her living will. But now the patient, presently incompetent, confused and perhaps scared, insists on the treatment. The conflict here is between the *past* wishes of the previously competent patient and the *present* wishes of the now incompetent patient. Which should have priority? To my knowledge, state living-will statutes ordinarily provide for a patient—whether competent or incompetent—to revoke a living will at any time. Thus the system essentially gives priority to the present wishes of the incompetent patient over the past wishes of the previously competent patient. But one might feel that this is not a satisfactory resolution of the issue, and some people have attempted to deal with this contingency by incorporating something like the following provision into their living wills: "And if I ever say, while incompetent, that I *do* want treatment, I hereby instruct you to disregard what I say."

CONCLUSION

I think we must say that difficult and unresolved problems attend the construction and implementation of advance directives, especially living wills. At the same time, these documents can be immensely valuable within the context of many people's lives. We should acknowledge the valuable role that advance directives can play; we should not lose sight of the associated problems.

NOTES

1 For one avenue of approach to the many problems associated with advance directives, see the series of articles in Special Supplement, "Advance Care Planning: Priorities for Ethical and Empirical Research," *Hastings Center Report,* 24:6 (1994), pp. S1–S36.

2 See, for example, Sheila T. Murphy et al., "Ethnicity and Advance Care Directives," *Journal of Law, Medicine & Ethics,* 24 (1996), pp. 108–117.

3 Norman Cantor presents one example of a very sophisticated, fully individualized document in "My Annotated Living Will," *Law, Medicine & Health Care,* 18:1–2 (1990), pp. 114–122.

4 Joanne Lynn, "Why I Don't Have a Living Will," *Law, Medicine, & Health Care,* 19:1–2 (1991), p. 104.

5 For one approach to this issue, see Dan W. Brock, "Trumping Advance Directives," Special Supplement, *Hastings Center Report,* 21:5 (1991), pp. S5–S6.

6 See, for example, Rebecca S. Dresser and John A. Robertson, "Quality of Life and Non-Treatment Decisions for Incompetent Patients: A Critique of the Orthodox Approach," *Law, Medicine, & Health Care,* 17 (1989), pp. 234–244.

7 For an extensive discussion of this issue, see Allen E. Buchanan and Dan W. Brock, *Deciding for Others: The Ethics of Surrogate Decision Making* (New York: Cambridge University Press, 1989), Chapter 3, "Advance Directives, Personhood, and Personal Identity.".

8 This case originally appeared in Thomas A. Mappes and David DeGrazia, eds., *Biomedical Ethics,* 4th ed. (New York: McGraw-Hill, 1996), pp. 637–638.

9 Nancy M.P. King discusses this problem in *Making Sense of Advance Directives,* rev. ed. (Wash., D.C.: Georgetown University Press, 1996), pp. 204–213.

THE CONSCIOUS INCOMPETENT PATIENT
Rebecca Dresser

Dresser provides a brief account of the *Wendland* case, in which the California Supreme Court refused to authorize the cessation of nutrition and hydration for a conscious but seriously brain-damaged man. In such cases (i.e., in cases involving conscious incompetent patients who are not terminally ill, in explicit contrast to cases involving permanently unconscious patients and cases involving terminally ill patients), Dresser points out, there seems to be an emerging legal consensus on the appropriateness of a very high evidentiary standard—the "clear and convincing evidence" standard. One especially notable result of this legal consensus is the following: In the absence of formal advance directives, prior statements by a patient indicating a "general aversion" to being maintained in a compromised state do not provide "clear and convincing evidence."

In 1995, the Michigan Supreme Court decided one of the landmark cases in end of life decisionmaking. *In re Martin* involved a man who had suffered severe brain damage in a car accident.[1] He was seriously debilitated and unable to make decisions, but he retained some awareness of his surroundings. Though he had no advance directive, before the accident he had said that he would not want to live if he became "dependent on people and machines." His wife wanted the feeding tube removed, but his mother and sister opposed this action. The Michigan court refused to permit withdrawal of the patient's feeding tube.

Six years later, faced with a strikingly similar set of facts, the California Supreme Court issued a similar ruling. In *Wendland v. Wendland,*[2] the court unanimously refused to authorize cessation of a severely brain-damaged patient's medical nutrition and hydration. The patient, Robert Wendland, had been injured in a car accident. He was conscious and able to engage in "clear, though inconsistent, interaction with his environment in response to simple commands." It was unclear whether Wendland understood these commands. He was paralyzed, incontinent, and dependent on a gastrostomy tube for nutrition and hydration. Physicians believed that there would be no further improvement in his condition.

Robert Wendland had no advance directive, but his wife, brother, and daughter all said that before the accident he had expressed strong views about life-sustaining treatment. When his father-in-law was close to death and being maintained on a respirator, Robert Wendland told his wife, Rose, "I would never want to live like that, and I wouldn't want my children to see me like that." When his brother worried that drinking and driving could leave Wendland "like a vegetable," Wendland responded, "whatever

you do, don't let that happen." His daughter reported that he had said, "if he could not be a provider for his family, if he could not do all the things that he enjoyed doing, . . . just basic things, feeding himself, talking, communicating, if he could not do those things, he would not want to live."

When Rose Wendland told the hospital that she wanted Robert's tube feeding stopped, the hospital ethics committee supported her request. Wendland's mother and sister disagreed, however, and obtained a restraining order preventing removal of the tube. The trial judge appointed Rose Wendland as Robert's conservator and later appointed an independent attorney as Robert's legal representative. The attorney eventually supported Rose Wendland's position. But the trial court ruled against them because the conservator had failed to supply clear and convincing evidence that Wendland, who was "not in a persistent vegetative state nor suffering from a terminal illness would, under the circumstances, want to die." Nor had she demonstrated by clear and convincing evidence that removing the tube would be in the patient's best interest.

Rose Wendland appealed the ruling and the intermediate appellate court reversed, based on its view that California law required physicians to implement whatever treatment decision the conservator thought would be in the patient's best interest, as long as that judgment was made in good faith. The California Supreme Court ruled against this interpretation of state law, however, and instead held that the relevant statutes required conservators to "make health care decisions for the conservatee in accordance with the conservatee's individual health-care instructions, if any, and other wishes to the extent known to the conservator." The court also said that if evidence regarding the patient's prior preferences is inadequate or unavailable, the conservator must decide in accordance with the patient's best interest.

Besides setting forth the substantive standards governing treatment decisions by conservators, the

Reprinted with permission of the author and the publisher from *Hastings Center Report,* vol. 32 (May–June 2002), pp. 9–10. Copyright © 2002 by The Hastings Center.

California Supreme Court established a high standard of proof for cases like *Wendland.* The court declared that a decision based on the patient's prior wishes or best interest must be supported by clear and convincing evidence, rather than the less demanding preponderance of the evidence. The court determined that the latter standard was acceptable when applied to terminally ill or permanently unconscious patients, but that the stricter standard should govern when conservators seek to forgo nutrition and hydration from conscious patients still able to perceive the discomfort and other symptoms that dehydration and starvation could produce. According to the court, applying a lower standard of proof to cases involving conscious patients could be unconstitutional because it would give inadequate protection to the patient's right to life and the state's interest in preserving life.

AN EMERGING CONSENSUS?

The California court cited as support for its ruling three other state supreme court decisions holding that clear and relatively precise evidence of a conscious, non-terminally ill, incompetent patient's prior wishes is necessary before nutrition and hydration may be forgone.[3] In response to Rose Wendland's argument that such a demanding evidentiary standard would improperly burden the individual's right to control future treatment, the court declared its agreement with the U.S. Supreme Court's statement in *Cruzan:* "The differences between the choice made *by* a competent person to refuse medical treatment, and the choice made *for* an incompetent person by someone else to refuse medical treatment, are so obviously different that the State is warranted in establishing rigorous procedures for the latter class of cases."[4] Moreover, the California court noted, the stringent evidentiary standard would be required only in cases involving conscious but incompetent patients who have no terminal illness and who failed to name a health care agent or complete a formal advance directive. Thus the impact of the clear and convincing evidence requirement on end of life decisions would be limited.

Robert Wendland died of pneumonia shortly before the California Supreme Court issued its opinion. If he had lived, however, the court would not have permitted clinicians to remove his feeding tube. According to the court, the evidence in the case failed to satisfy the clear and convincing standard. Robert Wendland's prior remarks were too general to indicate his clear desire to refuse treatment in his present circumstances. The judges refused "to define the extreme factual predicates that, if proved by clear and convincing evidence, might support a conservator's decision that withdrawing life support would be in the best interest of a conscious conservatee." Nevertheless, they were certain that the evidence in *Wendland* was insufficient to support the claim that the patient's quality of life was low enough to make withdrawing treatment in his best interest.

Wendland may signal a developing legal consensus. The class of patients described in *Wendland*—conscious incompetent patients—includes not only patients with brain injuries, but a much larger population of people with Alzheimer's disease and other forms of dementia. As the court observed, other state supreme courts considering end of life treatment for such patients have issued decisions resembling *Wendland.* In essence, the courts have refused to authorize cessation of treatment based on evidence of an individual's former general aversion to being maintained in a vegetative or other dependent state.

In *Wendland,* the California Supreme Court also focused on the experiential interests retained by conscious incompetent patients. According to the court, such patients have a stronger interest in avoiding a possibly burdensome non-treatment decision than do unconscious patients. To override this interest, at least one of two conditions must be met. There must be evidence that patients felt strongly enough about their non-treatment preferences to make a formal advance directive or to leave other specific instructions that they would not want treatment in their current situation. Alternatively, there must be persuasive evidence that maintaining life would impose pain or other serious experiential burdens that outweigh any positive experiences patients could gain from having their lives prolonged.

UNRESOLVED QUESTIONS

Since the 1970s, most ethicists and policymakers have regarded the competent individual's prior treatment preferences as the most defensible guide to decisionmaking for incompetent patients. This view gave rise to legislation and court decisions authorizing the cessation of treatment based on a person's general desire not to be maintained in a compromised state. But this legal approach was formulated in response to treatment questions involving patients in the persistent vegetative state or with illnesses expected to produce death in a relatively short time. *Wendland* and the other state supreme court decisions indicate that courts will demand greater justification to authorize nontreatment for conscious incompetent patients who are not terminally ill.

What remains uncertain is how courts will handle cases in which there is stronger evidence of a conscious incompetent patient's prior preferences for, or current interests in, having treatment stopped. For example, what if Robert Wendland had made a formal advance directive naming his wife as his treatment decisionmaker? Would the court have approved Rose Wendland's request to have the feeding tube removed? What if Robert Wendland had made

a directive refusing all forms of life support if he could not talk or feed himself? Would the court have authorized the treatment withdrawal? And what balance of burdens and benefits would satisfy the California Supreme Court's formulation of the best interest standard? What is the "extreme" fact situation that would make forgoing treatment in a conscious patient's best interest?

These will be the hard treatment questions facing courts, legislatures, and policymakers in the new century. With an increasing number of dementia patients and aging Baby Boomers seeking control over their future care, cases presenting such questions will inevitably arise. Morally defensible resolutions will demand a refined and expanded analysis of decisionmaking for these patients.

NOTES

1 *In re Martin,* 538 N.W.2d 399 (Mich. 1995).
2 *Wendland v. Wendland,* 110 Cal. Rptr. 2d 412 (Cal. 2001).
3 *In re Martin; In re Edna M. F.,* 563 N.W.2d 485 (Wis. 1997); *In re Conroy,* 486 A.2d 1209 (N.J. 1985).
4 *Cruzan v. Harmon,* 110 S. Ct. 2841, 2856 (1990).

ANNOTATED BIBLIOGRAPHY

Bernat, James L.: "A Defense of the Whole-Brain Concept of Death," *Hastings Center Report* 28 (March–April 1998), pp. 14–23. Bernat answers a collection of arguments directed against the whole-brain approach to the definition of death.

Cantor, Norman L.: "Twenty-Five Years After *Quinlan:* A Review of the Jurisprudence of Death and Dying," *Journal of Law, Medicine & Ethics* 29 (Summer 2001), pp. 182–196. In the first part of this wide-ranging review article, Cantor clarifies the options that are legally available to a competent patient vis-à-vis the dying process. In the second part, he clarifies the end-of-life options legally available to surrogates acting on behalf of formerly competent patients.

Celesia, Gastone G.: "Persistent Vegetative State: Clinical and Ethical Issues," *Theoretical Medicine* 18 (1997), pp. 221–236. Celesia clarifies the clinical diagnosis of persistent vegetative state (PVS) and identifies relevant factors in predicting outcomes for PVS patients. He also distinguishes five subgroups of PVS patients and makes suggestions about the level of treatment appropriate for members of each subgroup.

DeGrazia, David: "The Definition of Death," *Stanford Encyclopedia of Philosophy* (http://plato .stanford.edu). Focusing on philosophical dimensions of the debate over the definition of death. DeGrazia outlines and identifies leading arguments for and against the major contending standards before considering several more recent and radical proposals for understanding human death.

Dresser, Rebecca S., and John A. Robertson: "Quality of Life and Non-Treatment Decisions for Incompetent Patients: A Critique of the Orthodox Approach," *Law, Medicine & Health Care* 17

(Fall 1989), pp. 234–244. The authors argue against the orthodox approach to surrogate decision making, which emphasizes the desirability of advance directives and the priority of the substituted-judgment standard. Their principal complaint is that the orthodox approach allows an incompetent patient's past wishes to take priority over his or her present interests.

Fagerlin, Angela, and Carl E. Schneider: "Enough: The Failure of the Living Will," *Hastings Center Report* 34 (March–April 2004), pp. 30–42. Drawing extensively on empirical studies, Fagerlin and Schneider argue that policies designed to promote living wills are indefensible. They believe that several insoluble problems confront living wills.

Guidelines on the Termination of Life-Sustaining Treatment and the Care of the Dying: A Report by the Hastings Center (Bloomington: Indiana University Press, 1988). This document presents general guidelines on the decision-making process and other guidelines relevant to specific treatment modalities. Also included are guidelines on advance directives and the declaration of death.

Journal of the American Geriatrics Society 42 (August 1994). This issue features a collection of articles under the heading "Futility in Clinical Practice." Various aspects of the contemporary debate over medical futility are explored.

Kennedy Institute of Ethics Journal 14 (September 2004). This special issue contains a collection of articles under the heading "Death and Organ Procurement: Public Beliefs and Attitudes." Public opinion polls, clinical experience, and ethical perspectives are considered.

King, Nancy M. P.: *Making Sense of Advance Directives,* rev. ed. (Washington, DC: Georgetown University Press, 1996). In this useful book, King provides a comprehensive discussion of advance directives and the many issues associated with them.

Lynn, Joanne, ed.: *By No Extraordinary Means: The Choice to Forgo Life-Sustaining Food and Water* (Bloomington: Indiana University Press, 1986). This anthology provides a wide range of material on the issue of forgoing artificial nutrition and hydration.

Olick, Robert S.: *Taking Advance Directives Seriously: Prospective Autonomy and Decisions Near the End of Life* (Washington, DC: Georgetown University Press, 2001). Olick considers a number of challenges to advance directives and constructs an overall defense of their moral and legal weight.

President's Commission for the Study of Ethical Problems in Medicine and Biomedical and Behavioral Research: *Deciding to Forego Life-Sustaining Treatment* (1983). Chapter 4 of this valuable document provides material on the determination of incapacity (incompetence), surrogate decision making, and advance directives. Chapter 5 deals with patients who have permanently lost consciousness but are not "brain-dead." Chapter 6 considers seriously ill newborns, and Chapter 7 is concerned with resuscitation decisions.

———: *Defining Death* (1981). In this document, the commission provides an overall account of its deliberations leading to the recommendation that the Uniform Determination of Death Act be adopted in all states.

President's Council on Bioethics: *Controversies in the Determination of Death* (Washington, DC:, 2008), http://www.bioethics.gov. In this report, the council considers the criteria according to which an individual should be declared dead in light of life-sustaining technologies. This report examines the main lines of criticism and defense of a neurological standard and also explores the ethical concerns associated with the use of the traditional cardiopulmonary standard in the organ procurement practice known as "controlled donation after cardiac death."

Schneiderman, Lawrence J., Nancy S. Jecker, and Albert R. Jonsen: "Medical Futility: Its Meaning and Ethical Implications," *Annals of Internal Medicine* 112 (June 15, 1990), pp. 949–954. The authors distinguish between a quantitative and a qualitative sense of futility, and they assign an operational meaning to each sense. In a subsequent article—"Medical Futility: Response to Critiques," *Annals of Internal Medicine* 125 (October 15, 1996), pp. 669–674—the authors clarify and modify their original proposal and respond to several lines of criticism.

Shewmon, D. Alan: "Brain Death: Can it be Resuscitated?," *Hastings Center Report* 39 (March–April 2009), pp. 18–24. Shewmon reacts to *Controversies in the Determination of*

Death, a 2008 report of the President's Council on Bioethics. Although he praises the candor and clarity of the report, he remains unconvinced by the new rationale for a neurological criterion, favored by a majority of the council, which considers whether the organism continues to exist as a "functioning whole." Shewmon argues that the new rationale is ill-defined and unsupported.

Stone, Jim: "Advance Directives, Autonomy and Unintended Death," *Bioethics* 8 (July 1994), pp. 223–246. Stone argues that living wills are typically confused and dangerous documents: Not only do they often fail to culminate in the avoidance of unwanted medical treatments, but they also create a substantial risk that patients' lives will be ended in ways that were never intended. He also argues that health-care professionals often fail to distinguish living wills from DNR orders.

Veatch, Robert M.: "The Impending Collapse of the Whole-Brain Definition of Death," *Hastings Center Report* 23 (July–August 1993), pp. 18–24. Favoring a higher-brain approach to the definition of death, Veatch presents objections to the whole-brain approach and responds to a set of arguments commonly made against the higher-brain approach. He also argues for the incorporation of a "conscience clause" in definition-of-death statutes.

Youngner, Stuart J.: "Do-Not-Resuscitate Orders: No Longer Secret, but Still a Problem," *Hastings Center Report* 17 (February 1987), pp. 24–33. Youngner argues for the importance of (1) the improved documentation and specification of DNR orders; (2) the involvement of patient, family, and staff (including nurses) in DNR decisions; and (3) the regular (at least daily) review of a patient's DNR status. He also insists that DNR status does not entail medical or psychological abandonment.

———, Robert M. Arnold, and Renie Schapiro, eds.: *The Definition of Death: Contemporary Controversies* (Baltimore, MD: Johns Hopkins University Press, 1999). The articles in this useful collection address a wide range of issues associated with the definition and determination of death.

CHAPTER 6

SUICIDE, PHYSICIAN-ASSISTED SUICIDE, AND ACTIVE EUTHANASIA

INTRODUCTION

The mercy killing of patients, whether called "active euthanasia" (as it is here) or simply "euthanasia," is a topic of long-standing controversy in biomedical ethics. Can active euthanasia be morally justified? Should it be legalized? Parallel questions can be raised about physician-assisted suicide, a closely related topic that has also generated intense discussion. This chapter is designed in large part to deal with ethical questions about active euthanasia and physician-assisted suicide. Its point of departure, however, is a consideration of the morality of suicide, an issue whose relevance is not restricted to a medical context.

WHAT IS SUICIDE?

Clarity in discussions of the morality of suicide can be greatly enhanced by paying some attention to the concept of suicide. Consider two people, one saying that suicide is always immoral and the other saying that suicide is sometimes morally acceptable. It is possible that these two people are in substantive moral agreement and differ only with regard to an operating definition of *suicide*. One of them may hold that suicide is systematically immoral but say that a certain action is not suicide and is therefore morally acceptable, whereas the other may consider the same action suicide but consider it a morally acceptable form of suicide. The following cases and the accompanying analysis are presented in order to shed some measure of light on the concept of suicide.

(1) A woman, having despaired of achieving a satisfying life, leaps to her death from the top of a city skyscraper. (2) An elderly man dies from a massive overdose of sleeping

pills, leaving behind a note explaining that he is not bitter but that life seems to have passed him by. He has outlived his friends, he has no employment, he finds no enjoyment in his pastimes, and so forth. Both of these cases provide us with clear instances of suicide. In accordance with what might be called the standard definition of *suicide,* each of these cases is a suicide precisely because it features the *intentional termination of one's own life.* Consider a third case. (3) In time of war, a soldier is captured and subjected to torture. Feeling unable to resist any longer, but determined not to yield any information that would endanger the lives of his comrades, he hangs himself. This third case is noteworthy, in contrast to the first two, in that it features an other-directed rather than a self-directed motivation. Still, it seems to be a clear case of the intentional termination of one's own life. It is sometimes said that the self-killing in such cases is sacrificial rather than suicidal, but to deny that case 3 is a case of suicide is surely to abandon the standard definition of the term.

(4) A truck driver, foreseeing his own death, nevertheless steers his runaway truck into a concrete abutment to avoid hitting a schoolbus that has stopped on the roadway to discharge children. (5) In a somewhat similar and much discussed actual case, a certain Captain Oates fell ill and found himself physically unable to continue on with a party of explorers in the Antarctic. The explorers were struggling to find their way out of a blizzard. Captain Oates, determined to avoid further endangering his colleagues by hindering their progress, but unable to convince them to leave him to die, simply walked off to meet his death in the blizzard. One may feel some puzzlement as to whether cases 4 and 5 are to be identified as cases of suicide. As in case 3, the notion of sacrificial death may come to mind. Presumably, neither the truck driver nor Captain Oates wanted to die; each sacrificed his own life so that the lives of others might be protected. In contrast to case 3, however, it is plausible to say, in accordance with the standard definition, that cases 4 and 5 are not cases of suicide. In this view, it would be said that neither the truck driver nor Captain Oates *intentionally terminated* his life. While each initiated a chain of events that was foreseen as leading to his own death, neither initiated the chain of events because he desired to die; quite the contrary, he desired to attain some other objective—that is, the protection of others. Thus, the primary intention of the basic action (redirecting the truck, walking away from camp) was to protect others; one's own death, it is said, is foreseen but not intended.[1] Still, many would insist, contrary to the line of thought just developed, that both the truck driver and Captain Oates did intentionally terminate their lives. It was in their power to avoid their deaths, but they chose, seemingly in noble fashion, not to do so.

Consider one final case. (6) A Jehovah's Witness, as a matter of religious principle, refuses to consent to a blood transfusion and dies. Is this a case of suicide? This judgment turns, as does our judgment regarding cases 4 and 5, on the interpretation of the phrase *intentional termination.* The Jehovah's Witness, in many ways similar to the traditional Christian martyr, refuses to sacrifice religious principle and thereby brings about his or her own death. Those who say that case 6 is not a case of suicide point out that the Jehovah's Witness typically does not want to die. The Jehovah's Witness foresees but does not intend his or her own death. Those who say that case 6 is a case of suicide point out that, in effect, the avoidance of death is within the power of the Jehovah's Witness. Thus, in their view, choosing to refuse the blood transfusion constitutes an intentional termination of life.

Notice that, in certain circumstances, the refusal of life-sustaining treatment is undeniably suicide. Suppose a person in good health is accidentally injured and needs a routine surgical procedure in order to live (and fully recover). Suppose further that this person refuses medical intervention simply because he or she wants to die. In such a case, refusing life-sustaining treatment is simply a convenient way of committing suicide. The phrase *intentional termination,* however it is to be finally analyzed, clearly incorporates passive as well as active means. A person can commit suicide just as effectively by (passively) refusing to eat as by (actively) taking an overdose of drugs.

Ordinarily, the refusal of life-sustaining treatment by a terminally ill patient is not considered suicide—at least if the patient's death is reasonably imminent. Perhaps this is the case because the refusal of life-sustaining treatment in such cases is so naturally understood as a decision not to extend the dying process. On the other hand, consider a patient (not terminally ill) who is dissatisfied with the quality of life that has resulted from some incurable medical condition (e.g., paralysis) and refuses life-sustaining treatment for a treatable medical condition (e.g., pneumonia) that happens to arise. Is this not suicide?[2]

THE MORALITY OF SUICIDE

Under what conditions, if at all, is suicide morally acceptable? Classical literature on the morality of suicide provides a number of sources who issue a strong moral condemnation of suicide. St. Augustine, St. Thomas Aquinas, and Immanuel Kant are prominent examples. Augustine's arguments are dominantly theological in character, but Aquinas and Kant advance philosophical as well as religiously based arguments against suicide. According to Aquinas, suicide is to be condemned, not only because it violates our duty to God but also because it violates the natural law and, moreover, because it injures the community. Kant, in the first selection of this chapter, argues that suicide degrades human worth and is therefore always immoral. R. B. Brandt, in a very different vein, critically analyzes the most influential of the classical arguments against suicide and vigorously defends the view that suicide is not always immoral. This more liberal viewpoint, it is important to note, is not unprecedented in the classical literature on suicide. The Roman Stoic Seneca and the eighteenth-century Scottish philosopher David Hume are quite notable in their articulation and defense of such a view.

The more liberal view on the morality of suicide might be explicated in general terms as follows. Suicide is morally acceptable to the extent that it does no substantial damage to the interests of other individuals. Moreover, even in cases where suicide has some significant negative impact on others, no person is morally obliged to undergo extreme distress to prevent others from undergoing some smaller measure of discomfort, sadness, and so forth.

In his discussion, Brandt considers not only the morality of suicide but also the rationality of suicide. It is sometimes asserted that a suicidal intention is necessarily irrational and thus a symptom of mental illness and incompetence. In other words, it is impossible for a competent adult to have a suicidal intention. Although this point seems to be built into some psychiatric theories, many philosophers—and, today, many psychiatrists as well—consider it an implausible contention. Brandt, in particular, insists that suicide can be a rational choice, although he warns of the distorting effects that depression can exercise over human judgment.

THE MORALITY OF ACTIVE EUTHANASIA

There is both a narrow and a broad sense of *euthanasia.* The difference between the two is best understood by reference to the categories of killing and allowing to die, although the distinction between killing and allowing to die is itself a controversial one. Understood in the narrow sense, the category of euthanasia is limited to mercy *killing.* Thus, if a physician believes a terminally ill patient is better off dead and for that reason (mercifully) administers a lethal dose of a drug to the patient, this act is a paradigm of euthanasia. On the other hand, if a physician *allows a patient to die* (e.g., by withholding or withdrawing a respirator), this does not count as euthanasia. Although the narrow sense of euthanasia is becoming increasingly common, many writers still use the word *euthanasia* in the broad sense. Understood in the broad sense, the category of euthanasia encompasses both killing and allowing to die (on grounds of mercy). Of course, the underlying assumption in conceptualizing the withholding or withdrawal of treatment under the heading of euthanasia is that the physician withholds or withdraws life-sustaining treatment (mercifully) for the precise purpose of bringing about the patient's death. Those who use the broad sense of euthanasia typically distinguish between *active* euthanasia (i.e., killing) and *passive* euthanasia (i.e., allowing to die).

One other distinction is of central importance in discussions of euthanasia. *Voluntary* euthanasia proceeds in response to the (informed) request of a competent patient. *Nonvoluntary* euthanasia involves an individual who is incompetent to give consent. The possibility of nonvoluntary euthanasia might arise with regard to adults who have for any number of reasons (e.g., Alzheimer's disease) lost their decision-making capacity, and it might arise with regard to newborn infants or children. Both voluntary and nonvoluntary euthanasia may be further distinguished from *involuntary* euthanasia, which entails acting against the will or, at any rate, without the permission of a competent person. It is important to note, however, that some writers in biomedical ethics use the phrase *involuntary euthanasia* in referring to what has been identified here as nonvoluntary euthanasia.

If the voluntary/nonvoluntary distinction is combined with the active/passive distinction, four types of euthanasia can be distinguished: (1) voluntary active euthanasia, (2) nonvoluntary active euthanasia, (3) voluntary passive euthanasia, and (4) nonvoluntary passive euthanasia. Contemporary debate, however, focuses on the moral legitimacy of active euthanasia, especially voluntary active euthanasia. There is far less controversy about the moral legitimacy of passive euthanasia, whether voluntary or nonvoluntary. At any rate, the idea that it can be morally appropriate to withhold or withdraw life-sustaining treatment is firmly established, at least in the United States. This is not to say, of course, that there are no issues related to the specific conditions that must be satisfied in order for the withholding or withdrawal of life-sustaining treatment to be morally appropriate. (See Chapter 5 in this regard.)

James Rachels argues, in this chapter, for the moral legitimacy of active euthanasia. One of his central claims is that there is no morally significant distinction between killing and allowing to die. Daniel Callahan, by way of contrast, defends the coherence and moral importance of the distinction between killing and allowing to die. Callahan is opposed to active euthanasia and argues that killing patients is incompatible with the role of the physician in society. In his view, the power of the physician must be used "only to cure or comfort, never to kill." Dan W. Brock, in turn, rejects the idea that active euthanasia is incompatible with the fundamental professional commitments of a physician. Furthermore, in stating a case for the moral legitimacy of voluntary active euthanasia, Brock appeals to the centrality of two fundamental values—patient autonomy and patient well-being.

Those, such as Rachels, who argue for the moral legitimacy of active euthanasia usually emphasize considerations of humaneness. When the intent is to provide an overall defense of voluntary active euthanasia, the humanitarian appeal is typically conjoined with an appeal to the primacy of individual autonomy. Thus, the overall case for the moral legitimacy of voluntary active euthanasia incorporates two basic arguments: (1) It is cruel and inhumane to refuse the plea of a terminally ill person for his or her life to be mercifully ended in order to avoid future suffering and/or indignity. (2) Autonomous choice should be respected to the extent that it does not result in harm to others. Since no one is harmed—at least in typical cases—by terminally ill patients' undergoing active euthanasia, a decision to have one's life ended in this fashion should be respected.

Those who argue against the moral legitimacy of active euthanasia typically rest their case on one or all of the following claims: (1) Killing an innocent person is inherently wrong. (2) Killing is incompatible with the professional responsibilities of the physician. (3) Any systematic acceptance of active euthanasia would lead to detrimental social consequences (e.g., via a lessening of respect for human life). This third line of argument is the one that is typically most emphasized in discussions concerning the legalization of active euthanasia.

THE SUPREME COURT, PHYSICIAN-ASSISTED SUICIDE, AND TERMINAL SEDATION

Arguments for and against the moral legitimacy of physician-assisted suicide largely parallel the standard arguments for and against the moral legitimacy of voluntary active euthanasia, and one might wonder if there is a morally significant difference between these two practices. Physician-assisted suicide typically involves a physician in one or both of the following roles: (1) providing *information* to a patient about how to commit suicide in an effective manner and (2) providing the *means* necessary for an effective suicide (most commonly, by writing a prescription for a lethal amount of medication). Other modes of physician assistance in suicide might include providing moral support for the patient's decision, "supervising" the actual suicide, and helping the patient carry out the necessary physical actions. For example, a very frail patient might need a certain amount of physical assistance just to take pills.

In both physician-assisted suicide and voluntary active euthanasia, a physician plays an active role in bringing about the death of a patient. However, at face value, there is a difference between the two: In voluntary active euthanasia the physician ultimately kills the patient, whereas in physician-assisted suicide the patient ultimately kills himself or herself, albeit with the assistance of the physician. It is a controversial issue whether this difference in terms of ultimate causal agency can serve as a basis for the claim that there is a morally significant difference between physician-assisted suicide and voluntary active euthanasia.

An important development in the public debate over physician-assisted suicide took place in 1997, when the U.S. Supreme Court unanimously upheld the constitutionality of state statutes prohibiting physician-assisted suicide. In *Washington v. Glucksberg,* the Court rejected the claim that the Due Process Clause of the Fourteenth Amendment encompasses a fundamental right to physician-assisted suicide. In the companion case *Vacco v. Quill,* the Court rejected the claim that the Equal Protection Clause of the Fourteenth Amendment is violated by a state prohibiting physician-assisted suicide while at the same time permitting the withdrawal of life-sustaining treatment. In resolving this second case, the Court explicitly committed itself to the legitimacy and importance of drawing a distinction between assisting suicide and withdrawing life-sustaining treatment.

Each of the physician-assisted suicide cases was decided by a 9–0 vote, but the Court is not nearly so unified on the construction of the underlying issues as these unanimous votes might suggest. The Court's underlying fragmentation of viewpoint is reflected in a host of concurring opinions generated by the cases. Chief Justice William H. Rehnquist wrote the "Opinion of the Court" in each of the cases, but only four other justices actually concurred in these opinions, and one of these four, Justice Sandra Day O'Connor, also crafted a concurring opinion. Both of Chief Justice Rehnquist's opinions are reprinted in this chapter, as is the concurring opinion of Justice O'Connor. In another of this chapter's selections, David Orentlicher provides a commentary on the Supreme Court opinions on physician-assisted suicide. Orentlicher's analysis focuses on the Court's endorsement of the practice of *terminal sedation.*

The idea of terminal sedation naturally arises in those (presumably few) cases in which the severe pain or suffering of a terminally ill patient is resistant to established palliative techniques and can be alleviated only by *sedation into unconsciousness.* A frequent concomitant of terminal sedation, as actually practiced, is the withholding of nutrition and hydration. Thus, a patient who undergoes terminal sedation eventually dies either (1) as a result of the underlying disease or (2) from dehydration or starvation. Discussions of the ethics of terminal sedation frequently involve reference to the so-called Principle of Double Effect.[3] In accordance with this complex principle, a physician may never *intend* the death of a patient but may sometimes perform actions that *foreseeably* result in death. The principle is frequently cited as the underlying justification for providing a terminally ill patient with an adequate level of pain medication, even if the amount necessary to relieve pain is likely to hasten the patient's death (e.g., by depressing respiration).[4] In such a case, it is said, death can be understood as a foreseen but unintended consequence of providing the pain medication. Of course, those who are sympathetic to the tradition bound up with the Principle of Double Effect ordinarily reject physician-assisted suicide and active euthanasia on the grounds that these practices necessarily involve a physician in the intentional termination of a patient's life. But terminal sedation, it can be argued, is a morally acceptable practice precisely because the physician, in sedating the patient to unconsciousness, need intend only the relief of suffering, not the death of the patient. Orentlicher points out, however, that the Principle of Double Effect can justify only the sedation itself, not the withholding of nutrition and hydration.

PHYSICIAN-ASSISTED SUICIDE, ACTIVE EUTHANASIA, AND SOCIAL POLICY

Should active euthanasia be legalized? If so, in what form or forms and with what safeguards? Although active euthanasia is presently illegal in all fifty states and the District of Columbia, proposals for its legalization have been recurrently advanced. Most commonly, those proposals call for the legalization of *voluntary* active euthanasia.

There are some who consider active euthanasia in any form intrinsically immoral (sometimes on overtly religious grounds) and, for this reason, oppose the legalization of voluntary active euthanasia. Others are opposed to legalization because of their conviction that physicians in particular should not kill. Still others do not necessarily object to individual acts of voluntary active euthanasia but nevertheless stand opposed to any social policy that would permit its practice. The concern here is with the adverse social consequences of legalization. In this vein, it is alleged that vulnerable persons would be subject to abuse, that a disincentive for the availability of supportive services for the dying would be created, and that public trust and confidence in physicians would be undermined.

Another consequentialist concern is embodied in a frequently made "slippery-slope" argument: the legalization of voluntary active euthanasia would lead us down a slippery slope to the legalization of nonvoluntary (and perhaps involuntary) euthanasia. Those who support the legalization of voluntary active euthanasia recognize that some unfortunate consequences may result from legalization. However, they typically seek to establish that potential dangers are either overstated or can be minimized with appropriate safeguards.

Although arguments advanced against the legalization of physician-assisted suicide largely parallel those advanced against the legalization of voluntary active euthanasia, it is frequently argued that there is far less risk of abuse involved in the legalization of physician-assisted suicide. This point of view is embraced by Timothy E. Quill, Christine K. Cassel, and Diane E. Meier in one of this chapter's readings. In this particular reading, the three physicians recommend the legalization of physician-assisted suicide in accordance with a set of conditions they present.

A concrete model for the legalization of physician-assisted suicide has emerged in Oregon, where physician-assisted suicide is now legal. In November 1994, voters in Oregon approved by a margin of 51 to 49 percent a ballot initiative known as the Oregon Death with Dignity Act. This law survived constitutional challenges and ultimately went into effect on October 27, 1997; it also survived a second referendum in November 1997 in which Oregon voters opposed repeal by a margin of 60 to 40 percent. The law permits physicians in Oregon to prescribe lethal drugs for competent, terminally ill adult patients who want to end their own lives. One of the most important and distinctive features of the Oregon model is a mandatory "waiting period." In Oregon, a physician cannot provide a patient with a prescription for a lethal dose of medication until 15 days after the patient's initial request. The Oregon Death with Dignity Act is reprinted in this chapter in the form originally approved by Oregon voters.[5]

Consider, for a moment, some of the issues that might arise in specifying appropriate limits for the practice of physician-assisted suicide and/or voluntary active euthanasia. Would we want to restrict availability to patients who are terminally ill (according to some definition), to patients who are experiencing unbearable suffering (according to some definition), or to patients who are *both* terminally ill and experiencing unbearable suffering?[6] And if voluntary active euthanasia is at issue, would we want to insist that a patient be competent at the time he or she undergoes active euthanasia, or would we also want to allow for the possibility of active euthanasia in accordance with an advance directive?

Voluntary active euthanasia is a well-established practice in The Netherlands (see Appendix, Case 29). One of the interesting aspects of the Dutch system is its requirement that active euthanasia be available only if the patient is experiencing unbearable suffering (with no prospect of improvement), but there is no requirement that the patient be terminally ill. Another interesting feature of the Dutch system is its explicit acceptance of an advance-directive principle. That is, active euthanasia may be provided for patients who have become incompetent but who had clearly expressed their request for active euthanasia in a written declaration while competent.

In one of this chapter's readings, Franklin G. Miller et al. call for the legalization of both voluntary active euthanasia and physician-assisted suicide in accordance with a suggested regulatory scheme.[7] John Arras, in turn, argues strongly against the legalization of any form of physician-assisted death, a category that includes both voluntary active euthanasia and physician-assisted suicide. Arras's opposition to legalization is based on the strong likelihood of detrimental social consequences, especially a negative impact on vulnerable patients; in this regard he develops a two-pronged slippery-slope argument. According to another important point of view, since terminally ill patients are already free to refuse hydration and nutrition and thereby bring about death, there is no compelling need to legalize either voluntary active euthanasia or physician-assisted suicide. James L. Bernat, Bernard Gert, and R. Peter Mogielnicki give articulate voice to this viewpoint in their article in this chapter.

ACTIVE EUTHANASIA OF INFANTS AND THE GRONINGEN PROTOCOL IN THE NETHERLANDS

So far this introduction has discussed euthanasia and assisted suicide for adult patients. Distinctive ethical questions arise when the patient is a child or newborn infant. Before addressing active euthanasia involving infants—a topic on which this chapter includes a pair of readings—some background on passive euthanasia involving newborn infants will be helpful.

The selective nontreatment of severely impaired newborns is an issue that first entered the public consciousness in the early 1970s. In the 1980s, the issue gained an even higher profile. Media attention focused on a rash of "Baby Doe" cases (named after the pseudonym assigned to an infant who was the subject of a famous court case). In these cases, treatment was withheld from severely impaired newborns. The Reagan administration responded by introducing "Baby Doe" regulations.[8] As a result, the practice of selective nontreatment of severely impaired newborns has been subjected to intense scrutiny, with regard to both its legality and its morality.

In most of the developed world only passive euthanasia is permitted by law, regardless of the patient's age. The laws of most nations thus reflect the premise that it is never morally acceptable to take active steps to end the life of a severely impaired newborn. More precisely, these laws reflect the premise that it is never morally acceptable to end the life of a severely impaired newborn unless it would be morally acceptable to end the life of a normal infant under comparable conditions. Although caregivers are not required to prolong the life of a dying infant, they may not take active steps to end a life. Because active euthanasia is unlawful in most of the world, most moral disagreement about the treatment of severely impaired newborns concerns only the conditions under which treatment may be withheld, not the conditions under which lives may be actively ended.

A unique contrast is found in the Netherlands, where active euthanasia for competent persons over sixteen years old has been legal since 1985. In the Netherlands, the debate over infant euthanasia has recently expanded to include active euthanasia as well as passive. The basic moral question is: Under what conditions, if any, is it morally acceptable to take active steps to end the life of a severely impaired newborn? As noted, the dominant view throughout the world is that active euthanasia of infants is never permissible. A different view, beginning to receive consideration, is that it is morally acceptable to end the life of a severely impaired newborn if and only if death would be in the infant's best interests—that is, if and only if the infant would be better off dead. Defenders of this view are firmly committed to so-called quality-of-life judgments, but they systematically reject the contention that the hardship (emotional and/or financial) of caring for severely impaired newborns is a relevant factor in the decision to treat or not treat. A similar but somewhat less restrictive view would endorse ending the life of a severely impaired newborn if and only if there is no significant potential for a meaningful human existence.

In one of this chapter's selections two pediatricians, Eduard Verhagen and Pieter J.J. Sauer, espouse roughly the view just mentioned. They describe a protocol that they have developed—the *Groningen Protocol*—that reflects the idea that physicians should be permitted to end the life of an infant whose prognosis is poor and whose future promises unbearable suffering and low quality of life. The protocol includes various legal and ethical safeguards against abuse. First, the infant's parents must receive a full explanation of the condition and the infant's prognosis. Second, a team of physicians, including at least one doctor who is not directly involved in the infant's care, must also agree that active euthanasia is warranted. Third, the condition and prognosis must be clearly defined. Finally, the protocol requires that, after the infant has died, an outside legal body representing the state must determine if the decision was justified and if all necessary procedures were followed. The Groningen Protocol has been invoked in at least four cases since 2002. However, it remains highly controversial. It is criticized by pediatrician and bioethicist Alexander A. Kon in the final selection in this chapter. Kon understands the pressure that parents and caregivers feel to spare infants suffering. However, he argues that the Groningen Protocol uses unreliable judgments of future suffering and contradicts basic precepts of medical ethics such as informed consent and nonmaleficence. The risk of euthanizing an infant whose life would have been worth living, Kon insists, is too great for the protocol to be justified.

NOTES

1 The phrase "foreseen but not intended" derives from application of the Principle of Double Effect. This principle is explicitly discussed later in this Introduction.

2 See the Chapter 5 reading by Vicki Michel, "Suicide by Persons with Disabilities Disguised as the Refusal of Life-Sustaining Treatment."

3 For one useful articulation and critique of the Principle of Double Effect, see Timothy E. Quill, Rebecca Dresser, and Dan W. Brock, "The Rule of Double Effect—a Critique of Its Role in End-of-Life Decision Making," *New England Journal of Medicine* 337 (December 11, 1997), pp. 1768–1771.

4 Some commentators refer to the practice at issue here as *double-effect euthanasia.*

5 Further clarifications and small changes have subsequently been introduced in the language of the Oregon Death with Dignity Act. Current language can be accessed under "Legislative Statute" on the Oregon Department of Human Services home page (http://www.dhs.state.or.us/publichealth/chs/pas/pas.cfm). Also available on this site are annual statistical reports about the provision of physician-assisted suicide in Oregon. In 2003, 42 patients in Oregon used physician-assisted suicide to end their lives, compared to 38 who did so in 2002. On average, there are 31,000 deaths each year in Oregon.

6 For an argument to restrict availability (at least at the present time) to those who are terminally ill, see Martin Gunderson and David J. Mayo, "Restricting Physician-Assisted Death to the Terminally Ill," *Hastings Center Report* 30 (November–December 2000), pp. 17–23.

7 Miller's coauthors in this 1994 piece include Quill and Meier, whose views can be seen to have evolved from their 1992 article with Cassel. In this earlier article, Quill and Meier endorse the legalization of physician-assisted suicide but reject the legalization of voluntary active euthanasia.

8 The so-called final Baby Doe rule was published by the Department of Health and Human Services on April 15, 1985. For one interpretation of this rule, see Thomas H. Murray, "The Final, Anticlimactic Rule on Baby Doe," *Hastings Center Report* 15 (June 1985), pp. 5–9. For an alternative interpretation, see John C. Moskop and Rita L. Saldanha, "The Baby Doe Rule: Still a Threat," *Hastings Center Report* 16 (April 1986), pp. 8–14.

THE MORALITY OF SUICIDE

SUICIDE
Immanuel Kant

Kant issues a blanket moral condemnation of suicide: "Suicide is not permitted under any condition." However, on Kant's definition many acts that lead to one's death, and could be foreseen to do so, do not count as suicides. In his view, suicide is characterized by the intention to destroy oneself. Thus, a soldier who defends himself and his comrades to the death, rather than deserting them, is not guilty of suicide. Nor is one guilty of suicide whose reckless behavior leads, unintentionally, to a shortened life, although such a person is blameworthy for being reckless. Kant insists that suicide is self-contradictory, in the sense that the power of free will is used for its own destruction. In a related consideration, suicide is said to be a moral abomination because it degrades human worth. Kant also claims that suicide is rightly condemned on religious grounds.

OF DUTIES TO THE BODY, IN REGARD TO LIFE

We now come to the right that we have, to dispose over our life, and whether we have such a right. On the other side, there is the right to take care of our life. Let us note, for a start, that if the body belonged to life in a contingent way, not as a condition of life, but as a state of it, so that we could take it off if we wanted; if we could slip out of one body and enter another, like a country, then we could dispose over the body, it would then be subject to our free choice, albeit that in that case we would not be disposing over our life, but only over our state, over the movable goods, the chattels, that pertained to life. But now the body is the total condition of life, so that we have no other concept of our existence save that mediated by our body, and since the use of our freedom is possible only through the body, we see that the body constitutes a part of our self. So far, then, as anyone destroys his body, and thereby takes his own life, he has employed his choice to destroy the power of choosing itself; but in that case, free choice is in conflict with itself. If freedom is the condition of life, it cannot be employed to abolish life, since then it destroys and abolishes

From Immanuel Kant, *Lectures on Ethics,* edited and translated by Peter Heath, pp. 144–149. Copyright © 1997 by Cambridge University Press. Reprinted with the permission of Cambridge University Press.

itself; for the agent is using his life to put an end to it. Life is supposedly being used to bring about lifelessness, but that is a self-contradiction. So we already see in advance that man cannot dispose over himself and his life, though he certainly can over his circumstances. By means of his body, a man has power over his life; were he a spirit, he could not make away with his life; because nature has invested absolute life with an indestructibility, from which it follows that one cannot dispose over it, as though it were an end.

OF SUICIDE

Suicide can be considered under various aspects, from the blameworthy, the permissible and even the heroic point of view. At first it has a seeming air of being allowable and permitted. The defenders of this view argue that, so long as he does not infringe the rights of others, a man disposes freely over the earth's goods. So far as his body is concerned, he can dispose over it in many ways. He can have an abscess lanced, for example, or ignore a scar, have a limb amputated, etc., and is thus at liberty to do anything in regard to his body that seems to him expedient and useful. Should he not, then, be also entitled to take his life, if he sees that this is the most useful and expedient course for him? If he sees that he can in no way go on living and may thereby escape so much torment, misfortune and shame? Although it deprives him of a full lifetime, he nevertheless escapes at once in this way from every calamity. This appears to be a very telling argument. But let us, on the other hand, consider the action simply in itself, and not from the religious point of view. So long as we have the intention of preserving ourselves, we can, under such a condition, indeed dispose over our body. Thus a man can have his foot amputated, for example, insofar as it impedes him in life. So to preserve our person, we have disposition over our body; but the man who takes his own life is not thereby preserving his person; for if he disposes over his person, but not over his condition, he robs himself of that very thing itself. This is contrary to the supreme self-regarding duty, for the condition of all other duties is thereby abolished. It transcends all limits on the use of free choice, for the latter is only possible insofar as the subject exists.

Suicide can also come to have a plausible aspect, whenever, that is, the continuance of life rests upon such circumstances as may deprive that life of its value; when a man can no longer live in accordance with virtue and prudence, and must therefore put an end to his life from honourable motives. Those who defend suicide from this angle cite the example of Cato, who killed himself once he realized that, although all the people still relied on him, it would not be possible for him to escape falling into Caesar's hands; but as soon as he, the champion of freedom, had submitted, the rest would have thought: If Cato himself submits, what else are we to do? If he killed himself, however, the Romans might yet dedicate their final efforts to the defence of their freedom. So what was Cato to do? It seems, in fact, that he viewed his death as a necessity; his thought was: Since you can no longer live as Cato, you cannot go on living at all.

One must certainly admit of this example, that in such a case, where suicide is a virtue, there seems to be much to be said for it. It is also the one example that has given the world an opportunity of defending suicide. Yet it is also but one example of its kind. There have been many similar cases. Lucretia also killed herself, though from modesty and vengeful rage. It is assuredly a duty to preserve one's honour, especially for the fair sex, in whom it is a merit; but one should seek to save one's honour only inasmuch as it is not surrendered for selfish and voluptuous purposes; not, however, in such a case as this, for that did not apply to her. So she ought rather to have fought to the death in defence of her honour, and would then have acted rightly, and it would not have been suicide either. For to risk one's life against one's foes, and to observe the duty to oneself, and even to sacrifice one's life, is not suicide.

Nobody under the sun, no sovereign, can oblige me to commit suicide. The sovereign can certainly oblige the subject to risk his life against the foe for the fatherland, and even if he loses his life in doing so, it is not suicide, but depends on fate. And on the opposite side, it is again no preservation of life to be fearful and faint-hearted in the face of death, with which fate inevitably threatens us already. He who runs away to save his life from the enemy, and leaves all his comrades in the lurch, is a coward; but if he defends himself and his fellows to the death, that is no suicide, but is held to be noble and gallant; since, in and for itself, life is in no way to be highly prized, and I should seek to preserve my life only insofar as I am worthy to live. A distinction has to be made between a suicide and one who has lost his life to fate. He who shortens his life by intemperance, is certainly to blame for his lack of foresight, and his death can thus be imputed, indirectly, to himself; but not directly, for he did not intend to kill himself. It was not a deliberate death. For all our offences are either [due to fault] or [done with intent]. Now although there is no [intent] here, there is certainly [fault]. To such a one it can be said: You are yourself to blame for your death, but not: You are a suicide. It is the intention to destroy oneself that constitutes suicide. I must not, therefore, turn the intemperance that causes shortening of life into suicide, for if I raise intemperance to the level of suicide, the latter is thereby degraded in turn and reduced to intemperance.

There is a difference, therefore, between the imprudence in which a wish to live is still present, and the intention to do away with oneself. The most serious violations of the duties to oneself produce either revulsion with horror, and such is suicide, or revulsion with disgust, and such are the *crimina carnis*. Suicide evokes revulsion with horror, because everything in nature seeks to preserve itself: a damaged tree, a living body, an animal; and in man, then, is freedom, which is the highest degree of life, and constitutes the worth of it, to become now a *principium* for self-destruction? This is the most horrifying thing imaginable. For anyone who has already got so far as to be master, at any time, over his own life, is also master over the life of anyone else; for him, the door stands open to every crime, and before he can be seized he is ready to spirit himself away out of the world. So suicide evokes horror, in that a man thereby puts himself below the beasts. We regard a suicide as a carcase, whereas we feel pity for one who meets his end through fate.

The defenders of suicide try to push human freedom to the limit, which is flattering, and implies that persons are in a position to take their lives if they wish. So even well-meaning people defend it in this respect. There are many conditions under which life has to be sacrificed; if I cannot preserve it other than by violating the duties to myself, then I am bound to sacrifice it, rather than violate those duties; yet on the other hand, suicide is not permitted under any condition. Man has, in his own person, a thing inviolable; it is something holy, that has been entrusted to us. All else is subject to man, save only that he must not make away with himself. A being who existed of his own necessity could not possibly destroy himself; one who does not exist by such necessity sees his life as the condition of all else. He sees, and feels, that life has been entrusted to him, and if he now turns it against itself, it seems that he should recoil in trembling, at having thus violated the sacred trust assigned to him. That which a man can dispose over, must be a thing. Animals are here regarded as things; but man is not thing; so if, nevertheless, he disposes over his life, he sets upon himself the value of a beast. But he who takes himself for such, who fails to respect humanity, who turns himself into a thing, becomes an object of free choice for everyone; anyone, thereafter, may do as he pleases with him; he can be treated by others as an animal or a thing; he can be dealt with like a horse or dog, for he is no longer a man; he has turned himself into a thing, and so cannot demand that others should respect the humanity in him, since he has already thrown it away himself. Humanity, however, is worthy of respect, and even though somebody may be a bad man, the humanity in his person is en-

titled to respect. Suicide is not repulsive and forbidden because life is such a benefit, for in that case it is merely a question for each of us, whether he deem it to be a major good. By the rule of prudence, it would often be the best course, to remove oneself from the scene; but by the rule of morality it is not allowed under any condition, because it is the destruction of humanity, in that mankind is set lower than the beasts. In other respects, there is much in the world that is far higher than life. The observance of morality is far higher. It is better to sacrifice life than to forfeit morality. It is not necessary to live, but it is necessary that, so long as we live, we do so honourably; but he who can no longer live honourably is no longer worthy to live at all. We may at all times go on living, so long as we can observe the self-regarding duties, without doing violence to ourselves. But he who is ready to take his own life is no longer worthy to live. The pragmatic motivating-ground for living is happiness. Can I then take my life because I cannot live happily? No, there is no necessity that, so long as I live, I should live happily; but there is a necessity that, so long as I live, I should live honourably. Misery gives no man the right to take his life. For if we were entitled to end our lives for want of pleasure, all our self-regarding duties would be aimed at the pleasantness of life; but now the fulfilment of those duties demands the sacrifice of life.

Can heroism and freedom be met with, in the act of suicide? It is not good to practise sophistry from good intentions. Nor is it good to defend virtue or vice with sophistry. Even right-thinking people denounce suicide without giving the proper reasons. They say that there is great cowardice in it; but there are also suicides who display great *heroism,* such as Cato, Atticus and others. I cannot call such suicide cowardly. Anger, passion, and madness are in many cases the cause of suicide, which is why persons who have been saved from the attempt at it are affrighted at themselves, and do not venture it a second time. There was a period among the Greeks and Romans when suicide conferred honour, and hence, too, the Romans forbade their slaves to do away with themselves, because they belonged, not to themselves, but to their masters, and were therefore regarded as things, like any other animal. The Stoic declared suicide to be a gentle death for the sage, who leaves the world as he might go from a smoky room to another one, because he no longer cared to stay there. He departs from the world, not because he has no happiness in it, but because he despises it. As already mentioned, it is very flattering to a man to have the freedom to remove himself from the world if he so wishes. Indeed, there even seems to be something moral in it, for anyone who has the power to depart from the world when he pleases need be subject to nobody, and can be bound by nothing from telling the harshest truths to the greatest of tyrants; for the latter cannot compel him by any tortures, when he can rapidly make his exit from the world, just as a free man can go out of the country if he chooses. But this illusion disappears, if freedom can exist only through an immutable condition, which cannot be changed under any circumstances. This condition is that I do not employ my freedom against myself for my own destruction, and that I do not let it be limited by anything external. This is the noble form of freedom. I must not let myself be deterred from living by any fate or misfortune, but should go on living so long as I am a man and can live honourably. To complain of fate and misfortune dishonours a man. If Cato, under all the tortures that Caesar might have inflicted on him, had still adhered to his resolve with steadfast mind, that would have been noble; but not when he laid hands upon himself. Those who defend and teach the legitimacy of suicide inevitably do great harm in a republic. Suppose it were a general disposition that people cherished, that suicide was a right, and even a merit or honour; such people would be abhorrent to every-one. For he who so utterly fails to respect his life on principle can in no way be restrained from the most appalling vices; he fears no king and no torture.

But all such illusions are lost, if we consider suicide in regard to religion. We have been placed in this world for certain destinies and purposes; but a suicide flouts the intention of his creator. He arrives in the next world as one who has deserted his post, and must therefore be seen as a rebel against God. So long as we acknowledge this truth, that the preservation of our life is among God's purposes, we are in duty bound to regulate our free actions in accordance with it. We have neither right nor authority to do violence to our nature's preservative powers, or to upset the wisdom of her arrangements. This responsibility lies upon us until such time as God gives us His express command to depart this world.

Men are stationed here like sentries, and so we must not leave our posts until relieved by the beneficent hand of another. He is our proprietor, and we His property, and His providence ensures what is best for us: A bondman who is under the care of a kindly master invites punishment if he defies the latter's intentions.

Suicide, however, is impermissible and abhorrent, not because God has forbidden it; God has forbidden it, rather, because it is abhorrent. So all moralists must begin by demonstrating its inherent abhorrency. Suicide commonly occurs among those who have taken too much trouble over the happiness of life. For if someone has tasted the refinements of pleasure, and cannot always possess them, he falls into grief, worry and depression.

THE MORALITY AND RATIONALITY OF SUICIDE
R. B. Brandt

Operating on the assumption that suicide is to be understood as the intentional termination of one's own life, Brandt sets himself firmly against the view that suicide is always immoral. He critically analyzes, and finds wanting, various classes of arguments that have been advanced to support the alleged immorality of suicide: (1) theological arguments, (2) arguments from natural law, and (3) arguments to the effect that suicide necessarily harms other persons or society in general. Brandt does acknowledge that there is some obligation to refrain from committing suicide when that act would be injurious to others, but he insists that this obligation may often be overridden by other morally relevant considerations. Clearly, for Brandt, suicide is sometimes morally acceptable. He also insists that a person's decision to commit suicide may be quite rational, although he is careful to warn of potential errors in judgment. He concludes by analyzing the various factors that are relevant in establishing the moral obligation of other persons toward those who are contemplating suicide.

THE MORAL REASONS FOR AND AGAINST SUICIDE

[Assuming that there is suicide if and only if there is intentional termination of one's own life,] persons who say suicide is morally wrong must be asked which of two positions they are affirming: Are they saying that *every* act of suicide is wrong, *everything considered;* or are they merely saying that there is always *some* moral obligation—doubtless of serious weight—not to commit suicide, so that very often suicide is wrong, although it is possible that there are *countervailing considerations* which in particular situations make it right or even a moral duty? It is quite evident that the first position is absurd; only the second has a chance of being defensible.

In order to make clear what is wrong with the first view, we may begin with an example. Suppose an army pilot's single-seater plane goes out of control over a heavily populated area; he has the choice of staying in the plane and bringing it down where it will do little damage but at the cost of certain death for himself, and of bailing out and letting the plane fall where it will, very possibly killing a good many civilians. Suppose he chooses to do the former, and so, by our definition, commits suicide. Does anyone want to say that his action is morally wrong? Even Immanuel Kant, who opposed suicide in all circumstances, apparently would not wish to say that it is; he would, in fact, judge that this act is not one of suicide, for he says, "It is no suicide to risk one's life against one's enemies, and even to sacrifice it, in

order to preserve one's duties toward oneself."[1] St. Thomas Aquinas, in his discussion of suicide, may seem to take the position that such an act would be wrong, for he says, "It is altogether unlawful to kill oneself," admitting as an exception only the case of being under special command of God. But I believe St. Thomas would, in fact, have concluded that the act is right because the basic intention of the pilot was to save the lives of civilians, and whether an act is right or wrong is a matter of basic intention.[2]

In general, we have to admit that there are things with some moral obligation to avoid which, on account of other morally relevant considerations, it is sometimes right or even morally obligatory to do. There may be some obligation to tell the truth on every occasion, but surely in many cases the consequences of telling the truth would be so dire that one is obligated to lie. The same goes for promises. There is some moral obligation to do what one has promised (with a few exceptions); but, if one can keep a trivial promise only at serious cost to another person (i.e., keep an appointment only by failing to give aid to someone injured in an accident), it is surely obligatory to break the promise.

The most that the moral critic of suicide could hold, then, is that there is *some* moral obligation not to do what one knows will cause one's death; but he surely cannot deny that circumstances exist in which there are obligations to do things which, in fact, will result in one's death. If so, then in principle it would be possible to argue, for instance, that in order to meet my obligation to my family, it might be right for me to take my own life as the only way to avoid catastrophic hospital expenses in a terminal illness. Possibly the main point that critics of suicide on moral grounds would wish to make is that it is never right to take one's own life *for reasons of one's own personal welfare,* of any kind whatsoever. Some of the arguments used to support the immorality of suicide, however, are so framed that if they were supportable at all, they would prove that suicide is *never* moral.

One well-known type of argument against suicide may be classified as *theological.* St. Augustine and others urged that the Sixth Commandment ("Thou shalt not kill") prohibits suicide, and that we are bound to obey a divine commandment. To this reasoning one might first reply that it is arbitrary exegesis of the Sixth Commandment to assert that it was intended to prohibit suicide. The second reply is that if there is not some consideration which shows on the merits of the case that suicide is morally wrong, God had no business prohibiting it. It is true that some will object to this point, and I must refer them elsewhere for my detailed comments on the divine-will theory of morality.[3]

Another theological argument with wide support was accepted by John Locke, who wrote: ". . . Men being all the workmanship of one omnipotent and infinitely wise Maker; all the servants of one sovereign Master, sent into the world by His order and about His business; they are His property, whose workmanship they are made to last during His, not one another's pleasure . . . Every one . . . is bound to preserve himself, and not to quit his station wilfully. . . ."[4] And Kant: "We have been placed in this world under certain conditions and for specific purposes. But a suicide opposes the purpose of his Creator; he arrives in the other world as one who has deserted his post; he must be looked upon as a rebel against God. So long as we remember the truth that it is God's intention to preserve life, we are bound to regulate our activities in conformity with it. This duty is upon us until the time comes when God expressly commands us to leave this life. Human beings are sentinels on earth and may not leave their posts until relieved by another beneficent hand."[5] Unfortunately, however, even if we grant that it is the duty of human beings to do what God commands or intends them to do, more argument is required to show that God does *not* permit human beings to quit this life when their own personal welfare would be maximized by so doing. How does one draw the

requisite inference about the intentions of God? The difficulties and contradictions in arguments to reach such a conclusion are discussed at length and perspicaciously by David Hume in his essay "On Suicide," and in view of the unlikelihood that readers will need to be persuaded about these, I shall merely refer those interested to that essay.[6]

A second group of arguments may be classed as arguments *from natural law.* St. Thomas says: "It is altogether unlawful to kill oneself, for three reasons. First, because everything naturally loves itself, the result being that everything naturally keeps itself in being, and resists corruptions so far as it can. Wherefore suicide is contrary to the inclination of nature, and to charity whereby every man should love himself. Hence suicide is always a mortal sin, as being contrary to the natural law and to charity."[7] Here St. Thomas ignores two obvious points. First, it is not obvious why a human being is morally bound to do what he or she has some inclination to do. (St. Thomas did not criticize chastity.) Second, while it is true that most human beings do feel a strong urge to live, the human being who commits suicide obviously feels a stronger inclination to do something else. It is as natural for a human being to dislike, and to take steps to avoid, say, great pain, as it is to cling to life.

A somewhat similar argument by Immanuel Kant may seem better. In a famous passage Kant writes that the maxim of a person who commits suicide is "From self-love I make it my principle to shorten my life if its continuance threatens more evil than it promises pleasure. The only further question to ask is whether this principle of self-love can become a universal law of nature. It is then seen at once that a system of nature by whose law the very same feeling whose function is to stimulate the furtherance of life should actually destroy life would contradict itself and consequently could not subsist as a system of nature. Hence this maxim cannot possibly hold as a universal law of nature and is therefore entirely opposed to the supreme principle of all duty."[8] What Kant finds contradictory is that the motive of self-love (interest in one's own long-range welfare) should sometimes lead one to struggle to preserve one's life, but at other times to end it. But where is the contradiction? One's circumstances change, and, if the argument of the following section in this [paper] is correct, one sometimes maximizes one's own long-range welfare by trying to stay alive, but at other times by bringing about one's demise.

A third group of arguments, a form of which goes back at least to Aristotle, has a more modern and convincing ring. These are arguments to show that, in one way or another, a suicide necessarily does harm to other persons, or to society at large. Aristotle says that the suicide treats the *state* unjustly.[9] Partly following Aristotle, St. Thomas says: "Every man is part of the community, and so, as such, he belongs to the community. Hence by killing himself he injures the community."[10] Blackstone held that a suicide is an offense against the king "who hath an interest in the preservation of all his subjects," perhaps following Judge Brown in 1563, who argued that suicide cost the king a subject—"he being the head has lost one of his mystical members."[11] The premise of such arguments is, as Hume pointed out, obviously mistaken in many instances. It is true that Freud would perhaps have injured society had he, instead of finishing his last book, committed suicide to escape the pain of throat cancer. But surely there have been many suicides whose demise was not a noticeable loss to society; an honest man could only say that in some instances society was better off without them.

It need not be denied that suicide is often injurious to other persons, especially the family of a suicide. Clearly it sometimes is. But, we should notice what this fact establishes. Suppose we admit, as generally would be done, that there is some obligation not to perform any action which will probably or certainly be injurious to other people, the strength of the obligation being dependent on various factors, notably the seriousness of the expected injury. Then there is *some* obligation not to commit suicide, when that act would probably or certainly be injurious to other people. But, as we have already seen, many cases of *some* obligation to do something nevertheless are *not* cases of a duty to do that thing, *everything considered.* So it could sometimes be morally justified to commit suicide, even if the act will harm someone. Must a man with a terminal illness undergo excruciating pain because his death will cause his wife sorrow—when she will be caused sorrow a

month later anyway, when he is dead of natural causes? Moreover, to repeat, the fact that an individual has some obligation not to commit suicide when that act will probably injure other persons does not imply that, everything considered, it is wrong for him to do it, namely, that in all circumstances suicide *as such* is something there is some obligation to avoid.

Is there any sound argument, convincing to the modern mind, to establish that there is (or is not) *some moral obligation* to avoid suicide *as such,* an obligation, of course, which might be overridden by other obligations in some or many cases? (Captain Oates may have had a moral obligation not to commit suicide as such, but his obligation not to stand in the way of his comrades getting to safety might have been so strong that, everything considered, he was justified in leaving the polar camp and allowing himself to freeze to death.)

To present all the arguments necessary to answer this question convincingly would take a great deal of space. I shall, therefore, simply state one answer to it which seems plausible to some contemporary philosophers. Suppose it could be shown that it would maximize the long-run welfare of everybody affected if people were taught that there is a moral obligation to avoid suicide—so that people would be motivated to avoid suicide just because they thought it wrong (would have anticipatory guilt feelings at the very idea), and so that other people would be inclined to disapprove of persons who commit suicide unless there were some excuse. . . . One might ask: how could it maximize utility to mold the conceptual and motivational structure of persons in this way? To which the answer might be: feeling in this way might make persons who are impulsively inclined to commit suicide in a bad mood, or a fit of anger or jealousy, take more time to deliberate; hence, some suicides that have bad effects generally might be prevented. In other words, it might be a good thing in its effects for people to feel about suicide in the way they feel about breach of promise or injuring others, just as it might be a good thing for people to feel a moral obligation not to smoke, or to wear seat belts. However, it might be that negative moral feelings about suicide as such would stand in the way of action by those persons whose welfare really is best served by suicide and whose suicide is the best thing for everybody concerned.

WHEN A DECISION TO COMMIT SUICIDE IS RATIONAL FROM THE PERSON'S POINT OF VIEW

The person who is contemplating suicide is obviously making a choice between future world-courses; the world-course that includes his demise, say, an hour from now, and several possible ones that contain his demise at a later point. One cannot have precise knowledge about many features of the latter group of world-courses, but it is certain that they will all end with death some (possibly short) finite time from now.

Why do I say the choice is between *world-courses* and not just a choice between future life-courses of the prospective suicide, the one shorter than the other? The reason is that one's suicide has some impact on the world (and one's continued life has some impact on the world), and that conditions in the rest of the world will often make a difference in one's evaluation of the possibilities. One *is* interested in things in the world other than just oneself and one's own happiness.

The basic question a person must answer, in order to determine which world-course is best or rational for him to choose, is which he *would* choose under conditions of optimal use of information, when *all* of his desires are taken into account. It is not just a question of what we prefer *now,* with some clarification of all the possibilities being considered. Our preferences change, and the preferences of to-morrow (assuming we can know something about them) are just as legitimately taken into account in deciding what to do now as the preferences of today. Since any reason that can be given today for weighting heavily today's preference can be given tomorrow for weighting heavily tomorrow's preference, the preferences of any time-stretch have a rational claim to an equal vote. Now the importance of that fact is this: we often know quite well that our desires, aversions, and preferences may change after a short while. When a person is in a state of despair—perhaps brought about by a rejection in love or discharge from a long-held position—nothing but the thing he cannot have seems desirable; everything else is turned to ashes. Yet we know quite well that the passage of time is likely to reverse all this; replacements may be found or other types of things that are available to us may begin to look attractive. So, if we were to act on the preferences of today alone, when the emotion of despair seems more than we can stand, we might find death preferable to life; but, if we allow for the preferences of the weeks and years ahead, when many goals will be enjoyable and attractive, we might find life much preferable to death. So, if a choice of what is best is to be determined by what we want not only now but later (and later desires on an equal basis with the present ones)—as it should be—then what is the best or preferable world-course will often be quite different from what it would be if the choice, or what is best for one, were fixed by one's desires and preferences now.

Of course, if one commits suicide there are no future desires or aversions that may be compared with present ones and that should be allowed an equal vote in deciding what is best. In that respect the course of action that results in death is different from any other course of action we may undertake. I do not wish to suggest the rosy possibility that it is often or always reasonable to believe that next week "I shall be more interested in living than I am today, if today I take a dim view of continued existence." On the contrary, when a person is seriously ill, for instance, he may have no reason to think that the preference-order will be reversed—it may be that tomorrow he will prefer death to life more strongly.

The argument is often used that one can never be *certain* what is going to happen, and hence one is never rationally justified in doing anything as drastic as committing suicide. But we always have to live by probabilities and make our estimates as best we can. As soon as it is clear beyond reasonable doubt not only that death is now preferable to life, but also that it will be every day from now until the end, the rational thing is to act promptly.

Let us not pursue the question of whether it is rational for a person with a painful terminal illness to commit suicide; it is. However, the issue seldom arises, and few terminally ill patients do commit suicide. With such patients matters usually get worse slowly so that no particular time seems to call for action. They are often so heavily sedated that it is impossible for the mental processes of decision leading to action to occur; or else they are incapacitated in a hospital and the very physical possibility of ending their lives is not available. Let us leave this grim topic and turn to a practically more important problem: whether it is rational for persons to commit suicide for some reason other than painful terminal physical illness. Most persons who commit suicide do so, apparently, because they face a nonphysical problem that depresses them beyond their ability to bear.

Among the problems that have been regarded as good and sufficient reasons for ending life, we find (in addition to serious illness) the following: some event that has made a person feel ashamed or lose his prestige and status; reduction from affluence to poverty; the loss of a limb or of physical beauty; the loss of sexual capacity; some event that makes it seem impossible to achieve things by which one sets store; loss of a loved one; disappointment in love; the infirmities of increasing age. It is not to be denied that such things can be serious blows to a person's prospects of happiness.

Whatever the nature of an individual's problem, there are various plain errors to be avoided—errors to which a person is especially prone when he is depressed—in deciding whether, everything considered, he prefers a world-course containing his early demise to one in which his life continues to its natural terminus. Let us forget for a moment the relevance to the decision of preferences that he may have tomorrow, and concentrate on some errors that may infect his preference as of today, and for which correction or allowance must be made.

In the first place, depression, like any severe emotional experience, tends to primitivize one's intellectual processes. It restricts the range of one's survey of the possibilities. One thing that a rational person would do is compare the world-course containing his suicide with his *best* alternative. But his best alternative is precisely a possibility he may overlook if, in a depressed mood, he thinks only of how badly off he is and cannot imagine any way of improving his situation. If a person is disappointed in love, it is possible to adopt a vigorous plan of action that carries a good chance of acquainting him with someone he likes at least as well; and if old age prevents a person from continuing the tennis game with his favorite partner, it is possible to learn some

other game that provides the joys of competition without the physical demands.

Depression has another insidious influence on one's planning; it seriously affects one's judgment about probabilities. A person disappointed in love is very likely to take a dim view of himself, his prospects, and his attractiveness; he thinks that because he has been rejected by one person he will probably be rejected by anyone who looks desirable to him. In a less gloomy frame of mind he would make different estimates. Part of the reason for such gloomy probability estimates is that depression tends to repress one's memory of evidence that supports a nongloomy prediction. Thus, a rejected lover tends to forget any cases in which he has elicited enthusiastic response from ladies in relation to whom he has been the one who has done the rejecting. Thus his pessimistic self-image is based upon a highly selected, and pessimistically selected, set of data. Even when he is reminded of the data, moreover, he is apt to resist an optimistic inference.

Another kind of distortion of the look of future prospects is not a result of depression, but is quite normal. Events distant in the future feel small, just as objects distant in space look small. Their prospect does not have the effect on motivational processes that it would have if it were of an event in the immediate future. Psychologists call this the "goal-gradient" phenomenon; a rat, for instance, will run faster toward a perceived food box than a distant unseen one. In the case of a person who has suffered some misfortune, and whose situation now is an unpleasant one, this reduction of the motivational influence of events distant in time has the effect that present unpleasant states weigh far more heavily than probable future pleasant ones in any choice of world-courses.

If we are trying to determine whether we now prefer, or shall later prefer, the outcome of one world-course to that of another (and this is leaving aside the questions of the weight of the votes of preferences at a later date), we must take into account these and other infirmities of our "sensing" machinery. Since knowing that the machinery is out of order will not tell us what results it would give if it were working, the best recourse might be to refrain from making any decision in a stressful frame of mind. If decisions have to be made, one must recall past reactions, in a normal frame of mind, to outcomes like those under assessment. But many suicides seem to occur in moments of despair. What should be clear from the above is that a moment of despair, if one is seriously contemplating suicide, ought to be a moment of reassessment of one's goals and values, a reassessment which the individual must realize is very difficult to make objectively, because of the very quality of his depressed frame of mind.

A decision to commit suicide may in certain circumstances be a rational one. But a person who wants to act rationally must take into account the various possible "errors" and make appropriate rectification of his initial evaluations.

THE ROLE OF OTHER PERSONS

What is the moral obligation of other persons toward those who are contemplating suicide? The question of their moral blameworthiness may be ignored and what is rational for them to do from the point of view of personal welfare may be considered as being of secondary concern. Laws make it dangerous to aid or encourage a suicide. The risk of running afoul of the law may partly determine moral obligation, since moral obligation to do something may be reduced by the fact that it is personally dangerous.

The moral obligation of other persons toward one who is contemplating suicide is an instance of a general obligation to render aid to those in serious distress, at least when this can be done at no great cost to one's self. I do not think this general principle is seriously questioned by anyone, whatever his moral theory; so I feel free to assume it as a premise. Obviously the person contemplating suicide is in great distress of some sort; if he were not, he would not be seriously considering terminating his life.

How great a person's obligation is to one in distress depends on a number of factors. Obviously family and friends have special obligations to devote time to helping the prospective suicide—which others do not have. But anyone in this kind of distress has a moral claim on the time of any person who knows the situation (unless there are others more responsible who are already doing what should be done).

What is the obligation? It depends, of course, on the situation, and how much the second person knows about the situation. If the individual has

decided to terminate his life if he can, and it is clear that he is right in this decision, then, if he needs help in executing the decision, there is a moral obligation to give him help. On this matter a patient's physician has a special obligation, from which any talk about the Hippocratic oath does not absolve him. It is true that there are some damages one cannot be expected to absorb, and some risks which one cannot be expected to take, on account of the obligation to render aid.

On the other hand, if it is clear that the individual should not commit suicide, from the point of view of his own welfare, or if there is a presumption that he should not (when the only evidence is that a person is discovered unconscious, with the gas turned on), it would seem to be the individual's obligation to intervene, prevent the successful execution of the decision, and see to the availability of competent psychiatric advice and temporary hospitalization, if necessary. Whether one has a right to take such steps when a clearly sane person, after careful reflection over a period of time, comes to the conclusion that an end to his life is what is best for him and what he wants, is very doubtful, even when one thinks his conclusion a mistaken one; it would seem that a man's own considered decision about whether he wants to live must command respect, although one must concede that this could be debated.

The more interesting role in which a person may be cast, however, is that of adviser. It is often important to one who is contemplating suicide to go over his thinking with another, and to feel that a conclusion, one way or the other, has the support of a respected mind. One thing one can obviously do, in rendering the service of advice, is to discuss with the person the various types of issues discussed above, made more specific by the concrete circumstances of his case, and help him find whether, in view, say, of the damage his suicide would do to others, he has a moral obligation to refrain, and whether it is rational or best for him, from the point of view of his own welfare, to take this step or adopt some other plan instead.

To get a person to see what is the rational thing to do is no small job. Even to get a person, in a frame of mind when he is seriously contemplating (or perhaps has already unsuccessfully attempted) suicide, to recognize a plain truth of fact may be a major operation. If a man insists, "I am a complete failure," when it is obvious that by any reasonable standard he is far from that, it may be tremendously difficult to get him to see the fact. But there is another job beyond that of getting a person to see what is the rational thing to do; that is to help him *act* rationally, or *be* rational, when he has conceded what would be the rational thing.

How either of these tasks may be accomplished effectively may be discussed more competently by an experienced psychiatrist than by a philosopher. Loneliness and the absence of human affection are states which exacerbate any other problems; disappointment, reduction to poverty, and so forth, seem less impossible to bear in the presence of the affection of another. Hence simply to be a friend, or to find someone a friend, may be the largest contribution one can make either to helping a person be rational or see clearly what is rational for him to do; this service may make one who was contemplating suicide feel that there is a future for him which it is possible to face.

NOTES

1 Immanuel Kant, *Lectures on Ethics,* New York: Harper Torchbook (1963), p. 150.

2 See St. Thomas Aquinas, *Summa Theologica,* Second Part of the Second Part, Q. 64, Art. 5. In Article 7, he says: "Nothing hinders one act from having two effects, only one of which is intended, while the other is beside the intention. Now moral acts take their species according to what is intended, and not according to what is beside the intention, since this is accidental as explained above" (Q. 43, Art. 3: I–II, Q. 1, Art. 3, as 3). Mr. Norman St. John-Stevas, the most articulate contemporary defender of the Catholic view, writes as

follows: "Christian thought allows certain exceptions to its general condemnation of suicide. That covered by a particular divine inspiration has already been noted. Another exception arises where suicide is the method imposed by the state for the execution of a just death penalty. A third exception is *altruistic* suicide, of which the best known example is Captain Oates. Such suicides are justified by invoking the principles of double effect. The act from which death results must be good or at least morally indifferent; some other good effect must result: The death must not be directly intended or the real means to the good effect, and a grave reason must exist for adopting the course of action" [*Life, Death and the Law,* Bloomington, Ind.: Indiana University Press (1961), pp. 250–51]. Presumably the Catholic doctrine is intended to allow suicide when this is required for meeting strong moral obligations; whether it can do so consistently depends partly on the interpretation given to "real means to the good effect." Readers interested in pursuing further the Catholic doctrine of double effect and its implications for our problem should read Philippa Foot, "The Problem of Abortion and the Doctrine of Double Effect," *The Oxford Review,* 5:5–15 (Trinity 1967).

3 R. B. Brandt, *Ethical Theory,* Englewood Cliffs, N.J.: Prentice-Hall (1959), pp. 61–82.

4 John Locke, *Two Treatises of Government,* Ch. 2.

5 Kant, *Lectures on Ethics,* p. 154.

6 This essay appears in collections of Hume's works.

7 For an argument similar to Kant's, see also St. Thomas Aquinas, *Summa Theologica,* II, II, Q. 64, Art. 5.

8 Immanuel Kant, *The Fundamental Principles of the Metaphysic of Morals,* trans. H. J. Paton, London: The Hutchinson Group (1948), Ch. 2.

9 Aristotle, *Nicomachaean Ethics,* Bk. 5, Ch. 10, p. 1138a.

10 St. Thomas Aquinas, *Summa Theologica,* II, II, Q. 64, Art. 5.

11 Sir William Blackstone, *Commentaries,* 4:189; Brown in *Hales v. Petit,* I Plow. 253, 75 E.R. 387 (C. B. 1563). Both cited by Norman St. John-Stevas, *Life, Death and the Law,* p. 235.

THE MORALITY OF ACTIVE EUTHANASIA

ACTIVE AND PASSIVE EUTHANASIA
James Rachels

In this classic article, Rachels identifies the "conventional doctrine" on the morality of euthanasia as the doctrine that allows passive euthanasia but does not allow active euthanasia. He then argues that the conventional doctrine may be challenged for four reasons. First, active euthanasia is in many cases more humane than passive euthanasia. Second, the conventional doctrine leads to decisions concerning life and death on irrelevant grounds. Third, the doctrine rests on a distinction between killing and letting die that itself has no moral importance. Fourth, the most common argument in favor of the doctrine is invalid.

The distinction between active and passive euthanasia is thought to be crucial for medical ethics. The idea is that it is permissible, at least in some cases, to withhold treatment and allow a patient to die, but it is never permissible to take any direct action designed to kill the patient. This doctrine seems to be accepted by most doctors, and it is endorsed in a statement adopted by the House of Delegates of the American Medical Association on December 4, 1973:

> The intentional termination of the life of one human being by another—mercy killing—is contrary to that for which the medical profession stands and is contrary to the policy of the American Medical Association.
>
> The cessation of the employment of extraordinary means to prolong the life of the body when there is irrefutable evidence that biological death is imminent is the decision of the patient and/or his immediate family. The advice and judgment of the physician should be freely available to the patient and/or his immediate family.

However, a strong case can be made against this doctrine. In what follows I will set out some of the relevant arguments, and urge doctors to reconsider their views on this matter.

To begin with a familiar type of situation, a patient who is dying of incurable cancer of the throat is in terrible pain, which can no longer be satisfactorily alleviated. He is certain to die within a few days, even if present treatment is continued, but he does not want to go on living for those days since the pain is unbearable. So he asks the doctor for an end to it, and his family joins in the request.

Suppose the doctor agrees to withhold treatment, as the conventional doctrine says he may. The justification for his doing so is that the patient is in terrible agony, and since he is going to die anyway, it would be wrong to prolong his suffering needlessly. But now notice this. If one simply withholds treatment, it may take the patient longer to die, and so he may suffer more than he would if more direct action were taken and a lethal injection given. This fact

provides strong reason for thinking that, once the initial decision not to prolong his agony has been made, active euthanasia is actually preferable to passive euthanasia, rather than the reverse. To say otherwise is to endorse the option that leads to more suffering rather than less, and is contrary to the humanitarian impulse that prompts the decision not to prolong his life in the first place.

Part of my point is that the process of being "allowed to die" can be relatively slow and painful, whereas being given a lethal injection is relatively quick and painless. Let me give a different sort of example. In the United States about one in 600 babies is born with Down's syndrome. Most of these babies are otherwise healthy—that is, with only the usual pediatric care, they will proceed to an otherwise normal infancy. Some, however, are born with congenital defects such as intestinal obstructions that require operations if they are to live. Sometimes, the parents and the doctor will decide not to operate, and let the infant die. Anthony Shaw describes what happens then:

> . . . When surgery is denied [the doctor] must try to keep the infant from suffering while natural forces sap the baby's life away. As a surgeon whose natural inclination is to use the scalpel to fight off death, standing by and watching a salvageable baby die is the most emotionally exhausting experience I know. It is easy at a conference, in a theoretical discussion, to decide that such infants should be allowed to die. It is altogether different to stand by in the nursery and watch as dehydration and infection wither a tiny being over hours and days. This is a terrible ordeal for me and the hospital staff—much more so than for the parents who never set foot in the nursery.[1]

I can understand why some people are opposed to all euthanasia, and insist that such infants must be allowed to live. I think I can also understand why other people favor destroying these babies quickly and painlessly. But why should anyone favor letting "dehydration and infection wither a tiny being over hours and days"? The doctrine that says that a baby may be allowed to dehydrate and wither, but may not be given an injection that would end its life without suffering, seems so patently cruel as to require no further refutation. The strong language is not

Reprinted by permission from the *New England Journal of Medicine,* vol. 292, no. 2 (January 9, 1975), pp. 78–80.

intended to offend, but only to put the point in the clearest possible way.

My second argument is that the conventional doctrine leads to decisions concerning life and death made on irrelevant grounds.

Consider again the case of the infants with Down's syndrome who need operations for congenital defects unrelated to the syndrome to live. Sometimes, there is no operation, and the baby dies, but when there is no such defect, the baby lives on. Now, an operation such as that to remove an intestinal obstruction is not prohibitively difficult. The reason why such operations are not performed in these cases is, clearly, that the child has Down's syndrome and the parents and doctor judge that because of that fact it is better for the child to die.

But notice that this situation is absurd, no matter what view one takes of the lives and potentials of such babies. If the life of such an infant is worth preserving, what does it matter if it needs a simple operation? Or, if one thinks it better that such a baby should not live on, what difference does it make that it happens to have an unobstructed intestinal tract? In either case, the matter of life and death is being decided on irrelevant grounds. It is the Down's syndrome, and not the intestines, that is the issue. The matter should be decided, if at all, on that basis, and not be allowed to depend on the essentially irrelevant question of whether the intestinal tract is blocked.

What makes this situation possible, of course, is the idea that when there is an intestinal blockage, one can "let the baby die," but when there is no such defect there is nothing that can be done, for one must not "kill" it. The fact that this idea leads to such results as deciding life or death on irrelevant grounds is another good reason why the doctrine should be rejected.

One reason why so many people think that there is an important moral difference between active and passive euthanasia is that they think killing someone is morally worse than letting someone die. But is it? Is killing, in itself, worse than letting die? To investigate this issue, two cases may be considered that are exactly alike except that one involves killing whereas the other involves letting someone die. Then, it can be asked whether this difference makes any difference to the moral assessments. It is impor-

tant that the cases be exactly alike, except for this one difference, since otherwise one cannot be confident that it is this difference and not some other that accounts for any variation in the assessments of the two cases. So, let us consider this pair of cases:

In the first, Smith stands to gain a large inheritance if anything should happen to his six-year-old cousin. One evening while the child is taking his bath, Smith sneaks into the bathroom and drowns the child, and then arranges things so that it will look like an accident.

In the second, Jones also stands to gain if anything should happen to his six-year-old cousin. Like Smith, Jones sneaks in planning to drown the child in his bath. However, just as he enters the bathroom Jones sees the child slip and hit his head, and fall face down in the water. Jones is delighted; he stands by, ready to push the child's head back under if it is necessary, but it is not necessary. With only a little thrashing about, the child drowns all by himself, "accidentally," as Jones watches and does nothing.

Now Smith killed the child, whereas Jones "merely" let the child die. That is the only difference between them. Did either man behave better, from a moral point of view? If the difference between killing and letting die were in itself a morally important matter, one should say that Jones's behavior was less reprehensible than Smith's. But does one really want to say that? I think not. In the first place, both men acted from the same motive, personal gain, and both had exactly the same end in view when they acted. It may be inferred from Smith's conduct that he is a bad man, although that judgment may be withdrawn or modified if certain further facts are learned about him—for example, that he is mentally deranged. But would not the very same thing be inferred about Jones from his conduct? And would not the same further considerations also be relevant to any modification of this judgment? Moreover, suppose Jones pleaded, in his own defense, "After all, I didn't do anything except just stand there and watch the child drown. I didn't kill him; I only let him die." Again, if letting die were in itself less bad than killing, this defense should have at least some weight. But it does not. Such a "defense" can only be regarded as a grotesque perversion of moral reasoning. Morally speaking, it is no defense at all.

Now, it may be pointed out, quite properly, that the cases of euthanasia with which doctors are concerned are not like this at all. They do not involve personal gain or the destruction of normal, healthy children. Doctors are concerned only with cases in which the patient's life is of no further use to him, or in which the patient's life has become or will soon become a terrible burden. However, the point is the same in these cases: the bare difference between killing and letting die does not, in itself, make a moral difference. If a doctor lets a patient die, for humane reasons, he is in the same moral position as if he had given the patient a lethal injection for humane reasons. If his decision was wrong—if, for example, the patient's illness was in fact curable—the decision would be equally regrettable no matter which method was used to carry it out. And if the doctor's decision was the right one, the method used is not in itself important.

The AMA policy statement isolates the crucial issue very well; the crucial issue is "the intentional termination of the life of one human being by another." But after identifying this issue, and forbidding "mercy killing," the statement goes on to deny that the cessation of treatment is the intentional termination of life. This is where the mistake comes in, for what is the cessation of treatment, in these circumstances, if it is not "the intentional termination of the life of one human being by another"? Of course it is exactly that, and if it were not, there would be no point to it.

Many people will find this judgment hard to accept. One reason, I think, is that it is very easy to conflate the question of whether killing is, in itself, worse than letting die, with the very different question of whether most actual cases of killing are more reprehensible than most actual cases of letting die. Most actual cases of killing are clearly terrible (think, for example, of all the murders reported in the newspapers), and one hears of such cases every day. On the other hand, one hardly ever hears of a case of letting die, except for the actions of doctors who are motivated by humanitarian reasons. So one learns to think of killing in a much worse light than of letting die. But this does not mean that there is something about killing that makes it in itself worse than letting die, for it is not the bare difference between killing and letting die that makes the difference in

these cases. Rather, the other factors—the murderer's motive of personal gain, for example, contrasted with the doctor's humanitarian motivation—account for different reactions to the different cases.

I have argued that killing is not in itself any worse than letting die; if my contention is right, it follows that active euthanasia is not any worse than passive euthanasia. What arguments can be given on the other side? The most common, I believe, is the following:

> The important difference between active and passive euthanasia is that, in passive euthanasia, the doctor does not do anything to bring about the patient's death. The doctor does nothing, and the patient dies of whatever ills already afflict him. In active euthanasia, however, the doctor does something to bring about the patient's death: he kills him. The doctor who gives the patient with cancer a lethal injection has himself caused his patient's death; whereas if he merely ceases treatment, the cancer is the cause of the death.

A number of points need to be made here. The first is that it is not exactly correct to say that in passive euthanasia the doctor does nothing, for he does do one thing that is very important: he lets the patient die. "Letting someone die" is certainly different, in some respects, from other types of action—mainly in that it is a kind of action that one may perform by way of not performing certain other actions. For example, one may let a patient die by way of not giving medication, just as one may insult someone by way of not shaking his hand. But for any purpose of moral assessment, it is a type of action nonetheless. The decision to let a patient die is subject to moral appraisal in the same way that a decision to kill him would be subject to moral appraisal: it may be assessed as wise or unwise, compassionate or sadistic, right or wrong. If a doctor deliberately let a patient die who was suffering from a routinely curable illness, the doctor would certainly be to blame for what he had done, just as he would be to blame if he had needlessly killed the patient. Charges against him would then be appropriate. If so, it would be no defense at all for him to insist that he didn't "do anything." He would have done something very serious indeed, for he let his patient die.

Fixing the cause of death may be very important from a legal point of view, for it may determine whether criminal charges are brought against the doctor. But I do not think that this notion can be used to show a moral difference between active and passive euthanasia. The reason why it is considered bad to be the cause of someone's death is that death is regarded as a great evil—and so it is. However, if it has been decided that euthanasia—even passive euthanasia—is desirable in a given case, it has also been decided that in this instance death is no greater an evil than the patient's continued existence. And if this is true, the usual reason for not wanting to be the cause of someone's death simply does not apply.

Finally, doctors may think that all of this is only of academic interest—the sort of thing that philosophers may worry about but that has no practical bearing on their own work. After all, doctors must be concerned about the legal consequences of what they do, and active euthanasia is clearly forbidden by the law. But even so, doctors should also be concerned with the fact that the law is forcing upon them a moral doctrine that may well be indefensible, and has a considerable effect on their practices. Of course, most doctors are not now in the position of being coerced in this matter, for they do not regard themselves as merely going along with what the law requires. Rather, in statements such as the AMA policy statement that I have quoted, they are endorsing this doctrine as a central point of medical ethics. In that statement, active euthanasia is condemned not merely as illegal but as "contrary to that for which the medical profession stands," whereas passive euthanasia is approved. However, the preceding considerations suggest that there is really no moral difference between the two, considered in themselves (there may be important moral differences in some cases in their *consequences,* but, as I pointed out, these differences may make active euthanasia, and not passive euthanasia, the morally preferable option). So, whereas doctors may have to discriminate between active and passive euthanasia to satisfy the law, they should not do any more than that. In particular, they should not give the distinction any added authority and weight by writing it into official statements of medical ethics.

NOTE

1 Shaw A.: "Doctor, Do We Have a Choice?" *The New York Times Magazine,* January 30, 1972, p. 54.

KILLING AND ALLOWING TO DIE
Daniel Callahan

Callahan maintains that there is a valid distinction between killing and allowing to die, and he defends the distinction by reference to three overlapping perspectives— metaphysical, moral, and medical. In terms of a metaphysical perspective, Callahan emphasizes that the external world is distinct from the self and has its own causal dynamism. In terms of a moral perspective, he emphasizes the difference between *physical causality* and *moral culpability.* In conjunction with a medical perspective, he insists that killing patients is incompatible with the role of the physician in society.

. . . No valid distinction, many now argue, can be made between killing and allowing to die, or between an act of commission and one of omission. The standard distinction being challenged rests on the commonplace observation that lives can come to an end as the result of: (a) the direct action of another who becomes the cause of death (as in shooting a person), and (b) the result of impersonal forces

Reprinted with permission of the author and the publisher from *Hastings Center Report,* vol. 19 (January/February 1989), Special Supplement, pp. 5–6. © The Hastings Center.

where no human agent has acted (death by lightning, or by disease). The purpose of the distinction has been to separate those deaths caused by human action, and those caused by nonhuman events. It is, as a distinction, meant to say something about human beings and their relationship to the world. It is a way of articulating the difference between those actions for which human beings can be held rightly responsible, or blamed, and those of which they are innocent. At issue is the difference between physical causality, the realm of impersonal events, and moral culpability, the realm of human responsibility.

The challenges encompass two points. The first is that people can become equally dead by our omissions as well as our commissions. We can refrain from saving them when it is possible to do so, and they will be just as dead as if we shot them. It is our decision itself that is the reason for their death, not necessarily how we effectuate that decision. That fact establishes the basis of the second point: if we *intend* their death, it can be brought about as well by omitted acts as by those we commit. The crucial moral point is not how they die, but our intention about their death. We can, then, be responsible for the death of another by intending that they die and accomplish that end by standing aside and allowing them to die.

Despite these criticisms—resting upon ambiguities that can readily be acknowledged—the distinction between killing and allowing to die remains, I contend, perfectly valid. It not only has a logical validity but, no less importantly, a social validity whose place must be central in moral judgments. As a way of putting the distinction into perspective, I want to suggest that it is best understood as expressing three different, though overlapping, perspectives on nature and human action. I will call them the metaphysical, the moral, and the medical perspectives.

METAPHYSICAL

The first and most fundamental premise of the distinction between killing and allowing to die is that there is a sharp difference between the self and the external world. Unlike the childish fantasy that the

world is nothing more than a projection of the self, or the neurotic person's fear that he or she is responsible for everything that goes wrong, the distinction is meant to uphold a simple notion: there is a world external to the self that has its own, and independent, causal dynamism. The mistake behind a conflation of killing and allowing to die is to assume that the self has become master of everything within and outside of the self. It is as if the conceit that modern man might ultimately control nature has been internalized: that, if the self might be able to influence nature by its actions, then the self and nature must be one.

Of course that is a fantasy. The fact that we can intervene in nature, and cure or control many diseases, does not erase the difference between the self and the external world. It is as "out there" as ever, even if more under our sway. That sway, however great, is always limited. We can cure disease, but not always the chronic illness that comes with the cure. We can forestall death with modern medicine, but death always wins in the long run because of the innate limitations of the body, inherently and stubbornly beyond final human control. And we can distinguish between a diseased body and an aging body, but in the end if we wait long enough they always become one and the same body. To attempt to deny the distinction between killing and allowing to die is, then, mistakenly to impute more power to human action than it actually has and to accept the conceit that nature has now fallen wholly within the realm of human control. Not so.

MORAL

At the center of the distinction between killing and allowing to die is the difference between physical causality and moral culpability. To bring the life of another to an end by an injection kills the other directly; our action is the physical cause of the death. To allow someone to die from a disease we cannot cure (and that we did not cause) is to permit the disease to act as the cause of death. The notion of physical causality in both cases rests on the difference between human agency and the action of external nature. The ambiguity arises precisely because we can be morally culpable for killing someone (if we have no moral right to do so, as we would in self-defense) and no less culpable for allowing someone to die (if we have both the possibility and the obligation of keeping that person alive). Thus there are cases where, morally speaking, it makes no difference whether we killed or allowed to die; we are equally responsible. In those instances, the lines of physical causality and moral culpability happen to cross. Yet the fact that they can cross in some cases in no way shows that they are always, or even usually, one and the same. We can normally find the difference in all but the most obscure cases. We should not, then, use the ambiguity of such cases to do away altogether with the distinction between killing and allowing to die. The ambiguity may obscure, but does not erase, the line between the two.

There is one group of ambiguous cases that is especially troublesome. Even if we grant the ordinary validity between killing and allowing to die, what about those cases that combine (a) an illness that renders a patient unable to carry out an ordinary biological function (to breathe or eat on his own, for example), and (b) our turning off a respirator or removing an artificial feeding tube? On the level of physical causality, have we killed the patient or allowed him to die? In one sense, it is our action that shortens his life, and yet in another sense his underlying disease brings his life to an end. I believe it reasonable to say that, since his life was being sustained by artificial means (respirator or feeding tube) made necessary because of the fact that he had an incapacitating disease, his disease is the ultimate reality behind his death. But for its reality, there would be no need for artificial sustenance in the first place and no moral issue at all. To lose sight of the paramount reality of the disease is to lose sight of the difference between our selves and the outer world.

I quickly add, and underscore, a moral point: the person who, without good moral reason, turns off a respirator or pulls a feeding tube, can be morally culpable; that the patient has been allowed to die of his underlying condition does not morally excuse him. The moral question is whether we are obliged to continue treating a life that is being artificially sustained. To cease treatment may or may not be morally acceptable; but it should be understood, in either case, that the physical cause of death was the underlying disease.

MEDICAL

An important social purpose of the distinction between killing and allowing to die has been that of protecting the historical role of the physician as one who tries to cure or comfort patients rather than to kill patients. Physicians have been given special knowledge about the body, knowledge that can be used to kill or to cure. They are also given great privileges in making use of that knowledge. It is thus all the more important that physicians' social role and power be, and be seen to be, a limited power. It may be used only to cure or comfort, never to kill. They have not been given, nor should they be given, the power to use their knowledge and skills to bring life to an end. It would open the way for powerful misuse and, no less importantly, represent an intrinsic violation of what it has meant to be a physician.

Yet if it is possible for physicians to misuse their knowledge and power to kill people directly, are they thereby required to use that same knowledge always to keep people alive, always to resist a disease that can itself kill the patient? The traditional answer has been: not necessarily. For the physician's ultimate obligation is to the welfare of the patient, and excessive treatment can be as detrimental to that welfare as inadequate treatment. Put another way, the obligation to resist the lethal power of disease is limited—it ceases when the patient is unwilling to have it resisted, or where the resistance no longer serves the patient's welfare. Behind this moral premise is the recognition that disease (of some kind) ultimately triumphs and that death is both inevitable sooner or later and not, in any case, always the greatest human evil. To demand of the physician that he always struggle against disease, as if it was in his power always to conquer it, would be to fall into the same metaphysical trap mentioned above: that of assuming that no distinction can be drawn between natural and human agency.

A final word. I suggested [in an earlier discussion] that the most potent motive for active euthanasia and assisted suicide stems from a dread of the power of medicine. That power then seems to take on a drive of its own regardless of the welfare or wishes of patients. No one can easily say no—not physicians, not patients, not families. My guess is that happens because too many have already come to believe that it is their choice, and their choice alone, which brings about death; and they do not want to

exercise that kind of authority. The solution is not to erase the distinction between killing and allowing to die, but to underscore its validity and importance. We can bring disease as a cause of death back into the care of the dying.

VOLUNTARY ACTIVE EUTHANASIA
Dan W. Brock

In this excerpt from a much longer article, Brock argues that two fundamental ethical values support the ethical permissibility of voluntary active euthanasia. These values are individual self-determination (autonomy) and individual well-being, the same two values that support the consensus view that patients have a right to make decisions about life-sustaining treatment. Brock also argues that allowing physicians to perform euthanasia is not incompatible with the "moral center" of medicine.

. . . The central ethical argument for [voluntary active] euthanasia is familiar. It is that the very same two fundamental ethical values supporting the consensus on patient's rights to decide about life-sustaining treatment also support the ethical permissibility of euthanasia. These values are individual self-determination or autonomy and individual well-being. By self-determination as it bears on euthanasia, I mean people's interest in making important decisions about their lives for themselves according to their own values or conceptions of a good life, and in being left free to act on those decisions. Self-determination is valuable because it permits people to form and live in accordance with their own conception of a good life, at least within the bounds of justice and consistent with others doing so as well. In exercising self-determination people take responsibility for their lives and for the kinds of persons they become. A central aspect of human dignity lies in people's capacity to direct their lives in this way. The value of exercising self-determination presupposes some minimum of decision-making capacities or competence, which thus

limits the scope of euthanasia supported by self-determination; it cannot justifiably be administered, for example, in cases of serious dementia or treatable clinical depression.

Does the value of individual self-determination extend to the time and manner of one's death? Most people are very concerned about the nature of the last stage of their lives. This reflects not just a fear of experiencing substantial suffering when dying, but also a desire to retain dignity and control during this last period of life. Death is today increasingly preceded by a long period of significant physical and mental decline, due in part to the technological interventions of modern medicine. Many people adjust to these disabilities and find meaning and value in new activities and ways. Others find the impairments and burdens in the last stage of their lives at some point sufficiently great to make life no longer worth living. For many patients near death, maintaining the quality of one's life, avoiding great suffering, maintaining one's dignity, and ensuring that others remember us as we wish them to, become of paramount importance and outweigh merely extending one's life. But there is no single, objectively correct answer for everyone as to when, if at all, one's life becomes all things considered a burden and unwanted. If self-determination is a fundamental value, then the great variability among people on

Reprinted with permission of the author and the publisher from *Hastings Center Report,* vol. 22 (March/April 1992), pp. 11, 16. © The Hastings Center.

this question makes it especially important that individuals control the manner, circumstances, and timing of their dying and death.

The other main value that supports euthanasia is individual well-being. It might seem that individual well-being conflicts with a person's self-determination when the person requests euthanasia. Life itself is commonly taken to be a central good for persons, often valued for its own sake, as well as necessary for pursuit of all other goods within a life. But when a competent patient decides to forgo all further life-sustaining treatment then the patient, either explicitly or implicitly, commonly decides that the best life possible for him or her with treatment is of sufficiently poor quality that it is worse than no further life at all. Life is no longer considered a benefit by the patient, but has now become a burden. The same judgment underlies a request for euthanasia: continued life is seen by the patient as no longer a benefit, but now a burden. Especially in the often severely compromised and debilitated states of many critically ill or dying patients, there is no objective standard, but only the competent patient's judgment of whether continued life is no longer a benefit.

Of course, sometimes there are conditions, such as clinical depression, that call into question whether the patient has made a competent choice, either to forgo life-sustaining treatment or to seek euthanasia, and then the patient's choice need not be evidence that continued life is no longer a benefit for him or her. Just as with decisions about treatment, a determination of incompetence can warrant not honoring the patient's choice; in the case of treatment, we then transfer decisional authority to a surrogate, though in the case of voluntary active euthanasia a determination that the patient is incompetent means that choice is not possible.

The value or right of self-determination does not entitle patients to compel physicians to act contrary to their own moral or professional values. Physicians are moral and professional agents whose own self-determination or integrity should be respected as well. If performing euthanasia became legally permissible, but conflicted with a particular physician's reasonable understanding of his or her moral or professional responsibilities, the care of a patient who requested euthanasia should be transferred to another. . . .

. . . Permitting physicians to perform euthanasia, it is said, would be incompatible with their fundamental moral and professional commitment as healers to care for patients and to protect life. Moreover, if euthanasia by physicians became common, patients would come to fear that a medication was intended not to treat or care, but instead to kill, and would thus lose trust in their physicians. This position was forcefully stated in a paper by Willard Gaylin and his colleagues:

> The very soul of medicine is on trial. . . . This issue touches medicine at its moral center; if this moral center collapses, if physicians become killers or are even licensed to kill, the profession—and, therewith, each physician—will never again be worthy of trust and respect as healer and comforter and protector of life in all its frailty.

These authors go on to make clear that, while they oppose permitting anyone to perform euthanasia, their special concern is with physicians doing so:

> We call on fellow physicians to say that they will not deliberately kill. We must also say to each of our fellow physicians that we will not tolerate killing of patients and that we shall take disciplinary action against doctors who kill. And we must say to the broader community that if it insists on tolerating or legalizing active euthanasia, it will have to find non-physicians to do its killing.[1]

If permitting physicians to kill would undermine the very "moral center" of medicine, then almost certainly physicians should not be permitted to perform euthanasia. But how persuasive is this claim? Patients should not fear, as a consequence of permitting *voluntary* active euthanasia, that their physicians will substitute a lethal injection for what patients want and believe is part of their care. If active euthanasia is restricted to cases in which it is truly voluntary, then no patient should fear getting it unless she or he has voluntarily requested it. (The fear that we might in time also come to accept nonvoluntary, or even involuntary, active euthanasia is a slippery slope worry I address [in a later section].) Patients' trust of their physicians could be increased, not eroded, by knowledge that physicians will provide aid in dying when patients seek it.

Might Gaylin and his colleagues nevertheless be correct in their claim that the moral center of medicine would collapse if physicians were to become killers? This question raises what at the deepest level should be the guiding aims of medicine, a question that obviously cannot be fully explored here. But I do want to say enough to indicate the direction that I believe an appropriate response to this challenge should take. In spelling out above what I called the positive argument for voluntary active euthanasia, I suggested that two principal values—respecting patients' self-determination and promoting their well-being—underlie the consensus that competent patients, or the surrogates of incompetent patients, are entitled to refuse any life-sustaining treatment and to choose from among available alternative treatments. It is the commitment to these two values in guiding physicians' actions as healers, comforters, and protectors of their patients' lives that should be at the "moral center" of medicine, and these two values support physicians' administering euthanasia when their patients make competent requests for it.

What should not be at that moral center is a commitment to preserving patients' lives as such, without regard to whether those patients want their lives preserved or judge their preservation a benefit to them. . . .

REFERENCE

1 Willard Gaylin, Leon R. Kass, Edmund D. Pellegrino, and Mark Siegler, "Doctors Must Not Kill," *JAMA* 259 (1988): 2139–40.

THE SUPREME COURT, PHYSICIAN-ASSISTED SUICIDE, AND TERMINAL SEDATION

OPINION OF THE COURT IN *WASHINGTON V. GLUCKSBERG*
Chief Justice William H. Rehnquist

At issue in this case is the constitutionality of the State of Washington's ban on assisted suicide—in particular, whether it violates the Due Process Clause of the Fourteenth Amendment. Although the Supreme Court unanimously upholds Washington's assisted-suicide ban, the fact that this case has produced five separate concurring opinions indicates that the Court remains fragmented on the most appropriate way of constructing the underlying issues. Chief Justice Rehnquist, in this opinion joined by four other justices, rejects the contention (asserted by the Ninth Circuit Court of Appeals) that a competent, terminally ill adult can claim a constitutionally protected right to physician assistance in suicide. On his analysis, no such liberty interest is protected by the Due Process Clause of the Fourteenth Amendment; thus, no basis exists for a fundamental-right claim. It follows, he argues, that the constitutionality of Washington's assisted-suicide ban can be established merely by showing that the ban is rationally related to legitimate government interests. In order to display how this requirement is clearly met, the Chief Justice identifies and discusses the relevant state interests.

The question presented in this case is whether Washington's prohibition against "caus[ing]" or "aid[ing]" a suicide offends the Fourteenth Amendment to the United States Constitution. We hold that it does not.

It has always been a crime to assist a suicide in the State of Washington. In 1854, Washington's first

United States Supreme Court. 521 U.S. 702 (1997).

Territorial Legislature outlawed "assisting another in the commission of self-murder." Today, Washington law provides: "A person is guilty of promoting a suicide attempt when he knowingly causes or aids another person to attempt suicide." Wash. Rev. Code 9A.36.060(1) (1994). "Promoting a suicide attempt" is a felony, punishable by up to five years' imprisonment and up to a $10,000 fine. At the same time, Washington's Natural Death Act, enacted in 1979, states that the "withholding or withdrawal of life-sustaining treatment" at a patient's direction "shall not, for any purpose, constitute a suicide."

Petitioners in this case are the State of Washington and its Attorney General. Respondents Harold Glucksberg, M.D., Abigail Halperin, M.D., Thomas A. Preston, M.D., and Peter Shalit, M.D., are physicians who practice in Washington. These doctors occasionally treat terminally ill, suffering patients, and declare that they would assist these patients in ending their lives if not for Washington's assisted-suicide ban. In January 1994, respondents, along with three gravely ill, pseudonymous plaintiffs who have since died and Compassion in Dying, a nonprofit organization that counsels people considering physician-assisted suicide, sued in the United States District Court, seeking a declaration that Wash. Rev. Code 9A.36.060(1) (1994) is, on its face, unconstitutional. *Compassion in Dying v. Washington* (WD Wash. 1994).

The plaintiffs asserted "the existence of a liberty interest protected by the Fourteenth Amendment which extends to a personal choice by a mentally competent, terminally ill adult to commit physician-assisted suicide." Relying primarily on *Planned Parenthood v. Casey* (1992) and *Cruzan v. Director, Missouri Dept. of Health* (1990), the District Court agreed and concluded that Washington's assisted-suicide ban is unconstitutional because it "places an undue burden on the exercise of [that] constitutionally protected liberty interest." The District Court also decided that the Washington statute violated the Equal Protection Clause's requirement that "'all persons similarly situated. . . . be treated alike.'"

A panel of the Court of Appeals for the Ninth Circuit reversed, emphasizing that "[i]n the two hundred and five years of our existence no constitutional right to aid in killing oneself has ever been asserted and upheld by a court of final jurisdiction." *Compassion in Dying v. Washington* (1995). The Ninth Circuit reheard the case en banc, reversed the panel's decision, and affirmed the District Court. *Compassion in Dying v. Washington* (1996). Like the District Court, the en banc Court of Appeals emphasized our *Casey* and *Cruzan* decisions. The court also discussed what is described as "historical" and "current societal attitudes" toward suicide and assisted suicide, and concluded that "the Constitution encompasses a due process liberty interest in controlling the time and manner of one's death—that there is, in short, a constitutionally-recognized 'right to die.'" After "[w]eighing and then balancing" this interest against Washington's various interests, the court held that the State's assisted-suicide ban was unconstitutional "as applied to terminally ill competent adults who wish to hasten their deaths with medication prescribed by their physicians." The court did not reach the District Court's equal-protection holding. We granted certiorari and now reverse.

I

We begin, as we do in all due-process cases, by examining our Nation's history, legal traditions, and practices. In almost every State—indeed, in almost every western democracy—it is a crime to assist a suicide. The States' assisted-suicide bans are not innovations. Rather, they are longstanding expressions of the States' commitment to the protection and preservation of all human life. Indeed, opposition to and condemnation of suicide—and, therefore, of assisting suicide—are consistent and enduring themes of our philosophical, legal, and cultural heritages.

More specifically, for over 700 years, the Anglo-American common-law tradition has punished or otherwise disapproved of both suicide and assisting suicide. . . .

For the most part, the early American colonies adopted the common-law approach. . . . [For example,] Virginia . . . required ignominious burial for suicides, and their estates were forfeit to the crown.

Over time, however, the American colonies abolished these harsh common-law penalties. . . . [H]owever, . . . the movement away from the common law's harsh sanctions did not represent an acceptance of suicide; rather, . . . this change reflected the growing consensus that it was unfair to punish the suicide's family for his wrongdoing. . . . [C]ourts continued to condemn [suicide] as a grave public wrong.

That suicide remained a grievous, though non-felonious, wrong is confirmed by the fact that colonial and early state legislatures and courts did not retreat from prohibiting assisting suicide. . . . And the prohibitions against assisting suicide never contained exceptions for those who were near death. . . .

The earliest American statute explicitly to outlaw assisting suicide was enacted in New York in 1828. . . . By the time the Fourteenth Amendment was ratified, it was a crime in most States to assist a suicide. . . .

Though deeply rooted, the States' assisted-suicide bans have in recent years been reexamined and, generally, reaffirmed. Because of advances in medicine and technology, Americans today are increasingly likely to die in institutions, from chronic illnesses. Public concern and democratic action are therefore sharply focused on how best to protect dignity and independence at the end of life, with the result that there have been many significant changes in state laws and in the attitudes these laws reflect. Many States, for example, now permit "living wills," surrogate health-care decisionmaking, and the withdrawal or refusal of life-sustaining medical treatment. At the same time, however, voters and legislators continue for the most part to reaffirm their States' prohibitions on assisting suicide. . . .

. . . Against this backdrop of history, tradition, and practice, we now turn to respondents' constitutional claim.

II

The Due Process Clause guarantees more than fair process, and the "liberty" it protects includes more than the absence of physical restraint. The Clause also provides heightened protection against government interference with certain fundamental rights and liberty interests. In a long line of cases, we have held that, in addition to the specific freedoms protected by the Bill of Rights, the "liberty" specially protected by the Due Process Clause includes the rights to marry, to have children, to direct the education and upbringing of one's children, to marital privacy, to use contraception, to bodily integrity, and to abortion. We have also assumed, and strongly suggested, that the Due Process Clause protects the traditional right to refuse unwanted lifesaving medical treatment.

But we "ha[ve] always been reluctant to expand the concept of substantive due process because guideposts for responsible decisionmaking in this unchartered area are scarce and open-ended." By extending constitutional protection to an asserted right or liberty interest, we, to a great extent, place the matter outside the arena of public debate and legislative action. We must therefore "exercise the utmost care whenever we are asked to break new ground in this field," lest the liberty protected by the Due Process Clause be subtly transformed into the policy preferences of the members of this Court.

Our established method of substantive-due-process analysis has two primary features: First, we have regularly observed that the Due Process Clause specially protects those fundamental rights and liberties which are, objectively, "deeply rooted in this Nation's history and tradition" and "implicit in the concept of ordered liberty," such that "neither liberty nor justice would exist if they were sacrificed." Second, we have required in substantive-due-process cases a "careful description" of the asserted fundamental liberty interest. Our Nation's history, legal traditions, and practices thus provide the crucial "guideposts for responsible decision-making" that direct and restrain our exposition of the Due Process Clause. As we stated recently . . . , the Fourteenth Amendment "forbids the government to infringe . . . 'fundamental' liberty interests *at all,* no matter what process is provided, unless the infringement is narrowly tailored to serve a compelling state interest.". . .

Turning to the claim at issue here, the Court of Appeals stated that "[p]roperly analyzed, the first issue to be resolved is whether there is a liberty interest in determining the time and manner of one's death," or, in other words, "[i]s there a right to die?" Similarly, respondents assert a "liberty to choose how to die" and a right to "control of one's final days," and describe the asserted liberty as "the right to choose a humane, dignified death" and "the liberty to shape death." As noted above, we have a tradition of carefully formulating the interest at stake in substantive-due-process cases. For example, although *Cruzan* is often described as a "right to die" case, we were, in fact, more precise: we assumed that the Constitution granted competent persons a "constitutionally protected right to refuse lifesaving hydration and nutrition." The Washington statute at issue in this case prohibits "aid[ing] another person to attempt suicide," Wash. Rev. Code §9A.36.060(1) (1994), and, thus, the question before us is whether the "liberty" specially protected by the Due Process Clause includes a right to commit suicide which itself includes a right to assistance in doing so.

We now inquire whether this asserted right has any place in our Nation's traditions. Here, as discussed above, we are confronted with a consistent and almost universal tradition that has long rejected the asserted right, and continues explicitly to reject it today, even for terminally ill, mentally competent adults. To hold for respondents, we would have to reverse centuries of legal doctrine and practice, and strike down the considered policy choice of almost every State.

Respondents contend, however, that the liberty interest they assert *is* consistent with this Court's substantive-due-process line of cases, if not with this Nation's history and practice. Pointing to *Casey* and *Cruzan,* respondents read our jurisprudence in this area as reflecting a general tradition of "self-sovereignty" and as teaching that the "liberty" protected by the Due Process Clause includes "basic and intimate exercises of personal autonomy." According to respondents, our liberty jurisprudence, and the broad, individualistic principles it reflects, protects the "liberty of competent, terminally ill adults to make end-of-life decisions free of undue government interference." The question presented in this case, however, is whether the protections of the Due Process Clause include a right to commit suicide with another's assistance. With this "careful description" of respondents' claim in mind, we turn to *Casey* and *Cruzan.*

In *Cruzan,* we considered whether Nancy Beth Cruzan, who had been severely injured in an automobile accident and was in a persistive vegetative state, "ha[d] a right under the United States Constitution which would require the hospital to withdraw

life-sustaining treatment" at her parents' request. We began with the observation that "[a]t common law, even the touching of one person by another without consent and without legal justification was a battery." We then discussed the related rule that "informed consent is generally required for medical treatment." After reviewing a long line of relevant state cases, we concluded that "the common-law doctrine of informed consent is viewed as generally encompassing the right of a competent individual to refuse medical treatment." Next, we reviewed our own cases on the subject, and stated that "[t]he principle that a competent person has a constitutionally protected liberty interest in refusing unwanted medical treatment may be inferred from our prior decisions." Therefore, "for purposes of [that] case, we assume[d] that the United States Constitution would grant a competent person a constitutionally protected right to refuse lifesaving hydration and nutrition." We concluded that, notwithstanding this right, the Constitution permitted Missouri to require clear and convincing evidence of an incompetent patient's wishes concerning the withdrawal of life-sustaining treatment.

Respondents contend that in *Cruzan* we "acknowledged that competent, dying persons have the right to direct the removal of life-sustaining medical treatment and thus hasten death," and that "the constitutional principle behind recognizing the patient's liberty to direct the withdrawal of artificial life support applies at least as strongly to the choice to hasten impending death by consuming lethal medication." Similarly, the Court of Appeals concluded that "*Cruzan,* by recognizing a liberty interest that includes the refusal of artificial provision of life-sustaining food and water, necessarily recognize[d] a liberty interest in hastening one's own death."

The right assumed in *Cruzan,* however, was not simply deduced from abstract concepts of personal autonomy. Given the common-law rule that forced medication was a battery, and the long legal tradition protecting the decision to refuse unwanted medical treatment, our assumption was entirely consistent with this Nation's history and constitutional traditions. The decision to commit suicide with the assistance of another may be just as personal and profound as the decision to refuse unwanted medical treatment, but it has never enjoyed similar legal protection. Indeed, the two acts are widely and reasonably regarded as quite distinct. See *Quill v. Vacco* (1997). In *Cruzan* itself, we recognized that most States outlawed assisted suicide—and even more do today—and we certainly gave no intimation that the right to refuse unwanted medical treatment could be somehow transmuted into a right to assistance in committing suicide.

Respondents also rely on *Casey.* There, the Court's opinion concluded that "the essential holding of *Roe v. Wade* should be retained and once again reaffirmed." We held, first, that a woman has a right, before her fetus is viable, to an abortion "without undue interference from the State"; second, that States may restrict post-viability abortions, so long as exceptions are made to protect a woman's life and health; and third, that the State has legitimate interests throughout a pregnancy in protecting the health of the woman and the life of the unborn child. In reaching this conclusion, the opinion discussed in some detail this Court's substantive-due-process tradition of interpreting the Due Process Clause to protect certain fundamental rights and "personal decisions relating to marriage, procreation, contraception, family relationships, child rearing, and education," and noted that many of those rights and liberties "involv[e] the most intimate and personal choices a person may make in a lifetime."

The Court of Appeals, like the District Court, found *Casey* "'highly instructive'" and "'almost prescriptive'" for determining "'what liberty interest may inhere in a terminally ill person's choice to commit suicide'":

> Like the decision of whether or not to have an abortion, the decision how and when to die is one of "the most intimate and personal choices a person may make in a lifetime," a choice "central to personal dignity and autonomy."

. . . That many of the rights and liberties protected by the Due Process Clause sound in personal autonomy does not warrant the sweeping conclusion that any and all important, intimate, and personal decisions are so protected, and *Casey* did not suggest otherwise.

The history of the law's treatment of assisted suicide in this country has been and continues to be one of the rejection of nearly all efforts to permit it. That being the case, our decisions lead us to conclude that the asserted "right" to assistance in committing suicide is not a fundamental liberty interest protected by the Due Process Clause. The Constitution also requires, however, that Washington's assisted-suicide ban be rationally related to legitimate government interests. This requirement is unquestionably met here. As the court below recognized, Washington's assisted-suicide ban implicates a number of state interests.

First, Washington has an "unqualified interest in the preservation of human life." The State's prohibition on assisted suicide, like all homicide laws, both reflects and advances its commitment to this interest. This interest is symbolic and aspirational as well as practical:

> While suicide is no longer prohibited or penalized, the ban against assisted suicide and euthanasia shores up the notion of limits in human relationships. It reflects the gravity with which we view the decision to take one's own life or the life of another, and our reluctance to encourage or promote these decisions. New York State Task Force on Life and the Law, When Death is Sought: Assisted Suicide and Euthanasia in the Medical Context 131–132 (May 1994) (hereinafter New York Task Force).

Respondents admit that "[t]he State has a real interest in preserving the lives of those who can still contribute to society and enjoy life." The Court of Appeals also recognized Washington's interest in protecting life, but held that the "weight" of this interest depends on the "medical condition and the wishes of the person whose life is at stake." Washington, however, has rejected this sliding-scale approach and, through its assisted-suicide ban, insists that all persons' lives, from beginning to end, regardless of physical or mental condition, are under the full protection of the law. As we have previously affirmed, the States "may properly decline to make judgments about the 'quality' of life that a particular individual may enjoy." This remains true, as *Cruzan* makes clear, even for those who are near death.

Relatedly, all admit that suicide is a serious public-health problem, especially among persons in otherwise vulnerable groups. The State has an interest in preventing suicide, and in studying, identifying, and treating its causes.

Those who attempt suicide—terminally ill or not—often suffer from depression or other mental disorders. See New York Task Force 13–22, 126–128 (more than 95% of those who commit suicide had a major psychiatric illness at the time of death; among the terminally ill, uncontrolled pain is a "risk factor" because it contributes to depression). Research indicates . . . that many people who request physician-assisted suicide withdraw that request if their depression and pain are treated. The New York Task Force, however, expressed its concern that, because depression is difficult to diagnose, physicians and medical professionals often fail to respond adequately to seriously ill patients' needs. Thus, legal physician-assisted suicide could make it more difficult for the State to protect depressed or mentally ill persons, or those who are suffering from untreated pain, from suicidal impulses.

The State also has an interest in protecting the integrity and ethics of the medical profession. In contrast to the Court of Appeals' conclusion that "the integrity of the medical profession would [not] be threatened in any way by [physician-assisted suicide]," the American Medical Association, like many other medical and physicians' groups, has concluded that "[p]hysician-assisted suicide is fundamentally incompatible with the physician's role as healer." American Medical Association, Code of Ethics §2.211 (1994). And physician-assisted suicide could, it is argued, undermine the trust that is essential to the doctor-patient relationship by blurring the time-honored line between healing and harming.

Next, the State has an interest in protecting vulnerable groups—including the poor, the elderly, and disabled persons—from abuse, neglect, and mistakes. The Court of Appeals dismissed the State's concern that disadvantaged persons might be pressured into physician-assisted suicide as "ludicrous on its face." We have recognized, however, the real risk of subtle coercion and undue influence in end-of-life situations. Similarly, the New York Task

Force warned that "[l]egalizing physician-assisted suicide would pose profound risks to many individuals who are ill and vulnerable. . . . The risk of harm is greatest for the many individuals in our society whose autonomy and well-being are already compromised by poverty, lack of access to good medical care, advanced age, or membership in a stigmatized social group." New York Task Force 120. If physician-assisted suicide were permitted, many might resort to it to spare their families the substantial financial burden of end-of-life health-care costs.

The State's interest here goes beyond protecting the vulnerable from coercion; it extends to protecting disabled and terminally ill people from prejudice, negative and inaccurate stereotypes, and "societal indifference." The State's assisted-suicide ban reflects and reinforces its policy that the lives of terminally ill, disabled, and elderly people must be no less valued than the lives of the young and healthy, and that a seriously disabled person's suicidal impulses should be interpreted and treated the same way as anyone else's.

Finally, the State may fear that permitting assisted suicide will start it down the path to voluntary and perhaps even involuntary euthanasia. The Court of Appeals struck down Washington's assisted-suicide ban only "as applied to competent, terminally ill adults who wish to hasten their deaths by obtaining medication prescribed by their doctors." Washington insists, however, that the impact of the court's decision will not and cannot be so limited. If suicide is protected as a matter of constitutional right, it is argued, "every man and woman in the United States must enjoy it." The Court of Appeals' decision, and its expansive reasoning, provide ample support for the State's concerns. The court noted, for example, that the "decision of a duly appointed surrogate decision maker is for all legal purposes the decision of the patient himself," that "in some instances, the patient may be unable to self-administer the drugs and . . . administration by the physician . . . may be the only way the patient may be able to receive them," and that not only physicians, but also family members and loved ones, will inevitably participate in assisting suicide. Thus, it turns out that what is couched as a limited right to "physician-assisted suicide" is likely, in effect, a much broader license, which could prove extremely difficult to police and contain. Washington's ban on assisting suicide prevents such erosion. . . .

We need not weigh exactly the relative strengths of these various interests. They are unquestionably important and legitimate, and Washington's ban on assisted suicide is at least reasonably related to their promotion and protection. We therefore hold that Wash. Rev. Code §9A.36.060(1) (1994) does not violate the Fourteenth Amendment, either on its face or "as applied to competent, terminally ill adults who wish to hasten their deaths by obtaining medication prescribed by their doctors."

Throughout the Nation, Americans are engaged in an earnest and profound debate about the morality, legality, and practicality of physician-assisted suicide. Our holding permits this debate to continue, as it should in a democratic society. The decision of the en banc Court of Appeals is reversed. . . .

OPINION OF THE COURT IN *VACCO V. QUILL*
Chief Justice William H. Rehnquist

The issue raised by this case is whether the State of New York's ban on assisted suicide violates the Equal Protection Clause of the Fourteenth Amendment. Although the Supreme Court unanimously holds that New York's assisted-suicide ban does not violate the Equal Protection Clause, the fact that this case—like its companion case, *Washington v. Glucksberg* (1997)—has spawned multiple concurring opinions indicates that the Court remains fragmented on the most appropriate way of constructing the underlying issues. Chief Justice Rehnquist, in this opinion joined by four other justices, insists that it is "both important and logical" to draw a distinction between assisting suicide and withdrawing life-sustaining treatment. Thus, in his view, there is no basis for the contention (asserted by the Second Circuit Court of Appeals) that New York law—by prohibiting assisted suicide yet allowing the withdrawal of life-sustaining treatment—fails to "treat equally all competent persons who are in the final stages of fatal illness and wish to hasten their own deaths."

In New York, as in most States, it is a crime to aid another to commit or attempt suicide, but patients may refuse even lifesaving medical treatment. The question presented by this case is whether New York's prohibition on assisting suicide therefore violates the Equal Protection Clause of the Fourteenth Amendment. We hold that it does not.

Petitioners are various New York public officials. Respondents Timothy E. Quill, Samuel C. Klagsbrun, and Howard A. Grossman are physicians who practice in New York. They assert that although it would be "consistent with the standards of [their]

United States Supreme Court. 521 U.S. 793 (1997).

medical practice[s]" to prescribe lethal medication for "mentally competent, terminally ill patients" who are suffering great pain and desire a doctor's help in taking their own lives, they are deterred from doing so by New York's ban on assisting suicide. Respondents, and three gravely ill patients who have since died, sued the State's Attorney General in the United States District Court. They urged that because New York permits a competent person to refuse life-sustaining medical treatment, and because the refusal of such treatment is "essentially the same thing" as physician-assisted suicide, New York's assisted-suicide ban violates the Equal Protection Clause.

The District Court disagreed: "[I]t is hardly unreasonable or irrational for the State to recognize a difference between allowing nature to take its course, even in the most severe situations, and intentionally using an artificial death-producing device." The court noted New York's "obvious legitimate interests in preserving life, and in protecting vulnerable persons," and concluded that "[u]nder the United States Constitution and the federal system it establishes, the resolution of this issue is left to the normal democratic processes within the State."

The Court of Appeals for the Second Circuit reversed. The court determined that, despite the assisted-suicide ban's apparent general applicability, "New York law does not treat equally all competent persons who are in the final stages of fatal illness and wish to hasten their deaths," because "those in the final stages of terminal illness who are on life-support systems are allowed to hasten their deaths by directing the removal of such systems; but those who are similarly situated, except for the previous attachment of life-sustaining equipment, are not allowed to hasten death by self-administering prescribed drugs." In the court's view, "[t]he ending of life by [the withdrawal of life-support systems] is *nothing more nor less than assisted suicide*" (emphasis added). The Court of Appeals then examined whether this supposed unequal treatment was rationally related to any legitimate state interest, and concluded that "to the extent that [New York's statutes] prohibit a physician from prescribing medications to be self-administered by a mentally competent, terminally-ill person in the final stages of his terminal illness, they are not rationally related to any legitimate state interest." We granted certiorari and now reverse.

The Equal Protection Clause commands that no State shall "deny to any person within its jurisdiction the equal protection of the laws." This provision creates no substantive rights. Instead, it embodies a general rule that States must treat like cases alike but may treat unlike cases accordingly. If a legislative classification or distinction "neither burdens a fundamental right nor targets a suspect class, we will uphold [it] so long as it bears a rational relation to some legitimate end."

New York's statutes outlawing assisting suicide affect and address matters of profound significance to all New Yorkers alike. They neither infringe fundamental rights nor involve suspect classifications. These laws are therefore entitled to a "strong presumption of validity."

On their faces, neither New York's ban on assisting suicide nor its statutes permitting patients to refuse medical treatment treat anyone differently than anyone else or draw any distinctions between persons. *Everyone,* regardless of physical condition, is entitled, if competent, to refuse unwanted lifesaving medical treatment; *no one* is permitted to assist a suicide. Generally speaking, laws that apply evenhandedly to all "unquestionably comply" with the Equal Protection Clause.

The Court of Appeals, however, concluded that some terminally ill people—those who are on life-support systems—are treated differently than those who are not, in that the former may "hasten death" by ending treatment, but the latter may not "hasten death" through physician-assisted suicide. This conclusion depends on the submission that ending or refusing lifesaving medical treatment "is nothing more nor less than assisted suicide." Unlike the Court of Appeals, we think the distinction between assisting suicide and withdrawing life-sustaining treatment, a distinction widely recognized and endorsed in the medical profession and in our legal traditions, is both important and logical; it is certainly rational. ("When the basic classification is rationally based, uneven effects upon particular groups within a class are ordinarily of no constitutional concern.")

The distinction comports with fundamental legal principles of causation and intent. First, when a patient refuses life-sustaining medical treatment, he dies from an underlying fatal disease or pathology; but if a patient ingests lethal medication prescribed by a physician, he is killed by that medication.

Furthermore, a physician who withdraws, or honors a patient's refusal to begin, life-sustaining medical treatment purposefully intends, or may so intend, only to respect his patient's wishes and "to cease doing useless and futile or degrading things to the patient when [the patient] no longer stands to benefit from them." Assisted Suicide in the United States, Hearing before the Subcommittee on the Constitution of the House Committee on the Judiciary, 104th Cong., 2d Sess., 368 (1996) (testimony of Dr. Leon

R. Kass). The same is true when a doctor provides aggressive palliative care; in some cases, painkilling drugs may hasten a patient's death, but the physician's purpose and intent is, or may be, only to ease his patient's pain. A doctor who assists a suicide, however, "must, necessarily and indubitably, intend primarily that the patient be made dead." *Id.,* at 367. Similarly, a patient who commits suicide with a doctor's aid necessarily has the specific intent to end his or her own life, while a patient who refuses or discontinues treatment might not.

The law has long used actors' intent or purpose to distinguish between two acts that may have the same result. Put differently, the law distinguishes actions taken "because of" a given end from actions taken "in spite of" their unintended but foreseen consequences. ("When General Eisenhower ordered American soldiers onto the beaches of Normandy, he knew that he was sending many American soldiers to certain death. . . . His purpose, though, was to . . . liberate Europe from the Nazis.")

Given these general principles, it is not surprising that many courts, including New York courts, have carefully distinguished refusing life-sustaining treatment from suicide. . . .

Similarly, the overwhelming majority of state legislatures have drawn a clear line between assisting suicide and withdrawing or permitting the refusal of unwanted lifesaving medical treatment by prohibiting the former and permitting the latter. And "nearly all states expressly disapprove of suicide and assisted suicide either in statutes dealing with durable powers of attorney in health-care situations, or in 'living will' statutes." Thus, even as the States move to protect and promote patients' dignity at the end of life, they remain opposed to physician-assisted suicide.

New York is a case in point. The State enacted its current assisted-suicide statutes in 1965.[1] Since then, New York has acted several times to protect patients' common-law right to refuse treatment. In so doing, however, the State has neither endorsed a general right to "hasten death" nor approved physician-assisted suicide. Quite the opposite: The State has reaffirmed the line between "killing" and "letting die." More recently, the New York State Task Force on Life and the Law studied assisted suicide and euthanasia and, in 1994, unanimously recommended against legalization. When Death is Sought: Assisted Suicide and Euthanasia in the Medical Context vii (1994). In the Task Force's view, "allowing decisions to forego life-sustaining treatment and allowing assisted suicide or euthanasia have radically different consequences and meanings for public policy." *Id.,* at 146.

This Court has also recognized, at least implicitly, the distinction between letting a patient die and making that patient die. In *Cruzan v. Director, Mo. Dept. of Health* (1990), we concluded that "[t]he principle that a competent person has a constitutionally protected liberty interest in refusing unwanted medical treatment may be inferred from our prior decisions," and we assumed the existence of such a right for purposes of that case. But our assumption of a right to refuse treatment was grounded not, as the Court of Appeals supposed, on the proposition that patients have a general and abstract "right to hasten death," but on well established, traditional rights to bodily integrity and freedom from unwanted touching. In fact, we observed that "the majority of States in this country have laws imposing criminal penalties on one who assists another to commit suicide." *Cruzan* therefore provides no support for the notion that refusing life-sustaining medical treatment is "nothing more nor less than suicide."

For all these reasons, we disagree with respondents' claim that the distinction between refusing lifesaving medical treatment and assisted suicide is "arbitrary" and "irrational."[2] Granted, in some cases, the line between the two may not be clear, but certainty is not required, even were it possible. Logic and contemporary practice support New York's judgment that the two acts are different, and New York may therefore, consistent with the Constitution, treat them differently. By permitting everyone to refuse unwanted medical treatment while prohibiting anyone from assisting a suicide, New York law follows a longstanding and rational distinction.

New York's reasons for recognizing and acting on this distinction—including prohibiting intentional killing and preserving life; preventing suicide; maintaining physicians' role as their patients' healers; protecting vulnerable people from indifference, prejudice, and psychological and financial pressure

to end their lives; and avoiding a possible slide towards euthanasia—are discussed in greater detail in
our opinion in *Glucksberg, ante*. These valid and important public interests easily satisfy the constitutional requirement that a legislative classification
bear a rational relation to some legitimate end.

The judgment of the Court of Appeals is
reversed. . . .

NOTES

1 It has always been a crime, either by statute or under the
common law, to assist a suicide in New York.
2 Respondents also argue that the State irrationally
distinguishes between physician-assisted suicide and
"terminal sedation," a process respondents characterize as
"induc[ing] barbiturate coma and then starv[ing] the person

to death." Petitioners insist, however, that "'[a]lthough
proponents of physician-assisted suicide and euthanasia
contend that terminal sedation is covert physician-assisted
suicide or euthanasia, the concept of sedating
pharmacotherapy is based on informed consent and the
principle of double effect.'" Reply Brief for Petitioners 12
(quoting P. Rousseau, Terminal Sedation in the Care of
Dying Patients, 156 Archives Internal Med. 1785,
1785–1786 ([1996]). Just as a State may prohibit assisting
suicide while permitting patients to refuse unwanted
lifesaving treatment, it may permit palliative care related to
that refusal, which may have the foreseen but unintended
"double effect" of hastening the patient's death. See New
York Task Force, "When Death is Sought," at 163 ("It is
widely recognized that the provision of pain medication is
ethically and professionally acceptable even when the
treatment may hasten the patient's death, if the medication is
intended to alleviate pain and severe discomfort, not to
cause death").

CONCURRING OPINION IN *WASHINGTON V. GLUCKSBERG* AND *VACCO V. QUILL*

Justice Sandra Day O'Connor

In this concurring opinion, Justice O'Connor emphasizes that in both Washington
and New York there are presently no legal barriers to terminally ill patients' obtaining adequate pain-relieving medication, "even to the point of causing unconsciousness and hastening death." If terminally ill patients did not, in fact, have access to
such palliative care, she seems to suggest, there might be grounds for a different
conclusion regarding physician-assisted suicide.

Death will be different for each of us. For many, the
last days will be spent in physical pain and perhaps
the despair that accompanies physical deterioration
and a loss of control of basic bodily and mental functions. Some will seek medication to alleviate that
pain and other symptoms.

The Court frames the issue in *Washington v.
Glucksberg* as whether the Due Process Clause of
the Constitution protects a "right to commit suicide
which itself includes a right to assistance in doing
so," and concludes that our Nation's history, legal
traditions, and practices do not support the existence

of such a right. I join the Court's opinions because I
agree that there is no generalized right to "commit
suicide." But respondents urge us to address the narrower question whether a mentally competent person who is experiencing great suffering has a
constitutionally cognizable interest in controlling
the circumstances of his or her imminent death. I see
no need to reach that question in the context of the
facial challenges to the New York and Washington
laws at issue here. ("The Washington statute at issue
in this case prohibits 'aid[ing] another person to attempt suicide,' . . . and, thus, the question before us
is whether the 'liberty' specially protected by the
Due Process Clause includes a right to commit

United States Supreme Court. 521 U.S. 702 (1997).

suicide which itself includes a right to assistance in doing so"). The parties and *amici* agree that in these States a patient who is suffering from a terminal illness and who is experiencing great pain has no legal barriers to obtaining medication, from qualified physicians, to alleviate that suffering, even to the point of causing unconsciousness and hastening death. In this light, even assuming that we would recognize such an interest, I agree that the State's interests in protecting those who are not truly competent or facing imminent death, or those whose decisions to hasten death would not truly be voluntary, are sufficiently weighty to justify a prohibition against physician-assisted suicide.

Every one of us at some point may be affected by our own or a family member's terminal illness. There is no reason to think the democratic process will not strike the proper balance between the interests of terminally ill, mentally competent individuals who would seek to end their suffering and the State's interests in protecting those who might seek to end life mistakenly or under pressure. As the Court recognizes, States are presently undertaking extensive and serious evaluation of physician-assisted suicide and other related issues. In such circumstances, "the . . . challenging task of crafting appropriate procedures for safeguarding . . . liberty interests is entrusted to the 'laboratory' of the States . . . in the first instance."

In sum, there is no need to address the question whether suffering patients have a constitutionally cognizable interest in obtaining relief from the suffering that they may experience in the last days of their lives. There is no dispute that dying patients in Washington and New York can obtain palliative care, even when doing so would hasten their deaths. The difficulty in defining terminal illness and the risk that a dying patient's request for assistance in ending his or her life might not be truly voluntary justifies the prohibitions on assisted suicide we uphold here.

THE SUPREME COURT AND PHYSICIAN-ASSISTED SUICIDE: REJECTING ASSISTED SUICIDE BUT EMBRACING EUTHANASIA
David Orentlicher

Orentlicher analyzes the Supreme Court opinions on physician-assisted suicide in reference to the practice of *terminal sedation.* In Orentlicher's view, terminal sedation is often a form of euthanasia. Thus, he argues that the Court's acceptance of terminal sedation undermines the most important arguments against the legalization of assisted suicide. Moreover, Orentlicher contends, assisted suicide is ethically less problematic than terminal sedation.

In rejecting a constitutional right to physician-assisted suicide earlier this year,[1,2] the U.S. Supreme Court appeared to preserve the distinction between the withdrawal of life-sustaining treatment and assisted suicide or euthanasia. In fact, however, the Court undermined the distinction when it endorsed terminal sedation. Terminal sedation seems consistent with traditional medical care but often is a form of euthanasia. Moreover, it is a practice that is ethically more problematic than assisted suicide or voluntary euthanasia.

THE SUPREME COURT'S OPINIONS

In deciding against a right to assisted suicide, the Court faced the claim that such a right is necessary for some patients to ensure that they can avoid intolerable pain

Reprinted by permission of the publisher from *The New England Journal of Medicine,* vol. 337 (October 23, 1997), pp. 1236–1239. Copyright © 1997 Massachusetts Medical Society. All rights reserved.

in their final days. Although physical pain is almost always treatable, some pain cannot be relieved by analgesia. In response to this concern, hospice providers and other medical professionals assured the Court that even the most severe suffering could be alleviated by sedating the patient into unconsciousness. According to the brief of the American Medical Association, for example,

> The pain of most terminally ill patients can be controlled throughout the dying process without heavy sedation or anesthesia. . . . For a very few patients, however, sedation to a sleep-like state may be necessary in the last days or weeks of life to prevent the patient from experiencing severe pain.[3]

With this assurance from the medical profession, Justices Sandra Day O'Connor, Stephen Breyer, and Ruth Bader Ginsburg wrote in their concurring opinions that the case for a right to assisted suicide had not been made. If a right to assisted suicide turned on the need to relieve the suffering of patients, the alternative of terminal sedation made such a right unnecessary.[1,2]

An important question, then, is whether terminal sedation really is a good alternative to assisted suicide.

TERMINAL SEDATION

At the end of life, terminally ill patients may have intolerable pain, shortness of breath, delirium, or persistent vomiting that is refractory to the usual therapies.[4-7] Intolerable pain may be caused by several conditions, including cancer that has metastasized to the spine, intestinal obstruction, and headache due to massive intracerebral edema.[4] Intolerable shortness of breath can result from several conditions, too, including lung and other cancers, chronic obstructive lung disease, and congestive heart failure.[8] In cases of intolerable and refractory suffering, adequate relief can be obtained only by sedating the patient, often deeply. Although the frequency of intolerable and refractory symptoms is uncertain, studies have found them in 15 to 50 percent of terminally ill patients referred for palliative care.[4,9] With terminal sedation, opioids, benzodiazepines, barbiturates, neuroleptic

drugs, or combinations of these agents are used to sedate the patient.[4,10]

The sedation is maintained until the patient dies, usually within a few days, either from the underlying illness or from a second step that is typically part of terminal sedation—the withholding of nutrition and hydration. In most cases, terminal sedation shortens the patient's life by only hours to days, but it may shorten life by as much as several weeks.

At first glance, terminal sedation seems consistent with accepted practices. It is appropriate for physicians to treat the pain and other suffering of patients aggressively, even if doing so is likely to hasten death. On closer examination, however, terminal sedation at times is tantamount to euthanasia, or a kind of "slow euthanasia."[11]

TERMINAL SEDATION AS A FORM OF EUTHANASIA

In many cases, terminal sedation amounts to euthanasia because the sedated patient often dies from the combination of two intentional acts by the physician—the induction of stupor or unconsciousness and the withholding of food and water. Without these two acts, the patient would live longer before succumbing to illness.

It might be argued that death by terminal sedation is morally acceptable because death is due to the withdrawal of nutrition and hydration. As courts have consistently recognized,[12,13] it is ethically and legally permissible for patients to die because life-sustaining treatment has been discontinued.

Although death from dehydration or starvation during terminal sedation resembles death resulting from the withdrawal of treatment, it is in principle more like euthanasia. We permit the withdrawal of life-sustaining treatment while rejecting assisted suicide and euthanasia because, it is argued, the patient dies from the underlying disease, not from the active intervention of the physician.[1,13] A patient in a persistent vegetative state dies after the removal of a feeding tube because the patient's medical condition is responsible for the patient's inability to eat or drink. But this is not what happens in terminal sedation accompanied by the withholding of nutrition and hydration. In such cases, the patient dies from the induced stupor or coma. It is the physician-created state of diminished consciousness that renders the patient unable to eat, not the patient's underlying disease.

We might justify terminal sedation on the grounds that the patient's underlying disease creates the need for the sedation by causing the patient to ask for palliation. But that logic would also justify assisted suicide and euthanasia. In the case of assisted suicide or euthanasia, it is the patient's underlying disease that causes the patient to ask for a life-ending drug.

Proponents of terminal sedation might defend the practice by citing the principle of the double effect. According to that principle, physicians may take steps that might hasten the patient's death as long as the steps constitute a reasonable effort to treat the patient's suffering and the patient's death is not intended.[14] For example, it is permissible to give analgesics or sedatives to alleviate a patient's pain even if the drugs might halt the patient's breathing. However, the principle of the double effect justifies only the sedation that is part of terminal sedation. We cannot justify the withdrawal of food and water during terminal sedation, for that step does nothing to relieve the patient's suffering but only serves to bring about the patient's death. If it is argued that the withdrawal of food and water is a permissible act, then we are back to the previous response that it is permissible only because the patient's inability to eat or drink results from an underlying disease.

Terminal sedation is not only a type of euthanasia; it is also ethically more problematic than either assisted suicide or voluntary euthanasia. Terminal sedation poses the same risks of abuse as assisted suicide or euthanasia. At the same time, it serves fewer of the purposes of right-to-die law.

To see how terminal sedation carries the same risks as assisted suicide or euthanasia, we can consider a twist on the case of Janet Adkins, the woman with early Alzheimer's disease who became the first person to die with Dr. Jack Kevorkian's assistance. Let us assume that Ms. Adkins expressed her despair and her desire to consult Dr. Kevorkian to her personal physician. Suppose, further, that, in response, Ms. Adkins's physician suggested that she consider terminal sedation accompanied by the withholding of nutrition and hydration. If we are troubled by Ms. Adkins's suicide at the hands of Dr. Kevorkian, then we should be equally troubled if she had undergone terminal sedation at the hands of her personal physician. Like assisted suicide or euthanasia, terminal sedation can be provided to people whose illnesses are not yet serious or whose suffering results from a treatable depression. Moreover, like euthanasia, terminal sedation poses a risk of abuse that goes beyond the risks associated with assisted suicide. Assisted suicide requires the active participation of the patient;[15] terminal sedation, however, can be induced without the patient's consent or even the patient's knowledge. Accordingly, any incompetent patient could be terminally sedated.

Terminal sedation also serves fewer of the purposes of right-to-die law than assisted suicide or euthanasia. Although terminal sedation ensures a painless death, it forces patients to accept a dying process that is prolonged as compared with what it would be if assisted suicide or euthanasia were performed. Terminal sedation requires that patients linger in a state that may profoundly compromise their dignity and further distort the memory they leave behind. Terminal sedation also prevents patients from retaining some control over the timing and circumstances of their death, a control that may be critical to their psychological well-being.[16]

Because terminal sedation is often a type of euthanasia, the Court's acceptance of it undermines key objections to the legalization of assisted suicide. Many opponents of assisted suicide concede that it is morally acceptable in some circumstances, as when a person is suffering severe and intractable pain and will die shortly from metastatic cancer. However, these opponents argue, it will not be possible to limit assisted suicide to morally acceptable cases. Once we permit assisted suicide for some persons, we will have no principle that justifies denying it to other persons who claim great suffering.[17,18] Yet, if we can limit terminal sedation to appropriate cases, we can limit assisted suicide in the same way. By whatever criteria physicians use to decide when terminal sedation is appropriate therapy, they can also decide when assisted suicide is appropriate therapy.

The endorsement of terminal sedation undermines another key argument against legalizing assisted suicide. The distinction between the withdrawal of treatment and assisted suicide is often justified on the ground that, in the case of treatment withdrawal, the patient does not intend to die but intends only to be free of a burdensome medical treatment.[2,13] In requesting assisted suicide, it is argued, the patient seeks relief from suffering by choosing a "treatment" that is uniformly fatal. Yet when a patient agrees to deep sedation accompanied by the withholding of nutrition and hydration, the patient also chooses a treatment that is uniformly fatal. If intent is not relevant to terminal sedation, it is also not relevant to assisted suicide.

TERMINAL SEDATION VERSUS ASSISTED SUICIDE

If terminal sedation is essentially euthanasia in many cases, why did three concurring Supreme Court justices endorse the practice, and why did the five-justice majority expressly reject the claim that terminal sedation "is covert physician-assisted suicide"?[2]

The Court's decision suggests that it cares as much about why a patient wishes to die as about how a patient dies. In approving terminal sedation despite the fact that it amounts to euthanasia at times, the Court is essentially saying that the right to die primarily reflects a moral sentiment: that people who are dying and suffering intolerably should be allowed to die even if they cannot do so simply by refusing life-sustaining treatment.[19]

In addition, a right to terminal sedation may be necessary to protect a patient's right to refuse life-sustaining treatment. Without a right to terminal sedation, physicians would have to tell terminally ill patients who are experiencing intolerable and refractory suffering that they could be sedated for relief but that, once sedated, they could no longer have nutrition and hydration withheld or withdrawn. These patients would be forced to choose between obtaining relief from their suffering and retaining their right to refuse life-sustaining treatment. That would be an unfair choice to put to dying patients.

Although we can explain why the Court accepted terminal sedation, we still need to explain why the Court rejected the ethically better alternative

of assisted suicide. That decision appears to reflect considerations of symbolism. Although terminal sedation can effectively constitute euthanasia, it looks on the surface like a combination of the accepted practices of aggressive comfort care and withdrawal of treatment. Moreover, in practice, it appears to be limited to appropriate cases. No one is suggesting that physicians are administering terminal sedation to people who are not seriously ill or who really should be treated with psychological counseling and antidepressive drugs. In contrast, many suicides in this country are committed by people who are psychologically depressed but have no serious physical illness. The Court may have been concerned about the message it would send to these people if it permitted assisted suicide for terminally ill persons.

Nevertheless, the Court's deference to symbolic considerations creates its own problems of symbolism; assisted suicide is rejected only by embracing what is essentially euthanasia. Moreover, the symbolic benefits come at a substantial cost to patients. Patients who undergo terminal sedation are required to accept a form of death that may be less desirable for them and that is more vulnerable to abuse.

ACKNOWLEDGMENTS

I am indebted to Judy Failer, Ph.D., John Hansen-Flascben, M.D., and Timothy Quill, M.D., for their contributions.

REFERENCES

1 *Washington v. Glucksberg,* 117 S. Ct. 2258 (1997).
2 *Vacco v. Quill,* 117 S. Ct. 2293 (1997).
3 Brief of the American Medical Association, et al., as *amici curiae* in support of petitioners, at 6, *Washington v. Glucksberg,* 117 S. Ct. 2258 (1997) (No. 96–110).
4 Cherny N. I., Portenoy R. K. Sedation in the management of refractory symptoms: guidelines for evaluation and treatment. J Palliat Care 1994; 10(2):31–8.
5 Quill T. E., Brody R. V. 'You promised me I wouldn't die like this!': a bad death as a medical emergency. Arch Intern Med 1995; 155:1250–4.
6 Greene W. R., Davis W. H. Titrated intravenous barbiturates in the control of symptoms in patients with terminal cancer. South Med J 1991; 84:332–7.
7 Ramani S., Karnad A. B. Long-term subcutaneous infusion of midazolam for refractory delirium in terminal breast cancer. South Med J 1996; 89: 1101–3.

8 Reuben D. B., Mor V. Dyspnea in terminally ill cancer patients. Chest 1986;89:234–6.

9 Enck R. E. The medical care of terminally ill patients. Baltimore: Johns Hopkins University Press, 1994:166–72.

10 Truog R. D., Berde C. B., Mitchell C., Grier H. E. Barbiturates in the care of the terminally ill. N Engl J Med 1992; 327:1678–82.

11 Billings J. A, Block S. D. Slow euthanasia. J Palliat Care 1996; 12(4):21–30.

12 *Cruzan v. Director, Missouri Dept. of Health,* 497 U.S. 261 (1990).

13 *In re Conroy,* 486 A.2d 1209, 1224 (N.J. 1985).

14 Beauchamp T. L., Childress J. F. Principles of biomedical ethics. 4th ed. New York: Oxford University Press, 1994:206–11.

15 Angell M. The Supreme Court and physician-assisted suicide—the ultimate right. N Engl J Med 1997; 336:50–3.

16 Brock D. W. Voluntary active euthanasia. Hastings Cent Rep 1992; 22(2):10–22.

17 Callahan D. When self-determination runs amok. Hastings Cent Rep 1992; 22(2):52–5.

18 Kamisar Y. Against assisted suicide—even a very limited form. Univ Detroit Mercy Law Rev 1995; 72:735–69.

19 Orentlicher D. The legalization of physician-assisted suicide. N Engl J Med 1996; 335:663–7.

PHYSICIAN-ASSISTED SUICIDE, ACTIVE EUTHANASIA, AND SOCIAL POLICY

CARE OF THE HOPELESSLY ILL: PROPOSED CLINICAL CRITERIA FOR PHYSICIAN-ASSISTED SUICIDE

Timothy E. Quill, Christine K. Cassel, and Diane E. Meier

The authors oppose the legalization of voluntary (active) euthanasia but endorse the legalization of physician-assisted suicide as "the policy best able to respond to patients' needs and to protect vulnerable people." In an effort to clarify the conditions under which physician-assisted suicide should be permitted, they introduce a set of relevant criteria. In their view, there are six conditions that must be satisfied, and there is also a documentation requirement.

. . . Although physician-assisted suicide and voluntary euthanasia both involve the active facilitation of a wished-for death, there are several important distinctions between them.[1] In assisted suicide, the final act is solely the patient's, and the risk of subtle coercion from doctors, family members, institutions, or other social forces is greatly reduced.[2] The balance of power between doctor and patient is more nearly equal in physician-assisted suicide than in euthanasia. The physician is counselor and witness and makes the means available, but ultimately the patient must be the one to act or not act. In voluntary euthanasia, the physician both provides the means and carries out the final act, with greatly amplified power over the patient and an increased risk of error, coercion, or abuse.

In view of these distinctions, we conclude that legalization of physician-assisted suicide, but not of voluntary euthanasia, is the policy best able to respond to patients' needs and to protect vulnerable people. From this perspective, physician-assisted suicide forms part of the continuum of options for comfort care, beginning with the forgoing of life-sustaining therapy, including more aggressive symptom-relieving measures, and permitting physician-assisted suicide only if all other alternatives have failed and all criteria have been met. Active voluntary euthanasia is excluded from this continuum because of the risk of abuse it presents. We recognize that this exclusion is made at a cost to

Reprinted with permission of the publisher from the *New England Journal of Medicine,* vol. 327 (November 5, 1992), pp. 1381–1383.

competent, incurably ill patients who cannot swallow or move and who therefore cannot be helped to die by assisted suicide. Such persons, who meet agreed-on criteria in other respects, must not be abandoned to their suffering; a combination of decisions to forgo life-sustaining treatments (including food and fluids) with aggressive comfort measures (such as analgesics and sedatives) could be offered, along with a commitment to search for creative alternatives. We acknowledge that this solution is less than ideal, but we also recognize that in the United States access to medical care is currently too inequitable, and many doctor-patient relationships too impersonal, for us to tolerate the risks of permitting active voluntary euthanasia. We must monitor any change in public policy in this domain to evaluate both its benefits and its burdens.

We propose the following clinical guidelines to contribute to serious discussion about physician-assisted suicide. Although we favor a reconsideration of the legal and professional prohibitions in the case of patients who meet carefully defined criteria, we do not wish to promote an easy or impersonal process.[3] If we are to consider allowing incurably ill patients more control over their deaths, it must be as an expression of our compassion and concern about their ultimate fate after all other alternatives have been exhausted. Such patients should not be held hostage to our reluctance or inability to forge policies in this difficult area.

PROPOSED CLINICAL CRITERIA FOR PHYSICIAN-ASSISTED SUICIDE

Because assisted suicide is extraordinary and irreversible treatment, the patient's primary physician must ensure that the following conditions are clearly satisfied before proceeding. First, the patient must have a condition that is incurable and associated with severe, unrelenting suffering. The patient must understand the condition, the prognosis, and the types of comfort care available as alternatives. Although most patients making this request will be near death, we acknowledge the inexactness of such prognostications[4-6] and do not want to exclude arbitrarily persons with incurable, but not imminently terminal, progressive illnesses, such as amyotrophic lateral sclerosis or multiple sclerosis. When there is

considerable uncertainty about the patient's medical condition or prognosis, a second opinion or opinions should be sought and the uncertainty clarified as much as possible before a final decision about the patient's request is made.

Second, the physician must ensure that the patient's suffering and the request are not the result of inadequate comfort care. All reasonable comfort-oriented measures must at least have been considered, and preferably have been tried, before the means for a physician-assisted suicide are provided. Physician-assisted suicide must never be used to circumvent the struggle to provide comprehensive care or find acceptable alternatives. The physician's prospective willingness to provide assisted suicide is a legitimate and important subject to discuss if the patient raises the question, since many patients will probably find the possibility of an escape from suffering more important than the reality.

Third, the patient must clearly and repeatedly, of his or her own free will and initiative, request to die rather than continue suffering. The physician should understand thoroughly what continued life means to the patient and why death appears preferable. A physician's too-ready acceptance of a patient's request could be perceived as encouragement to commit suicide, yet it is important not to force the patient to "beg" for assistance. Understanding the patient's desire to die and being certain that the request is serious are critical steps in evaluating the patient's rationality and ensuring that all alternative means of relieving suffering have been adequately explored. Any sign of ambivalence or uncertainty on the part of the patient should abort the process, because a clear, convincing, and continuous desire for an end of suffering through death is a strict requirement to proceed. Requests for assisted suicide made in an advance directive or by a health care surrogate should not be honored.

Fourth, the physician must be sure that the patient's judgment is not distorted. The patient must be capable of understanding the decision and its implications. The presence of depression is relevant if it is distorting rational decision making and is reversible in a way that would substantially alter the situation. Expert psychiatric evaluation should be sought when the primary physician is inexperienced in the diagnosis and treatment of depression, or when there is uncertainty about the rationality of the request or the presence of a reversible mental disorder the treatment of which would substantially change the patient's perception of his or her condition.[7]

Fifth, physician-assisted suicide should be carried out only in the context of a meaningful doctor-patient relationship. Ideally, the physician should have witnessed the patient's previous illness and suffering. There may not always be a preexisting relationship, but the physician must get to know the patient personally in order to understand fully the reasons for the request. The physician must understand why the patient considers death to be the best of a limited number of very unfortunate options. The primary physician must personally confirm that each of the criteria has been met. The patient should have no doubt that the physician is committed to finding alternative solutions if at any moment the patient's mind changes. Rather than create a new subspecialty focused on death,[8] assistance in suicide should be given by the same physician who has been struggling with the patient to provide comfort care, and who will stand by the patient and provide care until the time of death, no matter what path is taken.[3]

No physician should be forced to assist a patient in suicide if it violates the physician's fundamental values, although the patient's personal physician should think seriously before turning down such a request. Should a transfer of care be necessary, the personal physician should help the patient find another, more receptive primary physician.

Sixth, consultation with another experienced physician is required to ensure that the patient's request is voluntary and rational, the diagnosis and prognosis accurate, and the exploration of comfort-oriented alternatives thorough. The consulting physician should review the supporting materials and should interview and examine the patient.

Finally, clear documentation to support each condition is required. A system must be developed for reporting, reviewing, and studying such deaths and clearly distinguishing them from other forms of suicide. The patient, the primary physician, and the consultant must each sign a consent form. A physician-assisted suicide must neither invalidate insurance policies nor lead to an investigation by the medical examiner or an unwanted autopsy. The primary physician, the medical consultant, and the family must be assured that if the conditions agreed on are satisfied in good faith, they will be free from criminal prosecution for having assisted the patient to die.

Informing family members is strongly recommended, but whom to involve and inform should be left to the discretion and control of the patient. Similarly, spiritual counseling should be offered, depending on the patient's background and beliefs. Ideally, close family members should be an integral part of the decision-making process and should understand and support the patient's decision. If there is a major dispute between the family and the patient about how to proceed, it may require the involvement of an ethics committee or even of the courts. It is to be hoped, however, that most of these painful decisions can be worked through directly by the patient, the family, and health care providers. Under no circumstances should the family's wishes and requests override those of a competent patient.

THE METHOD

In physician-assisted suicide, a lethal amount of medication is usually prescribed that the patient then ingests. Since this process has been largely covert and unstudied, little is known about which methods are the most humane and effective. If there is a change in policy, there must be an open sharing of information within the profession, and a careful analysis of effectiveness. The methods selected should be reliable and should not add to the patient's suffering. We must also provide support and careful monitoring for the patients, physicians, and families affected, since the emotional and social effects are largely unknown but are undoubtedly far-reaching.

Assistance with suicide is one of the most profound and meaningful requests a patient can make of a physician. If the patient and the physician agree that there are no acceptable alternatives and that all the required conditions have been met, the lethal medication should ideally be taken in the physician's presence. Unless the patient specifically requests it, he or she should not be left alone at the time of death. In addition to the personal physician, other health care providers and family members should be encouraged to be present, as the patient wishes. It is of the utmost importance not to abandon the patient at this critical moment.

The time before a controlled death can provide an opportunity for a rich and meaningful goodbye between family members, health care providers, and the patient. For this reason, we must be sure that any policies and laws enacted to allow assisted suicide do not require that the patient be left alone at the moment of death in order for the assisters to be safe from prosecution. . . .

REFERENCES

1 Weir R. F. The morality of physician-assisted suicide. Law Med Health Care 1992; 20:116–26.
2 Glover J. Causing death and saving lives. New York: Penguin Books, 1977:182–9.
3 Jecker N. S. Giving death a hand: when the dying and the doctor stand in a special relationship. J Am Geriatr Soc 1991; 39:831–5.
4 Poses R. M., Bekes C., Copare F. J., Scott W. E. The answer to "What are my chances, doctor?" depends on whom is asked: prognostic disagreement and inaccuracy for critically ill patients. Crit Care Med 1989; 17:827–33.
5 Charlson M. E. Studies of prognosis: progress and pitfalls. J Gen Intern Med 1987; 2:359–61.
6 Schonwetter R. S., Teasdale T. A., Storey P., Luchi R. J. Estimation of survival time in terminal cancer patients: an impedance to hospice admissions? Hospice J 1990; 6:65–79.
7 Conwell Y., Caine E. D. Rational suicide and the right to die—reality and myth. N Engl J Med 1991; 325:1100–3.
8 Benrubi G. I. Euthanasia—the need for procedural safeguards. N Engl J Med 1992; 326:197–9.

THE OREGON DEATH WITH DIGNITY ACT

This Oregon law permits physicians to prescribe lethal drugs for Oregon adult residents who are terminally ill and who want to end their own lives. In order for a patient to be eligible for such assistance, the attending physician must determine that the patient has a terminal disease—a diagnosis entailing that the patient is expected to die within six months—and a consulting physician must confirm this diagnosis. Prominent among the other stipulated requirements are the following: (1) The patient must make an initial oral request; reiterate the oral request after 15 days have passed; and also submit a written request, supported by two witnesses. (2) Before writing the prescription, the attending physician must wait at least 15 days after the patient's initial request and at least 48 hours after the written request. (3) The attending physician must fully inform the patient about the diagnosis, prognosis, and feasible alternatives, including comfort care, hospice care, and pain control. (4) Both the attending physician and the consulting physician must certify that the patient is "capable" (i.e., has decision-making capacity), is acting voluntarily, and has made an informed choice. (5) If either physician believes that the patient's judgment might be impaired (e.g., by depression), the patient must be referred for counseling.

Section 1: General Provisions

1.01 Definitions

The following words and phrases, whenever used in this Act, shall have the following meanings:

(1) "Adult" means an individual who is 18 years of age or older.

(2) "Attending physician" means the physician who has primary responsibility for the care of the patient and treatment of the patient's terminal disease.

(3) "Consulting physician" means a physician who is qualified by specialty or experience to make a professional diagnosis and prognosis regarding the patient's disease.

(4) "Counseling" means a consultation between a state licensed psychiatrist or psychologist

Oregon Revised Statutes, 1996 Supplement, 127.800-127.897.

and a patient for the purpose of determining whether the patient is suffering from a psychiatric or psychological disorder, or depression causing impaired judgment.

(5) "Health care provider" means a person licensed, certified, or otherwise authorized or permitted by the law of this State to administer health care in the ordinary course of business or practice of a profession, and includes a health care facility.

(6) "Incapable" means that in the opinion of a court or in the opinion of the patient's attending physician or consulting physician, a patient lacks the ability to make and communicate health care decisions to health care providers, including communication through persons familiar with the patient's manner of communicating if those persons are available. Capable means not incapable.

(7) "Informed decision" means a decision by a qualified patient, to request and obtain a prescription to end his or her life in a humane and dignified manner, that is based on an appreciation of the relevant facts and after being fully informed by the attending physician of:

    (a) his or her medical diagnosis;

    (b) his or her prognosis;

    (c) the potential risks associated with taking the medication to be prescribed;

    (d) the probable result of taking the medication to be prescribed;

    (e) the feasible alternatives, including, but not limited to, comfort care, hospice care and pain control.

(8) "Medically confirmed" means the medical opinion of the attending physician has been confirmed by a consulting physician who has examined the patient and the patient's relevant medical records.

(9) "Patient" means a person who is under the care of a physician.

(10) "Physician" means a doctor of medicine or osteopathy licensed to practice medicine by the Board of Medical Examiners for the State of Oregon.

(11) "Qualified patient" means a capable adult who is a resident of Oregon and has satisfied the requirements of this Act in order to obtain a prescription for medication to end his or her life in a humane and dignified manner.

(12) "Terminal disease" means an incurable and irreversible disease that has been medically confirmed and will, within reasonable medical judgment, produce death within six (6) months.

Section 2: Written Request for Medication to End One's Life in a Humane and Dignified Manner

2.01 Who may initiate a written request for medication

An adult who is capable, is a resident of Oregon, and has been determined by the attending physician and consulting physician to be suffering from a terminal disease, and who has voluntarily expressed his or her wish to die, may make a written request for medication for the purpose of ending his or her life in a humane and dignified manner in accordance with this Act.

2.02 Form of the written request

(1) A valid request for medication under this Act shall be in substantially the form described in Section 6 of this Act, signed and dated by the patient and witnessed by at least two individuals who, in the presence of the patient, attest that to the best of their knowledge and belief the patient is capable, acting voluntarily, and is not being coerced to sign the request.

(2) One of the witnesses shall be a person who is not:

    (a) A relative of the patient by blood, marriage or adoption;

    (b) A person who at the time the request is signed would be entitled to any portion of the estate of the qualified patient upon death under any will or by operation of law; or

    (c) An owner, operator or employee of a health care facility where the qualified patient is receiving medical treatment or is a resident.

(3) The patient's attending physician at the time the request is signed shall not be a witness.

(4) If the patient is a patient in a long term care facility at the time the written request is made, one of the witnesses shall be an individual

designated by the facility and having the qualifications specified by the Department of Human Resources by rule.

Section 3: Safeguards

3.01 Attending physician responsibilities

The attending physician shall:

(1) Make the initial determination of whether a patient has a terminal disease, is capable, and has made the request voluntarily;

(2) Inform the patient of:

    (a) his or her medical diagnosis;

    (b) his or her prognosis;

    (c) the potential risks associated with taking the medication to be prescribed;

    (d) the probable result of taking the medication to be prescribed;

    (e) the feasible alternatives, including, but not limited to, comfort care, hospice care and pain control.

(3) Refer the patient to a consulting physician for medical confirmation of the diagnosis, and for determination that the patient is capable and acting voluntarily;

(4) Refer the patient for counseling if appropriate pursuant to Section 3.03;

(5) Request that the patient notify next of kin;

(6) Inform the patient that he or she has an opportunity to rescind the request at any time and in any manner, and offer the patient an opportunity to rescind at the end of the 15 day waiting period pursuant to Section 3.06;

(7) Verify, immediately prior to writing the prescription for medication under this Act, that the patient is making an informed decision;

(8) Fulfill the medical record documentation requirements of Section 3.09;

(9) Ensure that all appropriate steps are carried out in accordance with this Act prior to writing a prescription for medication to enable a qualified patient to end his or her life in a humane and dignified manner.

3.02 Consulting physician confirmation

Before a patient is qualified under this Act, a consulting physician shall examine the patient and his or her relevant medical records and confirm, in writing, the attending physician's diagnosis that the patient is suffering from a terminal disease, and verify that the patient is capable, is acting voluntarily and has made an informed decision.

3.03 Counseling referral

If in the opinion of the attending physician or the consulting physician a patient may be suffering from a psychiatric or psychological disorder, or depression causing impaired judgment, either physician shall refer the patient for counseling. No medication to end a patient's life in a humane and dignified manner shall be prescribed until the person performing the counseling determines that the person is not suffering from a psychiatric or psychological disorder, or depression causing impaired judgment.

3.04 Informed decision

No person shall receive a prescription for medication to end his or her life in a humane and dignified manner unless he or she has made an informed decision as defined in Section 1.01(7). Immediately prior to writing a prescription for medication under this Act, the attending physician shall verify that the patient is making an informed decision.

3.05 Family notification

The attending physician shall ask the patient to notify next of kin of his or her request for medication pursuant to this Act. A patient who declines or is unable to notify next of kin shall not have his or her request denied for that reason.

3.06 Written and oral requests

In order to receive a prescription for medication to end his or her life in a humane and dignified manner, a qualified patient shall have made an oral request and a written request, and reiterate the oral request to his or her attending physician no less than fifteen (15) days after making the initial oral request. At the time the qualified patient makes his or her second oral request, the attending physician shall offer the patient an opportunity to rescind the request.

3.07 Right to rescind request

A patient may rescind his or her request at any time and in any manner without regard to his or her mental state. No prescription for medication under this Act may be written without the attending physician offering the qualified patient an opportunity to rescind the request.

3.08 Waiting periods

No less than fifteen (15) days shall elapse between the patient's initial and oral request and the writing of a prescription under this Act. No less than 48 hours shall elapse between the patient's written request and the writing of a prescription under this Act.

3.09 Medical record documentation requirements

The following shall be documented or filed in the patient's medical record:

(1) All oral requests by a patient for medication to end his or her life in a humane and dignified manner;

(2) All written requests by a patient for medication to end his or her life in a humane and dignified manner;

(3) The attending physician's diagnosis and prognosis, determination that the patient is capable, acting voluntarily and has made an informed decision.

(4) The consulting physician's diagnosis and prognosis, and verification that the patient is capable, acting voluntarily and has made an informed decision;

(5) A report of the outcome and determinations made during counseling, if performed;

(6) The attending physician's offer to the patient to rescind his or her request at the time of the patient's second oral request pursuant to Section 3.06; and

(7) A note by the attending physician indicating that all requirements under this Act have been met and indicating the steps taken to carry out the request, including a notation of the medication prescribed.

3.10 Residency requirement

Only requests made by Oregon residents, under this Act, shall be granted.

3.11 Reporting requirements

(1) The Health Division shall annually review a sample of records maintained pursuant to this Act.

(2) The Health Division shall make rules to facilitate the collection of information regarding compliance with this Act. The information collected shall not be a public record and may not be made available for inspection by the public.

(3) The Health Division shall generate and make available to the public an annual statistical report of information collected under Section 3.11(2) of this Act.

3.12 Effect on construction of wills, contracts and statutes

(1) No provision in a contract, will or other agreement, whether written or oral, to the extent the provision would affect whether a person may make or rescind a request for medication to end his or her life in a humane and dignified manner, shall be valid.

(2) No obligation owing under any currently existing contract shall be conditioned or affected by the making or rescinding of a request, by a person, for medication to end his or her life in a humane and dignified manner.

3.13 Insurance or annuity policies

The sale, procurement, or issuance of any life, health, or accident insurance or annuity policy or the rate charged for any policy shall not be conditioned upon or affected by the making or rescinding of a request, by a person, for medication to end his or her life in a humane and dignified manner. Neither shall a qualified patient's act of ingesting medication to end his or her life in a humane and dignified manner have an effect upon a life, health, or accident insurance or annuity policy.

3.14 Construction of Act

Nothing in this Act shall be construed to authorize a physician or any other person to end a patient's life by lethal injection, mercy killing or active euthanasia. Actions taken in accordance with this Act shall not, for any purpose, constitute suicide, assisted suicide, mercy killing or homicide, under the law.

Section 4: Immunities and Liabilities

4.01 Immunities

Except as provided in Section 4.02:

(1) No person shall be subject to civil or criminal liability or professional disciplinary action for participating in good faith compliance with this Act.

This includes being present when a qualified patient takes the prescribed medication to end his or her life in a humane and dignified manner.

(2) No professional organization or association, or health care provider, may subject a person to censure, discipline, suspension, loss of license, loss of privileges, loss of membership or other penalty for participating or refusing to participate in good faith compliance with this Act.

(3) No request by a patient for or provision by an attending physician of medication in good faith compliance with the provisions of this Act shall constitute neglect for any purpose of law or provide the sole basis for the appointment of a guardian or conservator.

(4) No health care provider shall be under any duty, whether by contract, by statute or by any other legal requirement to participate in the provision to a qualified patient of medication to end his or her life in a humane and dignified manner. If a health care provider is unable or unwilling to carry out a patient's request under this Act, and the patient transfers his or her care to a new health care provider, the prior health care provider shall transfer, upon request, a copy of the patient's relevant medical records to the new health care provider.

4.02 Liabilities

(1) A person who without authorization of the patient willfully alters or forges a request for medication or conceals or destroys a rescission of that request with the intent or effect of causing the patient's death shall be guilty of a Class A felony.

(2) A person who coerces or exerts undue influence on a patient to request medication for the purpose of ending the patient's life, or to destroy a rescission of such a request, shall be guilty of a Class A felony.

(3) Nothing in this Act limits further liability for civil damages resulting from other negligent conduct or intentional misconduct by any persons.

(4) The penalties in this Act do not preclude criminal penalties applicable under other law for conduct which is inconsistent with the provisions of this Act.

Section 5: Severability

5.01 Severability

Any section of this Act being held invalid as to any person or circumstance shall not affect the application of any other section of this Act which can be given full effect without the invalid section or application.

Section 6: Form of the Request

6.01 Form of the request

A request for a medication as authorized by this Act shall be in substantially the following form:

REQUEST FOR MEDICATION TO
END MY LIFE IN A HUMANE AND DIGNIFIED MANNER

I, _____, am an adult of sound mind.

I am suffering from _____, which my attending physician has determined is a terminal disease and which has been medically confirmed by a consulting physician.

I have been fully informed of my diagnosis, prognosis, the nature of medication to be prescribed and potential associated risks, the expected result, and the feasible alternatives, including comfort care, hospice care and pain control.

I request that my attending physician prescribe medication that will end my life in a humane and dignified manner.

INITIAL ONE:

_____ I have informed my family of my decision and taken their opinions into consideration.

_____ I have decided not to inform my family of my decision.

_____ I have no family to inform of my decision.

I understand that I have the right to rescind this request at any time.

I understand the full import of this request and I expect to die when I take the medication to be prescribed.

I make this request voluntarily and without reservation, and I accept full moral responsibility for my actions.

Signed: _____

Dated: _____

DECLARATION OF WITNESSES

We declare that the person signing this request:

(a) Is personally known to us or has provided proof of identity;

(b) Signed this request in our presence;

(c) Appears to be of sound mind and not under duress, fraud or undue influence;

(d) Is not a patient for whom either of us is attending physician.

_____ Witness 1/Date

_____ Witness 2/Date

NOTE: One witness shall not be a relative (by blood, marriage or adoption) of the person signing this request, shall not be entitled to any portion of the person's estate upon death and shall not own, operate or be employed at a health care facility where the person is a patient or resident. If the patient is an inpatient at a health care facility, one of the witnesses shall be an individual designated by the facility.

REGULATING PHYSICIAN-ASSISTED DEATH

Franklin G. Miller, Timothy E. Quill, Howard Brody, John C. Fletcher, Lawrence O. Gostin, and Diane E. Meier

The authors recommend legalization of physician-assisted death (a category that includes voluntary active euthanasia as well as physician-assisted suicide) in accordance with a regulatory scheme that they believe embodies adequate safeguards. In their view, physician-assisted death should be made available only to adults who retain decision-making capacity, but the practice should not be restricted solely to patients who are terminally ill; physician-assisted death should also be an available option for patients suffering from incurable, debilitating diseases. The authors insist that physician-assisted death must be considered a "treatment of last resort"—to be made available only if standard comfort-care measures fail to provide adequate relief from suffering. Certified palliative-care consultants, working in conjunction with regional palliative-care committees, are the cornerstone of the proposed regulatory scheme.

Reprinted by permission of the publisher from *The New England Journal of Medicine*, vol. 331 (July 14, 1994), pp. 119–123. Copyright © 1994 Massachusetts Medical Society. All rights reserved.

Public-opinion polls have consistently shown that approximately 60 percent of the American public favors legal reform allowing physician-assisted death as a last resort to end the suffering of competent patients.[1] Yet the voters in Washington State in 1991 and California in 1992 narrowly defeated referendums that would have permitted physicians to prescribe or administer lethal treatment to terminally ill patients. The lack of adequate safeguards to protect vulnerable patients and prevent abuse may have been an important factor in the rejection of these legislative proposals.[2] In this article we describe a policy of legalized physician-assisted death restricted to competent patients suffering from terminal illness or incurable, debilitating disease who voluntarily request to end their lives. Integral to this policy is a framework of regulation with safeguards that we believe are adequate to protect patients, preserve the professional integrity of physicians, and assure the public that voluntary physician-assisted death occurs only as a last resort.

Voluntary physician-assisted death serves the moral goals of relief of suffering and self-determination on the part of patients.[3-5] It becomes a permissible option when comfort care ceases to be effective for the terminally or incurably ill. ("Comfort care" refers to palliative and supportive treatment used in hospice programs and elsewhere.) Comfort care ought to be the standard medical treatment for patients who are suffering from a terminal illness or who have refused curative or life-sustaining treatment.[3] It is aimed at relieving symptoms, enhancing the quality and meaning of the patient's remaining life, and easing the process of dying. As a treatment of last resort, physician-assisted death becomes a legitimate option only after standard measures for comfort care have been found unsatisfactory by competent patients in the context of their own situation and values. Accordingly, the policy we recommend aims to promote comfort care and to permit voluntary physician-assisted death only in the relatively infrequent but troubling cases in which comfort care is inadequate. . . .

THE RATIONALE FOR REGULATION

Decisions about medical treatment are normally made in the privacy of the doctor-patient relationship.[6] Yet regulatory safeguards providing independent monitoring of medical decisions that involve physician-assisted death are necessary for two reasons. First, any treatment whose purpose is to cause death lies outside standard medical practice, which is defined here as medically indicated interventions aimed at promoting health and healing and alleviating the suffering of patients. Currently accepted standards of comfort care allow for the use of aggressive palliative treatment that may indirectly and unintentionally contribute to a patient's death.[3] However, standards of comfort care stop short of permitting death to be caused intentionally as a means of ending unrelievable suffering.

We regard physician-assisted death as a nonstandard medical practice reserved for extraordinary circumstances, when it is requested voluntarily by a patient whose suffering has become intolerable and who has no other satisfactory options. Although we argue that physician-assisted death should be permitted as a treatment of last resort, we do not claim that patients have a right to physician-assisted death, as they do to standard medical care. Physicians must carefully assess patients' requests for assistance in dying and thoroughly explore alternatives for comfort care.[7] In addition, they must consider their own values and willingness to participate in physician-assisted death. Because of the nonstandard nature of physician-assisted death, even when patients and physicians agree that there are no acceptable alternatives, regulatory oversight should be required.

The second reason for regulating physician-assisted death is the risk of abuse of vulnerable patients. In addition to the highly publicized and problematic assisted suicides in which Jack Kevorkian has participated, there is evidence of a relatively widespread secret practice of physician-assisted death in the United States, which is completely unregulated.[8] Voluntary physician-assisted death has been widely practiced in the Netherlands in recent years, although it remains technically illegal.[9] Studies indicate that Dutch physicians have provided lethal treatment to some suffering incompetent patients who have made no request to die.[10-12] The Dutch practice of physician-assisted death is carried out mainly in the privacy of the doctor-patient relationship, subject to guidelines that are not independently monitored.

The risks of abuse in the absence of regulatory safeguards might be greater in the United States than in the Netherlands because of the pressures for cost containment in our health care system, the burdens imposed on family members by the responsibility of caring for dying patients, and our cultural penchant for seeking technological solutions to complex medical and social problems. Therefore, an acceptable policy of legalized physician-assisted death must include independent monitoring to ensure that it is used only as a treatment of last resort in response to the voluntary requests of competent patients who are suffering from terminal or incurable illnesses.

LEGISLATION AS AN APPROPRIATE VEHICLE FOR REFORM

We believe that state legislation is the most appropriate means of expanding the options of suffering patients while establishing adequate safeguards, and of achieving greater clarity and fairness in policies concerning physician-assisted death. Legislators are elected and demonstrably accountable for their decisions. They also have the opportunity for the careful consideration of policy decisions through public hearings and debate. Accordingly, they can thoughtfully design laws and regulatory procedures to guide professional practice and safeguard against abuse.

Several attempts to legalize physician-assisted death have come in the form of state referendums. Though referendums epitomize democracy, they can be inadequate mechanisms for the development of complex public policy. Votes on referendums are subject to substantial influence by interest groups that can afford to spend large amounts of money on advertising. More important, the electorate can only approve or disapprove the proposed legislation but cannot alter its language. As demonstrated in Washington and California, referendums often offer simple solutions without careful attention to clear criteria, rigorous procedures, and adequate safeguards.

A federal district court judge recently held that a Washington State law prohibiting assisted suicide unconstitutionally interferes with liberty and privacy interests protected by the Fourteenth Amendment.[13] This case raises the question of whether the judicial branch of government might provide the impetus for reform. It is conceivable that reasoning applied to treatment-refusal cases could also be applied to physician-assisted death.[14,15] The chief disadvantage of judicial activism in this area is the difficulty courts may have in specifying detailed criteria and procedures to protect vulnerable patients. State legislatures are better positioned to design adequate safeguards for the appropriate use of physician-assisted death.

OBJECTIVES OF REGULATORY POLICY

We believe a policy regulating physician-assisted death should be designed with the following objectives: (1) to promote comfort care as standard treatment for dying patients; (2) to permit physician-assisted death only for competent patients suffering from terminal or incurable debilitating illnesses who voluntarily and repeatedly request to die; (3) to develop and promote practice guidelines for voluntary physician-assisted death aimed at making lethal treatment available only as a last resort for unrelievable suffering; (4) to provide independent and impartial oversight of decisions to pursue voluntary physician-assisted death without undue disruption of the doctor-patient relationship; (5) to provide a mechanism for prospective committee review of difficult or disputed cases; and (6) to ensure public accountability.

THE SCOPE OF LEGALIZED PHYSICIAN-ASSISTED DEATH

Our recommended policy reflects choices concerning two difficult issues: whether physician-assisted death should be limited to physician-assisted suicide, thus excluding voluntary, active euthanasia, and whether eligible patients must be only those for whom death is imminent or whether those who are not terminally ill but who suffer from incurable and debilitating conditions such as amyotrophic lateral sclerosis may also be considered eligible. We have opted for a liberal, inclusive policy with respect to these issues. To confine legalized physician-assisted death to assisted suicide unfairly discriminates against patients with unrelievable suffering who resolve to end their lives but are physically unable to do so. The method chosen is less important than the careful assessment that precedes assisted death. Limiting physician-assisted death to patients with terminal illness would deny this option of last resort to incurably, but not terminally, ill patients who make a rational decision to end their lives because of unremitting suffering. Physician-assisted death would be appropriate only after thorough consideration of potential ways to improve the patient's quality of life. We believe that the regulatory safeguards described below would minimize the risks associated with the legalization of physician-assisted death for patients who are not terminally ill and with the possibility of voluntary, active euthanasia.

OVERVIEW OF POLICY

The general responsibility for regulating physician-assisted death would be lodged with regional palliative-care committees. Case-specific oversight of decisions to undertake physician-assisted death would be provided by physicians certified as palliative-care consultants, who would report to the palliative-care committees. Treating physicians would be prohibited from providing lethal treatment without prior consultation and review by an independent, certified palliative-care consultant. The palliative-care committee would be available for prospective review in difficult or disputed cases.

In order to ensure that physician-assisted death is voluntary, which is the inviolable cornerstone of this policy, only adults with decision-making capacity should be eligible for physician-assisted death. Written or witnessed oral consent by the patient must be obtained. No physician would be obligated to participate in physician-assisted death. Treating physicians would be required to report death by assisted suicide or the administration of lethal treatment to the proper public authority. Physicians who provided lethal treatment without compliance with the legal requirements would be liable to professional sanctions and criminal penalties.

PALLIATIVE-CARE CONSULTANTS

Independent and impartial oversight by a certified palliative-care consultant is a vital safeguard in this proposed policy of legalized physician-assisted death. Palliative-care consultants would be physicians with experience in treating dying patients, who were knowledgeable about and committed to comfort care, skilled in the assessment of the decision-making capacity of patients suffering from terminal or incurable conditions, and well educated about the ethics of end-of-life decision making. In order to institute effective consultation, new programs for the training and certification of palliative-care consultants would need to be developed and implemented. We do not envision the creation of a new medical specialty devoted to palliative-care consultation. Rather, certified consultants would be practicing physicians who routinely care for severely ill and dying patients and spend part of their time in the role of palliative-care consultant. It is essential that these consultants, who would oversee decisions to perform physician-assisted death, be aware firsthand of the clinical reality faced by suffering patients and their physicians.

The requirement for oversight by a member of an approved panel of palliative-care consultants goes beyond the guidelines in the Netherlands and the referendum questions in Washington and California, which merely stipulated consultation with a physician other than the treating physician.[16] The goal is to require a rigorous, independent second opinion by an accountable expert in the light of the objectives of the regulatory policy.

Review by an independent palliative-care consultant would be required whenever a patient and a physician, after thorough deliberation, agreed to pursue the option of physician-assisted death. This consultative oversight would include the examination of medical records and interviews with the treating physician, the patient, and interested members of the patient's family. The consultant would review the patient's diagnosis and prognosis and explore whether the treating physician and patient had considered carefully all reasonable alternatives.[17] The process of consultation might lead to improved pain management or the use of other means of comfort care. The consultant would assess the voluntariness of the patient's request to die and the strength of his or her resolve, paying careful attention to the possibility of distorted thinking or undue pressure by others who might be burdened with caring for the patient. The consultant could request additional expert advice if there was uncertainty about the patient's competence or medical condition or about the adequacy of palliative measures.

Certified palliative-care consultants would have the authority to override agreements by patients and physicians to undertake physician-assisted death. The consultants would be required to prepare a reasoned and clearly articulated statement justifying their judgment that physician-assisted death was inappropriate. In addition, the patient and physician would have the right to appeal the consultant's judgment to the palliative-care committee. In all cases the palliative-care consultant would prepare a confidential written report that would be submitted to the palliative-care committee for retrospective monitoring. The palliative-care consultants would have the option of referring difficult or uncertain cases for prospective review to the palliative-care committees.

PALLIATIVE-CARE COMMITTEES

Regional palliative-care committees, made up of professional and lay members, would perform a variety of functions. The committees would develop, issue, and revise practice guidelines for physicians to supplement the legal requirements for physician-assisted death. For example, in order to avoid undue influence on vulnerable patients, the request for the consideration of lethal treatment must come from patients, and physicians should accede only after fully exploring the meaning of the patients' request to die and the available alternatives.[7]

The palliative-care committees would be responsible for educating clinicians and the public about methods of comfort care (including pain management), ethical standards of informed refusal and discontinuation of life-sustaining treatment, and the option of physician-assisted death. This educational activity would cover topics such as the law, practice guidelines, and the relevant regulations; how treating physicians should respond to requests by patients for the termination of life; methods of comfort care as an alternative to physician-assisted death; and effective methods of lethal treatment. The committees would engage in routine retrospective monitoring of cases of physician-assisted death, basing their review on reports filed by the palliative-care consultants. Finally, the committees would review prospectively difficult cases referred by palliative-care consultants and appeals from patients or their primary care physicians when their negotiated requests for physician-assisted death were disapproved by the palliative-care consultants.

BALANCING THE BENEFITS AND BURDENS OF REGULATION

The process of regulation should be aimed at striking a balance between competing imperatives. On the one hand, physician-assisted death should not be an easy way out for suffering patients and their physicians. On the other hand, oversight should not be so restrictive and onerous as to deprive patients of an adequate response to intolerable suffering.

It might be objected that the policy we recommend is unworkable because it is too cumbersome and intrusive. Such an objection might be justified in the case of a policy requiring mandatory prior committee review or a court hearing to authorize physician-assisted death. Review by a certified palliative-care consultant, however, seems comparable to other consultations by specialists. For a decision of this magnitude, an independent expert opinion is clearly desirable. Some patients and physicians might still feel burdened by such oversight, especially in difficult cases referred or appealed to the palliative-care committee. We believe that this is a price worth paying to protect vulnerable patients and to ensure public accountability. Critical to the success of this policy, however, would be the timely availability of palliative-care consultants, education that emphasized the sensitive nature of the oversight function, and scrupulous protection of confidentiality.

EVALUATIVE RESEARCH

Since there is no guarantee that the danger of abuse can be completely eliminated, a policy of regulating physician-assisted death should be viewed as experimental, and evaluative research should be built into any implementing legislation. Such research would be designed to determine and assess how physician-assisted death worked in practice, and to provide information helpful for modifying guidelines and procedures with the aim of improving the policy.

Two types of research would be desirable. First, to assess the effects of the policy, aggregate data should be collected and analyzed. These might include the number and disposition of cases reviewed by palliative-care consultants and palliative-care committees; the demographic characteristics and medical condition of patients requesting physician-assisted death; the location, methods, and circumstances of physician-assisted death; the attitudes of participating physicians and family members; the physicians' opinions of the regulatory process; and the long-term consequences for participants. Second, we recommend research into the personal and cultural meaning of physician-assisted death. In-depth interviews might be conducted with some patients, family members, treating physicians, and palliative-care consultants; researchers might witness the entire process of considering, reviewing, and providing physician-assisted death, subject to requirements of informed consent and confidentiality.

CONCLUSIONS

The ethical norms of relieving suffering and respecting patients' rights to self-determination support the permissibility of voluntary physician-assisted death as a last resort for terminally or incurably ill patients. The availability of the extraordinary option of lethal treatment, however, must be accompanied by careful regulation to minimize the risk of abuse. We recommend that physician-assisted death be legalized with adequate safeguards to protect vulnerable patients, preserve the professional integrity of physicians, and ensure accountability to the public. The policy we have outlined would ensure independent and impartial review of decisions to provide physician-assisted death in response to unrelievable suffering, without undue disruption of the doctor-patient relationship. We hope one or more states will decide democratically to expand the options for dying or incurably ill patients by implementing a policy that both promotes comfort care and permits voluntary physician-assisted death as a last resort.

REFERENCES

1 Blendon R. J., Szalay U. S., Knox R. A. Should physicians aid their patients in dying? The public perspective. JAMA 1992; 267:2658–62.

2 McGough P. M. Washington state initiative 119: the first public vote on legalizing physician-assisted death. Cambridge Q Healthcare Ethics 1993; 2: 63–7.

3 Quill T. E. Death and dignity. New York: W.W. Norton, 1993.

4 Brody H. Assisted death—a compassionate response to a medical failure. N Engl J Med 1992; 327:1384–8.

5 Miller F. G., Fletcher J. C. The case for legalized euthanasia. Perspect Biol Med 1993; 36:159–76.

6 Annas G. J., Glantz L. H., Mariner W. K. The right of privacy protects the doctor-patient relationship. JAMA 1990; 263:858–61.

7 Quill T. E. Doctor, I want to die. Will you help me? JAMA 1993; 270:870–3.

8 Meier D. E. Doctors' attitudes and experiences with physician-assisted death: a review of the literature. In: Humber J. M., Almeder R. F., Kasting G. A., eds. Physician-assisted death. Totowa, N.J.: Humana Press, 1994:5–24.

9 van der Maas P. J., van Delden J. J. M., Pijnenborg L., Looman C. W. N. Euthanasia and other medical decisions concerning the end of life. Lancet 1991; 338:669–74.

10 Gomez C. F. Regulating death. New York: Free Press, 1991.

11 ten Have H. A., Welie J. V. Euthanasia: normal medical practice? Hastings Cent Rep 1992; 22:34–8.

12 Pijnenborg L., van der Maas P. J., van Delden J. J. M., Looman C. W. N. Life-terminating acts without explicit request of patient. Lancet 1993; 341:1196–9.

13 Egan T. Federal judge says ban on suicide aid is unconstitutional. New York Times. May 5, 1994:A1.

14 Note: physician-assisted suicide and the right to die with assistance. Harvard Law Rev 1992; 105:2021.

15 Gostin L., Weir R. F. Life and death choices after Cruzan: case law and standards of professional conduct, Milbank Q. 1991; 69:143–73.

16 A dozen caveats concerning the discussion of euthanasia in the Netherlands. In: Battin M. P. The least worst death. New York: Oxford University Press, 1994:130–44.

17 Quill T. E., Cassel C. K., Meier D. E. Care of the hopelessly ill—proposed clinical criteria for physician-assisted suicide. N Engl J Med 1992; 327: 1380–4.

ON THE SLIPPERY SLOPE IN THE EMPIRE STATE: THE NEW YORK STATE TASK FORCE ON PHYSICIAN-ASSISTED DEATH

John D. Arras

Arras provides an account of the considerations that led the New York State Task Force on Life and the Law to oppose legalization of both physician-assisted suicide and active euthanasia. Although some members of the task force also based their opposition to legalization on other arguments, the entire membership agreed that the likely social consequences of legalization are sufficiently problematic to warrant strong opposition. Arras constructs the argument from social consequences as a "slippery-slope" argument, and he essentially distinguishes two prongs—each somewhat complex—in the overall argument. The first prong, based on an analysis of the logic of justification for legalization, focuses concern on the likelihood that any initial narrowly drawn policy for the legalization of physician-assisted death would lead to an expansion of the original boundaries. The second prong of the slippery-slope argument focuses concern on the strong likelihood that any system providing criteria for the availability of physician-assisted death would be abused. Arras also provides a brief exposition of the task force's call for "a positive program of clinical and social reform," and he concludes by offering a critical response to the regulatory scheme proposed by Miller et al. in the previous selection.

THE TASK FORCE AND ITS CONCLUSIONS

Created by Governor Mario Cuomo in 1984, the New York State Task Force on Life and the Law has provided ethical analysis and policy recommendations to the people and legislature of New York on a host of important issues in bioethics, including brain death, organ transplantation, surrogate parenting, and forgoing life-sustaining treatment. The Task Force is composed of 25 members drawn from a wide variety of professional affiliations and geographical locations within the state. The membership includes clergy representing all four great New York religions—i.e., Catholics, Jews, Protestants, and the ACLU—as well as physicians, nurses, social workers, attorneys, law professors, consumer advocates, and two philosopher/bioethicists (Professor Samuel Gorovitz of Syracuse University and, until recently, myself).

Reprinted with permission of the American Philosophical Association from *Newsletter on Philosophy and Medicine,* in *APA Newsletters,* vol. 95, no. 2, Spring 1996, pp. 80–83.

Although the Task Force had consistently displayed strong enthusiasm for the value of individual autonomy in its previous reports on DNR orders,[1] health care proxies,[2] and surrogate decision making,[3] it emphasized the limits of autonomy in its May 1994 report, *When Death Is Sought: Assisted Suicide and Euthanasia in the Medical Context.* In an extraordinary display of consensus within a non-partisan and strongly pluralistic group, the Task Force had unanimously agreed to retain the present legal and policy barriers to physician-assisted suicide (PAS) and active euthanasia.

In spite of their agreement to uphold the ban on PAS and active euthanasia, the members disagreed sharply over the rationale for this conclusion. One faction strongly condemned both practices as inherently immoral, as violations of the moral rule against killing the innocent. Another faction primarily objected to the fact that physicians were being called upon to do the killing. While conceding that killing the terminally ill or assisting in their suicides might not always be morally wrong for others to do, this group maintained that the participation of physicians in such practices would undermine their role as healers and fatally compromise the physician-patient relationship. Finally, a third faction, the one to which I belonged during my tenure with the Task Force, readily conceded that neither PAS nor active euthanasia were always morally wrong, whether practiced by ordinary citizens or by physicians. On the contrary, we believed that in certain rare instances early release from a painful or intolerably degrading existence might constitute both a positive good and an important exercise of personal autonomy for the individual. Indeed, several of us conceded that should such a terrible fate befall us, we would hope to find a thoughtful, compassionate, and courageous physician (such as Dr. Timothy Quill) to release us from our misery. But in spite of these important concessions, these members shrank from endorsing or regulating PAS and active euthanasia due to fears bearing on the social consequences of liberalization.

Notwithstanding these internal disagreements, the entire membership of the Task Force agreed that the law should not be changed. We also unanimously endorsed the reasoning of the third faction bearing on the dangers of the slippery slope. Because this reasoning proved decisive within the deliberations of the Task Force, I shall devote the remainder of this brief commentary to a fuller exposition of the argument from social consequences. This complex argument is not only important for understanding the position of the Task Force, but it is also crucial for evaluating some recent proposals for legalization and regulation.

MORALITY VERSUS POLICY

Crucial to the Task Force's analysis was the distinction between the morality of individual acts and the wisdom of social policy. Much of the debate in the popular media is driven by the depiction of especially dramatic and poignant instances of suffering humanity, desperate for release from the painful thrall of terminal illness. Quite understandably, many if not most of us are prompted to respond, "Should such a terrible fate ever befall me, I would certainly not want to suffer interminably; I would want the option of an early exit and the help of my trusted physician in securing it." The problem, however, lies in getting from such compelling individual

cases to social policy. The issue is not simply, "What would I want?", but rather what is the best social policy, all things considered. The Task Force warns that we cannot make this jump from individual case to policy without endangering the autonomy and the very lives of others, many of whom are numbered among our most vulnerable citizens.

THE WISH TO DIE AND THE FAILURE OF MEDICINE

The Task Force recognized that many people advocate legalization because they fear a loss of control at the end of life. They fear falling victim to the technological imperative; they fear dying in chronic and uncontrolled pain; and they fear the psychological suffering attendant upon the relentless disintegration of the self. All of these fears, it so happens, are eminently justified. As the SUPPORT study recently demonstrated with such depressing clarity, physicians routinely ignore the documented wishes of patients and all-too-often allow patients to die with uncontrolled pain.[4] Studies of cancer patients have shown that over 50% suffer from unrelieved pain. The Task Force found that uncontrolled pain, particularly when accompanied by feelings of hopelessness and untreated depression, is a significant contributing factor for suicide and suicidal ideation.

Clinical depression is another major factor. Depression accompanied by feelings of hopelessness is the strongest predictor of suicide for both individuals who are terminally ill and those who are not. Yet most doctors are not trained to notice depression, especially in complex cases such as the elderly suffering from terminal illness. And even when doctors succeed in diagnosing depression, they often do not successfully treat it with readily available medications in sufficient amounts.

The Task Force found that the vast majority of patients who request PAS or euthanasia are capable of being successfully treated both for their depression and their pain, and that when they receive adequate psychiatric and palliative care, their requests to die are usually withdrawn. In other words, patients given the requisite control over their lives and relief from depression and pain usually lose interest in PAS and euthanasia. This fact is of enormous importance for our evaluation of PAS and euthanasia as social policies, for if the root causes or motivations for assisted death can be successfully addressed for most patients through the delivery of technically competent and compassionate medicine, the case for changing the law loses much of its urgency.

But it does not, alas, lose all of its urgency. The Task Force recognized as well that a small percentage of patients suffer from conditions both physical and psychological that lie beyond the current reach of medicine and humane care. Some pain cannot be alleviated short of inducing a permanent state of unconsciousness in the patient; and some depression is unconquerable. For such unfortunate patients, the present law can represent an insuperable barrier to a dignified and decent death. While the Task Force expressed its compassion for the sufferings of such patients, its members were ultimately convinced that they could not be helped in a public way—i.e., be given publicly-sanctioned assistance in committing suicide—without endangering a far greater number of highly vulnerable patients.

In this sense, the Task Force members were painfully aware of the "tragic" nature of the choice confronting them. Whether they opted for a reaffirmation of the current legal restraints or for a policy of legitimation and regulation, there were bound to be victims. The victims of the current policy are easy to identify; they are on the news, the talk shows and the documentaries, and often on Dr. Kevorkian's roster of "patients." But who would be the victims of a more permissive policy? What exactly does the slippery slope argument amount to here?

AN "OPTION WITHOUT LIMITS"

The Task Force's first point is that a socially sanctioned practice of PAS would in all likelihood prove difficult, if not impossible, to cabin within its originally anticipated boundaries. The proponents of legalization usually begin with a wholesomely modest policy agenda, limiting their suggested reforms to a narrow and highly specified range of potential candidates and practices. "Give us PAS, not the more controversial practice of active euthanasia, for presently competent patients who are terminally ill and suffering unbearable pain." But the logic of the case for PAS, based as it is upon the twin pillars of patient autonomy and mercy, makes it highly unlikely

that society could stop with this modest proposal once it had ventured out on the slope. As numerous other critics have pointed out, if autonomy is the prime consideration, then additional constraints based upon terminal illness and/or unbearable pain would appear hard to justify. Indeed, if autonomy is crucial, the requirement of unbearable suffering would appear to be entirely subjective. Who is to say—other than the patient herself—how much suffering is too much? Likewise, the requirement of terminal illness seems an arbitrary standard against which to judge patients' own subjective evaluation of their quality of life. If my life is no longer worth living, why should a terminally ill cancer patient be granted PAS but not me, merely because my suffering is due to my "non-terminal" ALS or intractable psychiatric disorder?

Alternatively, if pain and suffering are deemed crucial to the justification of legalization, it is hard to see how the proposed barrier of contemporaneous consent of competent patients could withstand serious erosion. If the logic of PAS is at all similar to that of forgoing life-sustaining treatments—and we have every reason to think it so—then it would seem almost inevitable that a case would soon be made to permit PAS for incompetent patients who had left advance directives, followed by a "substituted judgment" test for patients who "would have wanted" PAS, and finally an "objective" test for patients (including newborns) whose best interests would be served by PAS or active euthanasia even in the absence of any subjective intent.

In the same way, the joint justifications of autonomy and mercy would combine to undermine the plausibility of a line drawn between PAS and active euthanasia. As the authors of one highly publicized proposal have come to see, the logic of justification for active euthanasia is identical to that of PAS.[5] Legalizing PAS while continuing to ban active euthanasia, would serve only to discriminate unfairly against patients who are suffering and wish to end their lives, but cannot do so because of some physical impairment. Surely these patients, it will be said, are "the worst off group" and therefore the most in need of the assistance of others who will do for them what they can no longer accomplish on their own.

None of these initial slippery slope considerations, it must be conceded, constitute knock-down objections to further liberalization of our laws and practices. It is not obvious, after all, that each of these highly predictable shifts—e.g., from terminal to "merely" incurable, from contemporaneous consent to best interests, and from PAS to active euthanasia—are patently immoral and unjustifiable. Still, in pointing out this likely slippage, the Task Force is calling on society to think about the likely consequences of taking the first tentative step onto the slope. If all of the extended practices predicted above pose substantially greater risks for vulnerable patients than the more highly circumscribed initial liberalization proposals, then we need to factor in these additional risks even as we ponder those more modest proposals.[6]

THE LIKELIHOOD OF ABUSE

The second prong of the slippery slope argument deployed by the Task Force argues that whatever criteria for justifiable PAS and active euthanasia are ultimately chosen, abuse of the system is highly likely to follow. In other words, patients who fall outside the ambit of our justifiable criteria will soon be candidates for death. This prong resembles what I have elsewhere called an "empirical slope"[7] argument, since it is based not on the close logical resemblance of concepts or justifications, but rather on an empirical prediction of what is likely to happen once we insert a particular social practice into our existing social system.

The Task Force made three assumptions about the requirements of any potentially justifiable social policy of PAS or active euthanasia. First, it would have to insist that all requests for death be voluntary; second, that all reasonable alternatives to PAS and active euthanasia must be explored before acceding to a patient's wishes; and third, a reliable system of reporting all cases must be established in order to effectively monitor these practices and respond to abuses. We argued that, given social reality as we know it, all three assumptions are problematic.

With regard to the voluntariness requirement, we contended that many requests would not be sufficiently voluntary. In addition to the subtlely coercive influences of physicians and family members, perhaps the most slippery aspect of this slope is the highly predictable failure of most physicians reliably to diagnose and treat reversible clinical depression, especially in the elderly population. As one geriatric psychiatrist testified, we now live in the "golden age" of treating depression but the "lead age" of diagnosing it.[8] We have the tools, but physicians are not adequately trained and motivated to use them. So unless dramatic changes are effected in the practice of medicine, we can predict with confidence that many instances of PAS and active euthanasia will constitute abuses of the original criterion of voluntariness.

As to the second requirement, given the abysmal track record of physicians in responding adequately to pain and suffering, we can also confidently predict that in many cases all reasonable alternatives will not have been exhausted. Instead of vigorously addressing the pharmacologic and psycho-social needs of such patients, physicians will no doubt continue to ignore, undertreat, or treat them in an impersonal manner. The result will be more depression, desperation, and requests for physician-assisted death from patients who could have been successfully treated. The root causes of this predictable lapse are manifold, but include such factors as the inaccessibility of decent primary care to over 37 million Americans, the appalling lack of training in palliative care even among primary care physicians and cancer specialists, discrimination in the delivery of pain control (and other medical treatments) on the basis of race and economic status, various myths shared by both physicians and patients about the supposed ill effects of pain medications, and restrictive state laws on access to opioids.

Finally, the Task Force doubts that any reporting system would be sufficiently effective to adequately monitor these practices. A great deal depends here on the extent to which patients and practitioners will regard these practices as essentially *private* matters to be discussed and acted upon within the privacy of the doctor-patient relationship. As the Dutch experience has conclusively demonstrated, physicians will be extremely loath to report instances of PAS and active euthanasia to public authorities, largely for fear of bringing the harsh glare of publicity upon families at times when privacy is most needed. The likely result of this lack of oversight will be society's inability to respond appropriately to disturbing incidents and long-term trends. In other words, the practice will not be as amenable to regulation as the proponents contend.

A PRUDENTIAL CONCLUSION

The Task Force's argument can be summed up, then, as follows:

1. The number of "genuine cases" justifying PAS and/or active euthanasia will be relatively small. Patients who receive good personal care, good pain relief, treatment for depression, and adequate psychosocial supports tend not to persist in a desire to die.

2. The social risks of legalization are serious and highly predictable. They include the expansion of these practices to nonvoluntary cases and the widespread failure to pursue readily available alternatives to suicide motivated by pain, depression, and hopelessness.

3. Rather than propose a momentous and dangerous policy shift for a relatively small number of "genuine cases"—a shift, by the way, that would surely involve a great deal of persistent social division and strife analogous to that involved in the abortion controversy—we should instead attempt to redirect the public debate toward a goal on which we can and should all agree—viz., the manifest and urgent need to reform the way we die in America. Instead of launching a highly divisive and dangerous campaign for PAS, why not attack the problem at its root with an ambitious program of reform in the areas of access to primary care and the education of physicians in palliative care? At least as far as the "slippery slope faction" within the Task Force is concerned, we should thus first see to it that every person in this country has access to adequate, affordable, and nondiscriminatory primary and palliative care. At the end of this long and arduous process, when we

finally have an equitable, effective, and compassionate health care system in place, we might well want to reopen the discussion of PAS and active euthanasia.

4. Finally, with regard to those few unfortunate patients who are truly beyond the pale of good palliative and psychiatric care, some Task Force members took limited solace from the fact that many such patients will still be able to find compassionate physicians who, like Dr. Quill, will ultimately be willing, albeit in fear and trembling, to "take small risks for patients [they] really care about." Such actions will continue to take place within the privacy of the patient-physician relationship, however, and will thus not threaten vulnerable patients and the social fabric to the extent that would result from full legalization and regulation. To be sure, this kind of continuing covert PAS will not be subject to regulation, but the mere threat of possible criminal sanctions and revocation of licensure will continue to serve as a powerful disincentive to abuse for the vast majority of physicians. Moreover, as we have seen, it is highly unlikely that the proposals for legalization would result in truly effective oversight.

A POSITIVE AGENDA

Instead of conceiving this as a choice between legalization/regulation, with all of their attendant risks, and the abandonment of patients to their pain and suffering, the Task Force thus recommends a positive program of clinical and social reform. On the clinical level, physicians must learn how better to listen to their patients, to unflinchingly engage them in sensitive discussions of their needs and the meaning of their requests for assisted death, to deliver appropriate palliative care, to distinguish fact from fiction in the ethics and law of pain relief, to diagnose and treat clinical depression, and, finally, to ascertain and respect their patients' wishes for control regarding the forgoing of life-sustaining treatments. On the social level, the Task Force perceives a need for major initiatives in medical and public education regarding pain control, in the sensitization of insurance companies and licensing agencies to issues of the quality of dying, and in the reform of state laws that currently hinder access to pain relieving medications.

A RECENT CHALLENGE

The Task Force's slippery slope argument has recently been indirectly challenged by the authors of an interesting new legislative proposal for regulation.[9] Two points about this proposal are worth briefly mentioning here before closing. First, the authors concede what some of them had explicitly denied in a previous proposal, viz., that the logic of the matter cannot effectively distinguish between PAS and active euthanasia on the one hand, and between terminal illness and ("merely") incurable conditions like ALS on the other. They should thus be commended for forthrightly identifying the crucial parameters of the issue for public debate.

Second, the authors propose an additional safeguard designed to address most of our "empirical slope" objections: viz., a requirement of independent and impartial oversight by a certified palliative-care consultant within a national network of palliative-care committees. Before any choice for death arrived at by patient and physician could be sanctioned within this proposed system, a certified consultant would have to review the patient's diagnosis and prognosis, the possibility of available but untried alternatives for palliative care, the voluntariness and strength of the patient's wish to die, and so on. Consultants would presumably all be well versed in the techniques of palliative care, the nuances of competency, bioethics and law, and in the lived reality of dying patients. Should a patient and/or physician disagree with the verdict of a consultant, they could appeal the case to the consultant's regional committee.

To be sure, this part of the proposal marks a significant improvement over past proposals and legislative ballot initiatives. The requirements that voluntariness and competency be verified by a skilled diagnostician/clinician, and that either PAS or active euthanasia be permitted only after the failure of all other reasonable alternatives, would both

go a long way toward providing serious safeguards and assuaging the Task Force's fears of an unalterably slippery slope. I for one, however, have a couple of reservations.

First, there is the lingering fear, expressed throughout the Task Force's report, that any legislative proposal would have to be implemented within the present context of deep and pervasive discrimination against the poor and members of minority groups. We have every reason to expect that a policy that worked tolerably well in an affluent community like Scarsdale might not work so well in a community like Bedford-Stuyvesant or Harlem. There is also reason to worry about any policy of PAS initiated within a growing system of managed care, capitation, and physician-incentives for delivering less care. Expert palliative care is no doubt an expensive and time-consuming proposition, requiring more rather than less time spent just talking with patients. It is highly doubtful that the context of physician-patient conversation within this new dispensation will be at all conducive to humane decisions untainted by subtle economic coercion.

Second, it must be noted that the impressive safeguards required by this proposal would entail significant costs in terms of privacy and autonomy for both patients and physicians. Even though these particular authors deny that their brief is based upon a "right to PAS"—which would itself be based upon the right to privacy in the same manner as abortion;[10]—they will have a hard time explaining this to patients whose appeals have been rejected by the palliative-care consultant and committee. Just as the elaborate paraphernalia of committee review of abortion decisions was swept aside by autonomy-driven judicial decisions in *Roe* v. *Wade* and *Doe* v. *Bolton* (1973), so here patients imbued with the rhetoric of autonomy will surely ask, "Who do these so-called 'consultants' and 'God-committees' think they are, passing judgment on the quality of my own very personal suffering?" And physicians, for their part, will surely be mightily offended by the implication that they cannot be trusted to handle these matters in a competent and sensitive way within the privacy of the physician-patient relationship without a new layer of intrusive and expensive bureaucracy. Indeed, to my mind, the biggest problem for the proponents of this plan would come, not from opponents of PAS on slippery slope grounds, but rather from patients and physicians eager, in the age of Newt, to cast off all remaining vestiges of state-sponsored bureaucracy. In short, the proposed regulations are plausible, at least in theory; but whether they could be sold to skeptical legislatures is a different and much more difficult question.

NOTES

1 *Do Not Resuscitate Orders,* April 1986.

2 *Life-Sustaining Treatment: Making Decisions and Appointing a Health Care Agent,* July 1987.

3 *When Others Must Choose: Deciding for Patients Without Capacity,* May 1992.

4 SUPPORT Principal Investigators, "A Controlled Trial to Improve Care for Seriously Ill Hospitalized Patients: The Study to Understand Prognoses and Preferences for Outcomes and Risks of Treatments (SUPPORT)," *JAMA* 274:20 (November 22/29): 1995. 1591–98.

5 See Timothy Quill, Christine Cassel, and Diane Meier, "Care of the Hopelessly Ill: Proposed Clinical Criteria for Physician-Assisted Suicide," *NEJM* 327:19 (Nov. 5, 1992): 1380–84, where the authors approve of PAS but disapprove of active euthanasia because it poses excessive social risks. Quill and Meier have subsequently conceded the untenability of this distinction in Franklin Miller et al., "Regulating Physician-Assisted Death," *NEJM* 331 (July 14, 1994): 119–123.

6 During the APA Eastern Division Session sponsored by the Committees on Philosophy and Medicine and Philosophy and Law (December 29, 1995) panel discussion, Professor

Dan Brock echoed the Dutch view. He held that if one is really concerned with the slippery slope, then allowing surrogates to forgo life-sustaining treatments for incompetents poses far greater risks to autonomy than a policy of physician-assisted death solidly based upon a requirement of the contemporaneous informed consent of the ill person. While Brock may be correct that our current practices surrounding surrogate decision making are subject to abuse and need to be hedged in with further safeguards, I believe that he seriously underestimates the social risks involved with PAS and euthanasia. One crucial dissimilarity between our current practice of forgoing life-sustaining treatment and physician-assisted death is that allowing the latter practice would surely implicate many more people in a hospital. The second crucial difference is that abolishing the firmly entrenched practice of surrogate decision making would throw the health care system into chaos and impose undignified deaths on vast numbers of incompetent patients, whereas continuing to withhold official sanction for physician-assisted death would, at worst, merely continue the status quo.

7 John Arras, "The Right to Die on the Slippery Slope," *Social Theory and Practice,* 8:3 (Fall 1982): 285–328.

8 Dr. Gary Kennedy of the Division of Geriatrics, Montefiore Medical Center, Albert Einstein College of Medicine.

9 Franklin Miller, Timothy Quill, Howard Brody, John Fletcher, Lawrence Gostin, and Diane Meier, "Regulating Physician-Assisted Death," *NEJM* 331 (July 14, 1994): 119–123.

10 See Ronald Dworkin, *Life's Dominion* (New York: Knopf, 1993) for an elegant and powerful restatement of the view that in a pluralistic society individuals should have rights against governmental interference with deeply personal "private choices," such as abortion and euthanasia.

PATIENT REFUSAL OF HYDRATION AND NUTRITION: AN ALTERNATIVE TO PHYSICIAN-ASSISTED SUICIDE OR VOLUNTARY ACTIVE EUTHANASIA

James L. Bernat, Bernard Gert, and R. Peter Mogielnicki

Bernat, Gert, and Mogielnicki focus attention on patient refusal of hydration and nutrition as a means whereby competent patients can effectively bring about their own death. They argue, based on the existing consensus that physicians are morally and legally required to honor the rational refusal of treatment by competent patients, that there is no need to legalize physician-assisted suicide or voluntary active euthanasia. Their basic point is that patient refusal of hydration and nutrition already provides a feasible (and much less problematic) alternative for patients who desire to shorten the dying process. In the course of developing their overall argument, the authors address a series of conceptual issues related to the distinction between killing and letting die. They also emphasize that the feasibility of patient refusal of hydration and nutrition as an alternative to physician-assisted suicide and voluntary active euthanasia depends upon further confirmation of the factual claim "that lack of hydration and nutrition does not cause unmanageable suffering in terminally ill patients."

Public and scholarly debates on legalizing physician-assisted suicide (PAS) and voluntary active euthanasia (VAE) have increased dramatically in recent years.[1-5] These debates have highlighted a significant moral controversy between those who regard PAS and VAE as morally permissible and those who do not. Unfortunately, the adversarial nature of this controversy has led both sides to ignore an alternative that avoids moral controversy altogether and has fewer associated practical problems in its implementation. In this article, we suggest that educating chronically and terminally ill patients about the feasibility of patient refusal of hydration and nutrition (PRHN) can empower them to control their own destiny without requiring physicians to reject the taboos on PAS and VAE that have existed for millennia. To be feasible, this alternative requires confirmation of the preliminary scientific evidence that death by starvation and dehydration need not be accompanied by suffering.

DEFINITIONS

Before proceeding, we will define several terms. Patients are *competent* to make a decision about their health care if they have the capacity to understand and appreciate all the information necessary to make a rational decision. Patient competence, freedom from coercion, and the receipt of adequate information from the physician are the elements of valid (informed) consent or refusal of treatment.[6,7]

A decision is *rational* if it does not produce harm to the patient (eg, death, pain, or disability) without an adequate reason (eg, to avoid suffering an equal or greater harm). It is rational to rank harms in different ways. For example, it is rational to rank

Reprinted with permission of the publisher from *Archives of Internal Medicine,* vol. 153 (December 27, 1993), pp. 2723–2728. Copyright © 1993, American Medical Association.

immediate death as worse than several months of suffering from a terminal disease; it is also rational to rank the suffering as worse than immediate death. We count as irrational only those rankings that result in the person suffering great harm and that would be rejected as irrational by almost everyone in the person's culture or subculture.[6,7]

Physician-assisted suicide occurs when the physician provides the necessary medical means for the patient to commit suicide, but death is not the direct result of the physician's act. In PAS, a physician accedes to the rational *request* of a competent patient to be provided with the necessary medical means for the patient to commit suicide. A suicide is *physician-assisted* if the physician's participation is a necessary but not sufficient component to the suicide. For example, a physician who complies with a dying patient's request to write a prescription for 100 pento-barbital tablets that the patient plans to swallow at a later time to commit suicide would be performing PAS.

Voluntary active euthanasia ("killing") occurs when a physician accedes to the rational *request* of a competent patient for some act by the physician to cause the death of the patient, which usually follows immediately on its completion. The physician's act in VAE is both necessary and sufficient to produce the patient's death. For example, a physician who complies with a dying patient's request to kill him mercifully with a lethal intravenous injection of pentobarbital sodium would be performing VAE.

Voluntary passive euthanasia ("letting die") occurs when a physician abides by the rational *refusal* of treatment by a competent patient with the knowledge that doing so will result in the patient dying sooner than if the physician had overruled the patient's refusal and had started or continued treatment. For example, when a physician complies with the refusal of a ventilator-dependent patient with motor neuron disease to receive further mechanical ventilatory support, and the patient dies as the result of extubation, this act is an example of voluntary passive euthanasia. Providing medical treatment to alleviate the pain and discomfort that normally accompanies extubation neither alters the fact that the physician is letting the patient die nor makes the act PAS. *Patient refusal of hydration and nutrition* is an example of voluntary passive euthanasia.

There are critical differences in the morality and legality of these acts. Physician-assisted suicide is legally prohibited in many jurisdictions, and there is a current controversy about whether it is moral. Voluntary active euthanasia is classified as criminal homicide and hence is strictly illegal in nearly every jurisdiction. Like PAS, its morality remains controversial. By contrast, there is no disagreement that physicians are morally and legally prohibited from overruling the rational refusal of therapy by a competent patient even when they know that death will result. There is also no disagreement that physicians are allowed to provide appropriate treatment for the pain and suffering that may accompany such refusals. In other words, physicians are morally and legally *required* to respect the competent patient's rational refusal of therapy, and they are morally and legally allowed to provide appropriate treatment for the pain and suffering involved. Physicians also are morally and legally required to abide by such refusals given as advance directives.[8]

CONFUSION CONCERNING KILLING VS LETTING DIE

Three areas of terminologic confusion that have clouded clear thinking about the morality of physician involvement in the care of the dying patient are (1) requests vs refusals by patients, (2) acts vs omissions by physicians, and (3) "natural" vs other causes of death.

PATIENTS' REQUESTS VS REFUSALS

Physicians are morally and legally required to honor a competent patient's rational *refusal* of therapy.[9-11] This requirement arises from the moral and legal prohibition against depriving a person of freedom and from the liberty-based right of a person to be left alone. In the medical context, it requires that the patient provide valid consent before any medical tests or treatments may be performed.

The moral and legal requirement to honor a refusal does not extend, however, to honoring a patient's *request* for specific therapy or other acts. Physicians should honor such requests or refuse to honor them on the basis of their professional judgment about the legal, moral, or medical appropriateness of doing so. A common example of the exercise of this freedom is physicians' refusal to prescribe requested narcotics in situations in which they judge narcotics to be inappropriate.

Confusion arises when the patient's refusal is framed misleadingly in terms resembling a request.[12] For example, a patient's "request" that no cardiopulmonary resuscitation be attempted is actually a refusal of permission for cardiopulmonary resuscitation. Similarly, written advance directives "requesting" the cessation or omission of other therapies are really refusals of treatment. Some writers have added to the confusion by simply talking of the patient's "choice" to forgo therapy as if there were no morally significant distinction between refusing and requesting.[12]

The distinction between requests and refusals has a critical importance in understanding the distinction between voluntary passive euthanasia (letting die) and VAE (killing). Patient *refusals* must be honored when they represent the rational decisions of competent patients even when physicians know death will result. There is no moral requirement to honor patient *requests* when physicians know death will result and there may be legal prohibitions against doing so.

PHYSICIANS' ACTS VS OMISSIONS

Some philosophers have misunderstood the definitions of VAE (killing) and passive euthanasia (letting die, including PRHN) and their moral significance by basing the distinction between killing and letting die on the distinction between acts and omissions.[13,14] In so doing, they have followed many physicians who have concentrated solely on what they themselves do (acts) or do not do (omissions) in distinguishing between killing and letting die. This way of distinguishing between killing and letting die creates a false moral distinction between a physician turning off intravenous feeding (act) and not replacing the intravenous solution container when it is empty (omission). When the distinction between killing and letting die is made in this way, it undermines legitimate medical and legal practice that permits allowing to die and does not permit killing.

This mistaken narrow focus on what the physician does or does not do without taking into account the larger context in which the physician acts or does not act can lead to the mistaken conclusion that PAS and VAE are really no different from voluntary passive euthanasia or "letting die." Recognition of the key role of whether or not the action is in response to the *patient's request* or the *patient's refusal* casts the issue in a clearer light.

As a matter of medical and legal practice, on the basis of a rational refusal of a competent patient, it is permitted either not to begin ventilatory therapy or to stop it; not to start treatment with antibiotics or to discontinue antibiotics; and not to start artificial hydration and nutrition or to cease them. All of these acts and omissions are morally and legally permitted when they result from a rational refusal by a competent patient. Indeed, it is misleading to say that these acts are morally and legally permitted, for they are morally and legally *required*. It is the rational refusal by a competent patient that is decisive here, not whether the physician acts or omits acting. It is the patient's refusal that makes the physician's acts and omissions "letting die" rather than "killing." Whether honoring this refusal requires the physician to act or omit acting is irrelevant. That is why those who base the distinction between killing and letting die on the distinction between acts and omissions mistakenly conclude that no morally relevant distinction exists.

'NATURAL' VS OTHER CAUSES OF DEATH

The term *natural*, as in "death by natural causes," has been another source of confusion. *Natural* is often used as a word of praise or, more generally, as a way of condoning something that otherwise would be considered unacceptable. Thus, voluntary passive euthanasia is often presented as acceptable because

it allows the patient to "die a natural death." Because the death was caused by the disease process, no person is assigned responsibility for the death. The freedom from responsibility for the patient's death is psychologically helpful for the physician. To make some state laws authorizing advance directives more acceptable to the public, they even have been labeled "natural death acts."

When death results from lack of hydration and nutrition, however, it is less plausible to say that "the death was caused by the disease process." Thus, someone must be assigned responsibility for the patient's death, and physicians wish to avoid this responsibility. A partial explanation for the misuse of technology to prolong dying unjustifiably may be an attempt by physicians to avoid this psychological responsibility. Physicians who recognize that patients have the authority to refuse any treatment, including hydration and nutrition, are more likely to avoid unjustified feelings of responsibility for their deaths.

Just as it is erroneous to think that the distinction between acts and omissions has any moral relevance, so it is erroneous to think that anything morally significant turns on the use of the terms *natural* or *cause*. What is morally significant is that the terminally ill patient is competent and has made a rational decision to refuse further treatment. Indeed, it is not even important whether what the patient has refused counts as treatment. If the patient has refused, the physician has no moral or legal authority to overrule that refusal. It is morally and legally irrelevant whether or not the resulting death is considered natural.

PATIENT REFUSAL OF HYDRATION AND NUTRITION

We maintain that a preferable alternative to legalization of PAS and VAE is for physicians to educate patients that they may refuse hydration and nutrition and that physicians will help them do so in a way that minimizes suffering. Chronically or terminally ill patients who wish to gain more control over their deaths can then refuse to eat and drink and refuse enteral or parenteral feedings or hydration. The failure of the present debate to include this alternative may be the result of the confusion discussed above, an erroneous assumption that thirst and hunger remain strong drives in terminal illness, and a misconception that failure to satisfy these drives causes intractable suffering.

The stereotypic image of a parched person on a desert crawling toward a mirage of water, and narrative accounts of otherwise healthy shipwrecked victims adrift without water, have contributed to the general notion that life-threatening dehydration is unbearable.[15,16] Although this is true in the above circumstances, it is the consensus of experienced physicians and nurses that terminally ill patients dying of dehydration or lack of nutrition do not suffer if treated properly. In fact, maintaining physiologic hydration and adequate nutrition is difficult in most seriously ill patients because intrinsic thirst and hunger are usually diminished or absent.

Throughout the 1980s, many thinkers expressed serious reservations about allowing withdrawal of hydration and nutrition to become acceptable medical practice. These reservations, however, were not based on any information about the discomfort or suffering experienced by patients under these circumstances. Rather, caregivers experienced psychologic distress due in part to the failure to understand the distinction between killing and letting die, and the social implications of withdrawing or withholding food and fluids, particularly because of its symbolism as communicating lack of caring.[17,18]

However, if the distinction between killing and letting die is based as it should be on patients' requests vs patients' refusals, these latter considerations lose their force. Now the crucial consideration becomes the degree of suffering associated with lack of hydration and nutrition. If the associated suffering is trivial, PRHN clearly has major advantages over PAS or VAE. Only if this suffering is unmanageable does the choice become more difficult. Scientific studies and anecdotal reports both suggest that dehydration and starvation in the seriously ill do not cause significant suffering. Physicians and particularly nurses have written many observational pieces describing peaceful and apparently comfortable deaths by starvation and dehydration.[19–21] Lay observers have corroborated these reports.[22]

Surprisingly, the scientific literature is incomplete on this matter. Systematic studies of the symptoms preceding death are hard to find, and those that do exist commonly do not separate suffering attributable to the underlying disease from suffering attributable to dehydration.[23–25] During World War II, metabolic studies of starvation and of fluid deprivation noted incidentally that the thirst experienced by normal healthy volunteers was typically "not actually uncomfortable" and characteristically was "quenched by an amount of water much less than was lost."[26,27]

A handful of laboratory studies and clinical trials are consistent with these older observational comments, but the picture is far from complete. Starvation is known to produce increased levels of acetoacetate, β-hydroxybutyrate, and acetone.[28] Other ketones (methyl butyl ketone and methyl heptyl ketone) have been shown to have an anesthetic action on isolated squid axons.[29] Depriving male Wistar rats of water and food for periods ranging from 24 to 72 hours has been shown to increase the levels of some endogenous opioids in the hypothalamus, although levels elsewhere in the brain and other organs decrease.[30] Healthy elderly men (over 65 years old) have been demonstrated to experience reduced thirst and associated symptoms during a 24-hour period of water deprivation and, when given ad libitum access to water to correct their dehydration, do so much more slowly than young healthy men.[31]

Observational data on the experience of terminally ill patients dying of dehydration have been recorded most recently in the hospice literature. This evidence suggests that the overwhelming majority of hospice deaths resulting from lack of hydration and nutrition can be managed such that the patients remain comfortable.[19,32–35] In a 1990 survey of 826 members of the (US) Academy of Hospice Physicians, 89% of hospice nurses and 86% of hospice physicians reported that their terminal patients who died by cessation of hydration and nutrition had peaceful and comfortable deaths.[36]

Taken in toto, the anecdotal reports, laboratory studies, and the observations of nurses and physicians who care for terminally ill patients suggest that lack of hydration and nutrition does not cause unmanageable suffering in terminally ill patients and may even have an analgesic effect. Clinical experience with severely ill patients suggests that the major symptom of dry mouth can be relieved by ice chips, methyl cellulose, artificial saliva, or small sips of water insufficient to reverse progressive dehydration.

BENEFITS OF PRHN OVER PAS AND VAE

Unlike PAS and VAE, PRHN is recognized by all as consistent with current medical, moral, and legal practices. It does not compromise public confidence in the medical profession because it does not require physicians to assume any new role or responsibility that could alter their roles of healer, caregiver, and counselor. It places the proper emphasis on the duty of physicians to care for dying patients, because these patients need care and comfort measures during the dying period. It encourages physicians to engage in educational discussions with patients and families about dying and the desirability of formulating clear advance directives.

Legalization of PAS or VAE would likely create unintended and harmful social pressures and expectations. Many elderly or chronically ill patients could feel "the duty to die." They would request euthanasia not on the basis of personal choice but because they believed that their families considered them a burden and expected them to agree to be killed. Furthermore, patients might sense pressure from their physicians to consider VAE as an alternative and agree because the physicians must know what is best for them.[37] The meaning of "voluntary" euthanasia thus could become corrupted, causing the elderly and chronically ill to become victimized.

Unlike the "duty to die" resulting from legalizing PAS or VAE, it is unlikely that patients choosing to die by PRHN would feel as much social pressure or expectations from family members to die earlier because of the duration of the process and the opportunity therein for reconsideration and family interaction. Furthermore, it is much less likely that there would be pressure from physicians or other health professionals. Additionally, the several-day interval before unconsciousness ensues from PRHN would permit time for appropriate mourning and good-byes to family and friends.

Physicians may experience psychological stress about the patient's refusal of hydration and nutri-

tion. Their moral and legal obligation to respect the treatment refusal should absolve some of the physician's discomfort. Physicians can seek no such solace in PAS or VAE because even if both were legalized, they would not be required. Physicians acceding to requests for PAS or VAE, even if it were legal, do so without legal or moral force compelling them to do so. This underscores the essential difference between passive euthanasia and PAS or VAE. It also lays bare the distress to be expected by physicians should they become involved with PAS and VAE in that they always will do so without an accompanying moral mandate.

Legalization of PAS or VAE would require the creation of a network of cumbersome legal safeguards to protect patients from abuse and misunderstanding or miscommunication. Despite such bureaucratic efforts, there would remain a risk that the practice of voluntary euthanasia would extend to involuntary cases, as has been alleged in the Dutch experience where VAE, although officially illegal, is permitted if physicians follow a series of judicial guidelines.[38,39] Furthermore, the safeguards would require the insinuation of courts, lawyers, and bureaucrats between the patient-family and the physician. The new legal requirements could have the effect of delaying the patient's death and generating unnecessary administrative complexity and expense.

Unlike PAS and VAE, PRHN is lawful already in most jurisdictions. Indeed, refusal of hydration and nutrition is listed as an option in commonly drafted advance directives in the United States. Communication errors, misunderstandings, and abuse are less likely with PRHN than with PAS or VAE and thus are less likely to result in an unwanted earlier death. The patient who refuses hydration and nutrition clearly demonstrates the seriousness and consistency of his or her desire to die. The several-day interval before the patient becomes unconscious provides time to reconsider the decision and for the family to accept that dying clearly represents the patient's wish. Furthermore, the process can begin immediately without first requiring legal approvals or other bureaucratic interventions. Thus, it may allow the patient to die faster than PAS or VAE, given the delays intrinsic to bureaucratic process.

THE PHYSICIAN'S ROLE IN PRHN

The current interest in legalizing PAS and VAE misplaces the emphasis of physicians' duties to their dying patients. Physicians should be more concerned about providing patients optimal terminal care than killing them or helping them kill themselves. Legalizing PAS would make it unnecessary for physicians to strive to maximize comfort measures in terminally ill patients and unnecessary for society to support research to improve the science of palliation.[12] By comparison, PRHN appropriately encourages the physician to attend to the medical treatment of dying patients.

The physician's traditional role has been summarized as "to cure sometimes, to relieve often, and to comfort always."[40] With PRHN, the physician can concentrate his or her energy on the last two of these three challenging tasks. In the modern era, this involves a number of important pragmatic matters worthy of review.

Terminal illness should be anticipated with all patients by education and offers of assistance in the design, completion, and implementation of advance directives for terminal care. Arrangements for appropriate home help and necessary nursing attendance must be addressed, as should appropriate means of avoiding well-intended but undesired resuscitation attempts by emergency medical technicians at the time of death. A pact should be made with the patient that the physician will do his or her best to minimize suffering during the dying process and will remain available to comfort the patient by physical presence as well as skillful treatment of symptoms, including pain, dyspnea, and dryness of the mouth.

Physicians caring for patients dying of PRHN have an important responsibility to provide adequate symptom control. Effective mouth care can relieve most of the unpleasant symptoms of thirst and mouth dryness. Physicians should be willing to prescribe narcotics and benzodiazepines in dosages sufficient to abate pain and other unpleasant sensations. They should not incorrectly limit the dosage of their prescriptions for fear of accelerating death; the intent should be to maintain adequate comfort during dying. The possibility of a hastened death as a complication of symptomatic treatment is an acceptable risk and does not count as PAS or VAE. There is evidence that adequate pain control in terminally ill cancer patients reduces the demand for PAS.[41] It is likely that adequate control of unpleasant symptoms during dying would also lessen demands for VAE.

There are several areas in PRHN where more work needs to be done. There remains a need for more systematic research on the phenomenology and pathophysiology of dying as a result of refusal of hydration and nutrition. Additional studies will help physicians understand the needs of dying patients and thereby ensure patient comfort throughout the dying process.

There needs to be societal acceptance that physicians have a moral duty to respect the rational wishes of competent, chronically ill but not terminally ill patients who wish to die by PRHN or other valid refusals of therapy. There is no reason why such patients should not have the same rights as the terminally ill to refuse life-sustaining therapies, including hydration and nutrition.[11] The American Academy of Neurology recently published a position statement asserting that chronically ill patients with severe paralysis and intact cognition, whether terminally ill or not, have the right to refuse life-sustaining therapy, including hydration and nutrition.[42,43]

The most pressing need is to dispel the myths about suffering caused by dehydration and to publicize as widely as possible to both physicians and their terminally ill patients the availability of PRHN as a means of shortening the dying process. Educational efforts should be directed to physicians, who are often ill-informed on this matter,[44] as well as to the general public. The emphasis on research and education on symptomatic treatments to relieve suffering during dying is fully compatible with the traditional and appropriate role of the physician as caregiver and comforter.

Since this manuscript was accepted for publication, other well-studied cases have been reported of comfortable deaths by patient refusal of hydration and nutrition.[45]

REFERENCES

1 Crigger B. J., ed. Dying well? a colloquy on euthanasia and assisted suicide. *Hastings Cent Rep.* 1992; 22:6–55.

2 Campbell C. S., Crigger B. J., eds. Mercy, murder, and morality: perspectives on euthanasia. *Hastings Cent Rep.* 1989; 19(suppl 1):1–32.

3 Pellegrino E. D. Doctors must not kill. *J Clin Ethics.* 1992; 3:95–102.

4 Quill T. E., Cassel C. K., Meier D. E. Care of the hopelessly ill: proposed clinical criteria for physician-assisted suicide. *N Engl J Med.* 1992; 327:1380–1384.

5 Brody H. Assisted death: a compassionate response to a medical failure. *N Engl J Med.* 1992; 327:1384–1388.

6 Culver C. M., Gert B. Basic ethical concepts in neurologic practice. *Semin Neurol.* 1984; 4:1–8.

7 Gert B., Culver C. M. Moral theory in neurologic practice. *Semin Neurol.* 1984; 4:9–14.

8 Gert B, Culver C. M. Distinguishing between active and passive euthanasia. *Clin Geriatr Med.* 1986; 2:29–36.

9 Culver C. M., Gert B. *Philosophy in Medicine: Conceptual and Ethical Issues in Medicine and Psychiatry.* New York, NY: Oxford University Press; 1982:20–64.

10 Gert B. *Morality: A New Justification of the Moral Rules.* New York, NY: Oxford University Press; 1988:282–303.

11 Meisel A. Legal myths about terminating life support. *Arch Intern Med.* 1991; 151:1497–1502.

12 Council on Ethical and Judicial Affairs, American Medical Association. Decisions near the end of life. *JAMA.* 1992; 267:2229–2233.

13 Rachels J. Active and passive euthanasia. *N Engl J Med.* 1975; 292:78–80.

14 Brock D. W. Voluntary active euthanasia. *Hastings Cent Rep.* 1992; 22:10–22.

15 Wolf A. V. *Thirst: Physiology of the Urge to Drink and Problems of Water Lack.* Springfield, IL: Charles C Thomas Publisher; 1958:208–252, 375–463.

16 Critchley M. *Shipwreck Survivors: A Medical Study.* London, England: Churchill Ltd; 1943:24–40.

17 Derr P. G. Why food and fluids can never be denied. *Hastings Cent Rep.* 1986; 16:28–30.

18 Callahan D. On feeding the dying. *Hastings Cent Rep.* 1983; 13:22.

19 Andrews M., Levine A. Dehydration in the terminal patient: perception of hospice nurses. *Am J Hospice Care.* 1989; 3:31–34.

20 Zerwekh J. The dehydration question. *Nursing.* 1983; 13:47–51.

21 Printz L. A. Terminal dehydration, a compassionate treatment. *Arch Intern Med.* 1992; 152:697–700.

22 Nearing H. *Loving and Leaving the Good Life.* Post Mills, Vt: Chelsea Green Publishing Co; 1992.

23 Mogielnicki R. P., Nelson W. A., Dulac J. A study of the dying process in elderly hospitalized males. *J Cancer Educ.* 1990; 5:135–145.

24 Billings J. Comfort measures for the terminally ill: is dehydration painful? *J Am Geriatr Soc.* 1985; 33:808–810.

25 Morris J. N., Suissa S., Sherwood S., et al. Last days: a study of the quality of life of terminally ill cancer patients. *J Chronic Dis.* 1986; 39:47–62.

26 Winkler A. W., Danowski T. S., Elkinton J. R., Peters J. P. Electrolyte and fluid studies during water deprivation and starvation in human subjects and the effect of ingestion of fish, of carbohydrates, and of salt solutions. *J Clin Invest.* 1944; 23:807–811.

27 Black D. A. K., McCance R. A., Young W. F. A study of dehydration by means of balance experiments. *J Physiol.* 1944; 102:406–414.

28 Owen O., Caprio S., Reichard G., et al. Ketosis of starvation: a revisit and new perspectives. *Clin Endocrinol Metab.* 1983; 12:359–379.

29 Elliott J. R., Haydon D. A., Hendry B. M. Anaesthetic action of esters and ketones: evidence for an interaction with the sodium channel protein in squid axons. *J Physiol.* 1984; 354: 407–418.

30 Majeed N. H., Lason W., Prewlocka B., et al. Brain and peripheral opioid peptides after changes in ingestive behavior. *Neuroendocrinology.* 1986; 42:267–272.

31 Phillips P. A., Rolls B. J., Ledingham J. G. G., et al. Reduced thirst after water deprivation in healthy elderly men. *N Engl J Med.* 1984; 311: 753–759.

32 Miller R. J., Albright P. G. What is the role of nutritional support and hydration in terminal cancer patients? *Am J Hospice Care.* 1989; 6:33–38.

33 Cox S. S. Is dehydration painful? *Ethics Med.* 1987; 12:1–2.

34 Lichter I, Hunt E. The last 48 hours of life. *J Palliat Care.* 1990; 6:7–15.

35 Miller R. J. Hospice care as an alternative to euthanasia. *Law Med Health Care.* 1992; 20:127–132.

36 Miller R. J. Nutrition and hydration in terminal disease. *J Palliat Care.* In press.

37 Kamisar Y. Some non-religious views against proposed 'mercy-killing' legislation. *Minn Law Rev.* 1958; 42:969–1042.

38 Benrubi G. I. Euthanasia: the need for procedural safeguards. *N Engl J Med.* 1992; 326:197–199.

39 Van der Maas P. J., van Delden J. J. M., Pijnenborg L, Looman C. W. N. Euthanasia and other medical decisions concerning the end of life. *Lancet.* 1991; 338:669–674.

40 Strauss M. B, ed. *Familiar Medical Quotations.* Boston, Mass: Little Brown & Co; 1968:410.

41 Foley K. M. The relationship of pain and symptom management to patient requests for physician-assisted suicide. *J Pain Symptom Management* 1991; 6:289–297.

42 American Academy of Neurology. Position statement: certain aspects of the care and management of profoundly and irreversibly paralyzed patients with retained consciousness and cognition. *Neurology.* 1993; 53:222–223.

43 Bernat J. L, Cranford R. E, Kittredge F. I. Jr, Rosenberg R. N. Competent patients with advanced states of permanent paralysis have the right to forgo life-sustaining therapy. *Neurology.* 1993; 43:224–225.

44 Ahronheim J. C., Gasner M. R. The sloganism of starvation. *Lancet.* 1990; 335:278–279.

45 Sullivan R. J. Accepting death without artificial nutrition or hydration. *J Gen Intern Med.* 1993; 8: 220–224.

THE GRONINGEN PROTOCOL—EUTHANASIA IN SEVERELY ILL NEWBORNS

Eduard Verhagen and Pieter J. J. Sauer

Dutch neonatologists Verhagen and Sauer describe a clinical protocol that they developed—known as the *Groningen Protocol*—for treating newborns with extremely poor prognoses. Some infants have a hopeless prognosis and are predicted to endure unbearable suffering, as in the most serious forms of spina bifida. The protocol, developed in consultation with a district attorney, permits physicians to end the infant's life through active means under some strict conditions: the parents must agree, on the basis of a thorough explanation of the condition and prognosis; a team of physicians, including at least one doctor who is not directly involved in the infant's care, must also agree; and the condition and prognosis must be clearly defined. After the infant has died, an outside legal body (typically the prosecutor's office) must determine if the decision was justified and if all necessary procedures were followed. The authors mention four cases in the Netherlands in which physicians in their practice group deliberately ended the life of a newborn, pursuant to the procedure. None of these physicians was prosecuted.

Of the 200,000 children born in the Netherlands every year, about 1000 die during the first year of life. For approximately 600 of these infants, death is preceded by a medical decision regarding the end of life. Discussions about the initiation and continuation of treatment in newborns with serious medical conditions are one of the most difficult aspects of pediatric practice. Although technological developments have provided tools for dealing with many consequences of congenital anomalies and premature birth, decisions regarding when to start and when to withhold treatment in individual cases remain very difficult to make. Even more difficult are the decisions regarding newborns who have serious disorders or deformities associated with suffering that cannot be alleviated and for whom there is no hope of improvement.

Suffering is a subjective feeling that cannot be measured objectively, whether in adults or in infants. But we accept that adults can indicate when

From *New England Journal of Medicine*, vol. 352, no. 10 (March 10, 2005), pp. 959–962. Copyright © 2005 Massachusetts Medical Society. All rights reserved.

their suffering is unbearable. Infants cannot express their feelings through speech, but they do so through different types of crying, movements, and reactions to feeding. Pain scales for newborns, based on changes in vital signs (blood pressure, heart rate, and breathing pattern) and observed behavior, may be used to determine the degree of discomfort and pain. Experienced caregivers and parents are able to evaluate the degree of suffering in a newborn, as well as the degree of relief afforded by medication or other measures. In the Netherlands, euthanasia for competent persons older than 16 years of age has been legally accepted since 1985. The question under consideration now is whether deliberate life-ending procedures are also acceptable for newborns and infants, despite the fact that these patients cannot express their own will. Or must infants with disorders associated with severe and sustained suffering be kept alive when their suffering cannot be adequately reduced?

In the Netherlands, as in all other countries, ending someone's life, except in extreme conditions, is considered murder. A life of suffering that cannot be alleviated by any means might be considered one of these extreme conditions. Legal control over euthanasia in newborns is based on physicians' own reports, followed by assessment by criminal prosecutors. To provide all the information needed for assessment and to prevent interrogations by police officers, we developed a protocol, known as the Groningen protocol, for cases in which a decision is made to actively end the life of a newborn. During the past few months, the international press has been full of blood-chilling accounts and misunderstandings concerning this protocol.

Infants and newborns for whom such end-of-life decisions might be made can be divided into three categories.[1] First, there are infants with no chance of survival. This group consists of infants who will die soon after birth, despite optimal care with the most current methods available locally. These infants have severe underlying disease, such as lung and kidney hypoplasia.

Infants in the second group have a very poor prognosis and are dependent on intensive care. These patients may survive after a period of intensive treatment, but expectations regarding their future condition are very grim. They are infants with severe brain abnormalities or extensive organ damage caused by extreme hypoxemia. When these infants can survive beyond the period of intensive care, they have an extremely poor prognosis and a poor quality of life.

Finally, there are infants with a hopeless prognosis who experience what parents and medical experts deem to be unbearable suffering. Although it is difficult to define in the abstract, this group includes patients who are not dependent on intensive medical treatment but for whom a very poor quality of life, associated with sustained suffering, is predicted. For example, a child with the most serious form of spina bifida will have an extremely poor quality of life, even after many operations. This group also includes infants who have survived thanks to intensive care but for whom it becomes clear after intensive treatment has been completed that the quality of life will be very poor and for whom there is no hope of improvement.

Deciding not to initiate or to withdraw life-prolonging treatment in newborns with no chance of survival is considered good practice for physicians in Europe and is acceptable for physicians in the United States. Most such infants die immediately after treatment has been discontinued.

Neonatologists in the Netherlands and the majority of neonatologists in Europe are convinced that intensive care treatment is not a goal in itself. Its aim is not only survival of the infant, but also an acceptable quality of life. Forgoing or not initiating life-sustaining treatment in children in the second group is acceptable to these neonatologists if both the medical team and the parents are convinced that treatment is not in the best interest of the child because the outlook is extremely poor.

Confronted with a patient in the third category, it is vital for the medical team to have as accurate a prognosis as possible and to discuss it with the parents. All possible measures must be taken to alleviate severe pain and discomfort. There are, however, circumstances in which, despite all measures taken, suffering cannot be relieved and no improvement can be expected. When both the parents and the physicians are convinced that there is an extremely poor prognosis, they may concur that death would be more humane than continued life. Under similar conditions, a person in the Netherlands who is older than 16 years of age can ask for euthanasia. Newborns, however, cannot ask for euthanasia, and such a request by parents, acting as the representatives of their child, is invalid under Dutch law. Does this mean that euthanasia in a newborn is always prohibited? We are convinced that life-ending measures can be acceptable in these cases under very strict conditions: the parents must agree fully, on the basis of a thorough explanation of the condition and prognosis; a team of physicians, including at least one who is not directly involved in the care of the patient, must agree; and the condition and prognosis must be very well defined. After the decision has been made and the child has died, an outside legal body should determine whether the decision was justified and all necessary procedures have been followed.

A national survey of neonatologists in the Netherlands has shown that each year there are 15 to 20 cases of euthanasia in newborn infants who would be categorized in the third group.[2] According to Dutch law, it is a doctor's duty to file a death certificate when a patient has died from natural causes. If a death is due to euthanasia, it cannot be certified as "natural." The doctor must inform the coroner, who inspects the body and, in turn, informs the district attorney, whose office reviews each case in light of the applicable laws or jurisprudence. The district attorney presents the case, together with his or her own opinion, to the College of Attorneys General, whose four members manage the national public prosecution department and provisionally decide whether or not to prosecute. The final decision is made by the minister of justice.

Two court cases, decided in the mid-1990s, regarding euthanasia in infants in the Netherlands provide some guidance for both judges and physicians. In the first case, a physician ended the life of a newborn who had an extreme form of spina bifida. In the second case, a physician ended the life of a newborn who had trisomy 13. Both cases involved a very limited life expectancy and extreme suffering that could not be alleviated. In their verdicts, the courts approved the procedures as meeting the requirements for good medical practice. Although these rulings have given some guidance, many organizations have repeatedly pleaded for clearer guidelines, arguing that a committee with multidisciplinary (medical, legal, and ethical) expertise would be more capable than judges of assessing such cases. Physicians would be expected to be much more willing to report procedures to such a committee than they are to report to a district attorney. The Dutch government, however, has neither created a committee nor offered other guidance, despite having promised repeatedly, since 1997, to do so.

Twenty-two cases of euthanasia in newborns have been reported to district attorneys' offices in the Netherlands during the past seven years. Recently, we were allowed to review these cases.[3] They all involved infants with very severe forms of spina bifida. In most cases (17 of the 22), a multidisciplinary spina bifida team was consulted. In the remaining five cases, at least two other independent medical experts were consulted. The physicians based their decisions on the presence of severe suf-

TABLE 1 Considerations Used to Support the Decision to End the Life of a Newborn in 22 Cases*

Consideration	No. of Cases (%)
Extremely poor quality of life (suffering) in terms of functional disability, pain, discomfort, poor prognosis, and hopelessness	22 (100)
Predicted lack of self-sufficiency	22 (100)
Predicted inability to communicate	18 (82)
Expected hospital dependency	17 (77)
Long life expectancy†	13 (59)

*Data are from Verhagen et al.[3]
†The burden of other considerations is greater when the life expectancy is long in a patient who is suffering.

fering without hope of improvement (see Table 1). The decisions were always made in collaboration with, and were fully approved by, both parents. The prosecutor used four criteria to assess each case: the presence of hopeless and unbearable suffering and a very poor quality of life, parental consent, consultation with an independent physician and his or her agreement with the treating physicians, and the carrying out of the procedure in accordance with the accepted medical standard. The conclusion in all 22 cases was that the requirements of careful practice were fulfilled. None of the physicians were prosecuted.

Given that the national survey indicated that such procedures are performed in 15 to 20 newborns per year, the fact that an average of three cases were reported annually suggests that most cases are simply not being reported. We believe that all cases must be reported if the country is to prevent uncontrolled and unjustified euthanasia and if we are to discuss the issue publicly and thus further develop norms regarding euthanasia in newborns. With that aim, we developed a protocol in 2002, in close collaboration with a district attorney. The protocol contains general guidelines and specific requirements related to the decision about euthanasia and its implementation. Five medical requirements must be fulfilled; other criteria are supportive, designed to clarify the decision and facilitate assessment (see Table 2). Following the protocol does not guarantee that the physician will not be prosecuted. Since implementing this protocol, our group has reported four cases in which we performed a deliberate life-ending procedure in a newborn. None have resulted in prosecution.

Dilemmas regarding end-of-life decisions for newborns with a very poor quality of life and presumably unbearable suffering and no hope of improvement are shared by physicians throughout the world. In the Netherlands, obligatory reporting with the aid of a protocol and subsequent assessment of euthanasia in newborns help us to clarify the decision-making process. This approach suits our legal and social culture, but it is unclear to what extent it would be transferable to other countries.

TABLE 2   The Groningen Protocol for Euthanasia in Newborns

Requirements that must be fulfilled

The diagnosis and prognosis must be certain

Hopeless and unbearable suffering must be present

The diagnosis, prognosis, and unbearable suffering must be confirmed by at least one independent doctor

Both parents must give informed consent

The procedure must be performed in accordance with the accepted medical standard

Information needed to support and clarify the decision about euthanasia

Diagnosis and prognosis

  Describe all relevant medical data and the results of diagnostic investigations used to establish the diagnosis

  List all the participants in the decision-making process, all opinions expressed, and the final consensus

  Describe how the prognosis regarding long-term health was assessed

  Describe how the degree of suffering and life expectancy were assessed

  Describe the availability of alternative treatments, alternative means of alleviating suffering, or both

  Describe treatments and the results of treatment preceding the decision about euthanasia

Euthanasia decision

  Describe who initiated the discussion about possible euthanasia and at what moment

  List the considerations that prompted the decision

  List all the participants in the decision-making process, all opinions expressed, and the final consensus

  Describe the way in which the parents were informed and their opinions

Consultation

  Describe the physician or physicians who gave a second opinion (name and qualifications)

  List the results of the examinations and the recommendations made by the consulting physician or physicians

Implementation

  Describe the actual euthanasia procedure (time, place, participants, and administration of drugs)

  Describe the reasons for the chosen method of euthanasia

Steps taken after death

  Describe the findings of the coroner

  Describe how the euthanasia was reported to the prosecuting authority

  Describe how the parents are being supported and counseled

  Describe planned follow-up, including case review, postmortem examination, and genetic counseling

REFERENCES

1 Sauer P. J. Ethical dilemmas in neonatology: recommendations of the Ethics Working Group of the CESP (Confederation of European Specialists in Paediatrics). Eur J Pediatr 2001; 160:364–8.

2 van der Heide A., van der Maas P. J., van der Wal G., et al. Medical end-of-life decisions made for neonates and infants in the Netherlands. Lancet 1997; 350:251–5.

3 Verhagen A. A. E., Sol J. J., Brouwer O. F., Sauer P. J. Actieve levensbeeindiging bij pasgeborenen in Nederland, Een analyse van alle meldingen van 1997–2004. Ned Tijdschr Geneeskd 2005; 149:183–8.

WE CANNOT ACCURATELY PREDICT THE EXTENT OF AN INFANT'S FUTURE SUFFERING: THE GRONINGEN PROTOCOL IS TOO DANGEROUS TO SUPPORT

Alexander A. Kon

Kon argues that the Groningen Protocol (defended in the previous selection) poses unacceptable risks and is incompatible with the ethical principle of nonmaleficence. Although he accepts that voluntary active euthanasia for terminally ill adults is ethically permitted, he distinguishes these adults from the newborns to whom the Groningen Protocol applies. First, he notes, an infant cannot give informed consent. Second, he claims, the protocol is intended to be used, and has been used, to end the lives of infants who are not terminally ill, but are simply deemed to have insufficient prospects for reasonable quality of life. Given that adults themselves often overestimate the suffering associated with serious medical disabilities, we cannot have confidence in judgments made about the future quality of life of a newborn, especially when our judgment is clouded by our desire to spare the infant presently visible suffering. Kon recognizes that some infants are, indeed, born with conditions that make their lives not worth living, but he denies that we can identify these infants with sufficient accuracy to justify a practice of actively euthanizing them. Rejecting the Groningen Protocol will lead some of these unlucky individuals to live lives that are not worth living, but using the protocol will lead to euthanizing some whose lives *would* have been worth living. The safer policy, he concludes, is to reject the protocol.

It is terrible to watch a child suffer. Like many others who care for children in the intensive care unit (ICU), I have too often witnessed what I considered to be intolerable suffering. Watching a dying child undergo painful procedures or anxiety-provoking interventions when there is no hope for cure or even providing prolongation of life with symptom improvement can be unbearable for care providers and parents. When medical interventions merely prolong dying and the care providers and parents agree that limiting or withdrawing life-prolonging measures is most consistent with the child's best interest, then doing so is appropriate and well-accepted. Indeed, most children who die in United States hospitals do so after life-prolonging interventions have been limited or withdrawn (Garros et al. 2003).

Also troubling to healthcare providers is performing invasive life-prolonging procedures on a child who is deemed to have no reasonable chance for a meaningful life. Although less well published, I have often heard physicians, nurses, and others in the ICU question whether it is reasonable to perform cardiac surgery on a child with severe chromosomal abnormalities, place a tracheostomy and surgical feeding tube in a child with profound neurodevelopmental delay, or even correct a tracheoesophageal fistula in a child with trisomy 21 (as was the question in the famed Baby Doe case). In such cases providers, and at times parents, question the appropriateness of invasive life-prolonging interventions.

The Groningen Protocol, however, goes one step further and creates a system whereby healthcare providers and parents may choose to terminate the life of a child based on the judgment that the child's future quality of life is so low that death is a better option than life. Like Jotkowitz and colleagues (Jotkowitz et al. 23), it is clear to me that the Dutch protocol has been used, and is meant to be used, solely for infants who are not terminally ill (Verhagen et al. 2005, Verhagen 2006, Verhagen and Sauer 2005). Although Manninen has argued that in some sense these children are terminally ill (Manninen 2006), because all children for whom the protocol has been employed had spina bifida, a non-terminal illness, and Verhagen et al. clearly articulate that the protocol is intended for non-terminally ill infants, it cannot be reasonably argued that the protocol covers dying children.

Although significant debate remains as to the ethical permissibility of voluntary active euthanasia (VAE) for adult patients, I will assume for this essay that VAE is ethically permissible. This assumption is not based on any notion that this debate has been resolved or that the arguments against VAE lack adequate foundation. Rather, I assume the permissibility of VAE because it seems impossible to justify the Groningen Protocol if one does not accept the permissibility of VAE. I argue, however, that even if one accepts as permissible VAE, the Groningen Protocol cannot be supported.

Because infants cannot express their wishes, and indeed cannot even conceive of wishes or judge what they believe to be in their best interest, decisions for neonates must be made by surrogate decision-makers. By choosing to euthanize the infant, parents and providers are therefore making a decision that it is in the infant's best interest to be euthanized. That is, they are deciding that the burdens of the infant's suffering outweigh the benefits of being alive, and therefore she would be better off dead than alive. Or, to put it another way, they judge that the infant's suffering is unbearable.

It has been well documented that many patients suffer tremendously at the end of life (Quill and Cassel 2003). We may therefore extrapolate that some patients not in the dying process also suffer tremendously. Some of these patients may indeed find their suffering to be unbearable, and may believe that death is a better option than life. For these patients, it may be that VAE is permissible because the patient himself or herself has weighed the benefits and burdens of life, and has determined that on balance the burdens of living with unbearable suffering outweigh the benefits of being alive. If some adult patients suffer so greatly that they believe that they would be better off dead than alive, than we may assume that for some children and infants with unbearable suffering it could be in their best interest to be euthanized.

The question we must answer under the Groningen Protocol is: Is *this* baby's suffering unbearable and will her future suffering be so great that it is in her best interest to have her life terminated? Suffering is inherently subjective. While we may be able to assess an infant's pain, anxiety, or discomfort, we cannot know the infant's perception of her pain, anxiety, or discomfort. Since the key question is not whether the patient is suffering but rather whether the patient is suffering *unbearably,* we can never be certain of our answer (Kon 2007).

As I have discussed elsewhere, there are many studies demonstrating that healthcare providers, parents, and the general public overestimate the burdens of living with a disability (Kon 2007). Indeed, many people who believe that they would never want to live with serious disability (e.g., quadriplegia) later believe that their life is fulfilling and very much worth living when faced with the reality of life with disability. Further, studies have demonstrated that even close family members and spouses are poor judges of the end of life choices of patients. These findings underscore the dangers of allowing others to decide when a patient's suffering is unbearable. Even if one concedes that for some small number of children it may be in their best interest to be euthanized, given the overwhelming data demonstrating that we (parents, health-care providers, and the general public) overestimate the burdens of living with a disability and generally undervalue the lives of persons with disabilities, we cannot support a system in which we make decisions regarding the unbearableness of the suffering of an infant. Based on these data, it is clear that if we accept the Groningen Protocol we would condemn to death many infants whose suffering is real but bearable.

Further, it seems impossible to adequately separate the parents' suffering from the suffering of the infant when making such a decision. Indeed, when employing the Groningen Protocol, physicians often administer a paralytic agent to the infant (Catlin and Novakovich 2008). Such an act cannot be grounded in the child's best interest since paralyzing the infant can only increase, not decrease, her suffering. Paralytic agents are used to make the death more palatable for the parents (Catlin and Novakovich 2008), and any act of terminating the life of an infant that employs interventions meant specifically to relieve the unease of someone other than the patient is unsupportable. If the sole objective is to act in the best interest of the infant, then there is no role for the use of paralytic agents.

It would seem that we are faced with a true ethical dilemma. On the one hand, if we use the Groningen Protocol to euthanize infants when we believe that their suffering is unbearable, we will certainly terminate the lives of some infants whose suffering is great but not unbearable. For these infants the benefits of being alive outweigh the burdens of their suffering, and in such cases one cannot classify the termination of life as euthanasia. Rather, in these cases terminating the child's life is simply killing (Kon 2007). On the other hand, if we continue the status quo and view euthanizing an infant as impermissible, we run the risk of condemning some infants to a life of unbearable suffering. Neither option is ideal, but which is more consistent with the tenets of medical practice? One of the fundamental principles of medicine is above all else, do no harm. Killing an infant for whom the benefits of living outweigh the burdens of her suffering may be the greatest harm a physician could ever inflict on a patient, and therefore we should not support any system that would allow this to occur. Therefore, on balance, we must not accept any protocol to actively terminate the life of an infant, particularly one who is neither dying nor terminally ill.

Perhaps the best solution, if one believes that VAE is ever permissible, is to provide infants who are not terminally ill with the best medical care possible. Support them fully and work diligently to minimize their suffering. As these infants grow into toddlers, then children, and eventually into adolescents, they will be increasingly able to assess their own suffering and communicate with parents and healthcare providers. If, as a child grows, she believes that her suffering is unbearable and she has decisional capacity (even if she lacks legal authority to consent), VAE may be permissible. If a child has such severe neurocognitive impairment that she lacks the ability to assess her own level of suffering, weigh the benefits and burdens of her life, and communicate that assessment, then it remains impermissible to terminate her life. While watching a child suffer may be unbearable for parents and healthcare providers, we cannot be certain that the child herself perceives the suffering as unbearable. Without a patient communicating her own subjective experience, actively terminating a child's life is not appropriate.

REFERENCES

Catlin, A., and Novakovich, R. 2008. The Groningen Protocol: What is it, how do the Dutch use it, and do we use it here? *Pediatric Nursing* 34(3): 247–51.

Garros, D., Rosychuk, R. J. and Cox, P. N. 2003. Circumstances surrounding end of life in a pediatric intensive care unit. *Pediatrics* 112(5): e371.

Jotkowitz, A. B., Glick, S., and Gesundheit, B. 2008. A case against justified non-voluntary active euthanasia. *American Journal of Bioethics* 8(11): 23–26.

Kon, A. A. 2007. Neonatal euthanasia is unsupportable: the Groningen protocol should be abandoned. *Theoretical Medicine and Bioethics* 28(5): 453–463.

Manninen, B. A. 2006. A case for justified non-voluntary active euthanasia: exploring the ethics of the Groningen Protocol. *Journal of Medical Ethics* 32(11): 643–651.

Quill, T. E., and Cassel, C. K. 2003. Professional organizations' position statement on physician-assisted suicide: A case for studied neutrality. *Annals of Internal Medicine* 138(3): 208–211.

Verhagen, A. A., Sol, J. J., Brouwer, O. F., and Sauer, P. J. 2005. Deliberate termination of life in newborns in The Netherlands; review of all 22 reported cases between 1997 and 2004. *Nederlands Tijdschrift Voor Geneeskunde* 149(4): 183–188.

Verhagen, E. 2006. End of life decisions in newborns in The Netherlands: Medical and legal aspects of the Groningen Protocol. *Medical Law* 25(2): 399–407.

Verhagen, E., and Sauer, P. J. 2005. The Groningen protocol—euthanasia in severely ill newborns. *New England Journal of Medicine* 352(10): 959–62.

ANNOTATED BIBLIOGRAPHY

Battin, Margaret Pabst: *Ethical Issues in Suicide* (Englewood Cliffs, NJ: Prentice Hall, 1995). In this useful book, Battin provides a comprehensive discussion of the traditional arguments concerning suicide. She also suggests an analysis of the concept of rational suicide, discusses suicide intervention as well as suicide facilitation, and considers the notion of suicide as a right. The book's final chapter provides a discussion of physician-assisted suicide.

_____, and David J. Mayo, eds.: *Suicide: The Philosophical Issues* (New York: St. Martin's Press, 1980). This valuable collection of articles includes material on the concept of suicide, the morality of suicide, and the rationality of suicide. There are also sections entitled "Suicide and Psychiatry" and "Suicide, Law, and Rights."

_____, Rosamond Rhodes, and Anita Silvers, eds.: *Physician-Assisted Suicide: Expanding the Debate* (New York: Routledge, 1998). The essays in Part Two of this extensive collection debate the projected impact of physician-assisted suicide on vulnerable patients. Part Three considers physician-assisted suicide in reference to the practice of medicine, Part Four provides contrasting viewpoints on the issue of legalization, and Part Five presents religious perspectives.

Beauchamp, Tom L.: "Suicide." In Tom Regan, ed., *Matters of Life and Death,* 3rd ed. (New York: McGraw-Hill, 1993), pp. 69–120. In this long essay, Beauchamp provides both a conceptual analysis of suicide and an evaluation of various moral views. He also discusses suicide intervention and assisted suicide.

_____: "The Right to Die as the Triumph of Autonomy," *Journal of Medicine and Philosophy* 31 (December 2006), pp. 643–654. Beauchamp, an early defender of the right to die, traces the history of the debate in courts, legislatures, public opinion, and the bioethics literature since the 1960s. He argues that this is a history of increasing sympathy for the right to die and an emerging victory for the value of autonomy in biomedical ethics.

Beck, Robert N., and John B. Orr, eds.: *Ethical Choice: A Case Study Approach* (New York: Free Press, 1970). Section 2 of this work is entitled "Suicide" and conveniently reprints several classical sources on suicide: Seneca, St. Augustine, St. Thomas Aquinas, Hume, and Schopenhauer.

Caplan, Arthur L., Robert H. Blank, and Janna C. Merrick, eds.: *Compelled Compassion: Government Intervention in the Treatment of Critically Ill Newborns* (Totowa, NJ: Humana Press, 1992). This book provides an extensive collection of material on the federal "Baby Doe" legislation.

Coleman, Carl H., and Alan R. Fleischman: "Guidelines for Physician-Assisted Suicide: Can the Challenge Be Met?" *Journal of Law, Medicine & Ethics* 24 (Fall 1996), pp. 217–224. Coleman and Fleischman survey various proposals for regulating physician-assisted suicide and argue against legalization of the practice.

Gomez, Carlos F.: *Regulating Death: Euthanasia and the Case of The Netherlands* (New York: Free Press, 1991). Gomez describes and criticizes the practice of (active) euthanasia in The Netherlands. He argues that the Dutch system is plagued with inadequate controls.

Hastings Center Report 22 (March–April 1992). This issue provides a collection of articles under the heading "Dying Well? A Colloquy on Euthanasia and Assisted Suicide." Several of the articles deal specifically with the practice of (active) euthanasia in The Netherlands. Also, Dan W. Brock offers an extensive defense of voluntary active euthanasia, which Daniel Callahan opposes in "When Self-Determination Runs Amok."

Hedberg, Katrina, David Hopkins, and Melvin Kohn: "Five Years of Legal Physician-Assisted Suicide in Oregon," *New England Journal of Medicine* 348 (March 6, 2003), pp. 961–964. The authors, on behalf of Oregon Public Health Services, present statistical data on the practice of physician-assisted suicide in Oregon during the first five years (1998–2002) subsequent to legalization.

Legemaate, Johan: "The Dutch Euthanasia Act and Related Issues," *Journal of Law and Medicine* 11 (February 2004), pp. 312–323. Legemaate provides a discussion of the 2002 Dutch Termination of Life on Request and Assisted Suicide Act. He sets this legislation in historical context and considers international reactions to it. The full text of the act itself is included as an appendix to the article.

Mayo, David J., and Martin Gunderson: "Vitalism Revitalized: Vulnerable Populations, Prejudice, and Physician-Assisted Death," *Hastings Center Report* 32 (July–August 2002), pp. 14–21. Mayo and Gunderson reject the argument that physician-assisted death should not be legalized because people with disabilities (and members of other vulnerable populations) would be coerced into choosing physician-assisted death. The authors contend that this argument ultimately depends upon medical vitalism, the indefensible view that life should be prolonged whenever possible.

McStay, Rob: "Terminal Sedation: Palliative Care for Intractable Pain, post *Glucksberg* and *Quill*," *American Journal of Law & Medicine* 29 (2003), pp. 45–76. McStay clarifies the legal basis of terminal sedation and describes how the debate about terminal sedation has played out among legal and medical commentators.

Miller, Franklin G., and Diane E. Meier: "Voluntary Death: A Comparison of Terminal Dehydration and Physician-Assisted Suicide," *Annals of Internal Medicine* 128 (April 1, 1998), pp. 559–562. Miller and Meier argue that terminal dehydration has some notable advantages over physician-assisted suicide.

_____, Howard Brody, and Timothy E. Quill: "Can Physician-Assisted Suicide Be Regulated Effectively?" *Journal of Law, Medicine & Ethics* 24 (Fall 1996), pp. 225–232. The authors provide a further defense of their view that mandatory, independent palliative-care consultation is the key procedural safeguard necessary for the effective regulation of physician-assisted suicide.

Paris, John J., Jeffrey Ferranti, and Frank Reardon: "From the Johns Hopkins Baby to Baby Miller: What Have We Learned from Four Decades of Reflection on Neonatal Cases?" *Journal of Clinical Ethics* 12 (Fall 2001), pp. 207–214. The authors provide commentary on a series of prominent cases involving nontreatment decisions for severely impaired infants.

Pellegrino, Edmund D.: "Doctors Must Not Kill," *Journal of Clinical Ethics* 3 (Summer 1992), pp. 95–102. Pellegrino contends (1) that the moral arguments in favor of (active) euthanasia are flawed, (2) that killing by physicians would seriously distort the healing relationship, and (3) that the social consequences of allowing such killing would be detrimental.

Prado, C. G.: *The Last Choice: Preemptive Suicide in Advanced Age,* 2nd ed. (Westport, CT: Praeger, 1998). Prado's basic claim is that it can be rational for an aging individual to commit suicide in order to avoid a demeaning decline. That is, he claims that suicide can be a rational choice even prior to the onset of unendurable mental or physical suffering.

Quill, Timothy E.: "Death and Dignity: A Case of Individualized Decision Making," *New England Journal of Medicine* 324 (March 7, 1991), pp. 691–694. Quill presents a brief account of a case, often referred to as "the case of Diane," in which he assisted in the suicide of one of his patients.

_____, and Margaret P. Battin, eds.: *Physician-Assisted Dying: The Case for Palliative Care and Patient Choice* (Baltimore, MD: Johns Hopkins University Press, 2004). In this edited volume, a group of physicians, ethicists, lawyers, and activists advocate legalizing physician-assisted dying for terminally ill patients who voluntarily request it. They examine ethical arguments concerning self-determination and the relief of suffering; analyze empirical data from Oregon and the Netherlands; describe their personal experiences as physicians, family members, and patients; assess the legal and ethical responsibilities of the physician; and discuss the role of pain, depression, faith, and dignity in this decision.

_____, Bernard Lo, and Dan W. Brock: "Palliative Options of Last Resort: A Comparison of Voluntarily Stopping Eating and Drinking, Terminal Sedation, Physician-Assisted Suicide, and Voluntary Active Euthanasia," *JAMA* 278 (December 17, 1977), pp. 2099–2104. The authors compare and contrast the four identified practices. Both a clinical analysis and an ethical analysis are presented. Also provided is a brief discussion of appropriate safeguards for hastening death by any of the methods under discussion.

Rachels, James: "Euthanasia." In Tom Regan, ed., *Matters of Life and Death,* 3rd ed. (New York: McGraw-Hill, 1993), pp. 30–68. In this long essay, Rachels evaluates (1) arguments for and against the morality of active euthanasia and (2) arguments for and against legalizing it. He concludes that active euthanasia is morally acceptable and should be legalized.

Steinbock, Bonnie, and Alastair Norcross, eds.: *Killing and Letting Die,* 2nd ed. (New York: Fordham University Press, 1994). This anthology provides a wealth of material on the distinction between killing and letting die.

Warnock, Mary, and Elisabeth Macdonald: *Easeful Death: Is There a Case for Assisted Dying?* (Oxford: Oxford University Press, 2008). The authors assess arguments for and against legalization of assisted suicide and euthanasia, drawing on the experience of Britain, the Netherlands, Belgium, and the United States. They ultimately conclude that the public is ready to embrace a more compassionate approach to assisted dying and that the dying themselves deserve a greater say in the timing and manner of their deaths.

Weir, Robert F.: *Selective Nontreatment of Handicapped Newborns: Moral Dilemmas in Neonatal Medicine* (New York: Oxford University Press, 1984). Weir surveys and critically analyzes a wide range of views (advanced by various pediatricians, attorneys, and ethicists) on the subject of selective nontreatment. He then presents and defends an overall policy for the guidance of decision making in this area.

Wolf, Susan M.: "Gender, Feminism, and Death: Physician-Assisted Suicide and Euthanasia." In Susan M. Wolf, ed., *Feminism & Bioethics: Beyond Reproduction* (New York: Oxford University Press, 1996), pp. 282–317. Wolf provides an analysis of physician-assisted suicide and (active) euthanasia in reference to the category of gender. She also constructs feminist counterarguments to standard arguments in support of these practices, which she considers dangerous to women.

CHAPTER 7

ABORTION AND EMBRYONIC STEM CELL RESEARCH

INTRODUCTION

The first object of concern in this chapter is the issue of the ethical (moral) acceptability of abortion. Some attention is then given to the social policy aspects of abortion, especially in conjunction with decisions made by the U.S. Supreme Court. Finally, attention is focused on the ethics of research on embryonic stem cells.

ABORTION: THE ETHICAL ISSUE

Discussions of the ethical acceptability of abortion often take for granted (1) an awareness of the various reasons that may be given for having an abortion and (2) a basic acquaintance with the biological development of a human fetus.

Reasons for Abortion   Why would a woman have an abortion? The following catalog, not meant to provide an exhaustive survey, is sufficient to demonstrate the wide range of potential reasons for abortion. (1) In certain extreme cases, if the fetus is allowed to develop normally and come to term, the pregnant woman herself will die. (2) In other cases, it is not the woman's life but her health, physical or mental, that will be severely endangered if the pregnancy is allowed to continue. (3) There are also cases in which the pregnancy will probably, or surely, produce a severely impaired child,[1] and (4) there are others in which the pregnancy is the result of rape or incest.[2] (5) There are instances in which the pregnant woman is unmarried and faces the social stigma of illegitimacy. (6) In other instances, having a child, or having another child, will be a substantial financial burden and the woman does not wish to endure pregnancy and childbirth only to give up her baby for adoption. (7) Certainly common, and perhaps most common of all, are those instances in which the woman does not wish to give up her baby for adoption, but pregnancy, childbirth, and/or childrearing will interfere with her happiness, the joint happiness of the couple, or the happiness of a family unit that already includes children. There are almost endless possibilities in this final category. For example, the woman may desire a professional career, a couple may be content and happy together and feel their relationship would be damaged by the intrusion of a child, and parents may have older children and not feel up to raising another child.

The Biological Development of a Human Fetus During the course of a human pregnancy, in the nine-month period from conception to birth, the entity resulting from conception undergoes a continual process of change and development. *Conception* takes place when a male germ cell (the spermatozoon) combines with a female germ cell (the ovum), resulting in a single cell (the single-cell zygote), which embodies the full genetic code, twenty-three pairs of chromosomes. The single-cell zygote, also commonly identified as a newly formed *embryo,* soon begins a process of cellular division. While continuing to grow and beginning to take shape, the embryo moves through the fallopian tube and then undergoes gradual *implantation* at the uterine wall. The process of implantation is complete about eight to ten days after conception. The embryonic period continues until the end of the eighth week, and it is during this period—subsequent to implantation—that organ systems and other recognizably human characteristics begin to undergo noticeable development; in particular, rudimentary electrical activity in the brain may be detectable as early as the end of the sixth week. From the end of the eighth week until birth, the developing entity is formally designated a *fetus.* (The term *fetus,* however, is commonly used as a general term to designate the developing entity, whatever its stage of development.) Two other points in the development of the fetus are especially noteworthy as relevant to discussions of abortion, but these points are usually identified by reference to gestational age as calculated not from conception but from the first day of the woman's last menstrual period. Accordingly, somewhere around the sixteenth to the eighteenth week there usually occurs *quickening,* the point at which the woman begins to feel the movements of the fetus. And somewhere around the twenty-second week, *viability* becomes a realistic possibility. Viability is the point at which the fetus is capable of surviving outside the womb.

With the facts of fetal development in clear view, it may be helpful to describe the various abortion procedures. First-trimester abortions were at one time performed by *dilation and curettage (D&C),* but that procedure was essentially replaced in the 1970s by *vacuum aspiration,* often referred to as *suction abortion.* D&C involves the stretching (dilation) of the cervix and the scraping (curettage) of the inner walls of the uterus. In vacuum aspiration, the fetus is sucked out of the uterus by means of a tube connected to a suction pump. Although standard vacuum aspiration cannot effectively be performed prior to about two months after a pregnant woman's last period, a related technique—*manual vacuum aspiration (MVA)*—now provides the possibility of much earlier surgical abortion. In MVA, ultrasound is used to locate the tiny (smaller than a pea) gestational sac, which is then removed with a hand-held vacuum syringe. The use of RU-486, a chemical method for the termination of early pregnancies, is discussed later in this introduction.

Abortions beyond the first trimester require procedures such as *dilation and evacuation (D&E), induction techniques,* or *hysterotomy.* In D&E, which is the abortion procedure commonly used in the early stages of the second trimester, a forceps is used to dismember the fetus within the uterus; the fetal remains are then withdrawn through the cervix. In one notable induction technique, a saline solution injected into the amniotic cavity induces labor, thereby expelling the fetus. Another important induction technique employs prostaglandins (hormonelike substances) to induce labor. Hysterotomy—in essence, a miniature caesarean section—is a major surgical procedure and is uncommonly employed in the United States.

A brief discussion of fetal development, together with a cursory survey of various reasons for abortion, has prepared the way for a formulation of the ethical issue of abortion in its broadest terms. *Up to what point of fetal development, if any, and for what reasons, if any, is abortion ethically acceptable?* Some hold that abortion is *never* ethically acceptable, or at most that it is acceptable only when necessary to save the life of the pregnant woman. This view is frequently termed the *conservative* view on abortion. Others hold that abortion is *always* ethically acceptable—at any point of fetal development and for any of the standard reasons. This view is frequently termed the *liberal* view on abortion. Still others are anxious to defend perspectives that are termed *moderate* views, holding that abortion is ethically acceptable up to a certain point of fetal development and/or holding that some reasons provide a sufficient justification for abortion whereas others do not.

THE CONSERVATIVE VIEW AND THE LIBERAL VIEW

The *moral status* of the fetus has been a pivotal issue in discussions of the ethical acceptability of abortion. To say that the fetus has full moral status is to say that it is entitled to the same degree of moral consideration deserved by more fully developed human beings, such as the writer and the reader of these words. Assigning full moral status to the fetus entails, in particular, that the fetus has a right to life that must be taken as seriously as the right to life of any other human being. On the other hand, to say that the fetus has no significant moral status is to say that it has no rights worth mentioning. In particular, it does not possess a significant right to life. Conservatives typically claim that the fetus has full moral status, and liberals typically claim that the fetus has no significant moral status. (Some moderates argue that the fetus has a subsidiary or *partial* moral status.) Since the fetus has no significant moral status, the liberal is prone to argue, it has no more right to life than a piece of tissue, such as an appendix, and an abortion is no more morally objectionable than an appendectomy. Since the fetus has full moral status, the conservative is prone to argue, its right to life must be respected with the utmost seriousness, and an abortion, except perhaps to save the life of a pregnant woman, is as morally objectionable as any other murder.

Discussions of the moral status of the fetus often refer directly to the biological development of the fetus and pose the question: At what point in the continuous development of the fetus does a human life exist? In the context of such discussions, *human* implies full moral status, *nonhuman* implies no significant moral status, and any notion of partial moral status is systematically excluded. To distinguish the human from the nonhuman, to "draw the line," and to do so in a nonarbitrary way, is the central matter of concern. A conservative on abortion typically holds that the line must be drawn at conception. Usually the conservative argues that conception is the only point at which the line can be nonarbitrarily drawn. Against attempts to draw the line at points such as implantation, quickening, viability, or birth, considerations of continuity in the development of the fetus are pressed. The conservative argues that a line cannot be securely drawn anywhere along the path of fetal development. It is said that the line will inescapably slide back to the point of conception to find objective support—by reference to the fact that the full genetic code is present subsequent to conception, whereas it is not present prior to conception.

With regard to drawing the line, a liberal typically contends that the fetus remains non-human even in its most advanced stages of development. The liberal, of course, does not mean to deny that a fetus is biologically a human fetus. Rather, the claim is that the fetus is not human in any morally significant sense; that is, the fetus has no significant moral status. This point is often made in terms of the concept of personhood. Mary Anne Warren, who defends the liberal view on abortion in one of this chapter's selections, argues that the fetus is not a person. She also contends that the fetus bears so little resemblance to a person that it cannot be said to have a significant right to life. It is important to notice, as Warren analyzes the concept of personhood, that even a newborn baby is not a person. This conclusion, as might be expected, prompts Warren to a consideration of the moral justifiability of infanticide, an issue closely related to the problem of abortion.

Although the conservative view on abortion is most commonly predicated on the straightforward contention that the fetus is a person from conception, at least two other lines of argument have been advanced in its defense. One conservative, advancing what might be labeled "the presumption argument," writes:

> In being willing to kill the embryo, we accept responsibility for killing what we must admit *may* be a person. There is some reason to believe it is—namely the *fact* that it is a living, human individual and the inconclusiveness of arguments that try to exclude it from the protected circle of personhood.
>
> *To be willing to kill what for all we know could be a person, is to be willing to kill it if it is a person.* And since we cannot absolutely settle if it is a person except by a metaphysical postulate, for all practical purposes we must hold that to be willing to kill the embryo is to be willing to kill a person.[3]

In accordance with this line of argument, although it may not be possible to show conclusively that the fetus is a person from conception, we must presume that it is. Another line of argument that has been advanced by some conservatives emphasizes the potential rather than the actual personhood of the fetus. Even if the fetus is not a person, it is said, there can be no doubt that it is a potential person. Accordingly, by virtue of its potential personhood, the fetus must be accorded a right to life. Warren, in response to this line of argument, argues that the potential personhood of the fetus provides no basis for the claim that it has a significant right to life.

The Roman Catholic church is a prominent proponent of the conservative view on abortion. In this chapter's first reading, Pope John Paul II gives voice to the Catholic tradition on the issue of abortion. In another reading in this chapter, Don Marquis argues for a conservative view on abortion, but he does not argue for what is commonly referred to as "the" conservative view on abortion. Whereas the standard conservative, such as John Paul II, is committed to a sanctity-of-life viewpoint, according to which the lives of all biologically human beings (assuming their moral innocence) are considered immune from attack, Marquis bases his opposition to abortion on a distinctive theory about the wrongness of killing. Although Marquis claims there is a strong moral presumption against abortion and although he clearly believes that the vast majority of abortions are seriously immoral, he is not committed to the standard conservative contention that the only possible exception is the case in which abortion is necessary to save the life of the pregnant woman.

MODERATE VIEWS

The conservative and liberal views, as explicated, constitute two extreme poles on the spectrum of ethical views on abortion. Each of the extreme views is marked by a formal simplicity. The conservative proclaims abortion to be immoral, irrespective of the stage of fetal development and irrespective of alleged justifying reasons. The one exception admitted by some conservatives is the case in which abortion is necessary to save the life of the pregnant woman.[4] The liberal proclaims abortion to be morally acceptable, irrespective of the stage of fetal development.[5] Moreover, there is no need to draw distinctions between those reasons that are sufficient to justify abortion and those that are not. No justification is needed. The moderate, in vivid contrast to both the conservative and the liberal, is unwilling either to condemn or to condone abortion in sweeping terms. Some abortions are morally justifiable; some are morally objectionable. In some moderate views, the stage of fetal development is a relevant factor in the assessment of the moral acceptability of abortion. In other moderate views, the alleged justifying reason is a relevant factor in the assessment of the moral acceptability of abortion. In still other moderate views, both the stage of fetal development and the alleged justifying reason are relevant factors in the assessment of the moral acceptability of abortion.

Moderate views have been developed in accordance with the following clearly identifiable strategies:

1. Moderation of the Conservative View   One strategy for generating a moderate view presumes the typical conservative contention that the fetus is a person (i.e., has full moral status) from conception. What is denied, however, is that we must accept to the moral impermissibility of abortion in *all* or nearly all cases. In a widely discussed article reprinted in this chapter, Judith Jarvis Thomson attempts to moderate the conservative view in just this way. For Thomson, even if it is presumed that the fetus is a person from conception, abortion is morally justified in a significant range of cases.

2. Moderation of the Liberal View   A second strategy for generating a moderate view presumes the liberal contention that the fetus has no significant moral status, even in the latest stages of pregnancy. What is denied, however, is that we must accept the moral permissibility of abortion in *all* cases. It might be said, in accordance with this line of thought, that abortion, even though it does not violate the rights of the fetus (which is presumed to have no rights), remains ethically problematic to the extent that negative social consequences flow from its practice. Such an argument seems especially forceful in the later stages of pregnancy, when the fetus increasingly resembles a newborn infant. It is argued that very late abortions have a brutalizing effect on those involved and, in various ways, lead to the breakdown of attitudes associated with respect for human life. Thus, the conclusion is that very late abortions cannot be morally justified in the absence of weighty reasons.

3. Moderation in Drawing the Line   A third strategy for generating a moderate view—in fact, a whole range of moderate views—is associated with drawing-the-line discussions. Whereas the conservative typically draws the line between human (full moral status) and nonhuman (negligible moral status) at conception and the liberal typically draws that line at birth (or even somewhat later), a moderate view may be generated by drawing the line somewhere between these two extremes. For example, one might draw the line at implantation, at the point where brain activity begins, at quickening, at viability, and so forth.[6] Whereas drawing the line at implantation would tend to generate a rather conservative moderate view, drawing the line at viability would tend to generate a rather liberal moderate view. Wherever the line is drawn, it is the burden of any such moderate view to show that the point specified is a nonarbitrary one. Once such a point has been specified, however, it might be argued that abortion is ethically acceptable before that point and ethically unacceptable after that point. Of course, further stipulations may be added in accordance with strategies 1 and 2.

4. Moderation in the Assignment of Moral Status A fourth strategy for generating a moderate view is dependent upon assigning the fetus some sort of *partial moral status*.[7] It would seem that anyone who defends a moderate view based on the concept of partial moral status must first of all face the problem of explicating the nature of such partial moral status. Second, and closely related, is the problem of showing how the interests of those with partial moral status (or perhaps the claims that can be made on their behalf) are to be weighed against the interests and rights of those who have full moral status. In one of the readings in this chapter, Margaret Olivia Little presents a unique, nuanced discussion of the morality of abortion. Her overall analysis is calculated to be responsive to the particular identities, commitments, and personal ideals of individual women who face abortion decisions, but the point of departure for her analysis can be understood as the claim that the fetus has some sort of partial moral status.

ABORTION AND SOCIAL POLICY

In the United States, the Supreme Court's decision in *Roe v. Wade* (1973) has been the focal point of the social policy debate over abortion. This case had the effect, for all practical purposes, of legalizing "abortion on request." The Court held that it was unconstitutional for a state to have laws prohibiting the abortion of a previable fetus. According to the *Roe* Court, a woman has a constitutionally guaranteed right to terminate a pregnancy (prior to viability), although a state, for reasons related to maternal health, may restrict the manner and circumstances in which abortions are performed subsequent to the end of the first trimester. The reasoning underlying the Court's holding in *Roe* can be found in the majority opinion reprinted in this chapter.

Since the action of the Court in *Roe* had the practical effect of establishing a woman's legal right to choose whether or not to abort, it was enthusiastically received by "pro-choice" forces. On the other hand, "pro-life" forces, committed to the conservative view on the morality of abortion, vehemently denounced the Court for "legalizing murder." In response to *Roe*, pro-life forces adopted a number of political strategies, several of which are discussed here.

Pro-life forces originally worked for the enactment of a constitutional amendment directly overturning *Roe*. The proposed "human life amendment"—declaring the personhood of the fetus—was calculated to achieve the legal prohibition of abortion, allowing an exception only for abortions necessary to save the life of a pregnant woman. Pro-life support also emerged for the idea of a constitutional amendment allowing Congress and/or each state to decide whether to restrict abortion. (If this sort of amendment were enacted, it would undoubtedly have the effect of prohibiting abortion or at least severely restricting it in a number of states.) Pro-choice forces reacted in strong opposition to these proposed constitutional amendments. In their view, any effort to achieve the legal prohibition of abortion represents an illicit attempt by one group—conservatives on abortion—to impose their moral views on those who have different views.

In 1980, pro-life forces were notably successful in working toward a more limited political aim, the cutoff of Medicaid funding for abortion. Medicaid is a social program designed to provide funds to pay for the medical care of impoverished people. At issue in *Harris v. McRae,* decided by the Supreme Court in 1980, was the constitutionality of the so-called Hyde amendment, legislation that had passed Congress with vigorous pro-life support. The Hyde amendment, in the version considered by the Court, restricted federal Medicaid funding to (1) cases in which the pregnant woman's life is endangered and (2) cases of rape and incest. The Court, in a five-to-four decision, upheld the constitutionality of the Hyde amendment. According to the Court, a woman's right to an abortion does not entail *the right to have society fund the abortion.* However, if there is no constitutional obstacle to the cutoff of Medicaid funding for abortion, the question remains whether society's refusal to fund the abortions of poor women is an ethically sound social policy. Considerations of social justice are often pressed by those who argue that it is not.

With the decision of the Supreme Court in *Webster v. Reproductive Health Services* (1989), pro-life forces celebrated a dramatic victory. Two crucial provisions of a Missouri statute were upheld. One provision bans the use of *public* facilities and *public* employees in the performance of abortions. Another requires physicians to perform tests to determine the viability of any fetus believed to be twenty weeks or older. From the perspective of pro-life forces, the Court's holding in *Webster* represented the first benefits of a long-term strategy to undermine *Roe v. Wade* by controlling (through the political process) the appointment of new Supreme Court justices. More important than the actual holding of the case was the fact that the Court had apparently indicated its willingness to abandon *Roe.* In *Planned Parenthood of Southeastern Pennsylvania v. Casey* (1992), however, the Court reaffirmed what it deemed the "essential holding" of *Roe:* that women have a constitutional right to obtain abortions prior to fetal viability, and to obtain postviability abortions when medically necessary to protect their lives or health. Although states may impose various requirements on women seeking previability abortions, such as twenty-four-hour waiting periods and mandated exposure to information about the procedure, such requirements must not constitute an "undue burden." The Court also abandoned what has come to be known as the trimester framework of *Roe,* noting that advances in neonatology had since rendered fetuses viable before the beginning of the third trimester.

The emergence of RU-486 (mifepristone), a drug developed in France, has further complicated the social policy debate over abortion in the United States. RU-486 can be taken as an "abortion pill" and, in combination with a second drug taken to induce contractions, effectively terminates early pregnancies.[8] Throughout the 1990s, pro-choice forces emphasized the importance of access to this private, nonsurgical form of abortion and worked to make RU-486 legally available in the United States. The drug first became legally available to pregnant women in the United States in September 2000, under a protocol approved by the Food and Drug Administration. Of course, pro-life forces bitterly oppose the legal availability of RU-486. They refer to the drug as a "human pesticide" and denounce its use as "chemical warfare on the unborn."

Another dimension of the social policy debate over abortion in the United States involves the use of a rare, late-term abortion procedure known medically as *intact dilation and extraction* (intact D&X). Opponents of the procedure commonly refer to it as "partial-birth abortion." Intact D&X, which is sometimes used for late second-trimester abortions and for third-trimester abortions, can be understood as a variation on the D&E procedure discussed earlier. In one of its forms, intact D&X involves the partial, feet-first delivery of a fetus, followed by extraction of the brain in order to collapse the skull, so that the head can then pass through the cervix. Whereas D&E results in a dismembered fetus, intact D&X results in an "intact" fetus. The history of legislative efforts to ban "partial-birth abortion" is already complex, as is the history of constitutional challenges to such bans. In *Stenberg v. Carhart* (2000), the U.S. Supreme Court struck down Nebraska's ban on "partial-birth abortion." At the time this case was decided, similar bans existed in about thirty states. Subsequently, Congress passed the Partial Birth Abortion Ban Act of 2003, which the Court upheld in *Gonzales v. Carhart* (2007), in a five-to-four opinion joined by the newest members, Justice Samuel Alito and Chief Justice John Roberts. In one of this chapter's readings, George J. Annas provides a rich account of the constitutional issues in *Stenberg* and *Carhart*.

EMBRYONIC STEM-CELL RESEARCH

A human embryo reaches the so-called *blastocyst* stage of its development about five days after fertilization. At the blastocyst stage, the embryo contains both an inner cell mass that would normally develop into a fetus and an outer layer of cells that would normally become part of the placenta. The cells making up the inner cell mass of the blastocyst are capable of developing into virtually any type of human cell or tissue. If these cells are extracted, they are identified as embryonic stem cells. Such cells are believed to have great value for various research applications, especially in connection with hoped-for therapies for many diseases and conditions, including Alzheimer's disease, diabetes, and spinal cord injury. Of course, deriving stem cells from a human embryo at the blastocyst stage entails the destruction of that embryo. Hence, subsequent to reports in 1998 of the first successful derivation of embryonic stem cells from human embryos, a firestorm of controversy erupted around the possibility of research on embryonic stem cells. At the center of this controversy is the ethics of research on embryonic stem cells, although a related policy issue is also prominent in the overall societal debate—that is, whether and to what extent federal funding should be provided for research on embryonic stem cells. Discussion in this chapter is largely restricted to the ethics of research on embryonic stem cells and does not directly engage the funding issue.

Obviously, the issue of the moral status of the early embryo is crucially implicated in discussions of the ethics of research on embryonic stem cells. If full moral status is attributed to the early embryo, then there would seem to be no ethical justification for the destruction of embryos necessary to derive embryonic stem cells for research purposes. On the other hand, if no significant moral status is attributed to the early embryo, there would seem to be no real problem with the derivation and use of embryonic stem cells for research purposes. In an excerpt included in this chapter, Jeff McMahan defends the latter view. He argues that you and I were never early embryos, and that destroying an early embryo does not kill someone like us. In his view, we do not begin to exist until the fetal brain develops the capacity for consciousness, between twenty-two and twenty-eight weeks. Although McMahan's position does not entail that creating and destroying embryos for research purposes is morally unproblematic, it removes the most obvious basis for claiming that early embryos have anything approaching the moral status of newborn infants.

Many commentators would, indeed, attribute some sort of partial or intermediate moral status to the early embryo. In their view, an embryo is entitled to some measure of respect corresponding to its intermediate moral status. Advocates of this approach differ among themselves, however, regarding whether or not the respect due to the early embryo is compatible with the creation and destruction of embryos for research purposes. Some argue that respect for embryos does not rule out the creation and destruction of embryos for research purposes, but requires only that embryos not be used for unimportant or frivolous purposes.[9] A contrasting view, given voice in this chapter by the President's Council on Bioethics, holds that if the early embryo is attributed an intermediate and developing moral status, this moral status will be the ground of a "special respect" for embryos, and this special respect must be understood as ruling out the creation of embryos solely for research applications that entail their very destruction. However, this view does not necessarily rule out the derivation of embryonic stem cells from already existing "spare" embryos—that is, embryos originally created for reproductive purposes but no longer needed.

In another of this chapter's readings, a document from the National Institutes of Health provides useful background information about so-called *pluripotent* stem cells and their potential therapeutic value. (Embryonic stem cells are the most prominent type of pluripotent stem cells.) The NIH document also provides background information on adult stem cells and their therapeutic potential. According to one important argument in the stem cell controversy, the potential therapeutic value of adult stem cells is so substantial that there is no compelling need for research on embryonic stem cells. This argument has gained some force in the wake of recent breakthroughs in which differentiated adult cells were genetically modified into a stem-cell-like state, resulting in *induced pluripotent stem cells*.[10] Many questions remain unanswered about the potential of these new cells, however, and many in the field argue that research using embryonic stem cells is still urgent and ethically defensible.

There is an important point at which the stem cell controversy intersects with the cloning controversy. The ethics of human reproductive cloning is fully discussed in Chapter 8, but it is essential at this time to explain the difference between *reproductive* cloning and *research* cloning. Both types of cloning involve somatic cell nuclear transfer (SCNT). In SCNT, the nucleus of a donor somatic cell is transferred into an egg cell whose nucleus has been extracted, and the overall result is the formation of a "cloned embryo." Reproductive cloning would involve the subsequent development of the cloned embryo, its implantation in the uterus of a woman, and the eventual birth of a human child, who would be a "clone" of the person who provided the original genetic material. Research cloning would involve the development of the embryo only to a certain stage, with the intention of studying its development or otherwise using it for research purposes.[11] One especially prominent possibility in this regard is allowing the cloned embryo to develop only to the blastocyst stage, then destroying it by extracting its stem cells. Thus, three important sources of embryonic stem cells can be identified: (1) "spare" embryos originally created for reproductive purposes by in vitro fertilization; (2) embryos expressly created for research purposes by in vitro fertilization; (3) cloned embryos expressly created for research purposes.

In *Human Cloning and Human Dignity: An Ethical Inquiry* (2002), the President's Council on Bioethics (PCB) considered both cloning to produce children (reproductive cloning) and cloning for biomedical research (research cloning).[12] Although members of the PCB unanimously agreed on the moral impermissibility of reproductive cloning, the group found itself deeply divided on the ethics of research cloning. Reflecting this deep division, the PCB presented in its report both "the moral case for cloning-for-biomedical-research," expressing the views of one segment of the council, and "the moral case against cloning-for-biomedical-research," expressing the views of the other segment. Only the latter section of the report is reprinted in this chapter.[13] According to those members of the PCB morally opposed to research cloning, it is morally indefensible to create any embryo, whether by cloning or by in vitro fertilization, solely for research purposes. This part of their argument is explicitly based on underlying claims about the moral status of the early embryo, but there are also other dimensions in their overall argument against research cloning. In particular, it is argued that research cloning would "open the door" for reproductive cloning.

NOTES

1 The first section of Chapter 8 provides an extensive discussion of prenatal diagnosis and selective abortion.

2 The expression *therapeutic abortion* suggests abortion for medical reasons. Accordingly, abortions corresponding to reasons 1, 2, and 3 are usually said to be therapeutic. More problematically, abortions corresponding to reason 4 have often been identified as therapeutic. Perhaps it is presumed that pregnancies resulting from rape or incest are traumatic and thus a threat to mental health. Alternatively, perhaps calling such an abortion "therapeutic" is just a way of indicating that it is thought to be justifiable.

3 Germain Grisez, *Abortion: The Myths, the Realities, and the Arguments* (New York: Corpus Books, 1970), p. 306.

4 In accordance with Roman Catholic moral teaching, the *direct* killing of innocent human life is forbidden. Hence, abortion is forbidden. Even if the pregnant woman's life is in danger, perhaps because her heart or kidney function is inadequate, abortion is impermissible. In two special cases, however, procedures resulting in the death of the fetus are allowable. In the case of an ectopic pregnancy, where the developing fetus is lodged in the fallopian tube, the fallopian tube may be removed. In the case of a pregnant woman with a cancerous uterus, the cancerous uterus may be removed. In these cases, the death of the fetus is construed as *indirect* killing, the foreseen but unintended by-product of a surgical procedure designed to protect the life of the woman. If the distinction between direct and indirect killing is a defensible one (and this is a controversial issue), it might still be suggested that the distinction is not rightly applied in the Roman Catholic view of abortion. For example, some critics contend that abortion may be construed as indirect killing—indeed, an allowable form of indirect killing—in at least all cases in which it is necessary to save the life of the pregnant woman. For one helpful exposition and critical analysis of the Roman Catholic position on abortion, see Daniel Callahan, *Abortion: Law, Choice and Morality* (New York: Macmillan, 1970), Chapter 12, pp. 409–447.

5 In considering the liberal contention that abortions are morally acceptable irrespective of the stage of fetal development, we should take note of an ambiguity in the concept of abortion. Does *abortion* refer merely to the termination of a pregnancy in the sense of detaching the fetus from the pregnant woman, or does it entail the death of the fetus as well? Whereas the abortion of a previable fetus entails its death, the "abortion" of a viable fetus by means of hysterotomy (a miniature caesarean section) does not entail the death of the fetus and would seem to be tantamount to the birth of a baby. With regard to the "abortion" of a *viable* fetus, liberals can defend the woman's right to detach the fetus from her body without contending that the woman has the right to insist on the death of the child.

6 L. W. Sumner argues that the line should be drawn at the point at which the fetus becomes sentient, that is, capable of feeling pleasure and pain: "It is likely that a fetus is unable to feel pleasure or pain at the beginning of the second trimester and likely that it is able to do so at the end of that trimester. If this is so, then the threshold of sentience, and thus also the threshold of moral standing, occurs sometime during the second trimester." L. W. Sumner, "Abortion," in Donald VanDeVeer and Tom Regan, eds., *Health Care Ethics: An Introduction* (Philadelphia: Temple University Press, 1987), p. 179. Jeff McMahan also considers the problem of determining the onset of consciousness/sentience in the developing fetus. "Most neurologists accept that the earliest point at which consciousness is possible is around the twentieth week of pregnancy. . . . It is, however, unlikely that consciousness becomes possible until at least another month—that is, until around the sixth month." Jeff McMahan, *The Ethics of Killing* (New York: Oxford University Press, 2002), p. 267.

7 Callahan embraces this approach in *Abortion: Law, Choice and Morality,* pp. 493–501.

8 RU-486 is not to be confused with the "morning after" pill. RU-486 dislodges an embryo already implanted in the uterus; the "morning after" pill prevents implantation (although it may also prevent ovulation and fertilization).

9 See, e.g., Bonnie Steinbock, "What Does 'Respect for Embryos' Mean in the Context of Stem Cell Research?," *Women's Health Issues* 10 (May/June 2000), pp. 127–30.

10 See Rob Stein, "Scientists Report Advance in Stem Cell Alternative," *Washington Post,* Sept. 26, 2008, p. A17.

11 Research cloning is sometimes called *therapeutic cloning* because the principal long-term aim underlying research on cloned embryos is the development of therapies for serious diseases and conditions.

12 This document is available on the council's website (www.bioethics.gov).

13 The corresponding section, located in Chapter 6 of the report, can be easily accessed at the council's website (see previous note).

THE MORALITY OF ABORTION

THE UNSPEAKABLE CRIME OF ABORTION
Pope John Paul II

Insisting that we must "call things by their proper name," Pope John Paul II identifies abortion as the *murder* of an innocent and defenseless human being. He considers some of the reasons ordinarily given to justify abortion and concludes that such reasons are never sufficient to justify the deliberate killing of an innocent human being. He then identifies several groups of people and claims that these groups, in various ways, share in the moral guilt associated with the practice of abortion. In the end, John Paul II argues that *from the moment of conception* a human being is a person or, at any rate, must be respected and treated as a person.

Among all the crimes which can be committed against life, procured abortion has characteristics making it particularly serious and deplorable. The Second Vatican Council defines abortion, together with infanticide, as an "unspeakable crime."[1]

But today, in many people's consciences, the perception of its gravity has become progressively obscured. The acceptance of abortion in the popular mind, in behaviour and even in law itself, is a telling sign of an extremely dangerous crisis of the moral sense, which is becoming more and more incapable of distinguishing between good and evil, even when the fundamental right to life is at stake. Given such a grave situation, we need now more than ever to have the courage to look the truth in the eye and to *call things by their proper name,* without yielding to convenient compromises or to the temptation of self-deception. In this regard the reproach of the Prophet

From *Evangelium Vitae,* encyclical letter of John Paul II, March 25, 1995. Reprinted with permission. © Libreria Editrice Vaticana, 00120 Città del Vaticano.

is extremely straightforward: "Woe to those who call evil good and good evil, who put darkness for light and light for darkness" (*Is* 5:20). Especially in the case of abortion there is a widespread use of ambiguous terminology, such as "interruption of pregnancy," which tends to hide abortion's true nature and to attenuate its seriousness in public opinion. Perhaps this linguistic phenomenon is itself a symptom of an uneasiness of conscience. But no word has the power to change the reality of things: procured abortion is *the deliberate and direct killing, by whatever means it is carried out, of a human being in the initial phase of his or her existence, extending from conception to birth.*

The moral gravity of procured abortion is apparent in all its truth if we recognize that we are dealing with murder and, in particular, when we consider the specific elements involved. The one eliminated is a human being at the very beginning of life. No one more absolutely *innocent* could be imagined. In no way could this human being ever be considered an aggressor, much less an unjust aggressor! He or she is *weak,* defenseless, even to the point of lacking that minimal form of defence consisting in the poignant power of a newborn baby's cries and tears. The unborn child is *totally entrusted* to the protection and care of the woman carrying him or her in the womb. And yet sometimes it is precisely the mother herself who makes the decision and asks for the child to be eliminated, and who then goes about having it done.

It is true that the decision to have an abortion is often tragic and painful for the mother, insofar as the decision to rid herself of the fruit of conception is not made for purely selfish reasons or out of convenience, but out of a desire to protect certain important values such as her own health or a decent standard of living for the other members of the family. Sometimes it is feared that the child to be born would live in such conditions that it would be better if the birth did not take place. Nevertheless, these reasons and others like them, however serious and tragic, *can never justify the deliberate killing of an innocent human being.*

As well as the mother, there are often other people too who decide upon the death of the child in the womb. In the first place, the father of the child may be to blame, not only when he directly pressures the woman to have an abortion, but also when he indirectly encourages such a decision on her part by leaving her alone to face the problems of pregnancy:[2] in this way the family is thus mortally wounded and profaned in its nature as a community of love and in its vocation to be the "sanctuary of life." Nor can one overlook the pressures which sometimes come from the wider family circle and from friends. Sometimes the woman is subjected to such strong pressure that she feels psychologically forced to have an abortion: certainly in this case moral responsibility lies particularly with those who have directly or indirectly obliged her to have an abortion. Doctors and nurses are also responsible, when they place at the service of death skills which were acquired for promoting life.

But responsibility likewise falls on the legislators who have promoted and approved abortion laws, and, to the extent that they have a say in the matter, on the administrators of the health-care centres where abortions are performed. A general and no less serious responsibility lies with those who have

encouraged the spread of an attitude of sexual permissiveness and a lack of esteem for motherhood, and with those who should have ensured—but did not—effective family and social policies in support of families, especially larger families and those with particular financial and educational needs. Finally, one cannot overlook the network of complicity which reaches out to include international institutions, foundations and associations which systematically campaign for the legalization and spread of abortion in the world. In this sense abortion goes beyond the responsibility of individuals and beyond the harm done to them, and takes on a distinctly social dimension. It is a most serious *wound* inflicted on society and its culture by the very people who ought to be society's promoters and defenders. As I wrote in my *Letter to Families,* "we are facing an immense threat to life: not only to the life of individuals but also to that of civilization itself."[3] We are facing what can be called a *"structure of sin"* *which opposes human life not yet born.*

Some people try to justify abortion by claiming that the result of conception, at least up to a certain number of days, cannot yet be considered a personal human life. But in fact, "from the time that the ovum is fertilized, a life is begun which is neither that of the father nor the mother; it is rather the life of a new human being with his own growth. It would never be made human if it were not human already. This has always been clear, and . . . modern genetic science offers clear confirmation. It has demonstrated that from the first instant there is established the programme of what this living being will be: a person, this individual person with his characteristic aspects already well determined. Right from fertilization the adventure of a human life begins, and each of its capacities requires time—a rather lengthy time—to find its place and to be in a position to act."[4] Even if the presence of a spiritual soul cannot be ascertained by empirical data, the results themselves of scientific research on the human embryo provide "a valuable indication for discerning by the use of reason a personal presence at the moment of the first appearance of a human life: how could a human individual not be a human person?"[5]

Furthermore, what is at stake is so important that, from the standpoint of moral obligation, the mere probability that a human person is involved would suffice to justify an absolutely clear prohibition of any intervention aimed at killing a human embryo. Precisely for this reason, over and above all scientific debates and those philosophical affirmations to which the Magisterium has not expressly committed itself, the Church has always taught and continues to teach that the result of human procreation, from the first moment of its existence, must be guaranteed that unconditional respect which is morally due to the human being in his or her totality and unity as body and spirit: "*The human being is to be respected and treated as a person from the moment of conception;* and therefore from that same moment his rights as a person must be recognized, among which in the first place is the inviolable right of every innocent human being to life."[6] . . .

NOTES

1 Pastoral Constitution on the Church in the Modern World *Gaudium et Spes,* 51: "Abortus necnon infanticidium nefanda sunt crimina."

2 Cf. John Paul II, Apostolic Letter *Mulieris Dignitatem* (15 August 1988), 14: *AAS* 80 (1988), 1686.

3 No. 21: *AAS* 86 (1994), 920.

4 Congregation for the Doctrine of the Faith, *Declaration on Procured Abortion* (18 November 1974), Nos. 12–13: *AAS* 66 (1974), 738.

5 Congregation for the Doctrine of the Faith, Instruction on Respect for Human Life in Its Origin and on the Dignity of Procreation *Donum Vitae* (22 February 1987), I, No. 1: *AAS* 80 (1988), 78–79.

6 *Ibid., loc. cit.,* 79.

ON THE MORAL AND LEGAL STATUS OF ABORTION
Mary Anne Warren

Warren, defending the liberal view on abortion, promptly distinguishes two senses of the term *human:* (1) One is *human in the genetic sense* when one is a member of the biological species *Homo sapiens.* (2) One is *human in the moral sense* when one is a full-fledged member of the moral community. Warren attacks the presupposition underlying the standard conservative argument against abortion—that the fetus is human in the moral sense. She contends that the moral community, the set of beings with full and equal moral rights, consists of all and only people (persons). (Thus, she takes the concept of personhood to be equivalent to the concept of humanity in the moral sense.) After analyzing the concept of a person, she concludes that there is no stage of fetal development at which a fetus resembles a person enough to have a significant right to life. She also argues that the fetus's *potential* for being a person does not provide a basis for the claim that it has a significant right to life. It follows, in her view, that a woman's right to obtain an abortion is absolute. Abortion is morally justified at any stage of fetal development, and no legal restrictions should be placed on a woman's right to abort. In a concluding postscript, Warren briefly assesses the moral justifiability of infanticide.

The question which we must answer in order to produce a satisfactory solution to the problem of the moral status of abortion is this: How are we to define the moral community, the set of beings with full and equal moral rights, such that we can decide whether a human fetus is a member of this community or not? What sort of entity, exactly, has the inalienable rights to life, liberty, and the pursuit of happiness? Jefferson attributed these rights to all *men,* and it may or may not be fair to suggest that he intended to

Reprinted by permission from vol. 57, no. 1, of *The Monist,* LaSalle, Illinois 61301. "Postscript on Infanticide" reprinted with permission of the author from *The Problem of Abortion,* second edition, edited by Joel Feinberg (Belmont, Calif.: Wadsworth, 1984).

attribute them *only* to men. Perhaps he ought to have attributed them to all human beings. If so, then we arrive, first, at [John] Noonan's problem of defining what makes a being human, and, second, at the equally vital question which Noonan does not consider, namely, What reason is there for identifying the moral community with the set of all human beings, in whatever way we have chosen to define that term?

1 ON THE DEFINITION OF "HUMAN"

One reason why this vital second question is so frequently overlooked in the debate over the moral status of abortion is that the term 'human' has two distinct, but not often distinguished, senses. This fact results in a slide of meaning, which serves to conceal the fallaciousness of the traditional argument that since (1) it is wrong to kill innocent human beings, and (2) fetuses are innocent human beings, then (3) it is wrong to kill fetuses. For if 'human' is used in the same sense in both (1) and (2) then, whichever of the two senses is meant, one of these premises is question-begging. And if it is used in two different senses then of course the conclusion doesn't follow.

Thus, (1) is a self-evident moral truth,[1] and avoids begging the question about abortion, only if 'human being' is used to mean something like 'a full-fledged member of the moral community.' (It may or may not also be meant to refer exclusively to members of the species *Homo sapiens.*) We may call this the *moral* sense of 'human.' It is not to be confused with what we call the *genetic* sense, i.e., the sense in which *any* member of the species is a human being, and no member of any other species could be. If (1) is acceptable only if the moral sense is intended, (2) is non-question-begging only if what is intended is the genetic sense.

In "Deciding Who is Human," Noonan argues for the classification of fetuses with human beings by pointing to the presence of the full genetic code, and the potential capacity for rational thought.[2] It is clear that what he needs to show, for his version of the traditional argument to be valid, is that fetuses are human in the moral sense, the sense in which it is analytically true that all human beings have full moral rights. But, in the absence of any argument showing that whatever is genetically human is also morally human, and he gives none, nothing more than genetic humanity can

be demonstrated by the presence of the human genetic code. And, as we will see, the *potential* capacity for rational thought can at most show that an entity has the potential for *becoming* human in the moral sense.

2 DEFINING THE MORAL COMMUNITY

Can it be established that genetic humanity is sufficient for moral humanity? I think that there are very good reasons for not defining the moral community in this way. I would like to suggest an alternative way of defining the moral community, which I will argue for only to the extent of explaining why it is, or should be, self-evident. The suggestion is simply that the moral community consists of all and only *people,* rather than all and only human beings,[3] and probably the best way of demonstrating its self-evidence is by considering the concept of personhood, to see what sorts of entity are and are not persons, and what the decision that a being is or is not a person implies about its moral rights.

What characteristics entitle an entity to be considered a person? This is obviously not the place to attempt a complete analysis of the concept of personhood, but we do not need such a fully adequate analysis just to determine whether and why a fetus is or isn't a person. All we need is a rough and approximate list of the most basic criteria of personhood, and some idea of which, or how many, of these an entity must satisfy in order to properly be considered a person.

In searching for such criteria, it is useful to look beyond the set of people with whom we are acquainted, and ask how we would decide whether a totally alien being was a person or not. (For we have no right to assume that genetic humanity is necessary for personhood.) Imagine a space traveler who lands on an unknown planet and encounters a race of beings utterly unlike any he has ever seen or heard of. If he wants to be sure of behaving morally toward these beings, he has to somehow decide whether they are people, and hence have full moral rights, or whether they are the sort of thing which he need not feel guilty about treating as, for example, a source of food.

How should he go about making this decision? If he has some anthropological background, he might look for such things as religion, art, and the manufacturing of tools, weapons, or shelters, since these factors have been used to distinguish our human from our prehuman ancestors, in what seems to be closer to the moral than the genetic sense of 'human.' And no doubt he would be right to consider the presence of such factors as good evidence that the alien beings were people, and morally human. It would, however, be overly anthropocentric of him to take the absence of these things as adequate evidence that they were not, since we can imagine people who have progressed beyond, or evolved without ever developing, these cultural characteristics.

I suggest that the traits which are most central to the concept of personhood, or humanity in the moral sense, are, very roughly, the following:

1. Consciousness (of objects and events external and/or internal to the being), and in particular the capacity to feel pain;

2. Reasoning (the *developed* capacity to solve new and relatively complex problems);

3. Self-motivated activity (activity which is relatively independent of either genetic or direct external control);

4. The capacity to communicate, by whatever means, messages of an indefinite variety of types, that is, not just with an indefinite number of possible contents, but on indefinitely many possible topics;

5. The presence of self-concepts, and self-awareness, either individual or racial, or both.

Admittedly, there are apt to be a great many problems involved in formulating precise definitions of these criteria, let alone in developing universally valid behavioral criteria for deciding when they apply. But I will assume that both we and our explorer know approximately what (1)–(5) mean, and that he is also able to determine whether or not they apply. How, then, should he use his findings to decide whether or not the alien beings are people? We needn't suppose that an entity must have *all* of these attributes to be properly considered a person; (1) and (2) alone may well be sufficient for personhood, and quite probably (1)–(3) are sufficient. Neither do we need to insist that any one of these criteria is *necessary* for personhood, although once again (1) and (2) look

like fairly good candidates for necessary conditions, as does (3), if 'activity' is construed so as to include the activity of reasoning.

All we need to claim, to demonstrate that a fetus is not a person, is that any being which satisfies *none* of (1)–(5) is certainly not a person. I consider this claim to be so obvious that I think anyone who denied it, and claimed that a being which satisfied none of (1)–(5) was a person all the same, would thereby demonstrate that he had no notion at all of what a person is—perhaps because he had confused the concept of a person with that of genetic humanity. If the opponents of abortion were to deny the appropriateness of these five criteria, I do not know what further arguments would convince them. We would probably have to admit that our conceptual schemes were indeed irreconcilably different, and that our dispute could not be settled objectively.

I do not expect this to happen, however, since I think that the concept of a person is one which is very nearly universal (to people), and that it is common to both proabortionists and antiabortionists, even though neither group has fully realized the relevance of this concept to the resolution of their dispute. Furthermore, I think that on reflection even the antiabortionists ought to agree not only that (1)–(5) are central to the concept of personhood, but also that it is a part of this concept that all and only people have full moral rights. The concept of a person is in part a moral concept; once we have admitted that *x* is a person we have recognized, even if we have not agreed to respect, *x*'s right to be treated as a member of the moral community. It is true that the claim that *x* is a *human being* is more commonly voiced as part of an appeal to treat *x* decently than is the claim that *x* is a person, but this is either because 'human being' is here used in the sense which implies personhood, or because the genetic and moral sense of 'human' have been confused.

Now if (1)–(5) are indeed the primary criteria of personhood, then it is clear that genetic humanity is neither necessary nor sufficient for establishing that an entity is a person. Some human beings are not people, and there may well be people who are not human beings. A man or woman whose consciousness has been permanently obliterated but who remains alive is a human being which is no longer a person; defective human beings, with no appreciable mental capacity, are not and presumably never will be people; and a fetus is a human being which is not yet a person, and which therefore cannot coherently be said to have full moral rights. Citizens of the next century should be prepared to recognize highly advanced, self-aware robots or computers, should such be developed, and intelligent inhabitants of other worlds, should such be found, as people in the fullest sense, and to respect their moral rights. But to ascribe full moral rights to an entity which is not a person is as absurd as to ascribe moral obligations and responsibilities to such an entity.

3 FETAL DEVELOPMENT AND THE RIGHT TO LIFE

Two problems arise in the application of these suggestions for the definition of the moral community to the determination of the precise moral status of a human fetus. Given that the paradigm example of a person is a normal adult human being, then (1) How like this paradigm, in particular how far advanced since conception, does a human being need to be before it begins to have a right to life by virtue, not of being fully a person as of yet, but of being *like* a person? and (2) To what extent, if any, does the fact that a fetus has the *potential* for becoming a person endow it with some of the same rights? Each of these questions requires some comment.

In answering the first question, we need not attempt a detailed consideration of the moral rights of organisms which are not developed enough, aware enough, intelligent enough, etc., to be considered people, but which resemble people in some respects. It does seem reasonable to suggest that the more like a person, in the relevant respects, a being is, the stronger is the case for regarding it as having a right to life, and indeed the stronger its right to life is. Thus we ought to take seriously the suggestion that, insofar as "the human individual develops biologically in a continuous fashion . . . the rights of a human person might develop in the same way."[4] But we must keep in mind that the attributes which are relevant in determining whether or not an entity is enough like a person to be regarded as having some of the same moral rights are no different from those which are relevant to determining whether or not it is fully a person—

i.e., are no different from (1)–(5)—and that being genetically human, or having recognizable human facial and other physical features, or detectable brain activity, or the capacity to survive outside the uterus, are simply not among these relevant attributes.

Thus it is clear that even though a seven- or eight-month fetus has features which make it apt to arouse in us almost the same powerful protective instinct as is commonly aroused by a small infant, nevertheless it is not significantly more personlike than is a very small embryo. It is *somewhat* more personlike; it can apparently feel and respond to pain, and it may even have a rudimentary form of consciousness, insofar as its brain is quite active. Nevertheless, it seems safe to say that it is not fully conscious, in the way that an infant of a few months is, and that it cannot reason, or communicate messages of indefinitely many sorts, does not engage in self-motivated activity, and has no self-awareness. Thus, in the *relevant* respects, a fetus, even a fully developed one, is considerably less personlike than is the average mature mammal, indeed the average fish. And I think that a rational person must conclude that if the right to life of a fetus is to be based upon its resemblance to a person, then it cannot be said to have any more right to life than, let us say, a newborn guppy (which also seems to be capable of feeling pain), and that a right of that magnitude could never override a woman's right to obtain an abortion, at any stage of her pregnancy.

There may, of course, be other arguments in favor of placing legal limits upon the stage of pregnancy in which an abortion may be performed. Given the relative safety of the new techniques of artificially inducing labor during the third trimester, the danger to the woman's life or health is no longer such an argument. Neither is the fact that people tend to respond to the thought of abortion in the later stages of pregnancy with emotional repulsion, since mere emotional responses cannot take the place of moral reasoning in determining what ought to be permitted. Nor, finally, is the frequently heard argument that legalizing abortion, especially late in the pregnancy, may erode the level of respect for human life, leading, perhaps, to an increase in unjustified euthanasia and other crimes. For this threat, if it is a threat, can be better met by educating people to the kinds of moral distinctions which we are making here than by limiting access to abortion (which limitation may, in its disregard for the rights of women, be just as damaging to the level of respect for human rights).

Thus, since the fact that even a fully developed fetus is not personlike enough to have any significant right to life on the basis of its personlikeness shows that no legal restrictions upon the stage of pregnancy in which an abortion may be performed can be justified on the grounds that we should protect the rights of the older fetus; and since there is no other apparent justification for such restrictions, we may conclude that they are entirely unjustified. Whether or not it would be *indecent* (whatever that means) for a woman in her seventh month to obtain an abortion just to avoid having to postpone a trip to Europe, it would not, in itself, be *immoral,* and therefore it ought to be permitted.

4 POTENTIAL PERSONHOOD AND THE RIGHT TO LIFE

We have seen that a fetus does not resemble a person in any way which can support the claim that it has even some of the same rights. But what about its *potential,* the fact that if nurtured and allowed to develop naturally it will very probably become a person? Doesn't that alone give it at least some right to life? It is hard to deny that the fact that an entity is a potential person is a strong prima facie reason for not destroying it; but we need not conclude from this that a potential person has a right to life, by virtue of that potential. It may be that our feeling that it is better, other things being equal, not to destroy a potential person is better explained by the fact that potential people are still (felt to be) an invaluable resource, not to be lightly squandered. Surely, if every speck of dust were a potential person, we would be much less apt to conclude that every potential person has a right to become actual.

Still, we do not need to insist that a potential person has no right to life whatever. There may well be something immoral, and not just imprudent, about wantonly destroying potential people, when doing so isn't necessary to protect anyone's rights. But even if a potential person does have some prima facie right to life, such a right could not possibly outweigh the right of a woman to obtain an abortion, since the rights of any actual person invariably outweigh those of any potential person, whenever the two conflict. Since this may not be immediately obvious in the case of a human fetus, let us look at another case.

Suppose that our space explorer falls into the hands of an alien culture, whose scientists decide to create a few hundred thousand or more human beings, by breaking his body into its component cells, and using these to create fully developed human beings, with, of course, his genetic code. We may imagine that each of these newly created men will have all of the original man's abilities, skills, knowledge, and so on, and also have an individual self-concept, in short that each of them will be a bona fide (though hardly unique) person. Imagine that the whole project will take only seconds, and that its chances of success are extremely high, and that our explorer knows all of this, and also knows that these people will be treated fairly. I maintain that in such a situation he would have every right to escape if he could, and thus to deprive all of these potential people of their potential lives; for his right to life outweighs all of theirs together, in spite of the fact that they are all genetically human, all innocent, and all have a very high probability of becoming people very soon, if only he refrains from acting.

Indeed, I think he would have a right to escape even if it were not his life which the alien scientists planned to take, but only a year of his freedom, or, indeed, only a day. Nor would he be obligated to stay if he had gotten captured (thus bringing all these people-potentials into existence) because of his own carelessness, or even if he had done so deliberately, knowing the consequences. Regardless of how he got captured, he is not morally obligated to remain in captivity for *any* period of time for the sake of permitting any number of potential people to come into actuality, so great is the margin by which one actual person's right to liberty outweighs whatever right to life even a hundred thousand potential people have. And it seems reasonable to conclude that the rights of a woman will outweigh by a similar margin whatever right to life a fetus may have by virtue of its potential personhood.

Thus, neither a fetus's resemblance to a person, nor its potential for becoming a person provides any basis whatever for the claim that it has any significant right to life. Consequently, a woman's right to protect her health, happiness, freedom, and even her life,[5] by terminating an unwanted pregnancy, will always override whatever right to life it may be appropriate to ascribe to a fetus, even a fully developed one. And thus, in the absence of any overwhelming social need for every possible child, the laws which restrict the right to obtain an abortion, or limit the period of pregnancy during which an abortion may be performed, are a wholly unjustified violation of a woman's most basic moral and constitutional rights.[6]

POSTSCRIPT ON INFANTICIDE, FEBRUARY 26, 1982

One of the most troubling objections to the argument presented in this article is that it may appear to justify not only abortion but infanticide as well. A newborn infant is not a great deal more personlike than a nine-month fetus, and thus it might seem that if late-term abortion is sometimes justified, then infanticide must also be sometimes justified. Yet most people consider that infanticide is a form of murder, and thus never justified.

While it is important to appreciate the emotional force of this objection, its logical force is far less than it may seem at first glance. There are many reasons why infanticide is much more difficult to justify than abortion, even though if my argument is correct neither constitutes the killing of a person. In this country, and in this period of history, the deliberate killing of viable newborns is virtually never justified. This is in part because neonates are so very *close* to being persons that to kill them requires a very strong moral justification—as does the killing of dolphins, whales, chimpanzees, and other highly personlike creatures. It is certainly wrong to kill such beings just for the sake of convenience, or financial profit, or "sport."

Another reason why infanticide is usually wrong, in our society, is that if the newborn's parents do not want it, or are unable to care for it, there are (in most cases) people who are able and eager to adopt it and to provide a good home for it. Many people wait years for the opportunity to adopt a child, and some are unable to do so even though there is every reason to believe that they would be good parents. The needless destruction of a viable infant inevitably deprives some person or persons of a source of great pleasure and satisfaction, perhaps severely impoverishing their lives. Furthermore, even if an infant is considered to be unadoptable (e.g., because of some extremely severe mental or physical handicap) it is still wrong in most cases to kill it. For most of us value the lives of infants, and would prefer to pay taxes to support orphanages and state institutions for the handicapped rather than to allow unwanted infants to be killed. So long as most people feel this way, and so long as our society can afford to provide care for infants which are unwanted or which have special needs that preclude home care, it is wrong to destroy any infant which has a chance of living a reasonably satisfactory life.

If these arguments show that infanticide is wrong, at least in this society, then why don't they also show that late-term abortion is wrong? After all, third trimester fetuses are also highly person like, and many people value them and would much prefer that they be preserved; even at some cost to themselves. As a potential source of pleasure to some family, a viable fetus is just as valuable as a viable infant. But there is an obvious and crucial difference between the two cases: once the infant is born, its continued life cannot (except, perhaps, in very exceptional cases) pose any serious threat to the woman's life or health, since she is free to put it up for adoption, or, where this is impossible, to place it in a state-supported institution. While she might prefer that it die, rather than being raised by others, it is not clear that such a preference would constitute a right on her part. True, she may suffer greatly from the knowledge that her child will be thrown into the lottery of the adoption system, and that she will be unable to ensure its well-being, or even to know whether it is healthy, happy, doing well in school, etc.: for the law generally does not permit natural parents to remain in contact with their children, once they are adopted by another family. But there are surely better ways of dealing with these problems than by permitting infanticide in such cases. (It might help, for instance, if the natural parents of adopted children could at least receive some information about their progress, without necessarily being informed of the identity of the adopting family.)

In contrast, a pregnant woman's right to protect her own life and health clearly outweighs other people's desire that the fetus be preserved—just as, when a person's life or limb is threatened by some wild animal, and when the threat cannot be removed without killing the animal, the person's right to self-protection outweighs the desires of those who would prefer that the animal not be harmed. Thus, while the moment of birth may not mark any sharp discontinuity in the degree to which an infant possesses a right to life, it does mark the end of the mother's absolute right to determine its fate. Indeed, if and when a late-term abortion could be safely performed without killing the fetus, she would have no absolute right to insist on its death (e.g., if others wish to adopt it or pay for its care), for the same reason that she does not have a right to insist that a viable infant be killed.

It remains true that according to my argument neither abortion nor the killing of neonates is properly considered a form of murder. Perhaps it is understandable that the law should classify infanticide as murder or homicide, since there is no other existing legal category which adequately or conveniently expresses the force of our society's disapproval of this action. But the moral distinction remains, and it has several important consequences.

In the first place, it implies that when an infant is born into a society which—unlike ours—is so impoverished that it simply cannot care for it adequately without endangering the survival of existing persons, killing it or allowing it to die is not necessarily wrong—provided that there is no *other* society which is willing and able to provide such care. Most human societies, from those at the hunting and gathering stage of economic development to the highly civilized Greeks and Romans, have permitted the practice of infanticide under such unfortunate circumstances, and I would argue that it shows a serious lack of understanding to condemn them as morally backward for this reason alone.

In the second place, the argument implies that when an infant is born with such severe physical anomalies that its life would predictably be a very short and/or very miserable one, even with the most heroic of medical treatment, and where its parents do not choose to bear the often crushing emotional, financial and other burdens attendant upon the artifi-

cial prolongation of such a tragic life, it is not morally wrong to cease or withhold treatment, thus allowing the infant a painless death. It is wrong (and sometimes a form of murder) to practice involuntary euthanasia on persons, since they have the right to decide for themselves whether or not they wish to continue to live. But terminally ill neonates cannot make this decision for themselves, and thus it is incumbent upon responsible persons to make the decision for them, as best they can. The mistaken belief that infanticide is always tantamount to murder is responsible for a great deal of unnecessary suffering, not just on the part of infants which are made to endure needlessly prolonged and painful deaths, but also on the part of parents, nurses, and other involved persons, who must watch infants suffering needlessly, helpless to end that suffering in the most humane way.

I am well aware that these conclusions, however modest and reasonable they may seem to some people, strike other people as morally monstrous, and that some people might even prefer to abandon their previous support for women's right to abortion rather than accept a theory which leads to such conclusions about infanticide. But all that these facts show is that abortion is not an isolated moral issue; to fully understand the moral status of abortion we may have to reconsider other moral issues as well, issues not just about infanticide and euthanasia, but also about the moral rights of women and of nonhuman animals. It is a philosopher's task to criticize mistaken beliefs which stand in the way of moral understanding, even when—perhaps especially when—those beliefs are popular and widespread. The belief that moral strictures against killing should apply equally to *all* genetically human entities, and *only* to genetically human entities, is such an error. The overcoming of this error will undoubtedly require long and often painful struggle; but it must be done.

NOTES

1 Of course, the principle that it is (always) wrong to kill innocent human beings is in need of many other modifications, e.g., that it may be permissible to do so to save a greater number of other innocent human beings, but we may safely ignore these complications here.

2 John Noonan, "Deciding Who Is Human," *Natural Law Forum,* 13 (1968), 135.

3 From here on, we will use 'human' to mean genetically human, since the moral sense seems closely connected to, and perhaps derived from, the assumption that genetic humanity is sufficient for membership in the moral community.

4 Thomas L. Hayes, "A Biological View," *Commonweal*, 85 (March 17, 1967), 677–78; quoted by Daniel Callahan, in *Abortion: Law, Choice and Morality* (London: Macmillan & Co., 1970).

5 That is, insofar as the death rate, for the woman, is higher for childbirth than for early abortion.

6 My thanks to the following people, who were kind enough to read and criticize an earlier version of this paper: Herbert Gold, Gene Glass, Anne Lauterbach, Judith Thomson, Mary Mothersill, and Timothy Binkley.

WHY ABORTION IS IMMORAL
Don Marquis

Marquis argues that abortion, with rare exceptions, is seriously immoral. He bases this conclusion on a theory that he presents and defends about the wrongness of killing. In his view, killing another adult human being is wrong precisely because the victim is deprived of all the value—"activities, projects, experiences, and enjoyments"—of his or her future. Since abortion deprives a typical fetus of a "future like ours," he contends, the moral presumption against abortion is as strong as the presumption against killing another adult human being.

The view that abortion is, with rare exceptions, seriously immoral has received little support in the recent philosophical literature. No doubt most philosophers affiliated with secular institutions of higher education believe that the anti-abortion position is either a symptom of irrational religious dogma or a conclusion generated by seriously confused philosophical argument. The purpose of this essay is to undermine this general belief. This essay sets out an argument that purports to show, as well as any argument in ethics can show, that abortion is, except possibly in rare cases, seriously immoral, that it is in the same moral category as killing an innocent adult human being.

This argument is based on a major assumption: If fetuses are in the same category as adult human beings with respect to the moral value of their lives, then the *presumption* that any particular abortion is immoral is exceedingly strong. Such a presumption could be overridden only by considerations more compelling than a woman's right to privacy. The defense of this assumption is beyond the scope of this essay.[1]

Furthermore, this essay will neglect a discussion of whether there are any such compelling considerations and what they are. Plainly there are strong candidates: abortion before implantation, abortion when the life of a woman is threatened by a pregnancy or abortion after rape. The casuistry of these hard cases will not be explored in this essay. The purpose of this essay is to develop a general argument for the claim that, subject to the assumption above, the overwhelming majority of deliberate abortions are seriously immoral. . . .

. . . A necessary condition of resolving the abortion controversy is a . . . theoretical account of the wrongness of killing. After all, if we merely believe, but do not understand, why killing adult human beings such as ourselves is wrong, how could we conceivably show that abortion is either immoral or permissible? . . .

In order to develop such an account, we can start from the following unproblematic assumption concerning our own case: it is wrong to kill *us*. Why is it wrong? Some answers can be easily eliminated. It might be said that what makes killing us wrong is that a killing brutalizes the one who kills. But the brutalization consists of being inured to the performance

Reprinted, as slightly modified by the author, with permission of the author and the publisher from the *Journal of Philosophy*, vol. 86 (April 1989).

of an act that is hideously immoral; hence, the brutalization does not explain the immorality. It might be said that what makes killing us wrong is the great loss others would experience due to our absence. Although such hubris is understandable, such an explanation does not account for the wrongness of killing hermits, or those whose lives are relatively independent and whose friends find it easy to make new friends.

A more obvious answer is better. What primarily makes killing wrong is neither its effect on the murderer nor its effect on the victim's friends and relatives, but its effect on the victim. The loss of one's life is one of the greatest losses one can suffer. The loss of one's life deprives one of all the experiences, activities, projects, and enjoyments that would otherwise have constituted one's future. Therefore, killing someone is wrong, primarily because the killing inflicts (one of) the greatest possible losses on the victim. To describe this as the loss of life can be misleading, however. The change in my biological state does not by itself make killing me wrong. The effect of the loss of my biological life is the loss to me of all those activities, projects, experiences, and enjoyments which would otherwise have constituted my future personal life. These activities, projects, experiences, and enjoyments are either valuable for their own sakes or are means to something else that is valuable for its own sake. Some parts of my future are not valued by me now, but will come to be valued by me as I grow older and as my values and capacities change. When I am killed, I am deprived both of what I now value which would have been part of my future personal life, but also what I would come to value. Therefore, when I die, I am deprived of all of the value of my future. Inflicting this loss on me is ultimately what makes killing me wrong. This being the case, it would seem that what makes killing *any* adult human being prima facie seriously wrong is the loss of his or her future.[2]

How should this rudimentary theory of the wrongness of killing be evaluated? It cannot be faulted for deriving an 'ought' from an 'is,' for it does not. The analysis assumes that killing me (or you, reader) is prima facie seriously wrong. The point of the analysis is to establish which natural property ultimately explains the wrongness of the killing, given that it is wrong. A natural property will ultimately explain the wrongness of killing, only if (1) the explanation fits with our intuitions about the matter and (2) there is no other natural property that provides the basis for a better explanation of the wrongness of killing. This analysis rests on the intuition that what makes killing a particular human or animal wrong is what it does to that particular human or animal. What makes killing wrong is some natural effect or other of the killing. Some would deny this. For instance, a divine-command theorist in ethics would deny it. Surely this denial is, however, one of those features of divine-command theory which renders it so implausible.

The claim that what makes killing wrong is the loss of the victim's future is directly supported by two considerations. In the first place, this theory explains why we regard killing as one of the worst of crimes. Killing is especially wrong, because it deprives the victim of more than perhaps any other crime. In the second place, people with AIDS or cancer who know they are dying believe, of course, that dying is a very bad thing for them. They believe that the loss of a future to them that they would otherwise have experienced is what makes their premature death a very bad thing for them. A better theory of the wrongness of killing would require a different natural property associated with killing which better fits with the attitudes of the dying. What could it be?

The view that what makes killing wrong is the loss to the victim of the value of the victim's future gains additional support when some of its implications are examined. In the first place, it is incompatible with the view that it is wrong to kill only beings who are biologically human. It is possible that there exists a different species from another planet whose members have a future like ours. Since having a future like that is what makes killing someone wrong, this theory entails that it would be wrong to kill members of such a species. Hence, this theory is opposed to the claim that only life that is biologically human has great moral worth, a claim which many anti-abortionists have seemed to adopt. This opposition, which this theory has in common with personhood theories, seems to be a merit of the theory.

In the second place, the claim that the loss of one's future is the wrong-making feature of one's being killed entails the possibility that the futures of some actual nonhuman mammals on our own planet are sufficiently like ours that it is seriously wrong to kill them also. Whether some animals do have the same right to life as human beings depends on adding to the account of the wrongness of killing some additional account of just what it is about my future or the futures of other adult human beings which makes it wrong to kill us. No such additional account will be offered in this essay. Undoubtedly, the provision of such an account would be a very difficult matter. Undoubtedly, any such account would be quite controversial. Hence, it surely should not reflect badly on this sketch of an elementary theory of the wrongness of killing that it is indeterminate with respect to some very difficult issues regarding animal rights.

In the third place, the claim that the loss of one's future is the wrong-making feature of one's being killed does not entail, as sanctity of human life theories do, that active euthanasia is wrong. Persons who are severely and incurably ill, who face a future of pain and despair, and who wish to die will not have suffered a loss if they are killed. It is, strictly speaking, the value of a human's future which makes killing wrong in this theory. This being so, killing does not necessarily wrong some persons who are sick and dying. Of course, there may be other reasons for a prohibition of active euthanasia, but that is another matter. Sanctity-of-human-life theories seem to hold that active euthanasia is seriously wrong even in an individual case where there seems to be good reason for it independently of public policy considerations. This consequence is most implausible, and it is a plus for the claim that the loss of a future of value is what makes killing wrong that it does not share this consequence.

In the fourth place, the account of the wrongness of killing defended in this essay does straightforwardly entail that it is prima facie seriously wrong to kill children and infants, for we do presume that they have futures of value. Since we do believe that it is wrong to kill defenseless little babies, it is important that a theory of the wrongness of killing easily account for this. Personhood theories of the wrongness of killing, on the other hand, cannot straightforwardly account for the wrongness of killing infants and young children. Hence, such theories must add special ad hoc accounts of the wrongness of killing the young. The plausibility of such ad hoc theories seems to be a function of how desperately one wants such theories to work. The claim that the primary wrong-making feature of a killing is the loss to the victim of the value of its future accounts for the wrongness of killing young children and infants directly; it makes the wrongness of such acts as obvious as we actually think it is. This is a further merit of this theory. Accordingly, it seems that this value of a future-like-ours theory of the wrongness of killing shares strengths of both sanctity-of-life and personhood accounts while avoiding weaknesses of both. In addition, it meshes with a central intuition concerning what makes killing wrong.

The claim that the primary wrong-making feature of a killing is the loss to the victim of the value of its future has obvious consequences for the ethics of abortion. The future of a standard fetus includes a set of experiences, projects, activities, and such which are identical with the futures of adult human beings and are identical with the futures of young children. Since the reason that is sufficient to explain why it is wrong to kill human beings after the time of birth is a reason that also applies to fetuses, it follows that abortion is prima facie seriously morally wrong.

This argument does not rely on the invalid inference that, since it is wrong to kill persons, it is wrong to kill potential persons also. The category that is morally central to this analysis is the category of having a valuable future like ours; it is not the category of personhood. The argument to the conclusion that abortion is prima facie seriously morally wrong proceeded independently of the notion of person or potential person or any equivalent. Someone may wish to start with this analysis in terms of the value of a human future, conclude that abortion is, except perhaps in rare circumstances, seriously morally wrong, infer that fetuses have the right to life, and then call fetuses "persons" as a result of their having the right to life. Clearly, in this case, the category of person is being used to state the *conclusion* of the analysis rather than to generate the *argument* of the analysis.

The structure of this anti-abortion argument can be both illuminated and defended by comparing it to what appears to be the best argument for the wrongness of the wanton infliction of pain on animals. This latter argument is based on the assumption that it is prima facie wrong to inflict pain on me (or you, reader). What is the natural property associated with the infliction of pain which makes such infliction wrong? The obvious answer seems to be that the infliction of pain causes suffering and that suffering is a misfortune. The suffering caused by the infliction of pain is what makes the wanton infliction of pain on me wrong. The wanton infliction of pain on other adult humans causes suffering. The wanton infliction of pain on animals causes suffering. Since causing suffering is what makes the wanton infliction of pain wrong and since the wanton infliction of pain on animals causes suffering, it follows that the wanton infliction of pain on animals is wrong.

This argument for the wrongness of the wanton infliction of pain on animals shares a number of structural features with the argument for the serious prima facie wrongness of abortion. Both arguments start with an obvious assumption concerning what it is wrong to do to me (or you, reader). Both then look for the characteristic or the consequence of the wrong action which makes the action wrong. Both recognize that the wrong-making feature of these immoral actions is a property of actions sometimes directed at individuals other than postnatal human beings. If the structure of the argument for the wrongness of the wanton infliction of pain on animals is sound, then the structure of the argument for the prima facie serious wrongness of abortion is also sound, for the structure of the two arguments is the same. The structure common to both is the key to the explanation of how the wrongness of abortion can be demonstrated without recourse to the category of person. In neither argument is that category crucial. . . .

Of course, this value of a future-like-ours argument, if sound, shows only that abortion is prima facie wrong, not that it is wrong in any and all circumstances. Since the loss of the future to a standard fetus, if killed, is, however, at least as great a loss as the loss of the future to a standard adult human being who is killed, abortion, like ordinary killing, could be justified only by the most compelling reasons. The loss of one's life is almost the greatest misfortune that can happen to one. Presumably abortion could be justified in some circumstances, only if the loss consequent on failing to abort would be at least as great. Accordingly, morally permissible abortions will be rare indeed unless, perhaps, they occur so early in pregnancy that a fetus is not yet definitely an individual. Hence, this argument should be taken as showing that abortion is presumptively very seriously wrong, where the presumption is very strong—as strong as the presumption that killing another adult human being is wrong. . . .

In this essay, it has been argued that the correct ethic of the wrongness of killing can be extended to fetal life and used to show that there is a strong presumption that any abortion is morally impermissible. If the ethic of killing adopted here entails, however, that contraception is also seriously immoral, then there would appear to be a difficulty with the analysis of this essay.

But this analysis does not entail that contraception is wrong. Of course, contraception prevents the actualization of a possible future of value. Hence, it follows from the claim that futures of value should be maximized that contraception is prima facie immoral. This obligation to maximize does not exist, however; furthermore, nothing in the ethics of killing in this paper entails that it does. The ethics of killing in this essay would entail that contraception is wrong only if something were denied a human future of value by contraception. Nothing at all is denied such a future by contraception, however.

Candidates for a subject of harm by contraception fall into four categories: (1) some sperm or other, (2) some ovum or other, (3) a sperm and an ovum separately, and (4) a sperm and an ovum together. Assigning the harm to some sperm is utterly arbitrary, for no reason can be given for making a sperm the subject of harm rather than an ovum. Assigning the harm to some ovum is utterly arbitrary, for no reason can be given for making an ovum the subject of harm rather than a sperm. One might attempt to avoid these problems by insisting that contraception deprives both the sperm and the ovum separately of a valuable future like ours. On this alternative, too many futures are lost. Contraception was supposed to be wrong, because it deprived us of one future of value, not two. One might attempt to avoid this problem by holding that contraception deprives the combination of sperm and ovum of a valuable future like ours. But here the definite article misleads. At the time of contraception, there are hundreds of millions of sperm, one (released) ovum and millions of possible combinations of all of these. There is no actual combination at all. Is the subject of the loss to be a merely possible combination? Which one? This alternative does not yield an actual subject of harm either. Accordingly, the immorality of contraception is not entailed by the loss of a future-like-ours argument simply because there is no nonarbitrarily identifiable subject of the loss in the case of contraception. . . .

The purpose of this essay has been to set out an argument for the serious presumptive wrongness of abortion subject to the assumption that the moral permissibility of abortion stands or falls on the moral status of the fetus. Since a fetus possesses a property, the possession of which in adult human beings is sufficient to make killing an adult human being wrong, abortion is wrong. This way of dealing with the problem of abortion seems superior to other approaches to the ethics of abortion, because it rests on an ethics of killing which is close to self-evident, because the crucial morally relevant property clearly applies to fetuses, and because the argument avoids the usual equivocations on 'human life,' 'human being,' or 'person.' The argument rests neither on religious claims nor on Papal dogma. It is not subject to the objection of "speciesism." Its soundness is compatible with the moral permissibility of euthanasia and contraception. It deals with our intuitions concerning young children.

Finally, this analysis can be viewed as resolving a standard problem—indeed, *the* standard problem—concerning the ethics of abortion. Clearly, it is wrong to kill adult human beings. Clearly, it is not wrong to end the life of some arbitrarily chosen single human cell. Fetuses seem to be like arbitrarily chosen human cells in some respects and like adult humans in other respects. The problem of the ethics of abortion is the problem of determining the fetal property that settles this moral controversy. The thesis of this essay is that the problem of the ethics of abortion, so understood, is solvable.

NOTES

1 Judith Jarvis Thomson has rejected this assumption in a famous essay, "A Defense of Abortion," *Philosophy and Public Affairs* 1, #1 (1971), 47–66.
2 I have been most influenced on this matter by Jonathan Glover, *Causing Death and Saving Lives* (New York: Penguin, 1977), ch. 3; and Robert Young, "What Is So Wrong with Killing People?" *Philosophy,* LIV, 210 (1979): 515–528.

A DEFENSE OF ABORTION[1]
Judith Jarvis Thomson

In an effort to moderate the conservative view, Thomson argues that the standard conservative claim about the moral impermissibility of abortion cannot be sustained even if (for the sake of argument) it is presumed that the fetus is a person from conception. Her central point is that the moral impermissibility of abortion does not follow simply from the admission that the fetus (as a person) has a right to life. In her view, the right to life is to be understood as the right not to be killed unjustly and does not entail the right to use another person's body. In cases where the pregnant woman has not extended to the fetus the right to use her body, most prominently in the case of rape, Thomson holds that abortion is not unjust killing and thus does not violate the fetus's right to life. Thomson acknowledges that there may be cases in which the fetus (presumed to be a person) has a right to the use of the pregnant woman's body and, thus, some cases where abortion would be unjust killing. She proceeds to distinguish between the moral demands of justice and the moral demands of decency. In some cases, she maintains, an abortion does no injustice (to the fetus) yet may be subject to moral criticism on the grounds that minimal standards of moral decency are transgressed.

Most opposition to abortion relies on the premise that the fetus is a human being, a person, from the moment of conception. The premise is argued for, but, as I think, not well. Take, for example, the most common argument. We are asked to notice that the development of a human being from conception through birth into childhood is continuous; then it is said that to draw a line, to choose a point in this development and say "before this point the thing is not a person, after this point it is a person" is to make an arbitrary choice, a choice for which in the nature of things no good reason can be given. It is concluded that the fetus is, or anyway that we had better say it is, a person from the moment of conception. But this conclusion does not follow. Similar things might be said about the development of an acorn into an oak tree, and it does not follow that acorns are oak trees, or that we had better say they are. Arguments of this form are sometimes called "slippery slope arguments"—the phrase is perhaps self-explanatory—and it is dismaying that opponents of abortion rely on them so heavily and uncritically.

I am inclined to agree, however, that the prospects for "drawing a line" in the development of the fetus look dim. I am inclined to think also that we shall probably have to agree that the fetus has already become a human person well before birth. Indeed, it comes as a surprise when one first learns how early in its life it begins to acquire human characteristics. By the tenth week, for example, it already has a face, arms and legs, fingers and toes; it has internal organs, and brain activity is detectable.[2] On the other hand, I think that the premise is false, that the fetus is not a person from the moment of conception. A newly fertilized ovum, a newly implanted clump of cells, is no more a person than an

Philosophy and Public Affairs, vol. 1, no. 1 (1971), pp. 47–50, 54–66. Copyright © 1971 by Princeton University Press. Reprinted by permission of Blackwell Publishing Ltd.

acorn is an oak tree. But I shall not discuss any of this. For it seems to me to be of great interest to ask what happens if, for the sake of argument, we allow the premise. How, precisely, are we supposed to get from there to the conclusion that abortion is morally impermissible? Opponents of abortion commonly spend most of their time establishing that the fetus is a person, and hardly any time explaining the step from there to the impermissibility of abortion. Perhaps they think the step too simple and obvious to require much comment. Or perhaps instead they are simply being economical in argument. Many of those who defend abortion rely on the premise that the fetus is not a person, but only a bit of tissue that will become a person at birth; and why pay out more arguments than you have to? Whatever the explanation, I suggest that the step they take is neither easy nor obvious, that it calls for closer examination than it is commonly given, and that when we do give it this closer examination we shall feel inclined to reject it.

I propose, then, that we grant that the fetus is a person from the moment of conception. How does the argument go from here? Something like this, I take it. Every person has a right to life. So the fetus has a right to life. No doubt the mother has a right to decide what shall happen in and to her body; everyone would grant that. But surely a person's right to life is stronger and more stringent than the mother's right to decide what happens in and to her body, and so outweighs it. So the fetus may not be killed; an abortion may not be performed.

It sounds plausible. But now let me ask you to imagine this. You wake up in the morning and find yourself back to back in bed with an unconscious violinist. A famous unconscious violinist. He has been found to have a fatal kidney ailment, and the Society of Music Lovers has canvassed all the available medical records and found that you alone have the right blood type to help. They have therefore kidnapped you, and last night the violinist's circulatory system was plugged into yours, so that your kidneys can be used to extract poisons from his blood as well as your own. The director of the hospital now tells you, "Look, we're sorry the Society of Music Lovers did this to you—we would never have permitted it if we had known. But still, they did it, and the violinist now is plugged into you. To unplug you would be to kill him. But never mind, it's only for nine months. By then he will have recovered from his ailment, and can safely be unplugged from you." Is it morally incumbent on you to accede to this situation? No doubt it would be very nice of you if you did, a great kindness. But do you *have* to accede to it? What if it were not nine months, but nine years? Or longer still? What if the director of the hospital says, "Tough luck, I agree, but you've now got to stay in bed, with the violinist plugged into you, for the rest of your life. Because remember this. All persons have a right to life, and violinists are persons. Granted you have a right to decide what happens in and to your body, but a person's right to life outweighs your right to decide what happens in and to your body. So you cannot ever be unplugged from him." I imagine you would regard this as outrageous, which suggests that something really is wrong with that plausible-sounding argument I mentioned a moment ago.

In this case, of course, you were kidnapped; you didn't volunteer for the operation that plugged the violinist into your kidneys. Can those who oppose abortion on the ground I mentioned make an exception for a pregnancy due to rape? Certainly. They can say that persons have a right to life only if they didn't come into existence because of rape; or they can say that all persons have a right to life, but that some have less of a right to life than others, in particular, that those who came into existence because of rape have less. But these statements have a rather unpleasant sound. Surely the question of whether you have a right to life at all, or how much of it you have, shouldn't turn on the question of whether or not you are the product of a rape. And in fact the people who oppose abortion on the ground I mentioned do not make this distinction, and hence do not make an exception in case of rape.

Nor do they make an exception for a case in which the mother has to spend the nine months of her pregnancy in bed. They would agree that would be a great pity, and hard on the mother; but all the same, all persons have a right to life, the fetus is a person, and so on. I suspect, in fact, that they would not make an exception for a case in which, miraculously enough, the pregnancy went on for nine years, or even the rest of the mother's life.

Some won't even make an exception for a case in which continuation of the pregnancy is likely to shorten the mother's life; they regard abortion as impermissible even to save the mother's life. Such cases are nowadays very rare, and many opponents of abortion do not accept this extreme view. . . .

[1] Where the mother's life is not at stake, the argument I mentioned at the outset seems to have a much stronger pull. "Everyone has a right to life, so the unborn person has a right to life." And isn't the child's right to life weightier than anything other than the mother's own right to life, which she might put forward as ground for an abortion?

This argument treats the right to life as if it were unproblematic. It is not, and this seems to me to be precisely the source of the mistake.

For we should now, at long last, ask what it comes to, to have a right to life. In some views having a right to life includes having a right to be given at least the bare minimum one needs for continued life. But suppose that what in fact *is* the bare minimum a man needs for continued life is something he has no right at all to be given? If I am sick unto death, and the only thing that will save my life is the touch of Henry Fonda's cool hand on my fevered brow, then all the same, I have no right to be given the touch of Henry Fonda's cool hand on my fevered brow. It would be frightfully nice of him to fly in from the West Coast to provide it. It would be less nice, though no doubt well meant, if my friends flew out to the West Coast and carried Henry Fonda back with them. But I have no right at all against anybody that he should do this for me. Or again, to return to the story I told earlier, the fact that for continued life that violinist needs the continued use of your kidneys does not establish that he has a right to be given the continued use of your kidneys. He certainly has no right against you that *you* should give him continued use of your kidneys. For nobody has any right to use your kidneys unless you give him such a right; and nobody has the right against you that you shall give him this right—if you do allow him to go on using your kidneys, this is a kindness on your part, and not something he can claim from you as his due. Nor has he any right against anybody else that *they* should give him continued use of your kidneys. Certainly he had no right against the Society of Music Lovers that they should plug him into you in the first place. And if you now start to unplug yourself, having learned that you will otherwise have to spend nine years in bed with him, there is nobody in the world who must try to prevent you, in order to see to it that he is given something he has a right to be given.

Some people are rather stricter about the right to life. In their view, it does not include the right to be given anything, but amounts to, and only to, the right not to be killed by anybody. But here a related difficulty arises. If everybody is to refrain from killing that violinist, then everybody must refrain from doing a great many different sorts of things. Everybody must refrain from slitting his throat, everybody must refrain from shooting him—and everybody must refrain from unplugging you from him. But does he have a right against everybody that they shall refrain from unplugging you from him? To refrain from doing this is to allow him to continue to use your kidneys. It could be argued that he has a right against us that *we* should allow him to continue to use your kidneys. That is, while he had no right against us that we should give him the use of your kidneys, it might be argued that he anyway has a right against us that we shall not now intervene and deprive him of the use of your kidneys. I shall come back to third-party interventions later. But certainly the violinist has no right against you that *you* shall allow him to continue to use your kidneys. As I said, if you do allow him to use them, it is a kindness on your part, and not something you owe him.

The difficulty I point to here is not peculiar to the right to life. It reappears in connection with all the other natural rights; and it is something which an adequate account of rights must deal with. For present purposes it is enough just to draw attention to it. But I would stress that I am not arguing that people do not have a right to life—quite to the contrary, it seems to me that the primary control we must place on the acceptability of an account of rights is that it should turn out in that account to be a truth that all persons have a right to life. I am arguing only that having a right to life does not guarantee having either a right to be given the use of or a right to be allowed continued use of another person's body—even if one needs it for life itself. So the right to life will not serve the opponents of abortion in the very simple and clear way in which they seem to have thought it would.

[2] There is another way to bring out the difficulty. In the most ordinary sort of case, to deprive someone of what he has a right to is to treat him unjustly. Suppose a boy and his small brother are jointly given a box of chocolates for Christmas. If the older boy takes the box and refuses to give his brother any of the chocolates, he is unjust to him, for the brother has been given a right to half of them. But suppose that, having learned that otherwise it means nine years in bed with that violinist, you unplug yourself from him. You surely are not being unjust to him, for you gave him no right to use your kidneys, and no one else can have given him any such right. But we have to notice that in unplugging yourself, you are killing him; and violinists, like everybody else, have a right to life, and thus in the view we were considering just now, the right not to be killed. So here you do what he supposedly has a right you shall not do, but you do not act unjustly to him in doing it.

The emendation which may be made at this point is this: the right to life consists not in the right not to be killed, but rather in the right not to be killed unjustly. This runs a risk of circularity, but never mind: it would enable us to square the fact that the violinist has a right to life with the fact that you do not act unjustly toward him in unplugging yourself, thereby killing him. For if you do not kill him unjustly, you do not violate his right to life, and so it is no wonder you do him no injustice.

But if this emendation is accepted, the gap in the argument against abortion stares us plainly in the face: it is by no means enough to show that the fetus is a person, and to remind us that all persons have a right to life—we need to be shown also that killing the fetus violates its right to life, i.e., that abortion is unjust killing. And is it?

I suppose we may take it as a datum that in a case of pregnancy due to rape the mother has not given the unborn person a right to the use of her body for food and shelter. Indeed, in what pregnancy could it be supposed that the mother has given the unborn person such a right? It is not as if there were unborn persons drifting about the world, to whom a woman who wants a child says "I invite you in."

But it might be argued that there are other ways one can have acquired a right to the use of another person's body than by having been invited to use it by that person. Suppose a woman voluntarily indulges in intercourse, knowing of the chance it will issue in pregnancy, and then she does become pregnant; is she not in part responsible for the presence, in fact the very existence, of the unborn person inside her? No doubt she did not invite it in. But doesn't her partial responsibility for its being there itself give it a right to the use of her body?[3] If so, then her aborting it would be more like the boy's taking away the chocolates, and less like your unplugging yourself from the violinist—doing so would be depriving it of what it does have a right to, and thus would be doing it an injustice.

And then, too, it might be asked whether or not she can kill it even to save her own life: If she voluntarily called it into existence, how can she now kill it, even in self-defense?

The first thing to be said about this is that it is something new. Opponents of abortion have been so concerned to make out the independence of the fetus, in order to establish that it has a right to life, just as its mother does, that they have tended to overlook the possible support they might gain from making out that the fetus is *dependent* on the mother, in order to establish that she has a special kind of responsibility for it, a responsibility that gives it rights against her which are not possessed by any independent person—such as an ailing violinist who is a stranger to her.

On the other hand, this argument would give the unborn person a right to its mother's body only if her pregnancy resulted from a voluntary act, undertaken in full knowledge of the chance a pregnancy might result from it. It would leave out entirely the unborn

person whose existence is due to rape. Pending the availability of some further argument, then, we would be left with the conclusion that unborn persons whose existence is due to rape have no right to the use of their mothers' bodies, and thus that aborting them is not depriving them of anything they have a right to and hence is not unjust killing.

And we should also notice that it is not at all plain that this argument really does go even as far as it purports to. For there are cases and cases, and the details make a difference. If the room is stuffy, and I therefore open a window to air it, and a burglar climbs in, it would be absurd to say, "Ah, now he can stay, she's given him a right to the use of her house—for she is partially responsible for his presence there, having voluntarily done what enabled him to get in, in full knowledge that there are such things as burglars, and that burglars burgle." It would be still more absurd to say this if I had had bars installed outside my windows, precisely to prevent burglars from getting in, and a burglar got in only because of a defect in the bars. It remains equally absurd if we imagine it is not a burglar who climbs in, but an innocent person who blunders or falls in. Again, suppose it were like this: people-seeds drift about in the air like pollen, and if you open your windows, one may drift in and take root in your carpets or upholstery. You don't want children, so you fix up your windows with fine mesh screens, the very best you can buy. As can happen, however, and on very, very rare occasions does happen, one of the screens is defective; and a seed drifts in and takes root. Does the person-plant who now develops have a right to the use of your house? Surely not—despite the fact that you voluntarily opened your windows, you knowingly kept carpets and upholstered furniture, and you knew that screens were sometimes defective. Someone may argue that you are responsible for its rooting, that it does have a right to your house, because after all you *could* have lived out your life with bare floors and furniture, or with sealed windows and doors. But this won't do—for by the same token anyone can avoid a pregnancy due to rape by having a hysterectomy, or anyway by never leaving home without a (reliable!) army.

It seems to me that the argument we are looking at can establish at most that there are *some* cases in which the unborn person has a right to the use of its mother's body, and therefore *some* cases in which abortion is unjust killing. There is room for much discussion and argument as to precisely which, if any. But I think we should sidestep this issue and leave it open, for at any rate the argument certainly does not establish that all abortion is unjust killing.

[3] There is room for yet another argument here, however. We surely must all grant that there may be cases in which it would be morally indecent to detach a person from your body at the cost of his life. Suppose you learn that what the violinist needs is not nine years of your life, but only one hour: all you need do to save his life is to spend one hour in that bed with him. Suppose also that letting him use your kidneys for that one hour would not affect your health in the slightest. Admittedly you were kidnapped. Admittedly you did not give anyone permission to plug him into you. Nevertheless it seems to me plain you *ought* to allow him to use your kidneys for that hour—it would be indecent to refuse.

Again, suppose pregnancy lasted only an hour, and constituted no threat to life or health. And suppose that a woman becomes pregnant as a result of rape. Admittedly she did not voluntarily do anything to bring about the existence of a child. Admittedly she did nothing at all which would give the unborn person a right to the use of her body. All the same it might well be said, as in the newly emended violinist story, that she *ought* to allow it to remain for that hour—that it would be indecent in her to refuse.

Now some people are inclined to use the term "right" in such a way that it follows from the fact that you ought to allow a person to use your body for the hour he needs, that he has a right to use your body for the hour he needs, even though he has not been given that right by any person or act. They may say that it follows also that if you refuse, you act unjustly toward him. This use of the term is perhaps so common that it cannot be called wrong; nevertheless it seems to me to be an unfortunate loosening of what we would do better to keep a tight rein on. Suppose that box of chocolates I mentioned earlier had not been given to both boys jointly, but was given only to the older boy. There he sits, stolidly eating his way through the box, his small brother watching enviously. Here we are likely to say "You ought not

to be so mean. You ought to give your brother some of those chocolates." My own view is that it just does not follow from the truth of this that the brother has any right to any of the chocolates. If the boy refuses to give his brother any, he is greedy, stingy, callous—but not unjust. I suppose that the people I have in mind will say it does follow that the brother has a right to some of the chocolates, and thus that the boy does act unjustly if he refuses to give his brother any. But the effect of saying this is to obscure what we should keep distinct, namely the difference between the boy's refusal in this case and the boy's refusal in the earlier case, in which the box was given to both boys jointly, and in which the small brother thus had what was from any point of view clear title to half.

A further objection to so using the term "right" that from the fact that A ought to do a thing for B, it follows that B has a right against A that A do it for him, is that it is going to make the question of whether or not a man has a right to a thing turn on how easy it is to provide him with it; and this seems not merely unfortunate, but morally unacceptable. Take the case of Henry Fonda again. I said earlier that I had no right to the touch of his cool hand on my fevered brow, even though I needed it to save my life. I said it would be frightfully nice of him to fly in from the West Coast to provide me with it, but that I had no right against him that he should do so. But suppose he isn't on the West Coast. Suppose he has only to walk across the room, place a hand briefly on my brow—and lo, my life is saved. Then surely he ought to do it, it would be indecent to refuse. Is it to be said "Ah, well, it follows that in this case she has a right to the touch of his hand on her brow, and so it would be an injustice in him to refuse"? So that I have a right to it when it is easy for him to provide it, though no right when it's hard? It's rather a shocking idea that anyone's rights should fade away and disappear as it gets harder and harder to accord them to him.

So my own view is that even though you ought to let the violinist use your kidneys for the one hour he needs, we should not conclude that he has a right to do so—we would say that if you refuse, you are, like the boy who owns all the chocolates and will give none away, self-centered and callous, indecent in fact, but not unjust. And similarly, that even supposing a case in which a woman pregnant due to rape ought to allow the unborn person to use her body for the hour he needs, we should not conclude that he has a right to do so; we should conclude that she is self-centered, callous, indecent, but not unjust, if she refuses. The complaints are no less grave; they are just different. However, there is no need to insist on this point. If anyone does wish to deduce "he has a right" from "you ought," then all the same he must surely grant that there are cases in which it is not morally required of you that you allow that violinist to use your kidneys, and in which he does not have a right to use them, and in which you do not do him an injustice if you refuse. And so also for mother and unborn child. Except in such cases as the unborn person has a right to demand it—and we were leaving open the possibility that there may be such cases—nobody is morally *required* to make large sacrifices, of health, of all other interests and concerns, of all other duties and commitments, for nine years, or even for nine months, in order to keep another person alive.

[4] We have in fact to distinguish between two kinds of Samaritan: the Good Samaritan and what we might call the Minimally Decent Samaritan. The story of the Good Samaritan, you will remember, goes like this:

> A certain man went down from Jerusalem to Jericho, and fell among thieves, which stripped him of his raiment, and wounded him, and departed, leaving him half dead.
>
> And by chance there came down a certain priest that way; and when he saw him, he passed by on the other side.
>
> And likewise a Levite, when he was at the place, came and looked on him, and passed by on the other side.
>
> But a certain Samaritan, as he journeyed, came where he was; and when he saw him he had compassion on him.
>
> And went to him, and bound up his wounds, pouring in oil and wine, and set him on his own beast, and brought him to an inn, and took care of him.
>
> And on the morrow, when he departed, he took out two pence, and gave them to the host, and said unto him, "Take care of him; and whatsoever thou spendest more, when I come again, I will repay thee."
> (Luke 10:30–35)

The Good Samaritan went out of his way, at some cost to himself, to help one in need of it. We are not told what the options were, that is, whether or not the priest and the Levite could have helped by doing less than the Good Samaritan did, but assuming they could have, then the fact they did nothing at all shows they were not even Minimally Decent Samaritans, not because they were not Samaritans, but because they were not even minimally decent.

These things are a matter of degree, of course, but there is a difference, and it comes out perhaps most clearly in the story of Kitty Genovese, who, as you will remember, was murdered while thirty-eight people watched or listened, and did nothing at all to help her. A Good Samaritan would have rushed out to give direct assistance against the murderer. Or perhaps we had better allow that it would have been a Splendid Samaritan who did this, on the ground that it would have involved a risk of death for himself. But the thirty-eight not only did not do this, they did not even trouble to pick up a phone to call the police. Minimally Decent Samaritanism would call for doing at least that, and their not having done it was monstrous.

After telling the story of the Good Samaritan, Jesus said "Go, and do thou likewise." Perhaps he meant that we are morally required to act as the Good Samaritan did. Perhaps he was urging people to do more than is morally required of them. At all events it seems plain that it was not morally required of any of the thirty-eight that he rush out to give direct assistance at the risk of his own life, and that it is not morally required of anyone that he give long stretches of his life—nine years or nine months—to sustaining the life of a person who has no special right (we were leaving open the possibility of this) to demand it.

Indeed, with one rather striking class of exceptions, no one in any country in the world is *legally* required to do anywhere near as much as this for anyone else. The class of exceptions is obvious. My main concern here is not the state of the law in respect to abortion, but it is worth drawing attention to the fact that in no state in this country is any man compelled by law to be even a Minimally Decent Samaritan to any person; there is no law under which charges could be brought against the thirty-eight who stood by while Kitty Genovese died. By contrast, in most states in this country women are compelled by law to be not merely Minimally Decent Samaritans, but Good Samaritans to unborn persons inside them. This doesn't by itself settle anything one way or the other, because it may well be argued that there should be laws in this country—as there are in many European countries—compelling at least Minimally Decent Samaritanism.[4] But it does show that there is a gross injustice in the existing state of the law. And it shows also that the groups currently working against liberalization of abortion laws, in fact working toward having it declared unconstitutional for a state to permit abortion, had better start working for the adoption of Good Samaritan laws generally, or earn the charge that they are acting in bad faith.

I should think, myself, that Minimally Decent Samaritan laws would be one thing, Good Samaritan laws quite another, and in fact highly improper. But we are not here concerned with the law. What we should ask is not whether anybody should be compelled by law to be a Good Samaritan, but whether we must accede to a situation in which somebody is being compelled—by nature, perhaps—to be a Good Samaritan. We have, in other words, to look now at third-party interventions. I have been arguing that no person is morally required to make large sacrifices to sustain the life of another who has no right to demand them, and this even where the sacrifices do not include life itself; we are not morally required to be Good Samaritans or anyway Very Good Samaritans to one another. But what if a man cannot extricate himself from such a situation? What if he appeals to us to extricate him? It seems to me plain that there are cases in which we can, cases in which a Good Samaritan would extricate him. There you are, you were kidnapped, and nine years in bed with that violinist lie ahead of you. You have your own life to lead. You are sorry, but you simply cannot see giving up so much of your life to the sustaining of his. You cannot extricate yourself, and ask us to do so. I should have thought that—in light of his having no right to the use of your body—it was obvious that we do not have to accede to your being forced to give up so much. We can do what you ask. There is no injustice to the violinist in our doing so.

[5] Following the lead of the opponents of abortion, I have throughout been speaking of the fetus merely as a person, and what I have been asking is whether or not the argument we began with, which proceeds only from the fetus' being a person, really does establish its conclusion. I have argued that it does not.

But of course there are arguments and arguments, and it may be said that I have simply fastened on the wrong one. It may be said that what is important is not merely the fact that the fetus is a person, but that it is a person for whom the woman has a special kind of responsibility issuing from the fact that she is its mother. And it might be argued that all my analogies are therefore irrelevant—for you do not have that special kind of responsibility for that violinist, Henry Fonda does not have that special kind of responsibility for me. And our attention might be drawn to the fact that men and women both *are* compelled by law to provide support for their children.

I have in effect dealt (briefly) with this argument in section [2] above; but a (still briefer) recapitulation now may be in order. Surely we do not have any such "special responsibility" for a person unless we have assumed it, explicitly or implicitly. If a set of parents do not try to prevent pregnancy, do not obtain an abortion, and then at the time of birth of the child do not put it out for adoption, but rather take it home with them, then they have assumed responsibility for it, they have given it rights, and they cannot *now* withdraw support from it at the cost of its life because they now find it difficult to go on providing for it. But if they have taken all reasonable precautions against having a child, they do not simply by virtue of their biological relationship to the child who comes into existence have a special responsibility for it. They may wish to assume responsibility for it, or they may not wish to. And I am suggesting that if assuming responsibility for it would require large sacrifices, then they may refuse. A Good Samaritan would not refuse—or anyway, a Splendid Samaritan, if the sacrifices that had to be made were enormous. But then so would a Good Samaritan assume responsibility for that violinist; so would Henry Fonda, if he is a Good Samaritan, fly in from the West Coast and assume responsibility for me.

[6] My argument will be found unsatisfactory on two counts by many of those who want to regard abortion as morally permissible. First, while I do argue that abortion is not impermissible, I do not argue that it is always permissible. There may well be cases in which carrying the child to term requires only Minimally Decent Samaritanism of the mother, and this is a standard we must not fall below. I am inclined to think it a merit of my account precisely that it does *not* give a general yes or a general no. It allows for and supports our sense that, for example, a sick and desperately frightened fourteen-year-old schoolgirl, pregnant due to rape, may *of course* choose abortion, and that any law which rules this out is an insane law. And it also allows for and supports our sense that in other cases resort to abortion is even positively indecent. It would be indecent in the woman to request an abortion, and indecent in a doctor to perform it, if she is in her seventh month, and wants the abortion just to avoid the nuisance of postponing a trip abroad. The very fact that the arguments I have been drawing attention to treat all cases of abortion, or even all cases of abortion in which the mother's life is not at stake, as morally on a par ought to have made them suspect at the outset.

Secondly, while I am arguing for the permissibility of abortion in some cases, I am not arguing for the right to secure the death of the unborn child. It is easy to confuse these two things in that up to a certain point in the life of the fetus it is not able to survive outside the mother's body; hence removing it from her body guarantees its death. But they are importantly different. I have argued that you are not morally required to spend nine months in bed, sustaining the life of that violinist; but to say this is by no means to say that if, when you unplug yourself, there is a miracle and he survives, you then have a right to turn round and slit his throat. You may detach yourself even if this costs him his life; you have no right to be guaranteed his death, by some other means, if unplugging yourself does not kill him. There are some people who will feel dissatisfied by this feature of my argument. A woman may be utterly devastated by the thought of a child, a bit of herself, put out for adoption and never seen or heard of again. She may therefore want not merely that the child be detached from her, but more, that it die. Some opponents of abortion are inclined to regard this as beneath contempt—thereby showing insensitivity to what is surely a powerful source of despair. All the same, I agree that the desire for the child's death is not one which anybody may gratify, should it turn out to be possible to detach the child alive.

At this place, however, it should be remembered that we have only been pretending throughout that the fetus is a human being from the moment of conception. A very early abortion is surely not the killing of a person, and so is not dealt with by anything I have said here.

NOTES

1 I am very much indebted to James Thomson for discussion, criticism, and many helpful suggestions.
2 Daniel Callahan, *Abortion: Law, Choice and Morality* (New York, 1970), p. 373. This book gives a fascinating survey of the available information on abortion. The Jewish tradition is surveyed in David M. Feldman, *Birth Control in Jewish Law* (New York, 1968), Part 5, the Catholic tradition in John T. Noonan, Jr., "An Almost Absolute Value in History," in *The Morality of Abortion,* ed. John T. Noonan, Jr. (Cambridge, Mass., 1970).
3 The need for a discussion of this argument was brought home to me by members of the Society for Ethical and Legal Philosophy, to whom this paper was originally presented.
4 For a discussion of the difficulties involved, and a survey of the European experience with such laws, see *The Good Samaritan and the Law,* ed. James M. Ratcliffe (New York, 1966).

THE MORALITY OF ABORTION
Margaret Olivia Little

Little argues that abortion is a morally weighty matter even if we put aside the claim that the fetus is a person. In her view, "burgeoning human life" matters morally; it has some degree of value (moral status) and, thus, to that extent is worthy of respect.

From this general starting point, Little explores the morality of abortion, paying special attention to two themes—motherhood and respect for creation—that often play a role in the thinking of women struggling with a decision to continue or end pregnancy. She explains how each of these themes adds a layer of complexity to a woman's decision to continue or end pregnancy, and she ultimately argues that personal decisions about the morality of abortion depend in part on the unique way in which individual women construct their fundamental identities, commitments, and personal ideals.

. . . Just as we cannot assume that abortion is monstrous if fetuses are persons, so too we cannot assume that abortion is empty of moral import if they are not. Given all the ink that has been spilt on arbitrating the question of fetal personhood, one might be forgiven for having thought so: on some accounts, decisions about whether to continue or end a pregnancy really are, from a moral point of view, just like decisions about whether to cut one's hair.

But as Ronald Dworkin (1993) has urged, to think abortion morally weighty does not require supposition that the fetus is a person, or even a creature with interests in continued life. Destruction of a Da Vinci painting, he points out, is not bad *for the painting*—the painting has no interests. Instead, it is regrettable because of the deep value it has. So, too, one of the reasons we might regard abortion as morally weighty does not have to do with its being bad *for the fetus*—a setback to its interests—for it may not satisfy the criteria of having interests. Abortion may be weighty, instead, because there is something precious and significant about germinating human life that deserves our deep respect. This, as Dworkin puts it, locates issues of abortion in a different neighborhood of our moral commitments: namely, the accommodation we owe to things of value. That an organism is a potential person may not make it a claims-bearer, but it does mean it has a kind of stature that is worthy of respect.

This intuition, dismissed by some as mere sentimentality, is, I think, both important and broadly held. Very few people regard abortion as the moral

equivalent of contraception. Most think a society better morally—not just by public health measures—if it regards abortion as a back-up to failed contraception rather than as routine birth control. Reasons adequate for contraception do not translate transparently as reasons adequate for abortion. Indeed, there is a telling shift in presumption: for most people, it takes no reason at all to justify contracepting; it takes *some* reason to justify ending a pregnancy. That a human life has now begun matters morally.

Burgeoning human life, we might put it, is *respectworthy*. This is why we care not just whether, but how, abortion is done—while crass jokes are made or with solemnity—and why we care how the fetal remains are treated. It is why the thought of someone aborting for genuinely trivial reasons—to fit into a favorite party dress, say—makes us morally queasy. Perhaps, most basically, it is why the thought of someone aborting with casual indifference fills us with misgiving. Abortion involves loss. Not just loss of the hope that various parties might have invested, but loss of something valuable in its own right. To respect something is to appreciate fully the value it has and the claims it presents to us; someone who aborts but never gives it a second thought has not exhibited genuine appreciation of the value and moral status of that which is now gone.

But if many share the intuition that early human life has a value deserving of respect, there is considerable disagreement about what that respect looks like. There is considerable conflict, that is, over what accommodation we owe to burgeoning human life. In part, of course, this is due to disagreement over the *degree* of value such life should be accorded: those for whom it is thoroughly modest will have very different views on issues, from abortion to stem-cell research, from those for whom it is transcendent. But this is only part of the story. Obscured by analogies to Da Vinci paintings, some of the most important sources of conflict, especially for the vast middle rank of moderates, ride atop rough agreement on "degree" of fetal value. If we listen to women's own struggles about when it is morally decent to end pregnancy, what we hear are themes about *motherhood* and *respect for creation*. These themes are enormously complex, I want to argue, for they enter stories on both sides of the ledger: for some women, as reasons to continue pregnancy, and, for others, as reasons to end it. Let me start with motherhood.

For many women who contemplate abortion, the desire to end pregnancy is not, or not centrally, a desire to avoid the nine months of pregnancy; it is to avoid what lies on the far side of those months—namely, motherhood. If gestation were simply a matter of rendering, say, somewhat risky assistance to help a burgeoning human life they have come across—if they could somehow render that assistance without thereby adding a member to their family—the decision faced would be a far different one. But gestation does not just allow cells to become a person; it turns one into a mother.

One of the most common reasons women give for wanting to abort is that they do not want to become a mother—now, ever, again, with this partner, or no reliable partner, with these few resources, or these many that are now, after so many years of mothering, slated finally to another cause (Hursthouse, 1987: ch. 8.4). Nor does adoption represent a universal solution. To give up a child would be for some a life-long trauma; others occupy fortunate circumstances that would, by their own lights, make it unjustified to give over a child for others to rear. Or again—and most frequently—she does not want to raise a child just now but knows that if she *does* carry the pregnancy to term, she will not *want* to give up the child for adoption. Gestation, she knows, is likely to reshape her heart and soul, transforming her into a mother emotionally, not just officially; and it is precisely that transformation she does not want to undergo. It is because continuing pregnancy brings with it this new identity and, likely, relationship, then, that many feel it legitimate to decline.

But pregnancy's connection to motherhood also enters the phenomenology of abortion in just the opposite direction. For some women, that it would be her child is precisely why she feels she must continue the pregnancy, even if motherhood is not what she desired. To be pregnant is to have one's potential child knocking at one's door: to abort is to turn one's back on it, a decision, many women say, that would haunt them forever. On this view, the desire to avoid motherhood, so compelling as a reason to use contraception, is uneasy grounds to abort: for once an embryo is on the scene, it is not about rejecting motherhood, it is about rejecting one's *child*. Not literally, of course, since there is no child yet extant to stand as the object of rejection. But the stance one should take to pregnancy, sought or not, is one of *acceptance:* when a potential family member is knocking at the door, one should move over, make room, and welcome her in.

These two intuitive stances represent just profoundly different ways of *gestalting* the situation of ending pregnancy. On the first view, abortion is closer to contraception: hardly equivalent, because it means the demise of something of value. But the desire to avoid the enterprise and identity of motherhood is an understandable and honorable basis for deciding to end a pregnancy. Given that there is no child yet on the scene, one does not owe special openness to the relationship that stands at the end of pregnancy's trajectory. On the second view, abortion is closer to exiting a parental relationship: hardly equivalent, for one of the key relata is not yet fully present. But one's decision about whether to continue the pregnancy already feels specially constrained; that one would be related to the resulting person exerts now some moral force. It would take especially grave reasons to refuse assistance here, for the norms of parenthood already have toehold. Assessing the moral status of abortion, it turns out, then, is not just about assessing the contours of generic respect owed to burgeoning human life, it is about assessing the salience of *impending relationship*. And this is an issue that functions in different ways for different women—and, sometimes, in one and the same woman.

In my own view, until the fetus is a person, we should recognize a moral prerogative to decline parenthood and end the pregnancy. Not because motherhood is necessarily a burden (though it can be), but because it so thoroughly changes what we might call one's fundamental *practical identity*. The enterprise of mothering restructures the self—changing the shape of one's heart, the primary commitments by which one lives one's life, the terms by which one judges one's life a success or a failure. If the enterprise is eschewed and one decides to give the child over to another, the identity of mother still changes the normative facts that are true of one, as there is now someone by whom one does well or poorly (see Ross, 1982). And either way—whether one rears the child or lets it go—to continue a pregnancy means that a piece of one's heart, as the saying goes, will forever walk outside one's body. As profound as the respect we should have for burgeoning human life, we should acknowledge moral prerogatives over identity-constituting commitments and enterprises as profound as motherhood.

Whether one agrees with this view or not, there is at any rate another layer of the moral story here. If women find themselves with different ways of *gestalting* the prospective relationship involved in pregnancy, it is in part because they have different identities, commitments, and ideals that such a prospect intersects with, commitments which, while permissibly idiosyncratic, are morally authoritative for *them*. If one woman feels already duty-bound by the norms of parenthood to nurture this creature, for example, it may be for the very good reason that, in an important personal sense, she already *is* its mother. She finds herself (perhaps to her surprise) with a maternal commitment to this creature. But taking on the identity of mother toward something just *is* to take on certain imperatives about its well-being as categorical. Her job is thus clear: it is to help this creature reach its fullest potential. For another woman, on the other hand, the identity of mother is yet to be taken on; it is tried on, perhaps accepted, but perhaps declined—in which case respect is owed, but love is saved, or confirmed, for others—other relationships, other projects, other passions.

And, again, if one woman feels she owes a stance of welcome to burgeoning human life that comes her way, it may be, not because she thinks such a stance authoritative for all, but because of the virtues around which her practical identity is now oriented: receptivity to life's agenda, for instance, or responsiveness to that which is most vulnerable. For another woman, the virtues to be exercised may tug in just the other direction: loyalty to treasured life plans, a commitment that it be she, not the chances of biology, that should determine her life's course, bolstering self-direction after a life too long ruled by serendipity and fate.

Deciding when it is morally decent to end a pregnancy, it turns out, is an admixture of settling impersonally or universally authoritative moral requirements, and of discovering and arbitrating—sometimes after agonizing deliberation, sometimes in a decision no less deep for its immediacy—one's own commitments, identity, and defining virtues.

A similarly complex story appears when we turn to the second theme. Another thread that appears in many women's stories in the face of unsought pregnancy is respect for the weighty responsibility involved in creating human life. Once again, it is a theme that pulls and tugs in different directions.

In its most familiar direction, it shows up in many stories of why an unsought pregnancy is continued. Many people believe that one's responsibility to nurture new life is importantly amplified if one is responsible for bringing about its existence in the first place. Just what it takes to count as responsible here is a point on which individuals diverge (whether voluntary intercourse with contraception is different from intercourse without use of birth control, and again from intentionally deciding to become pregnant at the IVF clinic). But triggering the relevant standard of responsibility for creation, it is felt, brings with it a heightened responsibility to nurture: it is disrespectful to create human life only to allow it to wither. Put more rigorously, one who is responsible for bringing about a creature that has intrinsic value in virtue of its potential to become a person has a special responsibility to enable it to reach that end state.

But the idea of respect for creation is also, if less frequently acknowledged, sometimes the reason why women are moved to *end* pregnancies. As Barbara Katz Rothman (1989) puts it, decisions to abort often represent, not a decision to destroy, but a refusal to create. Many people have deeply felt convictions about the circumstances under which they feel it right for them to bring a child into the world. Can it be brought into a decent world, an intact family, a society that can minimally respect its agency? These considerations may persist even after conception has taken place; for while the *embryo* has already been created, a person has not. Some women decide to abort, that is, not because they do not *want* the resulting child—indeed, they may yearn for nothing more, and desperately wish that their circumstances were otherwise—but because they do not think bringing a child into the world the right thing for them to do.

These are abortions marked by moral language. A woman wants to abort because she knows she could not give up a child for adoption but feels she could not give the child the sort of life, or be the sort of parent, she thinks a child *deserves;* a woman who would have to give up the child thinks it would be *unfair* to bring a child into existence already burdened by rejection, however well grounded its reasons; a woman living in a country marked by poverty and gender apartheid wants to abort because she decides it would be *wrong* for her to bear a daughter whose life, like hers, would be filled with so much injustice and hardship.

Some have thought that such decisions betray a simple fallacy: unless the child's life were literally going to be worse than non-existence, how can one abort out of concern for the future child? But the worry here is not that one would be imposing a *harm* on the child by bringing it into existence (as though children who are in the situations mentioned have lives that are not worth living). The claim is that bringing about a person's life in these circumstances would do violence to her ideals of creating and parenthood. She does not want to bring into existence a daughter she cannot love and care for, she does not want to bring into existence a person whose life will be marked by disrespect or rejection.

Nor does the claim imply judgment on women who *do* continue pregnancies in similar circumstances—as though there were here an obligation to abort. For the norms in question, once

again, need not be impersonally authoritative moral claims. Like ideals of good parenting, they mark out considerations all should be sensitive to, perhaps, but equally reasonable people may adhere to different variations and weightings. Still, they are normative for those who do have them; far from expressing mere matters of taste, the ideals one does accept carry an important kind of categoricity, issuing imperatives whose authority is not reducible to mere desire. These are, at root, issues about *integrity,* and the importance of maintaining integrity over one's participation in this enterprise precisely because it is so normatively weighty.

What is usually emphasized in the morality of abortion is the ethics of destruction, but there is a balancing ethics of creation. And for many people, conflict about abortion is a conflict *within* that ethics. On the one hand, we now have on hand an entity that has a measure of sanctity: that it has begun is reason to help it continue, perhaps especially if one has had a role in its procreation, which is why even early abortion is not normatively equivalent to contraception. On the other hand, not to end a pregnancy *is* to do something else, namely, to continue creating a person, and, for some women, pregnancy strikes in circumstances in which they cannot countenance that enterprise. For some, the sanctity of developing human life will be strong enough to tip the balance toward continuing the pregnancy; for others, their norms of respectful creation will hold sway. For those who believe that the norms governing creation of a person are mild relative to the normative telos of embryonic life, being a responsible creator means continuing to gestate, and doing the best one can to bring about the conditions under which that creation will be more respectful. For others, though, the normativity of fetal telos is mild and their standards of respectful creation high, and the lesson goes in just the other direction: it is a sign of respect not to continue creating when certain background conditions, such as a loving family or adequate resources, are not in place.

However one thinks these issues settle out, they will not be resolved by austere contemplation of the value of human life. They require wrestling with the rich meanings of creation, responsibility, and kinship. And these issues, I have suggested, are just as much issues about one's integrity as they are about what is impersonally obligatory. On many treatments of abortion, considerations about whether or not to continue a pregnancy are exhausted by preferences, on the one hand, and universally authoritative moral demands, on the other; but some of the most important terrain lies in between.

REFERENCES

Dworkin, R. (1993) *Life's Dominion: An Argument About Abortion, Euthanasia, and Individual Freedom*. New York: Alfred A. Knopf.

Hursthouse, R. (1987) *Beginning Lives*. Oxford: Open University Press.

Ross, S. L. (1982) Abortion and the death of the fetus. *Philosophy and Public Affairs,* 11:232–45.

Rothman, B. K. (1989) *Recreating Motherhood: Ideology and Technology in a Patriarchal Society*. New York: Norton.

ABORTION AND SOCIAL POLICY

MAJORITY OPINION IN *ROE V. WADE*
Justice Harry Blackmun

In this case, a pregnant single woman, suing under the fictitious name of Jane Roe, challenged the constitutionality of the existing Texas criminal abortion law. According to the Texas Penal Code, the performance of an abortion, except to save the life of the pregnant woman, constituted a crime that was punishable by a prison sentence of two to five years. At the time this case was finally resolved by the Supreme Court, abortion legislation varied widely from state to state. Some states, principally New York, had already legalized abortion on demand. Most other states, however, had legalized various forms of therapeutic abortion but had retained some measure of restrictive abortion legislation.

Justice Blackmun, writing an opinion concurred in by six other justices, argues that a woman's decision to terminate a pregnancy is encompassed by a *right to privacy*—but only up to a certain point in the development of the fetus. As the right to privacy is not an absolute right, it must yield at some point to the state's legitimate interests. Justice Blackmun contends that the state has a legitimate interest in protecting the health of the mother and that this interest becomes compelling at approximately the end of the first trimester in the development of the fetus. He also contends that the state has a legitimate interest in protecting potential life and that this interest becomes compelling at the point of viability.

It is . . . apparent that at common law, at the time of the adoption of our Constitution, and throughout the major portion of the 19th century, abortion was viewed with less disfavor than under most American statutes currently in effect. Phrasing it another way, a woman enjoyed a substantially broader right to terminate a pregnancy than she does in most States

United States Supreme Court; January 22, 1973. 410 U.S. 113, 93 S.Ct. 705.

today. At least with respect to the early stage of pregnancy, and very possibly without such a limitation, the opportunity to make this choice was present in this country well into the 19th century. Even later, the law continued for some time to treat less punitively an abortion procured in early pregnancy. . . .

Three reasons have been advanced to explain historically the enactment of criminal abortion laws in the 19th century and to justify their continued existence.

It has been argued occasionally that these laws were the product of a Victorian social concern to discourage illicit sexual conduct. Texas, however, does not advance this justification in the present case, and it appears that no court or commentator has taken the argument seriously. . . .

A second reason is concerned with abortion as a medical procedure. When most criminal abortion laws were first enacted, the procedure was a hazardous one for the woman. This was particularly true prior to the development of antisepsis. Antiseptic techniques, of course, were based on discoveries by Lister, Pasteur, and others first announced in 1867, but were not generally accepted and employed until about the turn of the century. Abortion mortality was high. Even after 1900, and perhaps until as late as the development of antibiotics in the 1940s, standard modern techniques such as dilation and curettage were not nearly so safe as they are today. Thus it has been argued that a State's real concern in enacting a criminal abortion law was to protect the pregnant woman, that is, to restrain her from submitting to a procedure that placed her life in serious jeopardy.

Modern medical techniques have altered this situation. Appellants and various *amici* refer to medical data indicating that abortion in early pregnancy, that is, prior to the end of first trimester, although not without its risk, is now relatively safe. Mortality rates for women undergoing early abortions, where the procedure is legal, appear to be as low as or lower than the rates for normal childbirth. Consequently, any interest of the State in protecting the woman from an inherently hazardous procedure, except when it would be equally dangerous for her to forego it, has largely disappeared. Of course, important state interests in the area of health and medical standards do remain. The State has a legitimate interest in seeing to it that abortion, like any other medical procedure, is performed under circumstances that insure maximum safety for the patient. This interest obviously extends at least to the performing physician and his staff, to the facilities involved, to the availability of after-care, and to adequate provision for any complication or emergency that might arise. The prevalence of high mortality rates at illegal "abortion mills" strengthens, rather than weakens, the State's interest in regulating the conditions under which abortions are performed. Moreover, the risk to the woman increases as her pregnancy continues. Thus the State retains a definite interest in protecting the woman's own health and safety when an abortion is performed at a late stage of pregnancy.

The third reason is the State's interest—some phrase it in terms of duty—in protecting prenatal life. Some of the argument for this justification rests on the theory that a new human life is present from the moment of conception. The State's interest and general obligation to protect life then extends, it is argued, to prenatal life. Only when the life of the pregnant mother herself is at stake, balanced against the life she carries within her, should the interest of the embryo or fetus not prevail. Logically, of course, a legitimate state interest in this area need not stand or fall on acceptance of the belief that life begins at conception or at some other point prior to live birth. In assessing the State's interest, recognition may be given to the less rigid claim that as long as at least *potential* life is involved, the State may assert interests beyond the protection of the pregnant woman alone.

Parties challenging state abortion laws have sharply disputed in some courts the contention that a purpose of these laws, when enacted, was to protect prenatal life. Pointing to the absence of legislative history to support the contention, they claim that most state laws were designed solely to protect the woman. Because medical advances have lessened this concern, at least with respect to abortion in early pregnancy, they argue that with respect to such abortions the laws can no longer be justified by any state interest. There is some scholarly support for this view of original purpose. The few state courts called upon to interpret their laws in the late 19th and early 20th centuries did focus on the State's interest in protecting the woman's health rather than in preserving the embryo and fetus. . . .

The Constitution does not explicitly mention any right of privacy. In a line of decisions, however, going back perhaps as far as *Union Pacific R. Co. v. Botsford* (1891), the Court has recognized that a right of personal privacy, or a guarantee of certain areas or zones of privacy, does exist under the constitution. In varying contexts the Court or individual Justices have indeed found at least the roots of that right in the First Amendment, . . . in the Fourth and Fifth Amendments . . . in the penumbras of the Bill of Rights . . . in the Ninth Amendment . . . or in the concept of liberty guaranteed by the first section of the Fourteenth Amendment. . . . These decisions make it clear that only personal rights that can be deemed "fundamental" or "implicit in the concept of ordered liberty," . . . are included in this guarantee of personal privacy. They also make it clear that the right has some extension to activities relating to marriage, . . . procreation, . . . contraception, . . . family relationships, . . . and child rearing and education. . . .

This right of privacy, whether it be founded in the Fourteenth Amendment's concept of personal liberty and restrictions upon state action, as we feel it is, or, as the District Court determined, in the Ninth Amendment's reservation of rights to the people, is broad enough to encompass a woman's decision whether or not to terminate her pregnancy. . . .

. . . [A]ppellants and some *amici* argue that the woman's right is absolute and that she is entitled to terminate her pregnancy at whatever time, in whatever way, and for whatever reason she alone chooses. With this we do not agree. Appellants' arguments that Texas either has no valid interest at all in regulating the abortion decision, or no interest strong enough to support any limitation upon the woman's sole determination, is unpersuasive. The Court's decisions recognizing a right of privacy also acknowledges that some state regulation in areas protected by that right is appropriate. As noted above, a state may properly assert important interests in safe guarding health, in maintaining medical standards, and in protecting potential life. At some point in pregnancy, these respective interests become sufficiently compelling to sustain regulation of the factors that govern the abortion decision. The privacy right involved, therefore, cannot be said to be absolute. . . .

We therefore conclude that the right of personal privacy includes the abortion decision, but that this right is not unqualified and must be considered against important state interests in regulation.

We note that those federal and state courts that have recently considered abortion law challenges have reached the same conclusion. . . .

Although the results are divided, most of these courts have agreed that the right of privacy, however

based, is broad enough to cover the abortion decision; that the right, nonetheless, is not absolute and is subject to some limitations; and that at some point the state interests as to protection of health, medical standards, and prenatal life, become dominant. We agree with this approach. . . .

The appellee and certain *amici* argue that the fetus is a "person" within the language and meaning of the Fourteenth Amendment. In support of this they outline at length and in detail the well-known facts of fetal development. If this suggestion of personhood is established, the appellant's case, of course, collapses, for the fetus' right to life is then guaranteed specifically by the Amendment. The appellant conceded as much on reargument. On the other hand, the appellee conceded on reargument that no case could be cited that holds that a fetus is a person within the meaning of the Fourteenth Amendment. . . .

All this, together with our observation, *supra*, that throughout the major portion of the 19th century prevailing legal abortion practices were far freer than they are today, persuades us that the word "person," as used in the Fourteenth Amendment, does not include the unborn. . . . Indeed, our decision in *United States v. Vuitch* (1971) inferentially is to the same effect, for we there would not have indulged in statutory interpretation favorable to abortion in specified circumstances if the necessary consequence was the termination of life entitled to Fourteenth Amendment protection.

. . . As we have intimated above, it is reasonable and appropriate for a State to decide that at some point in time another interest, that of health of the mother or that of potential human life, becomes significantly involved. The woman's privacy is no longer sole and any right of privacy she possesses must be measured accordingly.

Texas urges that, apart from the Fourteenth Amendment, life begins at conception and is present throughout pregnancy, and that, therefore, the State has a compelling interest in protecting that life from and after conception. We need not resolve the difficult question of when life begins. When those trained in the respective disciplines of medicine, philosophy, and theology are unable to arrive at any consensus, the judiciary, at this point in the development of man's knowledge, is not in a position to speculate as to the answer.

It should be sufficient to note briefly the wide divergence of thinking on this most sensitive and difficult question. There has always been strong support for the view that life does not begin until live birth. This was the belief of the Stoics. It appears to be the predominant, though not the unanimous, attitude of the Jewish faith. It may be taken to represent also the position of a large segment of the Protestant community, insofar as that can be ascertained; organized groups that have taken a formal position on the abortion issue have generally regarded abortion as a matter for the conscience of the individual and her family. As we have noted, the common law found greater significance in quickening. Physicians and their scientific colleagues have regarded that event with less interest and have tended to focus either upon conception or upon live birth or upon the interim point at which the fetus becomes "viable," that is, potentially able to live outside the mother's womb, albeit with artificial aid. Viability is usually placed at about seven months (28 weeks) but may occur earlier, even at 24 weeks. . . .

In areas other than criminal abortion the law has been reluctant to endorse any theory that life, as we recognize it, begins before live birth or to accord legal rights to the unborn except in narrowly defined situations and except when the rights are contingent upon live birth. . . . In short, the unborn have never been recognized in the law as persons in the whole sense.

In view of all this, we do not agree that, by adopting one theory of life, Texas may override the rights of the pregnant woman that are at stake. We repeat, however, that the State does have an important and legitimate interest in preserving and protecting the health of the pregnant woman, whether she be a resident of the State or a nonresident who seeks medical consultation and treatment there, and that it has still *another* important and legitimate interest in protecting the potentiality of human life. These interests are separate and distinct. Each grows in substantiality as the woman approaches term and, at a point during pregnancy, each becomes "compelling."

With respect to the State's important and legitimate interest in the health of the mother, the "com-

pelling" point, in the light of present medical knowledge, is at approximately the end of the first trimester. This is so because of the now established medical fact . . . that until the end of the first trimester mortality in abortion is less than mortality in normal childbirth. It follows that, from and after this point, a State may regulate the abortion procedure to the extent that the regulation reasonably relates to the preservation and protection of maternal health. Examples of permissible state regulation in this area are requirements as to the qualifications of the person who is to perform the abortion; as to the licensure of that person; as to the facility in which the procedure is to be performed, that is, whether it must be a hospital or may be a clinic or some other place of less-than-hospital status; as to the licensing of the facility; and the like.

This means, on the other hand, that, for the period of pregnancy prior to this "compelling" point, the attending physician, in consultation with his patient, is free to determine, without regulation by the State, that in his medical judgment the patient's pregnancy should be terminated. If that decision is reached, the judgment may be effectuated by an abortion free of interference by the State.

With respect to the State's important and legitimate interest in potential life, the "compelling" point is at viability. This is so because the fetus then presumably has the capability of meaningful life outside the mother's womb. State regulation protective of fetal life after viability thus has both logical and biological justifications. If the State is interested in protecting fetal life after viability, it may go so far as to proscribe abortion during that period except when it is necessary to preserve the life or health of the mother. . . .

To summarize and repeat:

1. A state criminal abortion statue of the current Texas type, that excepts from criminality only a life-saving procedure on behalf of the mother, without regard to pregnancy stage and without recognition of the other interests involved, is violative of the Due Process Clause of the Fourteenth Amendment.

   a. For the stage prior to approximately the end of the first trimester, the abortion decision and its effectuation must be left to the medical judgment of the pregnant woman's attending physician.

b. For the stage subsequent to approximately the end of the first trimester, the State, in promoting its interest in the health of the mother, may, if it chooses, regulate the abortion procedure in ways that are reasonably related to maternal health.

c. For the stage subsequent to viability the State, in promoting its interest in the potentiality of human life, may, if it chooses, regulate, and even proscribe, abortion except where it is necessary, in appropriate medical judgment, for the preservation of the life or health of the mother.

2. The State may define the term "physician," as it has been employed [here], to mean only a physician currently licensed by the State, and may proscribe any abortion by a person who is not a physician as so defined.

. . . The decision leaves the State free to place increasing restrictions on abortion as the period of pregnancy lengthens, so long as those restrictions are tailored to the recognized state interests. The decision vindicates the right of the physician to administer medical treatment according to his professional judgment up to the points where important state interests provide compelling justifications for intervention. Up to those points the abortion decision in all its aspects is inherently, and primarily, a medical decision, and basic responsibility for it must rest with the physician. If an individual practitioner abuses the privilege of exercising proper medical judgment, the usual remedies, judicial and intraprofessional, are available. . . .

THE SUPREME COURT AND ABORTION RIGHTS

George J. Annas

The bulk of this excerpt from a longer essay discusses the two U.S. Supreme Court cases that address an abortion procedure known medically as intact dilation and extraction: *Stenberg v. Carhart* (2000) and *Gonzales v. Carhart* (2007). Annas reviews the history of abortion rights in the U.S., noting that the qualified reaffirmation of *Roe v. Wade* (1973) in *Planned Parenthood v. Casey* (1992) led pro-life advocates to shift focus onto banning this rare and politically unpopular procedure, which they named "partial-birth abortion." Annas describes the relevant provisions of the Nebraska statute invalidated in *Stenberg* and the federal Partial Birth Abortion Act of 2003 that was upheld in *Carhart*. He emphasizes the role of Justice Anthony Kennedy, whose *Stenberg* dissent formed the basis for the majority opinion in *Carhart*. Annas also discusses in detail Justice Ruth Bader Ginsburg's *Carhart* dissent. Ginsburg laments the majority's failure to adhere to the precedents of *Casey* and *Stenberg,* and the fact that the *Carhart* Court upholds for the first time since *Roe* an abortion ban with no exception to protect the woman's health.

Since the Supreme Court's landmark 1973 abortion-rights decision in *Roe v. Wade,*[1] the law has taken the

From *New England Journal of Medicine*, vol. 356, no. 21 (May 24, 2007), pp. 2201–2207. Copyright © 2007 Massachusetts Medical Society. All rights reserved.

lead in defining the contours of the continuing public debate over reproductive liberty. Ever since then, abortion opponents have tried to make abortion more burdensome by limiting *Roe,* and these continuing challenges are the reason there have been so many Supreme Court decisions about abortion, including the Court's 1992 decision in *Planned Parenthood of Southeastern Pennsylvania v. Casey*,[2] which unexpectedly reaffirmed the core of *Roe*.

In the wake of *Casey*, political efforts to restrict abortion have switched to outlawing one specific medical procedure, which its opponents label "partial-birth abortion," and more than 30 states and the federal government have made it a crime to perform this procedure. In 2000, in *Stenberg v. Carhart*,[3] the Court ruled 5 to 4 that these laws are unconstitutional. In April 2007, also by a 5 to 4 vote, the Court reached the opposite conclusion in *Gonzales v. Carhart*.[4] This is the first time the Court has ever held that physicians can be prohibited from using a medical procedure deemed necessary by the physician to benefit the patient's health. The importance of the decision to physicians and their patients cannot be appreciated without an understanding of the constitutional law of reproductive liberty as it has developed during the past 40 years.

THE RIGHT TO PRIVACY

The first case to embrace the concept of reproductive liberty was *Griswold v. Connecticut*, in which the Court ruled in 1965 that a Connecticut statute criminalizing the use of contraceptives violated the constitutional right to privacy that married couples had in sexual relations.[5] Later, in 1972, the Court found that even outside marriage, a person had a "right to privacy . . . to be free from unwarranted governmental intrusion into matters so fundamentally affecting a person as the decision to bear or beget a child."[6]

The following year, in *Roe*, the Court struck down a Texas law that made it a crime for physicians to perform an abortion unless it was necessary to save the life of the patient; there were no exceptions for the woman's health. The Court held that women have a constitutional right of privacy that is fundamental and "broad enough to encompass a woman's decision . . . to terminate her pregnancy."[1] Because the right is fundamental, states that wish to restrict abortion rights were required to demonstrate a compelling interest to restrict the exercise of this right. The Court ruled that the state's interest in the life of the fetus became compelling only at the point of

viability, when the fetus can survive independently of its mother. Even after the point of viability, the state cannot favor the life of the fetus over the life or health of the pregnant woman. Under the right of privacy, physicians must be free to use their "medical judgment for the preservation of the life or health of the mother."[1] On the same day that the Court decided *Roe*, it also decided *Doe v. Bolton*,[7] in which the Court defined health very broadly:

> The medical judgment may be exercised in the light of all factors — physical, emotional, psychological, familial, and the woman's age — relevant to the well-being of the patient. All these factors may relate to health. This allows the attending physician the room he needs to make his best medical judgment.[7]

Roe and *Doe* together established that both physician and patient were protected by the constitutional right of privacy. In later cases, the Court continued to defer to the medical judgment of the attending physician. For example, in 1976 in *Planned Parenthood of Central Missouri v. Danforth*, the Court concluded that state legislatures could not determine when viability occurred; rather this "essentially medical concept . . . is, and must be, a matter for the judgment of the responsible attending physician."[8] By the end of the 1980s, a pattern in Court decisions could be discerned in which abortion regulations that significantly burdened a woman's decision, treated abortion differently from other similar medical or surgical procedures, interfered with the exercise of professional judgment by the attending physician, or were stricter than accepted medical standards were struck down by the Court.[9]

Privacy as a constitutional right became a one-word description of liberty to make decisions regarding marriage, procreation, contraception, sterilization, abortion, family relationships, child rearing, and sexual relationships free of governmental interference.[2,10]

THE RIGHT TO LIBERTY

One strategy to change *Roe* was to change the composition of the Supreme Court by appointing anti-*Roe* justices. Because of new justices on the Court in 1992, in *Casey*, the Court had its first real opportunity to overturn *Roe v. Wade.* Many Court observers thought it would. Instead, in an unusual procedure for the Court, three potentially anti-*Roe* justices, Justices Sandra Day O'Connor, David Souter, and Anthony Kennedy, joined together to write a joint opinion confirming the "core holding" of *Roe.* (They were joined in most of their opinion by two justices who would have simply upheld *Roe,* making this a 5-to-4 decision.) Most centrally, the authors of the joint opinion believed that although the pressure to overrule *Roe* has grown "more intense," doing so would severely and unnecessary damage the Court's legitimacy by undermining "the Nation's commitment to the rule of law."[2]

Specifically, the three justices wrote that they were reaffirming "*Roe*'s essential holding" that before the point of viability a woman has a right to choose abortion without undue state interference, that after the point of viability the state can restrict abortion "if the law contains exceptions for pregnancies which endanger the woman's life or health," and that "the state has legitimate interests from the outset of the pregnancy in protecting the health of the woman and the life of the fetus that may become a child." The Court applied these principles to uphold laws mandating much more detailed requirements for abortion, as well as a mandatory 24-hour waiting period, but struck down a spousal-notification requirement as an "undue burden." Thus, after *Casey, Roe* stood for the proposition that pregnant women have a "personal liberty" right ("privacy" went unmentioned) to choose to terminate their pregnancies before the point of viability and that the state cannot "unduly burden" such a right by erecting barriers that effectively prevent the exercise of that choice.[2,11] Of course, a major problem was definitional: burdensome regulations were acceptable, "unduly burdensome" ones were not—but it was not clear what qualified as which. Put another way, the state could demonstrate its concern for life by requiring that physicians make women seeking abortions jump through new and burdensome hoops (including offers of detailed and accurate information on abortion, the status of the fetus, adoption, sources of help for childbirth, and a 24-hour waiting period), as long as doing so did not "unduly burden" women by actually preventing them from being able to make a decision to have an abortion.

With the loss of all hope that the Court would overrule *Roe* wholesale, anti-*Roe* advocates switched strategies dramatically, focusing on criminalizing a specific procedure that they believed would horrify most Americans and that they labeled "partial-birth abortion." The first such bill passed Congress in 1996 and was vetoed by President Bill Clinton because the prohibition did not contain an exception for the health of the woman, as required by *Roe* and *Casey.* In 1997, this time with the support of the American Medical Association, the bill passed Congress again. President Clinton vetoed it, again for failure to contain a health exception.[12]

"PARTIAL-BIRTH ABORTION" AND THE STATES

Proponents of the ban took their cause to the individual states, a majority of which enacted substantially identical laws. In 2000, Nebraska's partial-birth abortion law reached the Supreme Court. The Nebraska law carried a penalty of up to 20 years in prison for physicians who performed the procedure. The law reads in relevant part:

> No partial-birth abortion shall be performed in this state, unless such a procedure is necessary to save the life of the mother whose life is endangered by a physical disorder, physical illness, or physical injury, including a life-endangering physical condition caused by or arising from the pregnancy itself.
>
> [A "partial-birth abortion" is] an abortion procedure in which the person performing the abortion partially delivers vaginally a living unborn child before killing the unborn child and completing the delivery. . . . [The statute further defines the phrase "partially delivers vaginally a living unborn child before killing the unborn child" as] deliberately and intentionally delivering into the vagina a living unborn child, or a substantial portion thereof, for the purpose of performing a procedure that the person performing such procedure knows will kill the unborn child and does kill the unborn child.[3]

This ban applies throughout pregnancy and has no exception to protect the woman's health, only to save her life. In a 5-to-4 opinion in *Stenberg v. Carhart,*[3,13] the Court found this law unconstitutional for two reasons. First, the description of the banned procedure was too close to dilation and evacuation (D&E), another procedure that was permitted and widely used for second-trimester abortions. Therefore, this law would discourage physicians from using the lawful procedure, which would place an undue burden on their patients. Second, the law failed to provide an exception for instances in which the procedure was deemed necessary by the physician to protect the woman's health, as required by *Roe* and *Casey*. Justice John Paul Stevens, in his concurring opinion, noted that the extreme anti-*Roe* rhetoric as exemplified in the partial-birth abortion debate obscured the fact that during the 27-year period since *Roe* was decided, the core holding of *Roe* "has been endorsed by all but 4 of the 17 Justices who have addressed the issue."[3]

A notable dissenting opinion was written by Justice Kennedy, who had specifically endorsed the core of *Roe* in *Casey*. Kennedy argued that the outlawing of "partial-birth abortion" was consistent with *Casey* because of the interest the state has throughout pregnancy in protecting the life of the fetus that may become a child. In his view, the banned procedure conflates abortion and childbirth in a way that "might cause the medical profession or society as a whole to become insensitive, even disdainful, to life, including life of the human fetus." He also argued that such a ban was not unduly burdensome to women because state legislatures can determine that specific medical procedures, like this one, are not medically necessary.[3]

"PARTIAL-BIRTH ABORTION" AND CONGRESS

Justice Stephen Breyer, the author of the *Stenberg* majority opinion, stated that a more precise law, with a health exception, could be constitutional.[3] In 2003, Congress passed a slightly revised law. It did not contain a health exception, but its preface did contain a declaration that the outlawed procedure was never medically necessary for the health of the woman. President Bush signed it into law on November 5, 2003. By the time the Court ruled on the constitutionality of this law in April 2007, in *Gonzales v. Carhart,* there were two important changes in the composition of the Court: a new chief justice, John Roberts, who replaced the

consistently anti-*Roe* Chief William Rehnquist, and Justice Samuel Alito, who replaced Justice Sandra Day O'Connor, who was consistently pro-*Roe* (as interpreted in *Casey*). The federal law provides that

(a) Any physician who, in or affecting interstate or foreign commerce, knowingly performs a partial birth abortion and thereby kills a human fetus shall be fined under this title or imprisoned not more than 2 years, or both. This subsection does not apply to a partial birth abortion that is *necessary to save the life of a mother* whose life is endangered by a physical disorder, physical illness, or physical injury, including a life-endangering physical condition caused by or arising from the pregnancy itself. . . .

(b) (1) The term "partial birth" abortion means an abortion in which the person performing the abortion

(A) *Deliberately and intentionally* vaginally delivers a living fetus until, in the case of a head-first presentation, the *entire fetal head is outside* the body of the mother, *or,* in the case of breech presentation, *any part of the fetal trunk past the navel is outside* the body of the mother, for the purpose of performing an overt act that the person knows will kill the partially delivered living fetus; and

(B) Performs the overt act, other than completion of delivery, that kills the partially delivered living fetus[4] [emphasis added].

The Court decided, 5 to 4, that this law was constitutional. Justice Kennedy wrote the majority opinion for himself, Justices Antonin Scalia and Clarence Thomas, and the two new justices. In it he substantially adopts his dissenting opinion in *Stenberg* as the Court's new majority opinion. Although he concludes that his decision is consistent with *Stenberg,* all three U.S. District courts and all three Courts of Appeal that had examined this federal law found it unconstitutional under the principles in *Casey* and *Stenberg,* primarily because of the vagueness of the definition and the lack of a health exception.[4]

As to the vagueness argument, Kennedy writes that the new law is no longer vague because it clarifies the distinction between the prohibited procedure (which he calls "intact D&E") and standard D&E abortions because the former requires the delivery of an intact fetus, whereas the latter requires "the removal of fetal parts that are ripped from the fetus as they are pulled through the cervix." In addition, the new federal law specifies fetal landmarks (e.g., the "navel") instead of the vague description of a "substantial portion" of the "unborn child."[4]

Since the law applies to fetuses both before and after the point of viability, Kennedy concedes that under *Casey* the law would be unconstitutional "if its purpose or effect is to place a substantial obstacle in the path of a woman seeking an abortion before the fetus attains viability."[4] Kennedy finds Congress's purpose is twofold: first, lawmakers wanted to "express respect for the dignity of human life" by outlawing "a method of abortion in which a fetus is killed just inches before completion of the birth process," because use of this procedure "will further coarsen society to the humanity of not only newborns, but of all vulnerable and innocent human life. . . ." Second, Congress wanted to protect medical ethics, finding that this procedure "confuses the medical, legal and ethical duties of physicians to preserve and promote life. . . ."[4]

The key to Kennedy's legal analysis is his conclusion that these reasons are constitutionally sufficient to justify the ban because under *Casey* "the State, from the inception of pregnancy, maintains its own regulatory interest in protecting the life of the fetus that may become a child [and this interest] cannot be set at naught by interpreting *Casey*'s requirement of a health exception so it becomes tantamount to allowing the doctor to choose the abortion method he or she might prefer."[4]

Kennedy then goes on to write that "respect for human life finds an ultimate expression in the bond of love the mother has for her child," and that "while no reliable data" exist on the subject, "it seems unexceptionable to conclude some women come to regret their choice to abort the infant life they once created and sustained. . . . Severe depression and loss of esteem can follow." Such regret, Justice Kennedy believes, can be caused or exacerbated if women later learn what the procedure entails, suggesting that physicians fail to describe it to patients because they "may prefer not to disclose precise details of the means [of abortion] that will be used. . . ."[4]

The final, important issue is whether the prohibition would "ever impose significant health risks on women" and whether physicians or Congress should make this determination. Kennedy picks Congress: "The law need not give abortion doctors unfettered choice in the course of their medical practice, nor should it elevate their status above other physicians in the medical community. . . . Medical uncertainty does not foreclose the exercise of legislative power in the abortion context any more than it does in other contexts."[4] Furthermore, Kennedy argues, the law does not impose an "undue burden" on women for another reason: alternative ways of killing a fetus have not been prohibited. In his words, "If the intact D&E procedure is truly necessary in some circumstances, it appears likely an injection that kills the fetus is an alternative under the Act that allows the doctor to perform the procedure."[4]

JUSTICE GINSBURG'S DISSENT

Writing for the four justices in the minority, Justice Ruth Bader Ginsburg observes, "Today's decision is alarming. It refuses to take *Casey* and *Stenberg* seriously. It tolerates, indeed applauds, federal intervention to ban nationwide a procedure found necessary and proper in certain cases by the American College of Obstetricians (ACOG). It blurs the line, firmly drawn in *Casey,* between previability and postviability abortions. And, for the first time since *Roe,* the Court blesses a prohibition with no exception safeguarding a woman's health."[4]

Ginsburg argues that the majority of the Court has overruled the conclusion in *Stenberg* that a health exception is required when "substantial medical authority supports the proposition that banning a particular abortion procedure could endanger women's health. . . ."[4] This conclusion, bolstered by evidence presented by nine professional organizations, including the ACOG, and conclusions by all three U.S. District Courts that heard evidence concerning the Act and its effects, directly contradicted the congressional declaration that "there is no credible medical evidence that partial-birth abortions are safe or are safer than other abortion procedures." Even Justice Kennedy agreed that Congress's finding was untenable.

Justice Ginsburg concludes that this leaves only "flimsy and transparent justifications" for upholding the ban. She rejects those justifications, arguing that the state's interest in "preserving and promoting fetal life" cannot be furthered by a ban that targets only a method of abortion and that cannot save "a single fetus from destruction" by its own terms but may put women's health at risk.[4] Ultimately, she believes that the decision rests entirely on the proposition, never before enshrined in a majority opinion and explicitly repudiated in *Casey,* that "ethical and moral concerns" unrelated to the government's interest in "preserving life" can overcome what had been considered fundamental rights of citizens.

The majority seeks to bolster its conclusion by describing pregnant women as in a fragile emotional state that physicians may take advantage of by withholding information about abortion procedures. Justice Ginsburg concludes that the majority's solution to this hypothetical problem is to "deprive women of the right to make an autonomous choice, even at the expense of their safety."[4] She continues, "This way of thinking [that men must protect women by restricting their choices] reflects ancient notions about women's place in the family and under the Constitution—ideas that have long since been discredited."[4]

Ginsburg further notes that the majority simply cannot contain its hostility to reproductive rights as articulated in *Roe* and *Casey,* calling physicians "abortion doctors," describing the fetus as an "unborn child" and as a "baby," labeling second-trimester abortions as "late term," and dismissing "the reasoned medical judgments of highly trained doctors . . . as 'preferences' motivated by 'mere convenience.'"[4]

Ginsburg makes two final points. First, although the Court invites a lawsuit to challenge the Act "as applied," it gives "no clue" as to how such a lawsuit should be brought. Surely, she asks, "the Court cannot mean that no suit to challenge the ban [based on how it affects an actual woman or her physician] may be brought until a woman's health is immediately jeopardized." Second, she argues that the opinion threatens to undercut the "rule of law" and the "principle of stare decisis," both of which the Court affirmed in *Casey,* concluding that, "A decision so at odds with our jurisprudence should not have staying power."[4] As described in *Casey,* stare decisis is a doctrine that obligates courts to follow the principles set forth in prior cases, called precedents, to assure continuity in the law, and precedents should not be abandoned under "political pressure" or as an "unprincipled emotional reaction."[2]

NOTES

1 Roe v. Wade, 410 U.S. 113 (1973).
2 Planned Parenthood of Southeastern Pennsylvania v. Casey, 505 U.S. 833 (1992).
3 Stenberg v. Carhart, 530 U.S. 914 (2000).
4 Gonzales v. Carhart, 2007 U.S. LEXIS 4338 (2007).
5 Griswold v. Connecticut, 381 U.S. 479 (1965).
6 Eisenstadt v. Baird, 405 U.S. 438 (1972).
7 Doe v. Bolton, 410 U.S. 179 (1973).
8 Planned Parenthood of Central Missouri v. Danforth, 428 U.S. 52 (1976).
9 Elias S., Annas G. J. Reproductive genetics and the law. Chicago: Year Book Medical, 1987:145–162.
10 Lawrence v. Texas, 539 U.S. 558 (2003).
11 Annas G. J. The Supreme Court, liberty, and abortion. N Engl J Med 1992; 327:651–4.
12 *Idem.* Partial-birth abortion, Congress, and the Constitution. N Engl J Med 1998; 339:279–83.
13 *Idem.* "Partial-birth abortion" and the Supreme Court. N Engl J Med 2001; 344:152–6.

EMBRYONIC STEM-CELL RESEARCH

STEM CELL BASICS

National Institutes of Health

This NIH document provides a basic understanding of stem cells and their prospective therapeutic uses. So-called *pluripotent* stem cells can be derived either from fetal tissue or earlier from human embryos at the blastocyst stage when *embryonic stem cells* become available. Pluripotent stem cells seem to have great therapeutic potential, but significant technological problems must be overcome for this potential to be realized. One recent breakthrough involves genetic modifications of specialized adult cells that cause them to become more like embryonic stem cells. This new type of cell is known as *induced pluripotent stem cells* (iPSCs). These cells have proven useful for drug development and the modeling of diseases. They promise some medical advantages over embryonic stem cells and invite few of the same ethical objections. Further research is needed to assess the safety and therapeutic potential of iPSCs.

I. INTRODUCTION: WHAT ARE STEM CELLS, AND WHY ARE THEY IMPORTANT?

Stem cells have the remarkable potential to develop into many different cell types in the body during early life and growth. In addition, in many tissues they serve as a sort of internal repair system, dividing essentially without limit to replenish other cells as long as the person or animal is still alive. When a stem cell divides, each new cell has the potential either to remain a stem cell or become another type of cell with a more specialized function, such as a muscle cell, a red blood cell, or a brain cell.

Stem cells are distinguished from other cell types by two important characteristics. First, they are unspecialized cells capable of renewing themselves through *cell division,* sometimes after long periods of inactivity. Second, under certain physiologic or experimental conditions, they can be induced to become tissue- or organ-specific cells with special functions. In some organs, such as the gut and bone marrow, stem cells regularly divide to repair and replace worn out or damaged tissues. In other organs, however, such as the pancreas and the heart, stem cells only divide under special conditions.

Until recently, scientists primarily worked with two kinds of stem cells from animals and humans: *embryonic stem cells* and non-embryonic *"somatic"* or *"adult"* stem cells. The functions and characteristics of these cells will be explained in this document. Scientists discovered ways to derive embryonic

stem cells from early mouse embryos nearly 30 years ago, in 1981. The detailed study of the biology of mouse stem cells led to the discovery, in 1998, of a method to derive stem cells from human embryos and grow the cells in the laboratory. These cells are called *human embryonic stem cells.* The embryos used in these studies were created for reproductive purposes through *in vitro fertilization* procedures. When they were no longer needed for that purpose, they were donated for research with the informed consent of the donor. In 2006, researchers made another breakthrough by identifying conditions that would allow some specialized adult cells to be "reprogrammed" genetically to assume a stem cell-like state. This new type of stem cell, called *induced pluripotent stem cells (IPSCs),* will be discussed in a later section of this document.

Stem cells are important for living organisms for many reasons. In the 3- to 5-day-old embryo, called a *blastocyst,* the inner cells give rise to the entire body of the organism, including all of the many specialized cell types and organs such as the heart, lung, skin, sperm, eggs and other tissues. In some adult tissues, such as bone marrow, muscle, and brain, discrete populations of adult stem cells generate replacements for cells that are lost through normal wear and tear, injury, or disease.

Given their unique regenerative abilities, stem cells offer new potentials for treating diseases such as diabetes and heart disease. However, much work remains to be done in the laboratory and the clinic to understand how to use these cells for *cell-based therapies* to treat disease, which is also referred to as *regenerative or reparative medicine.*

National Institutes of Health.

Laboratory studies of stem cells enable scientists to learn about the cells' essential properties and what makes them different from specialized cell types. Scientists are already using stem cells in the laboratory to screen new drugs and to develop model systems to study normal growth and identify the causes of birth defects.

Research on *stem cells* continues to advance knowledge about how an organism develops from a single cell and how healthy cells replace damaged cells in adult organisms. Stem cell research is one of the most fascinating areas of contemporary biology, but, as with many expanding fields of scientific inquiry, research on stem cells raises scientific questions as rapidly as it generates new discoveries.

II. WHAT ARE THE UNIQUE PROPERTIES OF ALL STEM CELLS?

Stem cells differ from other types of cells in the body. All stem cells—regardless of their source—have three general properties: 1) they are capable of dividing and renewing themselves for long periods; 2) they are unspecialized; and 3) they can give rise to specialized cell types.

Stem cells are capable of dividing and renewing themselves for long periods. Unlike muscle cells, blood cells, or nerve cells—which do not normally replicate themselves—stem cells may replicate many times, or *proliferate*. A starting population of stem cells that proliferates for many months in the laboratory can yield millions of cells. If the resulting cells continue to be unspecialized, like the parent stem cells, the cells are said to be capable of *long-term self-renewal*.

Scientists are trying to understand two fundamental properties of stem cells that relate to their long-term self-renewal:

1. Why can *embryonic stem cells* proliferate for a year or more in the laboratory without differentiating, but most non-embryonic stem cells (*adult stem cells*) cannot; and

2. What factors in living organisms normally regulate stem cell proliferation and self-renewal?

Discovering the answers to these questions may make it possible to understand how cell proliferation is regulated during normal embryonic development or during the abnormal *cell division* that leads to cancer. Such information would also enable scientists to grow embryonic and non-embryonic stem cells more efficiently in the laboratory.

The specific factors and conditions that allow stem cells to remain unspecialized are of great interest to scientists. It has taken many years of trial and error to learn to derive and maintain stem cells in the laboratory without them spontaneously differentiating into specific cell types. For example, it took two decades to learn how to grow *human embryonic stem cells* in the laboratory following the development of conditions for growing mouse stem cells. Therefore, [it is important to understand] the signals in a mature organism that cause a stem cell population to proliferate and remain unspecialized until the cells are needed. Such information is critical for scientists to be able to grow large numbers of unspecialized stem cells in the laboratory for further experimentation.

Stem cells are unspecialized. One of the fundamental properties of a stem cell is that it does not have any tissue-specific structures that allow it to perform specialized functions. For example, a stem cell cannot work with its neighbors to pump blood through the body (like a heart muscle cell), and it cannot carry oxygen molecules through the bloodstream (like a red blood cell). However, unspecialized stem cells can give rise to specialized cells, including heart muscle cells, blood cells, or nerve cells.

Stem cells can give rise to *specialized cells.* When unspecialized stem cells give rise to specialized cells, the process is called *differentiation*. While differentiating, the cell usually goes through several stages, becoming more specialized at each step. Scientists are just beginning to understand the signals inside and outside cells that trigger each step of the differentiation process. The internal *signals* are controlled by a cell's *genes,* which are interspersed across long strands of DNA, and carry coded instructions for all cellular structures and functions. The external signals for cell differentiation include chemicals secreted by other cells, physical contact with neighboring cells, and certain molecules in the *microenvironment*. The interaction of signals during differentiation causes the cell's DNA to acquire *epigenetic* marks that restrict DNA expression in the cell and can be passed on through cell division.

Many questions about stem cell differentiation remain. For example, are the internal and external signals for cell differentiation similar for all kinds of stem cells? Can specific sets of signals be identified that promote differentiation into specific cell types? Addressing these questions may lead scientists to find new ways to control stem cell differentiation in the laboratory, thereby growing cells or tissues that can be used for specific purposes such as *cell-based therapies* or drug screening.

Adult stem cells typically generate the cell types of the tissue in which they reside. For example, a blood-forming adult stem cell in the bone marrow normally gives rise to the many types of blood cells. It is generally accepted that a blood-forming cell in the bone marrow—which is called a *hematopoietic stem cell*—cannot give rise to the cells of a very different tissue, such as nerve cells in the brain. Experiments over the last several years have purported to show that stem cells from one tissue may give rise to cell types of a completely different tissue. This remains an area of great debate within the research community. This controversy demonstrates the challenges of studying adult stem cells and suggests that additional research using adult stem cells is necessary to understand their full potential as future therapies.

III. WHAT ARE EMBRYONIC STEM CELLS?

A. What stages of early embryonic development are important for generating embryonic stem cells?

Embryonic stem cells, as their name suggests, are derived from embryos. Most embryonic stem cells are derived from embryos that develop from eggs that have been fertilized *in vitro*—in an *in vitro fertilization* clinic—and then donated for research purposes with informed consent of the donors. They are *not* derived from eggs fertilized in a woman's body. The *embryos* from which *human embryonic stem cells* are derived are typically four or five days old and are a hollow microscopic ball of cells called the *blastocyst.* The blastocyst includes three structures: the *trophoblast,* which is the layer of cells that sur-

rounds the *blastocoel,* a hollow cavity inside the blastocyst; and the *inner cell mass,* which is a group of cells at one end of the blastocoel that develop into the embryo proper.

B. How are embryonic stem cells grown in the laboratory?

Growing cells in the laboratory is known as *cell culture.* Human embryonic stem cells are isolated by transferring the *inner cell mass* into a plastic laboratory culture dish that contains a nutrient broth known as *culture medium.* The cells divide and spread over the surface of the dish. The inner surface of the culture dish is typically coated with mouse embryonic skin cells that have been treated so they will not divide. This coating layer of cells is called a *feeder layer.* The mouse cells in the bottom of the culture dish provide the inner cell mass cells a sticky surface to which they can attach. Also, the feeder cells release nutrients into the culture medium. Researchers have devised ways to grow embryonic stem cells without mouse feeder cells. This is a significant scientific advance because of the risk that viruses or other macromolecules in the mouse cells may be transmitted to the human cells.

The process of generating an embryonic stem cell line is somewhat inefficient, so lines are not produced each time an inner cell mass is placed into a culture dish. However, if the plated inner cell mass cells survive, divide, and multiply enough to crowd the dish, they are removed gently and plated into several fresh culture dishes. The process of re-plating or *subculturing* the cells is repeated many times and for many months. Each cycle of subculturing the cells is referred to as a *passage.* Once the cell line is established, the original cells yield millions of embryonic stem cells. Embryonic stem cells that have proliferated in cell culture for six or more months without differentiating, are *pluripotent,* and appear genetically normal are referred to as an *embryonic stem cell line.* At any stage in the process, batches of cells can be frozen and shipped to other laboratories for further culture and experimentation.

If scientists can reliably direct the differentiation of embryonic stem cells into specific cell types, they may be able to use the resulting, differentiated cells to treat certain diseases in the future. Diseases that might be treated by transplanting cells generated from human embryonic stem cells include diabetes, traumatic spinal cord injury, Duchenne's muscular dystrophy, heart disease, and vision and hearing loss.

IV. WHAT ARE ADULT STEM CELLS?

An *adult stem cell* is thought to be an *undifferentiated* cell, found among differentiated cells in a tissue or organ that can renew itself and can differentiate to yield some or all of the major specialized cell types of the tissue or organ. The primary roles of adult stem cells in a living organism are to maintain and repair the tissue in which they are found. Scientists also use the term *somatic stem cell* instead of adult stem cell, where somatic refers to cells of the body (not the germ cells, sperm or eggs). Unlike *embryonic stem cells,* which are defined by their origin (the *inner cell mass* of the *blastocyst*), the origin of adult stem cells in some mature tissues is still under investigation.

Research on adult stem cells has generated a great deal of excitement. Scientists have found adult stem cells in many more tissues than they once thought possible. This finding has led researchers and clinicians to ask whether adult stem cells could be used for transplants. In fact, adult hematopoietic, or blood-forming, stem cells from bone marrow have been used in transplants for 40 years. Scientists now have evidence that stem cells exist in the brain and the heart. If the differentiation of adult stem cells can be controlled in the laboratory, these cells may become the basis of transplantation-based therapies.

The history of research on adult stem cells began about 50 years ago. In the 1950s, researchers discovered that the bone marrow contains at least two kinds of stem cells. One population, called *hematopoietic stem cells,* forms all the types of blood cells in the body. A second population, called *bone marrow stromal stem cells* (also called *mesenchymal stem cells,* or skeletal stem cells by some), were discovered a few years later. These non-hematopoietic stem cells make up a small proportion of the *stromal cell* population in the bone marrow, and can generate bone, cartilage, fat, cells that support the formation of blood, and fibrous connective tissue.

In the 1960s, scientists who were studying rats discovered two regions of the brain that contained dividing cells that ultimately become nerve cells. Despite these reports, most scientists believed that the adult brain could not generate new nerve cells. It was not until the 1990s that scientists agreed that the adult brain does contain stem cells that are able to generate the brain's three major cell types—*astrocytes* and *oligodendrocytes,* which are non-neuronal cells, and *neurons*, or nerve cells.

A. Where are adult stem cells found, and what do they normally do?

Adult stem cells have been identified in many organs and tissues, including brain, bone marrow, peripheral blood, blood vessels, skeletal muscle, skin, teeth, heart, gut, liver, ovarian epithelium, and testis. They are thought to reside in a specific area of each tissue (called a "stem cell niche"). In many tissues, current evidence suggests that some types of stem cells are pericytes, cells that compose the outermost layer of small blood vessels. Stem cells may remain quiescent (non-dividing) for long periods of time until they are activated by a normal need for more cells to maintain tissues, or by disease or tissue injury.

Typically, there is a very small number of stem cells in each tissue, and once removed from the body, their capacity to divide is limited, making generation of large quantities of stem cells difficult. Scientists in many laboratories are trying to find better ways to grow large quantities of adult stem cells in *cell culture* and to manipulate them to generate specific cell types so they can be used to treat injury or disease. Some examples of potential treatments include regenerating bone using cells derived from bone marrow stroma, developing insulin-producing cells for type 1 diabetes, and repairing damaged heart muscle following a heart attack with cardiac muscle cells.

B. What tests are used to identify adult stem cells?

Scientists often use one or more of the following methods to identify adult stem cells: (1) label the cells in a living tissue with molecular markers and then determine the specialized cell types they generate; (2) remove the cells from a living animal, label them in cell culture, and transplant them back into another animal to determine whether the cells replace (or "repopulate") their tissue of origin.

Importantly, it must be demonstrated that a single adult stem cell can generate a line of genetically identical cells that then gives rise to all the appropriate differentiated cell types of the tissue. To confirm experimentally that a putative adult stem cell is indeed a stem cell, scientists tend to show either that the cell can give rise to these genetically identical cells in culture, and/or that a purified population of these candidate stem cells can repopulate or reform the tissue after transplant into an animal.

In addition to reprogramming cells to become a specific cell type, it is now possible to reprogram adult somatic cells to become like embryonic stem cells (*induced pluripotent stem cells, iPSCs*) through the introduction of embryonic genes. Thus, a source of cells can be generated that are specific to the donor, thereby avoiding issues of histocompatibility, if such cells were to be used for tissue regeneration. However, as with embryonic stem cells, determination of the methods by which iPSCs can be completely and reproducibly committed to appropriate cell lineages is still under investigation.

C. What are the key questions about adult stem cells?

Many important questions about adult stem cells remain to be answered. They include:

How many kinds of adult stem cells exist, and in which tissues do they exist?

How do adult stem cells evolve during development and how are they maintained in the adult? Are they "leftover" embryonic stem cells, or do they arise in some other way?

Why do stem cells remain in an undifferentiated state when all the cells around them have differentiated? What are the characteristics of their "niche" that control their behavior?

Do adult stem cells have the capacity to transdifferentiate, and is it possible to control this process to improve its reliability and efficiency?

If the beneficial effect of adult stem cell transplantation is a trophic effect, what are the mechanisms? Is donor cell-recipient cell contact required, secretion of factors by the donor cell, or both?

What are the factors that control adult stem cell proliferation and differentiation?

What are the factors that stimulate stem cells to relocate to sites of injury or damage, and how can this process be enhanced for better healing?

V. WHAT ARE THE SIMILARITIES AND DIFFERENCES BETWEEN EMBRYONIC AND ADULT STEM CELLS?

Human embryonic and *adult stem cells* each have advantages and disadvantages regarding potential use for *cell-based regenerative therapies*. One major difference between adult and embryonic stem cells is their different abilities in the number and type of differentiated cell types they can become. *Embryonic stem cells* can become all cell types of the body because they are *pluripotent*. Adult stem cells are thought to be limited to differentiating into different cell types of their tissue of origin.

Embryonic stem cells can be grown relatively easily in culture. Adult stem cells are rare in mature tissues, so isolating these cells from an adult tissue is challenging, and methods to expand their numbers in *cell culture* have not yet been worked out. This is an important distinction, as large numbers of cells are needed for stem cell replacement therapies.

Scientists believe that tissues derived from embryonic and adult stem cells may differ in the likelihood of being rejected after transplantation. We don't yet know whether tissues derived from embryonic stem cells would cause transplant rejection, since the first Phase 1 clinical trial testing the safety of cells derived from hESCS has only recently been approved by the United States Food and Drug Administration (FDA).

Adult stem cells, and tissues derived from them, are currently believed less likely to initiate rejection after transplantation. This is because a patient's own cells could be expanded in culture, coaxed into assuming a specific cell type (*differentiation*), and then reintroduced into the patient. The use of adult stem cells and tissues derived from the patient's own adult stem cells would mean that the cells are less likely to be rejected by the immune system. This represents a significant advantage, as immune rejection can be circumvented only by continuous administration of immunosuppressive drugs, and the drugs themselves may cause deleterious side effects.

VI. WHAT ARE INDUCED PLURIPOTENT STEM CELLS?

Induced pluripotent stem cells (iPSCs) are adult cells that have been genetically reprogrammed to an embryonic stem cell–like state by being forced to express genes and factors important for maintaining the defining properties of embryonic stem cells. Although these cells meet the defining criteria for pluripotent stem cells, it is not known if iPSCs and embryonic stem cells differ in clinically significant ways. Mouse iPSCs were first reported in 2006, and human iPSCs were first reported in late 2007. Mouse iPSCs demonstrate important characteristics of pluripotent stem cells, including expressing stem cell markers, forming tumors containing cells from all three germ layers, and being able to contribute to many different tissues when injected into mouse embryos at a very early stage in development. Human iPSCs also express stem cell markers and are capable of generating cells characteristic of all three *germ layers*.

Although additional research is needed, iPSCs are already useful tools for drug development and modeling of diseases, and scientists hope to use them in transplantation medicine. Viruses are currently used to introduce the reprogramming factors into adult cells, and this process must be carefully controlled and tested before the technique can lead to useful treatments for humans. In animal studies, the virus used to introduce the stem cell factors sometimes causes cancers. Researchers are currently investigating non-viral delivery strategies. In any case, this breakthrough discovery has created a powerful new way to "de-differentiate" cells whose developmental fates had been previously assumed to be determined. In addition, tissues derived from iPSCs will be a nearly identical match to the cell donor and thus probably avoid rejection by the immune system. The iPSC strategy creates pluripotent stem cells that, together with studies of other types of pluripotent stem cells, will help researchers learn how to reprogram cells to repair damaged tissues in the human body.

VII. WHAT ARE THE POTENTIAL USES OF HUMAN STEM CELLS AND THE OBSTACLES THAT MUST BE OVERCOME BEFORE THESE POTENTIAL USES WILL BE REALIZED?

There are many ways in which human stem cells can be used in research and the clinic. Studies of *human embryonic stem cells* will yield information about the complex events that occur during human development. A primary goal of this work is to identify how *undifferentiated* stem cells become the differentiated cells that form the tissues and organs. Scientists know that turning *genes* on and off is central to this process. Some of the most serious medical conditions, such as cancer and birth defects, are due to abnormal *cell division* and *differentiation*. A more complete understanding of the genetic and molecular controls of these processes may yield information about how such diseases arise and suggest new strategies for therapy. Predictably controlling cell proliferation and differentiation requires additional basic research on the molecular and genetic signals that regulate cell division and specialization. While recent developments with iPS cells suggest some of the specific factors that may be involved, techniques must be devised to introduce these factors safely into the cells and control the processes that are induced by these factors.

Human stem cells could also be used to test new drugs. For example, new medications could be tested for safety on differentiated cells generated from human *pluripotent* cell lines. Other kinds of cell lines are already used in this way. Cancer cell lines, for example, are used to screen potential antitumor drugs. The availability of pluripotent stem cells would allow drug testing in a wider range of cell types. However, to screen drugs effectively, the conditions must be identical when comparing different drugs. Therefore, scientists will have to be able to precisely control the differentiation of stem cells into the specific cell type on which drugs will be tested. Current knowledge of the signals controlling differentiation falls short of being able to mimic these conditions precisely to generate pure populations of differentiated cells for each drug being tested.

Perhaps the most important potential application of human stem cells is the generation of cells and tissues that could be used for *cell-based therapies*. Today, donated organs and tissues are often used to replace ailing or destroyed tissue, but the need for transplantable tissues and organs far outweighs the available supply. Stem cells, directed to differentiate into specific cell types, offer the possibility of a renewable source of replacement cells and tissues to treat diseases including Alzheimer's diseases, spinal cord injury, stroke, burns, heart disease, diabetes, osteoarthritis, and rheumatoid arthritis.

For example, it may become possible to generate healthy heart muscle cells in the laboratory and then transplant those cells into patients with chronic heart disease. Preliminary research in mice and other animals indicates that *bone marrow stromal cells,* transplanted into a damaged heart, can have beneficial effects. Whether these cells can generate heart muscle cells or stimulate the growth of new blood vessels that repopulate the heart tissue, or help via some other mechanism is actively under investigation. For example, injected cells may repair by secreting growth factors, rather than actually incorporating into the heart. Promising results from animal studies have served as the basis for a small number of exploratory studies in humans. Other recent studies in *cell culture* systems indicate that it may be possible to direct the *differentiation* of embryonic stem cells or adult bone marrow cells into heart muscle cells.

In people who suffer from type 1 diabetes, the cells of the pancreas that normally produce insulin are destroyed by the patient's own immune system. New studies indicate that it may be possible to direct the differentiation of human embryonic stem cells in cell culture to form insulin-producing cells that eventually could be used in transplantation therapy for persons with diabetes.

To realize the promise of novel cell-based therapies for such pervasive and debilitating diseases, scientists must be able to manipulate stem cells so that they possess the necessary characteristics for successful differentiation, transplantation, and engraftment. The following is a list of steps in successful cell-based treatments that scientists will have to learn to control to bring such treatments to the clinic. To be useful for transplant purposes, stem cells must be reproducibly made to:

Proliferate extensively and generate sufficient quantities of tissue.

Differentiate into the desired cell type(s).

Survive in the recipient after transplant.

Integrate into the surrounding tissue after transplant.

Function appropriately for the duration of the recipient's life.

Avoid harming the recipient in any way.

Also, to avoid the problem of immune rejection, scientists are experimenting with different research strategies to generate tissues that will not be rejected.

To summarize, stem cells offer exciting promise for future therapies, but significant technical hurdles remain that will only be overcome through years of intensive research.

KILLING EMBRYOS FOR STEM CELL RESEARCH
Jeff McMahan

In this excerpt from a longer paper, McMahan considers the main moral objection to human embryonic stem cell research. This research involves killing human embryos, which are said to be essentially beings of the same sort that you and I are. This objection presupposes 1) that we once existed as early embryos and 2) that we had the same moral status then that we have now. McMahan challenges both those presuppositions, but in this excerpt he focuses on the first. He argues, based on widely accepted beliefs about monozygotic twinning (which produces identical twins), that early embryos may not even be human organisms, although he concedes that there is room for doubt on this point. More importantly, he denies that we are essentially human organisms, appealing to hypothetical cases of brain transplantation and actual cases involving conjoined twins. He concludes that we never existed as embryos, in which case killing an embryo does not kill someone like you or me but merely prevents one of us from existing.

Those who believe that the killing of human embryos is wrong typically support their view by claiming that embryos are innocent human beings, and that innocent human beings must be protected, not harmed or destroyed or used solely as a means of benefiting others. . . . Some reasons for believing that embryos are innocent human beings whom it is wrong to kill are religious in character. There are, however, two assumptions that I believe capture the essence of the religious concern but are also compatible with secular morality. I will focus my discussion on these. They are:

(1) The embryo is the earliest stage in the existence of someone like you or me. That is, we were once embryos.

(2) We have the same moral status at all times at which we exist. We mattered just as much when we were embryos as we do now.

I believe that both of these assumptions are false. . . . [T]he second assumption seems incompatible with the claim that many of the moral reasons why we have to treat an individual in certain ways and not treat that individual in other ways are given by that individual's intrinsic nature. If you were once an embryo, your nature was very different then from what it is now. It is reasonable to think that your moral status was correspondingly different, so that it may have been permissible to treat you then in ways that would be impermissible now. It seems implausible to suppose that radical changes in an individual's nature can never affect that individual's basic moral status.[1]

If you were never an embryo, however, the question of what your status was as an embryo cannot arise. My main aim in this essay is to offer

reasons for thinking that we were never embryos. I will focus on embryos at a very early stage in their development. The best time to intervene to derive stem cells by the traditional method that involves killing the embryo is a little less than a week after conception, when the embryo—or, technically, blastocyst—is five or six days old. I will therefore consider whether it is plausible to suppose that we were once six-day-old embryos. . . .

4. ARE SIX-DAY-OLD EMBRYOS HUMAN ORGANISMS?

Many people who believe that we were once embryos attempt to defend that view by claiming (1) that an embryo is a human organism in the earliest stage of its life and (2) that we are essentially human organisms. I believe, however, that the first of these claims is contentious and that the second is false. I will begin with the first. Although I do not think that it can be shown to be false that a six-day-old embryo is a human organism, I think that there is room for reasonable doubt about this. I will try to show what is at issue here.

There are two interpretations of what happens in the first fortnight after conception. The first treats the embryo as a human organism; the second does not. I will sketch them both and state the case for thinking that the second is more plausible.

According to the first interpretation, the successive cell divisions that follow the process of conception are events in the history of a single entity composed of various cells. This entity begins as one cell—the zygote—and continues to exist, as two cells, then four, and so on.

Yet it is unclear what makes all the various cells, considered synchronically or diachronically, parts of a single individual. They are all contiguous within a single extracellular membrane (the zona pellucida), but that alone does not make them a single entity any more than placing a number of marbles in a sack turns them into a single entity.

To consider whether the cells within the membrane of the early human embryo constitute a human organism, it is necessary to be clear about what a human organism is. I accept the familiar idea that a living human organism is an entity with human genes that is composed of various living parts that function together in an integrated way to sustain a single life, and that is not itself a part of another living biological entity.[2] (The last clause is necessary in order to exclude the implication that living human cells or organs are themselves human organisms.)

According to the second interpretation of the events in the first two weeks following conception, the cells that compose an embryo during this period do not yet serve sufficiently different functions to allow us to say that they are coordinated in the service of a single life. While each cell is itself alive, they are not together involved in processes that are constitutive of a further, higher-order life. During the first couple of weeks after conception, all that exists is a collection of qualitatively almost identical cells living within a single membrane. They are like marbles in a sack.

On this interpretation, the single-celled zygote is a single living entity, though not itself a human organism. When it divides, nothing but its constituent matter continues to exist. The zygote itself ceases to exist, as an ameba does when it divides, though in doing so it gives rise to two daughter cells. When they in turn divide, they too cease to exist. There is no individual that persists through these transformations. Only when there is sufficiently significant cell differentiation, so that different cells begin to serve different though coordinated functions that are identifiable as the regulative and self-preservative processes of a higher-order individual of which the cells are parts, do the cells together constitute a human organism. Only then is there a new and further life that is constituted by the integrated processes carried out by the various groups of differently functioning cells. Since significant cell differentiation is clearly identifiable at around two weeks after conception, it seems reasonable to treat that as the time at which a human organism begins to exist. For those who persist in thinking that a unique human

individual cannot exist until after the possibility of twinning has passed, it is perhaps significant that the time at which significant cell differentiation begins to occur coincides rather closely with the time at which twinning ceases to be possible.

This second interpretation may be disputed on the ground that the cells that compose the embryo are coordinated very early on, certainly before six days after conception.[3] There must, after all, be communication and coordination among them prior to significant differentiation, if only in order to ensure that different cell lines develop in different directions. Embryonic development would not get very far if all the cells decided, all at once, to specialize as skin cells.

This forceful objection helps to reveal what I think is fundamentally at issue in the dispute between proponents of these two different interpretations of what happens during the first two weeks after conception. Cellular specialization and intercellular coordination are matters of degree. Whether the cells within the zona pellucida constitute a human organism depends on whether they are differentiated and coordinated to a high enough degree to warrant the claim that their interactions constitute a higher-order life. But there is no objectively determinate degree of differentiation and coordination that is necessary and sufficient for the presence of a higher-order life. When we know all the facts about the various cells within the zona pellucida and their functions, we know all the basic facts there are to know. While there is no doubt a threshold along the spectrum of degrees of coordination beyond which it is undeniable that a collection of cells are functioning together to sustain a higher-order life, there may be, prior to that threshold, no objective fact about whether the cells together constitute on organism. Whether there is a human organism present may simply be underdetermined by the facts.

The question of when the level of differentiation and coordination becomes sufficient for the presence of a human organism is not a biological or scientific question but a metaphysical question. How we ought to answer it is a matter of overall coherence among our beliefs and concepts. Our answer should, for example, cohere with our beliefs about the end of life. If the minimal degree of cellular coordination that is present only a day or so after conception is sufficient for the existence of a living human organism, then it seems that we ought not to believe that brain death is the biological death of a human organism. For brain death is compatible with residual functioning among cells, tissues, and even organs that is far more extensive and highly coordinated than that found among the cells in a two-day-old or six-day-old embryo. Indeed, the level of coordination among the still-living parts of a brain-dead human organism that is given certain minimal forms of external support (such as mechanical ventilation) is immeasurably higher than that found among the cells in an early embryo, which is also dependent on life support from the maternal body. Thus, even most of those who reject brain death as the criterion of the biological death of a human organism, and embrace instead a criterion that is directly concerned with internally regulated integration among the organism's parts, would regard a once-living human organism as dead if it had no more coordination among its still-living parts than is present among the cells in a six-day-old embryo. This is one coherence-based reason for denying that such an embryo is a living human organism rather than a collection of cells that are each inner-directed along a path toward the formation of an organism.

Still, it may be best at this point to regard the question of when a human organism begins to exist as an open question. There is a strong case for the view that after about two weeks following conception there is sufficient differentiation and coordination among the cells in the zona pellucida to claim that together they constitute a higher-order life, the life of an organism. It is possible that before that point there is sufficient coordination to warrant the claim that the cells already constitute an organism. The best answer may well depend on facts about the cells and their relations with one another of which we are as yet unaware.

5. WE ARE NOT HUMAN ORGANISMS

No doubt it is odd to suppose that whether you existed at six days after conception depends on the degree to which a set of embryonic cells were coordinated with one another. Many people will be dismis-

sive of that idea and will accept as sturdy common sense that a human organism begins to exist at conception. Suppose this is right and two-day-old and six-day-old embryos are human organisms. Still, it follows that we were embryos only if we are essentially human organisms. I will argue that we are not.

Whether we are organisms is not a scientific question. There is no experiment that can be done to determine whether or not we are organisms, just as there is no experiment that could tell us whether a statue and the lump of bronze of which it is composed are one and the same thing or distinct substances. These are both metaphysical questions and must be settled by philosophical argument.

There are two arguments that I believe show that we cannot be human organisms. I will rehearse them only briefly here, as I have presented and developed each in more detail elsewhere (McMahan 2002, 31–39). The first appeals to a thought experiment, long familiar to students of philosophy, involving brain transplantation. (The thought experiment is actually more convincing if it involves transplantation only of the cerebrum and not of the entire brain. But for simplicity of exposition I will follow tradition and make it the entire brain.) Suppose that you and your identical twin are both involved in a terrible accident. Your brain is undamaged, but the rest of your body is so badly injured as to be moribund. Your identical twin's brain has been destroyed, but the rest of his or her body is undamaged. Exploiting new techniques that enable the proper neural connections to be made between your brain and your twin's body, your surgeons remove your twin's dead brain and transplant your perfectly functional brain in its place. Most of us believe that the person who then wakes up in that body is you. But if you were a human organism, you would now be the dead organism from which your brain was extracted, and the person who wakes up after the surgery would be your twin, now nicely equipped with a new brain.

Some people object to this argument because it depends on an example that is purely hypothetical. They think that we ought not to trust our intuitions about unrealistic cases. My second argument is not vulnerable to this objection, as it appeals to an actual phenomenon: dicephalus. Dicephalic twinning is a radically incomplete form of conjoined twinning in which two heads, each with its own brain and its own separate mental life, sit atop a single body. In some cases, there is very little duplication of organs below the neck; there is one circulatory system, one metabolic system, one reproductive system, and one immune system. In these cases, there are two persons but only one human organism. The two twins cannot both be the organism, because that would imply that they are not distinct individuals but one and the same person. Each twin's relation to the organism is the same; therefore there can be no reason to suppose that one of them is the organism while the other is not. It seems, therefore, that neither of them is identical with the organism. If dicephalic twins are essentially the same kind of thing that we are, then we are not organisms either.

But even if dicephalic twins were asymmetrically related to the organism as a whole, so that one twin had a much stronger claim to be the organism than the other, that could be sufficient to show that the other twin was clearly not the organism. But in that case there would be at least one person who was not identical to an organism. Unless that twin were essentially a different kind of entity from the rest of us, it would follow that we are not essentially organisms either.

There are in fact cases of highly asymmetric conjoined twins. In the phenomenon known as "craniopagus parasiticus," one conjoined twin is fully developed but the other, which is joined to the first at the head, has failed to develop a body and is thus, as the name suggests, a second head that draws life support from an organism to which it is attached but over which it exercises no control. There are only eleven recorded cases of this phenomenon, but two have occurred in the twenty-first century. In one case in Egypt, the second head was surgically removed, but the remaining twin died a little more than a year later from an infection of the brain. A BBC report comments that the "second head could smile and blink," but "whether it was capable of independent thought is unclear."[4] Whatever was true in this actual case, it seems possible that there could be a case in which the brain in the parasitic head would be fully developed and separate, thus forming a separate center of self-conscious, rational thought. That this is possible is suggested by the series of

experiments by Robert J. White in which various animals' heads were kept alive and fully conscious after being severed from the body, and by cases of high spinal cord transection. In such cases, the brain remains fully conscious if supplied with oxygenated blood even though it is otherwise actually or effectively unconnected with an organism. If there were a case of craniopagus parasiticus in which the parasitic head contained a fully developed brain, this would be a clear instance of a single organism supporting the existence of two distinct persons. Even if we were to claim that the person whose brain controlled the organism was identical with that organism, the person resident in the second head could not plausibly be identified with any organism. This again supports the view that individuals of the sort that you and I are cannot be essentially human organisms.

It might be objected to this argument that just as one of White's severed heads is itself an organism shorn of most of its nonessential parts, so the parasitic head in craniopagus parasiticus is also a distinct organism. But both these claims are false. A severed but living head with an external blood supply is not an organism but a surviving part, rather like an organ salvaged from a now-dead organism and kept alive pending transplantation. Similarly, a parasitic head is no more an organism than my head is.

If, however, we are not human organisms, then even if a human organism begins to exist at conception, it does not follow that we began to exist at that point. If you are not identical with the organism that supports your existence, it is possible that you began to exist in association with it at some point after it began to exist, whether that was at conception or a couple of weeks later. . . .

7. WHEN WE BEGIN TO EXIST

If we are neither human organisms nor souls, what kind of thing are we essentially, and when do things of our sort begin to exist? What I believe to be the best answer may emerge if you imagine yourself in the very early stages of progressive dementia. How long will you survive? You will be there as long as long as your brain continues to generate consciousness, and indeed as long as your brain retains the capacity to generate consciousness. As long as there is a subject of experiences present, or if it is possible to revive a subject of experiences in your body, then someone is present, and who might that be if not you?

But what if your brain altogether and irreversibly loses the capacity for consciousness? What remains? Suppose the organism that many people take to be you remains alive. If I am right that you are not and never were an organism, then that living organism cannot be you. It is hard to identify anything else that might be you. I think we should conclude that you ceased to exist along with the capacity for consciousness. That suggests that you are essentially an entity with the capacity for consciousness—a mind.

A human organism is conscious only by virtue of having a conscious part. We are that part. We are that which is nonderivatively the subject of consciousness. The label I use to describe what we essentially are is "embodied mind."

We coexist with our organisms throughout our lives, but our organisms begin to exist and are alive before we arrive on the scene, and they usually survive us, sometimes even remaining alive after we have ceased to be, as occurs, in my view, in persistent vegetative state. We begin to exist when the fetal brain develops the capacity for consciousness, which happens sometime between twenty-two and twenty-eight weeks after conception, when synapses develop among the neurons in the cerebral cortex. Only after the development of the capacity for consciousness is

there anyone who can be harmed, or wronged, by being killed. . . .

Acknowledgments I am very grateful for comments on this essay to Laura Grabel, Lori Gruen, and, especially, Alfonso Gómez-Lobo.

NOTES

1 [Ed. McMahan's arguments against the second assumption appear in sections of this paper not reproduced here]

2 This definition of a human organism implies that a zygote is not a human organism, even though it is genetically human and is an organism. The definition has this implication because it stipulates that at least some of a human organism's parts must be living, whereas the parts of a zygote are not thought to be separately alive. Those who believe that zygotes are human organisms could amend the definition by deleting the adjective "living."

3 I am much indebted to Alphonso Gómez-Lobo for pressing me on this, and for providing me with evidence of various forms and degrees of intercellular coordination that are manifest shortly after fertilization. He has persuaded me that, at a minimum, I should be more agnostic about the time at which a human organism begins to exist than I was in McMahan 2002, in which I argued for the second of the two interpretations discussed here.

4 See http://news.bbc.co.uk/2/hi/health/4285235.stm and http://news.bbc.co.uk/1/hi/world/4848164.stm (both last accessed on 22 October 2006).

REFERENCES

McMahan, Jeff. 2002. *The Ethics of Killing: Problems at the Margins of Life.* New York: Oxford University Press.

THE MORAL CASE AGAINST CLONING-FOR-BIOMEDICAL-RESEARCH
President's Council on Bioethics

In this selection, the President's Council on Bioethics (PCB) presents an overall argument against "cloning-for-biomedical-research." (Because the council was deeply divided on the ethics of research cloning, the views expressed here must be understood as the views of only one segment of the council's membership.) The argument has obvious application, among other things, to the use of cloned embryos as a source of embryonic stem cells, but a central strand in the overall argument—"what we owe to the embryo"—also entails that it is wrong to create any embryo, whether by in vitro fertilization or by cloning, solely for the purpose of harvesting its stem cells. The extensive commentary presented herein on the issue of the moral status of the early embryo includes the claim that the embryo has either full moral status (is "one of us") or has the sort of intermediate and developing moral status that would ground "special respect." In either case, the argument goes, the moral status of the embryo rules out the creation of embryos solely for research applications that entail their very destruction. A second major strand in the overall argument against cloning-for-biomedical-research involves an appeal to "the moral well-being of society as a whole." In this regard, concerns are expressed about (1) crossing the boundary from sexual to asexual reproduction, (2) "the complete instrumentalization of nascent human life," and (3) opening the door to even greater moral hazards, such as cloning-to-produce-children.

. . . Those of us who maintain—for both principled and prudential reasons—that cloning-for-biomedical-research *should not* be pursued . . . begin by acknowledging that substantial human goods might be gained from this research. Although it would be wrong to speak in ways that encourage false hope in those who are ill, as if a cure were likely in the near future, we who oppose such research take seriously its potential for one day yielding substantial (and perhaps unique) medical benefits. Even apart from more distant possibilities for advances in regenerative medicine, there are more immediate possibilities for progress in basic research and for developing models to study different diseases. All of us whose lives benefit enormously from medical advances that began with basic research know how great is our collective stake in continued scientific investigations. Only for very serious reasons—to avoid moral wrongdoing, to avoid harm to society, and to avoid foolish or unnecessary risks—should progress toward increased knowledge and advances that might relieve suffering or cure disease be slowed.

We also observe, however, that the realization of these medical benefits—like all speculative research and all wagers about the future—remains uncertain. There are grounds for questioning whether the proposed benefits of cloning-for-biomedical-research will be realized. And there may be other morally unproblematic ways to achieve similar scientific results and medical benefits. For example, promising results in research with nonembryonic and adult stem cells suggest that scientists may be able to make progress in regenerative medicine without engaging in cloning-

for-biomedical-research. We can move forward with other, more developed forms of human stem cell research and with animal cloning. We can explore other routes for solving the immune rejection problem or to finding valuable cellular models of human disease. Where such morally innocent alternatives exist, one could argue that the burden of persuasion lies on proponents to show not only that cloned embryo research is promising or desirable but that it is *necessary* to gain the sought-for medical benefits. Indeed, the Nuremberg Code of research ethics enunciates precisely this principle—that experimentation should be "such as to yield fruitful results for the good of society, *unprocurable by other methods or means of study*." Because of all the scientific uncertainties—and the many possible avenues of research—that burden cannot at present be met.

But, we readily concede, these same uncertainties mean that no one—not the scientists, not the moralists, and not the patients whose suffering we all hope to ameliorate—can know for certain which avenues of research will prove most successful. Research using cloned embryos may in fact, as we said above, yield knowledge and benefits unobtainable by any other means.

With such possible benefits in view, what reasons could we have for saying "no" to cloning-for-biomedical-research? Why not leave this possible avenue of medical progress open? Why not put the cup to our lips? In *The Winter's Tale*, Shakespeare has Leontes, King of Silicia, explain why one might not.[1]

There may be in the cup
A spider steep'd, and one may drink, depart,
And yet partake no venom, for his knowledge
Is not infected; but if one present

Reprinted from President's Council on Bioethics, *Human Cloning and Human Dignity: An Ethical Inquiry* (2002), pp. 150–165. Some notes omitted.

The abhorr'd ingredient to his eye, make known
How he hath drunk, he cracks his gorge, his sides
With violent hefts. I have drunk, and seen the spider.

To discern the spider in the cup is to see the moral reality of cloning-for-biomedical-research differently. It is to move beyond questions of immediately evident benefits or harms alone toward deeper questions about what an ongoing program of cloning-for-biomedical-research would mean. In part, this approach compels us to think about embryo research generally, but cloning (even for research purposes alone) raises its own special concerns, since only cloned embryos could one day become cloned children. We need to consider and articulate the reasons why, despite the possibility of great benefits, society should nevertheless turn away and not drink from this cup, and why the reasons for "drinking with limits" . . . are finally not persuasive.

. . . We differ, among ourselves, on the relative importance of the various arguments presented below. But we all agree that *moral objections to the research itself* and *prudential considerations about where it is likely to lead* suggest that we should oppose cloning-for-biomedical-research, albeit with regret.

A. WHAT WE OWE TO THE EMBRYO

The embryo is, and perhaps will always be, something of a puzzle to us. In its rudimentary beginnings, it is so unlike the human beings we know and live with that it hardly seems to be one of us; yet, the fact of our own embryonic origin evokes in us respect for the wonder of emerging new human life. Even in the midst of much that is puzzling and uncertain, we would not want to lose that respect or ignore what we owe to the embryo.

The cell synthesized by somatic cell nuclear transfer, no less than the fertilized egg, is a human organism in its germinal stage. It is not just a "clump of cells" but an integrated, self-developing whole, capable (if all goes well) of the continued organic development characteristic of human beings. To be sure, the embryo does not yet have, except in potential, the full range of characteristics that distinguish the human species from others, but one need not have those characteristics in evidence in order to

belong to the species. And of course human beings at some other stages of development—early in life, late in life, at any stage of life if severely disabled—do not forfeit their humanity simply for want of these distinguishing characteristics. We may observe different points in the life story of any human being—a beginning filled mostly with potential, a zenith at which the organism is in full flower, a decline in which only a residue remains of what is most distinctively human. But none of these points is itself the human being. That being is, rather, an organism with a continuous history. From zygote to irreversible coma, each human life is a single personal history.

But this fact still leaves unanswered the question of whether all stages of a human being's life have equal moral standing. Might there be sound biological or moral reasons for according the early-stage embryo only *partial* human worth or even none at all? If so, should such embryos be made available or even explicitly created for research that necessarily requires their destruction—especially if very real human good might come from it? Some of us who oppose cloning-for-biomedical-research hold that efforts to assign to the embryo a merely intermediate and developing moral status—that is, more humanly significant than other human cells, but less deserving of respect and protection than a human fetus or infant—are both biologically and morally unsustainable, and that the embryo is in fact fully "one of us": a human life in process, an equal member of the species *Homo sapiens* in the embryonic stage of his or her natural development. All of us who oppose going forward with cloning-for-biomedical-research believe that it is incoherent and self-contradictory for our colleagues . . . to claim that human embryos deserve "special respect" and to endorse nonetheless research that requires the creation, use, and destruction of these organisms, *especially when done routinely and on a large scale.*

The case for treating the early-stage embryo as simply the moral equivalent of all other human cells . . . is entirely unconvincing: it denies the continuous history of human individuals from zygote to fetus to infant to child; it misunderstands the meaning of potentiality—and, specifically, the difference between a "being-on-the-way" (such as a developing human embryo) and a "pile of raw materials," which has no definite potential and which might become anything at all; and it ignores the hazardous moral precedent that the routinized creation, use, and destruction of nascent human life would establish for other areas of scientific research and social life.

The more serious questions are raised—about individuality, potentiality, and "special respect"—by those who assign an intermediate and developing moral status to the human embryo, and who believe that cloned embryos can be used (and destroyed) for biomedical research while still according them special human worth.... But the arguments for this position—both biological and moral—are not convincing. For attempts to ground the special respect owed to a maturing embryo in certain of its developmental features do not succeed. And the invoking of a "special respect" owed to nascent human life seems to have little or no operative meaning once one sees what those who take this position are willing to countenance.

We are not persuaded by the argument that fourteen days marks a significant difference in moral status. Because the embryo's human and individual genetic identity is present from the start, nothing that happens later during the continuous development that follows—at fourteen days or any other time—is responsible for suddenly conferring a novel human individuality or identity. The scientific evidence suggests that the fourteen-day marker does not represent a biological event of moral significance; rather, changes that occur at fourteen days are merely the visibly evident culmination of more subtle changes that have taken place earlier and that are driving the organism toward maturity. Indeed, many advocates of cloning-for-biomedical-research implicitly recognize the arbitrariness of the fourteen-day line. The medical benefits to be gained by conducting research beyond the fourteen-day line are widely appreciated, and some people have already hinted that this supposed moral and biological boundary can be moved should the medical benefits warrant doing so. . . .

There are also problems with the claim that its capacity for "twinning" proves that the early embryo is not yet an individual or that the embryo's moral status is more significant after the capacity for twinning is gone. There is the obvious rejoinder that if one locus of moral status can become two, its moral standing does not thereby diminish but rather

increases. More specifically, the possibility of twinning does not rebut the individuality of the early embryo from its beginning. The fact that where "John" alone once was there are now both "John" and "Jim" does not call into question the presence of "John" at the outset. Hence, we need not doubt that even the earliest cloned embryo is an individual human organism in its germinal stage. Its capacity for twinning may simply be one of the characteristic capacities of an individual human organism at that particular stage of development, just as the capacity for crawling, walking, and running, or cooing, babbling, and speaking are capacities that are also unique to particular stages of human development. Alternatively, from a developmental science perspective, twinning may not turn out to be an intrinsic process within embryogenesis. Rather, it may be a response to a disruption of normal development from which the embryo recovers and then forms two. Twinning would thus be a testament to the resilience of self-regulation and compensatory repair within early life, not the lack of individuation in the early embryo. From this perspective, twinning is further testimony to the potency of the individual (in this case two) to fullness of form.

We are also not persuaded by the claim that in vitro embryos (whether created through IVF or cloning) have a lesser moral status than embryos that have been implanted into a woman's uterus, because they cannot develop without further human assistance. The suggestion that extra-corporeal embryos are not yet individual human organisms-on-the-way, but rather special human cells that acquire only through implantation the potential to become individual human organisms-on-the-way, rests on a misunderstanding of the meaning and significance of potentiality. An embryo is, by definition and by its nature, potentially a fully developed human person; its potential for maturation is a characteristic it *actually* has, and from the start. The fact that embryos have been created outside their natural environment—which is to say, outside the woman's body—and are therefore limited in their ability to realize their natural capacities, does not affect either the potential or the moral status of the beings themselves. A bird forced to live in a cage its entire life may never learn to fly. But this does not mean it is less of a bird, or that it lacks the immanent potentiality to fly on feathered wings. It means only that a caged bird—like an in vitro human embryo—has been deprived of its proper environment. There may, of course, be good human reasons to create embryos outside their natural environments—most obviously, to aid infertile couples. But doing so does not obliterate the moral status of the embryos themselves.

As we have noted, many proponents of cloning-for-biomedical-research (and for embryo research more generally) do not deny that we owe the human embryo special moral respect. Indeed, they have wanted positively to affirm it. But we do not understand what it means to claim that one is treating cloned embryos with special respect when one decides to create them intentionally for research that necessarily leads to their destruction. This respect is allegedly demonstrated by limiting such research—and therefore limiting the numbers of embryos that may be created, used, and destroyed—to only the most serious purposes: namely, scientific investigations that hold out the potential for curing diseases or relieving suffering. But this self-limitation shows only that our purposes are steadfastly high-minded; it does not show that the *means* of pursuing these purposes are *respectful of the cloned embryos* that are necessarily violated, exploited, and destroyed in the process. To the contrary, a true respect for a being would nurture and encourage it toward its own flourishing.

It is, of course, possible to have reverence for a life that one kills. This is memorably displayed, for example, by the fisherman Santiago in Ernest Hemingway's *The Old Man and the Sea,* who wonders whether it is a sin to kill fish even if doing so would feed hungry people. But it seems difficult to claim—even in theory but especially in practice—the presence of reverence once we run a stockyard or raise calves for veal—that is, once we treat the animals we kill (as we often do) simply as resources or commodities. In a similar way, we find it difficult to imagine that biotechnology companies or scientists who routinely engaged in cloning-for-biomedical-research would evince solemn respect for human life each time a cloned embryo was used and destroyed. Things we exploit even occasionally tend to lose their special value. It seems scarcely possible to

preserve a spirit of humility and solemnity while engaging in routinized (and in many cases corporately competitive) research that creates, uses, and destroys them.

The mystery that surrounds the human embryo is undeniable. But so is the fact that each human person began as an embryo, and that this embryo, once formed, had the unique potential to become a unique human person. This is the meaning of our embodied condition and the biology that describes it. If we add to this description a commitment to equal treatment—the moral principle that every human life deserves our equal respect—we begin to see how difficult it must be to suggest that a human embryo, even in its most undeveloped and germinal stage, could simply be used for the good of others and then destroyed. Justifying our intention of using (and destroying) human embryos for the purpose of biomedical research would force us either to ignore the truth of our own continuing personal histories from their beginning in embryonic life or to weaken the commitment to human equality that has been so slowly and laboriously developed in our cultural history.

Equal treatment of human beings does not, of course, mean identical treatment, as all parents know who have more than one child. And from one perspective, the fact that the embryo seems to amount to so little—seems to be little more than a clump of cells—invites us to suppose that its claims upon us can also not amount to much. We are, many have noted, likely to grieve the death of an embryo less than the death of a newborn child. But, then, we are also likely to grieve the death of an eighty-five-year-old father less than the death of a forty-five-year-old father. Perhaps, even, we may grieve the death of a newborn child less than the death of a twelve-year-old. We might grieve differently at the death of a healthy eighty-year-old than at the death of a severely demented eighty-year-old. Put differently, we might note how even the researcher in the laboratory may react with excitement and anticipation as cell division begins. Thus, reproductive physiologist Robert Edwards, who, together with Dr. Patrick Steptoe, helped produce Louise Brown, the first "test-tube baby," said of her: "The last time I saw her, she was just eight cells in a test-tube. She was beautiful then, and she's still beautiful now."[2] The embryo seems to amount to little; yet it has the capacity to become what to all of us seems very much indeed. There is a trajectory to the life story of human beings, and it is inevitable—and appropriate—that our emotional responses should be different at different points in that trajectory. Nevertheless, these emotions, quite naturally and appropriately different, would be misused if we calibrated the degree of respect we owe each other on the basis of such responses. In fact, we are obligated to try to shape and form our emotional responses—and our moral sentiments—so that they are more in accord with the moral respect we owe to those whose capacities are least developed (or those whom society may have wrongly defined as "non-persons" or "nonentities").

In short, how we respond to the weakest among us, to those who are nowhere near the zenith of human flourishing, says much about our willingness to envision the boundaries of humanity expansively and inclusively. It challenges—in the face of what we can know and what we cannot know about the human embryo—the depth of our commitment to equality. If from one perspective the fact that the embryo seems to amount to little may invite a weakening of our respect, from another perspective its seeming insignificance should awaken in us a sense of shared humanity. This was once our own condition. From origins that seem so little came our kin, our friends, our fellow citizens, and all human beings, whether known to us or not. In fact, precisely because the embryo seems to amount to so little, our responsibility to respect and protect its life correspondingly increases. As Hans Jonas once remarked, a true humanism would recognize "the inflexible principle that utter helplessness demands utter protection."[3]

B. WHAT WE OWE TO SOCIETY

Having acknowledged all that, we would miss something if we stopped with what is owed to the embryo—with the language of respect, claims, or rights. An embryo may seem to amount to little or nothing, but that very insignificance tests not the embryo's humanity but our own. Even those who are uncertain about the precise moral status of the human embryo—indeed, even those who believe that it has

only intermediate and developing status—have sound ethical-prudential reasons to refrain from using embryos for utilitarian purposes. Moreover, when the embryos to be used have been produced by cloning, there are additional moral dilemmas that go beyond the ethics of embryo research alone. There are principled reasons why people who *accept* research on leftover IVF embryos created initially for reproductive purposes should *oppose* the creation and use of cloned embryos explicitly for research. And there are powerful reasons to worry about where this research will lead us. All these objections have their ground not only in the embryo's character but also in our own, and in concern not only for the fate of nascent human life but for the moral well-being of society as a whole. *One need not believe the embryo is fully human to object vigorously to cloning-for-biomedical-research.*

We are concerned especially about three ways in which giving our moral approval to such research would harm the character of our common life and the way of life we want to transmit to future generations: (i) by crossing the boundary from sexual to asexual reproduction, in the process approving, whether recognized or not, genetic manipulation and control of nascent human life; (ii) by allowing and endorsing the complete instrumentalization of human embryos; and (iii) by opening the door to other—for some of us, far greater—moral hazards, such as cloning-to-produce-children or research on later-stage human embryos and fetuses.

1. Asexual Reproduction and the Genetic Manipulation of Embryos It is worth noting that human cloning—including cloning-for-biomedical-research itself and not simply cloning-to-produce-children—would cross a natural boundary between sexual and asexual reproduction, reducing the likelihood that we could either retrace our steps or keep from taking further steps. Cloning-for-biomedical-research and cloning-to-produce-children both begin with the same act of cloning: the production of a human embryo that is genetically virtually identical to its progenitor. The cloned embryo would therefore be the first human organism with a single genetic "parent" and, equally important, with a genetic constitution that is known and selected in advance. Both uses of cloning mark a significant leap in human power and human control over our genetic origins. Both involve deliberate genetic manipulation of nascent human life. It is, of course, precisely this genetic control that makes cloned embryos uniquely appealing and perhaps uniquely useful to those who seek to conduct research on them. But we should not be deceived about what we are agreeing to if we agree to start to clone: saying yes to cloned embryos in laboratories means saying yes *in principle* to an ever-expanding genetic mastery of one generation over the next.

2. The Complete Instrumentalization of Nascent Human Life By approving the production of cloned embryos for the sole purpose of research, society would transgress yet another moral boundary: that separating the different ways in which embryos might become available for human experimentation. It is one thing, as some have argued, to conduct research on leftover embryos from IVF procedures, which were created in attempts to have a child and, once no longer needed or wanted, are "destined" for destruction in any case. It is quite another to create embryos *solely* for research that will unavoidably and necessarily destroy them. Thus, for example, the National Bioethics Advisory Commission (in its report on stem cell research) reasoned that in circumstances where embryos were going to be discarded anyway, it did not undermine the moral respect owed to them if they were destroyed in one way (through research) rather than another (by being discarded when no longer wanted for IVF).[4] By contrast, the Commission reasoned that it was much harder to embrace the language of respect for the embryo if it were produced solely for purposes of research and, having been used, then destroyed. This argument maintained the following moral and practical distinction: that embryos created for reproduction but no longer desired could, with proper consent, be used as research subjects, but that embryos ought not be produced solely in order to be used as research subjects. So long as we oppose morally and may perhaps one day prohibit legally the production of cloned children, it is in the very nature of the case that cloned human embryos will not be acquirable as "spare" embryos left over from

attempts at reproduction. To the contrary, they will have to be produced solely and explicitly for the purpose of biomedical research, with no other end in view.

Some have argued that there is no significant moral difference between creating excess IVF embryos for reproduction *knowing in advance* that some will be discarded and creating cloned embryos for research *that leads necessarily* to their destruction. Because in both cases embryos are wittingly destroyed, there is, so the argument goes, no moral difference here.

When viewed simply in terms of the fates of embryos once they are created, the distinction between using leftover embryos and creating embryos solely for research may indeed be morally insignificant. But when viewed in terms of the different effects these two activities might have on the moral fabric of society—and the different moral dispositions of those who decide to produce embryos for these different purposes—the issue is more complex. In the eyes of those who create IVF embryos to produce a child, *every embryo,* at the moment of its creation, is *a potential child.* Even though more eggs are fertilized than will be transferred to a woman, each embryo is brought into being as an end in itself, not simply as a means to other ends. Precisely because one cannot tell which IVF embryo is going to reach the blastocyst stage, implant itself in the uterine wall, and develop into a child, the embryo "wastage" in IVF is more analogous to the embryo wastage in natural sexual intercourse practiced by a couple trying to get pregnant than it is to the creation and use of embryos that requires (without exception) their destruction.

Those who minimize or deny this distinction—between producing embryos hoping that one of them will become a child and producing embryos so that they can be used (and destroyed) in research—demonstrate the very problem we are worried about. Having become comfortable with seeing embryos as a means to noble ends (be it having a child or conducting biomedical research), they have lost sight of the fact that the embryos that we create as potential children are not means at all. Even those who remain agnostic about whether the human embryo is fully one of us should see the ways in which conducting such research would make us a different society: less humble toward that which we cannot fully understand, less willing to extend the boundaries of human respect ever outward, and more willing to transgress moral boundaries that we have, ourselves, so recently established, once it appears to be in our own interests to do so. We find it disquieting, even somewhat ignoble, to treat what are in fact seeds of the next generation as mere raw material for satisfying the needs of our own. Doing so would undermine the very prudence and humility to which defenders of limited embryo research often appeal: the idea that, while a human embryo may not be fully one of us, it is not humanly nothing and therefore should not be treated as a resource alone. But that is precisely what cloning-for-biomedical-research would do.

3. Opening the Door to Other Moral Hazards
This leads directly to our third concern—that the cloning of human embryos for research will open the door to additional (and to some of us, far greater) moral hazards. Human suffering from horrible diseases never comes to an end, and, likewise, our willingness to use embryonic life in the cause of research, once permitted, is also unlikely to find any natural stopping point. To set foot on this slope is to tempt ourselves to become people for whom the use of nascent human life as research material becomes routinized and everyday. That much is inherent in the very logic of what we would do in cloning-for-biomedical-research.

In addition, the reasons justifying production of cloned embryos for research can be predicted to expand. Today, the demand is for stem cells; tomorrow it may be for embryonic and fetal organs. . . . Should this prove to be the case, pressure will increase to grow cloned human blastocysts to later stages—either in the uteruses of suitably prepared animal hosts or (eventually) using artificial placenta-like structures in the laboratory—in order to obtain the more useful tissues. . . .

We should not be self-deceived about our ability to set limits on the exploitation of nascent life. What disturbs us today we quickly or eventually get used to; yesterday's repugnance gives way to tomorrow's endorsement. A society that already tolerates the destruction of fetuses in the second and third trimesters will hardly be horrified by embryo and fetus farming (including in animal wombs), if this should turn out to be helpful in the cure of dreaded diseases. . . .

Finally, if we accept even limited uses of cloning-for-biomedical-research, we significantly increase the likelihood of cloning-to-produce-children. The technique will gradually be perfected and the cloned embryos will become available, and those who would be interested in producing cloned children will find it much easier to do so. The only way to prevent this from happening would be to prohibit, by law, the implantation of cloned embryos for the purpose of producing children. To do so, however, the government would find itself in the unsavory position of designating a class of embryos that it would be a felony not to destroy. It would *require,* not just permit, the destruction of cloned embryos—which seems to us the very opposite of showing such cloned embryos "special respect.". . .

NOTES

1 Brian Appleyard calls attention to this passage in his book, *Brave New Worlds: Staying Human in the Genetic Future* (New York: Viking, 1998).
2 Cited in Kass, L. "The Meaning of Life—in the Laboratory," *The Public Interest,* No. 146, pp. 45–46, Winter 2002.
3 Jonas, H. "Philosophical Reflections on Experimenting With Human Subjects" in *Readings on Ethical and Social Issues in Biomedicine,* ed. Richard W. Wertz (Prentice-Hall, 1973), p. 32.
4 National Bioethics Advisory Commission, *Ethical Issues in Human Stem Cell Research,* volume I, p. 53. Bethesda, MD: Government Printing Office, 1999.

ANNOTATED BIBLIOGRAPHY

Boonin, David: *A Defense of Abortion* (Cambridge: Cambridge University Press, 2003). Boonin contends (1) that the fetus does not acquire a right to life until the onset of organized cortical brain activity, which on his reading of the evidence occurs sometime between the 25th and 32nd week; and (2) that, even if the fetus had a right to life as early as conception, it would not follow from that fact that most abortions are morally impermissible. Indeed, he argues more positively, most abortions are morally permissible.

Brody, Baruch: "On the Humanity of the Foetus." In Robert L. Perkins, ed., *Abortion: Pro and Con* (Cambridge, MA: Schenkman, 1974), pp. 69–90. Brody critically examines various proposals for "drawing the line" on the humanity of the fetus, ultimately suggesting that the most defensible view would draw the line at the point where fetal brain activity begins.

Dwyer, Susan, and Joel Feinberg, eds.: *The Problem of Abortion,* 3rd ed. (Belmont, CA: Wadsworth, 1997). This useful anthology features a wide range of articles on the moral justifiability of abortion. Also included is an extensive bibliography.

Hansen, J.-E. S.: "Embryonic Stem Cell Production Through Therapeutic Cloning Has Fewer Ethical Problems than Stem Cell Harvest from Surplus IVF Embryos," *Journal of Medical Ethics* 28 (April 2002), pp. 86–88. Hansen argues that an IVF embryo clearly lacks human moral status and a cloned embryo even more clearly lacks human moral status.

Harman, Elizabeth: "Creation Ethics: The Moral Status of Early Fetuses and the Ethics of Abortion," *Philosophy and Public Affairs* 28 (1999), pp. 310–324. Harman challenges the assumption that all fetuses at the same stage of development have the same moral status, arguing that a fetus that will be brought to term has moral status, while one that will be aborted does not.

Kamm, F. M.: *Creation and Abortion: A Study in Moral and Legal Philosophy* (Oxford: Oxford University Press, 1992). A major deontologist defends a right to abortion based on premises similar to Judith Thomson's and arguing from her own intuitive responses to hypothetical cases.

Kuflik, Arthur: "The 'Future Like Ours' Argument and Human Embryonic Stem Cell Research," *Journal of Medical Ethics* 34 (June 2008), pp. 417–421. Kuflik argues that Don Marquis's "future like ours" argument against abortion response provides no argument against using embryos in stem cell research.

Langerak, Edward A.: "Abortion: Listening to the Middle," *Hastings Center Report* 9 (October 1979), pp. 24–28. Langerak suggests a theoretical framework for a moderate view that incorporates two "widely shared beliefs": (1) that there is something about the fetus *itself* that makes abortion morally problematic and (2) that late abortions are significantly more problematic than early abortions.

Mills, Eugene: "The Egg and I: Conception, Identity, and Abortion," *Philosophical Review* 117 (July 2008), pp. 323–348. Mills maintains that each of us originated not at the moment of biological conception, but either before or after. On this basis he defends a conditional conclusion: if aborting pregnancies involving single-cell zygotes is immoral, then so are contraception and abstinence.

Noonan, John T., Jr.: "An Almost Absolute Value in History." In John T. Noonan, Jr., ed., *The Morality of Abortion: Legal and Historical Perspectives* (Cambridge, MA: Harvard University Press, 1970), pp. 51–59. In this well-known statement of the conservative view on the morality of abortion, Noonan argues that conception is the only objectively based and nonarbitrary point at which to "draw the line" between the nonhuman and the human.

Outka, Gene: "The Ethics of Human Stem Cell Research," *Kennedy Institute of Ethics Journal* 12 (June 2002), pp. 175–213. Outka surveys and analyzes various views on the ethics of human stem cell research. He ultimately argues that research on "excess" embryos can be justified by appeal to the "nothing is lost" principle, but the creation of embryos solely for research purposes cannot be justified.

Pojman, Louis P., and Francis J. Beckwith, eds.: *The Abortion Controversy: 25 Years After Roe v. Wade: A Reader,* 2nd ed. (Belmont, CA: Wadsworth, 1998). The articles in this long anthology are organized under eight headings, including "Evaluations of *Roe v. Wade,*" "Personhood Arguments on Abortion," and "Feminist Arguments on Abortion."

President's Council on Bioethics, *Monitoring Stem Cell Research* (2004). Chapter 2 of this report provides a description of "current federal law and policy." Chapter 3 presents an analysis of "recent developments in the ethical and policy debates," and Chapter 4 offers an account of "recent developments in stem cell research and therapy."

Ross, Steven L.: "Abortion and the Death of the Fetus," *Philosophy and Public Affairs* 11 (Summer 1982), pp. 232–245. Ross draws a distinction between abortion as the termination of pregnancy and abortion as the termination of the life of the fetus. He proceeds to defend abortion in the latter sense, insisting that it is justifiable for a woman to desire not only the termination of pregnancy but also the death of the fetus.

Ruse, Michael, and Christopher A. Pynes: *The Stem Cell Controversy: Debating the Issues* (Amherst, NY: Prometheus, 2003). This anthology offers sections on (1) the science of stem cells, (2) medical cures and promises, (3) moral issues, (4) religious issues, and (5) policy issues.

Sherwin, Susan: *No Longer Patient: Feminist Ethics and Health Care* (Philadelphia: Temple University Press, 1992). In Chapter 5 of this book (pp. 99–116), Sherwin presents an analysis of abortion that reflects her commitment to feminist ethics.

Steinbock, Bonnie: *Life Before Birth: The Moral and Legal Status of Embryos and Fetuses* (New York: Oxford University Press, 1992). Steinbock argues in Chapter 1 for "the interest view" of moral status—that is, the claim that "all and only beings who have interests have moral status." In Chapter 2, she provides an analysis of abortion.

Stone, Jim: "Why Potentiality Matters," *Canadian Journal of Philosophy* 17 (December 1987), pp. 815–830. Stone argues that a fetal right to life can be effectively grounded in the fact that a fetus is *potentially* an adult human being.

Strong, Carson: *Ethics in Reproductive and Perinatal Medicine: A New Framework* (New Haven, CT: Yale University Press, 1997). In Chapter 3, Strong argues for the view that the moral standing of the fetus progressively increases in strength as fetal development proceeds.

Tong, Rosemarie: *Feminist Approaches to Bioethics: Theoretical Reflections and Practical Applications* (Boulder, CO: Westview Press, 1997). In Chapter 6, Tong contrasts feminist and nonfeminist perspectives on abortion. She also distinguishes among various feminist approaches.

Tooley, Michael: *Abortion and Infanticide* (New York: Oxford University Press, 1983). In this long book, Tooley defends the liberal view on the morality of abortion. He insists that the question of the morality of abortion cannot be satisfactorily resolved "in isolation from the questions of the morality of infanticide and of the killing of nonhuman animals."

CHAPTER 8

GENETICS
AND HUMAN
REPRODUCTION

INTRODUCTION

With the rapid advance of knowledge and techniques in human genetics and the biology of human reproduction, a number of complex and troubling ethical issues have arisen. This chapter is designed to address some of the most important of these issues.

GENETIC DISEASE AND THE LANGUAGE OF GENETICS

Tay-Sachs disease is one prominent example of a genetic disease.[1] This disease, which most commonly affects Jewish children of Eastern European heritage, is characterized by progressive neurological degeneration and death in early childhood. Although a child afflicted with Tay-Sachs disease has the disease by virtue of his or her genetic inheritance, the child's parents do not have the disease. (Those afflicted with Tay-Sachs disease do not survive to reproduce.) The parents are *carriers*. Tay-Sachs carriers are those persons who have one normal gene and one variant, or defective, gene (the Tay-Sachs gene) at the same location on paired chromosomes. The Tay-Sachs gene is *recessive*. When it is paired with a normal gene, as is the case with the carrier, the normal gene is dominant. As a result, the carrier does not manifest the disease. However, if a child inherits the Tay-Sachs gene from both parents, then the child will be afflicted with Tay-Sachs disease.

Since Tay-Sachs disease is traceable to a recessive gene, it is said to be a recessive disease. Moreover, it is said to be an autosomal recessive disease; the word *autosomal* simply indicates that the defective genes are located on a pair of chromosomes other than the sex chromosomes. Furthermore, in the language of genetics, Tay-Sachs carriers are said to be in the *heterozygous* state, whereas a child afflicted with Tay-Sachs disease is said to be in the *homozygous* state, with regard to the Tay-Sachs gene. Carriers, having the Tay-Sachs gene paired with a different (normal) gene, are heterozygous with regard to the Tay-Sachs gene. The afflicted child, having two copies of the Tay-Sachs gene, is homozygous. The carrier is sometimes termed a "heterozygote"; the afflicted child, a "homozygote."

According to the (Mendelian) laws of heredity, when two carriers of a gene associated with an autosomal recessive disease produce offspring, there is one chance in four (25 percent) that their child will be afflicted with the genetic disease in question. There are two chances in four (50 percent) that their child will be, like them, a carrier. Finally, there is one chance in four (25 percent) that their child will be free both of the disease and of the carrier status.

Sickle-cell anemia is, like Tay-Sachs disease, a well-known autosomal recessive disease. Most commonly affecting people of African descent, sickle-cell anemia is characterized by acute episodes of pain (e.g., in the abdomen, chest, or joints) and exhibits a range of severity. There have been some notable treatment advances, but, at present, the average life expectancy for victims of sickle-cell anemia is less than 50. An estimated 10 percent of African Americans carry the sickle-cell gene.[2] As is characteristic of autosomal recessive diseases, if two carriers of the sickle-cell gene produce offspring, there is one chance in four (25 percent) that their child will be afflicted with sickle-cell anemia.

Cystic fibrosis provides one further example of an autosomal recessive disease. In the United States, since about 1 in 30 Caucasians carries the cystic fibrosis gene, about 1 in 900 Caucasian couples will be a carrier-carrier pairing and thus be at risk (one chance in four) of producing offspring with the disease. At present, although hopes are high for therapeutic advances, the median age of death for victims of cystic fibrosis is not much over 30. The disease is primarily characterized by a dysfunction of the exocrine glands. This dysfunction results in abnormal amounts of mucus, which can obstruct organ passages and produce intense pulmonary and digestive distress.

Huntington's disease provides a leading example of a genetic disease in the category of autosomal *dominant* diseases. Typically, the symptoms of Huntington's disease emerge only in the prime of life, between the ages of 35 and 50. It is characterized by mental and physical deterioration, leading to death within several years. The defective gene responsible for Huntington's disease is a dominant one. If a person has the defective gene, that person will eventually fall victim to the disease. Moreover, for any offspring of a person carrying the defective gene, there is one chance in two (50 percent) that the gene will be inherited.

In contrast to autosomal genetic diseases, some genetic diseases are linked to mutant genes located on the sex chromosomes. Prominent among the genetic diseases in this latter category are the so-called *X-linked diseases.* Hemophilia, a well-known disease characterized by uncontrollable bleeding, is a leading example of an X-linked disease. Of the 46 chromosomes that constitute the normal complement of genetic material in human beings, there are two sex chromosomes. A female has two X chromosomes, and a male has one X and one Y chromosome. In human reproduction, if the sperm fertilizing the egg provides an X chromosome, the child will be female. If the sperm fertilizing the egg provides a Y chromosome, the child will be male. (The egg always provides an X chromosome.) Hemophilia is a *recessive* X-linked disease. A female, therefore, will have the disease of hemophilia only if she has the mutant gene on both of her X chromosomes. If a female has one normal gene and one mutant gene, however, she will be a carrier. Since a male has only one X chromosome, if he has the mutant gene associated with hemophilia, he will have the disease. On the assumption that a female carrier mates with a male who is free of the disease, there is no risk that their female children will have the disease. Female children will inherit a normal gene from their father and thus themselves be free of the disease, although there is one chance in two (50 percent) that they will inherit their mother's mutant gene and be, like her, a carrier. In contrast, there is one chance in two (50 percent) that male children (of a female carrier and a disease-free male) will have the disease of hemophilia.

PRENATAL DIAGNOSIS AND SELECTIVE ABORTION

A number of techniques are presently employed for the detection of chromosomal abnormalities, many genetic diseases, and certain serious anatomical abnormalities in the fetus in utero. Among these techniques, amniocentesis and chorionic villi sampling (CVS) are the most prominent, although ultrasound is also of great importance. Ultrasound is a non-invasive technique that produces a visual representation of the developing fetus, thereby allowing the detection of many anatomical abnormalities.

In amniocentesis, a needle is inserted through a pregnant woman's abdomen, and a sample of the amniotic fluid surrounding the fetus is withdrawn. Diagnostic testing of fetal cells in the amniotic fluid makes it possible to detect the presence of various genetic diseases in the fetus. Also detectable, via chromosomal analysis, are conditions associated with an abnormal number of chromosomes or an abnormal arrangement of chromosomes. Down syndrome, for example, is associated with the presence of an extra chromosome, namely, three instead of two number 21 chromosomes. Amniocentesis can also be employed for the detection of neural-tube defects (anencephaly and spina bifida). In this case, a positive diagnosis rests on the presence of increased levels of alphafetoprotein in the amniotic fluid.

Amniocentesis, first introduced in the late 1960s, has achieved wide acceptance among physicians as a relatively low-risk medical procedure. However, it is not ordinarily performed before the 15th or 16th week of gestation, and selective abortion must await the results of diagnostic testing, which may not be available until the 20th week or so. Since second-trimester abortions are more problematic (medically, psychologically, socially, and perhaps morally) than first-trimester abortions, a procedure capable of combining the prenatal diagnostic value of amniocentesis with the possibility of first-trimester abortion is much to be preferred, assuming, of course, that risk factors are within acceptable limits. Chorionic villi sampling (CVS), a procedure developed in Europe and first introduced in the United States in 1983, is now established as an alternative to amniocentesis in the detection of genetic diseases and chromosomal abnormalities. In CVS, a procedure that can be performed in the first trimester, usually around the 10th week, a small amount of tissue is extracted from the placenta, and the results of diagnostic testing on this tissue are typically available about seven days later. However, the risk of miscarriage is apparently somewhat greater for CVS than for amniocentesis.

Since prenatal diagnosis is ordinarily undertaken with an eye toward selective abortion, the practice of prenatal diagnosis clearly confronts us with one particular aspect of the more general problem of abortion, as discussed in Chapter 7. (There is also a close link with the problem of the treatment of impaired newborns, as discussed in Chapter 5.) Is the practice of selective abortion, on grounds of genetic defect, ethically acceptable? Leon R. Kass, in one of this chapter's selections, abstracts from the problem of abortion in general and argues specifically against the practice of selective (genetic) abortion. Kass's arguments resonate strongly with a viewpoint usually identified today as the *disability rights critique* of prenatal diagnosis and selective abortion.[3] Advocates of the disability rights critique claim, among other things, that the selection against disability embodied in selective abortion is a form of discrimination. Whether the disability rights critique of prenatal diagnosis and selective abortion can ultimately be sustained is a matter that continues to provoke intense debate.

MORALITY AND REPRODUCTIVE RISK

One important ethical issue associated with human genetics has to do with the morality of reproduction under circumstances of genetic risk. Laura M. Purdy argues, in this chapter, that it is morally wrong to reproduce when there is a high risk of serious genetic disease. In particular, she considers the case of Huntington's disease. If it is justifiable to maintain that there is a moral obligation of the sort that Purdy outlines, we may find ourselves once more faced with the problem of prenatal diagnosis and selective abortion. Clearly, in cases where prenatal diagnosis is available (e.g., Huntington's disease, Tay-Sachs disease, sickle-cell anemia, cystic fibrosis), selective abortion offers a means of sidestepping the risk of serious genetic disease.

Closely associated with the issue of the morality of reproduction under circumstances of genetic risk is another ethical issue, the justifiability of the use of coercive measures to achieve social control over individual reproductive decisions. It is one thing to say that certain reproductive choices are immoral and quite another to say that coercive measures for the control of reproductive choices are justified. Such coercive controls as compulsory sterilization and mandatory amniocentesis followed by forced abortion are widely rejected as invasive of fundamental rights. Mandatory screening programs for the identification of carriers, while surely less invasive than other coercive measures, are also viewed with suspicion by most commentators.

REPRODUCTIVE TECHNOLOGIES AND THE TREATMENT OF INFERTILITY

Human reproduction, as it naturally occurs, is characterized by sexual intercourse, tubal fertilization, implantation in the uterus, and subsequent in utero gestation. The expression *reproductive technologies* can be understood as applicable to an array of technical procedures that would replace the various steps in the natural process of reproduction, to a lesser or greater extent.[4]

Artificial insemination (also called assisted insemination) is a procedure that replaces sexual intercourse as a means of achieving tubal fertilization. Artificial insemination has long been available, primarily as a means of overcoming infertility on the part of a male, usually a husband. It is sometimes possible for a husband's infertility to be overcome by artificial insemination with the sperm of the *husband* (AIH). More often, at least in the past, a couple has found it necessary to turn to artificial insemination with the sperm of a *donor* (AID).[5] AID can also be employed when it has been established that the husband carries a mutant gene that would place a couple's offspring at genetic risk. Moreover, it has been suggested, most prominently in the work of the well-known geneticist Hermann J. Muller, that AID be voluntarily employed as a way of achieving the aims of positive eugenics.[6] Muller recommended the formation of sperm banks that would collect and store the sperm of men judged to be "outstanding" in various ways. His idea was that any "enlightened" couple desiring a child would have recourse to one of these banks in order to arrange for the wife's artificial insemination. Another controversial use of AID is its use by unmarried women. Probably even more controversial is the use of artificial insemination within the context of a surrogacy arrangement. In the most typical case, a wife's infertility motivates a couple to seek out a so-called surrogate mother. The surrogate agrees to be artificially inseminated with the husband's sperm, in order to bear a child for the couple.

In vitro fertilization (IVF) literally means "fertilization in glass." The sperm of a husband (or a donor) is united, in a laboratory, with the ovum of a wife (or a donor). Whereas artificial insemination is a technically simple procedure, in vitro fertilization followed by embryo transfer (to the uterus for implantation) is a system of reproductive technology that features a high degree of technical sophistication. The first documented "test-tube baby," Louise Brown, was born in England in July 1978. Her birth was the culmination of years of collaboration between a gynecologist, Patrick Steptoe, and an embryologist, Robert Edwards. This pioneering team developed methods of obtaining mature eggs from a woman's ovaries (via a minor surgical procedure called a laparoscopy), effectively fertilizing eggs in the laboratory, cultivating them to the eight-cell stage, and then transferring a developing embryo to the uterus for implantation.

Reproductive centers throughout the United States now provide in vitro procedures for the treatment of infertility, although success rates continue to be somewhat disappointing. Since it is now possible, with the use of fertility drugs, to harvest a crop of mature eggs (perhaps ten or so) from a woman's ovaries, embryos are sometimes frozen (e.g., at the eight-cell stage) and then selectively thawed at appropriate times over a period of several months in an effort to achieve a successful implantation. Of course, the freezing of embryos may lead to other problems—for example, how to deal with frozen embryos no longer needed. However, the freezing of unfertilized eggs, which at face value may seem preferable to the freezing of embryos, has proven to be technically more difficult.

In vitro fertilization followed by embryo transfer is a system of reproductive technology that replaces not only sexual intercourse but also tubal fertilization in the natural process of reproduction. But consider also the future possibility of dispensing with implantation and in utero gestation as well. There seems to be no theoretical obstacle to totally artificial gestation, which would take place within the confines of an artificial womb. If *ectogenesis,* the process of artificial gestation, becomes a reality, then the combination of in vitro fertilization and ectogenesis would constitute a system of reproductive technology in which each element in the natural process of reproduction has been effectively replaced. At the present time, however, in vitro fertilization (accompanied by embryo transfer) is seen primarily as a means of overcoming certain forms of infertility—for example, infertility due to obstruction of the fallopian tubes.

One notable spinoff of IVF technology is a procedure called gamete intrafallopian transfer (GIFT). In this procedure, eggs are obtained as they would be for IVF, but instead of fertilization in vitro, the eggs are placed together with sperm in the fallopian tube (or tubes), where it is hoped that fertilization will take place in vivo (i.e., in the living situation). A closely related procedure is called zygote intrafallopian transfer (ZIFT). In ZIFT, a single-cell zygote, which is the product of in vitro fertilization, is transferred to the fallopian tube.

Intracytoplasmic sperm injection (ICSI), another spinoff of IVF technology, is a technique that was first developed in 1992. Now widely used in clinical practice, it was originally introduced to address problems of male infertility. In ICSI, a single sperm is injected into an egg to achieve fertilization in a laboratory dish. Even a man with a very low sperm count can become a biological father by the use of this technique, thereby allowing a couple to avoid the problems associated with the use of donor sperm in order to combat male infertility. At present, however, there are unresolved safety concerns about the use of ICSI, as there are about the use of IVF itself. These and related safety concerns are addressed in some detail by the President's Council on Bioethics in a selection reprinted in this chapter. In this selection, the council also presents a very useful account of state-of-the-art practice with regard to IVF and closely related procedures.

In contrast to a woman whose infertility can be traced to fallopian tube obstruction, consider a woman whose ovaries are either absent or nonfunctional. Since she has no ova, she cannot produce genetic offspring. If her uterus is functional, however, there is no biological obstacle to her bearing a child. Let us suppose that she wants to bear a child that is her husband's genetic offspring. Her problem can be addressed by some form of *egg donation*.[7] The most obvious possibility in this regard is in vitro fertilization of a donor egg with the husband's sperm, followed by embryo transfer to the wife.

In the case just discussed, a woman has a functional uterus but nonfunctional ovaries. Consider now the converse case—a woman has functional ovaries but a nonfunctional uterus. Perhaps she has had a hysterectomy. She is capable of becoming the *genetic* but not the *gestational* mother of a child. Now, suppose that she and her husband desire a child "of their own." This situation gives rise to the possibility of a surrogacy arrangement somewhat different from the kind predicated upon artificial insemination. In this case, in vitro fertilization could be employed to fertilize the wife's egg with the husband's sperm. The embryo could then be transferred to the uterus of a surrogate, who would agree to bear the child for the couple. The surrogate would then be the gestational but not the genetic mother of the child.

REPRODUCTIVE TECHNOLOGIES: ETHICAL CONCERNS

To what extent, if at all, is it ethically acceptable to employ the various reproductive technologies just described? Numerous ethical concerns have been expressed about these technologies, and a brief survey of the most prominent of these concerns should prove helpful.

Much of the ethical opposition to artificial insemination derives from religious views. AID especially has been attacked on the grounds that it illicitly separates procreation from the marriage relationship. Inasmuch as AID introduces a third party (the sperm donor) into a marriage relationship, it has been called a form of adultery. Even AIH, which cannot be accused of separating procreation from the marriage relationship, has not uniformly escaped attack. Some religious ethicists have gone so far as to contend that procreation is morally illicit whenever it is not the product of personal lovemaking. Although these sorts of objections frequently recur in discussions of egg donation, in vitro fertilization, and other reproductive technologies, they seem to have little force for those who do not share the basic worldview from which they proceed.

Some of the ethical opposition to in vitro fertilization (and related technologies) is based on the perceived "unnaturalness" of the procedure. Closely related is the charge that the procedure depersonalizes or dehumanizes procreation. Further, in this same vein, complaints are made against the "manufacture" and "commodification" of children. Another recurrent argument against in vitro fertilization is that its acceptance by society will lead to the acceptance of more and more objectionable developments in reproductive technology (e.g., ectogenesis).

In addition to arguments advanced in support of a wholesale rejection of in vitro fertilization, a number of concerns having a more limited scope can be identified. Some commentators have been quite willing to endorse the use of in vitro fertilization and embryo transfer within the framework of a marital relationship but object to any third-party involvement—that is, sperm or egg donation, embryo donation, and surrogate motherhood. Other critics object primarily to a frequent concomitant of in vitro procedures—the discarding of embryos considered unneeded or unsuitable for implantation. Those who consider even an early embryo a person (in the sense of having full moral status) are especially vocal on this score, and they also register a vigorous complaint against the use of surplus embryos for research purposes (see the stem cell discussion in Chapter 7), although they often endorse the idea of donating surplus embryos to another couple for attempted implantation. Of course, those who embrace a very different view of the moral status of the early embryo will typically argue that there is no ethical problem with either discarding surplus embryos or using them for research purposes.

Two readings in this chapter focus directly on the ethics of IVF.[8] Peter Singer provides a defense of IVF by countering many of the standard arguments against it. Susan Sherwin, in a very different spirit, works out a critique of IVF based on her commitment to feminist ethics. From a feminist point of view, she maintains, IVF is morally problematic for a number of closely related reasons. Although there is a diversity of views in the feminist community about the ethics of IVF, many feminists believe that the availability of IVF and other reproductive technologies is at best a mixed blessing for women.

In one of this chapter's readings, The New York State Task Force on Life and the Law presents an overall survey of ethical perspectives on reproductive technology. In another reading, Thomas H. Murray argues that the alternative reproductive practices made possible by contemporary technologies will not pass moral inspection if they fail to cohere with values at the core of family life. He is opposed in particular to the intrusion of marketplace values into the realm of family life. Thus, he is opposed to the *commercialization* of third-party involvement in reproduction, although he is not opposed to noncommercial third-party involvement. In Murray's view, payment for gamete donation (whether sperm or egg) is morally unsound, as is payment for the services of a surrogate mother.

Much of the ethical opposition to surrogate motherhood can be traced to (1) concerns about psychosocial problems likely to arise for the child who is born as a result of a surrogacy arrangement and (2) concerns that the practice will have a negative impact on family structure. However, as Murray's analysis makes clear, additional concerns can be raised about the practice of *commercial* surrogacy.

At present, the legal status of commercial surrogacy contracts varies from state to state, and legislatures have taken various approaches in attempting to deal with the social policy aspects of surrogacy. One option is for a state simply to recognize commercial surrogacy contracts as valid and legally enforceable. Another option is for the state to prohibit commercial surrogacy contracts altogether. Bonnie Steinbock argues, in this chapter, against the legal prohibition of surrogacy contracts, although she insists on the importance of state regulation. In her view, commercial surrogacy contracts should be permitted only if provision is made for a "waiting period" subsequent to birth. During this period, the surrogate would have the opportunity to change her mind about surrendering her parental rights.

In the celebrated Baby M case (see Appendix, Case 38), the "surrogate" was both the genetic and gestational mother of a child. Other cases involve purely gestational surrogates—that is, women who have agreed to carry a child for a couple, each of whom is a genetic parent. Here the surrogate is the gestational but not the genetic mother of a child. If this type of surrogacy agreement breaks down, the following issue arises: Should we identify the genetic mother or the gestational mother as the child's legal mother?

HUMAN CLONING

With the announcement in February 1997 of the successful cloning of a sheep in Scotland, much attention has been focused on the prospect of human cloning.[9] Accordingly, the following sequence of events can be imagined. A mature human egg will be obtained from a woman and enucleated in a laboratory—that is, the nucleus of the egg cell will be removed. Meanwhile, a somatic cell from an adult human being (who might be anyone, including the woman who has provided the egg) will be obtained and enucleated. The extracted nucleus, which contains the donor's heretofore unique genotype (assuming the donor is not an identical twin), will then be inserted into the egg cell, and the renucleated egg will be activated, so that it will develop in the way that a newly fertilized egg ordinarily develops.[10] Embryo transfer (not necessarily into the uterus of the woman from whom the original egg was obtained) and subsequent in utero gestation will then lead to the birth of a human "clone." In contrast to offspring resulting from sexual reproduction, where the resultant genotype is the result of contributions by two parents, the clone will have the same genotype as his or her "parent."[11]

The type of cloning just described, somatic cell nuclear transfer (SCNT), is the focal point of concern in contemporary debates about the ethics of human cloning. Another important process, less dramatic than SCNT, is also considered by many commentators to be a type of cloning. This process involves the splitting of a very early embryo (e.g., at the eight-cell stage) and thus the formation of duplicate embryos. The embryo-splitting type of cloning is not technically difficult, and because it does not necessarily result in a "time lag" between identical twins in the way that SCNT does, many commentators consider it less problematic than SCNT. It may be important to realize, however, that embryo splitting followed by implantation of some embryos and freezing of others for later implantation would, in fact, lead to identical twins of different ages.

Many of the ethical concerns that can be raised about human cloning are continuous with concerns that have been raised about other reproductive technologies, but the prospect of human cloning also seems to confront us with some distinctive ethical concerns. In one of this chapter's selections, Leon R. Kass constructs four lines of argument against human cloning and maintains that it is deeply unethical. Also in this chapter, Thomas H. Murray expresses some serious reservations about human cloning. Robert Wachbroit presents a very different point of view on the ethics of human cloning. His arguments are calculated to defend human cloning in response to the various concerns raised by its critics.

Two presidential commissions have explicitly confronted the possibility of human (SCNT) cloning. In 1997, the National Bioethics Advisory Commission submitted its report *Cloning Human Beings*. In concluding that it is morally unacceptable "at this time" for anyone to attempt to create a child by cloning, the commission placed special emphasis on safety concerns. The commission's central recommendation was that federal legislation be enacted to prohibit anyone from attempting to create a child via cloning, although it also recommended incorporation of a sunset clause calculated to ensure that Congress would reconsider after three to five years whether a ban was still needed. No legislative action was forthcoming in response to commission recommendations. In 2002, the President's Council on Bioethics submitted its report *Human Cloning and Human Dignity: An Ethical Inquiry*.[12] The council considered both cloning-to-produce-children (reproductive cloning) and cloning-for-biomedical-research (research cloning). (The distinction between reproductive and research cloning is articulated in the Introduction to Chapter 7, in conjunction with the discussion of embryonic stem cells.) Members of the council unanimously agreed that reproductive cloning is morally unacceptable and unanimously recommended that Congress ban all attempts at reproductive cloning. The council also recommended a four-year national moratorium (that is, a temporary ban) on research cloning, although in this case only 10 of the 17 voting members of the council favored the moratorium. At the date of this writing (Fall 2009), political wrangling over the stem-cell issue has stymied any leg-islative action by Congress.

PREIMPLANTATION GENETIC DIAGNOSIS

Preimplantation genetic diagnosis (PGD) is a procedure that has emerged against the back-ground of IVF technology. In PGD, embryos produced by IVF can be analyzed for chro-mosomal abnormalities and selected genetic diseases *before* implantation is attempted. The most common form of PGD involves extracting one or two cells from the preimplantation embryo, often around the eight-cell stage. Testing of these extracted cells allows affected embryos to be identified and discarded. Embryos that are unaffected are available for im-plantation. Couples at risk for the transmission of genetic disease sometimes choose IVF and PGD in order to avoid the problem of selective abortion that is associated with prena-tal diagnosis during pregnancy. Some of the issues raised by the use of PGD to screen out embryos with chromosomal abnormality or genetic disease are continuous with issues raised by the practice of prenatal diagnosis and selective abortion. In particular, both prac-tices feature a selection process against disability that advocates of the disability rights cri-tique allege to be discriminatory. Of course, many commentators reject this claim of discrimination and argue for the ethical acceptability of both practices. Is PGD ethically preferable to prenatal diagnosis and selective abortion? The answer to this question surely depends in part on the issue of the moral status of the preimplantation embryo vis-à-vis the moral status of the developing fetus.

Although the standard medical use of PGD is to select against embryos with chromo-somal or genetic disorders, other possible uses can be identified. In one of this chapter's readings, John A. Robertson surveys these various uses, both medical and nonmedical. Nonmedical uses of PGD are especially controversial. These uses include selecting em-bryos on the basis of gender (sex) and selecting embryos for desired traits (e.g., perfect pitch). In a closely related reading in this chapter, the President's Council on Bioethics con-siders whether it is likely that significant demand will emerge for PGD in order to select embryos for desired traits. In the course of its analysis, the council effectively clarifies a number of practical problems confronting this possible extension of PGD use.

GENETIC ENGINEERING, GENE THERAPY, AND ENHANCEMENT

Two important distinctions are involved in discussions of the ethics of genetic engineering (intervention, manipulation). *Therapeutic* genetic engineering, commonly called "gene ther-apy," involves interventions directed at the cure of disease. *Nontherapeutic* genetic engi-neering, often called "enhancement engineering," involves interventions directed at the enhancement of human traits (e.g., height) and capabilities (e.g., memory). *Somatic-cell* ge-netic interventions involve introducing modifications into nonreproductive cells (e.g., blood cells), so that the resultant changes are not passed on to future generations. *Germ-line* ge-netic interventions involve introducing modifications into sperm, ova, or preimplantion em-bryos, so that the resultant changes are passed on to future generations. By reference to these two distinctions, four categories of genetic engineering can be distinguished: (1) somatic-cell gene therapy, (2) germ-line gene therapy, (3) somatic-cell enhancement (nontherapeu-tic) engineering, and (4) germ-line enhancement (nontherapeutic) engineering.

It may be possible in the foreseeable future to cure a wide range of genetic diseases (e.g., cystic fibrosis and hemophilia) by the genetic manipulation of somatic cells. It is also hoped that somatic-cell gene therapy will eventually provide effective treatment for such diseases as cancer and cardiovascular disease. Despite the complaint that any use of genetic engineering places human beings in the role of "playing God," the continued development and use of somatic-cell gene therapy is widely endorsed and relatively uncontroversial—that is, in theory. In practice, progress in the development of somatic-cell gene therapy has been mostly disappointing, and numerous ethical and policy issues are associated with the conduct of clinical trials. Some of these issues are highlighted in this chapter by Sophia Kolehmainen, in conjunction with her discussion of the tragic case of Jesse Gelsinger, an eighteen-year-old male who died in 1999 as a result of his participation in a gene therapy clinical trial. Gelsinger's case anticipated some similar cases from 2000, in which patients suffering from severe combined immunodeficiencies (SCIDs) were successfully treated with gene therapy. These cases were widely celebrated as the first real successes of the therapy, but they were followed by the unfortunate realization in 2002 that two of ten patients who had been successfully treated had developed leukemia as a side-effect of the treatment.[13]

There is extensive debate about the ethical acceptability of both germ-line gene therapy and enhancement engineering in any form. In one of this chapter's selections, LeRoy Walters and Julie Gage Palmer review the arguments commonly made for and against the use of germ-line gene therapy. Their analysis culminates in an endorsement of germ-line gene therapy, at least in principle. In another selection, Michael J. Sandel argues that genetic enhancement technologies threaten to reduce our appreciation for the arbitrary, "unbidden" character of natural gifts and to damage the sense of social solidarity between the fortunate and the less fortunate. A more positive view of the ethics of enhancement engineering is offered by Dan W. Brock in the final selection of this chapter.

NOTES

1 Discussion of genetic disease in this section is limited to *Mendelian* diseases—that is, those produced by a single-gene defect. Polygenetic (or multigenetic) diseases are produced by the interaction of several genes, and many common diseases (e.g., cancer and cardiovascular disease) are the product of genetic predisposition (involving multiple genes) in combination with environmental factors.

2 A single copy of the sickle-cell gene is believed to make the carrier more resistant to malaria, an advantage especially in tropical climates.

3 For one helpful articulation of the disability rights critique of prenatal diagnosis and selective abortion, see Erik Parens and Adrienne Asch, "The Disability Rights Critique of Prenatal Genetic Testing: Reflections and Recommendations," in Erik Parens and Adrienne Asch, eds., *Prenatal Testing and Disability Rights* (Washington, DC: Georgetown University Press, 2000), pp. 3–43.

4 A broader conception of *reproductive technologies* would encompass other forms of technical assistance calculated to aid the process of reproduction—for example, the use of "fertility drugs" to stimulate ovulation.

5 More recently, the problem of male infertility has been effectively addressed by ICSI, a procedure discussed in a subsequent paragraph.

6 See, for example, Hermann J. Muller, "Means and Aims in Human Genetic Betterment," in T. M., Sonneborn, ed., *The Control of Human Heredity and Evolution* (New York: Macmillan, 1965), pp. 100–122. Roughly, positive eugenics aims at enhancing the genetic heritage of the species, whereas negative eugenics aims at preventing deterioration of the gene pool. However, use of the word *eugenics* is frequently attended with much confusion. So-called eugenics programs have usually featured elements of government coercion, but eugenics need not be understood as entailing coercion.

7 Egg donation might also be considered when a woman's own ova would place her offspring at risk for genetic disease.

8 In another reading already mentioned, "Assisted Reproduction," the President's Council on Bioethics contributes—at least indirectly—to an overall understanding of the ethics of IVF.

9 In this section, "human cloning" refers to *reproductive* cloning, not *research* cloning. (See the Introduction to Chapter 7.)

10 In the case of Dolly, the first cloned sheep, an entire somatic cell was fused with an enucleated egg by means of an electric current.

11 Strictly speaking, the clone's genotype will be almost identical to the genotype of the "parent." Mitochondrial DNA in the enucleated egg cell will also make a small contribution to the clone's genotype.

12 This valuable document is available on the council's website (http://www.bioethics.gov).

13 See Marina Cavazzana-Calvo et al., "The Future of Gene Therapy: Balancing the Risks and the Benefits of Clinical Trials," *Nature* 427 (February 2004), pp. 779–81.

REPRODUCTIVE RISK, PRENATAL DIAGNOSIS, AND SELECTIVE ABORTION

IMPLICATIONS OF PRENATAL DIAGNOSIS FOR THE HUMAN RIGHT TO LIFE
Leon R. Kass

Setting aside a discussion of the moral problem of abortion in general, Kass focuses on some of the ethical difficulties associated with the abortion of fetuses known by amniocentesis to be genetically defective. He maintains that the practice of *genetic* abortion, inasmuch as it involves a qualitative assessment of fetuses, represents a threat to the "radical moral equality of all human beings." As a result of the practice of genetic abortion, Kass suggests, we will be inclined to take a more negative view of those who are genetically defective or otherwise "abnormal." Thus, we will be inclined to treat them in a second-class manner. Moreover, he contends, to commit ourselves to the practice of genetic abortion is to reflect acceptance of a very dangerous principle, that "defectives should not be born."

It is especially fitting on this occasion to begin by acknowledging how privileged I feel and how pleased I am to be a participant in this symposium. I suspect that I am not alone among the assembled in considering myself fortunate to be here. For I was conceived after antibiotics yet before amniocentesis, late enough to have benefited from medicine's ability to prevent and control fatal infectious diseases, yet early enough to have escaped from medicine's ability to prevent me from living to suffer from my genetic diseases. To be sure, my genetic vices are, as far as I know them, rather modest, taken individually—myopia, asthma and other allergies, bilateral forefoot adduction, bowleggedness, loquaciousness, and pessimism,

From *Ethical Issues in Human Genetics,* edited by Bruce Hilton et al. (Kluwer Academic/Plenum Publishers, 1973). Reprinted with kind permission from Springer Science and Business Media.

plus some four to eight as yet undiagnosed recessive lethal genes in the heterozygous condition—but, taken together, and if diagnosable prenatally, I might never have made it.

Just as I am happy to be here, so am I unhappy with what I shall have to say. Little did I realize when I first conceived the topic, "Implications of Prenatal Diagnosis for the Human Right to Life," what a painful and difficult labor it would lead to. More than once while this paper was gestating, I considered obtaining permission to abort it, on the grounds that, by prenatal diagnosis, I knew it to be defective. My lawyer told me that I was legally in the clear, but my conscience reminded me that I had made a commitment to deliver myself of this paper, flawed or not. Next time, I shall practice better contraception.

Any discussion of the ethical issues of genetic counseling and prenatal diagnosis is unavoidably haunted by a ghost called the morality of abortion. This ghost I shall not vex. More precisely, I shall not vex the reader by telling ghost stories. However, I would be neither surprised nor disappointed if my discussion of an admittedly related matter, the ethics of aborting the genetically defective, summons that hovering spirit to the reader's mind. For the morality of abortion is a matter not easily laid to rest, recent efforts to do so notwithstanding. A vote by the legislature of the State of New York can indeed legitimatize the disposal of fetuses, but not of the moral questions. But though the questions remain, there is likely to be little new that can be said about them, and certainly not by me.

Yet before leaving the general question of abortion, let me pause to drop some anchors for the discussion that follows. Despite great differences of opinion both as to what to think and how to reason about abortion, nearly everyone agrees that abortion is a moral issue.[1] What does this mean? Formally, it means that a woman seeking or refusing an abortion can expect to be asked to justify her action. And we can expect that she should be able to give reasons for her choice other than "I like it" or "I don't like it." Substantively, it means that, in the absence of good reasons for intervention, there is some presumption in favor of allowing the pregnancy to continue once it has begun. A common way of expressing this presumption is to say that "the fetus has a right to continued life."[2] In this context, disagreement concerning the moral permissibility of abortion concerns what rights (or interests or needs), and whose, override (take precedence over, or outweigh) this fetal "right." Even most of the "opponents" of abortion agree that the mother's right to live takes precedence, and that abortion to save her life is permissible, perhaps obligatory. Some believe that a woman's right to determine the number and spacing of her children takes precedence, while yet others argue that the need to curb population growth is, at least at this time, overriding.

Hopefully, this brief analysis of what it means to say that abortion is a moral issue is sufficient to establish two points. First, that the fetus is a living thing with some moral claim on us not to do it violence, and therefore, second, that justification must be given for destroying it.

Turning now from the general questions of the ethics of abortion, I wish to focus on the special ethical issues raised by the abortion of "defective" fetuses (so-called "abortion for fetal indications"). I shall consider only the cleanest cases, those cases where well-characterized genetic diseases are diagnosed with a high degree of certainty by means of amniocentesis, in order to side-step the added moral dilemmas posed when the diagnosis is suspected or possible, but unconfirmed. However, many of the questions I shall discuss could also be raised about cases where genetic analysis gives only a statistical prediction about the genotype of the fetus, and also about cases where the defect has an infectious or chemical rather than a genetic cause (e.g., rubella, thalidomide).

My first and possibly most difficult task is to show that there is anything left to discuss once we have agreed not to discuss the morality of abortion in general. There is a sense in which abortion for genetic defect is, after abortion to save the life of the mother, perhaps the most defensible kind of abortion. Certainly, it is a serious and not a frivolous reason for abortion, defended by its proponents in sober and rational speech—unlike justifications based upon the false notion that a fetus is a mere part of a woman's body, to be used and abused at her pleasure. Standing behind genetic abortion are serious and well-intentioned people, with reasonable ends in view: the prevention of genetic diseases, the elimination of suffering in families, the preservation of precious financial and medical resources, the protection of our genetic heritage. No profiteers, no sexploiters, no racists. No arguments about the connection of abortion with promiscuity and licentiousness, no perjured testimony about the mental health of the mother, no arguments about the seriousness of the population problem. In short, clear objective data, a worthy cause, decent men and women. If abortion, what better reason for it?

Yet if genetic abortion is but a happily wagging tail on the dog of abortion, it is simultaneously the nose of a camel protruding under a rather different tent. Precisely because the quality of the fetus is central to the decision to abort, the practice of genetic abortion has implications which go beyond those raised by abortion in general. What may be at stake here is the belief in the radical moral equality of all human beings, the belief that all human beings possess equally and independent of merit certain fundamental rights, one among which is, of course, the right to life.

To be sure, the belief that fundamental human rights belong equally to all human beings has been but an ideal, never realized, often ignored, sometimes shamelessly. Yet it has been perhaps the most powerful moral idea at work in the world for at least two centuries. It is this idea and ideal that animates most of the current political and social criticism around the globe. It is ironic that we should acquire the power to detect and eliminate the genetically unequal at a time when we have finally succeeded in removing much of the stigma and disgrace previously attached to victims of congenital illness, in providing them with improved care and support, and in preventing, by means of education, feelings of guilt on the part of their parents. One might even wonder whether the development of amniocentesis and prenatal diagnosis may represent a backlash against these same humanitarian and egalitarian tendencies in the practice of medicine, which, by helping to sustain to the age of reproduction persons with genetic disease has itself contributed to the increasing incidence of genetic disease, and with it, to increased pressures for genetic screening, genetic counseling, and genetic abortion.

No doubt our humanitatian and egalitarian principles and practices have caused us some new difficulties, but if we mean to weaken or turn our backs on them, we should do so consciously and thoughtfully. If, as I believe, the idea and practice of genetic abortion points in that direction, we should make ourselves aware of it. . . .

GENETIC ABORTION AND THE LIVING DEFECTIVE

The practice of abortion of the genetically defective will no doubt affect our view of and our behavior toward those abnormals who escape the net of detection and abortion. A child with Down's syndrome or with hemophilia or with muscular dystrophy born at a time when most of his (potential) fellow sufferers were destroyed prenatally is liable to be looked upon by the community as one unfit to be alive, as a second-

class (or even lower) human type. He may be seen as a person who need not have been, and who would not have been, if only someone had gotten to him in time.

The parents of such children are also likely to treat them differently, especially if the mother would have wished but failed to get an amniocentesis because of ignorance, poverty, or distance from the testing station, or if the prenatal diagnosis was in error. In such cases, parents are especially likely to resent the child. They may be disinclined to give it the kind of care they might have before the advent of amniocentesis and genetic abortion, rationalizing that a second-class specimen is not entitled to first-class treatment. If pressed to do so, say by physicians, the parents might refuse, and the courts may become involved. This has already begun to happen.

In Maryland, parents of a child with Down syndrome refused permission to have the child operated on for an intestinal obstruction present at birth. The physicians and the hospital sought an injunction to require the parents to allow surgery. The judge ruled in favor of the parents, despite what I understand to be the weight of precedent to the contrary, on the grounds that the child was Mongoloid, that is, had the child been "normal," the decision would have gone the other way. Although the decision was not appealed to and hence not affirmed by a higher court, we can see through the prism of this case the possibility that the new powers of human genetics will strip the blindfold from the lady of justice and will make official the dangerous doctrine that some men are more equal than others.

The abnormal child may also feel resentful. A child with Down syndrome or Tay-Sachs disease will probably never know or care, but what about a child with hemophilia or with Turner's syndrome? In the past decade, with medical knowledge and power over the prenatal child increasing and with parental authority over the postnatal child decreasing, we have seen the appearance of a new type of legal action, suits for wrongful life. Children have brought suit against their parents (and others) seeking to recover damages for physical and social handicaps inextricably tied to their birth (e.g., congenital deformities, congenital syphilis, illegitimacy). In some of the American cases, the courts have recognized the justice of the child's claim (that he was injured due to parental negligence), although they have so far refused to award damages, due to policy considerations. In other countries, e.g., in Germany, judgments with compensation have gone for the plaintiffs. With the spread of amniocentesis and genetic abortion, we can only expect such cases to increase. And here it will be the soft-hearted rather than the hard-hearted judges who will establish the doctrine of second-class human beings, out of compassion for the mutants who escaped the traps set out for them.

It may be argued that I am dealing with a problem which, even if it is real, will affect very few people. It may be suggested that very few will escape the traps once we have set them properly and widely, once people are informed about amniocentesis, once the power to detect prenatally grows to its full capacity, and once our "superstitious" opposition to abortion dies out or is extirpated. But in order even to come close to this vision of success, amniocentesis will have to become part of every pregnancy—either by making it mandatory, like the test for syphilis, or by making it "routine medical practice," like the Pap smear. Leaving aside the other problems with universal amniocentesis, we could expect that the problem for the few who escape is likely to be even worse precisely because they will be few.

The point, however, should be generalized. How will we come to view and act toward the many "abnormals" that will remain among us—the retarded, the crippled, the senile, the deformed, and the true mutants—once we embark on a program to root out genetic abnormality? For it must be remembered that we shall always have abnormals—some who escape detection or whose disease is undetectable *in utero,* others as a result of new mutations, birth injuries, accidents, maltreatment, or disease—who will require our care and protection. The existence of "defectives" cannot be fully prevented, not even by totalitarian breeding and weeding programs. Is it not likely that our principle with respect to these people will change from "We try harder" to "Why accept second best?" The idea of "the unwanted because abnormal child" may become a self-fulfilling

prophecy, whose consequences may be worse than those of the abnormality itself.

GENETIC AND OTHER DEFECTIVES

The mention of other abnormals points to a second danger of the practice of genetic abortion. Genetic abortion may come to be seen not so much as the prevention of genetic disease, but as the prevention of birth of defective or abnormal children—and, in a way, understandably so. For in the case of what other diseases does preventive medicine consist in the elimination of the patient-at-risk? Moreover, the very language used to discuss genetic disease leads us to the easy but wrong conclusion that the afflicted fetus or person *is* rather than *has* a disease. True, one is partly defined by his genotype, but only partly. A person is more than his disease. And yet we slide easily from the language of possession to the language of identity, from "He has hemophilia" to "He is a hemophiliac," from "She has diabetes" through "She is diabetic" to "She is a diabetic," from "The fetus has Down syndrome" to "The fetus is a Down's." This way of speaking supports the belief that it is defective persons (or potential persons) that are being eliminated, rather than diseases.

If this is so, then it becomes simply accidental that the defect has a genetic cause. Surely, it is only because of the high regard for medicine and science, and for the accuracy of genetic diagnosis, that genotypic defectives are likely to be the first to go. But once the principle, "Defectives should not be born," is established, grounds other than cytological and biochemical may very well be sought. Even ignoring racialists and others equally misguided—of course, they cannot be ignored—we should know that there are social scientists, for example, who believe that one can predict with a high degree of accuracy how a child will turn out from a careful, systematic study of the socio-economic and psycho-dynamic environment into which he is born and in which he grows up. They might press for the prevention of socio-psychological disease, even of "criminality," by means of prenatal environmental diagnosis and abortion. I have heard rumor that a crude, unscientific form of eliminating potential "phenotypic defectives" is already being practiced in some cities, in that submission to abortion is allegedly being made a condition for the receipt of welfare payments. "Defectives should not be born" is a principle without limits. We can ill-afford to have it established.

Up to this point, I have been discussing the possible implications of the practice of genetic abortion for our belief in and adherence to the idea that, at least in fundamental human matters such as life and liberty, all men are to be considered as equals, that for these matters we should ignore as irrelevant the real qualitative differences amongst men, however important these differences may be for other purposes. Those who are concerned about abortion fear that the permissible time of eliminating the unwanted will be moved forward along the time continuum, against newborns, infants, and children. Similarly, I suggest that we should be concerned lest the attack on gross genetic inequality in fetuses be advanced along the continuum of quality and into the later stages of life.

I am not engaged in predicting the future; I am not saying that amniocentesis and genetic abortion will lead down the road to Nazi Germany. Rather, I am suggesting that the principles underlying genetic abortion simultaneously justify many further steps down that road. The point was very well made by Abraham Lincoln:

> If A can prove, however conclusively, that he may, of right, enslave B—Why may not B snatch the same argument and prove equally, that he may enslave A?
>
> You say A is white, and B is black. It is color, then; the lighter having the right to enslave the darker? Take care. By this rule, you are to be slave to the first man you meet with a fairer skin than your own.
>
> You do not mean color exactly? You mean the whites are intellectually the superiors of the blacks, and, therefore have the right to enslave them? Take care again. By this rule, you are to be slave to the first man you meet with an intellect superior to your own.

> But, say you, it is a question of interest; and, if you can make it your interest, you have the right to enslave another. Very well. And if he can make it his interest, he has the right to enslave you.[3]

Perhaps I have exaggerated the dangers; perhaps we will not abandon our inexplicable preference for generous humanitarianism over consistency. But we should indeed be cautious and move slowly as we give serious consideration to the question "What price the perfect baby?"[4] . . .

NOTES

1 This strikes me as by far the most important inference to be drawn from the fact that men in different times and cultures have answered the abortion question differently. Seen in this light, the differing and changing answers themselves suggest that it is a question not easily put under, at least not for very long.

2 Other ways include: one should not do violence to living or growing things; life is sacred; respect nature; fetal life has value; refrain from taking innocent life; protect and preserve life. As some have pointed out, the terms chosen are of different weight, and would require reasons of different weight to tip the balance in favor of abortion. My choice of the "rights" terminology is not meant to beg the questions of whether such rights really exist, or of where they come from. However, the notion of a "fetal right to life" presents only a little more difficulty in this regard than does the notion of a "human right to life," since the former does not depend on a claim that the human fetus is already "human." In my sense of terms "right" and "life," we might even say that a dog or fetal dog has a "right to life," and that it would be cruel and immoral for a man to go around performing abortions even on dogs for no good reason.

3 Lincoln, A. (1854). In *The Collected Works of Abraham Lincoln,* R. P. Basler, editor. New Brunswick, New Jersey, Rutgers University Press, Vol. II, p. 222.

4 For a discussion of the possible biological rather than moral price of attempts to prevent the birth of defective children see Motulsky, A. G., G. R. Fraser, and J. Felsenstein (1971). In Symposium on Intra-uterine Diagnosis, D. Bergsma, editor. *Birth Defects: Original Article Series,* Vol. 7, No. 5. Also see Neel, J. (1972). In *Early Diagnosis of Human Genetic Defects: Scientific and Ethical Considerations,* M. Harris, editor. Washington, D.C., U.S. Government Printing Office, pp. 366–380.

GENETICS AND REPRODUCTIVE RISK:
CAN HAVING CHILDREN BE IMMORAL?
Laura M. Purdy

Purdy argues that it can be morally wrong to reproduce in circumstances of genetic risk, most clearly in cases where there is a high risk of serious genetic disease. In developing her overall argument, she is committed to the view that we have a duty to try to provide a *minimally satisfying life* for our children. Much of Purdy's analysis focuses on Huntington's disease, and she emphasizes how the emergence of reliable genetic testing has opened up new possibilities for those at risk of passing on the disease.

Is it morally permissible for me to have children?[1] A decision to procreate is surely one of the most significant decisions a person can make. So it would seem that it ought not to be made without some moral soul-searching.

There are many reasons why one might hesitate to bring children into this world if one is concerned about their welfare. Some are rather general, like the deteriorating environment or the prospect of poverty. Others have a narrower focus, like continuing civil war in Ireland, or the lack of essential social support for child-rearing persons in the United States. Still others may be relevant only to individuals at risk of passing harmful diseases to their offspring.

There are many causes of misery in this world, and most of them are unrelated to genetic disease. In the general scheme of things, human misery is most efficiently reduced by concentrating on noxious social and political arrangements. Nonetheless, we shouldn't ignore preventable harm just because it is confined to a relatively small corner of life. So the question arises: can it be wrong to have a child because of genetic risk factors?[2]

Unsurprisingly, most of the debate about this issue has focused on prenatal screening and abortion: much useful information about a given fetus can be made available by recourse to prenatal testing. This fact has meant that moral questions about reproduction have become entwined with abortion politics, to the detriment of both. The abortion connection has made it especially difficult to think about whether it is wrong to prevent a child from coming into being since doing so might involve what many people see as wrongful killing; yet there is no necessary link between the two. Clearly, the existence of genetically compromised children can be prevented not only by aborting already existing fetuses but also by preventing conception in the first place.

Worse yet, many discussions simply assume a particular view of abortion, without any recognition of other possible positions and the difference they make in how people understand the issues. For example, those who object to aborting fetuses with genetic problems often argue that doing so would undermine our conviction that all humans are in some important sense equal.[3] However, this position rests on the assumption that conception marks the point at which humans are endowed with a right to life. So aborting fetuses with genetic problems looks morally the same as killing "imperfect" people without their consent.

This position raises two separate issues. One pertains to the legitimacy of different views on abortion. Despite the conviction of many abortion activists to the contrary, I believe that ethically respectable views can be found on different sides of the debate, including one that sees fetuses as developing humans without any serious moral claim on continued life. There is no space here to address the details, and doing so would be once again to fall into the trap of letting the abortion question swallow up all others. Fortunately, this issue need not be resolved here. However, opponents of abortion need to face the fact that many thoughtful individuals do not *see* fetuses as moral persons. It follows that their reasoning process and hence the implications of their decisions are radically different from those envisioned by opponents of prenatal screening and abortion. So where the latter see genetic abortion as murdering people who just don't measure up, the former see it as a way to prevent the development of persons who are more likely to live miserable lives. This is consistent with a world view that values persons equally and holds that each deserves high quality of life. Some of those who object to genetic abortion appear to be oblivious to these psychological and logical facts. It follows that the nightmare scenarios they paint for us are beside the point: many people simply do not share the assumptions that make them plausible.

How are these points relevant to my discussion? My primary concern here is to argue that conception can sometimes be morally wrong on grounds of genetic risk, although this judgment will not apply to those who accept the moral legitimacy of abortion and are willing to employ prenatal screening and selective abortion. If my case is solid, then those who oppose abortion must be especially careful not to conceive in certain cases, as they are, of course, free to follow their conscience about abortion. Those like myself who do not see abortion as murder have more ways to prevent birth.

HUNTINGTON'S DISEASE

There is always some possibility that reproduction will result in a child with a serious disease or handicap. Genetic counselors can help individuals determine whether they are at unusual risk and, as the Human Genome Project rolls on, their knowledge will increase by quantum leaps. As this knowledge becomes available, I believe we ought to use it to determine whether possible children are at risk *before* they are conceived.

I want in this paper to defend the thesis that it is morally wrong to reproduce when we know there is a high risk of transmitting a serious disease or defect. This thesis holds that some reproductive acts are wrong, and my argument puts the burden of proof on those who disagree with it to show why its conclusions can be overridden. Hence it denies that people should be free to reproduce mindless of the

consequences.[4] However, as moral argument, it should be taken as a proposal for further debate and discussion. It is not, by itself, an argument in favor of legal prohibitions of reproduction.[5]

There is a huge range of genetic diseases. Some are quickly lethal; others kill more slowly, if at all. Some are mainly physical, some mainly mental; others impair both kinds of function. Some interfere tremendously with normal functioning, others less. Some are painful, some are not. There seems to be considerable agreement that rapidly lethal diseases, especially those, like Tay-Sachs, accompanied by painful deterioration, should be prevented even at the cost of abortion. Conversely, there seems to be substantial agreement that relatively trivial problems, especially cosmetic ones, would not be legitimate grounds for abortion.[6] In short, there are cases ranging from low risk of mild disease or disability to high risk of serious disease or disability. Although it is difficult to decide where the duty to refrain from procreation becomes compelling, I believe that there are some clear cases. I have chosen to focus on Huntington's Disease to illustrate the kinds of concrete issues such decisions entail. However, the arguments presented here are also relevant to many other genetic diseases.[7]

The symptoms of Huntington's Disease usually begin between the ages of thirty and fifty. It happens this way:

> Onset is insidious. Personality changes (obstinacy, moodiness, lack of initiative) frequently antedate or accompany the involuntary choreic movements. These usually appear first in the face, neck, and arms, and are jerky, irregular, and stretching in character. Contractions of the facial muscles result in grimaces; those of the respiratory muscles, lips, and tongue lead to hesitating, explosive speech. Irregular movements of the trunk are present; the gait is shuffling and dancing. Tendon reflexes are increased. . . . Some patients display a fatuous euphoria; others are spiteful, irascible, destructive, and violent. Paranoid reactions are common. Poverty of thought and impairment of attention, memory, and judgment occur. As the disease progresses, walking becomes impossible, swallowing difficult, and dementia profound. Suicide is not uncommon.[8]

The illness lasts about fifteen years, terminating in death.

Huntington's Disease is an autosomal dominant disease, meaning that it is caused by a single defective gene located on a non-sex chromosome. It is passed from one generation to the next via affected individuals. Each child of such an affected person has a fifty percent risk of inheriting the gene and thus of eventually developing the disease, even if he or she was born before the parent's disease was evident.[9]

Until recently, Huntington's Disease was especially problematic because most affected individuals did not know whether they had the gene for the disease until well into their childbearing years. So they had to decide about childbearing before knowing whether they could transmit the disease or not. If, in time, they did not develop symptoms of the disease, then their children could know they were not at risk for the disease. If unfortunately they did develop symptoms, then each of their children could know there was a fifty percent chance that they, too, had inherited the gene. In both cases, the children faced a period of prolonged anxiety as to whether they would develop the disease. Then, in the 1980s, thanks in part to an energetic campaign by Nancy Wexler, a genetic marker was found that, in certain circumstances, could tell people with a relatively high degree of probability whether or not they had the gene for the disease.[10] Finally, in March 1993, the defective gene itself was discovered.[11] Now individuals can find out whether they carry the gene for the disease, and prenatal screening can tell us whether a given fetus has inherited it. These technological developments change the moral scene substantially.

How serious are the risks involved in Huntington's Disease? Geneticists often think a ten percent risk is high.[12] But risk assessment also depends on what is at stake: the worse the possible outcome the more undesirable an otherwise small risk seems. In medicine, as elsewhere, people may regard the same result quite differently. But for devastating diseases like Huntington's this part of the judgment should be unproblematic: no one wants a loved one to suffer in this way.[13]

There may still be considerable disagreement about the acceptability of a given risk. So it would be difficult in many circumstances to say how we should respond to a particular risk. Nevertheless, there are good grounds for a conservative approach, for it is reasonable to take special precautions to avoid very bad consequences, even if the risk is small. But the possible consequences here *are* very bad: a child who may inherit Huntington's Disease has a much greater than average chance of being subjected to severe and prolonged suffering. And it is one thing to risk one's own welfare, but quite another to do so for others and without their consent.

Is this judgment about Huntington's Disease really defensible? People appear to have quite different opinions. Optimists argue that a child born into a family afflicted with Huntington's Disease has a reasonable chance of living a satisfactory life. After all, even children born of an afflicted parent still have a fifty percent chance of escaping the disease. And even if afflicted themselves, such people will probably enjoy some thirty years of healthy life before symptoms appear. It is also possible, although not at all likely, that some might not mind the symptoms caused by the disease. Optimists can point to diseased persons who have lived fruitful lives, as well as those who seem genuinely glad to be alive. One is Rick Donohue, a sufferer from the Joseph family disease: "You know, if my mom hadn't had me, I wouldn't be here for the life I have had. So there is a good possibility I will have children."[14] Optimists therefore conclude that it would be a shame if these persons had not lived.

Pessimists concede some of these facts, but take a less sanguine view of them. They think a fifty percent risk of serious disease like Huntington's appallingly high. They suspect that many children born into afflicted families are liable to spend their youth in dreadful anticipation and fear of the disease. They expect that the disease, if it appears, will be perceived as a tragic and painful end to a blighted life. They point out that Rick Donohue is still young, and has not experienced the full horror of his sickness. It is also well-known that some young persons have such a dilated sense of time that they can hardly envision themselves at thirty or forty, so the prospect of pain at that age is unreal to them.[15]

More empirical research on the psychology and life history of sufferers and potential sufferers is clearly needed to decide whether optimists or pessimists have a more accurate picture of the experiences of individuals at risk. But given that some will surely realize pessimists' worst fears, it seems unfair to conclude that the pleasures of those who deal best with the situation simply cancel out the suffering of those others when that suffering could be avoided altogether.

I think that these points indicate that the morality of procreation in situations like this demands further investigation. I propose to do this by looking first at the position of the possible child, then at that of the potential parent.

POSSIBLE CHILDREN AND POTENTIAL PARENTS

The first task in treating the problem from the child's point of view is to find a way of referring to possible future offspring without seeming to confer some sort of morally significant existence upon them. I will follow the convention of calling children who might be born in the future but who are not now conceived "possible" children, offspring, individuals, or persons.

Now, what claims about children or possible children are relevant to the morality of childbearing in the circumstances being considered? Of primary importance is the judgment that we ought to try to provide every child with something like a minimally satisfying life. I am not altogether sure how best to formulate this standard but I want clearly to reject the view that it is morally permissible to conceive individuals so long as we do not expect them to be so miserable that they wish they were dead.[16] I believe that this kind of moral minimalism is thoroughly unsatisfactory and that not many people would really want to live in a world where it was the prevailing standard. Its lure is that it puts few demands on us, but its price is the scant attention it pays to human well-being.

How might the judgment that we have a duty to try to provide a minimally satisfying life for our children be justified? It could, I think, be derived fairly straightforwardly from either utilitarian or contractarian theories of justice, although there is no space here for discussion of the details. The net result of such analysis would be the conclusion that neglecting this duty would create unnecessary unhappiness or unfair disadvantage for some persons.

Of course, this line of reasoning confronts us with the need to spell out what is meant by "minimally satisfying" and what a standard based on this concept would require of us. Conceptions of a minimally satisfying life vary tremendously among societies and also within them. *De Rigueur* in some circles are private music lessons and trips to Europe, while in others providing eight years of schooling is a major accomplishment. But there is no need to consider this complication at length here since we are concerned only with health as a prerequisite for a minimally satisfying life. Thus, as we draw out what such a standard might require of us, it seems reasonable to retreat to the more limited claim that parents should try to ensure something like normal health for their children. It might be thought that even this moderate claim is unsatisfactory since in some places debilitating conditions are the norm, but one could circumvent this objection by saying that parents ought to try to provide for their children health normal for that culture, even though it may be inadequate if measured by some outside standard.[17] This conservative position would still justify efforts to avoid the birth of children at risk for Huntington's Disease and other serious genetic diseases in virtually all societies.[18]

This view is reinforced by the following considerations. Given that possible children do not presently exist as actual individuals, they do not have a right to be brought into existence, and hence no one is maltreated by measures to avoid the conception of a possible person. Therefore, the conservative course that avoids the conception of those who would not be expected to enjoy a minimally satisfying life is at present the only fair course of action. The alternative is a laissez-faire approach which brings into existence the lucky, but only at the expense of the unlucky. Notice that attempting to avoid the creation of the unlucky does not necessarily lead to *fewer* people being brought into being; the question boils down to taking steps to bring those with better prospects into existence, instead of those with worse ones.

I have so far argued that if people with Huntington's Disease are unlikely to live minimally satisfying lives, then those who might pass it on should not have genetically related children. This is consonant with the principle that the greater the danger of serious problems, the stronger the duty to avoid them. But this principle is in conflict with what people think of as the right to reproduce. How might one decide which should take precedence?

Expecting people to forego having genetically related children might seem to demand too great a sacrifice of them. But before reaching that conclusion we need to ask what is really at stake. One reason for wanting children is to experience family life, including love, companionship, watching kids grow, sharing their pains and triumphs, and helping to form members of the next generation. Other reasons emphasize the validation of parents as individuals within a continuous family line, children as a source of immortality, or perhaps even the gratification of producing partial replicas of oneself. Children may also be desired in an effort to prove that one is an adult, to try to cement a marriage or to benefit parents economically.

Are there alternative ways of satisfying these desires? Adoption or new reproductive technologies can fulfil many of them without passing on known genetic defects. Replacements for sperm have been available for many years via artificial insemination by donor. More recently, egg donation, sometimes in combination with contract pregnancy,[19] has been used to provide eggs for women who prefer not to use their own. Eventually it may be possible to clone individual humans, although that now seems a long way off. All of these approaches to avoiding the use of particular genetic material are controversial and have generated much debate. I believe that tenable moral versions of each do exist.[20]

None of these methods permits people to extend both genetic lines, or realize the desire for immortality or for children who resemble both parents; nor is it clear that such alternatives will necessarily succeed in proving that one is an adult, cementing a marriage, or providing economic benefits. Yet, many people feel these desires strongly. Now, I am sympathetic to William James's dictum regarding desires: "Take any demand, however slight, which any creature, however weak, may make. Ought it not, for its own sole sake be satisfied? If not, prove why not."[21] Thus a world where more desires are satisfied is generally better than one where fewer

are. However, not all desires can be legitimately satisfied since, as James suggests, there may be good reasons—such as the conflict of duty and desire—why some should be overruled.

Fortunately, further scrutiny of the situation reveals that there are good reasons why people should attempt—with appropriate social support—to talk themselves out of the desires in question or to consider novel ways of fulfilling them. Wanting to see the genetic line continued is not particularly rational when it brings a sinister legacy of illness and death. The desire for immortality cannot really be satisfied anyway, and people need to face the fact that what really matters is how they behave in their own lifetime. And finally, the desire for children who physically resemble one is understandable, but basically narcissistic, and its fulfillment cannot be guaranteed even by normal reproduction. There are other ways of proving one is an adult, and other ways of cementing marriages—and children don't necessarily do either. Children, especially prematurely ill children, may not provide the expected economic benefits anyway. Nongenetically related children may also provide benefits similar to those that would have been provided by genetically related ones, and expected economic benefit is, in many cases, a morally questionable reason for having children.

Before the advent of reliable genetic testing, the options of people in Huntington's families were cruelly limited. On the one hand, they could have children, but at the risk of eventual crippling illness and death for them. On the other, they could refrain from childbearing, sparing their possible children from significant risk of inheriting this disease, perhaps frustrating intense desires to procreate—only to discover, in some cases, that their sacrifice was unnecessary because they did not develop the disease. Or they could attempt to adopt or try new reproductive approaches.

Reliable genetic testing has opened up new possibilities. Those at risk who wish to have children can get tested. If they test positive, they know their possible children are at risk. Those who are opposed to abortion must be especially careful to avoid conception if they are to behave responsibly. Those not opposed to abortion can responsibly conceive children, but only if they are willing to test each fetus and abort those who carry the gene. If individuals at risk test negative, they are home free.

What about those who cannot face the test for themselves? They can do prenatal testing and abort fetuses who carry the defective gene. A clearly positive test also implies that the parent is affected, although negative tests do not rule out that possibility. Prenatal testing can thus bring knowledge that enables one to avoid passing the disease to others, but only, in some cases, at the cost of coming to know with certainty that one will indeed develop the disease. This situation raises with peculiar force the question of whether parental responsibility requires people to get tested.

Some people think that we should recognize a right "not to know." It seems to me that such a right could be defended only where ignorance does not put others at serious risk. So if people are prepared to forego genetically related children, they need not get tested. But if they want genetically related children then they must do whatever is necessary to ensure that affected babies are not the result. There is, after all, something inconsistent about the claim that one has a right to be shielded from the truth, even if the price is to risk inflicting on one's children the same dread disease one cannot even face in oneself.

In sum, until we can be assured that Huntington's Disease does not prevent people from living a minimally satisfying life, individuals at risk for the disease have a moral duty to try not to bring affected babies into this world. There are now enough options available so that this duty needn't frustrate their reasonable desires. Society has a corresponding duty to facilitate moral behavior on the part of individuals. Such support ranges from the narrow and concrete (like making sure that medical testing and counseling is available to all) to the more general social environment that guarantees that all pregnancies are voluntary, that pronatalism is eradicated, and that women are treated with respect regardless of the reproductive options they choose.

NOTES

1 This paper is loosely based on "Genetic Diseases: Can Having Children Be Immoral?" originally published in *Genetics Now,* ed. John L. Buckley (Washington, DC: University Press of America, 1978) and subsequently anthologized in a number of medical ethics texts. Thanks to Thomas Mappes and David DeGrazia for their helpful suggestions about updating the paper.

2 I focus on genetic considerations, although with the advent of AIDS the scope of the general question here could be expanded. There are two reasons for sticking to this relatively narrow formulation. One is that dealing with a smaller chunk of the problem may help us think more clearly, while realizing that some conclusions may nonetheless be relevant to the larger problem. The other is the peculiar capacity of some genetic problems to affect ever more individuals in the future.

3 For example, see Leon Kass, "Implications of Prenatal Diagnosis for the Human Right to Life," *Ethical Issues in Human Genetics,* eds. Bruce Hilton et al. (New York: Plenum Press, 1973).

4 This is, of course, a very broad thesis. I defend an even broader version in "Loving Future People," *Reproduction, Ethics and the Law,* ed. Joan Callahan (Bloomington: Indiana University Press, forthcoming).

5 Why would we want to resist legal enforcement of every moral conclusion? First, legal action has many costs, costs not necessarily worth paying in particular cases. Second, legal enforcement would tend to take the matter in question out of the realm of debate and treat it as settled. But in many cases, especially where mores or technology are rapidly evolving, we don't want that to happen. Third, legal enforcement would undermine individual freedom and decision-making capacity. In some cases, the ends envisioned are important enough to warrant putting up with these disadvantages, but that remains to be shown in each case.

6 Those who do not see fetuses as moral persons with a right to life may nonetheless hold that abortion is justifiable in these cases. I argue at some length elsewhere that lesser defects can cause great suffering. Once we are clear that there is nothing discriminatory about failing to conceive particular possible individuals, it makes sense, other things being equal, to avoid the prospect of such pain if we can. Naturally, other things rarely are equal. In the first place, many problems go undiscovered until a baby is born. Secondly, there are often substantial costs associated with screening programs. Thirdly, although women should be encouraged to consider the moral dimensions of routine pregnancy, we do not want it to be so fraught with tension that it becomes a miserable experience. (See "Loving Future People.")

7 It should be noted that failing to conceive a single individual can affect many lives: in 1916, nine hundred and sixty-two cases could be traced from six seventeenth-century arrivals in America. See Gordon Rattray Taylor, *The Biological Time Bomb* (New York, 1968), p. 176.

8 *The Merck Manual* (Rahway, NJ: Merck, 1972), pp. 1363, 1346. We now know that the age of onset and severity of the disease is related to the number of abnormal replications of the glutamine code on the abnormal gene. See Andrew

Revkin, "Hunting Down Huntington's," *Discover,* December 1993, p. 108.

9 Hymie Gordon, "Genetic Counseling," *JAMA,* Vol. 217, n. 9 (August 30, 1971), p. 1346.

10 See Revkin, "Hunting Down Huntington's," pp. 99–108.

11 "Gene for Huntington's Disease Discovered," *Human Genome News,* Vol. 5, n. 1 (May 1993), p. 5.

12 Charles Smith, Susan Holloway, and Alan E. H. Emery, "Individuals at Risk in Families—Genetic Disease," *Journal of Medical Genetics,* Vol. 8 (1971), p. 453.

13 To try to separate the issue of the gravity of the disease from the existence of a given individual, compare this situation with how we would assess a parent who neglected to vaccinate an existing child against a hypothetical viral version of Huntington's.

14 *The New York Times,* September 30, 1975, p. 1, col. 6. The Joseph family disease is similar to Huntington's Disease except that symptoms start appearing in the twenties. Rick Donohue was in his early twenties at the time he made this statement.

15 I have talked to college students who believe that they will have lived fully and be ready to die at those ages. It is astonishing how one's perspective changes over time, and how ages that one once associated with senility and physical collapse come to seem the prime of human life.

16 The view I am rejecting has been forcefully articulated by Derek Parfit, *Reasons and Persons* (Oxford: Oxford University Press, 1984). For more discussion, see "Loving Future People."

17 I have some qualms about this response since I fear that some human groups are so badly off that it might still be wrong for them to procreate, even if that would mean great changes in their cultures. But this is a complicated issue that needs its own investigation.

18 Again, a troubling exception might be the isolated Venezuelan group Nancy Wexler found where, because of in-breeding, a large proportion of the population is affected by Huntington's. See Revkin, "Hunting Down Huntington's."

19 Or surrogacy, as it has been popularly known. I think that "contract pregnancy" is more accurate and more respectful of women. Eggs can be provided either by a woman who also gestates the fetus or by a third party.

20 The most powerful objections to new reproductive technologies and arrangements concern possible bad consequences for women. However, I do not think that the arguments against them on these grounds have yet shown the dangers to be as great as some believe. So although it is perhaps true that new reproductive technologies and arrangements shouldn't be used lightly, avoiding the conceptions discussed here is well worth the risk. For a series of viewpoints on this issue, including my own "Another Look at Contract Pregnancy," see Helen B. Holmes, *Issues in Reproductive Technology I: An Anthology* (New York: Garland Press, 1992).

21 *Essays in Pragmatism,* ed. A. Castell (New York, 1948), p. 73.

REPRODUCTIVE TECHNOLOGIES

IVF: THE SIMPLE CASE

Peter Singer

Singer identifies seven distinct objections that have been made to the use of in vitro fertilization (IVF) even in the "simple case"—a case in which a married couple is infertile, only eggs and sperm provided by the couple are involved, and all resulting embryos are transferred to the wife's uterus. He takes some of these objections more seriously than others but ultimately concludes that none should "count against going ahead" with IVF in the simple case.

The so-called simple case of IVF is that in which a married, infertile couple use an egg taken from the wife and sperm taken from the husband, and all embryos created are inserted into the womb of the wife. This case allows us to consider the ethics of IVF in itself, without the complications of the many other issues that can arise in different circumstances. Then we can go on to look at these complications separately.

THE TECHNIQUE

The technique itself is now well known and is fast becoming a routine part of infertility treatment in many countries. The infertile woman is given a hormone treatment to induce her ovaries to produce more than one egg in her next cycle. Her hormone levels are carefully monitored to detect the precise moment at which the eggs are ripening. At this time the eggs are removed. This is usually done by laparoscopy, a minor operation in which a fine tube is inserted into the woman's abdomen and the egg is sucked out up the tube. A laparoscope, a kind of periscope illuminated by fiber optics, is also inserted into the abdomen so that the surgeon can locate the place where the ripe egg is to be found. Instead of laparoscopy, some IVF teams are now using ultrasound techniques, which eliminate the need for a general anesthetic.

Once the eggs have been collected they are placed in culture in small glass dishes known as petri dishes, not in test tubes despite the popular label of "test-tube babies." Sperm is then obtained from the male partner by means of masturbation and placed with the egg. Fertilization follows in at least 80 percent of the ripe eggs. The resulting embryos are allowed to cleave once or twice and are usually transferred to the woman some 48 to 72 hours after fertilization. The actual transfer is done via the vagina and is a simple procedure.

It is after the transfer, when the embryo is back in the uterus and beyond the scrutiny of medical science, that things are most likely to go wrong. Even with the most experienced IVF teams, the majority of embryos transferred fail to implant in the uterus. One pregnancy for every five transfers is currently considered to be a good working average for a competent IVF team. Many of the newer teams fail to achieve anything like this rate. Nevertheless, there are so many units around the world now practicing IVF that thousands of babies have been produced as a result of the technique. IVF has ceased to be experimental and is now a routine, if still "last resort" method of treating some forms of infertility.

OBJECTIONS TO THE SIMPLE CASE

There is some opposition to IVF even in the simple case. The most frequently heard objections are as follows:

1. IVF is unnatural.

2. IVF is risky for the offspring.

3. IVF separates the procreative and the conjugal aspects of marriage and so damages the marital relationship.

4. IVF is illicit because it involves masturbation.

5. Adoption is a better solution to the problem of childlessness.

6. IVF is an expensive luxury and the resources would be better spent elsewhere.

7. IVF allows increased male control over reproduction and hence threatens the status of women in the community.

We can deal swiftly with the first four of these objections. If we were to reject medical advances on the grounds that they are "unnatural" we would be rejecting modern medicine as a whole, for the very purpose of the medical enterprise is to resist the ravages of nature which would otherwise shorten our lives and make them much less pleasant. If anything is in accordance with the nature of our species, it is the application of our intelligence to overcome adverse situations in which we find ourselves. The application of IVF to infertile couples is a classic example of this application of human intelligence.

The claim that IVF is risky for the offspring is one that was argued with great force before IVF became a widely used technique. It is sufficient to note that the results of IVF so far have happily refuted these fears. The most recent Australian figures, for example, based on 934 births, indicate that the rate of abnormality was 2.7%, which is very close to the national average of 1.5%. When we take into account the greater average age of women seeking IVF, as compared with the childbearing population as a whole, it does not seem that the *in vitro* technique itself adds to the risk of an abnormal offspring. This view is reinforced by the fact that the abnormalities were all ones that arise with the ordinary method of reproduction; there have been no new "monsters" produced by IVF.[1] Perhaps we still cannot claim with statistical certainty that the risk of defect is no higher with IVF than with the more common method of conception; but if the risk is higher at all, it would appear to be only very slightly higher, and still within limits which may be considered acceptable.

The third and fourth objections have been urged by spokesmen for certain religious groups, but they are difficult to defend outside the confines of particular religions. Few infertile couples will take seriously the view that their marital relationship will be damaged if they use the technique which offers them the best chance of having their own child. It is in any case extraordinarily paternalistic for anyone else to tell a couple that they should not use IVF because it will harm their marriage. That, surely, is for them to decide.

The objection to masturbation comes from a similar source and can be even more swiftly dismissed. Religious prohibitions on masturbation are taboos from past times which even religious spokesmen are beginning to consider outdated. Moreover, even if one could defend a prohibition on masturbation for sexual pleasure—perhaps on the (very tenuous) ground that sexual activity is wrong unless it is directed either toward procreation or toward the strengthening of the bond between marriage partners—it would be absurd to extend a prohibition with that kind of rationale to a case in which masturbation is being used in the context of a marriage and precisely in order to make reproduction possible. (The fact that some religions do persist in regarding masturbation as wrong, even in these circumstances, is indicative of the folly of an ethical system based on absolute rules, irrespective of the circumstances in which those rules are being applied, or the consequences of their application.)

OVERPOPULATION AND THE ALLOCATION OF RESOURCES

The next two objections, however, deserve more careful consideration. In an overpopulated world in which there are so many children who cannot be properly fed and cared for, there is something incongruous about using all the ingenuity of modern medicine to create more children. And similarly, when there are so many deaths caused by preventable diseases, is there not something wrong with the priorities which lead us to develop expensive techniques for overcoming the relatively less serious problem of infertility?

These objections are sound to the following extent: in an ideal world we would find loving families for unwanted children before we created additional children; and in an ideal world we would clear up all the preventable ill-health and malnutrition-related diseases before we went on to tackle the problem of infertility. But is it appropriate to ask, of IVF alone, whether it can stand the test of measurement against what we would do in an ideal world? In an ideal world, none of us would consume more than our fair share of resources. We would not drive expensive cars while others die for the lack of drugs costing a few cents. We would not eat a diet rich in wastefully produced animal products while others cannot get enough to nourish their bodies. We cannot demand more of infertile couples than we are ready to demand of ourselves. If fertile couples are free to have large families of their own, rather than adopt destitute children from overseas, infertile couples must also be free to do what they can to have their own families. In both cases, overseas adoption, or perhaps the adoption of local children who are unwanted because of some impairment, should be considered; but if we are not going to make this compulsory in the former case, it should not be made compulsory in the latter.

There is a further question: to what extent do infertile couples have a right to assistance from community medical resources? Again, however, we must not single out IVF for harsher treatment than we give to other medical techniques. If tubal surgery is available and covered by one's health insurance, or is offered as part of a national health scheme, then why should IVF be treated any differently? And if infertile couples can get free or subsidized psychiatry to help them overcome the psychological problems of infertility, there is something absurd about denying them free or subsidized treatment which could overcome the root of the problem, rather than the symptoms. By today's standards, after all, IVF is not an inordinately expensive medical technique; and there is no country, as far as I know, which limits its provision of free or subsidized health care to those cases in which the patient's life is in danger. Once we extend medical care to cover cases of injury, incapacity, and psychological distress, IVF has a strong claim to be included among the range of free or subsidized treatments available.

THE EFFECT ON WOMEN

The final objection is one that has come from some feminists. In a recently published collection of essays by women titled *Test-Tube Women: What Future for Motherhood?,* several contributors are suspicious of the new reproductive technology. None is more hostile than Robyn Rowland, an Australian sociologist, who writes:

> Ultimately the new technology will be used for the benefit of men and to the detriment of women. Although technology itself is not always a negative development, the real question has always been—who controls it? Biological technology is in the hands of men.[2]

And Rowland concludes with a warning as dire as any uttered by the most conservative opponents of IVF:

> What may be happening is the last battle in the long war of men against women. Women's position is most precarious . . . we may find ourselves without a product of any kind with which to bargain. For the history of "mankind" women have been seen in terms of their value as childbearers. We have to ask, if that last power is taken and controlled by men, what role is envisaged for women in the new world? Will women become obsolete? Will we be fighting to retain or reclaim the right to bear children—has patriarchy conned us once again? I urge you sisters to be vigilant.[2]

I can see little basis for such claims. For a start, women have figured quite prominently in the leading IVF teams in Britain, Australia, and the United States: Jean Purdy was an early colleague of Edwards and Steptoe in the research that led to the birth of Louise Brown; Linda Mohr has directed the development of embryo freezing at the Queen Victoria Medical Centre in Melbourne; and in the United States Georgeanna Jones and Joyce Vargyas have played leading roles in the groundbreaking clinics in Norfolk, Virginia, and at the University of Southern California, respectively. It seems odd for a feminist to neglect the contributions these women have made.

Even if one were to grant, however, that the technology remains predominantly in male hands, it has to be remembered that it was developed in response to the needs of infertile couples. From inter-

views I have conducted and meetings I have attended, my impression is that while both partners are often very concerned about their childlessness, in those cases in which one partner is more distressed than the other by this situation, that partner is usually the woman. Feminists usually accept that this is so, attributing it to the power of social conditioning in a patriarchal society; but the origin of the strong female desire for children is not really what is in question here. The question is: in what sense is the new technology an instrument of male domination over women? If it is true that the technology was developed at least as much in response to the needs of women as in response to the needs of men, then it is hard to see why a feminist should condemn it.

It might be objected that whatever the origins of IVF and no matter how benign it may be when used to help infertile couples, the further development of techniques such as ectogenesis—the growth of the embryo from conception totally outside the body, in an artificial womb—will reduce the status of women. Again, it is not easy to see why this should be so. Ectogenesis will, if it is ever successful, provide a choice for women. Shulamith Firestone argued several years ago in her influential feminist work *The Dialectic of Sex*[3] that this choice will remove the fundamental biological barrier to complete equality. Hence Firestone welcomed the prospect of ectogenesis and condemned the low priority given by our male-dominated society to research in this area.

Firestone's view is surely more in line with the drive to sexual equality than the position taken by Rowland. If we argue that to break the link between women and childbearing would be to undermine the status of women in our society, what are we saying about the ability of women to obtain true equality in other spheres of life? I am not so pessimistic about the abilities of women to achieve equality with men across the broad range of human endeavor. For that reason I think women will be helped, rather than harmed, by the development of a technology which makes it possible for them to have children without being pregnant. As Nancy Breeze, a very differently inclined contributor to the same collection of essays, puts it:

> Two thousand years of morning sickness and stretch marks have not resulted in liberation for women or

children. If you should run into a Petri dish, it could turn out to be your best friend. So rock it; don't knock it![4]

So to sum up this discussion of the ethics of the simple case of IVF: the ethical objections urged against IVF under these conditions are not strong. They should not count against going ahead with IVF when it is the best way of overcoming infertility and when the infertile couple are not prepared to consider adoption as a means of overcoming their problem. There is, admittedly, a serious question about how much of the national health budget should be allocated to this area. But then, there are serious questions about the allocation of resources in other areas of medicine as well.

REFERENCES

1 Abstract. Proceedings of the Fifth Scientific Meeting of the Fertility Society of Australia, Adelaide, Dec 2–6, 1986.
2 Rowland R. Reproductive technologies: The final solution to the woman question? In: Arditti R., Klein R. D., Minden S., eds., Test-tube women: What future for motherhood? London: Pandora, 1984.
3 Firestone S. The dialectic of sex. New York: Bantam, 1971.
4 Breeze N. Who is going to rock the petri dish? In: Arditti R., Klein R. D., Minden S., eds, Test-tube women: What future for motherhood? London: Pandora, 1984.

FEMINIST ETHICS AND IN VITRO FERTILIZATION
Susan Sherwin

Sherwin outlines the nature of feminist ethics and provides a feminist critique of in vitro fertilization (IVF). She maintains that IVF is morally problematic for a number of closely related reasons, including the following: (1) Although the desires of infertile couples for access to IVF are understandable and worthy of sympathetic regard, such desires themselves emerge from social arrangements and cultural values that are deeply oppressive to women; (2) IVF technology gives the appearance of providing women with increased reproductive freedom but in reality threatens women with a significant decrease of reproductive freedom. Sherwin also insists that those who find themselves in moral opposition to IVF have a responsibility to support medical and social developments that would reduce the perceived need of couples for IVF.

Many authors from all traditions consider it necessary to ask why it is that some couples seek [IVF] technology so desperately. Why is it so important to so many people to produce their 'own' child? On this question, theorists in the analytic tradition seem to shift to previously rejected ground and suggest that this is a natural, or at least a proper, desire. Englehardt, for example, says, 'The use of technology in the fashioning of children is integral to the goal of rendering the world congenial to persons.'[1] Bayles more cautiously observes that 'A desire to beget for its own sake . . . is probably irrational'; nonetheless, he immediately concludes, 'these techniques for fulfilling that desire have been found ethically permissible.'[2] R. G. Edwards and David Sharpe state the case most strongly: 'the desire to have children must be among the most basic of human instincts, and denying it can lead to considerable psychological and social difficulties.'[3] Interestingly, although the recent pronouncement of the Catholic Church assumes that 'the desire for a child is natural,'[4] it denies that a couple has a right to a child: 'The child is not an object to which one has a right.'[5]

Reprinted with permission of the author and the publisher from *Canadian Journal of Philosophy,* Supplementary Volume 13 (1987), pp. 276–284.

Here, I believe, it becomes clear why we need a deeper sort of feminist analysis. We must look at the sort of social arrangements and cultural values that underlie the drive to assume such risks for the sake of biological parenthood. We find that the capitalism, racism, sexism, and elitism of our culture have combined to create a set of attitudes which views children as commodities whose value is derived from their possession of parental chromosomes. Children are valued as privatized commodities, reflecting the virility and heredity of their parents. They are also viewed as the responsibility of their parents and are not seen as the social treasure and burden that they are. Parents must tend their needs on pain of prosecution, and, in return, they get to keep complete control over them. Other adults are inhibited from having warm, stable interactions with the children of others—it is as suspect to try to hug and talk regularly with a child who is not one's own as it is to fondle and hang longingly about a car or a bicycle which belongs to someone else—so those who wish to know children well often find they must have their own.

Women are persuaded that their most important purpose in life is to bear and raise children; they are told repeatedly that their life is incomplete, that they are lacking in fulfillment if they do not have children. And, in fact, many women do face a barren existence without children. Few women have access to meaningful, satisfying jobs. Most do not find themselves in the centre of the romantic personal relationships which the culture pretends is the norm for heterosexual couples. And they have been socialized to be fearful of close friendships with others—they are taught to distrust other women, and to avoid the danger of friendship with men other than their husbands. Children remain the one hope for real intimacy and for the sense of accomplishment which comes from doing work one judges to be valuable.

To be sure, children can provide that sense of self-worth, although for many women (and probably for all mothers at some times) motherhood is not the romanticized satisfaction they are led to expect. But there is something very wrong with a culture where childrearing is the only outlet available to most women in which to pursue fulfillment. Moreover, there is something wrong with the ownership theory of children that keeps other adults at a distance from children. There ought to be a variety of close relationships possible between children and adults so that we all recognize that we have a stake in the well-being of the young, and we all benefit from contact with their view of the world.

In such a world, it would not be necessary to spend the huge sums on designer children which IVF requires while millions of other children starve to death each year. Adults who enjoyed children could be involved in caring for them whether or not they produced them biologically. And, if the institution of marriage survives, women and men would marry because they wished to share their lives together, not because the men needed someone to produce heirs for them and women needed financial support for their children. That would be a world in which we might have reproductive freedom of choice. The world we now live in has so limited women's options and self-esteem, it is legitimate to question the freedom behind women's demand for this technology, for it may well be largely a reflection of constraining social perspectives.

Nonetheless, I must acknowledge that some couples today genuinely mourn their incapacity to produce children without IVF and there are very significant and unique joys which can be found in producing and raising one's own children which are not accessible to persons in infertile relationships. We must sympathize with these people. None of us shall live to see the implementation of the ideal cultural values outlined above which would make the demand for IVF less severe. It is with real concern that some feminists suggest that the personal wishes of couples with fertility difficulties may not be compatible with the overall interests of women and children.

Feminist thought, then, helps us to focus on different dimensions of the problem than do other sorts of approaches. But, with this perspective, we still have difficulty in reaching a final conclusion on whether to encourage, tolerate, modify, or restrict this sort of reproductive technology. I suggest that we turn to the developing theories of feminist ethics for guidance in resolving this question.[6]

In my view, a feminist ethics is a moral theory that focuses on relations among persons as well as on individuals. It has as a model an inter-connected social fabric, rather than the familiar one of isolated, independent atoms; and it gives primacy to bonds among people rather than to rights to independence. It is a theory that focuses on concrete situations and persons and not on free-floating abstract actions.[7] Although many details have yet to be worked out, we can see some of its implications in particular problem areas such as this.

It is a theory that is explicitly conscious of the social, political, and economic relations that exist among persons; in particular, as a feminist theory, it attends to the implications of actions or policies on the status of women. Hence, it is necessary to ask questions from the perspective of feminist ethics in addition to those which are normally asked from the perspective of mainstream ethical theories. We must view issues such as this one in the context of the social and political realities in which they arise, and resist the attempt to evaluate actions or practices in isolation (as traditional responses in biomedical ethics often do). Thus, we cannot just address the question of IVF per se without asking how IVF contributes to general patterns of women's oppression. As Kathryn Pyne Addelson has argued about abortion,[8] a feminist perspective raises questions that are inadmissible within the traditional ethical frameworks, and yet, for women in a patriarchal society, they are value questions of greater urgency. In particular, a feminist ethics, in contrast to other approaches in biomedical ethics, would take seriously the concerns just reviewed which are part of the debate in the feminist literature.

A feminist ethics would also include components of theories that have been developed as 'feminine ethics,' as sketched out by the empirical work of Carol Gilligan.[9] (The best example of such a theory is the work of Nel Noddings in her influential book *Caring*.)[10] In other words, it would be a theory that gives primacy to interpersonal relationships and woman-centered values such as nurturing, empathy, and co-operation. Hence, in the case of IVF, we must care for the women and men who are so despairing about their infertility as to want to spend the vast sums and risk the associated physical and emotional costs of the treatment, in pursuit of 'their own children.' That is, we should, in Noddings' terms, see

their reality as our own and address their very real sense of loss. In so doing, however, we must also consider the implications of this sort of solution to their difficulty. While meeting the perceived desires of some women—desires which are problematic in themselves, since they are so compatible with the values of a culture deeply oppressive to women—this technology threatens to further entrench those values which are responsible for that oppression. A larger vision suggests that the technology offered may, in reality, reduce women's freedom and, if so, it should be avoided.

A feminist ethics will not support a wholly negative response, however, for that would not address our obligation to care for those suffering from infertility; it is the responsibility of those who oppose further implementation of this technology to work toward the changes in the social arrangements that will lead to a reduction of the sense of need for this sort of solution. On the medical front, research and treatment ought to be stepped up to reduce the rates of peral sepsis and gonorrhea which often result in tubal blockage, more attention should be directed at the causes and possible cures for male infertility, and we should pursue techniques that will permit safe reversible sterilization providing women with better alternatives to tubal ligation as a means of fertility control; these sorts of technology would increase the control of many women over their own fertility and would be compatible with feminist objectives. On the social front, we must continue the social pressure to change the status of women and children in our society from that of breeder and possession respectively; hence, we must develop a vision of society as community where all participants are valued members, regardless of age or gender. And we must challenge the notion that having one's wife produce a child with his own genes is sufficient cause for the wives of men with low sperm counts to be expected to undergo the physical and emotional assault such technology involves.

Further, a feminist ethics will attend to the nature of the relationships among those concerned. Annette Baier has eloquently argued for the importance of developing an ethics of trust,[11] and I believe a feminist ethics must address the question of the degree of trust appropriate to the relationships involved. Feminists have noted that women have little reason to trust the medical specialists who offer to respond to their reproductive desires, for commonly women's interests have not come first from the medical point of view.[12] In fact, it is accurate to perceive feminist attacks on reproductive technology as expressions of the lack of trust feminists have in those who control the technology. Few feminists object to reproductive technology per se; rather they express concern about who controls it and how it can be used to further exploit women. The problem with reproductive technology is that it concentrates power in reproductive matters in the hands of those who are not directly involved in the actual bearing and rearing of the child; i.e., in men who relate to their clients in a technical, professional, authoritarian manner. It is a further step in the medicalization of pregnancy and birth which, in North America, is marked by relationships between pregnant women and their doctors which are very different from the traditional relationships between pregnant women and midwives. The latter relationships fostered an atmosphere of mutual trust which is impossible to replicate in hospital deliveries today. In fact, current approaches to pregnancy, labour, and birth tend to view the mother as a threat to the fetus who must be coerced to comply with medical procedures designed to ensure delivery of healthy babies at whatever cost necessary to the mother. Frequently, the fetus-mother relationship is medically characterized as adversarial and the physicians choose to foster a sense of alienation and passivity in the role they permit the mother. However well IVF may serve the interests of the few women with access to it, it more clearly serves the interests (be they commercial, professional, scholarly, or purely patriarchal) of those who control it.

Questions such as these are a puzzle to those engaged in the traditional approaches to ethics, for they always urge us to separate the question of evaluating the morality of various forms of reproductive technology in themselves, from questions about particular uses of that technology. From the perspective of a feminist ethics, however, no such distinction can be meaningfully made. Reproductive technology is not an abstract activity, it is an activity done in particular contexts and it is those contexts which must be addressed.

Feminist concerns [make] clear the difficulties we have with some of our traditional ethical concepts; hence, feminist ethics directs us to rethink our basic ethical notions. Autonomy, or freedom of choice, is not a matter to be determined in isolated instances, as is commonly assumed in many approaches to applied ethics. Rather it is a matter that involves reflection on one's whole life situation. The freedom of choice feminists appeal to in the abortion situation is freedom to define one's status as childbearer, given the social, economic, and political significance of reproduction for women. A feminist perspective permits us to understand that reproductive freedom includes control of one's sexuality, protection against coerced sterilization (or iatrogenic sterilization, e.g., as caused by the Dalkon Shield), and the existence of a social and economic network of support for the children we may choose to bear. It is the freedom to redefine our roles in society according to our concerns and needs as women.

In contrast, the consumer freedom to purchase technology, allowed only to a few couples of the privileged classes (in traditionally approved relationships), seems to entrench further the patriarchal notions of woman's role as childbearer and of heterosexual monogamy as the only acceptable intimate relationship. In other words, this sort of choice does not seem to foster autonomy for women on the broad scale. IVF is a practice which seems to reinforce sexist, classist, and often racist assumptions of our culture; therefore, on our revised understanding of freedom, the contribution of this technology to the general autonomy of women is largely negative.

We can now see the advantage of a feminist ethics over mainstream ethical theories, for a feminist analysis explicitly accepts the need for a political component to our understanding of ethical issues. In this, it differs from traditional ethical theories and it also differs from a simply feminine ethics approach, such as the one Noddings offers, for Noddings seems to rely on individual relations exclusively and is deeply suspicious of political alliances as potential threats to the pure relation of caring. Yet, a full understanding of both the threat of IVF, and the alternative action necessary should we decide to reject IVF, is possible only if it includes a political dimension reflecting on the role of women in society.

From the point of view of feminist ethics, the primary question to consider is whether this and other forms of reproductive technology threaten to reinforce the lack of autonomy which women now experience in our culture—even as they appear, in the short run, to be increasing freedom. We must recognize that the interconnections among the social forces oppressive to women underlie feminists' mistrust of this technology which advertises itself as increasing women's autonomy.[13] The political perspective which directs us to look at how this technology fits in with general patterns of treatment for women is not readily accessible to traditional moral theories, for it involves categories of concern not accounted for in those theories—e.g., the complexity of issues which makes it inappropriate to study them in isolation from one another, the role of oppression in shaping individual desires, and potential differences in moral status which are connected with differences in treatment.

It is the set of connections constituting women's continued oppression in our society which inspires feminists to resurrect the old slippery slope arguments to warn against IVF. We must recognize that women's existing lack of control in reproductive matters begins the debate on a pretty steep incline. Technology with the potential to further remove control of reproduction from women makes the slope very slippery indeed. This new technology, though offered under the guise of increasing reproductive freedom, threatens to result, in fact, in a significant decrease in freedom, especially since it is a technology that will always include the active involvement of designated specialists and will not ever be a private matter for the couple or women concerned.

Ethics ought not to direct us to evaluate individual cases without also looking at the implications of our decisions from a wide perspective. My argument is that a theory of feminist ethics provides that wider perspective, for its different sort of methodology is sensitive to both the personal and the social dimensions of issues. For that reason, I believe it is the only ethical perspective suitable for evaluating issues of this sort.

NOTES

1 H. Tristram Englehardt, *The Foundations of Bioethics* (Oxford: Oxford University Press 1986), 239.

2 Michael Bayles, *Reproductive Ethics* (Englewood Cliffs, NJ: Prentice-Hall 1984) 31.

3 Robert G. Edwards and David J. Sharpe, 'Social Values and Research in Human Embryology,' *Nature* 231 (May 14, 1971), 87.

4 Joseph Card Ratzinger and Alberto Bovone, 'Instruction on Respect for Human Life in Its Origin and on the Dignity of Procreation: Replies to Certain Questions of the Day' (Vatican City: Vatican Polyglot Press 1987), 33.

5 Ibid., 34.

6 Many authors are now working on an understanding of what feminist ethics entail. Among the Canadian papers I am familiar with are Kathryn Morgan's 'Women and Moral Madness,' Sheila Mullett's 'Only Connect: The Place of Self-Knowledge in Ethics,' both in this volume, and Leslie Wilson's 'Is a Feminine Ethics Enough?' *Atlantis* (forthcoming).

7 Susan Sherwin, 'A Feminist Approach to Ethics,' *Dalhousie Review* 64, 4 (Winter 1984–85) 704–13.

8 Kathryn Pyne Addelson, 'Moral Revolution,' in Marilyn Pearsall, ed., *Women and Values* (Belmont, CA: Wadsworth 1986), 291–309.

9 Carol Gilligan, *In a Different Voice* (Cambridge, MA: Harvard University Press 1982).

10 Nel Noddings, *Caring* (Berkeley: University of California Press 1984).

11 Annette Baier, 'What Do Women Want in a Moral Theory?' *Nous* 19 (March 1985) 53–64, and 'Trust and Antitrust,' *Ethics* 96 (January 1986) 231–60.

12 Linda Williams presents this position particularly clearly in her invaluable work 'But What Will They Mean for Women? Feminist Concerns About the New Reproductive Technologies,' No. 6 in the *Feminist Perspective* Series, CRIAW.

13 Marilyn Frye vividly describes the phenomenon of interrelatedness which supports sexist oppression by appeal to the metaphor of a bird cage composed of thin wires, each relatively harmless in itself, but, collectively, the wires constitute an overwhelming barrier to the inhabitant of the cage. Marilyn Frye, *The Politics of Reality: Essays in Feminist Theory* (Trumansburg, NY: The Crossing Press 1983), 4–7.

ETHICAL DEBATES ABOUT INFERTILITY AND ITS TREATMENT

The New York State Task Force on Life and the Law

In this reading, a chapter reprinted from a much longer report on assisted reproductive technologies, the task force begins by clarifying the issues involved in debates about how to define *infertility*. The task force then organizes the contemporary debate about the use of assisted reproductive technologies by distinguishing among three groups of commentators. One group of commentators is opposed to any use of assisted reproductive technology. A second group, emphasizing the importance of autonomous choice, is committed to the claim that individuals have a right to use the entire range of assisted reproductive technologies. A third group argues that the right to use assisted reproductive technologies is sometimes outweighed by competing societal interests. The task force concludes its discussion by considering different perspectives on the question of whether children can be harmed by the very technologies that allow them to be born.

With an increasing number of physicians now providing assisted reproductive technologies (ARTs) and more infertile people opting for these services, many segments of society seem already to have concluded that assisted reproduction is a reasonable response to fertility problems. According to some commentators, this conclusion reflects an assumption that those who are infertile will, and perhaps should, want to find a way to create a child who is genetically, or at least gestationally, related to them. Yet, some have challenged the wisdom of this assumption, criticizing societal pressures on women to achieve biological motherhood at all costs and expressing concern about both the risks and the limited success rates of the technologies involved.

This chapter reviews the debate over the appropriateness of using assisted reproduction as a response to infertility. The ethical implications of particular aspects of the practice of assisted reproduction are discussed in Part II of this report.

DEFINING INFERTILITY

Discussions of the appropriateness of using assisted reproduction as a response to infertility often begin with debates about how to define infertility. Many

The New York State Task Force on Life and the Law, *Assisted Reproductive Technologies: Analysis and Recommendations for Public Policy* (April 1998), Chapter 3, pp. 95–104.

commentators, as well as advocacy organizations representing infertile individuals, characterize infertility as a disease. These commentators argue that "diseases are physical or mental conditions of an organism that result in deviations from normal species function,"[1] and, at least for those who desire biological children, infertility is a deviation from normal function.[2] Noting that infertility can be caused by a range of physical conditions, they define the disease of infertility as "the result of specific physical dysfunctions in the reproductive organs and/or other bodily systems, including such conditions as congenital malformations of the reproductive organs, endometriosis, hormonal imbalances, and immunologic factors."[3] Some commentators argue that because infertility "adversely affects a basic and important human capacity,"[4] and because some people experience it as distressing and limiting, it should be assigned "a relatively high priority with respect to other disease states."[5]

A number of feminist commentators object to the characterization of infertility as a disease requiring medical treatment. They believe that society's approach to infertility is distorted by viewing it as an illness to be solved, rather than as a physical difference that people may or may not wish to take steps to affect.[6] As one commentator observes, "Medicalizing subfertility with the help of procreative technologies sets up norms: bodily norms, behavioral norms, ethical norms."[7] Once infertility is viewed as a medical condition, this commentator argues, the infertile woman is expected to obtain treatment to "normalize her into pregnancy."[8] Other commentators are also critical of the societal emphasis on treatment for infertility, noting that infertility specialists expect their patients to "pursue all available treatments," not acknowledging any difference in kind among the treatments or the possibility that medical treatment may not be the most reasonable solution for a particular patient.[9]

These critics also argue that the term "treatment" misrepresents what actually happens in assisted reproduction. In their view, assisted reproduction does not treat infertility but, instead, bypasses it. In fact, they argue, many of the women who are "treated" by the use of assisted reproduction do not suffer from any physical difference of their own, but are being treated for "a rather unusual 'disease' "—sterility—"that exists in another person, a male partner."[10]

Other commentators maintain that there are many instances in medicine when treatment does not cure the condition or disease but instead "modifies its expression," enabling the patient to achieve a desired goal.[11] As one commentator argues, "The fact that [ARTs] do not correct infertility, but only allow a person to overcome the functional deficit of the disease does not mean that their use is not medical treatment for a disease. Many medical and rehabilitative treatments, including many that are standardly covered by health care insurance, do not correct the underlying condition, but only correct for its attendant disability."[12] For example, just as assisted reproduction enables an infertile person to reproduce without restoring that person's fertility, glasses enable a visually-impaired person to see, insulin enables a diabetic to live, and a hearing aid enables a hearing-impaired person to hear, all without correcting the underlying medical problem.

One commentator proposes that infertility should be described as a disability rather than a disease. This nomenclature acknowledges both the inherently social nature of the problem and the fact that medical treatment may be an appropriate response.[13] This commentator maintains that characterizing infertility as a disability rather than a disease broadens the types of responses one will consider. In the case

of a disease, medical treatment is almost always viewed as the answer. In the case of a disability, medical treatment could cure or bypass the disability, but there are also "equally important non-medical ways of managing disability, ways that address the handicapping effects of the disability—like learning sign language, having wheelchair ramps, adopting babies."[14]

While the debate about how to define infertility may seem like a matter of semantics, commentators argue that the definition significantly affects both individual and societal responses. Some people note that unless infertility is viewed as a disease, it will be difficult to justify the provision of insurance coverage for assisted reproductive services, which could make these procedures accessible to many more infertile people.[15] Other people maintain that calling infertility a disease leads to the conclusion that medical treatment is the only proper response to the inability to conceive a child. In their view, this attitude reinforces society's expectation that all women will procreate and thus makes it more difficult for women to define themselves in other ways.[16] However, some commentators argue that the relevant question is not whether infertility is a disease, but whether particular responses to infertility are themselves appropriate. Even if infertility services "do not treat an illness or disease," these commentators maintain, they may be an appropriate use of medical services because they "relieve the misfortune of an impediment to the satisfaction of a desire for a 'good' in life not otherwise available."[17]

ASSISTED REPRODUCTION AS A RESPONSE TO INFERTILITY

Secular and religious commentators have expressed differing opinions on the appropriateness of using assisted reproduction as a response to infertility.[18] While some commentators oppose all ARTs, others defend the individual's right to use the entire range of available technologies. A third group supports the use of at least some of the technologies, but believes that in some cases their use must be limited to protect the interests of any children who might result and of society.

Opposition to Assisted Reproduction Some commentators reject assisted reproduction as a misguided solution to infertility. They maintain that making babies in a laboratory is a "degradation of parenthood."[19] One commentator, for example, argues that it is wrong to create a baby in a laboratory because it takes the creation of a child out of the marital relationship and inserts the practice of medicine and technology where it does not belong. He also argues that assisted reproduction is the "thin edge of the wedge," which will inevitably lead to the broader manipulation of genetic material in the laboratory and the utilization of science to create the perfect child.[20] According to this commentator, "Medical practice loses its way into an entirely different human activity—manufacture (which most wants to satisfy desires)—if it undertakes either to produce a child without curing infertility as a condition or to produce simply the desired sort of child."[21] Another commentator expresses a similar concern that assisted reproduction could lead to undesirable scientific advances. "The decisions we must now make," he notes, "may very well help to determine whether human beings will eventually be produced in laboratories. Once the genies let the babies into the bottle, it may be impossible to get them out again."[22]

Many of these commentators express particular concern about the impact of assisted reproduction on the way in which children are valued. They fear that "the child conceived through reproductive techniques becomes a means to an end of adult happiness, vanity, or obsession with genetic lineage."[23] Their concern is that the child will be viewed not as an invaluable and unique treasure but rather as a product valued for its cost and ostensible quality. Worried that children will be seen as just another product to be manufactured, bought, and sold, these commentators ask whether children are "more likely to flourish in a culture where making children is governed by the same rules that govern the making of automobiles or VCRs."[24]

Some commentators believe that the high cost of assisted reproduction will turn children into commodities from which parents will demand certain performance and perfection. The unattractive, slow, or disabled child will become unacceptable, in much the same way that a defective product is unacceptable and usually returned. These commentators are particularly concerned about the use of assisted re-production to prevent the creation of children with undesirable traits. While most commentators do not object to pre-implantation genetic testing or sex selection to avoid the transmission of genetic diseases, many object to these practices when they are used for "morally frivolous reasons."[25]

Some feminists also oppose the use of assisted reproduction but for different reasons. Echoing their criticism of viewing infertility as a disease, they argue that assisted reproduction represents yet another attempt by male doctors to dominate women's bodies, and that it reinforces the view of women as primarily mothers. "Although [in vitro fertilization] appears to offer more choices and hence more freedom to women," states one commentator, "in fact it threatens to undermine women's freedom in the long run. It does this both by reinforcing sex-role stereotypes in which a woman's worth is dependent upon her reproductive capacity and also by reinforcing the power of men in the reproductive sphere."[26] These commentators argue that we live in a society in which "to choose to be childless is still socially disapproved and to be childless in fact is to be stigmatized as selfish and uncaring. In such a situation, to offer the hope of becoming a mother to a childless woman is a coercive offer."[27] They believe that the very existence of technology that allows some infertile women to give birth to a genetically, or at least gestationally, related child pushes all infertile women, and women with infertile partners, to continue trying to reproduce despite the odds, rather than coming to terms with their infertility.[28]

Other commentators have raised objections to ARTs because of concerns that they "reflect and reinforce the racial hierarchy in America."[29] As one commentator notes, although black women have higher infertility rates than white women,[30] "one of the most striking features of the new reproduction is that it is used almost exclusively by white people."[31] She maintains that, in addition to the high cost of infertility treatment, this racial disparity results from deliberate efforts by physicians to steer black women away from assisted reproduction.[32] She also argues that the desire among some white people to have a genetically related child reflects a long tradition of efforts "to preserve white racial purity."[33]

Assisted Reproduction: An Autonomous Right

At the other end of the spectrum are those who believe that decisions about the use of assisted reproduction should be left to the individuals involved, with the state playing only a limited regulatory role.[34] These commentators believe that all forms of assisted reproduction can be acceptable as long as the individuals utilizing them behave responsibly. As one notes, "In vitro fertilization and techniques that allow us to study and control human reproduction are morally neutral instruments for the realization of profoundly important human goals, which are bound up with the realization of the good of others: children for infertile parents and greater health for the children that will be born."[35] These commentators dispute the contention that children created through assisted reproduction will inevitably be treated as commodities, arguing that "the critical issue is not whether something involves monetary exchange as one of its aspects, but whether it is treated as reducible solely to its monetary features."[36]

The position of these commentators is based in large part on a determination that individuals have a right to procreate, and that this right includes a right to procreate non-coitally.[37] Although the Supreme Court has not explicitly recognized an affirmative constitutional right to procreate, as opposed to the more limited right to avoid procreation, most commentators assume that such a right exists, at least within marriage.[38] This assumption is based in part on a strong tradition in this country "of regarding questions of reproduction and family life as private matters."[39]

In the case of assisted reproduction, many commentators argue that this tradition of procreative liberty and privacy requires respect for autonomy as the guiding principle for all decision making. As such, they support the regulation of assisted reproduction only when its purpose is to protect autonomous choice and prevent coercion. In general, they conclude that the best way to achieve these goals is through the process of informed consent. For a patient considering assisted reproduction, commentators suggest that informed consent should include counseling that provides complete information about the likelihood of success, the risks and costs of the procedure, and medical and lifestyle al-

ternatives available to the patient.[40] They also support state efforts to improve the quality of care available, as long as regulations "do not limit access to medically appropriate treatment."[41] In addition, they endorse regulations that provide uniform reporting of success rates of particular treatments and particular programs to protect the interests of patients as consumers.[42]

Some feminist commentators have adopted this autonomy-based view of assisted reproduction.[43] They believe that assisted reproduction increases women's reproductive freedom by expanding their choices about when to reproduce and allowing them to do so without a partner of the opposite sex.[44] They emphasize that with adequate informed consent women can be protected from exploitation by the commercial assisted reproduction market.[45] Some of these commentators believe that a technological solution to infertility is particularly appropriate in light of the fact that many women are infertile as a result of technological developments such as intrauterine devices and drugs such as diethylstilbestrol (DES). They conclude that "the drive to make use of the new reproductive technologies derives not simply from the fact of infertility, nor from its apparent increase, but from the social and medical circumstances under which infertility has been sustained."[46]

A Middle Ground In the middle are those commentators who believe that individuals have a right to choose assisted reproduction to enable them to create a family but that other interests may outweigh this right in certain circumstances. Commentators taking this position stress that procreative liberty, like other individual rights, is not an absolute and must always be balanced against the well-being of society and the best interests of existing children and the children who may be born as a result of ARTs.[47] They urge society to proceed cautiously, particularly when the technologies will have significant ramifications for people other than the individual or couple trying to reproduce.[48]

These commentators emphasize that the use of ARTs implicates important societal interests. Society has an interest in the impact of assisted reproduction on future generations, the effect on societal resources, and the implications for the value attached to human life. Society must also be concerned with the principle of beneficence, which emphasizes the impact of actions on others, in contrast to autonomy, which is concerned only with the protection of individual choice. As one commentator notes, "A commitment to the creation of a just society requires that an individual desire for genetically related children cannot be held up as an end commanding significant government resources and energy if as a 'good' it encourages the exploitation of vulnerable persons or fosters negative attitudes towards persons or groups of persons."[49]

Commentators taking this middle position recognize some of the concerns raised by opponents of assisted reproduction, particularly the risk that children will come to be viewed as commodities rather than individuals to be valued in their own right. In addition, many of these commentators express particular concern about third party participants in assisted reproduction, especially egg donors and surrogates, who may undergo significant medical risks without any possibility of direct benefit.[50] In general, however, these commentators conclude that the risks involved in assisted reproduction should be addressed by limiting or regulating particular practices rather than by prohibiting the use of the technologies entirely.

Some of these commentators emphasize the consequences of assisted reproduction for societal fairness or distributive justice. They ask whether substantial sums should be spent on assisted reproduction when there are children already born who need homes and infertile low-income women who cannot afford assisted reproduction but might benefit from money spent on preventive health measures or other forms of treatment.[51] These commentators maintain that concerted efforts to prevent infertility are at least as important, if not more so, than the continuing pursuit of new technological ways to bypass the infertile condition.[52]

Critics of the current emphasis on ARTs also note that while these technologies may be beneficial to a small, elite group of women who have the time and financial resources to pursue them, women as a social group would benefit much more if those resources were used to address breast cancer, AIDS, and the poverty that kills and maims many women and children. As one commentator notes, "The issue should not be increasing access to experimental, costly, and debilitating technologies but rather implementing priorities that prevent maternal morbidity and infant mortality as well as ensure basic access to nutrition, sanitation, prenatal care, and the prevention of disease."[53]

Harm to Children as the Critical Factor For many commentators, determining the best interests of children is the primary factor in assessing the appropriateness of particular types of ARTs.[54] The debate about the effect of assisted reproduction on the children who are created raises complex philosophical questions about whether children can be harmed by the technologies that allow them to be born.

Some commentators maintain that assisted reproduction can never harm the children who result because without assisted reproduction the children would not exist. As one commentator concludes, "Risking damage to offspring would not seem to wrong the offspring if it were not possible for them to be conceived or born without undergoing the risk of damage."[55] According to these commentators, this position is reflected in state court decisions refusing to recognize the tort of "wrongful life," which would allow an infant to recover damages from a physician who negligently failed to inform the infant's parents of fetal defects which, if known, might have prompted the parents to terminate the pregnancy that led to the infant's birth.[56]

Those who maintain that children can be harmed by the use of assisted reproduction respond that creating a child under certain circumstances can be wrong even if after birth the child would prefer life to nonexistence.[57] As one commentator notes, "Even if we cannot ascribe a preference for nonexistence to the child, surely we can say that this life is so awful that no one could possibly wish it for the child."[58] These commentators argue that "in deciding whether to have children, people should not only be concerned with their own interests in reproducing. They must think also, and perhaps primarily, of the welfare of the children they will bear. They should ask themselves, 'What kind of life is my child likely to have?'"[59]

According to several commentators, the claim that children cannot be harmed by assisted reproduction unless their life is worse than nonexistence reflects a failure to distinguish between the interests of existing children and those of children not yet conceived. One commentator argues that the view that children cannot be harmed by the technologies that allow them to exist "assumes that children with an interest in existing are waiting in a spectral world of nonexistence where their situation is less desirable than it would be were they released into this world."[60] This assumption is wrong, she argues, because unlike death, nonexistence before life is "neither good nor bad."[61] In comparison to such a state, a life of substantial suffering can indeed be harmful, even if a person already alive would prefer that life to no existence at all. Participants in a workshop on the ethics of reproductive medicine similarly concluded that "no one is ever harmed by not being born at all, by not being implanted into someone's uterus, but one can be very badly harmed if brought into the world with a lethal and terrible disease."[62]

Some commentators argue that it should not matter whether children can technically be "harmed" by the use of technologies that allow them to be born, because the use of those technologies can be "wrongful" even if they do not cause direct harm. One commentator, for example, maintains that when assisted reproduction leads to the birth of a child with a disease or disability that is serious but not so debilitating that the child would prefer never to have been born, it is possible to conclude that "the action is wrong, although the person who suffers the handicap is not harmed." Such "nonharmful wrongs," he concludes, might constitute "legitimate and possibly sufficient grounds for restricting procreative liberty."[63]

Those commentators who believe that children can be harmed by the use of assisted reproduction acknowledge the difficulty of determining the type of risks to a child that would make a decision to procreate ethically problematic. Noting the cultural variability of concepts of health, one commentator argues that such judgments must take into account "the nature of the disorder from which the child would suffer, the circumstances into which the child would be brought, and the ameliorative resources available for that child."[64] Ultimately, she argues,

the question to be determined is whether the child will be born with an "inadequate opportunity for health."[65] Another commentator similarly argues that the relevant question is whether the child will be born "in circumstances where there is not a decent minimum opportunity for development."[66]

NOTES

1 D. W. Brock, "Funding New Reproductive Technologies: Should They Be Included in Health Insurance Benefit Packages?" in *New Ways of Making Babies: The Case of Egg Donation,* ed. C. B. Cohen (Bloomington: Indiana University Press, 1996), 213, 224.

2 Ibid., 225.

3 RESOLVE, *Ethical Issues Related to Medical Treatment of Infertility* (Somerville, MA: RESOLVE, 1995), 4.

4 A. L. Caplan, "The Ethics of In Vitro Fertilization," *Primary Care* 13 (1986): 241, 249–250.

5 Ibid., 250.

6 J. G. Raymond, *Women as Wombs* (San Francisco: Harper, 1993), 2.

7 H. L. Nelson, "Dethroning Choice: Analogy, Personhood, and the New Reproductive Technologies," *Journal of Law, Medicine and Ethics* 23 (1995): 129, 133.

8 Ibid.

9 P. Lauritzen, *Pursuing Parenthood: Ethical Issues in Assisted Reproduction* (Bloomington: Indiana University Press, 1993), xiv–xv.

10 Raymond, 2–3.

11 R. G. Edwards, "Fertilization of Human Eggs in Vitro: A Defense," in *The Ethics of Reproductive Technology,* ed. K. D. Alpern (New York: Oxford University Press, 1992), 75.

12 Brock, "Funding," 225.

13 B. K. Rothman, *Recreating Motherhood* (New York: Norton, 1989), 143.

14 Ibid., 144.

15 For a discussion of the ethical debates surrounding insurance coverage for assisted reproduction, see Chapter 17, pages 433–435. [The chapter citation here, as in subsequent notes, refers to the task force report *Assisted Reproductive Technologies* (April 1998).]

16 P. Lauritzen, "What Price Parenthood?" *Hastings Center Report* 20, no. 2 (1990): 40.

17 J. Spike and J. Greenlaw, "Case Study: Ethics Consultation," *Journal of Law, Medicine and Ethics* 22 (1994): 348.

18 For a discussion of religious perspectives on assisted reproduction, see The New York State Task Force on Life and the Law, *Assisted Reproductive Technologies: Analysis and Recommendations for Public Policy* (April 1998), Chapter 4.

19 L. R. Kass, "Making Babies—The New Biology and the Old Morality," *Public Interest* 26 (1972): 49.

20 P. Ramsey, "Shall We 'Reproduce'? II; Rejoinders and Future Forecast," *Journal of the American Medical Association* 220 (1972): 1481.

21 Ibid., 1482.

22 L. R. Kass, "The Meaning of Life—In the Laboratory," in *The Ethics of Reproductive Technology,* 108.

23 M. M. Schultz, "Reproductive Technology and Intent-Based Parenthood: An Opportunity for Gender Neutrality," *Wisconsin Law Review* (1990): 297, 334.

24 T. H. Murray, "New Reproductive Technologies and the Family," in *New Ways of Making Babies,* 62.

25 Schultz, 364. For further discussion of pre-implantation genetic testing and sex selection, see New York State Task Force on Life and the Law, *Assisted Reproductive Technologies,* Chapter 7, pages 165–169.

26 K. Lebacqz, "Feminism and Bioethics: An Overview," *Second Opinion* 17, no. 2 (1991): 11.

27 Lauritzen, "What Price Parenthood?" 40 (describing feminist positions).

28 M. A. Warren, "IVF and Women's Interests: An Analysis of Feminist Concerns," *Bioethics* 2 (1988): 37, 45.

29 D. E. Roberts, "Race and the New Reproduction," *Hastings Law Journal* 47 (1996): 935, 937.

30 Ibid., 939.

31 Ibid., 937.

32 Ibid., 940.

33 Ibid., 943.

34 Ethics Committee of the American Fertility Society, "Ethical Considerations of Assisted Reproductive Technologies," *Fertility and Sterility* 62, Supplement 1 (1994): 13S.

35 H. T. Engelhardt, Jr., *The Foundations of Bioethics* (New York: Oxford University Press, 1986), 241.

36 Schultz, "Reproductive Technology," 336.

37 J. A. Robertson, "Embryos, Families, and Procreative Liberty: The Legal Structure of the New Reproduction," *Southern California Law Review* 59 (1986): 939, 960.

38 See New York State Task Force on Life and the Law, *Assisted Reproductive Technologies,* Chapter 6, pages 135–137.

39 A. M. Capron, "The New Reproductive Possibilities: Seeking a Moral Basis for Concerted Action in a Pluralistic Society," *Law, Medicine and Health Care* (1984): 193.

40 J. A. Nisker, "A User-Friendly Framework for Exploration of Ethical Issues in Reproductive Medicine," *Assisted Reproduction Reviews* 5 (1995): 273.

41 RESOLVE, *Statements of Principle* (Somerville, MA: RESOLVE, 1995).

42 Ibid.

43 Warren, "IVF and Women's Interests," 41–42.

44 Brock, "Funding," 222.

45 Raymond, *Women as Wombs,* 88; Warren, 38–39.

46 J. H. Hollinger, "From Coitus to Commerce: Legal and Social Consequences of Noncoital Reproduction," *Journal of Law Reform* 18 (1985): 865, 876.

47 Lauritzen, *Pursuing Parenthood,* 66–67; C. B. Cohen, "Unmanaged Care: The Need to Regulate New Reproductive Technologies in the United States," *Bioethics* 11 (1997): 348, 360 ("The reproductive interests of those who are subfertile must be weighed against the harm and wrong that fulfilling those interests might do to the resulting children, to third party participants, to those persons themselves, and to society.").

48 Lauritzen, *Pursuing Parenthood,* 67.

49 M. A. Ryan, "The Argument for Unlimited Procreative Liberty: A Feminist Critique," *Hastings Center Report* 20, no. 4 (1990): 6, 12.

50 See New York State Task Force on Life and the Law, *Assisted Reproductive Technologies,* Chapter 10, page 243.

51 Ryan, "A Feminist Critique," 12; Roberts, "Race," 948; E. Bartholet, *Family Bonds: Adoption and the Politics of Parenting* (Boston: Houghton Mifflin, 1993), 36–37.

52 Warren, "IVF and Women's Interests," 49.

53 Raymond, *Women as Wombs,* 137.

54 C. B. Cohen, "'Give Me Children or I Shall Die!' New Reproductive Technologies and Harm to Children," *Hastings Center Report* 26, no. 2 (1996): 19, 26.

55 Robertson, "Embryos," 988; see also J. A. Robertson, *Children of Choice: Freedom and the New Reproductive Technologies* (Princeton: Princeton University Press, 1994), 75–76.

56 See, e.g., *Becker v. Schwartz,* 46 N.Y.2d 401, 386 N.E.2d 807 (1978). A few courts have allowed such claims. See *Procanik v. Cillo,* 478 A.2d 722 (N.J. 1984); *Harbeson v. Parke-Davis,* 656 P.2d 483 (Wash. 1983); *Turpin v. Sortini,* 643 P.2d 954 (Cal. 1982).

57 B. Steinbock and R. McClamrock, "When Is Birth Unfair to the Child?" *Hastings Center Report* 24, no. 6 (1994): 15.

58 B. Steinbock, *Life Before Birth* (New York: Oxford University Press, 1992), 120.

59 Steinbock and McClamrock, 17.

60 Cohen, "Give Me Children," 21.

61 Ibid., 23.

62 B. Steinbock, "Workshop Summary: Ethics of Reproductive Medicine: Responsibilities and Challenges," *Assisted Reproduction Reviews* 7 (1997): 39.

63 D. W. Brock, "Book Review: *Children of Choice: Freedom and the New Reproductive Technologies,*" *Texas Law Review* 74 (1995): 187, 204–205.

64 Cohen, "Give Me Children," 25.

65 Ibid., 24.

66 C. Strong, *Ethics in Reproductive and Perinatal Medicine: A New Framework* (New Haven: Yale University Press, 1997), 92.

ASSISTED REPRODUCTION

President's Council on Bioethics

In this selection, the President's Council on Bioethics begins by providing a rich description of state-of-the-art practice in the field of "assisted reproduction," understanding by that phrase IVF and closely related procedures. Next, the council expresses concern about "the intersection of two key factors": (1) Technologies in the field of assisted reproduction are sometimes introduced into clinical practice without adequate testing; (2) The vulnerability of patients suffering from infertility may lead them to take undue risks. Finally, the council surveys the risk factors associated with assisted reproduction, first in reference to the children born as a result of these technologies, then in reference to the women who choose to use them.

I. TECHNIQUES AND PRACTICES

Most methods of assisted reproduction involve five discrete phases: (1) collection and preparation of gametes; (2) fertilization; (3) transfer of an embryo or multiple embryos to a woman's uterus; (4) pregnancy; and (5) delivery and birth. We will discuss each phase separately. . . .

A. Collection and Preparation of Gametes The precursors of human life are the gametes: sperm and ova. Parents seeking to conceive through assisted reproduction usually provide their own gametes. In the United States in the year 2001, 75.2 percent of the ART [assisted reproductive technology] cycles undertaken used never-frozen, non-donor ova or embryos and another 13.7 percent used frozen non-donor ova or embryos. Of the remaining 11.1 percent of cycles using donor embryos, the breakdown is as follows: 3.2 percent of the embryos were previously cryopreserved, and 8 percent were not.[1] . . .

Acquiring ova for use in artificial reproduction is significantly more onerous, painful, and risky than acquiring sperm (though its risks are still low in absolute terms). In the normal course of ovulation, one mature oocyte is produced per menstrual cycle. However in assisted reproduction—to increase the probability of success—many more ova are typi-

cally retrieved and fertilized. Thus, the ova source (who is usually also the gestational mother) undergoes a drug-induced process intended to stimulate her ovaries to produce many mature oocytes in a single cycle. This procedure, commonly referred to as "superovulation," requires the daily injection of a synthetic gonadatropin analog, accompanied by frequent monitoring using blood tests and ultrasound examinations. This treatment begins midway through the previous menstrual cycle and continues until just before ova retrieval. The synthetic gonadatropin analogs give the clinician greater control over ovarian stimulation and prevent premature release of the ova. . . .

When blood testing and ultrasound monitoring suggest that the ova are sufficiently mature, the clinician attempts to harvest them. This is typically achieved by ultrasound-guided transvaginal aspiration. In this procedure, a needle guided by ultrasound is inserted through the vaginal wall and into the mature ovarian follicles. An ovum is withdrawn (along with some fluid) from each follicle. This is an outpatient procedure. Risks and complications are low, but may include accidental puncture of nearby organs such as the bowel, ureter, bladder, or blood vessels, as well as the typical risks accompanying outpatient surgery (for example, risks related to administration of anesthesia, infection, etc.).

Once sperm and ova have been collected, they are cultured and treated to maximize the probability of success. . . .

Reprinted from President's Council on Bioethics, *Reproduction & Responsibility: The Regulation of New Biotechnologies* (2004), Chapter 2. Many notes omitted.

B. Fertilization Once the ova and sperm have been properly prepared, the clinician attempts to induce fertilization—the union of sperm and ovum culminating in the fusion of their separate pronuclei and the initiation of a new, integrated, self-directing organism. It is common practice to attempt to fertilize all available ova.[2] Fertilization can be achieved through a number of means including (1) "classical" IVF, (2) gamete intrafallopian transfer (GIFT), (3) intracytoplasmic sperm injection (ICSI). . . .

IVF is the most common method of artificial fertilization. In 2001, it was used by 99 percent of ART patients. As noted previously, both sperm and ovum are cultured to maximize the probability of fertilization. The ova are examined and rated for maturity in an effort to calculate the optimal time for fertilization. They are usually placed in a tissue culture medium and left undisturbed for two to twenty-four hours. . . . Once the gametes are adequately prepared, thousands of tiny droplets of sperm are placed in the culture medium containing a single ovum. After 24 hours, each of the oocytes is examined to determine whether fertilization has occurred.

GIFT was introduced in 1984 as an alternative to standard IVF. Today, attempts at fertilization via GIFT are rare. In 2001, they accounted for less than 1 percent of all attempts at fertilization used by ART patients. As the name suggests, fertilization using GIFT occurs within the woman's body. Ovarian stimulation and retrieval are performed in the same manner as in IVF. In a single procedure, ova are retrieved, combined with the sperm outside the body, and then transferred back into the fallopian tube where it is hoped that fertilization itself will occur. . . .

A new and increasingly popular technique for fertilization is intracytoplasmic sperm injection. As the name implies, with ICSI, ovum-sperm fusion is accomplished not by chance, but by injecting a single sperm directly into an oocyte. . . . A single sperm is selected and drawn into a thin pipette from which it is injected into the cytoplasm of the ovum cell.

ICSI is indicated in cases of severe male-factor infertility, in which male patients have either malformed sperm or an abnormally low sperm count. ICSI is also ideal for patients whose sperm would not otherwise penetrate the exterior of an oocyte. ICSI was used in 49.2 percent of all ART cycles in 2001. However, 42.2 percent of those ICSI cycles were undertaken by couples *without* male-factor infertility. The growing popularity of this technique most likely has to do with the wish to increase the control over, and success rates for, fertilization: ICSI, unlike standard IVF, guarantees the entrance of a single sperm directly into a single egg. . . .

Because in many cases not all embryos are transferred in each cycle, cryopreservation of embryos has become an integral part of ART.[3] . . . A recently reported study by the Society for Assisted Reproductive Technology and RAND estimates that 400,000 embryos are in cryostorage in the United States.[4]

Most ART patients do not receive cryopreserved embryos. In 2001, only 14 percent of all ART cycles involved transfer of frozen embryos. The rate of live births for cycles using cryopreserved embryos is significantly lower than it is for never-frozen embryos (23.4 percent versus 33.4 percent). Experts estimate that only 65 percent of frozen embryos survive the thawing process. There are, however, incentives for couples to use cryopreserved embryos; doing so eliminates the cost and effort of further oocyte retrieval. This can decrease the cost of a future cycle by roughly $6,000. . . . Cryopreservation also reduces pressure to implant all embryos at once, thus reducing the risk of high-order multiple pregnancies.

C. Transfer . . . Typically, the embryos are transferred on the second or third day after fertilization, at the four- to eight-cell stage. To maximize the probability of implantation, some clinicians cultivate embryos until the blastocyst stage (five days after fertilization) before transferring them to the uterus. . . .

Once the embryos have been selected and prepared, they are transferred into the uterus. The total number of embryos transferred per cycle varies, usually according to the age of the recipient. For women under 35, the average number of never-frozen embryos transplanted per transfer procedure was 2.8. For women 35 to 37, 38 to 40, and 41 to 42, the average numbers of never-frozen embryos transplanted per transfer procedure were, respectively, 3.1, 3.4, and 3.7. . . .

Typically embryos are transferred into the uterus using a catheter. The catheter is inserted through the woman's cervix and the embryos are injected into her uterus (along with some amount of the culture fluid). This procedure does not require anesthesia. Following injection, the patient must lie still for at least one hour. While the transfer procedure is regarded as simple, different practitioners tend to achieve different outcomes.

An alternative method of embryo transfer is zygote intrafallopian transfer (ZIFT). In ZIFT, the embryo is placed (via laparoscopy) directly into the fallopian tube, rather than into the uterus. In this way, it is similar to the transfer of gametes in GIFT. Some individuals opt for ZIFT on the theory that it enhances the likelihood of implantation, given that the embryo matures en route to the uterus, presumably as it would in natural conception and implantation. Additionally, many patients prefer ZIFT to GIFT because the process of fertilization and early development of the embryo may be monitored. However, ZIFT remains a rare choice, accounting for 0.8 percent of all ART cycles in 2001.

D. Pregnancy Successful implantation of an embryo in the uterine lining marks the beginning of pregnancy. In 2001, 32.8 percent of the ART cycles undertaken resulted in clinical pregnancy.[5] This number varied according to patient age. . . .

Multiple gestations are common among pregnancies facilitated by assisted reproductive technologies. The rate of multiple-fetus pregnancies from ART cycles using never-frozen, nondonor ova or embryos in 2001 was 36.7 percent. For the same time period, the multiple infant birth rate in the United States was 3 percent. The extraordinarily high rate of multiple pregnancies resulting from assisted reproduction is almost entirely attributable to the transfer of multiple embryos per cycle.

In an effort to reduce the risks of multiple pregnancy, practitioners sometimes employ a procedure termed "fetal reduction," the reduction in the number of fetuses in utero by selective abortion. Fetuses are selected for destruction based on size, position, and viability (in the clinician's judgment). The clinician, using ultrasound for guidance, inserts a needle through the mother's abdomen (transabdominal

multifetal reduction) through the uterine wall. The clinician then administers a lethal injection to the heart of the selected fetus—typically potassium chloride. The dead fetus's body decomposes and is resorbed. To be effective, transabdominal multifetal reduction must be performed at ten to twelve weeks' gestation. In an alternative procedure, transvaginal multifetal reduction, a needle is inserted through the vagina. Transvaginal multifetal reduction must be performed between six and eight weeks gestation (eight weeks is recommended).

E. Delivery In 2001, for never-frozen nondonor ova or embryos, the overall rate of live births per cycle[6] was 27 percent (33.4 percent live births per transfer).[7] Among these pregnancies, 82.2 percent resulted in live births. Of these resulting 21,813 live births, 35.8 percent were multiple infant births (32 percent twins and 3.8 percent triplets or more). . . .

F. Disposition of Unused Embryos As mentioned above, in many cases of ART there are in vitro embryos that remain untransferred following a successful cycle. There are five possible outcomes for such an embryo: (1) it may remain in cryostorage until transferred into the mother's uterus in a future ART cycle; (2) it may be donated to another person or couple seeking to initiate a pregnancy; (3) it may be donated for purposes of research; (4) it may remain in cryostorage indefinitely; or (5) it may be thawed and destroyed. . . .

II. ETHICAL CONSIDERATIONS

The development and practice of assisted reproductive technologies have yielded great goods. They have relieved the suffering of many who are afflicted with infertility, helping them to conceive biologically related children. Yet these activities also raise a variety of ethical issues. Some concern the well-being of the participants in assisted reproduction. . . .

The intersection of two key factors—patient vulnerability and novel (in some cases untested) technology—defines much of the arena of concern. First, assisted reproduction is generally practiced on patients who are experiencing great emotional strain. When it succeeds it can be a source of great joy—as it has been for tens of thousands of parents each year. But success is far from universal, especially for older patients; and even when it happens, the process and the circumstances surrounding it can be difficult to bear. Those suffering from infertility often come to practitioners of assisted reproduction after prolonged periods of failure and dismay. This vulnerability may lead some individuals to take undue risks (such as to insist on transferring an unduly large number of embryos). The occasional irresponsible clinician may even pressure patients to take such risks, for the sake of improving his reportable success rates.

Second, some assisted reproductive technologies have been used in clinical practice without prior rigorous testing in primates or studies of long-term outcomes. IVF itself was performed on at least 1,200 women before it was reported to have been performed on chimps, although it had been extensively investigated in rabbits, hamsters, and mice. The same is true for ICSI. The reproductive use of ICSI was first introduced by Belgian researchers in 1992. Two years later, relying on a two-study review of safety and efficacy, ASRM (The American Society for Reproductive Medicine) declared ICSI to be a "clinical" rather than "experimental" procedure. Yet the first nonhuman primate conceived by ICSI was born only in 1997 and the first successful ICSI procedure in mice was reported in 1995. Absent long-term studies of the children conceived using ICSI or other novel procedures, it is unclear to what extent these alterations in the ART process affect the health and development of the children so conceived. . . .

A. Well-Being of the Child The central figure in the process of assisted reproduction, directly affected by every action taken but incapable of consenting to such actions, is the child born with the aid of ART. Each intervention or stage in the ART process might affect this child's health and well-being: gamete retrieval and preparation, fertilization, embryo culture, embryo transfer, pregnancy, and of course birth. . . .

There have been very few comprehensive or long-term studies of the health and well-being of children born using ART, although more than 170,000 such children have been born in the United States. The fact that no major investigation or public study has yet been called for in this area might suggest that there is no discernible health crisis in assisted reproduction, as does the fact that demand for ART has grown substantially and continuously since its inception. At the same time, however, our ability to know this with certainty is limited, both because of the absence of major longitudinal studies of the well-being of children born using different assisted reproduction techniques, and because the oldest person conceived through ART is only in her mid-twenties.

Some recent studies have associated various birth defects and developmental difficulties with the uses of various technologies and practices of assisted reproduction. None of these studies provide a causal link between ART and the dysfunctions observed, and some commentators have taken issue with some of the methodologies used. Nevertheless, these findings have raised some concerns. One such study concluded that children conceived by assisted reproduction are twice as likely to suffer major birth defects as children conceived without such assistance.[8] Other recent studies have reached similar conclusions. Additional studies have associated the use of assisted reproduction technologies with a higher incidence of diseases and malformations, including Beckwith-Wiedemann syndrome (BWS),[9] . . .

While many are concerned about the increased risk to children suggested by these studies, the overall incidence of such harms is low enough that infertile couples have not been deterred in their efforts to conceive using IVF or ICSI. Indeed, ART clinicians (and in some cases the authors of these studies) advise their patients that such data should not dissuade them from pursuing infertility treatment.

ICSI has raised concerns among some observers largely for the very reasons that it has proven so successful as a means of fertilization: ICSI circumvents the ovum's natural barrier against sperm otherwise incapable of insemination. Some suspect that removing this barrier may permit a damaged sperm (for example, aneuploid or with damaged DNA) to fertilize an ovum, resulting in spontaneous abortion or harm to the resulting child. Some male ART patients have a gene mutation or a chromosomal deletion that renders them infertile. Yet, if a sperm can be retrieved from these patients, they may be able to conceive a child via ICSI, possibly passing along the genetic abnormality to the resulting child. . . .

It is a matter of concern that there have been few longitudinal studies analyzing the long-term effects of ICSI on the children born with its aid. The Belgian group that pioneered ICSI has collected a database that details neonatal outcome and congenital malformations in children conceived through ICSI. But there do not seem to be any ongoing or published studies of this kind investigating the long-term effects of ICSI beyond the neonatal stage. . . .

Multiple gestations, far more common in the context of assisted reproduction than in natural conception, have a higher incidence of adverse impacts on the health of the children born. Such pregnancies greatly increase the risk of prenatal death. Multiple pregnancies are also more likely to lead to premature birth; and prematurity is associated with myriad health problems including serious infection, respiratory distress syndrome, and heart defects. One in ten children born following high-order pregnancies dies before one year of age. Children born following a multiple pregnancy are at greater risk for such disabilities as blindness, respiratory dysfunction, and brain damage. Moreover, infants born following such a pregnancy tend to have an extremely low birthweight, which is itself associated with a number of health problems, including some that manifest themselves only later in life, such as hypertension, cardiac disease, stroke, and osteoporosis in middle age. Interestingly, the higher incidence of low birthweight may not be limited to infants born from multiple pregnancies. According to recent studies, singletons born with the aid of ART tend to have an abnormally high incidence of prematurity and low birthweight.

So-called "fetal reduction" aims to reduce the problems associated with multiple pregnancy. But fetal reduction is itself potentially associated with a number of adverse effects on the children who remain following the procedure. . . .

Taken together, the significance of these various studies is uncertain. They raise a broad range of concerns, but the scale of the research has been limited. In many cases, there are observed correlations between ART and a higher incidence of certain health problems in the resulting children. But in most studies, there is no demonstrable causal relationship between a particular facet of ART and the undesirable health effect. Infertile individuals seeking assisted reproduction may be disproportionately afflicted with heritable disorders, and these may in part account for the higher incidence of birth and developmental abnormalities in ART children compared to those conceived in vivo. The results are therefore still preliminary. The need seems clear for more data to determine what risks, if any, different assisted reproduction techniques present to the well-being of the future child. Moreover, in cases where ART is the only available means for individuals or couples to conceive a biologically related child, it is an important ethical and social question what level of increased risk can be privately justified by patients and doctors, and what level of increased risk should be publicly justified by society as a whole, especially should the society bear the costs of caring for any resulting health problems.

B. Well-Being of Women in the ART Process Another concern is for the well-being of the women who participate directly in the process of assisted reproduction.

Aside from the discomforts and burdens of ovarian stimulation and monitoring, there are also some risks attached to hormonal stimulation. One such risk is "ovarian hyperstimulation syndrome," characterized by dramatic enlargement of the ovaries and fluid imbalances that can be (in extreme cases) life threatening. Complications can include rupture of the ovaries, cysts, and cancers. The reported incidence of severe ovarian hyperstimulation syndrome is between 0.5 and 5.0 percent. Additionally, adverse side effects of the hormones administered during superovulation have included memory loss, neurological dysfunction, cardiac disorders, and even sudden death. There do not appear to be any studies on the incidence of such side effects. . . .

Multiple pregnancies are far more common following ART, owing especially to the practice of transferring multiple embryos but also to the higher incidence of spontaneous twinning with any single embryo. Multiple pregnancies pose greater risks to mothers than do singleton pregnancies. A woman carrying multiple fetuses has a greater chance of suffering from high blood pressure, anemia, or pre-eclampsia. Because multiple-gestation pregnancies are generally more taxing on the mother's body, they are likelier to aggravate pre-existing medical conditions. Moreover, such pregnancies expose the woman to higher risks of uterine rupture, placenta previa, or abruption. . . .

NOTES

1 Centers for Disease Control and Prevention (CDC), *2001 Assisted Reproductive Technology Success Rates, National Summary and Fertility Clinic Reports,* Atlanta, Georgia: Government Printing Office, 2003, p. 14. [Subsequent figures cited for 2001 also derive from this document.]

2 The number of ova collected depends on a number of variables, including the donor's age, health, and other factors. In some cases, ten or more ova are fertilized in a single cycle.

3 There is not yet a reliable method of freezing unfertilized ova. This is perhaps due to their large size and high water content. Additionally, it seems that freezing an ovum toughens the zona pellucida in a way that can inhibit sperm penetration.

4 Hoffman, D., et al., "Cryopreserved Embryos in the United States and Their Availability for Research," *Fertility and Sterility* 79: 1063–1069 (2003).

5 This statistic is for never-frozen, nondonor ova or embryos—the most common approach in 2001.

6 A "cycle" is initiated when a woman begins the process of superovulation and monitoring. (CDC Report, p. 4.) Not all cycles result in successful ova collection, fertilization, transfer, pregnancy, or birth.

7 There seems to be a negative association between cryopreservation and implantation. For all pregnancies initiated using frozen, nondonor embryos, the success rate was 20.3 percent live births per transfer. . . .

8 Hansen, M., et al., "The Risk of Major Birth Defects After Intracytoplasmic Sperm Injection and In Vitro Fertilization," *The New England Journal of Medicine* 346: 725 (2002). Specifically, among the children in the study conceived by IVF, 9 percent were diagnosed with a major birth defect or defects by the age of one year. Among children conceived using ICSI, the rate was 8.6 percent. The incidence of such abnormalities among children in the study who were conceived by natural means was 4.2 percent.

9 Researchers at Johns Hopkins University noted that among the patients listed in the 1994 Beckwith-Wiedemann registry, IVF conception was six times more common than in the general population. That is, 4.6 percent of the patients in the registry were conceived through IVF, as compared with 0.8 percent of the national population. Children with BWS have symptoms that can include an abnormally large tongue (which can cause respiratory difficulties), abdominal wall defects (including umbilical hernia and protrusion of intestine or other abdominal organs from the child's navel), low blood sugar, lethargy, poor feeding, seizures, and enlargement of organs and some tissues. BWS sufferers are predisposed to Wilms' tumor, hepatoblastoma, neuroblastoma, and other cancers. Despite their findings, JHU researchers suggested that parents should not alter their plans to use IVF. See, for example, DeBaun, M. R., et al., "Association of in vitro fertilization with Beckwith-Wiedemann syndrome and epigenetic alterations of LIT_1 and H_{19}," *American Journal of Human Genetics* 72: 156–160 (2003).

GAMETE DONATION AND SURROGACY

FAMILIES, THE MARKETPLACE, AND VALUES: NEW WAYS OF MAKING BABIES

Thomas H. Murray

Murray argues that alternative reproductive practices should be judged morally unacceptable to the extent that they fail to cohere with or threaten to undermine values at the core of family life. He argues explicitly against a competing framework of moral analysis, according to which reproductive liberty and marketplace values are of overriding significance. Indeed, Murray argues against any intrusion of marketplace values into the realm of family life. He is not opposed to third-party involvement in reproduction, but he is opposed to the *commercialization* of such involvement. Thus, he objects to commercial surrogacy, and he objects to the practice of paying men for providing their sperm and paying women for providing their ova.

... The values embedded in certain alternative reproductive practices form a constellation that aligns poorly with other values at the heart of family life. Two contrasting images of values and relationships within families illustrate the point.

The champion of procreative liberty celebrates control and choice and portrays decisions about whether and how to acquire children as similar to decisions to acquire other new entities, only more important than most. If choice is valued in selecting a new appliance, all the more should it be valued in selecting a new child. If we are permitted to make voluntary agreements to spend our money to obtain new objects, all the more important to allow us similar freedom of contract and commerce to obtain new children, with one caveat: the children should not be harmed.

The other image is harder to label. It sees a role for values like control and choice within families but insists that these are not the principal values for which we make families; it is aware of the tension between unbridled liberty and control, on the one hand, and the values at the core of family life, on the other. It is vigilant against the encroachment of marketplace values into the family sphere because it recognizes that in commercial relationships the goal is to purchase a good or service, not to deepen the relationship, whereas all that is most valuable in family life centers on nurturing relationships.[1] Potential ways of adding children to the family must be scrutinized to assure that they will not undermine the values sought in family life, now or in the long run.[2]

In a defense of cloning human embryos, John Robertson, an ardent exponent of reproductive liberty, argues that couples wishing to "adopt" (his word) an embryo that is a clone of already living children should know all they want to know about those children. He says, "The right of adoptive parents to receive as full information as possible about the children whom they seek to adopt is increasingly recognized. There is no reason why the same principle should not apply to embryo 'adoptions.' Even though the couple seeking the embryos will be

choosing embryos on the basis of expected characteristics, such a choice is neither invalid nor immoral."[3] A couple, that is, may exercise quality control through choice.

The emphasis here on control and choice does not fit well with our understanding of families. Good families are characterized more by acceptance than control. Furthermore, families are the preeminent realm of unchosen obligations. We may choose our spouses (although a persuasive argument could be made that for most of us this choice bears scarce resemblance to the model of rational, autonomous, carefully considered decision making). We may choose to have a child, but—unless we are "adopting" one of Robertson's cloned embryos—we do not choose to have this *particular* child, with its interests, moods, and manners. And as offspring, we certainly did not choose our parents. Yet most of us would agree that we do have moral obligations to our parents, as well as to our spouses and children. An interesting problem for an ethics that enshrines autonomous choice as the fundamental requirement for moral obligation is this: How do you explain the enormously powerful web of moral obligations that supports family life, despite the only partly chosen or wholly unchosen nature of those relationships?

Some of the new reproductive practices require enlisting third parties. Women or men supply gametes, couples provide embryos, and women gestate their own or someone else's fetus. Justifying the involvement of third parties usually builds on the values of choice and control and invokes liberty. The question immediately arises, Why would any third party agree to participate in another couple's effort to have a child? For many people the answer is obvious: money. Robertson states the case bluntly: "If collaborative reproduction is viewed positively, reproduction contracts become the instruments of reproductive freedom."[4] He acknowledges the implication of this view:

Legal liberty allows persons to treat each other as means to reproductive ends, with their negotiating ability and other resources determining the fate of future offspring. The extracorporeal embryo, that potent symbol of human life, becomes subject to the vagaries of a market that drives people to buy or sell reproductive factors and services. Yet such freedom also allows people to determine and satisfy their welfare more efficaciously than by government prescription. In liberal society, the invisible hand of procreative preference must be allowed to flourish, despite the qualms of those who think it debases our humanity.[5]

Freedom equals the right to make a contract, to welcome, in Robertson's memorable paraphrase of Adam Smith, "the invisible hand of procreative preference." The price we pay for that freedom, including a market for human embryos, is the necessary cost of liberty, or so Robertson argues. With admirable tenacity, Robertson leads us down the reproductive path paved by the values of the market—individual liberty, choice, personal preference, contract, and commercialization. We are now in a position to see where we have arrived—and what beautiful, perhaps fragile, shoots have been bulldozed in the rush to build this particular highway.

The difference between the two images is clearest in their responses to surrogate motherhood for pay. How does a paid surrogate childbearer explain to her other children what has happened? Does she say, "Mommy loves her children so much that she wants to give another woman a chance to have her own children to love"? Does she add, "Oh, by the way, it also lets us buy groceries/pay off the mortgage/go to Disney World/finish the third floor"? What do her children think about their own security? Their relationship with their parents? What have they learned about the nature of the parent-child relationship? Have they learned that it is subject to the same harsh rules of supply and demand as any other commodity? Will such doubts make them more secure, contribute to their emotional development?

What of the surrogate herself? David H. Smith observes that the surrogate contract signed by Mary Beth Whitehead, biological mother of the famous Baby M, gave striking power over Mrs. Whitehead to William Stern, her fetus's biological father. Indeed, the contract gave Mr. Stern "rights Whitehead's husband would not have had if he and Whitehead had engendered a child." Smith grants the appeal of such control to the Sterns, but he worries about the "status they impose upon the surrogate, whose entire life is subordinated to 'the delivery of a product' for another."[6] He considers the analogy of surrogacy to slavery, admitting that there are important dissimilarities but insisting that "surrogacy is like slavery in the absence of reciprocity, in the fact that one person becomes what Aristotle called an 'animated tool' of another, serving simply as a means to another's end."[7]

We need to think not only about the impact on those directly and immediately involved but also about the values, practices, and institutions that affect families now and in the future. Are children likely to flourish in a culture where making children is governed by the same rules that govern the making of automobiles or VCRs? Or is their flourishing more assured in a culture where making children, and matching children with nurturing adults, is treated as a sphere separate from the marketplace, a sphere governed by the ethics of gift and relationship, not contract and commerce?

My claim is not that a market in children, embryos, or gametes violates some abstract principle in the noumenal realm. Rather, it is that given the sort of creatures we humans are, our patterns of psychosocial development, our needs at different stages of our lives—given these facts, certain values, institutions, and practices support our mutual flourishing better than others. Specifically, the values of the marketplace are ill suited for nurturing the values, institutions, and practices that support the flourishing of children and adults within families.

A market in gametes, or even in offspring, might not be a moral and social problem for other sorts of creatures for whom rationality is preeminent. But such a market is a threat for us humans who need affection, trust, and, above all, intimate and enduring relationships in order to flourish.

Note that I did not say that those hypothetical beings for whom a reproductive market might be acceptable were more *rational*—only that for them rationality is preeminent. What would it take for us humans to be most rational in understanding the ethical and policy implications of alternative means of reproduction? It would make no sense whatsoever to ignore what sort of creatures we really are, what circumstances are most conducive to our mutual flourishing. No doubt, there is disagreement about just what institutions and practices are the most likely to support our flourishing. But responsible practical moral reasoning cannot wish such matters away. We cannot honestly pretend to resolve these questions with a strictly moral or legal argument—an appeal to individual autonomy or reproductive liberty, for example. We must take into account factual as well as moral considerations in our practical moral judgments.

Some reproductive alternatives are more troubling than others. For a variety of reasons, a man might produce some normal sperm but not be able to place enough of them in a good position to reach an ovum ready for fertilization. Artificially inseminating a woman with her husband's sperm, for example, strikes most people as eminently acceptable. (The Roman Catholic church is an exception to this general chorus of approval.) Using another man's sperm is more complicated morally.

The usual practice in the United States, known as artificial insemination by donor, or AID, is a misnomer. The "donor" is usually paid for his sperm, making him a sperm vendor. I think this is a serious confusion, not a minor semantic quibble. Calling the supplier of sperm a donor invokes the realm of gifts, and with it the sphere of family and friendship. In commercial sperm banks, the vendors are actually anonymous strangers, paid for their "product" and then sent away, with presumably no more interest in what happens to it subsequently than a seller of office supplies has with what happens to his or her Post-it notes™. Some men who sell or donate sperm discover later that they care about what has happened to it.[8] This is evidence that the market is a poor description of what transpires when gametes are transferred from one party to another. Because the market fails as a description, it is unlikely to be a faithful guide to ethical understanding as well.

So far, discussions about the ethics of alternative reproduction in the United States have paid scant attention to the practice of paying for sperm. The prospect of a man sitting in a booth and ejaculating into a container is the source of many jokes. But if I am correct about the dangers of the values of the market intruding on the sphere of the family, then AIV—artificial insemination by vendor—

should make us uneasy. Not because of any sexual squeamishness, but because commerce in this realm may threaten what is genuinely valuable within it. Using gametes provided by another man raises other morally relevant difficulties.[9] Even if, as seems likely, those are outweighed by the good of creating new parent-child relationships, we should be concerned about the impact of commercializing the practice.

Suppose we stopped paying for sperm and instead asked men to be genuine donors. Would that create a shortage of sperm? There are reasons to believe that it would not. First, several countries find an adequate number of such volunteers.[10] Second, there is the analogy with blood. In the United States it used to be assumed that you could only obtain an adequate supply of whole blood by paying individuals for it, or by offering them some other advantage. That assumption was false. People give blood because they are convinced other persons need it and they do not have to undergo great inconvenience to make a donation.[11] Like donations of blood, donations of sperm can assuage an important form of human suffering.

Whatever moral difficulties we find in a market for sperm, they are magnified in the market for ova because of the much greater physical risks involved. There are fewer healthy ova available for treating infertility than there are women who want them. Getting healthy ova to use in in vitro fertilization (IVF) and related procedures is a much more elaborate and invasive procedure than what is required to obtain sperm. The woman who will be the source of these eggs typically takes hormones that stimulate her ovaries to ripen multiple eggs, which must then be removed by aspiration or laparoscopy. Why would a woman go through such an ordeal? In many instances, the woman is a genuine donor, providing an egg for a relative or a friend. In other cases, the woman receives money. Compensating the supplier is fine, according to the American Fertility Society's "Guidelines for Gamete Donation: 1993." The guidelines say that "donors should be compensated for the direct and indirect expenses associated with their participation, their inconvenience and time, and to some degree, for the risk and discomfort undertaken."[12] One proposal calculates that with all the interviewing, testing, examinations, the procedure itself, and a full day to recover, an egg donation takes fifty-six hours of a woman's time. Assuming that men are paid $25 an hour for sperm, the authors of this proposal conclude that a woman should "receive $1,400 for her time alone, exclusive of any compensation for travel, risk, or inconvenience."[13] They ask, "Since it is standard to compensate men for sperm donation, shouldn't the policy be equal pay for equal time?"[14] A survey of infertility programs found that women who were paid for their ova received an average of $1,548, with a range from $750 to $3,500.[15]

MARKET VALUES AND THE VALUES OF FAMILY LIFE

"Equal pay for equal work" sums it up well. Paying individuals for their biological products makes them vendors, not donors. And it places the interactions between the parties squarely in the marketplace. Markets are built on the premise that individuals are rational pursuers of their own satisfaction and that choice and control are preeminent values. Market enthusiasts claim that the more things we allow the market to distribute, the better off we are. In practice, most market proponents recognize that some things should not be bought and sold. But the moral logic of some market advocates encompasses even children.[16] Explanations of why we should not allow children to be bought and sold often rely on two kinds of arguments: either that children have intrinsic moral value or worth and that such things should never be bought, sold, or owned; or that the consequences for children will be bad. I want to suggest a different line of argument.

The key errors in market analyses of the sphere of the family are a faulty set of presuppositions coupled to a dry, shrunken conception of human flourishing. The presuppositions include the notion that people are best understood as rational, isolated individuals in selfish pursuit of their own satisfaction, with the values of choice and control preeminent. There are problems with each piece of this model of human life. The emphasis on the *rational* underesti-

mates the importance of the emotional in human life. The emphasis on the *isolated individual* discounts the great significance of relationships for people's flourishing. The assumption that people's motivations are essentially *selfish* fails to comprehend the complexity of human motivation, especially in the sphere of family life. . . . The celebration of *control* and *choice* fails to acknowledge the very limited role these values play in family life, indeed that a disproportionate emphasis on either can destroy families.

If children flourish best in stable, loving families, then we harm them by promoting a view of human relationship that equates the decision to initiate such a relationship with the decision to buy a widescreen television or a medium-priced car. If adults flourish best in enduring, warm relationships and if caring for children also contributes to the flourishing of adults, then we should encourage practices and policies that support such relationships. To the extent that the dry view of human flourishing implicit in marketplace values shrinks our perceptions and undermines our support for family life, it threatens not merely children but adults as well.

I am not arguing that marketplace values are linked in some tight logical or mechanistic way so that where one is present the others follow inexorably. Rather, I am claiming that they form a mutually supportive web of compatible considerations. The focus on rational individuals seeking the maximum of satisfaction for themselves supports choice and control as values. The same focus tends to evaluate all things—objects, entertainments, other people—according to how well they satisfy the individual's desires. I like crusty bread, so I chose a bread machine with that feature; you like hazel eyes and curly black hair, so should you choose your children by those characteristics?

WHAT DIFFERENCE DOES IT MAKE?

If we set aside the moral framework of contract and market in favor of one more in tune with what we value about families, how would we regard alternative methods of reproduction? Most significant would be a shift in how we frame the moral question. The currently fashionable way to think about such matters is to place individual liberty and choice on one side of the balance and the harms caused on the other side. Robertson uses this strategy frequently and skillfully. His analysis of surrogacy provides a typical example.[17] Robertson emphasizes the voluntary nature of the agreement between the paying couple and the paid surrogate. He looks at potential harms to the couple and the surrogate as unlikely, not that different from other things we already tolerate, and in any event a consequence of their own free choice.

The child-product of the surrogacy contract is a more difficult story. But not much more difficult. The prospect of harms to such children could be dismissed as implausible or unproved, or as not so different from other practices we tolerate anyway, especially adoption. The parallel with harms to the adults involved in surrogacy ends there. Robertson, like other defenders of commercial surrogacy, cannot use the child's fictitious "consent" to justify any harms that might come to it. But he has another strategy. The child, he argues, benefits because "but for the surrogacy contract, this child would not exist at all. . . . [E]ven if the child does suffer identity problems, as adopted children often do . . . this child has benefited, or at least has not been wronged, for without the surrogate arrangement, she would not have been born at all."[18]

Try now to imagine some novel method of bringing children into the world which this way of framing the issues would condemn, as long as the adults participating did so freely. Cloning human embryos? No problem. Cloning embryos, freezing some and thawing them out later for implantation in someone else? Still no problem. Implanting an aborted fetus's ovary, with its millions of yet-unripe eggs, into a woman's body, so that she might become pregnant with that fetus's ova? It is difficult to see how anyone who frames the argument as Robertson and other enthusiasts do could make a strong objection to the practice. Who is harmed? Not the woman who chose to abort the fetus and gave her consent to using its ovaries. Certainly not the woman or her spouse who wants this supply of healthy ova. As for any children born from these eggs, who could prove they would have been better off never existing?

Would it matter if the reason the woman desired the fetal ovary was her own infertility, or because she is thirty-five and wanted to avoid the increased risk of birth defects that comes from older eggs? Or that she and her spouse wanted children with blue eyes, or some other genetically linked characteristics? I doubt that Robertson or most other supporters of reproductive alternatives would embrace such bizarre practices. But, it is also hard to see how, given the way they structure the ethical balancing, they could argue persuasively against them. You would have to demonstrate harms of such magnitude and certainty to individuals who have not, by their own choice, accepted the risks, that they overwhelm the powerful presumption in favor of liberty. Robertson, for one, looks with favor on doing genetic screening on and then freezing embryos while a woman is young, "until education, career, or relationship goals are worked out. They can then be transferred to the woman when there is a lower risk of a handicapped birth than if fertilization occurred shortly before implantation."[19]

What of healthy fertile women, who want to have their own genetic child, but do not want to go through pregnancy? Robertson believes that "surrogacy for convenience . . . may turn out to be more acceptable if it proves to be an effective way for women to combine work and reproduction. . . . As long as surrogate interests are protected, an optimal situation for all might result from surrogacy for convenience, if one accepts the change in the concept of mother that it would appear to entail."[20] This is precisely the inexorable moral logic of the marketplace, a logic that sweeps everything before it, deterred only by compelling evidence of serious, direct harm to those who have not consented by virtue of their own participation. As for the children thus created, we would have to prove that they would have been better off never being born.

New York State's Task Force on Life and the Law argues that the way the question is framed essentially dictates the answer because it presupposes that the children in question already exist. The task force suggests an alternative framing: whether, given the disadvantages of commercial surrogacy for future children, the practice should be permitted in the first place.[21] We should extend the task force's question and ask if these alternative means of creating children support or interfere with what we value in family and parenthood. Would they, on balance, create not just individual parent-child relationships but the kind of relationships that foster mutuality, loyalty, and love; relationships that endure, that survive the inevitable occasions when the relationship is causing a great deal more pain than pleasure? Beyond individual relationships, would they help build social attitudes and institutions that support the flourishing of children and adults within families?

I am suspicious of practices such as paying gamete suppliers or surrogate childbearers that thrust the values of the market into the heart of the family. It would be ridiculous to argue that all children born of such arrangements are irreparably damaged, or their relationships with their rearing parents warped. But I do not think it is silly to worry about the effect such practices have on our intimate relationships more generally and on parent-child relationships in particular. Unreflective ideological commitments can and do lead us astray, away from what we genuinely and deeply value. The attitudes and institutions that provide the absolutely necessary cultural support for what we value can be eroded, so gradually that we scarcely notice.

I agree with Robertson and other proponents of new reproductive arrangements about the enormous importance of children in the lives of adults. We both want to promote social practices that match children with nurturing adults. But where he regards contract and commercialization as "the instruments of reproductive freedom," I view them as, at best, threats and, at worst, inimical to the values families are meant to promote. They should be our culture's last resort, if we allow resort to them at all. Cultural meanings are shared creations, and their protection, or change, a shared project.

There is enough reason for concern to throw the burden of proof back onto the shoulders of proponents of marketplace values in reproduction. Show us that the practices you advocate do not threaten what we value about family life and that reasonable alternatives are lacking. Artificial insemination by vendor, for example, would not be justifiable because a nonmarket alternative exists—genuine donors.

To protect the few against the tyranny of the majority, the law may have to permit in the name of liberty some practices that we believe are unwise. But our moral vision must remain clear. If commercializing reproductive practices threatens cultural meanings and institutions, then our respect for political liberty does not require us to welcome such practices. Some commentators argue that procreative liberty is a fundamental constitutional right. Under our constitution, the government must have a compelling purpose to justify interfering with a fundamental constitutional right. But other experts disagree with the claim that our reproductive rights encompass practices such as gestation for pay. Alex Capron and Margaret Radin conclude that the "claim that the right to privacy protects surrogacy may be more plausible for noncommercial than for commercial surrogacy; even if the Constitution should be understood as including a right to bear a child for someone else, it should not be interpreted as including a right to be paid for it."[22] They argue that there is no obstacle in the Constitution to prevent a community from banning commercial surrogacy agencies, brokers, or advertising. I believe that we should prohibit commercial surrogacy.

There is another kind of surrogacy—gift surrogacy. A woman who is willing to bear her sister's or best friend's child out of loyalty and affection is acting in harmony with the values we prize in families. I would urge caution on the part of everyone involved, but I see what she is doing as an act of generosity, an extraordinary gift. Despite the outward physiological similarity between surrogacy-for-love and surrogacy-for-pay, the meanings of the two acts could not be more different. The former builds on a relationship of affection to create new affectionate relationships. The latter transmutes the creation of a child into a commercial transaction—a sort of reverse alchemy, turning gold into dross. . . .

. . . The uncritical celebration of procreative liberty and other marketplace values in reproduction is indeed a threat to what we value about families. Reproductive alternatives need to be examined in the light of those same values.

NOTES

1 Even incursions of the market as simple as children's allowances must be handled carefully. See Viviana Zelizer, *Pricing the Priceless Child* (New York: Basic Books, 1985).

2 David H. Smith makes a related distinction. In a discussion of surrogacy, he describes alternative "ways of thinking about a woman's relationship to a child she bears and indeed to her own reproductive processes. In one of these perspectives the relationship between self and reproductive involvement is extrinsic and contingent. Pregnancy is viewed externally and objectively as a temporary state one is in for any one of a number of reasons. The self calculates its reasons for pregnancy, mode and form of personal involvement. . . . Another perspective on body is also possible: I identify myself with my body. I not only control it, but I have to listen to it. . . . I have embodied involvements with others, involvements that are constitutive of me as a self. These constitutive, involving embodiments are clearest in our relations with our parents and our children." Smith, "Wombs for Rent, Selves for Sale?" *Journal of Contemporary Health Law and Policy* 4 (1988): 30–31.

3 John A. Robertson, "The Question of Human Cloning," *Hastings Center Report* (March 1994): 6–14.

4 Robertson, "Embryos, Families and Procreative Liberty: The Legal Structure of the New Reproduction," *Southern California Law Review* 59, no. 5 (1986): 1031. Robertson's commitment to reproductive liberty is clear in both the title and the text of his book, *Children of Choice: Freedom and the New Reproductive Technologies* (Princeton: Princeton University Press, 1994). In it he restates his guiding principle: "I propose that procreative liberty be given presumptive priority in all conflicts, with the burden on opponents of any particular technique to show that harmful effects from its use justify limiting procreative choice" (p. 16).

5 Ibid., 1040.

6 Smith, "Wombs for Rent, Selves for Sale?" 33.

7 Ibid., 34.

8 See K. R. Daniels, "Semen Donors: Their Motivations and Attitudes to Their Offspring," *Journal of Reproductive and Infant Psychology* 7 (1989): 121–127, and R. Rowland, "Attitudes and Opinions of Donors on an Artificial Insemination by Donor (AID) Programme," *Clinical Reproduction and Fertility* 2 (1983): 249–259.

9 Paul Lauritzen, *Pursuing Parenthood* (Bloomington: Indiana University Press, 1993).

10 Ken R. Daniels and Karyn Taylor, "Secrecy and Openness in Donor Insemination," *Politics and the Life Sciences* 12, no. 2 (1993): 155–170, confirm that Australia and New Zealand rely on genuine donors. In the same issue of the journal, Jacques Lansac affirms that France uses only sperm donors, not vendors ("One Father Only: Donor Insemination and CECOS in France," pp. 185–186).

11 Alvin W. Drake, Stan N. Finkelstein, and Harvey M. Sapolsky, *The American Blood Supply* (Cambridge: MIT Press, 1982).

12 American Fertility Society, "Guidelines for Gamete Donation: 1993," *Fertility and Sterility, Supplement 1* 59, no. 2 (1993): 5S–9S, 6S; sec. VI.A.

13 Machelle M. Seibel and Ann Kiessling, "Compensating Egg Donors: Equal Pay for Equal Time?" *New England Journal of Medicine* 328, no. 10 (1993): 737.

14 Ibid.

15 Andrea Mechanick Braverman, "Survey Results on the Current Practice of Ovum Donation," *Fertility and Sterility* 59, no. 6 (1993): 1216–1220.

16 In a famous article, Landes and Posner consider "some tentative and reversible steps toward a free baby market in order to determine experimentally the social costs and benefits of using the market in this area." "The Economics of the Baby Shortage," *Journal of Legal Studies,* 7, no. 2 (1978): 347.

17 John A. Robertson, "Surrogate Mothers: Not So Novel After All," *Hastings Center Report* 13, no. 5 (1983): 28–34.

18 Ibid., 29.

19 Robertson, "Embryos, Families and Procreative Liberty," 1030.

20 Ibid.

21 New York State Task Force on Life and the Law, *Surrogate Parenting: Analysis and Recommendations for Public Policy* (1988). The task force concluded unanimously that public policy ought to discourage surrogate parenting and proposed legislation to ban fees to surrogates or brokers and to void surrogacy contracts. Their response to the argument that children born under surrogacy arrangements are better off because otherwise they would not have been born at all is as follows:

> But this argument assumes the very factor under deliberation—the child's conception and birth. The assessment for public policy occurs prior to conception when the surrogate arrangements are made. The issue then is not whether a particular child should be denied life, but whether children should be conceived in circumstances that would place them at risk. The notion that children have an interest in being born prior to their conception and birth is not embraced in other public policies and should not be assumed in the debate on surrogate parenting. (p. 120)

I am grateful to John Arras for pointing out this argument to me.

22 Alexander M. Capron and Margaret J. Radin, "Choosing Family Law Over Contract Law as a Paradigm for Surrogate Motherhood," *Law, Medicine & Health Care* 16, nos. 1–2 (1988): 34, 40.

SURROGATE MOTHERHOOD AS PRENATAL ADOPTION
Bonnie Steinbock

Steinbock maintains that commercial surrogacy contracts should not be prohibited by the state. She argues that it is unjustifiably paternalistic for the state to ban surrogacy in an effort to protect the potential surrogate from a choice that may later be regretted. She also argues that concerns about a negative psychological impact on potential offspring are insufficient to warrant an outright ban. Moreover, in her view, commercial surrogacy is neither inherently exploitive nor inconsistent with human dignity. In dealing with the charge that commercial surrogacy amounts to baby selling, she insists that payment to the surrogate can be understood as compensation for "the risks, sacrifice, and discomfort the surrogate undergoes during pregnancy." Although Steinbock considers the legal prohibition of surrogacy contracts to be incompatible with a proper regard for the value of individual freedom, she believes that the practice of surrogacy should be regulated by the state. In particular, she would insist that surrogacy contracts be structured so as to allow the surrogate a postnatal waiting period, during which she would be free to change her mind and keep the child. (Steinbock makes several references to the Baby M case; for the facts of this case, see Appendix, Case 38.)

The recent [1986] case of "Baby M" has brought surrogate motherhood to the forefront of American attention. Ultimately, whether we permit or prohibit surrogacy depends on what we take to be good reasons for preventing people from acting as they wish. A growing number of people want to be, or hire, surrogates; are there legitimate reasons to prevent them? Apart from its intrinsic interest, the issue of surrogate motherhood provides us with an opportunity to examine different justifications for limiting individual freedom.

. . . I examine claims that surrogacy is ethically unacceptable because it is exploitive, inconsistent with human dignity, or harmful to the children born of such arrangements. I conclude that these reasons justify restrictions on surrogate contracts, rather than an outright ban. . . .

SHOULD SURROGACY BE PROHIBITED?

On June 27, 1988, Michigan became the first state to outlaw commercial contracts for women to bear children for others.[1] Yet making a practice illegal does not necessarily make it go away: witness black-market adoption. The legitimate concerns that support a ban on surrogacy might be better served by careful regulation. However, some practices, such as slavery, are ethically unacceptable, regardless of how carefully regulated they are. Let us consider the arguments that surrogacy is intrinsically unacceptable.

Paternalistic Arguments These arguments against surrogacy take the form of protecting a potential surrogate from a choice she may later regret. As an argument for banning surrogacy, as opposed to providing safeguards to ensure that contracts are freely and knowledgeably undertaken, this is a form of paternalism.

At one time, the characterization of a prohibition as paternalistic was a sufficient reason to reject it. The pendulum has swung back, and many people are willing to accept at least some paternalistic restrictions on freedom. Gerald Dworkin points out that even Mill made one exception to his otherwise absolute rejection of paternalism: he thought that no one should be allowed to sell himself into slavery, because to do so would be to destroy his future autonomy.

From *Law, Medicine, and Health Care,* vol. 16 (Spring 1988). Reprinted with permission of the author and the publisher (American Society of Law, Medicine & Ethics).

This provides a narrow principle to justify some paternalistic interventions. To preserve freedom in the long run, we give up the freedom to make certain choices, those that have results that are "far-reaching, potentially dangerous and irreversible."[2] An example would be a ban on the sale of crack. Virtually everyone who uses crack becomes addicted and, once addicted, a slave to its use. We reasonably and willingly give up our freedom to buy the drug, to protect our ability to make free decisions in the future.

Can a Dworkinian argument be made to rule out surrogacy agreements? Admittedly, the decision to give up a child is permanent, and may have disastrous effects on the surrogate mother. However, many decisions may have long-term, disastrous effects (e.g., postponing childbirth for a career, having an abortion, giving a child up for adoption). Clearly we do not want the state to make decisions for us in all these matters. Dworkin's argument is rightly restricted to paternalistic interferences that protect the individual's autonomy or ability to make decisions in the future. Surrogacy does not involve giving up one's autonomy, which distinguishes it from both the crack and selling-oneself-into-slavery examples. Respect for individual freedom requires us to permit people to make choices they may later regret.

Moral Objections . . . We must all agree that a practice that exploits people or violates human dignity is immoral. However, it is not clear that surrogacy is guilty on either count.

Exploitation The mere fact that pregnancy is *risky* does not make surrogate agreements exploitive, and therefore morally wrong. People often do risky things for money; why should the line be drawn at undergoing pregnancy? The usual response is to compare surrogacy and kidney-selling. The selling of organs is prohibited because of the potential for coercion and exploitation. But why should kidney-selling be viewed as intrinsically coercive? A possible explanation is that no one would do it, unless driven by poverty. The choice is both forced and dangerous, and hence coercive.

The situation is quite different in the case of the race-car driver or stuntman. We do not think that they are *forced* to perform risky activities for money:

they freely choose to do so. Unlike selling one's kidneys, these are activities that we can understand (intellectually, anyway) someone choosing to do. Movie stuntmen, for example, often enjoy their work, and derive satisfaction from doing it well. Of course they "do it for the money," in the sense that they would not do it without compensation; few people are willing to work "for free." The element of coercion is missing, however, because they enjoy the job, despite the risks, and could do something else if they chose.

The same is apparently true of most surrogates. "They choose the surrogate role primarily because the fee provides a better economic opportunity than alternative occupations, but also because they enjoy being pregnant and the respect and attention that it draws."[3] Some may derive a feeling of self-worth from an act they regard as highly altruistic: providing a couple with a child they could not otherwise have. If these motives are present, it is far from clear that the surrogate is being exploited. Indeed, it seems objectionally paternalistic to insist that she is.

Human Dignity It may be argued that even if womb-leasing is not necessarily exploitive, it should still be rejected as inconsistent with human dignity. But why? As John Harris points out, hair, blood, and other tissue is often donated or sold; what is so special about the uterus?[4]

Human dignity is more plausibly invoked in the strongest argument against surrogacy, namely, that it is the sale of a child. Children are not property, nor can they be bought or sold. It could be argued that surrogacy is wrong because it is analogous to slavery, and so is inconsistent with human dignity.

However, there are important differences between slavery and a surrogate agreement. The child born of a surrogate is not treated cruelly or deprived of freedom or resold; none of the things that make slavery so awful are part of surrogacy. Still, it may be thought that simply putting a market value on a child is wrong. Human life has intrinsic value; it is literally priceless. Arrangements that ignore this violate our deepest notions of the value of human life. It is profoundly disturbing to hear in a television documentary on surrogacy the boyfriend of a surrogate say, quite candidly, "We're in it for the money."

[The trial court judge in the Baby M case] accepted the premise that producing a child for money denigrates human dignity, but he denied that this happens in a surrogate agreement. Ms. Whitehead was not paid for the surrender of the child to the father: she was paid for her willingness to be impregnated and carry Mr. Stern's child to term. The child, once born, is his biological child. "He cannot purchase what is already his."[5]

This is misleading, and not merely because Baby M is as much Ms. Whitehead's child as Mr. Stern's. It is misleading because it glosses over the fact that the surrender of the child was part—indeed, the whole point—of the agreement. If the surrogate were paid merely for being willing to be impregnated and carrying the child to term, then she would fulfill the contract upon giving birth. She could take the money *and* the child. Mr. Stern did not agree to pay Ms. Whitehead merely to *have* his child, but to provide him with a child. The New Jersey Supreme Court held that this violated New Jersey's laws prohibiting the payment or acceptance of money in connection with adoption.

One way to remove the taint of baby-selling would be to limit payment to medical expenses associated with the birth or incurred by the surrogate during pregnancy (as is allowed in many jurisdictions, including New Jersey, in ordinary adoptions). Surrogacy could be seen, not as baby-selling, but as a form of adoption. Nowhere did the Supreme Court find any legal prohibition against surrogacy when there is no payment, and when the surrogate has the right to change her mind and keep the child. However, this solution effectively prohibits surrogacy, since few women would become surrogates solely for self-fulfillment or reasons of altruism.

The question, then, is whether we can reconcile paying the surrogate, beyond her medical expenses, with the idea of surrogacy as prenatal adoption. We can do this by separating the terms of the agreement, which include surrendering the infant at birth to the biological father, from the justification for payment. The payment should be seen as compensation for the risks, sacrifice, and discomfort the surrogate undergoes during pregnancy. This means that if, through no fault on the part of the surrogate, the baby is stillborn, she should still be paid in full, since she has

kept her part of the bargain. (By contrast, in the Stern-Whitehead agreement, Ms. Whitehead was to receive only $1,000 for a stillbirth).[6] If, on the other hand, the surrogate changes her mind and decides to keep the child, she would break the agreement, and would not be entitled to any fee or to compensation for expenses incurred during pregnancy. . . .

. . . There are sound moral and policy . . . reasons to provide a postnatal waiting period in surrogate agreements. As the Baby M case makes painfully clear, the surrogate may underestimate the bond created by gestation and the emotional trauma caused by relinquishing the baby. Compassion requires that we acknowledge these findings, and not deprive a woman of the baby she has carried because, before conception, she underestimated the strength of her feelings for it. Providing a waiting period, as in ordinary postnatal adoptions, will help protect women from making irrevocable mistakes, without banning the practice.

Some may object that this gives too little protection to the prospective adoptive parents. They cannot be sure that the baby is theirs until the waiting period is over. While this is hard on them, a similar burden is placed on other adoptive parents. If the absence of a guarantee serves to discourage people from entering surrogacy agreements, that is not necessarily a bad thing, given all the risks inherent in such contracts. In addition, this requirement would make stricter screening and counseling of surrogates essential, a desirable side-effect.

Harm to Others Paternalistic and moral objections to surrogacy do not seem to justify an outright ban. What about the effect on the offspring of such contracts? We do not yet have solid data on the effects of being a "surrogate child." Any claim that surrogacy creates psychological problems in the children is purely speculative. But what if we did discover that such children have deep feelings of worthlessness from learning that their natural mothers deliberately created them with the intention of giving them away? Might we ban surrogacy as posing an unacceptable risk of psychological harm to the resulting children?

Feelings of worthlessness are harmful. They can prevent people from living happy, fulfilling lives. However, a surrogate child, even one whose life is miserable because of these feelings, cannot claim to have been harmed by the surrogate agreement. Without the agreement, the child would never have existed. Unless she is willing to say that her life is not worth living because of these feelings, that she would be better off never having been born, she cannot claim to have been harmed by being born of a surrogate mother.

Elsewhere I have argued that children can be *wronged* by being brought into existence, even if they are not, strictly speaking, *harmed*.[7] They are wronged if they are deprived of the minimally decent existence to which all citizens are entitled. We owe it to our children to see that they are not born with such serious impairments that their most basic interests will be doomed in advance. If being born to a surrogate is a handicap of this magnitude, comparable to being born blind or deaf or severely mentally retarded, then surrogacy can be seen as wronging the offspring. This would be a strong reason against permitting such contracts. However, it does not seem likely. Probably the problems arising from surrogacy will be like those faced by adopted children and children whose parents divorce. Such problems are not trivial, but neither are they so serious that the child's very existence can be seen as wrongful.

If surrogate children are neither harmed nor wronged by surrogacy, it may seem that the argument for banning surrogacy on grounds of its harmfulness to the offspring evaporates. After all, if the children themselves have no cause for complaint, how can anyone else claim to reject it on their behalf? Yet it seems extremely counter-intuitive to suggest that the risk of emotional damage to the children born of such arrangements is not even relevant to our deliberations. It seems quite reasonable and proper—even morally obligatory—for policymakers to think about the possible detrimental effects of new reproductive technologies, and to reject those likely to create physically or emotionally damaged people. The explanation for this must involve the idea that it is wrong to bring people into the world in a harmful condition, even if they are not, strictly speaking, harmed by having been brought into existence. Should evidence emerge that surrogacy produces

children with serious psychological problems, that would be a strong reason for banning the practice.

There is some evidence on the effect of surrogacy on the other children of the surrogate mother. One woman reported that her daughter, now seventeen, who was eleven at the time of the surrogate birth, "is still having problems with what I did, and as a result she is still angry with me." She explains: "Nobody told me that a child could bond with a baby while you're still pregnant. I didn't realize then that all the times she listened to his heartbeat and felt his legs kick that she was becoming attached to him."[8]

A less sentimental explanation is possible. It seems likely that her daughter, seeing one child given away, was fearful that the same might be done to her. We can expect anxiety and resentment on the part of children whose mothers give away a brother or sister. The psychological harm to these children is clearly relevant to a determination of whether surrogacy is contrary to public policy. At the same time, it should be remembered that many things, including divorce, remarriage, and even moving to a new neighborhood, create anxiety and resentment in children. We should not use the effect on children as an excuse for banning a practice we find bizarre or offensive.

CONCLUSION

There are many reasons to be extremely cautious of surrogacy. I cannot imagine becoming a surrogate, nor would I advise anyone else to enter into a contract so fraught with peril. But the fact that a practice is risky, foolish, or even morally distasteful is not sufficient reason to outlaw it. It would be better for the state to regulate the practice, and minimize the potential for harm, without infringing on the liberty of citizens.

NOTES

1 *New York Times,* June 28, 1988, A20.
2 Gerald Dworkin, "Paternalism," in R. A. Wasserstrom, ed., *Morality and the Law* (Belmont, Cal.: Wadsworth, 1971); reprinted in J. Feinberg and H. Gross, eds., *Philosophy of Law,* 3d ed. (Belmont, Cal.: Wadsworth, 1986), 265.
3 John Robertson, "Surrogate Mothers: Not So Novel After All," *Hastings Center Report,* 13, no. 5 (1983): 29; citing P. Parker, "Surrogate Mother's Motivations: Initial Findings," *American Journal of Psychiatry,* 140 (1983): 1.

4 J. Harris, *The Value of Life* (London: Routledge & Kegan Paul, 1985), 144.

5 *In re Baby "M,"* 217 N. J. Super. 372, 525 A.2d 1157 (1987).

6 George Annas, "Baby M: Babies (and Justice) for Sale," *Hastings Center Report,* 17, no. 3 (1987): 14.

7 Bonnie Steinbock, "The Logical Case for 'Wrongful Life,'" *Hastings Center Report,* 16, no. 2 (1986): 15.

8 "Baby M Case Stirs Feelings of Surrogate Mothers," *New York Times,* March 2, 1987, B1.

HUMAN CLONING

CLONING OF HUMAN BEINGS
Leon R. Kass

In this testimony presented to the National Bioethics Advisory Commission (NBAC), Kass urges the commission to declare human cloning deeply unethical and to recommend a legal ban. Calling attention to the widespread sense of repugnance elicited by the prospect of human cloning, he advances four lines of argument against its use. These arguments are based on (1) considerations related to the ethics of experimentation, (2) concerns about identity and individuality, (3) the dangers of transforming procreation into manufacture, and (4) the negative impact upon our understanding of what it means to have children.

Mr. Chairman, Members of the Commission.

I am deeply grateful for the opportunity to present some of my thoughts about the ethics of human cloning, by which I mean precisely—the production of cloned human beings. This topic has occupied me off and on for over 30 years; it was the subject of one of my first publications in bioethics 25 years ago. Since that time, we have in some sense been softened up to the idea of human cloning—through movies, cartoons, jokes, and intermittent commentary in the mass media, occasionally serious, more often lighthearted. We have become accustomed to new practices in human reproduction—in vitro fertilization, embryo manipulation, and surrogate pregnancy—and, in animal biotechnology, to transgenic animals and a burgeoning science of genetic engineering. Changes in the broader culture make it now more difficult to express a common, respectful understanding of sexuality, procreation, nascent life, and the meaning of motherhood, fatherhood, and the links between the generations. In a world whose

once-given natural boundaries are blurred by technological change and whose moral boundaries are seemingly up for grabs, it is, I believe, much more difficult than it once was to make persuasive the still compelling case against human cloning. As Raskolnikov put it, "Man gets used to everything—the beast!"

Therefore, the first thing of which I want to persuade you is not to be complacent about what is here at issue. Human cloning, though in some respects continuous with previous reproductive technologies, also represents something radically new, both in itself and in its easily foreseeable consequences. The stakes here are very high indeed. Let me exaggerate, but in the direction of the truth: You have been asked to give advice on nothing less than whether human procreation is going to remain human, whether children are going to be made rather than begotten, and whether it is a good thing, humanly speaking, to say yes to the road which leads (at best) to the dehumanized rationality of Brave New World. If I could persuade you of nothing else, it would be this: What we have here is not business as usual, to be fretted about for a while but finally to be given our seal of

Testimony presented to the National Bioethics Advisory Commission. March 14, 1997, Washington, D.C.

approval, not least because it appears to be inevitable. Rise to the occasion, address the subject in all its profundity, and advise as if the future of our humanity may hang in the balance.

"Offensive." "Grotesque." "Revolting." "Repugnant." "Repulsive." These are the words most commonly heard these days regarding the prospect of human cloning. Such reactions one hears both from the man or woman in the street and from the intellectuals, from believers and atheists, from humanists and scientists. Even Dolly's creator, Dr. Wilmot, has said he "would find it offensive" to clone a human being. People are repelled by many aspects of human cloning: The prospect of mass production of human beings, with large clones of lookalikes, compromised in their individuality; the idea of father-son or mother-daughter twins; the bizarre prospects of a woman giving birth to a genetic copy of herself, her spouse, or even her deceased father or mother; the creation of embryonic genetic duplicates of oneself, to be frozen away in case of later need for homologous organ transplantation; the narcissism of those who would clone themselves, the arrogance of others who think they know who deserves to be cloned or which genotype any child-to-be should be thrilled to receive; the Frankensteinian hubris to create human life and increasingly to control its destiny; man playing at being God. Almost no one sees any compelling reason for human cloning; almost everyone anticipates its possible misuses and abuses. Many feel oppressed by the sense that there is nothing we can do to prevent it from happening. This makes the prospect all the more revolting.

Revulsion is surely not an argument, and some of yesterday's repugnances are today calmly accepted. But in crucial cases, repugnance is often the emotional bearer of deep wisdom, beyond reason's power fully to articulate it. Can anyone really give an argument fully adequate to the horror which is father-daughter incest (even with consent) or having sex with animals or eating human flesh, or even just raping or murdering another human being? Would anyone's failure to give full rational justification for his revulsion at these practices make that revulsion ethically suspect? Not at all. In my view, our repugnance at human cloning belongs in this category. We are repelled by the prospect of cloning human beings

not because of the strangeness or novelty of the undertaking, but because we intuit and feel, immediately and without argument, the violation of things we rightfully hold dear. I doubt very much whether I can give the proper rational voice to this horror, but in the remarks that follow I will try. But please consider seriously that this may be one of those instances about which the heart has its reasons that reason cannot adequately know.

I will raise four kinds of objections: the ethics of experimentation; identity and individuality; fabrication and manufacture; despotism and the violation of what it means to have children.

First, any attempt to clone a human being would constitute an unethical experiment upon the resulting child-to-be. As the animal experiments indicate, there is grave risk of mishaps and deformities. Moreover, one cannot presume a future cloned child's consent to be a clone, even a healthy one. Thus, we cannot ethically get to know even whether or not human cloning is feasible.

I understand, of course, the philosophical difficulty of trying to compare life with defects against non-existence. But common sense tells us that it is irrelevant. It is surely true that people can harm and even maim children in the very act of conceiving them, say, by paternal transmission of the HIV virus or maternal transmission of heroin dependence. To do so intentionally, or even negligently, is inexcusable and clearly unethical.

Second, cloning creates serious issues of identity and individuality. The cloned person may experience concerns about his distinctive identity not only because he will be in genotype and appearance identical to another human being, but, in this case, it will be to a twin who might be his "father" or "mother"—if one can still call them that. What would be the psychic burdens of being the "child" or "parent" of your twin? Moreover, the cloned individual will be saddled with a genotype that has already lived. He will not be fully a surprise to the world: people are likely always to compare his performances in life with that of his alter ego. True, his nurture and circumstance in life will be different; genotype is not exactly destiny. But one must also expect parental and other efforts to shape this new life after the original—or at least to view the child with the original version firmly in mind. For why else did they clone from the star basketball player, mathematician, and beauty queen—or even dear old Dad—in the first place?

Genetic distinctiveness not only symbolizes the uniqueness of each human life and the independence of its parents that each human child rightfully attains. It can also be an important support for living a worthy and dignified life. Such arguments apply with great force to any large-scale replication of human individuals. But they are, in my view, sufficient to rebut even the first attempts to clone a human being. One must never forget that these are human beings upon whom our eugenic or merely playful fantasies are to be enacted.

Third, human cloning would represent a giant step toward turning begetting into making, procreation into manufacture (literally, something "hand made"), a process already begun with in vitro fertilization and genetic testing of embryos. With cloning, not only is the process in hand, but the total genetic blueprint of the cloned individual is selected and determined by the human artisans. To be sure, subsequent development is still according to natural processes; and the resulting children will still be recognizably human. But we here would be taking a major step into making man himself simply another one of the man-made things. Human nature becomes merely the last part of nature to succumb to the technological project, which turns all of nature into raw material at human disposal, to be homogenized by our rationalized technique according to the subjective prejudices of the day.

How does begetting differ from making? In natural procreation, we two human beings come together, complementarily male and female, to give existence to another being who is formed, exactly as we were, by what we are—living, hence perishable, hence aspiringly erotic human beings. But in clonal reproduction, and in the more advanced forms of manufacture to which it leads, we give existence to a being not by what we are but by what we intend and design. As with any product of our making, no matter how excellent, the artificer stands above it, not as an equal but as a superior, transcending it by his will and creative prowess. Scientists who clone animals make it perfectly clear that they are engaged

in instrumental making; the animals are, from the start, designed as means to serve rational human purpose. In human cloning, scientists and prospective "parents" would be adopting the same technocratic mentality to human children: human children would be their artifacts. Such an arrangement is profoundly dehumanizing, no matter how good the product. Mass-scale cloning of the same individual makes the point vividly; but the violation of human equality, freedom, and dignity are present even in a single planned clone.

Finally, and perhaps most important, the practice of human cloning by nuclear transfer—like other anticipated forms of genetic engineering of the next generation—would enshrine and aggravate a profound and mischief-making misunderstanding of the meaning of having children and of the parent-child relationship. When a couple now chooses to procreate, the partners are saying yes to the emergence of new life in its novelty, are saying yes not only to having a child but also, tacitly, to having whatever child this child turns out to be. Whether we know it or not, we are thereby also saying yes to our own finitude and mortality, to the necessity of our replacement and the limits of our control. In this ubiquitous way of nature, to say yes to the future by procreating means precisely that we are relinquishing our grip, even as we thereby take up our own share in what we hope will be the immortality of human life and the human species. This means that our children are not our children: They are not our property, they are not our possessions. Neither are they supposed to live our lives for us, or anyone else's life but their own. To be sure, we seek to guide them on their way, imparting to them not just life but nurture, love, and a way of life; to be sure, they bear our hopes that they will surpass us in goodness and happiness, enabling us in small measure to transcend our own limitations. But their genetic distinctiveness and independence is the natural foreshadowing of the deep truth that they have their own and never-before-enacted life to live. Though sprung from a past, they take an uncharted course into the future.

Much mischief is already done by parents who try to live vicariously through their children; children are sometimes compelled to fulfill the broken dreams of unhappy parents; John Doe, Jr. or the III is under the burden of having to live up to his forebear's name. But in cloning, such overbearing parents take at the start a decisive step which contradicts the entire meaning of the open and forward-looking nature of parent-child relations. The child is given a genotype that has already lived, with full expectation that this blueprint of a past life ought to be controlling of the life that is to come. Cloning is inherently despotic, for it seeks to make one's children or someone else's children after one's own image (or an image of one's choosing) and their future according to one's will. In some cases, the despotism may be mild and benevolent, in others, mischievous and downright tyrannical. But despotism—the control of another through one's will—it will unavoidably be.

What then should we do? We should declare human cloning deeply unethical in itself and dangerous in its likely consequences. In so doing, we shall have the backing of the overwhelming majority not only of our fellow Americans, but of the human race—including, I believe, most practicing scientists. Next, we should do all that we can to prevent human cloning from happening, by an international legal ban if possible, by a unilateral national ban, at a minimum. Scientists can, of course, secretly undertake to violate such a law, but they will at least be deterred by not being able to stand up proudly to claim the credit for their technological bravado and success. Such a ban on human cloning will not harm the progress of basic genetic science and technology; on the contrary, it will reassure the public that scientists are happy to proceed without violating the deep ethical norms and intuitions of the human community.

The President has given this Commission a glorious opportunity. In a truly unprecedented way, you can strike a blow for the human control of the technological project, for wisdom, prudence, and human dignity. The prospect of human cloning, so repulsive to contemplate, in fact provides the occasion—as well as the urgent necessity—of deciding whether we shall be slaves of unregulated progress, and ultimately its artifacts, or whether we shall remain free human beings who guide our technique toward the enhancement of human dignity. To seize the occasion, we—you—must, as the late Paul Ramsey said, "raise the ethical questions with a serious and not a frivolous conscience. A man of frivolous conscience announces that there are ethical quandaries ahead that we must urgently consider before the future catches up with us. By this he often means that we need to devise a new ethics that will provide the rationalization for doing in the future what men are bound to do because of new actions and interventions science will have made possible. In contrast a man of serious conscience means to say in raising urgent ethical questions that there may be some things that men should never do. The good things that men do can be made complete only by the things they refuse to do."

EVEN IF IT WORKED, CLONING WOULDN'T BRING HER BACK

Thomas H. Murray

Murray argues that we must face several "hard truths" about human cloning. One of these hard truths is that cloning—at least at this stage of technological development—does not produce healthy, normal offspring. The other hard truths he identifies are asserted in opposition to the idea that if cloning did produce healthy offspring, parents could sensibly use it to replace a dead child.

Eleven days ago, as I awaited my turn to testify at a congressional hearing on human reproductive cloning, one of five scientists on the witness list took the microphone. Brigitte Boisselier, a chemist working with couples who want to use cloning techniques to create babies, read aloud a letter from "a father,

Reprinted with permission of the author from *The Washington Post,* April 8, 2001.

(Dada)." The writer, who had unexpectedly become a parent in his late thirties, describes his despair over his 11-month-old son's death after heart surgery and 17 days of "misery and struggle." The room was quiet as Boisselier read the man's words: "I decided then and there that I would never give up on my child. I would never stop until I could give his DNA—his genetic make-up—a chance."

I listened to the letter writer's refusal to accept the finality of death, to his wish to allow his son another opportunity at life through cloning, and I was struck by the futility and danger of such thinking. I had been asked to testify as someone who has been writing and teaching about ethical issues in medicine and science for more than 20 years; but I am also a grieving parent. My 20-year-old daughter's murder, just five months ago, has agonizingly reinforced what I have for years argued as an ethicist: Cloning can neither change the fact of death nor deflect the pain of grief.

Only four years have passed since the birth of the first cloned mammal—Dolly the sheep—was announced and the possibility of human cloning became real. Once a staple of science fiction, cloning was now the stuff of scientific research. A presidential commission [the National Bioethics Advisory Commission], of which I am a member, began to deliberate the ethics of human cloning; scientists disavowed any interest in trying to clone people; and Congress held hearings but passed no laws. A moratorium took hold, stable except for the occasional eruption of self-proclaimed would-be cloners such as Chicago-based physicist Richard Seed and a group led by a man named Rael who claims that we are all clones of alien ancestors.

Recently, Boisselier, Rael's chief scientist, and Panos Zavos, an infertility specialist in Kentucky, won overnight attention when they proclaimed that they would indeed create a human clone in the near future. The prospect that renegade scientists might try to clone humans reignited the concern of lawmakers, which led to the recent hearings before the House Energy and Commerce subcommittee on oversight and investigations.

Cloning advocates have had a difficult time coming up with persuasive ethical arguments. Indulging narcissism—so that someone can create many Mini-Me's—fails to generate much support

for their cause. Others make the case that adults should have the right to use any means possible to have the child they want. Their liberty trumps everything else; the child's welfare barely registers, except to avoid a life that would be worse than never being born, a standard akin to dividing by zero—no meaningful answer is possible. The strategy that has been the most effective has been to play the sympathy card—and who evokes more sympathy than someone who has lost a child?

Sadly, I'm in a position to correct some of these misunderstandings. I'm not suggesting that my situation is the same as that of the letter's author. Not better. Not worse. Simply different. His son was with him for less than a year, our daughter for 20; his son died of disease in a hospital; Emily, daughter to Cynthia and me, sister to Kate and Matt, Nicky and Pete, was reported missing from her college campus in early November. Her body was found more than five weeks later. She had been abducted and shot.

As I write those words, I still want to believe they are about someone else, a story on the 11 o'clock news. Cynthia and I often ask each other, how can this be our life? But it is our life and Emily, as a physical, exuberant, loving presence, is not in the same way a part of it anymore. Death changes things and, I suspect, the death of a child causes more wrenching grief than any other death. So I am told; so my experience confirms.

I want to speak, then, to the author of that letter, father to father, grieving parent to grieving parent; and to anyone clinging to unfounded hope that cloning can somehow repair the arbitrariness of disease, unhappiness and death. I have nothing to sell you, I don't want your money, and I certainly don't want to be cruel. But there are hard truths here that some people, whether through ignorance or self-interest, are obscuring.

The first truth is that cloning does not result in healthy, normal offspring. The two scientific experts on animal cloning who shared the panel with Boisselier reported the results of the cattle, mice and other mammals cloned thus far: They have suffered staggering rates of abnormalities and death; some of the females bearing them have been injured and some have died. Rudolf Jaenisch, an expert on mouse cloning at MIT's Whitehead Institute for Biomedical Research, told the subcommittee that he did not believe there was a single healthy cloned mammal in existence—not even Dolly, the sheep that started it all, who is abnormally obese.

Scientists do not know why cloning fails so miserably. One plausible explanation begins with what we already know—that as the cells of an embryo divide and begin to transform into the many varieties of tissue that make up our bodies, most of the genes in each cell are shut down, leaving active only those that the cell needs to perform its specific role. A pancreatic islet cell, for example, needs working versions of the genes that recognize when a person needs the hormone insulin, then cobble it together and shunt it into the bloodstream. All of that individual's other genetic information is in that islet cell, but most of it is chemically locked, like an illegally parked car immobilized by a tire boot.

To make a healthy clone, scientists need to unlock every last one of those tire boots in the cell that is to be cloned. It is not enough to have the genes for islet cells; every gene will be needed sometime, somewhere. Unless and until scientists puzzle out how to restore all the genes to their original state, we will continue to see dead, dying and deformed clones.

You do not need to be a professional bioethicist, then, to see that trying to make a child by cloning, at this stage in the technology, would be a gross violation of international standards protecting people from overreaching scientists, a blatant example of immoral human experimentation.

Some scientists claim they can avoid these problems. Zavos, who spoke at the hearing, has promised to screen embryos and implant only healthy ones. But Zavos failed to give a single plausible reason to believe that he can distinguish healthy from unhealthy cloned embryos.

Now for the second truth: Even if cloning produced a healthy embryo, the result would not be the same person as the one whose genetic material was used. Each of us is a complex amalgam of luck, experience and heredity. Where in the womb an embryo burrows, what its mother eats or drinks, what stresses she endures, her age—all these factors shape the developing fetus. The genes themselves conduct an intricately choreographed dance, turning on and off, instructing other genes to do the same in response to their interior rhythms and to the pulses of the world outside. How we become who we are remains a mystery.

About the only thing we can be certain of is that we are much more than the sum of our genes. As I said in my testimony, perhaps the best way to extinguish the enthusiasm for human cloning would be to clone Michael Jordan. Michael II might well have no interest in playing basketball but instead long to become an accountant. What makes Michael I great is not merely his physical gifts, but his competitive fire, his determination, his fierce will to win.

Yet another hard truth: Creating a child to stand in for another—dead—child is unfair. No child should have to bear the oppressive expectation that he or she will live out the life denied to his or her idealized genetic avatar. Parents may joke about their specific plans for their children; I suspect their children find such plans less amusing. Of course, we should have expectations for our children: that they be considerate, honest, diligent, fair and more. But we cannot dictate their temperament, talents or interests. Cloning a child to be a reincarnation of someone else is a grotesque, fun-house mirror distortion of parental expectations.

Which brings me to the final hard truth: There is no real escape from grief.

Cynthia and I have fantasized about time running backward so that we could undo Emily's murder. We would give our limbs, our organs, our lives to bring her back, to give her the opportunity to live out her dream of becoming an Episcopal priest, of retiring as a mesmerizing old woman sitting on her porch on Cape Cod, surrounded by her grandchildren and poodles.

But trying to recreate Emily from her DNA would be chasing an illusion. Massive waves of sorrow knock us down, breathless; we must learn to live with them. When our strength returns we stagger to our feet, summon whatever will we can, and do what needs to be done. Most of all we try to hold each other up. We can no more wish our grief away than King Canute could stem the ocean's tide.

So I find myself wanting to say to the letter writer, and to the scientists who offer him and other sorrowing families false hope: There are no technological fixes for grief; cloning your dear dead son will not repair the jagged hole ripped out of the tapestry of your life. Your letter fills me with sadness for you and your wife, not just for the loss of your child but also for the fruitless quest to quench your grief in a genetic replica of the son you lost. It would be fruitless even—especially—if you succeeded in creating a healthy biological duplicate. But there is little chance of that.

Emily lived until a few months shy of her 21st birthday. In those years our lives became interwoven in ways so intricate that I struggle for words to describe how Cynthia and I now feel. We were fortunate to have her with us long enough to see her become her own person, to love her whole-heartedly and to know beyond question that she loved us. Her loss changes us forever. Life flows in one direction; science cannot reverse the stream or reincarnate the dead.

The Emily we knew and loved would want us to continue to do what matters in our lives, to love each other, to do good work, to find meaning. Not to forget her, ever: We are incapable of that. Why would we want to? She was a luminous presence in our family, an extraordinary friend, a promising young philosopher. And we honor her by keeping her memory vibrant, not by trying to manufacture a genetic facsimile. And that thought makes me address the letter's author once more: I have to think that your son, were he able to tell you, would wish for you the same.

GENETIC ENCORES: THE ETHICS OF HUMAN CLONING
Robert Wachbroit

Wachbroit constructs a series of arguments in response to the various concerns raised by critics of human cloning. First of all, because Wachbroit believes that many such concerns are based on false beliefs about genetic influence, he argues directly against the view identified as genetic determinism. He then addresses concerns raised about the interests and rights of human clones; his conclusion is that concerns about the negative impact of cloning on those produced by this process are not sufficient to sustain a moral objection to cloning. Next, in attempting to minimize concerns about the social consequences of the cloning process, Wachbroit compares cloning with two closely related technologies—assisted reproductive technologies and genetic engineering—and he concludes that in some ways cloning is actually less problematic than these other two technologies. Finally, Wachbroit considers the reasons that might motivate the use of cloning to create a child, and he responds to the argument that a permissive social policy regarding cloning essentially constitutes an endorsement of a narcissitic motivation for having children.

The successful cloning of an adult sheep, announced in Scotland this past February [1997], is one of the most dramatic recent examples of a scientific discovery becoming a public issue. During the last few months, various commentators—scientists and theologians, physicians and legal experts, talk-radio hosts and editorial writers—have been busily responding to the news, some calming fears, others raising alarms about the prospect of cloning a human being. At the request of the President, the National Bioethics Advisory Commission (NBAC) held hearings and prepared a report on the religious, ethical, and legal issues surrounding human cloning. While declining to call for a permanent ban on the practice, the Commission recommended a moratorium on

Reprinted with permission of the publisher from *Report from the Institute for Philosophy & Public Policy,* vol. 17, no. 4, Fall 1997, pp. 1–7.

efforts to clone human beings, and emphasized the importance of further public deliberation on the subject.

An interesting tension is at work in the NBAC report. Commission members were well aware of "the widespread public discomfort, even revulsion, about cloning human beings." Perhaps recalling the images of Dolly the ewe that were featured on the covers of national news magazines, they noted that "the impact of these most recent developments on our national psyche has been quite remarkable." Accordingly, they felt that one of their tasks was to articulate, as fully and sympathetically as possible, the range of concerns that the prospect of human cloning had elicited.

Yet it seems clear that some of these concerns, at least, are based on false beliefs about genetic influence and the nature of the individuals that would be produced through cloning. Consider, for instance, the fear that a clone would not be an "individual" but merely a "carbon copy" of someone else—an automaton of the sort familiar from science fiction. As many scientists have pointed out, a clone would not in fact be an identical *copy,* but more like a delayed identical *twin.* And just as identical twins are two separate people—biologically, psychologically, morally and legally, though not genetically—so, too, a clone would be a separate person from her non-contemporaneous twin. To think otherwise is to embrace a belief in genetic determinism—the view that genes determine everything about us, and that environmental factors or the random events in human development are insignificant.

The overwhelming scientific consensus is that genetic determinism is false. In coming to understand the ways in which genes operate, biologists have also become aware of the myriad ways in which the environment affects their "expression." The genetic contribution to the simplest physical traits, such as height and hair color, is significantly mediated by environmental factors (and possibly by stochastic events as well). And the genetic contribution to the traits we value most deeply, from intelligence to compassion, is conceded by even the most enthusiastic genetic researchers to be limited and indirect.

It is difficult to gauge the extent to which "repugnance" toward cloning generally rests on a belief in genetic determinism. Hoping to account for the fact that people "instinctively recoil" from the prospect of cloning, James Q. Wilson wrote, "There is a natural sentiment that is offended by the mental picture of identical babies being produced in some biological factory." Which raises the question: once people learn that this picture is mere science fiction, does the offense that cloning presents to "natural sentiment" attenuate, or even disappear? Jean Bethke Elshtain cited the nightmare scenarios of "the man and woman on the street," who imagine a future populated by "a veritable army of Hitlers, ruthless and remorseless bigots who kept reproducing themselves until they had finished what the historic Hitler failed to do: annihilate us." What happens, though, to the "pity and terror" evoked by the topic of cloning when such scenarios are deprived (as they deserve to be) of all credibility?

Richard Lewontin has argued that the critics' fears—or at least, those fears that merit consideration in formulating public policy—dissolve once genetic determinism is refuted. He criticizes the NBAC report for excessive deference to opponents of human cloning, and calls for greater public education on the scientific issues. (The Commission in fact makes the same recommendation, but Lewontin seems unimpressed.) Yet even if a public education campaign succeeded in eliminating the most egregious misconceptions about genetic influence, that wouldn't settle the matter. People might continue to express concerns about the interests and rights of human clones, about the social and moral consequences of the cloning process, and about the possible motivations for creating children in this way.

INTERESTS AND RIGHTS

One set of ethical concerns about human clones involves the risks and uncertainties associated with the current state of cloning technology. This technology has not yet been tested with human subjects, and scientists cannot rule out the possibility of mutation or other biological damage. Accordingly, the NBAC report concluded that "at this time, it is morally unacceptable for anyone in the public or private sector, whether in a research or clinical setting, to attempt to create a child using somatic cell nuclear transfer cloning." Such efforts, it said, would pose "unacceptable risks to the fetus and/or potential child."

The ethical issues of greatest importance in the cloning debate, however, do not involve possible failures of cloning technology, but rather the consequences of its success. Assuming that scientists were able to clone human beings without incurring the risks mentioned above, what concerns might there be about the welfare of clones?

Some opponents of cloning believe that such individuals would be wronged in morally significant ways. Many of these wrongs involve the denial of what Joel Feinberg has called "the right to an open future." For example, a child might be constantly compared to the adult from whom he was cloned, and thereby burdened with oppressive expectations. Even worse, the parents might actually limit the child's opportunities for growth and development: a child cloned from a basketball player, for instance, might be denied any educational opportunities that were not in line with a career in basketball. Finally, regardless of his parents' conduct or attitudes, a child might be burdened by the *thought* that he is a copy and not an "original." The child's sense of self-worth or individuality or dignity, so some have argued, would thus be difficult to sustain.

How should we respond to these concerns? On the one hand, the existence of a right to an open future has a strong intuitive appeal. We are troubled by parents who radically constrict their children's possibilities for growth and development. Obviously, we would condemn a cloning parent for crushing a child with oppressive expectations, just as we might condemn fundamentalist parents for utterly isolating their children from the modern world, or the parents of twins for inflicting matching wardrobes and rhyming names. But this is not enough to sustain an objection to cloning itself. Unless the claim is that cloned parents cannot help but be oppressive, we would have cause to say they had wronged their children only because of their subsequent, and avoidable, sins of bad parenting—not because they had chosen to create the child in the first place. (The possible reasons for making this choice will be discussed below.)

We must also remember that children are often born in the midst of all sorts of hopes and expectations; the idea that there is a special burden associated with the thought "There is someone who is genetically just like me" is necessarily speculative. Moreover, given the falsity of genetic determinism, any conclusions a child might draw from observing the person from whom he was cloned would be uncertain at best. His knowledge of his future would differ only in degree from what many children already know once they begin to learn parts of their family's (medical) history. Some of us knew that we would be bald, or to what diseases we might be susceptible. To be sure, the cloned individual might know more about what he or she could become. But because our knowledge of the effect of environment on development is so incomplete, the clone would certainly be in for some surprises.

Finally, even if we were convinced that clones are likely to suffer particular burdens, that would not be enough to show that it is wrong to create them. The child of a poor family can be expected to suffer specific hardships and burdens, but we don't thereby conclude that such children shouldn't be born. Despite the hardships, poor children can experience parental love and many of the joys of being alive: the deprivations of poverty, however painful, are not decisive. More generally, no one's life is entirely free of some difficulties or burdens. In order for these considerations to have decisive weight, we have to be able to say that life doesn't offer any compensating benefits. Concerns expressed about the welfare of human clones do not appear to justify such a bleak assessment. Most such children can be expected to have lives well worth living; many of the imagined harms are no worse than those faced by children acceptably produced by more conventional means. If there is something deeply objectionable about cloning, it is more likely to be found by examining implications of the cloning process itself, or the reasons people might have for availing themselves of it.

CONCERNS ABOUT PROCESS

Human cloning falls conceptually between two other technologies. At one end we have the assisted reproductive technologies, such as in vitro fertilization, whose primary purpose is to enable couples to produce a child with whom they have a biological connection. At the other end we have the emerging technologies of genetic engineering—specifically, gene transplantation technologies—whose primary purpose is to produce a child that has certain traits. Many proponents of cloning see it as part of the first technology: cloning is just another way of providing a couple with a biological child they might otherwise be unable to have. Since this goal and these other technologies are acceptable, cloning should be acceptable as well. On the other hand, many opponents of cloning see it as part of the second technology: even though cloning is a transplantation of an entire nucleus and not of specific genes, it is nevertheless an attempt to produce a child with certain traits. The deep misgivings we may have about the genetic manipulation of offspring should apply to cloning as well.

The debate cannot be resolved, however, simply by determining which technology to assimilate cloning to. For example, some opponents of human cloning see it as continuous with assisted reproductive technologies; but since they find those technologies objectionable as well, the assimilation does not indicate approval. Rather than argue for grouping cloning with one technology or another, I wish to suggest that we can best understand the significance of the cloning process by comparing it with these other technologies, and thus broadening the debate.

To see what can be learned from such a comparative approach, let us consider a central argument that has been made against cloning—that it undermines the structure of the family by making identities and lineages unclear. On the one hand, the relationship between an adult and the child cloned from her could be described as that between a parent and offspring. Indeed, some commentators have called cloning "asexual reproduction," which clearly suggests that cloning is a way of generating *descendants*. The clone, on this view, has only one biological parent. On the other hand, from the point of view of genetics, the clone is a *sibling*, so that cloning is more accurately described as "delayed twinning" rather than as asexual reproduction. The clone, on this view, has two biological parents, not one—they are the same parents as those of the person from whom that individual was cloned.

Cloning thus results in ambiguities. Is the clone an offspring or a sibling? Does the clone have one biological parent or two? The moral significance of these ambiguities lies in the fact that in many societies, including our own, lineage identifies responsibilities. Typically, the parent, not the sibling, is responsible for the child. But if no one is unambiguously the parent, so the worry might go, who is responsible for the clone? Insofar as social identity is based on biological ties, won't this identity be blurred or confounded?

Some assisted reproductive technologies have raised similar questions about lineage and identity. An anonymous sperm donor is thought to have no parental obligations toward his biological child. A surrogate mother may be required to relinquish all parental claims to the child she bears. In these cases, the social and legal determination of "who is the parent" may appear to proceed in defiance of profound biological facts, and to subvert attachments that we as a society are ordinarily committed to upholding. Thus, while the *aim* of assisted reproductive technologies is to allow people to produce or raise a child to whom they are biologically connected, such technologies may also involve the creation of social ties that are permitted to override biological ones.

In the case of cloning, however, ambiguous lineages would seem to be less problematic, precisely because no one is being asked to relinquish a claim on a child to whom he or she might otherwise acknowledge a biological connection. What, then, are the critics afraid of? It does not seem plausible that someone would have herself cloned and then hand the child over to her parents, saying, "You take care of her! She's *your* daughter!" Nor is it likely that, if the cloned individual did raise the child, she would suddenly refuse to pay for college on the grounds that this was not a sister's responsibility. Of course, policymakers should address any confusion in the social or legal assignment of responsibility resulting from cloning. But there are reasons to think that this would be *less* difficult than in the case of other reproductive technologies.

Similarly, when we compare cloning with genetic engineering, cloning may prove to be the less troubling of the two technologies. This is true even though the dark futures to which they are often alleged to lead are broadly alike. For example, a recent *Washington Post* article examined fears that the development of genetic enhancement technologies might "create a market in preferred physical traits." The reporter asked, "Might it lead to a society of DNA haves and have-nots, and the creation of a new underclass of people unable to keep up with the genetically fortified Joneses?" Similarly, a member of the National Bioethics Advisory Commission expressed concern that cloning might become "almost a preferred practice," taking its place "on the continuum of providing the best for your child." As a consequence, parents who chose to "play the lottery of old-fashioned reproduction would be considered irresponsible."

Such fears, however, seem more warranted with respect to genetic engineering than to cloning. By offering some people—in all probability, members of the upper classes—the opportunity to acquire desired traits through genetic manipulation, genetic engineering could bring about a biological reinforcement (or accentuation) of existing social divisions. It is hard enough already for disadvantaged children to compete with their more affluent counterparts, given the material resources and intellectual opportunities that are often available only to children of privilege. This unfairness would almost certainly be compounded if genetic manipulation came into the picture. In contrast, cloning does not bring about "improvements" in the genome: it is, rather, a way of *duplicating* the genome—with all its imperfections. It wouldn't enable certain groups of people to keep getting better and better along some valued dimension.

To some critics, admittedly, this difference will not seem terribly important. Theologian Gilbert Meilaender, Jr., objects to cloning on the grounds that children created through this technology would be "designed as a product" rather than "welcomed as a gift." The fact that the design process would be more selective and nuanced in the case of genetic engineering would, from this perspective, have no moral significance. To the extent that this objection reflects a concern about the commodification of human life, we can address it in part when we consider people's reasons for engaging in cloning.

REASONS FOR CLONING

This final area of contention in the cloning debate is as much psychological as it is scientific or philosophical. If human cloning technology were safe and widely available, what use would people make of it? What reasons would they have to engage in cloning?

In its report to the President, the Commission imagined a few situations in which people might avail themselves of cloning. In one scenario, a husband and wife who wish to have children are both carriers of a lethal recessive gene:

> Rather than risk the one in four chance of conceiving a child who will suffer a short and painful existence, the couple considers the alternatives: to forgo rearing children; to adopt; to use prenatal diagnosis and selective abortion; to use donor gametes free of the recessive trait; or to use the cells of one of the adults and attempt to clone a child. To avoid donor gametes and selective abortion, while maintaining a genetic tie to their child, they opt for cloning.

In another scenario, the parents of a terminally ill child are told that only a bone marrow transplant can save the child's life. "With no other donor available, the parents attempt to clone a human being from the cells of the dying child. If successful, the new child will be a perfect match for bone marrow transplant, and can be used as a donor without significant risk or discomfort. The net result: two healthy children, loved by their parents, who happen [sic] to be identical twins of different ages."

The Commission was particularly impressed by the second example. That scenario, said the NBAC report, "makes what is probably the strongest possible case for cloning a human being, as it demonstrates how this technology could be used for lifesaving purposes." Indeed, the report suggests that it would be a "tragedy" to allow "the sick child to die because of a moral or political objection to such cloning." Nevertheless, we should note that many people would be morally uneasy about the use of a minor as a donor, regardless of whether the child were a result of cloning. Even if this unease is justifiably overridden by other concerns, the "transplant scenario" may not present a more compelling case for cloning than that of the infertile couple desperately seeking a biological child.

Most critics, in fact, decline to engage the specifics of such tragic (and presumably rare) situations. Instead, they bolster their case by imagining very different scenarios. Potential users of the technology, they suggest, are narcissists or control freaks—people who will regard their children not as free, original selves but as products intended to meet more or less rigid specifications. Even if such people are not genetic determinists, their recourse to cloning will indicate a desire to exert all possible influence over what "kind" of child they produce.

The critics' alarm at this prospect has in part to do, as we have seen, with concerns about the psychological burdens such a desire would impose on the clone. But it also reflects a broader concern about the values expressed, and promoted, by a society's reproductive policies. Critics argue that a society that enables people to clone themselves thereby endorses the most narcissistic reason for having children—to perpetuate oneself through a genetic encore. The demonstrable falsity of genetic determinism may detract little, if at all, from the strength of this motive. Whether or not clones will have a grievance against their parents for producing them with this motivation, the societal indulgence of that motivation is improper and harmful.

It can be argued, however, that the critics have simply misunderstood the social meaning of a policy that would permit people to clone themselves even in the absence of the heartrending exigencies described in the NBAC report. This country has developed a strong commitment to reproductive autonomy. (This commitment emerged in response to the dismal history of eugenics—the very history that is sometimes invoked to support restrictions on cloning.) With the exception of practices that risk coercion and exploitation—notably baby-selling and commercial surrogacy—we do not interfere with people's freedom to create and acquire children by almost any means, for almost any reason. This policy does not reflect a dogmatic libertarianism. Rather, it recognizes the extraordinary personal importance and private character of reproductive decisions, even those with significant social repercussions.

Our willingness to sustain such a policy also reflects a recognition of the moral complexities of parenting. For example, we know that the motives people have for bringing a child into the world do not necessarily determine the manner in which they raise him. Even when parents start out as narcissists, the experience of childrearing will sometimes transform their initial impulses, making them caring,

respectful, and even self-sacrificing. Seeing their child grow and develop, they learn that she is not merely an extension of themselves. Of course, some parents never make this discovery; others, having done so, never forgive their children for it. The pace and extent of moral development among parents (no less than among children) is infinitely variable. Still, we are justified in saying that those who engage in cloning will not, by virtue of this fact, be immune to the transformative effects of parenthood—even if it is the case (and it won't always be) that they begin with more problematic motives than those of parents who engage in the "genetic lottery."

Moreover, the nature of parental motivation is itself more complex than the critics often allow. Though we can agree that narcissism is a vice not to be encouraged, we lack a clear notion of where pride in one's children ends and narcissism begins. When, for example, is it unseemly to bask in the reflected glory of a child's achievements? Imagine a champion gymnast who takes delight in her daughter's athletic prowess. Now imagine that the child was actually cloned from one of the gymnast's somatic cells. Would we have to revise our moral assessment of her pleasure in her daughter's success? Or suppose a man wanted to be cloned and to give his child opportunities he himself had never enjoyed. And suppose that, rightly or wrongly, the man took the child's success as a measure of his own untapped potential—an indication of the flourishing life he might have had. Is *this* sentiment blamable? And is it all that different from what many natural parents feel?

CONCLUSION

Until recently, there were few ethical, social, or legal discussions about human cloning via nuclear transplantation, since the scientific consensus was that such a procedure was not biologically possible. With the appearance of Dolly, the situation has changed. But although it now seems more likely that human cloning will become feasible, we may doubt that the practice will come into widespread use.

I suspect it will not, but my reasons will not offer much comfort to the critics of cloning. While the technology for nuclear transplantation advances, other technologies—notably the technology of genetic engineering—will be progressing as well. Human genetic engineering will be applicable to a wide variety of traits; it will be more powerful than cloning, and hence more attractive to more people. It will also, as I have suggested, raise more troubling questions than the prospect of cloning has thus far.

SOURCES

National Bioethics Advisory Commission, "Cloning Human Beings: Report and Recommendations" (June 9, 1997).

James Q. Wilson, "The Paradox of Cloning," *Weekly Standard* (May 26, 1997).

Jean Bethke Elshtain, "Ewegenics," *New Republic* (March 31, 1997).

R. C. Lewontin, "The Confusion Over Cloning," *New York Review of Books* (October 23, 1997).

Leon Kass, "The Wisdom of Repugnance," *New Republic* (June 2, 1997).

Susan Cohen, "What Is a Baby? Inside America's Unresolved Debate About the Ethics of Cloning," *Washington Post Magazine* (October 12, 1997).

Rick Weiss, "Genetic Enhancements' Thorny Ethical Traits," *Washington Post* (October 12, 1997).

PREIMPLANTATION GENETIC DIAGNOSIS

EXTENDING PREIMPLANTATION GENETIC DIAGNOSIS: MEDICAL AND NON-MEDICAL USES

John A. Robertson

Robertson surveys the established, emerging, and prospective uses of preimplantation genetic diagnosis (PGD), emphasizing the distinction between medical and non-medical uses. PGD has principally been used to screen out embryos with aneuploidy (i.e., chromosomal abnormality) and Mendelian disease (i.e., genetic disease produced by a single-gene defect). As Robertson explains, newer medical uses include screening embryos for cancer susceptibility and late onset disorders, as well as HLA matching for existing children. He considers all of these medical uses of PGD to be ethically acceptable. Turning his attention to possible nonmedical uses of PGD, he identifies a series of factors that he considers relevant to their ethical assessment. Robertson applies his suggested ethical scheme in some detail to two nonmedical uses of PGD: (1) selection on the basis of gender and (2) selection for a perfect-pitch gene, should such a gene exist and be identified. He argues that the case against PGD for gender (sex) selection of a first child is much stronger than the case against gender selection for subsequent children in order to achieve gender "balance" in the family. His analysis also suggests that the case for allowing couples to use PGD to select for perfect pitch is fairly strong.

Debate about new reproductive technologies often cites preimplantation genetic diagnosis (PGD)—the technique by which early human embryos are genetically screened for selection for transfer to the uterus—as a practice that needs close ethical, legal, and social scrutiny. The use of PGD is growing, as are

Reprinted with permission of the publisher from *Journal of Medical Ethics*, vol. 29 (August 2003), pp. 213–216 © 2003 BMJ Publishing Group & Institute of Medical Ethics.

the indications for it. This article describes medical and non-medical extensions of PGD, and discusses the ethical, legal, and policy issues which they raise.

PGD AND ITS PREVALENCE

PGD has been available since 1990 for testing of aneuploidy in low prognosis in vitro fertilisation (IVF) patients, and for single gene and X linked diseases in at-risk couples. One cell (blastomere) is removed from a cleaving embryo and tested for the genetic or chromosomal condition of concern. Some programmes analyse polar bodies extruded from oocytes during meiosis, rather than blastomeres.[1] Cells are then either karyotyped to identify chromosomal abnormalities, or analysed for single gene mutations and linked markers.

Physicians have performed more than 3000 clinical cycles of PGD since 1990, with more than 700 children born as a result. The overall pregnancy rate of 24% is comparable to assisted reproductive practices which do not involve embryo or polar body biopsy.[1] Four centres (Chicago, Livingston (New Jersey), Bologna, and Brussels) accounted for nearly all the reported cases. More than 40 centres worldwide offer the procedure, however, including other centres in the United States and Europe, four centres in London and centres in the eastern Mediterranean, Southeast Asia, and Australia.

More than two-thirds of PGD has occurred to screen out embryos with chromosomal abnormalities in older IVF patients and in patients with a history of miscarriage. About 1000 cycles have involved single gene mutational analysis.[1] Mutational analysis requires additional skills beyond karyotyping for aneuploidies, including the ability to conduct the multiplex polymerase chain reaction (PCR) of the gene of interest and related markers.

Several new indications for PGD single gene mutational analysis have recently been reported. New uses include PGD to detect mutations for susceptibility to cancer and for late onset disorders such as Alzheimer's disease.[2, 3] In addition, parents with children needing hematopoietic stem cell transplants have used PGD to ensure that their next child is free of disease and a good tissue match for an existing child.[4] Some persons are also requesting PGD for gender selection for both first and later born children, and others have speculated that selection of embryos for a variety of non-medical traits is likely in the future.

PGD is ethically controversial because it involves the screening and likely destruction of embryos, and the selection of offspring on the basis of expected traits. While persons holding right to life views will probably object to PGD for any reason, those who view the early embryo as too rudimentary in development to have rights or interests see no principled objection to all PGD. They may disagree, however, over whether particular reasons for PGD show sufficient respect for embryos and potential offspring to justify intentional creation and selection of embryos. Donation of unwanted embryos to infertile couples reduces this problem somewhat, but there are too few such couples to accept all unwanted embryos, and in any event, the issue of selecting offspring traits remains.

Although ethical commentary frequently mentions PGD as a harbinger of a reproductive future of widespread genetic selection and alteration of prospective offspring, its actual impact is likely to be quite limited.[5, 6] Even with increasing use the penetrance of PGD into reproductive practice is likely to remain a very small percentage of the 150,000-plus cycles of IVF performed annually throughout the world. Screening for susceptibility and late onset diseases is limited by the few diseases for which single gene predispositions are known. Relatively few parents will face the need to conceive another child to provide an existing child with matched stem cells. Nor are nonmedical uses of PGD, other than for gender, likely to be practically feasible for at least a decade or more. Despite the limited reach of PGD, the ethical, legal, and policy issues that new uses raise, deserve attention.

NEW MEDICAL USES

New uses of PGD may be grouped into medical and non-medical categories. New medical uses include not only screening for rare Mendelian diseases, but also for susceptibility conditions, late onset diseases, and HLA matching for existing children.

Embryo screening for susceptibility and late onset conditions are logical extensions of screening for serious Mendelian diseases. For example, using PGD to screen out embryos carrying the p53 or BRCA1&2 mutations prevent the birth of children who would face a greatly increased lifetime risk of cancer, and hence require close monitoring, prophylactic surgery, or other preventive measures. PGD for highly penetrant adult disorders such as Alzheimer's or Huntington's disease prevents the birth of a child who will be healthy for many years, but who in her late thirties or early forties will experience the onset of progressive neurological disease leading to an early death.

Although these indications do not involve diseases that manifest themselves in infancy or childhood, the conditions in question lead to substantial health problems for offspring in their thirties or forties.[7] Avoiding the birth of children with those conditions thus reflects the desire of parents to have offspring with good prospects for an average life span. If PGD is accepted to exclude offspring with early onset genetic diseases, it should be accepted for later onset conditions as well.

PGD for adult onset disorders does mean that a healthy child might then be born to a person with those conditions who is likely to die or become incompetent while the child is dependent on her.[8] But that risk has been tolerated in other cases of assisted reproduction, such as intrauterine insemination with sperm of a man who is HIV positive, IVF for women with cystic fibrosis, and use of gametes stored prior to cancer therapy. As long as competent caregivers will be available for the child, the likely death or disability of a parent does not justify condemning or stopping this use, anymore than that reproduction by men going off to war should be discouraged.

A third new medical indication—HLA matching to an existing child—enables a couple to have their next child serve as a matched hematopoietic stem cell donor for an existing sick child. It may also ensure that the new child does not also suffer from that same disease. The availability of PGD, however, should not hinge on that fact, as the Human Fertilisation and Embryology Authority, in the UK, now requires.[9] A couple that would coitally conceive a child to be a tissue donor should be free to use PGD to make sure that that child will be a suitable match, regardless of whether that child is also at risk for genetic disease. Parents who choose PGD for this purpose are likely to value the new child for its own sake, and not only for the stem cells that it will make available. They do not use the new child as a "mere means" simply because they have selected HLA matched embryos for transfer.[10, 11]

NON-MEDICAL USES OF PGD

More ethically troubling has been the prospect of using PGD to screen embryos for genes that do not relate to the health of resulting children or others in the family. Many popular accounts of PGD assume that it will eventually be used to select for such non-medical traits as intelligence, height, sexual orientation, beauty, hair and eye colour, memory, and other factors.[5, 6] Because the genetic basis of those traits is unknown, and in any case is likely to involve many different genes, they may not be subject to easy mutational analysis, as Mendelian disease or susceptibility conditions are. Aside from gender, which is identifiable through karyotyping, it is unrealistic to think that non-medical screening for other traits, with the possible exception of perfect pitch, will occur anytime soon.

Still, it is useful to consider the methodology that ethical assessment of non-medical uses of PGD, if available, should follow. The relevant questions would be whether the proposed use serves valid reproductive or rearing interests; whether those interests are sufficient to justify creating and destroying embryos; whether selecting for a trait will harm resulting children; whether it will stigmatise existing persons, and whether it will create other social harms.

To analyse how these factors interact, I discuss PGD for sex selection and for children with perfect pitch. Similar issues would arise with PGD for sexual orientation, for hair and eye color, and for intelligence, size, and memory.

PGD for Gender Selection The use of medical technology to select the sex of offspring is highly controversial because of the bias against females which it usually reflects or expresses, and the resulting social disruptions which it might cause. PGD for gender selection faces the additional problem of appearing to be a relatively weak reason for creating and selecting embryos for discard or transfer.

The greatest social effects of gender selection arise when the gender of the first child is chosen. Selection for first children will overwhelmingly favour males, particularly if one child per family population policies apply. If carried out on a large scale, it could lead to great disparities in the sex ratio of the population, as has occurred in China and India through the use of ultrasound screening and abortion.[12, 13] PGD, however, is too expensive and inaccessible to be used on a wide scale for sex selection purposes. Allowing it to be used for the first child is only marginally likely to contribute to societal sex ratio imbalances. But its use is likely to reflect cultural notions of male privilege and may reinforce entrenched sexism toward women.

The use of PGD to choose a gender opposite to that of an existing child or children is much less susceptible to a charge of sexism. Here a couple seeks variety or "balance" in the gender of offspring because of the different rearing experiences that come with rearing children of different genders. Psychologists now recognise many biologically based differences between male and female children, including different patterns of aggression, learning, and spatial recognition, as well as hormonal differences.[14, 15] It may not be sexist in itself to wish to have a child or children of each gender, particularly if one has two or more children of the same gender.

Some feminists, however, would argue that any attention to the gender of offspring is inherently sexist, particularly when social attitudes and expectations play such an important role in constructing sex role expectations and behaviours.[16] Other feminists find the choice of a child with a gender different from existing children to be morally defensible as long as "the intention and consequences of the practice are not sexist," which is plausibly the case when gender variety in children is sought.[17] Desiring the different rearing experiences with boys and girls does not mean that the parents, who have already had children of one gender, are sexists or likely to value unfairly one or the other gender.[18]

Based on this analysis the case is weak for allowing PGD for the first child, but may be acceptable for gender variety in a family. With regard to the first child, facilitating preferences for male firstborns carries a high risk of promoting sexist social mores. It may also strike many persons as too trivial a concern to meet shared notions of the special respect due pre-implantation embryos. A proponent of gender selection, however, might argue that cultural preferences for firstborn males should be tolerated, unless a clearer case of harm has been shown. If PGD is not permitted, pregnancy and abortion might occur instead.

The case for PGD for gender variety is stronger because the risk of sexism is lessened. A couple would be selecting the gender of a second or subsequent children for variety in rearing experiences, and not out of a belief that one gender is privileged

over another. Gender selection in that case would occur without running the risks of fostering sexism and hurting women.[18]

The question still arises whether the desire for gender variety in children, even if not sexist, is a strong enough reason to justify creating and discarding embryos. The answer depends on how strong an interest that is. No one has yet marshalled the evidence showing that the need or desire for gender variety in children is substantial and important, or whether many parents would refrain from having another child if PGD for gender variety were not possible. More evidence of the strength and prevalence of this need would help in reaching a conclusion. If that case is made, then PGD for gender variety might be acceptable as well.[19]

The ethics committee of the American Society of Reproductive Medicine (ASRM) has struggled with these issues in a series of recent opinions. It initially addressed the issue of PGD for gender selection generally, and found that it "should be discouraged" for couples not going through IVF, and "not encouraged" for couples who were, but made no distinction between PGD for gender selection of first and later children.[20] Subsequently, it found that *preconception* gender selection would be acceptable for purposes of gender variety but not for the first child.[18]

Perceiving these two positions to be inconsistent, a doctor who wanted to offer PGD for gender selection inquired of the ethics committee why preconception methods for gender variety, which lacked 100% certainty, were acceptable but PGD, which guaranteed that certainty, was not. Focusing only on the sexism and gender discrimination issue, the chair of the ethics committee, in a widely publicised letter, found that PGD for gender balancing would be acceptable.[21] When the full committee reconsidered the matter, it concluded that it had not yet received enough evidence that the need for gender variety was so important in families that it justified creating and discarding embryos for that purpose.[19] In the future if such evidence was forthcoming then PGD for gender variety might also be acceptable.

What might constitute such evidence? One source would be families with two or more children of one gender who very much would like to have another child but only if they could be sure that it would be a child of the gender opposite of existing children. Given the legitimacy of wanting to raise children of both genders, reasonable persons might find that this need outweighs the symbolic costs of creating and discarding embryos for that purpose.

Another instance would be a case in which a couple has had a girl, but now wants a boy in order to meet cultural norms of having a male heir or a male to perform funeral rituals or play other cultural roles. An IVF programme in India is now providing PGD to select male offspring as the second child of couples who have already had a daughter.[22] Because of the importance of a male heir in India, those couples might well consider having an abortion if pregnant with a female fetus (even though illegal in India for that purpose). In that setting PGD for gender selection for gender variety appears to be justified.

PGD for Perfect Pitch Perfect or "absolute" pitch is the ability to identify and recall musical notes from memory.[23] Although not all great or successful musicians have perfect pitch, a large number of them do. Experts disagree over whether perfect pitch is solely inborn or may also be developed by early training, though most agree that a person either has it or does not. It also runs in families, apparently in an autosomal dominant pattern.[23] The gene or genes coding for this capacity have not, however, been mapped, much less sequenced. Because genes for perfect pitch may also relate to the genetic basis for language or other cognitive abilities, research to find that gene may be forthcoming.

Once the gene for perfect pitch or its linked markers are identified, it would be feasible to screen embryos for those alleles, and transfer only those embryos that test positive. The prevalence of those genes is quite low (perhaps three in 100) in the population, but high in certain families.[23] Thus only persons from those families who have a strong interest in the musical ability of their children would be potential candidates for PGD for perfect pitch. Many of them are likely to take their chances with coital conception and exposure of the child to music at an early age. Some couples, however, may be willing to undergo IVF and PGD to ensure musical

ability in their child. Should their request be accepted or denied?

As noted, the answer to this question depends on the importance of the reproductive choice being asserted, the burdens of the selection procedure, its impact on offspring, and its implications for deselected groups and society generally. The strongest case for the parents is if they persuasively asserted that they would not reproduce unless they could select that trait, and they have a plausible explanation for that position. Although the preference might appear odd to some, it might also be quite understandable in highly musical families, particularly ones in which some members already have perfect pitch. Parents clearly have the right to instill or develop a child's musical ability after birth. They might reasonably argue that they should have that right before birth as well.

If so, then creating and discarding embryos for this purpose should also be acceptable. If embryos are too rudimentary in development to have inherent rights or interests, then no moral duty is violated by creating and destroying them.[24] Some persons might think that doing so for trivial or unimportant reasons debases the inherent dignity of all human life, but having a child with perfect pitch will not seem trivial to parents seeking this technique. Ultimately, the judgment of triviality or importance of the choice within a broad spectrum rests with the couple. If they have a strong enough preference to seek PGD for this purpose and that preference rationally relates to understandable reproductive goals, then they have demonstrated its great importance to them. Only in cases unsupported by a reasonable explanation of the need—for example, perhaps creating embryos to pick eye or hair colour, should a person's individual assessment of the importance of creating embryos be condemned or rejected.

A third relevant factor is whether musical trait selection is consistent with respect for the resulting child. Parents who are willing to undergo the costs and burdens of IVF and PGD to have a child with perfect pitch may be so overly invested in the child having a musical career that they will prevent it from developing its own personality and identity. Parents, however, are free to instill and develop musical ability once the child is born, just as they are entitled to instill particular religious views. It is difficult to say that they cross an impermissible moral line of risk to the welfare of their prospective child in screening embryos for this purpose. Parents are still obligated to provide their child with the basic education and care necessary for any life plan. Wanting a child to have perfect pitch is not inconsistent with parents also wanting their child to be well rounded and equipped for life in other contexts.

A fourth factor, impact on deselected groups, is much less likely to be an issue in the case of perfect pitch because there is no stigma or negative association tied to persons without that trait. Persons without perfect pitch suffer no stigma or opprobrium by the couple's choice or public acceptance of it, as is arguably the case with embryo selection on grounds of gender, sexual orientation, intelligence, strength, size, or other traits. Nor is PGD for perfect pitch likely to perpetuate unfair class advantages, as selection for intelligence, strength, size, or beauty might.

A final factor is the larger societal impact of permitting embryo screening for a non-medical condition such as perfect pitch. A valid concern is that such a practice might then legitimise embryo screening for other traits as well, thus moving us toward a future in which children are primarily valued according to the attractiveness of their expected characteristics. But that threat is too hypothetical to justify limiting what are otherwise valid exercises of parental choice. It is highly unlikely that many traits would be controlled by genes that could be easily tested in embryos. Gender is determined by the chromosome, and the gene for pefect pitch, if ever found, would be a rare exception to the multifactorial complexity of such traits. Screening embryos for perfect pitch, if otherwise acceptable, should not be stopped simply because of speculation about what might be possible several decades from now.

PGD for Other Non-Medical Traits The discussion of PGD for perfect pitch illustrates the issues that would arise if single gene analysis became possible for other traits, such as sexual orientation, hair or eye colour, or height, intelligence, size, strength, and memory. In each case the ethical assessment depends on an evaluation of the importance of the

choice to the parents and whether that choice plausibly falls within societal understandings of parental needs and choice in reproducing and raising children. If so, it should usually be a sufficient reason to create and screen embryos. The effect on resulting offspring would also be of key moral importance. Whether selection carries a public or social message about the worth of existing groups should also be addressed.

Applying this methodology might show that some instances of non-medical selection are justified, as we have seen with embryo selection for gender variety and perhaps for having a child with perfect pitch. The acceptability of PGD to select other non-medical traits will depend on a careful analysis of the relevant ethical factors, and social acceptance of much greater parental rights to control the genes of offspring than now exists.

CONCLUSION

Although new indications are emerging for PGD, it is likely to remain a small part of reproductive practice for some time to come. Most new indications serve legitimate medical purposes, such as screening for single gene mutations for late onset disorders or susceptibility to cancer. There is also ethical support for using PGD to assure that a child is an HLA match with an existing child.

More controversial is the use of PGD to select gender or other non-medical traits. As with medical uses, the acceptability of non-medical screening will depend upon the interests served and the effects of using PGD for those purposes. Speculations about potential future non-medical uses should not restrict new uses of PGD which are otherwise ethically acceptable.

ACKNOWLEDGMENT

Professor Robertson was supported by the Ethical, Legal, and Social Issues Program of the National Institute of Human Genome Research, US National Institutes of Health (USA).

REFERENCES

1 International Working Group on Preimplantation Genetics. Preimplantation genetic diagnosis: Experience of 3000 clinical cycles. Report of the 11th annual meeting, May 15, 2001. *Reprod Biomedicine Online* 2001; 3:49–53.

2 Verlinsky Y., Rechitsky S., Verlinsky O., *et al.* Preimplantation diagnosis of P53 tumor suppressor gene mutations. *Reprod Biomedicine Online* 2001; 2:102–5.

3 Verlinsky Y., Rechitsky S., Schoolcraft W., *et al.* Preimplantation diagnosis for fanconi anemia combined with HLA matching. *JAMA* 2001; 285:3130–3.

4 Verlinsky Y., Rechitsky S., Verlinsky O., *et al.* Preimplantation diagnosis for early-onset alzheimer's disease caused by V717L mutation. *JAMA* 2002; 283:1018–21.

5 Fukuyama F. *Our postmodern future: consequences of the biotechnology revolution.* New York: Farrar, Strauss, & Giroux, 2002.

6 Stock G. *Redesigning humans: our inevitable genetic future.* New York: Houghton Mifflin, 2002.

7 Simpson J. L. Celebrating preimplantation genetic diagnosis of p53 mutations in Li-Fraumeni syndrome. *Reprod Biomedicine Online* 2001; 3: 2–3.

8 Towner D., Loewy R. S., Ethics of preimplantation diagnosis for a woman destined to develop early-onset Alzheimer disease. *JAMA* 2002; 283:1038–40.

9 Human Fertilisation and Embryology Authority. *Opinion of the ethics committee. Ethical issues in the creation and selection of preimplantation embryos to produce tissue donors.* London: HFEA, 2001 Nov 22.

10 Pennings G., Schots S., Liebaers I. Ethical considerations on preimplantation genetic diagnosis for HLA typing to match a future child as a donor of haematopoietic stem cells to a sibling. *Hum Reprod* 2002; 17:534–8.

11 Robertson J. A., Kahn J., Wagner J. Conception to obtain hematopoietic stem cells. *Hastings Cent Rep* 2002; 32:34–40.

12 Sen A. More than 100 million women are missing. *New York Review of Books* 1990; 37:61–8.

13 Eckholm E. Desire for sons drives use of prenatal scans in China. *The New York Times* 2002 Jun 21:A3.

14 Jaccoby E. E., Jacklin C. N., *The psychology of sex differences.* Palo Alto: Stanford University Press, 1974.

15 Robertson J. A., Preconception gender selection. *Am J Bioeth* 2001; 1:2–9.

16 Grubb A., Walsh P., Gender-vending II. *Dispatches* 1994; 1:1–3.

17 Mahowald M. B., *Genes, women, equality.* New York: Oxford University Press, 2000: 121.

18 American Society of Reproductive Medicine, Ethics Committee. Preconception gender selection for nonmedical reasons. *Fertil Steril* 2001; 75:861–4.

19 Robertson J. A., Sex selection for gender variety by preimplantation genetic diagnosis. *Fert Steril* 2002; 78:463.

20 American Society of Reproductive Medicine, Ethics Committee. Sex selection and preimplantation genetic diagnosis. *Fertil Steril* 1999; 72:595–8.

21 Kolata G. Society approves embryo selection. *The New York Times* 2001 Sept 26:A14.

22 Malpani A., Malpani A., Modi D., Preimplantation sex selection for family balancing in India. *Hum Reprod* 2002; 17:11–12.

23 Blakeslee S. Perfect pitch: the key may lie in the genes. *The New York Times* 1990 Nov 30:1.

24 American Society of Reproductive Medicine, Ethics Committee. Ethical considerations of assisted reproductive technologies. *Fertil Steril* 1994; 62(suppl):32–7S.

SELECTING EMBRYOS FOR DESIRED TRAITS

President's Council on Bioethics

In this brief passage, the President's Council on Bioethics considers whether it is likely that significant demand will emerge for preimplantation genetic diagnosis (PGD) to select embryos *for* desired traits, in contrast to the established practice of using PGD to select *against* embryos with genetic or chromosomal disorders. In the council's view, several practical problems confront this possible extension of PGD use, making it unlikely that the use of PGD to select embryos for desired traits will "become widespread in the forseeable future." Still, the council argues, there are reasons to believe that "the use of this approach toward 'better children' might well become the practice of at least a significant minority."

... [T]he possibility of genetic enhancement of children through embryo selection cannot be easily dismissed. This approach ... would not introduce new genes but would merely select positively among those that occur naturally. It depends absolutely on IVF, as augmented by the screening of the early embryos for the presence (or absence) of the desired genetic markers, followed by the selective transfer of those embryos that pass muster. This would amount to an "improvement-seeking" extension of the recently developed practice of preimplantation genetic diagnosis (PGD), now in growing use as a way to detect the presence or absence of genetic or chromosomal abnormalities *before* the start of a pregnancy.

As currently practiced, PGD works as follows: Couples at risk for having a child with a chromosomal or genetic disease undertake IVF to permit embryo screening before transfer, obviating the need for later prenatal diagnosis and possible abortion. A dozen or more eggs are fertilized and the embryos are grown to the four-cell or the eight-to-ten-cell stage. One or two of the embryonic cells (blastomeres) are removed for chromosomal analysis and genetic testing. Using a technique called polymerase chain reaction to amplify the tiny amount of DNA in the blastomere, researchers are able to detect the presence of genes responsible for one or more genetic disorders.[1] Only the embryos free of the genetic or chromosomal determinants for the disorders under scrutiny are made eligible for transfer to the woman to initiate a pregnancy.

The use of IVF and PGD to move from disease avoidance to baby improvement is conceptually simple, at least in terms of the techniques of screening, and would require no change in the procedure. Indeed, PGD has already been used to serve two goals unrelated to the health of the child-to-be: to preselect the sex of a child, and to produce a child who could serve as a compatible bone-marrow or umbilical-cord-blood donor for a desperately ill sibling. (In the former case, chromosomal analysis of the blastomere identifies the embryo's sex; in the latter case, genetic analysis identifies which embryos are immunocompatible with the needy recipient.) It is certainly likely that blastomere testing can be adapted to look for specific genetic variants at *any* locus of the human genome. And even without knowing the precise function of specific genes, statistical correlation of the presence of certain genetic variants with certain phenotypic traits (say, with an increase in IQ points or with perfect pitch) could lead to testing for these genetic variants, with selection following on this basis. As Dr. Francis Collins, director of the National Human Genome Research Institute, noted in his presentation to the Council, the time may soon arrive in which PGD is practiced for the purpose of selecting embryos with desired genotypes, even in the absence of elevated risk of particular genetic disorders.[2] Dr. Yury Verlinsky, director of the Reproductive Genetics Institute in Chicago, has recently predicted that soon "there will be no IVF without PGD."[3] Over the years, more and more traits will presumably become identifiable with the aid of PGD, including desirable genetic markers for intelligence, musicality, and so on, as well as undesirable markers for obesity, nearsightedness, color-blindness,[4] etc.

Yet, as Dr. Collins also pointed out to the Council, there are numerous practical difficulties with this scenario. For one thing, neither of the parents may carry the genetic variant they are most interested in selecting for. Also, selecting for highly polygenic traits would require screening a large number of embryos in order to find one that had the desirable complement. With only a dozen or so embryos to choose from, it will not be possible to optimize for the many necessary variants.[5]

The practice of PGD and selective transfer is still quite new, and fewer than 10,000 children have been born with its aid. How likely or widespread such a practice might become is difficult to predict. As we have already indicated, a number of practical issues would need to be addressed before PGD could be extended to permit selection of desirable traits beyond the absence of genetic disorders. First are questions of possible harm caused by removing blastomeres for testing (up to a sixth or even a quarter of the embryo's cells are taken). Although current evidence (from limited practice) suggests that the procedure inflicts neither any immediately visible harm on the early embryos, nor any obvious harm on

Reprinted from President's Council on Bioethics, *Beyond Therapy: Biotechnology and the Pursuit of Happiness* (2003), pp. 40–44.

the child that results, more attention to long-term risks to the child born following PGD is needed before many people would consider using it for "improvement" purposes only. Because many of the desirable human phenotypic traits are very likely polygenic, the contribution of any single gene identifiable by blastomere testing is likely to be small, and the likelihood of finding all the "desired" genetic variants in a single embryo is exponentially smaller still. Testing for multiple genetic variants using the DNA from a single blastomere is likely to be limited—for a time—by the quantities of DNA available, the sensitivity of the genetic tests, and the ability to perform multiple tests on the same sample. But it seems only a matter of time before techniques are perfected that will permit simultaneous screening of IVF embryos for multiple genetic variants. And should some of the "desirable" genes come grouped in clusters, selection for at least some desired traits might well be possible.

Finally, even if PGD could be used successfully to select an embryo with a number of desirable genetic variants, there is simply no guarantee that the child born after this procedure would grow up with the desired traits. The interplay of nature and nurture (genes and environment) in human development is too complex and too little understood to make such results predictable. Given that IVF combined with PGD is an inconvenient and expensive alternative to normal procreation, and given that success is doubtful at best, the purely elective use of this procedure seems unlikely to become widespread in the foreseeable future. . . .

Nevertheless, we think it would be imprudent to ignore completely this approach to "better children." More and more people are turning to assisted reproduction technologies (ART): in parts of western Europe, roughly five percent of all births involve ART; in the United States, it is roughly one percent and climbing, as the average maternal age of childbirth keeps rising and family size keeps declining. More and more people are using IVF not merely to overcome infertility but to screen and select embryos free of certain genetic defects. Women who plan to delay childbearing are being encouraged to consider early removal and cryopreservation of their own youthful ovarian tissue, to be reintroduced into their bodies at sites easily accessible for egg harvesting when they decide to have children. Other novel methods of obtaining supplies of eggs for IVF—possibly including deriving them in bulk from stem cells[6]—would make the procedure less burdensome, and would, in theory, permit the creation of a large enough population of embryos to make screening for polygenic traits feasible.

The anticipated vast extension of genetic screening will make many more couples aware of the risks they run in natural reproduction, and they may choose to turn to IVF to reduce them—especially if obtaining eggs became easy. Once more and more couples start screening embryos for disease-related concerns, and once scientists have identified those genes that correlate with various admirable traits, the anticipated expansion of improved and more precise screening techniques might enable users of IVF to screen for "desirable genes" as well. People already using PGD to screen for disease markers might seek information also about other traits, as they have with sex or histocompatibility. And if, once screening becomes automated, its cost comes down, or if society decides to reimburse for PGD (regarding it as less expensive than the care of genetically diseased children), the use of this approach toward "better children" might well become the practice of at least a significant minority. Under these circumstances, should genuine and significant improvements be achieved for a few highly desired attributes (say, in maximum lifespan . . .), one can easily imagine that there would be an increased demand for the practice, inconvenient or not. In the meantime, we would do well to consider the ethical implications not only of such future prospects but also of our current practices that make use of genetic knowledge.

NOTES

1 Although scientists are able to identify thousands of human genes and their variants, the fact that at present blastomere testing is done on the minute quantity of DNA present in one or two cells limits the reach of PGD in any given embryo to a handful of genetic variants. However, ongoing research on techniques for whole genome amplification will likely permit PGD in the future to test simultaneously for hundreds or even thousands of genetic variants in the same embryo. Of course, because of the complex relationship between genes and traits, the mere ability to screen for multiple

genetic variants in no way guarantees that numerous phenotypic traits will soon be detectable.

2 Collins, F., "Genetic Enhancements: Current and Future Prospects," Presentation at the December 2002 meeting of the President's Council on Bioethics, Washington, D.C. Transcript available on the Council's website at www.bioethics.gov.

3 Mandavilli, A., "Fertility's new frontier takes shape in the test tube," *Nature Medicine* 9(8): 1095, 2003.

4 Color-blindness, a single-gene defect, can already be screened for.

5 If, for example, a desired trait required the concurrence of only seven specific genetic alleles and (to take the simplest case) there were only two alternate variants of each gene, one would need (on the average) 128 embryos (and even more eggs) to get the full complement (2 to the seventh power). . . . Today, in the average IVF cycle, twelve to fifteen eggs are obtained by superovulation, and roughly only half make it to the stage where screening could occur. Of course, if the oocyte supply could be increased, say by deriving oocytes from embryonic stem cells, this problem might be soluble.

6 Hübner, K., et al., "Derivation of oocytes from mouse embryonic stem cells," *Science* 300(5620): 1251–1256, 2003.

THE DANGEROUS PROMISE OF GENE THERAPY
Sophia Kolehmainen

Kolehmainen discusses the tragic case of Jesse Gelsinger, a young man who volunteered for a 1999 gene therapy protocol and died as a result of his participation. In Kolehmainen's view, the Gelsinger case pointedly illustrates the need for more effective regulation and oversight of gene therapy research. In this regard, she considers problems associated with (1) the safety of gene therapy protocols, (2) commercial interests in gene therapy, and (3) the recruitment of research subjects for gene therapy protocols.

In the mid-1980s scientists began to extol the promises of gene therapy. Conceptually (and if you consider the world only at the sub-microscopic level), gene therapy is a logical, straightforward solution to genetic disease: if a gene seems to be causing a disease, then to cure the disease scientists must remove the "bad" gene, and substitute or add a "good" gene. The reality is much more complex. Scientists have faced hurdles at every step of the gene therapy process as the multiple relationships among genes and between genes, disease, proteins, and the immune system (to name just a few of the relevant factors) have undermined the simplicity of the theory and added to the already difficult technicalities of inserting new genes into humans. Though more than three hundred gene therapy protocols, involving more than four thousand patients, have been approved for human trials in the United States, gene therapy has yet to fulfil its promise of curing any genetic disease.

On September 17th, 1999, 18-year-old Jesse Gelsinger died as a result of his voluntary participation in a gene-therapy experiment, becoming the first known human victim of this technology. Jesse's experience illuminates important elements in gene therapy that should make government agencies, scientists, and the public take the need to regulate and oversee this technology very seriously.

Jesse had a rare genetic disease, known as ornithine transcarbamylase (OTC) deficiency, which affected his ability to rid his body of ammonia, a usual, but toxic, breakdown product of protein. In

From *GeneWatch*, vol. 13, no. 1 (February 2000). Reprinted with permission of *GeneWatch*, the magazine of the Council for Responsible Genetics.

healthy individuals, as proteins are broken down, enzymes in the liver rid the body of the ammonia. People who have OTC (usually males, as the associated gene appears to be located on the X chromosome, making it much rarer for women, who have two X chromosomes, to have the condition) lack the enzymes needed to rid the body of ammonia, and so the ammonia builds up in the blood, can travel to the brain, and, in extreme cases, lead to coma, brain damage and death.

In its severest form, OTC induces coma and usually brain damage just seventy-two hours after birth. One half of children with OTC die in their first month of life, and half of the rest die before their fifth birthday. Jesse had a mild form of the disease because some of his enzymes were functioning normally. He was therefore able to control the disease with diet and drugs, though he needed to take 32 pills a day. However, as long as he stuck to the restrictive diet and drug regimen, Jesse was not sick.

The experimental protocol for which Jesse volunteered had no chance of providing him, or any of the other volunteers, with any benefit. It was designed only to test the safety of a treatment that would be used on babies with the fatal form of OTC. The scientists who designed the protocol at the University of Pennsylvania's Institute for Gene Therapy, Dr. James Wilson and Dr. Mark Batshaw, believed that OTC could be surmounted with gene therapy. They hoped to infuse babies who had OTC with genes that would help them produce the missing enzymes. In order to get these genes into the patient's cells, Dr. Wilson developed a weakened cold virus (known as adenovirus) which was designed to enter the cells as any virus would, but, instead of delivering disease, it was supposed to deliver the corrective OTC gene. Wilson and Batshaw hoped that the infusion of adenovirus and corrective genes could be used to reduce infant fatalities by controling the high levels of ammonia in babies with OTC immediately after birth.

Wilson and Batshaw worked together to develop the protocol and, in 1995, they submitted their OTC protocol to the National Institute of Health's (NIH) Recombinant DNA Advisory Committee (RAC) and the Food and Drug Administration (FDA) for review and approval, as is required for all human experiments involving gene therapy. Their human gene therapy trial called for 18 patients with OTC in six groups of three, to receive increasing doses of the genetically altered adenovirus carrying the corrective OTC gene. The adenovirus-OTC infusion was to be delivered to the patients through a catheter into an artery that leads directly to the liver. The goal of the trial was to find the maximum tolerated dose of adenovirus and OTC: high enough to work, and low enough to avoid serious side effects.

Jesse found out about the trial from his pediatric geneticist when he was seventeen and, though he wanted to sign up right away, regulations required him to wait until his eighteenth birthday. Four days after his eighteenth birthday, Jesse was at the University of Pennsylvania meeting with Dr. Raper, the surgeon in charge of patient and medical care for the gene therapy trial. Jesse was deemed eligible for the study and assigned to the final test subject group— the group that would receive the highest dose of adenovirus. At the time, the researchers believed that in the worst case, the trial might result in an inflamed liver. When Jesse was to begin the experiment on September 13, 1999, he traveled to Pennsylvania from Arizona by himself; his father had made plans to fly out later for the liver biopsy—the procedure that was considered to carry the most serious risk.

On September 13, 1999 Dr. Raper injected 30 milliliters of the adenovirus with the corrective OTC gene into Jesse's bloodstream. That evening Jesse was sick with a fever of 104.5 degrees. Dr. Raper was not particularly concerned because other patients in the study had had a similar reaction. By the morning of September 14, however, Jesse seemed disoriented and exhibited signs of jaundice—a condition which usually results from either liver failure or blood clotting, both of which would be serious for an individual with a liver already weakened by OTC. That evening, Jesse had dangerously high ammonia levels in his blood and was in a coma. Jesse's father arrived on the morning of September 15th. Later that day Jesse's lungs began to fail and he went into kidney failure the next day. According to the physicians, Jesse's severe immune system reaction led to multiple-organ-system failure and he died on September 17th, 1999, four days after the gene-therapy injection.

THE SAFETY OF GENE THERAPY

Human gene therapy trials raise the question of how safe an experiment must be before it is ethical to try it on humans. Prior to the human protocol, Batshaw and Wilson had done animal studies to help prove that OTC gene therapy was ready for human trial. They cited more than twenty experiments on mice to prove the efficacy of the treatment, and twelve safety studies in mice, Rhesus monkeys and baboons.

In Wilson and Batshaw's early animal experiments with adenovirus, several Rhesus monkeys died after intense immune system reactions like Jesse's to high doses of adenovirus. Wilson then experimented with the adenovirus itself, removing different combinations of its DNA to make it safer. Wilson believed that the adenovirus variation he used in the human protocol was significantly less toxic than the one which caused the death of the monkeys. The U. Penn researchers also decided to reduce the highest dose to be used in the human trial two-hundredfold from that used in the animal experiments.

In addition to safety measures suggested by the animal experiments, the mandatory review of human gene therapy experiments by the FDA and RAC is supposed to add another level of precaution. However, critics of this process have often stated that the current regulatory framework—review by the NIH's RAC and approval by the FDA—creates an ineffectual review process. When Wilson and Batshaw first presented their protocol for review by the RAC, both of the RAC scientists reviewing the protocol had reservations about approving it. They felt that the protocol was too dangerous to test on asymptomatic individuals as it was the first time heavy doses of adenovirus would be injected directly into the bloodstream and the experiment had no chance of lasting benefit to the human subjects. However, continued negotiations between the federal reviewers (including RAC and FDA officials) and the University of Pennsylvania scientists resulted in approval of the protocol.

Following the report of Jesse Gelsinger's death, and subsequent revelations of six other deaths in gene therapy experiments in New York and Massachusetts, the National Institute of Health (NIH) RAC convened a three-day public inquiry into Jesse's death, the conduct of gene therapy research, and the

safety of using adenovirus. The inquiry was covered in the media, and attended by officials of the FDA, the University of Pennsylvania scientists, other gene therapy researchers, and family and friends of Jesse Gelsinger.

In what was described as a tumultuous exchange on the first day of the inquiry, the FDA argued that Jesse's liver was not functioning well enough at the time of the infusion of adenovirus, and he should not have been eligible for the study; that the Pennsylvania scientists had violated FDA regulations by failing to report information about patients who had experienced serious side effects that could have ended the trial; and that the informed consent document that Jesse signed deviated from the one approved by the agency when it reviewed the protocol. The new consent form had made no mention of the severe immune system responses to adenovirus that led to the deaths of the monkeys.

Dr. Wilson and the scientists from the University of Pennsylvania countered that they had no evidence from human or animal testing that could have foretold Jesse's death; and that at the time Jesse enrolled in the study he was eligible. On the second day of the inquiry, the University of Pennsylvania stated that they still could not explain Jesse's death, though they had found some evidence in his bone marrow of another virus which might have increased his susceptibility to the effects of the adenovirus.

On January 21, 2000, the FDA indefinitely shut down human gene therapy experiments at the University of Pennsylvania, citing "numerous serious deficiencies" in ensuring patient safety, and issued a report detailing 18 specific violations. This action by the FDA halted eight experiments at Dr. Wilson's Institute for Gene Therapy at the University of Pennsylvania, including five active clinical trials. The trials will remain "on-hold" until the Institute responds formally to the FDA's report, and convinces the FDA that it can properly follow the federal rules designed to ensure the safety of study volunteers.

The human gene therapy trials at the University of Pennsylvania were not the only trials affected by the inquiry into Jesse's death. The FDA also suspended enrollment in gene therapy trials for advanced liver cancer patients being run by the Schering-Plough Corporation of Madison, NJ and the University of California San Francisco. The Schering-Plough trials were using high doses of adenovirus in the liver and researchers there had also found evidence of serious side effects from the use of adenovirus in gene therapy.

Since the news of Jesse's death was first brought to the attention of government regulators and the public in September 1999, further evidence of serious risks to patient safety in other gene therapy experiments has come to light. In response to reminders sent out by regulators, the NIH received 691 reports of "serious adverse events" in gene therapy experiments, and although the current regulatory structure requires researchers to promptly notify the NIH as problems arise, 652 of the reports had never been presented to the NIH. Reports from at least two gene therapy trials revealed that volunteers had died during the course of the experiments. The scientists in both cases decided that the deaths were not related to the gene therapy treatment. However, their reports indicate that, in fact, they cannot conclusively say what caused the deaths of some of the volunteers.

CORPORATE INTERESTS IN GENE THERAPY

In addition to questions of safety, the massive amount of corporate interest in the development of gene therapy technology raises questions that can only be addressed with diligent oversight. Intense commercial interest in gene therapy may create conflicts between business decisions and medical decisions.

In the case of the gene therapy trial that led to Jesse's death, Dr. James Wilson, the head of the Institute for Gene Therapy at the University of Pennsylvania, also owns a private company called Genovo Inc., which he founded in 1992. Genovo has the rights to any discoveries made by Wilson at his University of Pennsylvania lab. Through this arrangement, Genovo has access to Wilson's discoveries, at the same time minimizing its business risks as the company can let the lab run the clinical trials prior to deciding to invest. The NIH further reduced Genovo's risk and maximized the company's benefits by funding the OTC trial in which Jesse took

part. Genovo also has a financial stake in the adenovirus variation Wilson developed and tested on Jesse in the human gene therapy trial, which would have been very marketable if it had been successful.

In addition, BIOGEN, a Cambridge-based biotechnology company, has paid Genovo thirty-seven million dollars since 1995 for the right to eventually market any liver and lung related therapies developed by Genovo. Genovo shares the money from BIOGEN with Dr. Wilson's Institute at U.Penn, and in fact the Biogen money accounts for twenty percent of the Institute's budget. The Genovo-Biogen deal (which is up for renewal this year) calls for Genovo to make progress in moving gene therapy toward a marketable product.

In August, 1999, Genovo entered into an agreement with GENZYME (another Cambridge-based biotech company), to develop liver-directed gene therapy for metabolic disorders.

Wilson has stated many times that his business interests do not influence his judgment during trials and, also, that his involvement in gene therapy is not about money, but about "leadership, notoriety, and accomplishment." Even so, the existence of the financial stakes and relationships described above, which seem to be typical in the gene therapy research industry, require vigilant oversight to ensure that the medical decisions, as much as possible, are based on considerations of health and not money.

WILLING AND ABLE VOLUNTEERS

The intense corporate interest in human gene therapy becomes even more disturbing when considered in conjunction with the fact that people are literally lining up to be test subjects for clinical trials. Gene therapy gives promise to people who are desperately searching for hope. It is a technology marketed as a cure for genetic disease—diseases which often lead to suffering which is entirely unjustifiable. If a friend or a family member had a genetic disease, and you watched him or her suffer without respite or chance of cure, wouldn't you jump at any opportunity to end that? This scenario raises serious concerns since it puts a most vulnerable and well-meaning group of people at serious risk without adequate protections.

One of the most important questions Wilson and Batshaw faced in designing their human trial of OTC gene therapy was determining who were the appropriate test subjects for their research. Initially, they believed that the protocol should be tried on infants with severe OTC, as the therapy was designed specifically for these babies. But Arthur Caplan, the resident bioethics expert at the University of Pennsylvania, disagreed. He stated that it would be unethical to experiment with sick babies because the parents of dying infants are too stressed to be able to give informed consent.

Consequently, Wilson and Batshaw decided to use stable adults for the protocol—men like Jesse who had the disease but were surviving with drugs and diet, and women who carry the gene linked to OTC. This shift from dying infants to stable adults meant that people who were living with their disease and benefiting from conventional treatments were put at risk in situations which would not produce any benefit for them.

The NIH/RAC hearings after Jesse's death also made public the fact that some of the volunteers for this study were recruited in a coercive manner—using Internet sites and newsletters which detailed the promise of the therapy if it worked and which stressed the need for human subjects. This type of information, placed where it would be seen by a population sensitive to the problems of living with a genetic disease raises further issues about getting truly informed and voluntary subjects for human experimentation.

Human gene therapy experimentation raises many issues. The promise of the technology is represented as very great and the reality of it is very dangerous, that human gene therapy must be seriously and cautiously evaluated. Without increased and more effective oversight, Jesse's death could be the first of many in gene therapy. Though Jesse's participation in the human trial did not provide him or the infants with OTC with any benefit, it did perhaps lead to something even more important in this field. Jesse's death has forced researchers and government officials to reappraise the current framework and structure of gene therapy research, to reexamine informed consent procedures, and to take public responsibility for their actions.

GERM-LINE GENE THERAPY
LeRoy Walters and Julie Gage Palmer

Walters and Palmer begin by presenting four scenarios in which germ-line gene therapy, if it were available, would be very useful. Their subsequent analysis of the ethics of germ-line gene therapy is based on the assumption that effective (and safe) germ-line intervention methods will eventually be developed. Surveying the major ethical arguments for and against germ-line gene therapy, the authors identify and articulate five arguments in support of germ-line gene therapy and eight arguments against it. Ultimately supportive of germ-line gene therapy, Walters and Palmer explicitly endorse three of the five 'pro' arguments and offer replies to the eight 'con' arguments.

. . . It should be recognized that the various alternatives for approaching genetic disease have differing

effects on the germ line of the treated patient. Standard medical therapies, like somatic cell gene therapy, are somatic treatments and do not correct genetic defects in a patient's germ line. They may allow patients to live and to reproduce, passing on genetic mistakes which, without treatment, would not be perpetuated. Preimplantation and prenatal selection, like somatic medicine, may also result in a higher incidence of germ-line genetic defects because, unless they employ selective discard and selective abortion of unaffected carriers, both strategies increase the number of carriers of genetic defects that are born.

Successful germ-line gene replacement, on the other hand, will not perpetuate genetic mistakes. It will not only cure the patient at hand; it will also prevent the disease in question from arising in that patient's descendants. Applied to heterozygous carriers on a large scale, it could theoretically eliminate chosen disease-causing genes from the human gene pool.

As long as germ-line gene therapy must be performed on human zygotes or embryos one at a time after in vitro fertilization, it is likely to remain an expensive technology with limited use. Only if a technique is developed for performing gene replacement or gene repair within the reproductive cells of human adults—perhaps through the injection of highly refined vectors that "home in" only on those cells (or their precursors in males)—are we likely to see the widespread diffusion of germ line genetic intervention for disease prevention. . . .

FOR WHAT CLINICAL SITUATIONS WILL GERM-LINE GENE THERAPY BE PROPOSED?

It is difficult to predict the precise context in which germ-line gene therapy will first be considered. Tables 1 through 4 show four scenarios where the issue of germ-line intervention may at least be discussed at some point in the future.

TABLE 1 Mode of Inheritance 1

Both the wife and the husband are afflicted with a recessive genetic disorder. That is, both have two copies of the same malfunctioning gene at a particular site in their chromosomes. Therefore, all of their offspring are likely to be affected with the same genetic disorder.

TABLE 2 Mode of Inheritance 2

Both the wife and the husband are carriers of a recessive genetic disorder. That is, each has one copy of a properly functioning and one copy of a malfunctioning gene at a particular site in their chromosomes. Following Mendel's laws, 25% of the couple's offspring are likely to be "normal," 50% are likely to be carriers like their parents, and 25% are likely to be afflicted with the genetic disorder.

TABLE 3 Disease Condition 1

A diagnosable genetic disorder results in major, irreversible damage to the brains of affected fetuses during the first trimester of pregnancy. There is no known method for making genetic repairs in the uterus during pregnancy. If any genetic repair is to be made, it must be completed before the embryo begins its intrauterine development.

TABLE 4 Disease Condition 2

A diagnosable genetic disorder affects many different cell types in many different parts of the bodies of patients affected by the disorder. Somatic cell gene therapy that targets a particular cell type is therefore unlikely to be successful in combating the disorder. Therefore, germ-line gene therapy delivered early enough to affect *all* cell types may be the only feasible way to prevent disease in a particular future person.

The kind of situation described in Table 1 is likely to arise as medical care succeeds in prolonging the lives of people with genetic disorders such as sickle cell disease or cystic fibrosis. If somatic cell gene therapy is employed in significant numbers of people afflicted with recessive genetic diseases, some of those people's somatic cells will be able to function normally, but their reproductive cells will remain unchanged, thus assuring that they will be carriers of genetic disease to the next generation. If two such phenotypically cured people marry and have children, all or almost all of their children will be afflicted with the disease which their parents had. Each succeeding generation of these children will need somatic cell gene therapy for the treatment of their disease.

Table 2 sketches a scenario frequently encountered by genetic counselors. In this case, germ-line genetic intervention could be viewed as an alternative to prenatal diagnosis and selective abortion of affected fetuses or to preimplantation diagnosis and the selective discard of affected early embryos. A couple might also elect germ-line genetic intervention in order to avoid producing children who are *carriers* of genetic defects, even if the children are not themselves afflicted with genetic disease. The parents would know that children who are carriers may one day face precisely the kind of difficult reproductive decisions that they as parents are facing.

In the type of case outlined in Table 3, somatic cell gene therapy might be effective if one could deliver it to the developing embryo and fetus during the earliest stages of pregnancy, that is, shortly after the embryo has implanted in the uterus. However, there is no known method of administering intrauterine therapy to an early first-trimester embryo, and a deferral of treatment until the second or third trimester would probably allow irreversible damage to occur. Preimplantation treatment, which would almost certainly affect the future germ-line cells as well as the future somatic cells, could be the only feasible approach to producing children who are not brain damaged, especially for couples who reject the alternative of selectively discarding early embryos.[1]

The scenario presented in Table 4 may be especially relevant to the development of particular kinds of cancers as a result of inborn genetic factors and subsequent mutations. For example, about 40% of people with a cancer of the retina called *retinoblastoma* transmit a dominant gene for this disorder to their children. In patients with this germ-line type of retinoblastoma, somatic mutational events that occur after birth seem to activate the cancer-causing gene and can result in multiple types of cancer developing in different cell types within the patient's body. For example, a kind of cancer called *osteogenic sarcoma* frequently develops later in life in patients who have been successfully treated for retinoblastoma.[2] With germ-line retinoblastoma, the only effective antidote to the development of multiple types of cancers may be early germ-line gene therapy that effectively repairs *all* of the cells in a developing embryo.[3]

THE NEEDED TECHNOLOGICAL BREAKTHROUGH: GENE REPLACEMENT OR GENE REPAIR

As we noted earlier in this chapter [of *The Ethics of Human Gene Therapy*], the current technique for somatic-cell gene therapy relies on rather imprecise methods of gene addition. For safe and effective germ-line gene therapy, it seems likely that a more precisely targeted method of gene replacement or gene repair will be necessary. The most obvious reason for preferring gene replacement is that gene addition in embryos would result in their (later-developing) sperm or egg cells containing *both* the malfunctioning and the properly functioning genes. Thus, one undesirable effect of researchers' treating present or future reproductive cells by gene addition is that the researchers would be directly contributing to an increase in the number of malfunctioning genes in future generations. In addition, if any of the germ-line disorders are dominant, as retinoblastoma seems to be, then only gene replacement is likely to eradicate the deleterious effects of the malfunctioning gene.

MAJOR ETHICAL ARGUMENTS IN FAVOR OF GERM-LINE GENE THERAPY

In this and the following section we will analyze the major ethical arguments[4] for and against germ-line gene therapy.[5] For this analysis we will make the optimistic assumption that germ-line intervention methods will gradually be refined until they reach the point where gene replacement or gene repair is technically feasible and able to be accomplished in more than 95% of attempted gene transfer procedures. Thus, the following analysis presents the arguments for and against germ-line intervention under the most favorable conditions for such intervention.

A first argument in favor of germ-line intervention is that it may be the only way to prevent damage to particular biological individuals when that damage is caused by certain kinds of genetic defects. This argument is most closely related to the last two scenarios presented above. That is, only genetic modifications introduced into preimplantation embryos are likely to be early enough to affect all of the important cell types (as in retinoblastoma), or to reach a large enough fraction of brain cells, or to be in time to prevent irreversible damage to the developing embryo. In these circumstances the primary intent of gene therapy would, or at least could, be to provide gene therapy for the early embryo. A side effect of the intervention would be that all of the embryonic cells, including the reproductive cells that would later develop, would be genetically modified.[6]

A second moral argument for germ-line genetic intervention might be advanced by parents. It is that they wish to spare their children and grandchildren from either (1) having to undergo somatic cell gene therapy if they are born affected with a genetic defect or (2) having to face difficult decisions regarding possibly transmitting a disease-related gene to their own children and grandchildren. In our first scenario, admittedly a rare case, two homozygous parents who have a genetic disease know in advance that all of their offspring are likely to be affected with the same genetic disease. In the second scenario, there is a certain probability that the parents' offspring will be affected or carriers. An assumption lying behind this second argument is that parents should enjoy a realm of moral and legal protection when they are making good-faith decisions about the health of their children. Only if their decisions are clearly adverse to the health interests of the children should moral criticism or legal intervention be considered.

A third moral argument for germ-line intervention is more likely to be made by health professionals, public-health officials, and legislators casting a wary eye toward the expenditures for health care. This argument is that, from a social and economic point of view, germ-line intervention is more efficient than repeating somatic cell gene therapy generation after generation. From a medical and public health point of view, germ-line intervention fits better with the increasingly preferred model of disease prevention and health promotion. In the very long run, germ-line intervention, if applied to both affected individuals and asymptomatic carriers of serious genetic defects, could have a beneficial effect on the human gene pool and the frequency of genetic disease.[7]

A fourth argument refers to the roles of researchers and health professionals. As a general rule, researchers deserve to have the freedom to explore new modes of treating and/or preventing human disease.[8] To be sure, moral rules set limits on how this research is conducted. For example, animals involved in the preclinical stages of the research should be treated humanely. In addition, the human subjects involved in the clinical trials should be treated with respect. When and if germ-line gene therapy is someday validated as a safe and effective intervention, health care providers should be free to, and may have a moral obligation to, offer it to their patients as a possible treatment. This freedom is based on the professional's general obligation to seek out and offer the best possible therapeutic alternatives to patients and society's recognition of a sphere in which health professionals are at liberty to exercise their best judgment on behalf of their patients.

A fifth and final argument in favor of germ-line gene therapy is that this kind of intervention best accords with the health professions' healing role and with the concern to protect rather than penalize individuals who have disabilities. This argument is not simply a plea for protecting all embryos and fetuses from the time of fertilization forward. Both authors of this book [*The Ethics of Human Gene Therapy*] think that abortion is morally justifiable in certain circumstances. However, prenatal diagnosis followed by selective abortion and preimplantation diagnosis followed by selective discard seem to us to be uncomfortable and probably discriminatory halfway technologies that should eventually be replaced by effective modes of treatment. The options of selective abortion and selective discard essentially say to prospective parents, "There is nothing effective that the health care system has to offer. You may want to give up on this fetus or embryo and try again." To people with disabilities that are diagnosable at the prenatal or preimplantation stages of development the message of selective abortion and selective discard may seem more threatening. That message may be read as, "If we health professionals and prospective parents had known you were coming, we would have terminated your development and attempted to find or create a nondisabled replacement."

This argument is not intended to limit the legal access of couples to selective abortion in the case of serious health problems for the fetus. We support such access. Rather, it is an argument about what the long-term goal of medicine and society should be. In our view, that long-term goal should be to prevent disability and disease wherever possible. Where prevention is not possible, the second-best alternative is a cure or other definitive remedy. In cases where neither prevention nor cure is possible, our goal should be to help people cope with disability and disease while simultaneously seeking to find a cure.

MAJOR ARGUMENTS AGAINST GERM-LINE GENE THERAPY

First, if the technique has unanticipated negative effects, those effects will be visited not only on the recipient of the intervention himself or herself but also on all of the descendants of that recipient. This argument seems to assume that a mistake, once made, could not be corrected, or at least that the mistake might not become apparent until the recipient became the biological parent of at least one child. For that first child, at least, the negative effects could be serious, as well as uncorrectable.

Second, some critics of germ-line genetic intervention argue that this technique will never be necessary because of available alternative strategies for preventing the transmission of diagnosable genetic diseases. Specifically, critics of germ-line gene therapy have sometimes suggested that preimplantation diagnosis and the selective discard of affected embryos might be a reasonable alternative to the high-technology, potentially risky attempt to repair genetic defects in early human embryos. Even without in vitro fertilization and preimplantation diagnosis, the option of prenatal diagnosis and selective abortion is available for many disorders. According to this view, these two types of selection, before embryos or fetuses have reached the stage of viability, are effective means for achieving the same goal.

The third argument is closely related to the second: this technique will always be an expensive option that cannot be made available to most couples, certainly not by any publicly funded health care system. Therefore, like in vitro fertilization for couples attempting to overcome the problem of infertility,

germ-line gene therapy will be available only to wealthy people who can afford to pay its considerable expense on their own.

The fourth argument builds on the preceding two: precisely because germ-line intervention will be of such limited utility in preventing disease, there will be strong pressures to use this technique for genetic enhancement at the embryonic stage, when it could reasonably be expected to make a difference in the future life prospects of the embryo. Again in this case, only the affluent would be able to afford the intervention. However, if enhancement interventions were safe and efficacious, the long-term effect of such germ-line intervention would probably be to exacerbate existing differences between the most-well-off and the least-well-off segments of society.

Fifth, even though germ-line genetic intervention aims in the long run to treat rather than to abort or discard, the issue of appropriate respect for preimplantation embryos and implanted fetuses will nonetheless arise in several ways. After thoroughgoing studies of germ-line intervention have been conducted in nonhuman embryos, there will undoubtedly be a stage at which parallel studies in human embryos will be proposed. The question of human embryo research was recently studied by a committee appointed by the director of the National Institutes of Health.[9] Although the committee specifically avoided commenting on germ-line intervention, its recommendation that certain kinds of human embryo research should be continued and that such research should be funded by NIH provoked considerable controversy. Critics of the committee's position would presumably also oppose the embryo research that would be proposed to prepare the way for germ-line gene therapy in humans.[10] Their principal argument would be that the destruction or other harming of preimplantation embryos in research is incompatible with the kind of respect that should be shown to human embryos.

Even after the research phase of germ-line genetic intervention is concluded, difficult questions about the treatment of embryos will remain. For example, preimplantation diagnosis may continue to involve the removal of one or two totipotential cells from a four- to eight-cell embryo. While the moral status of totipotential human embryonic cells has received scant attention in bioethical debates, there is at least a plausible argument that a totipotential cell, once separated from the remainder of a preimplantation embryo, is virtually equivalent to a zygote; that is, under favorable conditions it could develop into an embryo, a fetus, a newborn, and an adult. This objection to the destruction of totipotential embryonic cells will only be overcome if a noninvasive genetic diagnostic test for early embryos (like an x-ray or a CT scan) can be developed. Further, even if a noninvasive diagnostic test is available, as we have noted above, a postintervention diagnostic test will probably be undertaken with each embryo to verify that the intervention has been successful. Health professionals and prospective parents will probably be at least open to the possibility of selective discard or selective abortion if something has gone radically wrong in the intervention procedure. Thus, germ-line genetic intervention may remain foreclosed as a moral option to those who are conscientiously opposed to any action that would directly terminate the life of a preimplantation embryo or a fetus.

The sixth argument points to potential perils of concentrating great power in the hands of human beings. According to this view, the technique of germ-line intervention would give human beings, or a small group of human beings, too much control over the future evolution of the human race. This argument does not necessarily attribute malevolent intentions to those who have the training that would allow them to employ the technique. It implies that there are built-in limits that humans ought not to exceed, perhaps for theological or metaphysical reasons, and at least hints that corruptibility is an ever-present possibility for the very powerful.

The seventh argument explicitly raises the issue of malevolent use. If one extrapolates from Nazi racial hygiene programs, this argument asserts, it is likely the germ-line intervention will be used by unscrupulous dictators to produce a class of superior human beings. The same techniques could be also used in precisely the opposite way, to produce human-like creatures who would willingly perform the least-attractive and the most-dangerous work for a society. According to this view, Aldous Huxley's *Brave New World* should be updated, for modern molecular biology provides tyrants with tools for modifying human beings that Huxley could not have imagined in 1932.

The eighth and final argument against germ-line genetic intervention is raised chiefly by several European authors who place this argument in the context of human rights.[11] According to these commentators, human beings have a moral right to receive from their parents a genetic patrimony that has not been subjected to artificial tampering. Although the term "tampering" is not usually defined, it seems to mean any intentional effort to introduce genetic changes into the germ line, even if the goal is to reduce the likelihood that a genetic disease will be passed on to the children and grandchildren of a particular couple. The asserted right to be protected against such tampering may be a slightly different formulation of the sixth argument noted above—namely, that there are built-in limits, embedded in the nature of things, beyond which not even the most benevolent human beings should attempt to go.

A BRIEF EVALUATION OF THE ARGUMENTS

In our view, the effort to cure and prevent serious disease and premature death is one of the noblest of all human undertakings. For this reason the first pro argument—that germ-line intervention may be the only way to treat or prevent certain diseases—seems to us to be of overriding importance. We also find the third pro argument to be quite strong, that a germ-line correction, if demonstrated to be safe and effective, would be more efficient than repeated applications of somatic cell gene therapy. In addition, the final pro argument about the overall mission of the health professions and about society's approach to disabilities seems to us to provide a convincing justification for the germ-line approach, when gene replacement is available.

Our replies to the objections raised by critics of germ-line intervention are as follows:

1. *Irreversible mistakes.* While we acknowledge that mistakes may be made in germ-line gene therapy, we think that the same sophisticated techniques that were employed to introduce the new genes will be able to be

used to remove those genes or to compensate for their presence in some other way. Further, in any sphere of innovative therapy, a first step into human beings must be taken at some point.

2. *Alternative strategies.* Some couples, perhaps even most couples, will choose the alternative strategies of selective abortion or selective discard. In our view, a strategy of attempting to prevent or treat potential disease or disability in the particular biological individual accords more closely with the mission of the health sciences and shows greater respect for children and adults who are afflicted with disease or disability.

3. *High cost, limited availability.* It is too early to know what the relative cost of germ-line intervention will be when the technique is fully developed. In addition, the financial costs and other personal and social harms of preventable diseases will need to be compared with the financial costs of germ-line gene therapy. It is at least possible that this new technology could become widely diffused and available to many members of society.

4. *Use for enhancement.* Prudent social policy should be able to set limits on the use of germ-line genetic intervention. Further, some enhancements of human capabilities may be morally justifiable, especially when those enhancements are health related. We acknowledge that the distribution of genetic enhancement is an important question for policy makers. (The issue of enhancement is discussed in greater detail in [Chapter 4 of *The Ethics of Human Gene Therapy*].)

5. *Human embryos.* In our view, research with early human embryos that is directed toward the development of germ-line gene therapy is morally justifiable in principle. Further, we acknowledge the potential of a totipotential cell but think that the value of a genetic diagnosis outweighs the value of such a cell. We also accept that, if a serious error is made in germ-line gene therapy, ter-

minating the life of the resulting embryo or fetus may be morally justifiable. In short, there is a presumption in favor of fostering the continued development of human embryos and fetuses, but that presumption can in our view be overridden by other considerations like serious harm to the developing individual or others and the needs of preclinical research.

6. *Concentration of power.* We acknowledge that those who are able to use germ-line intervention will have unprecedented ability to introduce precise changes into the germ lines of particular individuals and families. However, in our view, it is better for human beings to possess this ability and to use it for constructive purposes like preventing disease in families than not to possess the ability. The central ethical question is public accountability by the scientists, health providers, and companies that will be involved with germ-line intervention. Such accountability presupposes transparency about the use of the technology and an ongoing monitoring process aimed at preventing its misuse.

7. *Misuse by dictators.* This objection focuses too much attention on technology and too little on politics. There is no doubt that bona fide tyrants have existed in the 20th century and that they have made use of all manner of technologies—whether the low-tech methods of surgical sterilization or the annihilation of concentration camp inmates with poison gas or high-tech weapons like nuclear warheads and long-range missiles—to terrify and to dominate. However, the best approach to preventing the misuse of genetic technologies may not be to discourage the development of the technologies but rather to preserve and encourage democratic institutions that can serve as an antidote to tyranny. A second possible reply to the tyrannical misuse objection is that germ-line intervention requires a long lead time, in order to allow the offspring produced to grow to

adulthood. Tyrants are often impatient people and are likely to prefer the more instantaneous methods of propaganda, intimidation, and annihilation of enemies to the relatively slow pace of germ-line modification.

8. *Human rights and tampering.* It is a daunting task to imagine what the unborn and as-yet-unconceived generations of people coming after us will want.[12] Even more difficult is the effort to ascribe rights to [future] human beings. Insofar as we can anticipate the needs and wants of future generations, we think that any reasonable future person would prefer health to serious disease and would therefore welcome a germ-line intervention in his or her family line that effectively prevented cystic fibrosis from being transmitted to him or her. In our view, such a person would not regard this intervention as tampering and would regard as odd the claim that his or her genetic patrimony has been artificially tampered with. Cystic fibrosis was not a part of his or her family's heritage that the future person was eager to receive or to claim. . . .

NOTES

1 It is perhaps worth noting that researchers performing somatic-cell gene therapy have carefully avoided diseases and subtypes of diseases that affect mental functioning. One thinks, for example, of Lesch-Nyhan syndrome, of certain subtypes of Gaucher disease and Hunter syndrome, of Tay-Sachs disease, and of metachromatic leukodystrophy.

2 We owe the suggestion of retinoblastoma as a candidate disorder to Kevin FitzGerald, S. J. We are also indebted to Nelson A. Wivel for information on the genetics of retinoblastoma. See Nelson A. Wivel and LeRoy Walters, "Germ-Line Gene Modification and Disease Prevention: Some Medical and Ethical Perspectives," *Science* 262(5133): 533–538; 22 October 1993. See also Stephen H. Friend et al., "A Human DNA Segment with Properties of the Gene That Predisposes to Retinoblastoma and Osteosarcoma," *Nature* 323(6089): 643–646; 16 October 1986; and Ei Matsunaga, "Hereditary Retinoblastoma: Host Resistance and Second Primary Tumors," *Journal of the National Cancer Institute* 65(1): 47–51; July 1980.

3 Although the genetics of the germ-line p53 gene mutation are more complex than the genetics of the germ-line

mutation that causes retinoblastoma, p53 may turn out to be another important tumor suppressor gene to which the same comments apply. On the germ-line p53 mutation, see Frederick P. Li et al., "Recommendations on Predictive Testing for Germ Line p53 Mutations Among Cancer-Prone Individuals," *Journal of the National Cancer Institute* 84(15): 1156–1160; 5 August 1992; and Curtis C. Harris and Monica Hollstein, "Clinical Implications of the *p53* Tumor-Suppressor Gene," *New England Journal of Medicine* 329(18): 1318–1327; 28 October 1993.

4 Eric T. Juengst, "Germ-Line Gene Therapy: Back to Basics," *Journal of Medicine and Philosophy* 16(6): 589–590; December 1991.

5 Burke K. Zimmerman, "Human Germ-Line Therapy: The Case for Its Development and Use," *Journal of Medicine and Philosophy* 16(6): 596–598; December 1991.

6 For a detailed discussion of and justification for germ-line intervention in this setting, see Marc Lappé, "Ethical Issues in Manipulating the Human Germ Line," *Journal of Medicine and Philosophy* 16(6): 621–639; December 1991.

7 As noted above, already in 1962 Joshua Lederberg was arguing against H. J. Muller's proposals for improving the human gene pool through programs of "voluntary germinal choice" by appealing to the prospect of rapid, global genetic intervention by means of germ-line gene therapy. See Joshua Lederberg, "Biological Future of Man," in Gordon Wolstenholme, ed., *Man and His Future* (London: J. & A. Churchill, 1963), pp. 265 and 269.

8 On the general issue of the freedom of scientific inquiry, see Loren R. Graham, "Concerns About Science and Attempts to Regulate Inquiry," *Daedalus* 107(2): 1–21; Spring 1978.

9 National Institutes of Health, Human Embryo Research Panel, *Report* (Bethesda, MD: NIH, 27 September 1994).

10 See, for example, the following critiques of human embryo research: "The Inhuman Use of Human Beings," *First Things* 49: 17–21; January 1995; Dianne N. Irving, "Testimony Before the NIH Human Embryo Research Panel," *Linacre Quarterly* 61(4): 82–89; November 1994; and Kevin O'Rourke, "Embryo Research: Ethical Issues," *Health Care Ethics USA* 2(4): 2–3; Fall 1994.

11 Alex Mauron and Jean-Marie Thévoz, "Germ-Line Engineering: A Few European Voices," *Journal of Medicine and Philosophy* 16(6): 654–655; December 1991.

12 There is a rather substantial literature on this topic. See, for example, Ruth Faden, Gail Geller, and Madison Powers, eds., *AIDS, Women and the Next Generation* (New York: Oxford University Press, 1991); LeRoy Walters, "Ethical Issues in Maternal Serum Alpha-Fetoprotein Testing and Screening: A Reappraisal," in Mark I. Evans et al., eds., *Fetal Diagnosis and Therapy: Science, Ethics and the Law* (Philadelphia: J. B. Lippincott, 1989), pp. 54–60; and Lori B. Andrews et al., eds., *Assessing Genetic Risks: Implications for Health and Social Policy: Report* (Washington, DC: National Academy Press, 1994).

GENETIC ENHANCEMENT

MASTERY AND GIFT
Michael J. Sandel

In this chapter of his recent book, Sandel argues that genetic enhancement threatens to reduce our appreciation for what he calls the "gifted" character of human abilities and achievements. If we lose this appreciation, he claims, it will transform for the worse three important features of our moral lives: humility, responsibility, and solidarity. As opportunities for genetic self-improvement emerge, we will cease to view our talents as gifts for which we are indebted, seeing them instead as achievements for which we are responsible. Professional athletes already feel pressure to use stimulants and steroids to enhance performance. Prospective parents are already blamed for having children with genetic disabilities if they failed to screen for these traits. The burden on parents will grow, commensurately, as they are presented with more opportunities to shape the genetic inheritance of their offspring. Sandel worries that, as each individual becomes more responsible for his or her fate, our sense of solidarity with those less fortunate than ourselves may diminish. If we lose the sense that nature's gifts are arbitrary, then we may come to believe that the wealthy are wealthy because they are more deserving than the poor. Thus, the pursuit of genetic perfection threatens norms of unconditional parental love, the celebration of natural talents, humility in the face of privilege, and a willingness to share the blessings of good fortune through social institutions.

The problem with eugenics and genetic engineering is that they represent the one-sided triumph of willfulness over giftedness, of dominion over reverence, of molding over beholding. But why, we may wonder, should we worry about this triumph? Why not shake off our unease with enhancement as so much superstition? What would be lost if biotechnology dissolved our sense of giftedness?

HUMILITY, RESPONSIBILITY, AND SOLIDARITY

From the standpoint of religion, the answer is clear: To believe that our talents and powers are wholly our own doing is to misunderstand our place in creation, to confuse our role with God's. But religion is not the only source of reasons to care about giftedness. The moral stakes can also be described in secular terms. If the genetic revolution erodes our appreciation for the gifted character of human powers and achievements, it will transform three key features of our moral landscape—humility, responsibility, and solidarity.

In a social world that prizes mastery and control, parenthood is a school for humility. That we care deeply about our children, and yet cannot choose the kind we want, teaches parents to be open to the unbidden. Such openness is a disposition worth affirming, not only within families but in the wider world as well. It invites us to abide the unexpected, to live with dissonance, to rein in the impulse to control. A *Gattaca*-like world, in which parents became accustomed to specifying the sex and genetic traits of their children, would be a world inhospitable to the unbidden, a gated community writ large.

The social basis of humility would also be diminished if people became accustomed to genetic self-improvement. The awareness that our talents

Reprinted with permission of the publisher from *The Case Against Perfection: Ethics in the Age of Genetic Engineering* by Michael J. Sandel, pp. 85–100. Cambridge, Mass.: The Belknap Press of Harvard University Press. Copyright © 2007 by Michael J. Sandel.

and abilities are not wholly our own doing restrains our tendency toward hubris. If bioengineering made the myth of the "self-made man" come true, it would be difficult to view our talents as gifts for which we are indebted rather than achievements for which we are responsible. (Genetically enhanced children would of course remain indebted rather than responsible for their traits, though their debt would run more to their parents and less to nature, chance, or God.)

It is sometimes thought that genetic enhancement erodes human responsibility by overriding effort and striving. But the real problem is the explosion, not the erosion, of responsibility. As humility gives way, responsibility expands to daunting proportions. We attribute less to chance and more to choice. Parents become responsible for choosing, or failing to choose, the right traits for their children. Athletes become responsible for acquiring, or failing to acquire, the talents that will help their team win.

One of the blessings of seeing ourselves as creatures of nature, God, or fortune is that we are not wholly responsible for the way we are. The more we become masters of our genetic endowments, the greater the burden we bear for the talents we have and the way we perform. Today when a basketball player misses a rebound, his coach can blame him for being out of position. Tomorrow the coach may blame him for being too short.

Even now, the growing use of performance-enhancing drugs in professional sports is subtly transforming the expectations players have for one another. In the past when a starting pitcher's team scored too few runs to win, he could only curse his bad luck and take it in stride. These days, the use of amphetamines and other stimulants is so widespread that players who take the field without them are criticized for "playing naked." A recently retired major league outfielder told *Sports Illustrated* that some pitchers blame teammates who play unenhanced: "If the starting pitcher knows that you're going out there naked, he's upset that you're not giving him [everything] you can. The big-time pitcher wants to make sure you're beaning up before the game."[1]

The explosion of responsibility, and the moral burdens it creates, can also be seen in changing norms that accompany the use of prenatal genetic

testing. Once, giving birth to a child with Down syndrome was considered a matter of chance; today many parents of children with Down syndrome or other genetic disabilities feel judged or blamed.[2] A domain once governed by fate has now become an arena of choice. Whatever one believes about which, if any, genetic conditions warrant terminating a pregnancy (or selecting against an embryo, in the case of preimplantation genetic diagnosis), the advent of genetic testing creates a burden of decision that did not exist before. Prospective parents remain free to choose whether to use prenatal testing and whether to act on the results. But they are not free to escape the burden of choice that the new technology creates. Nor can they avoid being implicated in the enlarged frame of moral responsibility that accompanies new habits of control.

The Promethean impulse is contagious. In parenting as in sports, it unsettles and erodes the gifted dimension of human experience. When performance-enhancing drugs become commonplace, unenhanced ballplayers find themselves "playing naked." When genetic screening becomes a routine part of pregnancy, parents who eschew it are regarded as "flying blind" and are held responsible for whatever genetic defect befalls their child.

Paradoxically, the explosion of responsibility for our own fate, and that of our children, may diminish our sense of solidarity with those less fortunate than ourselves. The more alive we are to the chanced nature of our lot, the more reason we have to share our fate with others. Consider the case of insurance. Since people do not know whether or when various ills will befall them, they pool their risk by buying health insurance and life insurance. As life plays itself out, the healthy wind up subsidizing the unhealthy, and those who live to a ripe old age wind up subsidizing the families of those who die before their time. The result is mutuality by inadvertence. Even without a sense of mutual obligation, people pool their risks and resources, and share one another's fate.

But insurance markets mimic the practice of solidarity only insofar as people do not know or control their own risk factors. Suppose genetic testing advanced to the point where it could reliably predict each person's medical history and life expectancy.

Those confident of good health and long life would opt out of the pool, causing premiums to skyrocket for those destined for ill health. The solidaristic aspect of insurance would disappear as those with good genes fled the actuarial company of those with bad ones.

The concern that insurance companies would use genetic data to assess risks and set premiums recently led the U.S. Senate to vote to prohibit genetic discrimination in health insurance.[3] But the bigger danger, admittedly more speculative, is that genetic enhancement, if routinely practiced, would make it harder to foster the moral sentiments that social solidarity requires.

Why, after all, do the successful owe anything to the least advantaged members of society? One compelling answer to this question leans heavily on the notion of giftedness. The natural talents that enable the successful to flourish are not their own doing but, rather, their good fortune—a result of the genetic lottery.[4] If our genetic endowments are gifts, rather than achievements for which we can claim credit, it is a mistake and a conceit to assume that we are entitled to the full measure of the bounty they reap in a market economy. We therefore have an obligation to share this bounty with those who, through no fault of their own, lack comparable gifts.

Here, then, is the connection between solidarity and giftedness: A lively sense of the contingency of our gifts—an awareness that none of us is wholly responsible for his or her success—saves a meritocratic society from sliding into the smug assumption that success is the crown of virtue, that the rich are rich because they are more deserving than the poor.

If genetic engineering enabled us to override the results of the genetic lottery, to replace chance with choice, the gifted character of human powers and achievements would recede, and with it, perhaps, our capacity to see ourselves as sharing a common fate. The successful would become even more likely than they are now to view themselves as self-made and self-sufficient, and hence wholly responsible for their success. Those at the bottom of society would be viewed not as disadvantaged, and so worthy of a measure of compensation, but as simply unfit, and so worthy of eugenic repair. The meritocracy, less chastened by chance, would become harder, less

forgiving. As perfect genetic knowledge would end the simulacrum of solidarity in insurance markets, perfect genetic control would erode the actual solidarity that arises when men and women reflect on the contingency of their talents and fortunes.

OBJECTIONS

My argument against enhancement is likely to invite at least two objections: Some may complain that it is overly religious; others may object that it is unpersuasive in consequentialist terms. The first objection asserts that to speak of a gift presupposes a giver. If this is true, then my case against genetic engineering and enhancement is inescapably religious.[5] I argue, to the contrary, that an appreciation for the giftedness of life can arise from either religious or secular sources. While some believe that God is the source of the gift of life, and that reverence for life is a form of gratitude to God, one need not hold this belief in order to appreciate life as a gift or to have reverence for it. We commonly speak of an athlete's gift, or a musician's, without making any assumption about whether or not the gift comes from God. What we mean is simply that the talent in question is not wholly the athlete's or the musician's own doing; whether he has nature, fortune, or God to thank for it, the talent is an endowment that exceeds his control.

In a similar way, people often speak of the sanctity of life, and even of nature, without necessarily embracing the strong metaphysical version of that idea. For example, some hold with the ancients that nature is sacred in the sense of being enchanted, or inscribed with inherent meaning, or animated by divine purpose; others, in the Judeo-Christian tradition, view the sanctity of nature as deriving from God's creation of the universe; and still others believe that nature is sacred simply in the sense that it is not a mere object at our disposal, open to any use we may desire. These various understandings of the sacred all insist that we value nature and the living beings within it as more than mere instruments; to act otherwise displays a lack of reverence, a failure of respect. But this moral mandate need not rest on a single religious or metaphysical background.

It might be replied that nontheological notions of sanctity and gift cannot ultimately stand on their own but must lean on borrowed metaphysical assumptions they fail to acknowledge. This is a deep and difficult question that I cannot attempt to resolve here.[6] It is worth noting, however, that liberal thinkers from Locke to Kant to Habermas accept the idea that freedom depends on an origin or standpoint that exceeds our control. For Locke, our life and liberty, being inalienable rights, are not ours to give away (through suicide or selling ourselves into slavery). For Kant, though we are the authors of the moral law, we are not at liberty to exploit ourselves or to treat ourselves as objects any more than we may do so to other persons. And for Habermas . . . our freedom as equal moral beings depends on having an origin beyond human manipulation or control. We can make sense of these notions of inalienable and inviolable rights without necessarily embracing religious conceptions of the sanctity of human life. In a similar way, we can make sense of the notion of giftedness, and feel its moral weight, whether or not we trace the source of the gift to God.

The second objection construes my case against enhancement as narrowly consequentialist, and finds it wanting, along the following lines: Pointing to the possible effects of bioengineering on humility, responsibility, and solidarity may be persuasive to those who prize those virtues. But those who care more about gaining a competitive edge for their children or themselves may decide that the benefits to be gained from genetic enhancement outweigh its allegedly adverse effects on social institutions and moral sentiments. Moreover, even assuming that the desire for mastery is bad, an individual who pursues it may achieve some redeeming moral good—a cure for cancer, for example. So why should we assume that the "bad" of mastery necessarily outweighs the good it can bring about?[7]

To this objection I reply that I do not mean to rest the case against enhancement on consequentialist considerations, at least not in the usual sense of the term. My point is not that genetic engineering is objectionable simply because the social costs are likely to outweigh the benefits. Nor do I claim that people who bioengineer their children or themselves are necessarily motivated by a desire for mastery, and that this motive is a sin no good result could possibly outweigh. I am suggesting instead that the moral stakes in the enhancement debate are not fully captured by the familiar categories of autonomy and rights, on the one hand, and the calculation of costs and benefits, on the other. My concern with enhancement is not as individual vice but as habit of mind and way of being.[8]

The bigger stakes are of two kinds. One involves the fate of human goods embodied in important social practices—norms of unconditional love and an openness to the unbidden, in the case of parenting; the celebration of natural talents and gifts in athletic and artistic endeavors; humility in the face of privilege, and a willingness to share the fruits of good fortune through institutions of social solidarity. The other involves our orientation to the world that we inhabit, and the kind of freedom to which we aspire.

It is tempting to think that bioengineering our children and ourselves for success in a competitive society is an exercise of freedom. But changing our nature to fit the world, rather than the other way around, is actually the deepest form of disempowerment. It distracts us from reflecting critically on the world, and deadens the impulse to social and political improvement. Rather than employ our new genetic powers to straighten "the crooked timber of humanity,"[9] we should do what we can to create social and political arrangements more hospitable to the gifts and limitations of imperfect human beings.

THE PROJECT OF MASTERY

In the late 1960s, Robert L. Sinsheimer, a molecular biologist at the California Institute of Technology, glimpsed the shape of things to come. In an article entitled "The Prospect of Designed Genetic Change," he argued that freedom of choice would vindicate the new genetics, and set it apart from the discredited eugenics of old. "To implement the older eugenics of Galton and his successors would have required a massive social program carried out over many generations. Such a program could not have been initiated without the consent and cooperation of a major fraction of the population, and would have been continuously subject to social control. In contrast, the new eugenics could, at least in principle, be implemented on a quite individual basis, in one generation, and subject to no existing restrictions."[10]

According to Sinsheimer, the new eugenics would be voluntary rather than coerced, and also more humane. Rather than segregate and eliminate the unfit, it would improve them. "The old eugenics would have required a continual selection for breeding of the fit, and a culling of the unfit. The new eugenics would permit in principle the conversion of all the unfit to the highest genetic level."[11]

Sinsheimer's paean to genetic engineering caught the heady, Promethean self-image of the age. He wrote hopefully of rescuing "the losers in that chromosomal lottery that so firmly channels our human destinies," including not only those born with genetic defects but also "the 50 million 'normal' Americans with an IQ of less than 90." But he also saw that something bigger was at stake than improving upon nature's "mindless, age-old throw of dice." Implicit in the new technologies of genetic intervention was a new, more exalted place for human beings in the cosmos. "As we enlarge man's freedom, we diminish his constraints and that which he must accept as given." Copernicus and Darwin had "demoted man from his bright glory at the focal point of the universe," but the new biology would restore his pivotal role. In the mirror of our new genetic knowledge, we would see ourselves as more than a link in the chain of evolution: "We can be the agent of transition to a whole new pitch of evolution. This is a cosmic event."[12]

There is something appealing, even intoxicating, about a vision of human freedom unfettered by the given. It may even be the case that the allure of that vision played a part in summoning the genomic age into being. It is often assumed that the powers of enhancement we now possess arose as an inadvertent by-product of biomedical progress—the genetic revolution came, so to speak, to cure disease, but stayed to tempt us with the prospect of enhancing our performance, designing our children, and perfecting our nature. But that may have the story backward. It is also possible to view genetic engineering as the ultimate expression of our resolve to see ourselves astride the world, the masters of our nature. But that vision of freedom is flawed. It threatens to banish our appreciation of life as a gift, and to leave us with nothing to affirm or behold outside our own will.

NOTES

1 Tom Verducci, "Getting Amped: Popping Amphetamines or Other Stimulants Is Part of Many Players' Pregame Routine," *Sports Illustrated,* June 3, 2002, p. 38.

2 See Amy Harmon, "The Problem with an Almost-Perfect Genetic World," *New York Times,* November 20, 2005; Amy Harmon, "Burden of Knowledge: Tracking Prenatal Health," *New York Times,* June 20, 2004; Elizabeth Weil, "A Wrongful Birth?" *New York Times,* March 12, 2006. On the moral complexities of prenatal testing generally, see Erik Parens and Adrienne Asch, eds., *Prenatal Testing and Disability Rights* (Washington, DC: Georgetown University Press, 2000).

3 See Laurie McGinley, "Senate Approves Bill Banning Bias Based on Genetics," *Wall Street Journal,* October 15, 2003, p. D11.

4 See John Rawls, *A Theory of Justice* (Cambridge, MA: Harvard University Press, 1971), pp. 72–75, 102–105.

5 This challenge to my argument has been posed, from different points of view, by Carson Strong, in "Lost in Translation," *American Journal of Bioethics* 5 (May–June 2005): 29–31, and by Robert P. George, in discussion at a meeting of the President's Council on Bioethics, December 12, 2002 (transcript at *http://www.bioethics.gov/transcripts/ deco2/session4.html*).

6 For illuminating discussion of the way modern self-understandings draw in complex ways on unacknowledged moral sources, see Charles Taylor, *Sources of the Self* (Cambridge, MA: Harvard University Press, 1989).

7 See Frances M. Kamm, "Is There a Problem with Enhancement?" *American Journal of Bioethics* 5 (May–June 2005): 1–10. Kamm, in a thoughtful critique of an earlier version of my argument, construes what I call the "drive" or "disposition" to mastery as a desire or motive of individual agents, and argues that acting on such a desire would not render enhancement impermissible.

8 I am indebted to the discussion of this point by Patrick Andrew Thronson in his undergraduate honors thesis, "Enhancement and Reflection: Korsgaard, Heidegger, and the Foundations of Ethical Discourse," Harvard University, December 3, 2004; see also Jason Robert Scott, "Human Dispossession and Human Enhancement," *American Journal of Bioethics* 5 (May–June 2005): 27–28.

9 See Isaiah Berlin, "John Stuart Mill and the Ends of Life," in Berlin, *Four Essays on Liberty* (London: Oxford University Press, 1969), p. 193, quoting Kant: "Out of the crooked timber of humanity no straight thing was ever made."

10 Robert L. Sinsheimer, "The Prospect of Designed Genetic Change," *Engineering and Science Magazine,* April 1969 (California Institute of Technology). Reprinted in Ruth F. Chadwick, ed., *Ethics, Reproduction and Genetic Control* (London: Routledge, 1994), pp. 144–145.

11 Ibid., p. 145.

12 Ibid., pp. 145–146.

GENETIC ENGINEERING

Dan W. Brock

Brock defends the prospective use of genetic engineering to enhance human traits and functions against various moral objections. He rejects the idea that genetic engineering (of an embryo) would change the fundamental identity of an individual in a way that the efforts of parents to develop the capacities of their children by manipulating environmental factors do not. He also rejects the idea that the treatment of disease is objectively beneficial for an individual in a way that enhancement of normal function would not be. Brock acknowledges that some enhancements of normal human traits and functions would be beneficial only within a limited range. He also briefly considers whether there is any justified basis to the moral concern that the use of genetic engineering to enhance particular human capacities would transform and devalue the associated human activities. Next, he argues that any moral assessment of genetic engineering for purposes of enhancement must take account of *who* is employing the relevant genetic technology (e.g., whether it is government or parents), and he concludes his analysis by acknowledging that the use of genetic engineering to enhance capacities that would confer competitive advantages on recipients raises serious issues about fairness and equality of opportunity.

In June 2000 government and industry groups jointly announced that the goal of the worldwide Human Genome Project (HGP) to map and sequence the entire human genome had essentially been completed. Of course, enormous work still lay ahead to understand the specific genes that contribute to human disease and disability, much less to the multitude of complex physical, cognitive, emotional, and behavioral traits of normal humans. No one can confidently predict the rate at which that understanding will be achieved in the future nor the ultimate limits on it. The way in which genes interact with other genes and with different environments only multiplies what we still for the most part do not yet understand. But, despite how much remains to be learned, we have already made great strides in beginning to understand the genetic bases of human nature. Much of the initial work in the HGP has focused on a search for the specific genetic contributions to human disease and disability. The gene has been identified, and tests for it developed, that allow prediction with a very high

degree of certainty of whether an individual will develop Huntington's chorea, an adult-onset, single gene disease that leads to devastating neurological deterioration and death over a period of years. In other cases, genes have been identified, and tests for them developed, that only increase individuals' risks of developing diseases like breast cancer.

At present, this new information still allows only limited and relatively crude control over the genetic inheritance of our progeny. A couple who know from family history or other means that one or both are at risk of passing on a particular genetic disease to their children can test for their risk of doing so before conception. If a risk is found to be present, various means, such as sperm or egg donation, *in vitro* fertilization (IVF), pre-implantation embryo testing, or forgoing conception, are now available to avoid transmission of the genetic disease to future children. After conception, testing of the fetus is sometimes possible to determine whether it carries the gene or genes for the disease, and the parents can then decide whether to abort an affected fetus. While such testing is now possible for only a quite limited number of diseases or disabilities for which there is a significant genetic component, we can expect

Reprinted with permission of the publisher from *A Companion to Applied Ethics* (2003), edited by R. G. Frey and Christopher Heath Wellman, pp. 356–357, 361–367. Copyright © 2003 by Blackwell Publishing Ltd. Reproduced with permission from Blackwell Publishing Ltd.

these capacities to continue to expand rapidly in the future. Moreover, the capacity to detect deleterious genes is likely to be combined with new abilities for *in utero* therapeutic interventions or genetic manipulations to correct for the deleterious gene(s). Thus, we can expect that advances in genetic knowledge and technology will increase our ability to prevent or to reduce the prevalence of disease caused in significant part by deleterious genes.

It is not just much disease, however, but virtually all normal human traits that have some significant genetic basis. The same advances in genetic knowledge and technology that will enable us to prevent disease will ultimately enable us to undertake interventions to manipulate the genes underlying normal traits and functions and to enhance those traits and functions in the absence of any disease or disability; it may become possible to manipulate genes to enhance normal intelligence or memory, immune responses to many human diseases, physical strength or dexterity, and life expectancy, to take only a few examples. Thus, we face the prospect of being able to take control over and to design human nature and the nature of our progeny. What was once in the hands of God or the natural lottery will come increasingly within deliberate human choice and control. This [essay] is about some of the ethical issues we can expect to face when we gain that control.

In the limited space available here, I will not pursue the technical means by which these genetic interventions will likely occur. While some bases for them are already in place, how they will develop is speculative and uncertain at this time and while some of the ethical concerns will be specific to particular technical means as they develop over time, most of the deepest ethical concerns do not turn on the specific technical details of genetic interventions. I will understand "genetic engineering" here to mean the deliberate alteration or addition of genes in a human embryo; this includes somatic cell genetic interventions that affect only the subject of the intervention as well as germ cell interventions where the changes will be passed on to the progeny of the subject of the intervention. This means that our current means noted above of preventing the passing on of genetic disease are not instances of genetic engineering as I will understand it here. . . .

USE OF GENETIC ENGINEERING TO ENHANCE NORMAL FUNCTION

To use genetic engineering . . . to seek to prevent genetic diseases and the suffering and disabilities that they cause does not seem morally wrong and may sometimes be morally required. This is in keeping with efforts in medicine more generally to prevent or treat disease and the suffering and disability it causes. However, many people worry that the use of genetic engineering to enhance normal function in persons who are without disease raises fundamentally different and deeper moral concerns than the medical use of genetic engineering. Yet what could be wrong with parents using the technology of genetic engineering if it becomes available to improve their children's lives and opportunities? Parents are generally regarded as having permission, and in some cases an obligation, to produce the best children they can. They are expected, for example, to keep their children as healthy as possible. If genetic techniques gave parents a way to enhance their children's immune systems, and the intervention posed only risks comparable to vaccination, should parents not be free, or even required in some cases, to use them? Parents invest time, efforts, and resources in developing athletic talents, intellectual abilities, and prudential or moral virtues in their children. If parents have great leeway in attempting to produce the best children they can, according to their own view of what is best, why not extend this liberty to genetic means?

ENVIRONMENTAL VERSUS GENETIC CHANGES

Some opponents of genetic engineering mistakenly see it as changing the fundamental identity of a person in a way that parents' environmental efforts do not. They see parental efforts as environmental in helping to develop the capacities their children already have, as bringing out the potential that is already there. In contrast, genetic interventions are seen as changing children in some more fundamental way, making them different from who they otherwise would have been. But this contrast is problematic. When parents use their control over environmental factors to "bring out the best" in their children, they modify phenotype. Given their children's geno-types, the range of traits and capabilities—both physical and behavioral—that constitute the pheno-type of the child we see and interact with is very much a result of the environment that parents and others create. There is no pre-existing and fixed best in the child that is brought out by parental manipu-lation of environmental causes; such manipulation has enormous effects in shaping and determining phenotype. Why not then add to parents' arsenal of methods whatever genetic interventions make it eas-ier to accomplish their goals for their children?

Part of what disturbs many people is the mis-taken belief that genetic interventions modify the essence or identity of the individual, whereas envi-ronmental interventions only modify accidental fea-tures and leave identity unchanged. The idea seems to be that genetic interventions result in a new indi-vidual, whereas environmental interventions merely modify the same individual. But our genes do not constitute our identity in any deep sense. Suppose the operation of our immune system could be en-hanced or our eye color changed by a genetic inter-vention. We would not be inclined to muse: "I wonder who I would have been if my parents had not altered my immune system or eye color in this way?" We might have very different responses if they altered genes that produced major changes in aspects of the self that we consider central to our sense of self or personal identity. For each of us, it is particular elements of our phenotype, such as being intelligent, compassionate, or witty, not every aspect of our genotype, that we take to be central to our conceptions of self and to our essence as a particular individual. These traits are produced by interactions between our genotype and our environment and nei-ther means of altering them is more fundamental.

WHEN ARE ENHANCEMENTS BENEFITS?

Treatment of disease that restores normal human function is typically and uncontroversially assumed to benefit persons. One source of moral concern and unease about genetic engineering is whether enhanc-ing individuals' normal human traits would in fact be beneficial for them. In *Brave New World,* Aldous

Huxley (1946) imagined engineering some persons to have limited abilities and aspirations, and to be happy doing menial jobs in society. While this might be beneficial for the society, it was morally objec-tionable in exploiting those individuals for the ben-efit of the rest of society. Morally acceptable genetic engineering of individuals should, certainly in the great majority of cases, plausibly be of benefit to those individuals from their own perspective.

Are treatments of disease objectively good for a person in respects in which enhancements are not? For example, treatment that prevents paraplegia seems uncontroversially and objectively beneficial to anyone, whereas enhancement of a capacity to ex-cel in athletics or play a musical instrument may only be beneficial for a person with interests in these activities. However, this is not a contrast between genetic engineering used for treatment versus en-hancement, but rather a contrast between abilities that are all-purpose means, useful in virtually any plan of life, and abilities useful in some plans of life but not in many others. Some enhancements of ca-pacities like memory or the ability to focus attention on tasks for extended periods of time would likewise be useful in nearly any plan of life, whereas treat-ment, for example, of a disease that impairs fine mo-tor skills might be very important to a pianist but of little importance to a person who did not make sig-nificant use of those skills. There is no systematic contrast between treatment of disease and enhance-ment of normal function that makes the former ob-jectively beneficial in a way the latter is not.

THE MAGNITUDE OF ENHANCEMENT

If disease is understood roughly as a condition caus-ing an adverse deviation in normal species function, however, treatment that prevents or treats disease and so maintains or restores normal function will be at least prima facie beneficial for a person. More-over, the attaining of normal function provides a rough stopping point for successful treatment. On the other hand, in the use of genetic engineering for enhancement, the limits of possible changes in peo-ple's genetic inheritance are more open-ended both in the capacities that might be enhanced and in the degree to which the capacities might be improved;

there is no obvious end-point to potential enhancements comparable to the role normal function plays with treatment. How much stronger or smarter or more memory should we aim at?

It might seem that the more a desirable trait is enhanced by genetic engineering the better, but that would be a mistake for at least two reasons. First, some enhancements would only be beneficial within a limited range because of how the enhanced capacity or trait would interact with the individual's other capacities or traits. For example, enhancing some forms of memory beyond a limited range might so interfere with other forms of memory or other cognitive processes as to be, overall, undesirable instead of a benefit. The second reason why some enhancements would only be beneficial within a limited range is that beyond that range individuals would become unsuited for human social life. For example, there are well-known social benefits to being tall. That is why growth hormone—a pharmacological intervention—that raised a normal individual's height to several inches above the norm might be a beneficial enhancement. But there are limits to how much of an increase in height would be beneficial. To grow to be 9 ft tall, certainly not now possible with growth hormone, would be on balance harmful in nearly any human society because our social world is constructed for persons whose height rarely reaches beyond 7 ft at most. One would literally become, in a physical respect, unfit for human company. And if the change were still more dramatic, as in the case of Gulliver in Lilliput, it could become hard to see the individual still as a member of the same species. Many changes in human features and capacities by genetic engineering would only be beneficial within some range, and public policy could quite appropriately regulate its use to ensure that it stays within the beneficial range.

THE MEANS USED FOR ENHANCEMENT

Is it morally important that genetic engineering is the means used to enhance human capacities? Of course, means may vary in various morally important ways, such as the risks they carry, but is there something about genetic manipulation itself that raises moral worries? Many people admire others who have developed skills and abilities through long hard effort that they would not admire when the means used was genetic engineering. Moreover, sometimes a valued activity is defined in part by the means it employs, not just by the end at which it aims. It was a great achievement several years ago when IBM's computer "Big Blue" beat the then world chess champion Gary Kasparov. But it surely was a very different achievement from the one in which a human challenger recently beat Kasparov. And suppose an IBM engineer who designed Big Blue's program and implemented the moves it chose claimed that he was the new world chess champion. Here, means make all the difference in the chess skills and successes with which the engineer should be credited. In many valued human activities, the means of acquiring the capacities are as much valued and admired as the performance itself. Opponents of genetic engineering on these grounds will need to show that enhancing particular human capacities by genetic engineering as opposed to other means transforms and devalues important activities that employ those capacities.

WHO IS USING GENETIC ENGINEERING?

It will often be morally important who is using genetic engineering technologies to enhance a particular capacity. I believe the most important differences are between three cases: first, when government employs or strongly encourages their use; second, when individuals use them on others, most importantly parents on their children; third, when individuals use them to enhance their own capacities (strictly, this last would not be genetic engineering as defined above, but genetic interventions may become possible later than the embryo stage of development). The most obvious difference is between the first two cases and the third, since the first two raise the issue of the justification of some persons acting to affect someone else; for example, it is widely held that individuals are justified in taking risks for themselves that they would not be justified in imposing on others. Less obvious, but at least as important, are the different degrees and forms of neutrality about what is a good life that are properly expected from the state, from parents toward their children, and from individuals in their own lives.

In liberal democracies, it is widely held that the state should seek to be neutral between different comprehensive conceptions of a good life that its citizens may hold. This liberal neutrality places substantial limits on governmental action to employ, encourage, or require the use of genetic engineering that would only be beneficial in some specific conceptions of a good life. The genetic engineering compatible with this liberal state neutrality is roughly that which enhances what John Rawls (1971) called primary goods, that is, general purpose means useful in a wide variety of, if not virtually all, plans of life. Placing fluoride in the water supply is justified on these grounds: enhancing resistance to tooth decay is beneficial no matter what one's particular plan of life. Enhancing memory by genetic engineering might be as well.

Consider now parents' use of genetic engineering for their children. Whoever has primary responsibility for raising children—in most societies, parents—must have substantial discretion in the values they impart and the particular capacities they seek to develop and enhance in their children. There are moral limits, however, on parents' authority to enhance their children's capacities, whether by genetic engineering or other means, as the following case illustrates. Suppose parents put their 7-year-old daughter into an intensive tennis training program to develop her potential to become a professional tennis player; whether wise or not, parents are generally accepted to have the right to do this. But suppose the parents also proposed to withdraw her from school because they believed her education was interfering with her tennis training. Public policy, quite properly, would not permit them to do so because, although it might enhance her tennis skills, it would be at the cost of severely limiting or neglecting many other capacities and opportunities she would otherwise have later to choose and pursue other, different, life plans. Parents do not have an unlimited moral right to shape their children and their children's capacities at the cost of denying them a reasonable array of opportunities to select and pursue their own conception of a good life as they mature and develop the capacities to make those choices. Children have what Joel Feinberg (1980) has called a right to an "open future," which is derivative from the more

fundamental right of adults to self-determination in making significant choices about their lives for themselves and according to their own values or conception of a good life. Disagreements will arise, of course, about the extent or scope of a child's right to an open future and what would violate that right, but the right places significant limits on the use of genetic engineering by parents for their children.

If individuals could use genetic engineering for themselves, neither of these forms of neutrality would be required because their doing so would be an exercise, not an infringement, of self-determination or autonomy. Public policy might legitimately seek to ensure that such choices are well informed, particularly when there are significant and irreversible risks, but it should not substitute its own judgments about when genetic engineering would be desirable for the voluntary, informed judgments of competent adults. As a general matter, we have seen that who would be using genetic engineering could be important for the moral justification of that use.

IMPACT OF GENETIC ENGINEERING ON FAIRNESS AND INEQUALITY

I want finally to provide what I believe is the most important example of the moral issues public policy will face in responding to widespread new capacities for genetic engineering that enhances normal capacities. The problem arises when an enhancement by genetic engineering would confer a substantial competitive or positional advantage on its recipient, thereby strengthening an individual's position relative to others in competitions for scarce roles or benefits. If the genetic engineering is expensive and distributed on the basis of an ability to pay for it, then only the economically well off will get it. This will raise concerns about fairness and equality of opportunity, specifically whether those who cannot afford genetic engineering have a fair opportunity to compete for the benefit against those whose capacities to compete have been enhanced by genetic engineering. Imagine that the children of the higher socioeconomic classes not only have the social advantages they now typically have, but that they also have certification that their intelligence, memory, immune system, and capacity to concentrate attention on tasks for extended periods of time have all been enhanced by genetic engineering. This would be a very significant advantage in work and other contexts; it would likely significantly increase inequality and would raise serious issues of fairness and equality of opportunity for public policy. Public policy could reasonably regulate the use of genetic engineering that would unfairly increase inequality, but there would be an important moral complication in doing so, quite apart from generating the necessary political will to do so.

Many real enhancements that may become possible through genetic engineering will in part confer positional or competitive advantages, but will in part confer non-competitive or intrinsic benefits as well. Take the example of enhancing individuals' capacities to focus their attention more intensely for significant periods of time on a particular task or activity. Many adults with no disease or deficit now use the drug Ritalin for this purpose. This would confer a significant advantage in work contexts. But it would also increase individuals' intrinsic satisfactions from activities like listening to music, watching films or sunsets, and so forth, none of which are competitive benefits that make anyone else worse off. The quandary for public policy is that concerns about fairness and equality of opportunity would support limits on this use of genetic engineering, but these limits would at the same time deny individuals the opportunity of gaining significant, non-competitive benefits in their lives.

Public policy will face other difficult issues in responding to new capacities for genetic engineering, including regulation of competitive enhancements that would be self-defeating if widely used and regulation of the risks that will be inherent in their use. Whether used for treatment of disease or for enhancement, genetic engineering in humans should take place only after careful evaluation to ensure that its risks are justified by its potential benefits—this will be especially important for any germ-line interventions. But the potential long-term adverse impact on inequality and fairness may well prove to be the greatest challenge.

The moral and policy issues that will likely be raised in the future by new capacities to employ genetic engineering to prevent disease and disability and to enhance normal human capacities will ultimately concern how we are to shape our nature as humans. Some people will condemn any such interventions as "playing God," but I believe the potential for human benefit makes any general moral bar to their use unjustified. What I have tried to do in this [essay] is to articulate some of the moral and policy issues that we must confront if we are to use genetic engineering wisely, safely, and ethically.

ACKNOWLEDGMENTS

This [essay] draws heavily on Brock (1998) and Buchanan et al. (2000).

REFERENCES

Brock, D. W. (1998) Enhancement of human function: Some distinctions for policy makers. In E. Parens (ed.), *Technologies for the Enhancement of Human Capacities.* Washington, DC: Georgetown University Press.

Buchanan, A. E., Brock, D. W., Daniels, N., and Wikler, D. (2000) *From Chance to Choice: Genetics and Justice.* Cambridge: Cambridge University Press.

Feinberg, J. (1980) The child's right to an open future. In W. Aiken and H. LaFollette (eds.), *Whose Child? Children's Rights, Parental Authority, and State Power.* Totowa, NJ: Rowman and Littlefield.

Rawls, J. (1971) *A Theory of Justice.* Cambridge, MA: Harvard University Press.

ANNOTATED BIBLIOGRAPHY

Adams, Harry: "A Human Germline Modification Scale," *Journal of Law, Medicine & Ethics* 32 (Spring 2004), pp. 164–173. Adams suggests the following categories as a framework for the assessment of possible germ-line modifications, whether therapeutic in nature or enhancements: (1) those that should be prohibited, (2) those that should be available to everyone, (3) those that may be available to anyone with adequate resources, and (4) those that should be mandatory for everyone.

Alpern, Kenneth D., ed.: *The Ethics of Reproductive Technology* (New York: Oxford University Press, 1992). This anthology is designed to address both normative and conceptual questions associated with innovations in human reproduction—both technological innovations (e.g., IVF) and social innovations (e.g., surrogate motherhood).

Boss, Judith A.: *The Birth Lottery: Prenatal Diagnosis and Selective Abortion* (Chicago: Loyola University Press, 1993). The first two chapters of this book provide useful factual information on genetic disorders and prenatal diagnostic procedures. In later chapters, Boss examines various proposed justifications for selective abortion and ultimately concludes that the practice cannot be justified.

Botkin, Jeffrey R.: "Ethical Issues and Practical Problems in Preimplantation Genetic Diagnosis," *Journal of Law, Medicine & Ethics* 26 (Spring 1998), pp. 17–28. Botkin discusses the risks, limitations, and costs of PGD, clarifies the purposes that the procedure might serve, and provides an analysis of the ethical issues raised by the procedure.

Brock, Dan W.: "An Assessment of the Ethical Issues Pro and Con," in *Cloning Human Beings: Report and Recommendations of the National Bioethics Advisory Commission* (Rockville, MD: NBAC, June 1997), Volume II, Section E, pp. 1–23. This valuable paper provides an overall survey of the moral arguments for and against human cloning.

Buchanan, Allen, Dan W. Brock, Norman Daniels, and Daniel Wikler: *From Chance to Choice: Genetics and Justice* (Cambridge: Cambridge University Press, 2000). The authors examine a wide range of ethical issues associated with the use of genetic technologies.

Burley, Justine, and John Harris, eds.: *A Companion to Genethics* (Oxford: Blackwell, 2002). Philosophers and writers in other disciplines address ethical issues surrounding the completion of the Human Genome Project. Topics addressed include genetic screening, gene therapy, privacy, cloning, workplace issues, and social justice.

Cameron, C., and R. Williamson: "Is There an Ethical Difference Between Preimplantation Genetic Diagnosis and Abortion?" *Journal of Medical Ethics* 29 (2003), pp. 90–92. The authors argue that PGD and implantation of an unaffected embryo, while allowing affected embryos to die, is ethically preferable to prenatal diagnosis and selective abortion.

Cohen, Cynthia B., ed.: *New Ways of Making Babies: The Case of Egg Donation* (Bloomington: Indiana University Press, 1996). This collection includes a set of articles addressing the ethical and policy issues associated with egg donation.

Damelio, Jennifer, and Kelly Sorensen: "Enhancing Autonomy in Paid Surrogacy," *Bioethics* 22 (June 2008), pp. 269–277. The authors discuss the economic and educational vulnerability of gestational surrogates and consider arguments for a ban on commercial surrogacy, ultimately rejecting such a ban in favor of state-mandated education for prospective surrogates aimed at informing them and enhancing their autonomy.

Journal of Medicine and Philosophy 16 (December 1991). This issue features a series of articles under the general title of "Human Germ-Line Engineering." A wide range of arguments for and against germ-line gene therapy can be found in the various articles.

Kennedy Institute of Ethics Journal 15 (March 2005). This special issue on "Justice and Genetic Enhancement" includes seven papers exploring a variety of issues relating to social justice and genetic enhancement, including inequality, access, risk, and global justice.

Klotzko, Arlene Judith, ed.: *The Cloning Sourcebook* (New York: Oxford University Press, 2001). Part I of this anthology deals with the science of cloning, Part II considers the context of cloning, Part III is dedicated to the ethics of cloning, and Part IV addresses policy issues.

Lauritzen, Paul: *Pursuing Parenthood: Ethical Issues in Assisted Reproduction* (Bloomington: Indiana University Press, 1993). Lauritzen considers the ethics of AIH, IVF, donor insemination (AID), and surrogate motherhood. His final chapter is entitled "The Myth and Reality of Current Adoption Practice."

Law, Medicine & Health Care 16 (Spring/Summer 1988). This special issue is entirely dedicated to surrogate motherhood. Articles are organized under the headings of (1) civil liberties, (2) ethics, and (3) women's autonomy. Material is also provided on the case of Baby M.

New York State Task Force on Life and the Law: *Assisted Reproductive Technologies: Analysis and Recommendations for Public Policy* (April 1998). This report provides a wealth of information about the various reproductive technologies used in clinical practice. Clinical, legal, and policy issues are identified, and analysis of these issues culminates in an extensive set of conclusions and recommendations.

Nussbaum, Martha C., and Cass R. Sunstein, eds.: *Clones and Clones: Facts and Fantasies About Human Cloning* (New York: W. W. Norton, 1998). Writers from a wide range of disciplines, including scientists, legal scholars, psychoanalysts, and literary critics discuss the social and ethical aspects of human cloning.

Overall, Christine: *Ethics and Human Reproduction: A Feminist Analysis* (Boston: Allen & Unwin, 1987). Overall embraces a feminist perspective on reproductive ethics and contrasts a feminist approach with nonfeminist and antifeminist approaches. She discusses sex preselection in Chapter 2, surrogate motherhood in Chapter 6, and artificial reproduction in Chapter 7.

Parens, Erik, and Adrienne Asch, eds.: *Prenatal Testing and Disability Rights* (Washington, DC: Georgetown University Press, 2000). This valuable collection of articles provides divergent viewpoints on the various claims associated with the disability rights critique of prenatal diagnosis and selective abortion.

Pence, Gregory E.: *Who's Afraid of Human Cloning?* (Lanham, MD: Rowman & Littlefield, 1998). Pence constructs an overall case for the moral acceptability of human cloning.

Purdy, Laura M.: "Surrogate Mothering: Exploitation or Empowerment?" *Bioethics* 3 (January 1989), pp. 18–34. Purdy argues against the view that surrogate mothering is necessarily immoral. She acknowledges the danger that surrogate mothering could deepen the exploitation of women but also insists that surrogacy has the potential to empower women.

Robertson, John A.: *Children of Choice: Freedom and the New Reproductive Technologies* (Princeton, NJ: Princeton University Press, 1994). Emphasizing the importance of procreative freedom, Robertson provides an analysis of the ethical, legal, and social issues associated with various reproductive technologies. He considers IVF in Chapter 5; sperm donation, egg donation, and gestational surrogacy in Chapter 6; and the selection and shaping of offspring characteristics in Chapter 7.

Sparrow, Robert: "Cloning, Parenthood, and Genetic Relatedness," *Bioethics* 20 (November 2006), pp. 308–318. Sparrow argues that cloning can never create the kind of genetic relationship that is required for a couple to be the parents of a cloned child. He concludes that cloning could not serve as an ethically viable medical procedure to overcome infertility.

Tong, Rosemarie: *Feminist Approaches to Bioethics: Theoretical Reflections and Practical Applications* (Boulder, CO: Westview Press, 1997). Chapter 7 of this book provides discussions of artificial insemination and IVF. Chapter 8 provides a discussion of surrogacy. Chapter 9 includes discussions of prenatal diagnosis and gene therapy.

Walters, LeRoy, and Julie Gage Palmer: *The Ethics of Human Gene Therapy* (New York: Oxford University Press, 1997). This useful book provides chapters on somatic-cell gene therapy, germline gene therapy, and enhancement engineering.

CHAPTER 9

SOCIAL JUSTICE AND ACCESS TO HEALTH CARE

INTRODUCTION

Although significant health-care reform may be forthcoming, at the time of this writing American health care is a terrible mess. Over 46 million Americans, about 16 percent of the population, lack health insurance; millions more are underinsured.[1] Those lacking health insurance face serious consequences. The Institute of Medicine puts it bluntly: "Uninsured children and adults suffer worse health outcomes and die sooner than those with insurance."[2] Moreover, an estimated 18,000 unnecessary deaths occur every year in the United States due to lack of insurance.[3] A further consequence for many families is threatened financial security. Meanwhile, the cost of forgoing needed medical services is huge: an estimated $65–130 billion per year,[4] more than what some experts regard as necessary to cover all the uninsured.[5]

Other features of American health care are also dispiriting. Despite not covering nearly one of every six Americans, we spend *far* more on health care per capita (over $7000 in 2009)—including the uninsured—and as a fraction of gross domestic product (16 percent) than do citizens of any other country; and despite the enormous, unsustainable expenditure on health care, the United States ranks twenty-ninth in infant mortality, forty-eighth in life expectancy, and nineteenth out of nineteen industrialized nations in avoiding preventable deaths.[6] For many years, health care costs have risen faster than wages and general inflation. Meanwhile, insured patients frequently complain that insurance companies restrict their choice of doctors and impose seemingly excessive bureaucratic hassles. On the whole, the American public is deeply dissatisfied with its health-care system.[7] Such facts as these give the lie to the oft-repeated canard, "American health care is the best in the world." On the contrary, American health care is in urgent need of overhaul—and, arguably, overhaul far more extensive than President Barack Obama's plan, some version of which Congress appears likely to pass.

What shape would appropriate reform take? More fundamentally, what should we expect of a health-care system? Perhaps the most commonly accepted goals of a health-care system and, therefore, of health-care reform are the following: universal insurance coverage, cost controls, comprehensiveness of benefits, freedom of choice and freedom from hassle for patients, and high quality of care.

As already noted, the United States is far from achieving universal coverage, with one-sixth of its population lacking health insurance and many more Americans underinsured. Importantly, the health-care reform plans currently being debated, assuming one becomes law, will greatly expand health care coverage but will not achieve universal coverage.[8] By contrast, every other industrialized country provides universal health-care coverage.

As for controlling costs, the United States has done poorly. Consider these figures, which compare American spending with the spending of other countries whose health care systems we will examine in this chapter. In 2003 (the last year for which we could find reliable comparative data), the United States spent $5635 per person on health care for a total of 15 percent of its GDP. Compare those data with those for the other countries, *all of which provide universal coverage:* Great Britain: $2231 and 7.7 percent; Canada: $3003 and 9.9 percent; Germany: $2996 and 11.1 percent; and France: $2903 and 10.1 percent. With these disparities in expenditure, it can hardly be claimed that the United States is controlling health care costs well. Of these nations, moreover, only Great Britain—which spends relatively little per capita but is in the process of significant reform—has a higher rate of average health-care inflation from 1993–2003; health-care inflation in Canada, Germany, and France is considerably lower than in the United States.[9]

Turning now to the goals of comprehensiveness of benefits and patient freedom, we find further bleak comparisons. The articles discussing the health care systems of Canada, Great Britain, Germany, and France that are reprinted in this chapter demonstrate that residents of those countries are insured for a wider array of health benefits than those enjoyed by most Americans, especially those covered by poor private plans and, of course, those who have no insurance. Moreover, while (insured) Americans long enjoyed considerable freedom in choosing doctors, hospitals, and the like, managed care has imposed some significant restrictions on patient choice. (*Managed care* may be defined as an approach to health care that combines health insurance and the delivery of a broad range of integrated health care services for some group of enrollees, paying for those services prospectively from an estimated limited budget.[10]) Moreover, while for decades the administrative complexity of American health care has been criticized for greatly inconveniencing patients, managed care has in many instances exacerbated this problem with additional layers of complexity. By comparison, the systems of countries that provide universal coverage generally extend more freedom of choice to patients while imposing less inconvenience.

What about the quality of care? Is this not the pride of the American system? It may be that American prowess in high-technology medicine is second to none. But one could argue that most people need good basic care more than they need high-technology virtuosity, and persons lacking insurance or covered by relatively weak private plans or public programs commonly receive substandard care. Also sobering is the estimated 98,000 American deaths per year due to medical error.[11] Here is a blunt assessment from Ezekiel J. Emanuel, an oncologist and political philosopher who previously headed the Department of Bioethics at the National Institutes of Health and currently advises the White House on health policy:

> Yet despite these fantastic sums of money being spent, the health status of America's citizens looks sickly when measured against the tallies in other industrialized countries. Our infant mortality rate is twice as high as that of Japan, Sweden, and Norway, even among

whites. We have lower life expectancy than the Japanese, French, Canadians, and Germans. Even among adults who reach age 60, Americans expect to live another 16.6 years while in other industrialized countries the average is another 19.1 years. Annually, we lose a higher percentage of lives to the ravages of diabetes than people in other developed nations, perhaps because, when compared to Europeans and Australians, fewer Americans have a regular physician. Fewer American patients hospitalized with heart attacks or pneumonia receive recommended care than patients in other countries. And only 49 percent of Americans receive screening and preventive care compared to 80 percent in many other countries.[12]

There is, indeed, much evidence that the quality of American health care is not as high as Americans seem inclined to believe.[13]

Some of the difficulties of the American approach to health care can be understood in terms of its experience with managed care and its reliance on market forces. The nonprofit group health plans of a generation ago—the earliest health maintenance organizations (HMOs)—rightly claimed to provide high-quality care while reducing costs by emphasizing prevention and health maintenance within a coordinated system of care. But today the for-profit managed care organizations (MCOs) that dominate American health care are mainly responsive to the bottom line—that is, to maximizing profits. Having much higher turnover of patients than old-fashioned HMOs, they do not find it so economically advantageous to invest in patients' lifetime wellness. Meanwhile, although the basic purpose of health insurance is to spread risk broadly among a population, thereby protecting everyone (especially the less fortunate), today's dominant MCOs try to avoid covering people who are sick or likely to get sick and try to minimize the costs of treating individuals they do cover. One wonders whether the logic of insurance is really compatible with the logic of Wall Street.

Consequently, the American experiment of allowing the free market to determine the shape of health-care finance and delivery has failed to yield progress in connection with the basic goals of health care. Longstanding reluctance to involve the government in significant overhaul of the system has entailed piecemeal initiatives that increase expenditures without improving the efficiency of the overall system. Examples include the Health Insurance Portability and Accountability Act (HIPAA) of 1996, which makes it easier for those who change jobs or become unemployed to retain coverage, and the 1997 States Children's Health Insurance Program (SCHIP), which has reduced the number of uninsured children.

Because most Americans are disadvantaged by the health-care status quo, it should not be surprising that, as reflected in polls, the American public has long favored substantial health-care reform. For example, a 2003 *Washington Post* poll found 80 percent of respondents to regard the achievement of universal coverage more important than holding down taxes.[14] A 2004 survey by the American Hospital Association found that affordable health care had emerged as the country's second leading concern, that 69 percent of citizens were willing to pay more in taxes to secure universal coverage, and even that 54 percent of Republicans (who are traditionally less interested in health-care reform) would be willing to do so.[15] A Kaiser Family Foundation poll in 2008 found roughly two thirds of the public to agree that the federal government should guarantee health care for Americans who lack insurance, even if this means raising taxes.[16] When Obama was elected to the presidency in November 2008, he apparently had most of the public's support to initiate substantial health-care reform. Although American interest in reform might be obscured by opponents' angry outbursts at town meetings in 2009 (a phenomenon fueled in part by misinformation disseminated by commentators and politicians hostile to reform), polls continue to show that most Americans favor either reforms like those currently being debated in Congress or more extensive reforms.[17]

If, as seems likely at the time of this writing, a reform bill passes and becomes law, then health care coverage will significantly expand in the United States. But the issue of health-care reform will not go away, for at least these reasons: the reforms under consideration will not achieve universal coverage; they will not adequately control costs; and they will leave in place serious problems involving comprehensiveness, patient freedom, and quality. Further reform will be an issue.

So far we have discussed the possibility of reform through the lens of widely accepted goals for health care. But what does *justice* require of a health-care system? What do other moral values such as efficiency (utility), liberty, and care add to the moral evaluation of health-care systems and possible reforms of a particular system such as ours? How have other nations expressed their sense of justice and other moral values in their health-care systems? What sort of health-care reform should the United States adopt either in the short term or down the temporal road? This chapter explores these and related questions.

JUSTICE, RIGHTS, AND SOCIETAL OBLIGATIONS

Does society have a moral obligation to ensure that everyone has access to at least some level of health-care services? In other words, is the popular goal of universal access morally sound? If so, what level of care is the appropriate standard? For example, should society ensure access to all needed services, or should only basic care or some other array of services be guaranteed? Answering such questions requires an understanding of various conceptions of justice as well as other possible bases of societal obligations regarding health care.

Justice, Liberty, Equality, and the Right to Health Care Three broad *conceptions* or *visions* of justice dominate social-political theory: libertarian, socialist, and liberal. These conceptions or visions are sometimes sharpened into specific *theories* of justice. Two moral values, liberty and equality, are of key importance. (Utility also plays a role insofar as everyone agrees that efficiency is an important value. But utility does not unambiguously favor one of the three basic approaches.) The *libertarian* conception of justice holds liberty to be the ultimate moral ideal; the *socialist* conception of justice takes social equality to be the ultimate moral ideal; and the *liberal* conception tries to combine equality and liberty into one moral ideal.

The Libertarian Conception of Justice On a libertarian view, persons are understood as owning themselves, their labor, and whatever they appropriately acquire through their labor. Accordingly, persons have moral rights to life, liberty, and property, which any just society must recognize and respect. As libertarianism is usually interpreted, these rights are conceived of as *negative* rights or rights of noninterference: If A has a right to X, no one should prevent A from pursuing X or deprive A of X. On this view, the sole function of government is to protect the individual's life, liberty, and property against force, theft, and fraud. Providing for the welfare of those who cannot or will not provide for themselves is not a morally justifiable function of government. To make such provisions, the government would have to take from some against their will in order to give to others. This is perceived as an unjustifiable limitation on individual liberty. Individuals, again, own themselves and the labor they exert. It follows, for the libertarian, that individuals have the right to whatever income or wealth their labor can earn in a free marketplace, and no one has the right forcibly to take part of that income to provide goods for other persons. The only exceptions to this principle concern those goods—such as the protection afforded by a police force—that are necessary to protect people's negative rights from being violated by others.[18]

The Socialist Conception of Justice A direct challenge to libertarians comes from those who defend the socialist conception of justice. Although socialist views differ in many respects, one common element is a commitment to social equality, however specified, and to government or collective measures furthering that equality. Since social equality is the ultimate value, limitations on individual liberty that are necessary to promote equality are seen as justified. Socialists challenge libertarian views on the primacy of liberty in at least two ways. First, they defend their ideal of social equality. (Their arguments take different forms and need not concern us here.) Second, they assert the meaninglessness of rights of noninterference to those who lack adequate food, health care, and so forth. For those who lack the money needed to buy food and health care needed to sustain life, the libertarian right to life is an empty sham. Liberty rights, such as the right to exchange goods freely, are meaningless to those who cannot exercise such rights because of severe economic or material limitations. Where libertarians stress freedom from government interference, socialists stress the government's obligation to promote the welfare of its citizens by ensuring that their most important needs are met. Where libertarians stress *negative rights,* socialists stress *positive rights*—that is, rights to be provided with certain things. Where libertarians criticize socialism for the limitations it imposes on liberty, socialism criticizes libertarianism for allowing gross inequalities among those who are "equally human."

The Liberal Conception of Justice Liberals reject the libertarian conception of justice for failing to include what liberals perceive as a fundamental moral concern: the requirement that those who have more than enough must help those in need. Like the socialist, the liberal recognizes the extent to which economic constraints can limit the exercise of negative rights by those lacking economic means. The liberal, however, is likely to perceive more of the negative rights asserted by libertarianism as extremely important; while some socialists agree with liberals that civil liberties (e.g., freedom of speech) are very important, liberals generally place more importance than socialists do on, for instance, the value of economic liberty or noninterference. At the same time, liberals defend institutions that provide for the basic needs of disadvantaged members of society. Not opposing all social and economic inequalities, they differ among each other concerning both the morally acceptable extent of those inequalities and their justification. A utilitarian liberal, for example, might hold that inequalities are justified to the extent that they increase the total amount of good in society. A different approach is taken by liberal philosopher John Rawls, who maintains that inequalities in the distribution of primary social goods (e.g., income, opportunities) are justified only if they benefit everyone in society, especially the least advantaged.[19] The primary concern here is not with the total amount of good in society but with the good of the least advantaged.

Theories of Justice and a Right to Health Care What, if anything, can be inferred from theories of justice regarding the possible existence of a moral right to health care? Allen

Buchanan in this chapter asks this question in regard to both a libertarian and a liberal theory of justice. After discussing the libertarian approach as exemplified in the work of Robert Nozick, Buchanan points out that for the libertarian, there is no moral right to health care and no societal obligation to provide it. (Note that a right to health care as an entitlement to be provided some good would be a *positive* right.) Citing Rawls's view as an example of a liberal position, Buchanan explains Rawls's central principles of justice before speculating about their implications regarding what constitutes justice in health care. According to Buchanan, the implications of Rawls's theory for a right to health care are far from clear.[20]

Buchanan also discusses the stance a utilitarian might take regarding a right to health care. He has in mind rule-utilitarianism, which (as explained in Chapter 1) can support the assertion of certain rights. In rule-utilitarianism, the correct conception of justice and of related moral rights is the one whose application maximizes the net amount of good in society. Buchanan examines some of the implications of a utilitarian approach for a right to health care and the scope of any such right.

In another reading in this chapter, Kai Nielsen argues from a socialist position in defending a right to health care based on a view of justice whose fundamental principle is moral equality. He interprets the principle of moral equality to mean that everyone's life matters equally. On this account, any society committed to moral equality must make publicly funded medical treatment of the same quality and extent available to all.

Societal Obligations or Commitments to Provide Health Care Some arguments supporting a societal obligation to provide health care do not involve the claim that individuals have a *right* to health care. These arguments often appeal to considerations of beneficence as well as considerations of the special nature of health care needs, a strategy adopted by the President's Commission for the Study of Ethical Problems in Medicine and Biomedical and Behavioral Research.[21] In its influential report, the Commission asserts that society has an obligation to ensure that every citizen has access to adequate health care without being subject to excessive burdens. This assertion is grounded in (1) the special moral significance of health care, (2) the fact that many health care needs are undeserved, and (3) the implausibility of expecting everyone to be able to meet their needs using their own resources when theses needs are so unpredictable, costly, and unevenly distributed among people. Because the Commission contends only that society has an obligation to ensure universal access to an *adequate* level of care, its view is consistent with a two-tier medical system in which the wealthy can purchase additional services beyond what is available to everyone.

Other arguments support a societal obligation to provide health care without assuming a right to health care. One approach focuses on what universal access to health care (or lack thereof) expresses about a society's character. No decent and compassionate society, according to this line of thinking, could fail to provide health care to its members when it has the financial resources to do so. This argument amounts to an appeal to *virtue;* someone advancing such an argument might not even use the term *societal obligation* (since virtue ethics downplays the concept of obligation), preferring instead to speak of *appropriate societal commitments*. A similar argument could be developed from the perspective of *the ethics of care:* A caring society would commit itself to guaranteeing adequate health care to its people, thereby strengthening the social bonds among them. (See Chapter 1 for discussions of virtue ethics and the ethics of care.)

RATIONING, MANAGED CARE, AND HEALTH CARE
REFORM IN THE UNITED STATES

In the United States, policy decisions about the allocation of health-care resources are regularly made by Congress, state legislatures, managed-care organizations, and other health-insurance companies, plans, and programs. These decisions are often said to involve *rationing*. Though the term "rationing" is used in several ways, it may be broadly understood for our purposes as involving choices within a particular area of biomedicine concerning the relative weight to be given to competing needs. For example, concerning the allocation of public funds, should the funding of prenatal care take precedence over the funding of heart transplants? One sense of rationing is that of *denying* individuals services they need or want because of limited resources. (The strongly negative connotations of this sense of rationing are sometimes exploited by opponents to health care reform when they accuse a proposed reform of rationing.) It is in this sense of rationing that some commentators assert that the American system currently rations by the ability to pay; persons lacking adequate health insurance or sufficient funds are often denied health care they need or want. Especially when health care costs are rising quickly, a commonly asked question is whether more explicit forms of rationing should be accepted.

Whether or not such explicit rationing should be accepted, it occurs regularly in the context of managed care. Indeed, the topics of rationing and managed care are inextricably connected in American health care. As explained earlier, managed care combines health insurance and the delivery of integrated medical services for a population of enrollees, financing the care from an estimated, limited budget. Thus, within a managed-care plan, money devoted to costly, marginally effective treatments is simply not available for other purposes. Because not every possible treatment that might benefit enrollees (patients) can be funded within the limited budget, managed care plans need to make decisions about what sorts of services to cover, whether to cover a particular treatment in a particular case, or both. American managed care is currently dominated by *for-profit* MCOs, creating further pressure to ration. Money taken for profits cannot be devoted to services for patients, effectively shrinking the economic pie from which all patients must eat.

Debates about appropriate criteria for rationing (e.g., effects on quality of life, likelihood of forestalling death) and about how to implement a rationing plan are fueled by the assumption that rationing is inevitable or necessary. When the term "rationing" is used to refer to the withholding of care that certain patients need, or strongly believe they need, such rationing may be difficult to justify in the absence of a persuasive case for its necessity. What is not really disputable is that some rationing in this sense must occur in any health-care system. It is inconceivable that any real-world health-care system could operate without setting some limits on what care will be funded, because demand for services will always exceed what the system can reasonably afford. All health-care systems must, at the very least, limit access to exorbitant care of dubious benefit such as "last-chance therapies" available only in clinical trials.[22]

While some rationing will always be necessary in a health-care system, what is more disputable is whether a particular kind of service must be rationed within a particular system. Disagreement about whether a particular medical service ought to be withheld, or its supply significantly limited, may naturally trace to disagreement about whether this service provides any significant benefit. Yet, even if two people agree on the matter of benefit, they may disagree on whether the medical service in question should be rationed due to differing views on another matter: whether changes in the relevant insurance program or in the health-care system as a whole might make that service affordable. Perhaps cost savings through a more efficient health-care program or system would permit the provision of services that now appear unaffordable due to inefficiency. Therefore, just as the topics of rationing and managed care are inextricably linked in the present context of American health care, both topics are closely tied to the issue of health-care reform in the United States.

Insofar as the topic of health-care reform concerns the entire health-care system, it is, in a sense, more fundamental—and for this reason more important—than the topics of rationing and managed care. Accordingly, the present chapter includes an extensive section on the topic of health-care reform in the United States (and none on the specific topics of rationing or managed care). Because the discussion of American health-care reform can be informed by the experience of other countries that have relatively successful health-care systems, the section on American reform proposals is preceded by a section with discussions of the health-care systems of Canada, Great Britain, Germany, and France.

Before turning to the experiences of these other countries, and then to proposals for reforming American health care, we need to revisit the status quo. The American health-care system features a mix of private and public elements. A large proportion of the American population has some form of private health insurance, commonly obtained as a benefit from employers. Federal funds provide insurance for people over 65 (Medicare) and, in combination with state funds, for those below a certain income level (Medicaid and SCHIPs), though income thresholds vary greatly from state to state. In addition, specific groups, such as veterans and military personnel, are directly cared for in hospitals operated by the government. As noted previously, over 46 million Americans today have neither private nor public health insurance. As also noted, MCOs have become a primary force in health insurance. Not only do they dominate the private insurance market; many enrollees in public programs such as Medicare and Medicaid are strongly encouraged to sign up with MCOs. On the whole, the American health-care system has fared rather poorly in terms of the basic goals of health care. Hence the calls for reform and the current debate in Congress.

Assuming some sort of health-care reform is morally imperative, for what system of health-care delivery and finance should we aim? What models are available? Several models (e.g., market reforms, single-payer finance, managed competition) will be considered in the final section of this chapter. But inasmuch as American society seems significantly pluralistic with respect to theories of social justice, it is fair to ask whether there is a reasonable standpoint from which to evaluate competing models for reform. It would seem that there is. While Americans differ significantly with respect to theories of justice, they agree much more on the appropriate goals of health care. These can serve as benchmarks for evaluating reform proposals. Moreover, the experience of other nations with various health-care systems can furnish relevant evidence regarding what sorts of systems can achieve basic goals and what sorts of approaches are unlikely to do so. With this in mind, let us turn our attention to the health care systems of Canada, Great Britain, Germany, and France.

SYSTEMS OF HEALTH-CARE DELIVERY AND FINANCE: FOUR INTERNATIONAL PERSPECTIVES

The Canadian System The Canadian single-payer (i.e., publicly funded) approach can be understood as a form of managed care.[23] It combines insurance and the delivery of integrated health-care services for a population of enrollees (the residents of a particular province), paying for those services prospectively from a limited budget (in the form of medical expenditure caps). But in Canadian-style managed care—known as Medicare—universal coverage is achieved while costs are controlled by a greatly streamlined form of administration and the absence of profiteering within the public system.

Canada is just one of numerous industrial countries with single-payer systems affording universal access to health care. While spending considerably less per capita on health care than the United States does ($3003 versus $5635 in 2003), Canada provides high-quality care and achieves health indices that are comparable to, or slightly better than, those of its southern neighbor. Significantly, Canada provides a fairly comprehensive package of health-care services for its citizens, covering inpatient and ambulatory care, long-term care for the chronically disabled elderly, and psychiatric services. Only some provinces cover dental services, chiropractic care, optometric services, and prescription drugs. The administrative simplicity of the Canadian system allows it to spend only about one-eighth of every health-care dollar on administration, while the United States spends about one-quarter of each dollar for this purpose. The United States has more than 1000 different payers. Most of them, as part of the private sector, must advertise, determine patient eligibility, elaborate restrictions on coverage, conduct patient-by-patient utilization reviews, try to collect on bad debts, and pay huge executive salaries, while seeking a profit. In contrast, Canada funds almost all of its care through the federal and provincial governments. Patients are rarely billed. Providers are either paid a fixed sum for each patient enrolled in their practices—a *capitation* approach to payment—or they submit simple, standardized forms and get paid on a *fee-for-service* basis. While some private insurance companies offer elective services not covered by the universal Medicare plan (e.g., cosmetic surgery), the role of private insurance is marginal, due in part to the illegality of private companies' providing the same services as are offered in the universal Medicare package.

Canadians and others familiar with this single-payer system generally agree that it provides universal access to high-quality health services in a cost-effective manner that affords extensive patient freedom. Pressures to reduce costs, however, are a reality that actually led to *decreased* public expenditures for several years in the 1990s, generating concerns about not meeting some health needs. There have also been, over the years, complaints about lengthy waits in line for elective services. While the vast majority of Canadians would not trade their health care system for the American system, according to polls, patient satisfaction with Canadian medicine appears to have declined some in recent years.

In a reading reprinted here, Raisa Berlin Deber provides a descriptive overview of the Canadian health-care system with special emphasis on its history, structure, and current challenges. She offers this perspective on the performance of the Canadian system as well as its difficulties: "In all industrial nations, health care seems to be perennially in crisis; however, access and quality in Canada are relatively high, spending relatively well controlled, and satisfaction high, though declining." The Canadian experience with health care offers several lessons for the United States, according to Deber. Prominent among these lessons is that (1) single-payer systems can avoid bloated bureaucracies and achieve universal coverage less expensively than pluralistic funding approaches, and (2) they avoid the fragmentation of health-care markets for the simple reason that everyone is insured as a matter of law.

The British Approach A distinct model of health-care delivery and finance is found in Great Britain. Founded shortly after World War II, the British National Health Service (NHS) immediately provided all British citizens equitable access to health care. Importantly, private care and insurance were not abolished. British citizens may choose to pay for private insurance and their tax contributions fund the NHS. Between 11 and 12 percent of the population have private insurance policies. Meanwhile, unlike their Canadian counterparts, British physicians may provide a particular type of medical service both within the public system and outside of it, and private insurance companies may cover services that are provided in the NHS. As Donald W. Light explains in an article reprinted here, the prerogative of British physicians to maintain their private practices after the NHS was created was crucial to winning their allegiance to a new, universal, publicly-financed system. Since its creation, the NHS has received its share of criticisms, but no substantial proportion of the public has ever called for its abolition.

Some further details about how the system operates may be helpful. First, the benefits offered by the NHS are even more comprehensive than those offered by Canada. In addition to inpatient, ambulatory, and long-term care, the NHS covers dental services, prescription drugs (with a copay), psychiatric care, chiropractic care, and optometric services. At the same time, the system controls costs in part by more aggressively limiting the supply of medical services and equipment (e.g., limiting the supply of dialysis machines). As a single-payer system, the NHS also saves a great deal through simplified administration. NHS physicians have traditionally either received salaries or a lump sum for assuming the care of particular patients; recently, other payment methods (e.g., "pay for performance") have been experimented with. Another means of controlling costs has been limiting patients' choice of primary care physicians, whose referrals are generally needed to see specialists. On the whole, British patients' freedom of choice is probably comparable to that of many American patients insured by MCOs (though it is clearly greater than that of uninsured Americans) while British patients typically encounter less bureaucratic inconvenience.

British health-care expenditures have been a double-edged sword. On the one hand, cost controls have been remarkably successful. Providing one indication are certain comparative figures mentioned earlier: 2003 per capita health spending in Great Britain was only $2231 as compared with $3003 in Canada, $2996 in Germany, and $5635 in the United States. On the other hand, the system has arguably undersupplied health care, causing long waits for routine surgeries and failing to update infrastructure sufficiently as buildings and equipment become outdated—or at least that was the humble picture until recently. As Light puts it in his article, "Tony Blair and his ministers … have moved toward the [very] difficult position of admitting that the NHS has been starved of funds for years and raising the national health insurance tax to fund the largest increases in history." Thus, health spending is on the rise in Great Britain—and more rapidly than in most nations[24]—even though the total British expenditure remains very moderate by European standards and remains less than half of what Americans spend per capita.

According to Light, the British health-care experience suggests a number of lessons for Americans who are interested in reform. First, health care should be "free at the point of service" because copayments and deductibles create inequities and barriers to care without being cost-effective. Second, universal health care should be funded through income taxes, which is by far the most efficient way to collect the needed funds. Third, primary care should be emphasized and supported while specialists should be paid at the same rates, so that young doctors will be encouraged to pursue the specialty they find most satisfying and at which they excel. Finally, prescription drug prices should be controlled while genuine breakthroughs in drug development (as opposed to redundant "me too" drugs) are rewarded.

The German Model A third model for financing and delivering health care is offered by Germany. German health care is not a single-payer system. Rather, as Christa Altenstetter explains in an article reprinted here, the federal government "operates as supervisor, enabler, facilitator, and monitor." The most distinctive feature of this system is its "sickness funds." These nonprofit, semi-private organizations together offer coverage to all citizens. Sickness funds set premiums based on one's ability to pay and not on risk factors such as occupational hazards or one's health history; both employers and employees pay into the funds. About one-tenth of the population either opts for alternative coverage from for-profit insurance companies—which offer more amenities but not additional medical services—or, in the case of civil servants, enjoys governmental insurance. Members of sickness funds choose their own physicians. The medical coverage includes inpatient and ambulatory care, prescription drugs, dental services, psychiatric services, and chiropractic and optometric care; coverage also includes cash benefits in special circumstances (e.g., maternity, necessary travel, burials). At the same time, long-term care for the chronically disabled elderly is means-tested and some services require modest copayments. Rationing is essentially a non-issue.

In order to contain costs, the system's financing has always featured global budgeting, including controls on the prices and volume of services, equipment, and products. Additionally, hospital doctors and nurses are salaried. Such cost control measures have been fairly successful: Per capita spending on health care in Germany, while somewhat high by European standards, is comparable to that in Canada and well below the American average. Considering its success in maintaining universal coverage and high quality of care while minimizing rationing, German cost controls represent a notable achievement. At the same time, difficulties that have long confronted the system include a glut of doctors and weak integration between primary care and hospital care.

One important transformation in German health care is the result of 1993 legislation that gave Germans the right to choose among a range of sickness funds, rather than being assigned to one, resulting in a form of managed competition: Funds compete with each other, but do so within national restrictions such as fee schedules for paying health-care professionals, specific salary agreements, and standards on what types of care funds must cover. Perhaps the most conspicuous consequence of the 1993 legislation is that the number of sickness funds decreased from about one thousand in 1993 to fewer than five hundred within five years as less competitive funds sought safety in mergers.[25]

Among the lessons that German health care may offer to the United States, two (suggested by Altenstetter's analysis) are particularly noteworthy. First, single-payer systems do not provide the only means for achieving the basic goals of health care: universal access, cost controls, comprehensiveness of benefits, patient freedom, and high quality of care; something along the lines of German "sickness funds" is another viable approach. Second, simultaneous achievement of these goals is extremely unlikely unless the federal government assumes a major role in organizing the system, setting standards, controlling costs, and monitoring performance—all within a structure that guarantees health insurance for all.

The French Approach Ranked first among all nations in a 2000 World Health Organization study,[26] the French health-care system has more in common with the German approach than with the Canadian and British single-payer systems. As Victor G. Rodwin and Claude Le Pen put it in their article reprinted in this chapter:

> French policymakers typically view their NHI [national health insurance] as a realistic compromise between Britain's National Health Service, which they believe requires too

much rationing and offers insufficient choice, and the mosaic of subsystems in the United States, which they consider socially irresponsible because 15 percent of the population younger than 65 years of age has no health insurance.

In France, all residents are automatically enrolled with an insurance fund based on their occupational status; 90 percent of the population takes out supplementary insurance to cover benefits not covered in the NHI such as dental and optometric care. But it took from 1928, when the NHI was founded, to 2000 for the system to evolve to the point of covering 100 percent of the population. The French system combines universal coverage with a public-private mix of inpatient and ambulatory care. It is dominated by fee-for-service private practice for ambulatory care and public hospitals for acute care. Unlike in some forms of managed care, there are no gatekeepers limiting access to specialists and particular hospitals; patient choice of providers is very extensive. While patients share costs in a system mostly financed by payroll taxes, government general-revenue funds, and some coinsurance, they are not subject to deductibles.

Although somewhat costly by European standards, French health care has achieved universal coverage—with mostly high quality care and extensive benefits—while spending at much lower than American levels. Since 1996, Parliament has set national spending targets each year, helping to contain costs. As in Germany, rationing is essentially a non-issue in France. And, as one commentator put it, "Despite their reputation for guzzling red wine and eating fatty cheese, French people have for years enjoyed a longer life expectancy then their counterparts in the United States, currently at 80.98 years compared with 78.11."[27] But, in France, as Rodwin and Le Pen explain, access to care is no longer perceived as a sufficient goal, given that the quality of health services is not uniform among social classes and geographical regions—a problem exacerbated by patients' wide freedom of navigation throughout the system. Accordingly, a 2004 law, in addition to raising taxes, sought to implement a kind of state-led managed care characterized by electronic medical records, practice guidelines, and encouragement to use primary care physicians as gate-keepers. The intention of this reform is to modernize the health sector and improve quality while controlling costs.

French health care might offer the United States several lessons. Some are common to all four countries under consideration in this discussion—for example, the importance of governmental leadership in organizing the system. Perhaps the most distinctively French lesson is that the major goals of health care can be achieved incrementally over time.

Broadening the American Perspective The variety of health-care systems around the world all face significant financial and other challenges. As Americans continue to reflect on the shape of their own health-care system, and how it might be improved, reflections will improve by being well-informed. Surprisingly, many discussions in the United States assume that the major goals of health care, such as those discussed in this introduction, cannot be achieved in a harmonious way. Indeed, Americans often assume that achieving universal coverage and reasonable cost controls are incompatible. These common assumptions are myths, as evidence from around the world amply demonstrates. While no system is free of significant difficulties, widely accepted goals of health care are achievable.

The chances are good that by the time this textbook appears in print, the U.S. Congress will have passed, and President Obama will have signed into law, some substantial reforms of the American health-care system. But the reforms under consideration are incapable of achieving universal coverage and will leave in place most of the current cost-ineffective system—including excessively high costs for prescription medications; the socially regressive tax exemption for employment-based insurance; enormous expenditures diverted to administration, advertising, and profit-making; along with the means-tested public programs, Medicaid and SCHIP, which have much higher overhead costs than Medicare. So, no matter what happens in the next few years, the question of appropriate health-care reform will remain with us. Let us therefore turn to various proposals for reform.

REFORM PROPOSALS FOR THE UNITED STATES

Market Reforms In a reading reprinted here, the American Medical Association (AMA) proposes insurance market regulations, including guaranteed insurance renewability and "modified community rating" (in which only age and gender, not health status, affect premium rates). These features, the AMA contends, would encourage "consumers" to remain longer with the same insurers, lowering the latter's administrative costs with the eventual result of lower premiums.

Tax Credits A tax credit for the purchase of health insurance is a sum that can be subtracted from the tax one owes. Refundable tax credits, a measure proposed along with market reforms by the AMA, would permit those who owe no income tax to receive a government payment that could be spent on health insurance. One way to ensure funds for tax credits would be to end the federal income tax exclusion of employer-provided insurance, an exemption that costs the government well over $100 billion of tax revenues annually. The tax exclusion is also regressive, for it exempts those fortunate enough to have insurance through their work from paying progressive income taxes on the value of their premiums.[28]

Individual Mandates These would legally require adults who lack health insurance to purchase it for themselves and their dependents or pay a fine. The reform bills currently being debated by Congress include an individual mandate.

Employer Mandates This measure would require employers to "play or pay": either provide health insurance for their workers or pay into a fund that would cover those not otherwise insured.

Incremental Expansion of Existing Public Sector Programs This strategy would enlarge Medicare, Medicaid, and/or SCHIP to expand coverage. The current reform bills under discussion by Congress include plans for a massive expansion of Medicaid for the poor. Although a proponent of this approach might favor demoting the private-insurance industry from prominence—which would clear the ground for expanded public programs to merge and cover all Americans, effectively creating a single-payer system—most proponents prefer to leave private insurance largely in place. This is the case in President Obama's approach.

Managed Competition This strategy, familiar from President Clinton's reform proposal in 1993, might be combined with individual and employer mandates. A leading option is to adopt the Federal Employees Health Benefits (FEHB) model. While the federal government organizes and manages the system that insures nine million employees and their families, competing health plans provide the insurance. Private fee-for-service insurance and more integrated delivery systems (such as HMOs) offer packages of benefits at varying premiums. Plans that are approved compete for enrollees among federal workers, who may enroll in any competing plan. One current reform proposal is to permit all Americans to enroll in any of these plans.

Two leading proponents of the managed competition approach, Ezekiel J. Emanuel and Victor Fuchs—whose proposal is described in a reading reprinted here—recommend a national, quasi-governmental, nonpartisan commission to administer the system and recommend levels of funding and insurance benefits to Congress. Emanuel and Fuchs also call for vouchers as a mechanism. On their approach, every American under 65 would obtain a voucher that would guarantee and pay for the health benefits offered by a competing health plan. Individuals would be able to select any qualified plan while remaining free to purchase services beyond those provided by the plan. Funding for the vouchers would come from an earmarked, value-added tax, tying benefit levels to tax rates so as to motivate fiscally prudent decisions about the extent of services vouchers would cover. Employer-based insurance, according to the authors, would likely fade away over time, and means-tested programs such as Medicaid and SCHIP would be eliminated. Once the voucher plan was under way, no one would be added to Medicare, so that program would phase out over time as well.

Single-Payer Finance Earlier we were introduced to the concept of single-payer finance with the examples of Canada and Great Britain. Both countries provide universal health coverage funded by tax funds. A key assumption motivating this approach is that the least costly way to achieve universal coverage while promoting patient freedom and a high quality of care is to provide health insurance to all citizens (and perhaps other residents) as a matter of legal fiat and to pay for that coverage through public funds. In a reading reprinted here, David U. Himmelstein and Steffie Woolhandler defend precisely that assumption. They argue, more specifically, that savings on administrative overhead along with the elimination of profiteering would offset the expense of achieving universal coverage to a comprehensive array of benefits. Thus, they conclude, the United States could adopt a single-payer system of health care finance without raising overall health expenditures.

In another article reprinted in this chapter, Ezekiel J. Emanuel contends that health reform embracing a single-payer approach, notwithstanding some undeniable advantages, would be plagued by these shortcomings: (1) The reform would preserve our outdated system of delivering health care without reliable means of assessing and improving quality; (2) While saving greatly on administrative costs, the total costs of this approach—including those of unchecked fraud and abuse—would likely be great; (3) There would be no viable means of stemming health-care inflation over time; and (4) The new system would be vulnerable to politicized decision-making about funding and coverage. In the final reading of this chapter, David DeGrazia defends single-payer finance, canvassing evidence for its cost-effectiveness and replying to criticisms such as those advanced by Emanuel, while suggesting its merger with managed competition. The system he proposes may be seen as occupying a middle ground between single-payer systems as ordinarily conceived (represented by Himmelstein and Woolhandler) and the sort of voucher approach favored by Emanuel and Fuchs.

NOTES

1 U.S. Census Bureau, *Income, Poverty, and Health Insurance Coverage in the United States: 2005* (Washington, DC: Government Printing Office, 2006), p. 20.

2 Institute of Medicine, "Insuring America's Health: Principles and Recommendations" (Washington, DC: National Academies of Science, 2004), http://www.iom.edu/Object.File/Master/17/732/Uninsured6-EnglishFINAL.pdf.

3 Institute of Medicine, "Insuring America's Health: Principles and Recommendations," January 4, 2004, press release.

4 Institute of Medicine, *Hidden Costs, Value Lost* (Washington, DC: National Academies Press, 2003), p. 112.

5 See, e.g., Julius B. Richmond and Rashi Fein, *The Health Care Mess* (Cambridge, MA: Harvard University Press, 2005), p. 233.

6 See, e.g., Gerard Anderson et al., "Health Spending in the United States and the Rest of the Industrialized World," *Health Affairs* 24 (4) (2005): 903–914; Peter Aldhous and Jim Giles, "Money Alone Won't Cure What's Ailing America's Healthcare," *New Scientist* (1 August 2009), p. 7; and Ceci Connolly, "U.S. 'Not Getting What We Pay For,'" *The Washington Post* (November 30, 2008), pp. A1, A6.

7 See, e.g., Employee Benefit Research Institute, "2006 Health Confidence Survey: Dissatisfaction with Health Care System Doubles since 1998," *EBRI Notes* 27 (11) (2006), www.ebri.org, and ABC News/USA Today/Kaiser Family Foundation Health Care Poll, www.usatoday.com/news/health/2006-10-15-health-poll1.htm.

8 The plan does not guarantee coverage by law but rather "requires" individuals without coverage to purchase it or face a fine. The state of Massachusetts adopted essentially the same approach with this predictable result: considerably expanded, but much less than universal, coverage. See Steffie Woolhandler and David U. Himmelstein, "The New Massachusetts Health Reform: Half a Step Forward and Three Steps Back," *Hastings Center Report* 36 (5) (2006), pp. 19–21.

9 The data in this paragraph come from Gerard F. Anderson et al., "Health Care Spending and Use of Information Technology in OECD Countries," *Health Affairs* 25 (May-June 2006), pp. 819–831.

10 Allen E. Buchanan, "Managed Care: Rationing Without Justice, But Not Unjustly," *Journal of Health Politics, Policy and Law* 23 (August 1998), p. 618.

11 Linda T. Kohn, Janet M. Corrigan, and Molla S. Donaldson (eds.), *To Err is Human: Building a Safer Health System* (Washington, DC: National Academy Press, 2000).

12 *Healthcare, Guaranteed* (New York: Public Affairs, 2008), pp. 1–2.

13 See, e.g., G. Schieber, J.-P. Poullier, and L. Greenwald, "Health System Performance in OECD Countries: 1980–1992," *Health Affairs* 13 (4) (1994), pp. 100–112; Karen Donelan et al., "The Cost of Health System Change: Public Discontent in Five Nations," *Health Affairs* 18 (3) (1999), pp. 206–216; Gerard Anderson et al., "Health Spending and Outcomes: Trends in OECD Countries, 1960–1998," *Health Affairs* 19 (3) (2000), pp. 150–157; Peter S. Hussey et al., "How Does the Quality of Care Compare in Five Countries?" *Health Affairs* 23 (3) (2004); and Karen E. Lasser et al., "Access to Care, Health Status, and Health Disparities in the United States and Canada," *American Journal of Public Health* 96 (2006), pp. 1300–1307.

14 Washington Post-ABC News Poll, *The Washington Post* (October 20, 2003), p. A17.

15 American Hospital Association, "AHA National and Selected Statewide Surveys" (a Powerpoint presentation available at www.aha.org/aha_app/jsp-aha/search/results.jsp?), p. 4.

16 Kaiser Family Foundation, "Kaiser Public Opinion Spotlight: Public Opinion on the Uninsured" (www.kff.org/spotlight/uninsured/upload/spotlight_Oct08).

17 Several recent polls and other indications of American interest in health care reform are discussed in Ron Wyden and Bob Bennett, "Finally, Fixing Health Care: What's Different Now?" *Health Affairs* 27 (May/June 2008), pp. 689–692.

18 This paragraph has characterized libertarianism as it is normally understood. In recent decades, a distinct version of libertarianism known as *left* libertarianism—in contrast to what is now sometimes called *right* libertarianism, as just discussed—has become recognized in social-political theory. While the two factions agree fully on the idea of self-ownership, they have different understandings of property rights. Right libertarians hold that resources may be appropriated by whoever first discovers them and "mixes her labor" with them—without others' consent and with no compensation to others. Left libertarians, in contrast, maintain that unappropriated resources belong to everyone. Thus, those who claim rights over natural resources may be required to compensate others for the value of those rights, providing a basis for egalitarian redistribution of wealth or resources. For an introduction to the distinction between right and left

libertarianism, see Peter Vallentyne, "Libertarianism," *Stanford Encyclopedia of Philosophy* (www.plato.stanford.edu; first published September 5, 2002). On left libertarianism in particular, see Peter Vallentyne and Hillel Steiner, eds., *The Origins of Left Libertarianism* (New York: Palgrave, 2000).

19 John Rawls, *A Theory of Justice* (Cambridge, MA: Harvard University Press, 1971).

20 Philosophers have, in fact, emphasized different elements in Rawls's theory of justice in spelling out consequences for health care allocation. See, e.g., Ronald M. Green, "Health Care and Justice in Contract Theory Perspective," in Robert M. Veatch and Roy Branson, eds., *Ethics and Health Policy* (Cambridge, MA: Ballinger, 1976), pp. 111–126; Normal Daniels, "Health Care Needs and Distributive Justice," *Philosophy and Public Affairs* 10 (spring 1981), pp. 146–179; and David DeGrazia, "Grounding a Right to Health Care in Self-Respect and Self-Esteem," *Public Affairs Quarterly* 5 (October 1991), pp. 301–318.

21 President's Commission for the Study of Ethical Problems in Medicine and Biomedical and Behavioral Research, *Securing Access to Health Care* (Washington, DC: Government Printing Office, 1983).

22 Leonard Fleck, "Rationing: Don't Give Up," *Hastings Center Report* 32 (March-April 2002), pp. 35–36.

23 Pat Armstrong, "Managing Care the Canadian Way," *Humane Health Care International* 13 (spring 1997), pp. 13–14.

24 Data are provided by the Organisation for Economic Cooperation and Development (www.oecd.org).

25 Lawrence D. Brown and Volker E. Amelung, "'Manacled Competition': Market Reforms in German Health Care," *Health Affairs* 18 (3) (1999), pp. 76–91.

26 World Health Report 2000 (www.who.int/whr/2000/en).

27 Edward Cody, "For French, U.S. Health Debate Hard to Imagine," *Washington Post* (September 22, 2009) (www.washingtonpost.com/wp-dyn/content/article/2009/09/22).

28 Alliance for Health Reform, "Health Care Coverage in America" (www.CoverTheUninsured.org).

JUSTICE, RIGHTS, AND SOCIETAL OBLIGATIONS

JUSTICE: A PHILOSOPHICAL REVIEW
Allen Buchanan

Buchanan begins by setting out three theoretical approaches to justice: (1) a utilitarian approach, (2) Rawls's theory of justice as fairness, and (3) Nozick's libertarian theory. He confronts each position with several questions about health care. These questions deal with a right to health care, the relative importance of health care or health-care needs vis-à-vis other goods or needs, the relative importance of various forms of health care, and the compatibility of our current health-care system with the demands of justice. Buchanan concludes that none of the three theoretical approaches provides clear answers to all the questions raised and that the application of each depends upon numerous unavailable empirical premises. This leaves a great deal of work to be done in developing an account of justice in health care.

INTRODUCTION

The past decade has seen the burgeoning of bioethics and the resurgence of theorizing about justice. Yet until now these two developments have not been as mutually enriching as one might have hoped. Bioethicists have tended to concentrate on micro issues (moral problems of individual or small group decision making), ignoring fundamental moral questions about the macro structure within which the micro issues arise. Theorists of justice have advanced very general principles but have typically neglected to show how they can illuminate the particular problems we face in health care and other urgent areas.

Micro problems do not exist in an institutional vacuum. The parents of a severely impaired newborn and the attending neonatologist are faced with

From *Justice and Health Care*, edited by Earl Shelp, pp. 3–21.

the decision of whether to treat the infant aggressively or to allow it to die because neonatal intensive care units now exist which make it possible to preserve the lives of infants who previously would have died. Neonatal intensive care units exist because certain policy decisions have been made which allocated certain social resources to the development of technology for sustaining defective newborns rather than for preventing birth defects. Limiting moral inquiry to the micro issues supports an unreasoned conservatism by failing to examine the health care institutions within which micro problems arise and by not investigating the larger array of institutions of which the health care sector is only one part. Since not only particular actions but also policies and institutions may be just or unjust, serious theorizing about justice forces us to expand the narrow focus of the micro approach by raising fundamental queries about the background social, economic, and political institutions from which micro problems emerge.

On the other hand, the attention to individual cases which dominates contemporary bioethics can provide a much needed concrete focus for refining and assessing competing theories of justice. The adequacy or inadequacy of a moral theory cannot be determined by inspecting the principles which constitute it. Instead, rational assessment requires an ongoing process in which general principles are revised and refined through confrontation with the rich complexity of our considered judgments about particular cases, while our judgments about particular cases are gradually structured and modified by our provisional acceptance of general principles. Since our considered judgments about particular cases may often be more sensitive and sure than our assessments of abstract principles, careful attention to accurately described, concrete moral situations is essential for theorizing about justice.

Further, it is not just that the problems of bioethics provide one class of test cases for theories of justice among others: the problems of bioethics are among the most difficult and pressing issues with which a theory of justice must cope. It appears, then, that the continued development of both bioethics and of theorizing about justice in general requires us to explore the problems of justice in health care. In this essay I hope to contribute to that enterprise by first providing a sketch of three major theories of justice and by then attempting to ascertain some of their implications for moral problems in health care.

THEORIES OF JUSTICE

Utilitarianism Utilitarianism purports to be a comprehensive moral theory, of which a utilitarian theory of justice is only one part. There are two main types of comprehensive utilitarian theory: Act and Rule Utilitarianism. Act Utilitarianism defines rightness with respect to particular acts: an act is right if and only if it maximizes utility. Rule Utilitarianism defines rights with respect to rules of action and makes the rightness of particular acts depend upon the rules under which those acts fall. A rule is right if and only if general compliance with that rule (or with a set of rules of which it is an element) maximizes utility, and a particular action is right if and only if it falls under such a rule.

Both Act and Rule Utilitarianism may be versions of either Classic or Average Utilitarianism. Classic Utilitarianism defines the rightness of acts or rules as maximization of *aggregate* utility; Average Utilitarianism defines rightness as maximization of utility *per capita*. The aggregate utility produced by an act or by general compliance with a rule is the sum of the utility produced for each individual affected. Average utility is the aggregate utility divided by the number of individuals affected. 'Utility' is defined as pleasure, satisfaction, happiness, or as the realization of preferences, as the latter are revealed through individuals' choices.

The distinction between Act and Rule Utilitarianism is important for a utilitarian theory of justice, since the latter must include an account of when *institutions* are just. Thus, institutional rules may maximize utility even though those rules do not direct individuals as individuals or as occupants of institutional positions to maximize utility in a case by case fashion. For example, it may be that a judicial system which maximizes utility will do so by including rules which prohibit judges from deciding a case according to their estimates of what would maximize utility in that particular case. Thus the utilitarian justification of a particular action or decision may not be that it maximizes utility, but rather that it falls under some rule of an institution or set of institutions which maximizes utility.[1]

Some utilitarians, such as John Stuart Mill, hold that principles of justice are the most basic moral principles because the utility of adherence to them is especially great. According to this view, utilitarian principles of justice are those utilitarian moral principles which are of such importance that they may be *enforced,* if necessary. Some utilitarians, including Mill perhaps, also hold that among the utilitarian principles of justice are principles specifying individual rights, whether the latter are thought of as enforceable claims which take precedence over appeals to what would maximize utility in the particular case. Indeed, some contemporary rights theorists such as Ronald Dworkin define a (justified) right claim as one which takes precedence over mere appeals to what would maximize utility.

A utilitarian moral theory, then, can include rights principles which themselves prohibit appeals to utility maximization, so long as the justification of those principles is that they are part of an institutional system which maximizes utility. In cases where two or more rights principles conflict, considerations of utility may be invoked to determine which rights principles are to be given priority. Utilitarianism is incompatible with rights only if rights exclude appeals to utility maximization at all levels of justification, including the most basic institutional level. Rights founded ultimately on considerations of utility may be called *derivative,* to distinguish them from rights in the *strict* sense.

Utilitarianism is the most influential version of teleological moral theory. A moral theory is teleological if and only if it defines the good independently of the right and defines the right as that which maximizes the good. Utilitarianism defines the good as happiness (satisfaction, etc.), independently of any account of what is morally right, and then defines the right as that which maximizes the good (either in the particular case or at the institutional level). A moral theory is *deontological* if and only if it is not a teleological theory, i.e., if and only if it either does not define the good independently of the right or does not define the right as that which maximizes the good. Both the second and third theories of justice we shall consider are deontological theories.

John Rawls's Theory: Justice as Fairness In *A Theory of Justice* Rawls pursues two main goals. The first is to set out a small but powerful set of principles of justice which underlie and explain the considered moral judgments we make about particular actions, policies, laws, and institutions. The second is to offer a theory of justice superior to Utilitarianism. These two goals are intimately related for Rawls because he believes that the theory which does a better job of supporting and accounting for our considered judgments is the better theory, other things being equal. The principles of justice Rawls offers are as follows:

1. The principle of greatest equal liberty: Each person is to have an equal right to the most extensive system of equal basic liberties compatible with a similar system of liberty for all ([6], pp. 60, 201–205).

2. The principle of equality of fair opportunity: Offices and positions are to be open to all under conditions of equality of fair opportunity—persons with similar abilities and skills are to have equal access to offices and positions ([6], pp. 60, 73, 83–89).[2]

3. The difference principle: Social and economic institutions are to be arranged so as to benefit maximally the worst off ([6], pp. 60, 75–83).[3]

The basic liberties referred to in (1) include freedom of speech, freedom of conscience, freedom from arbitrary arrest, the right to hold personal property, and freedom of political participation (the right to vote, to run for office, etc.).

Since the demands of these principles may conflict, some way of ordering them is needed. According to Rawls, (1) is *lexically prior* to (2) and (2) is *lexically prior* to (3). A principle 'P' is lexically prior to a principle 'Q' if and only if we are first to satisfy all the requirements of 'P' before going on to satisfy the requirements of 'Q.' Lexical priority allows no trade-offs between the demands of conflicting principles: the lexically prior principle takes absolute priority.

Rawls notes that "many kinds of things are said to be just or unjust: not only laws, institutions, and social systems, but also particular actions . . . decisions, judgments and imputations. . . ." ([6], p. 7). But he insists that the primary subject of justice is the *basic structure* of society because it exerts a pervasive and profound influence on individuals' life prospects. The basic structure is the entire set of major political, legal, economic, and social institutions. In our society the basic structure includes the Constitution, private ownership of the means of production, competitive markets, and the monogamous family. The basic structure plays a large role in distributing the burdens and benefits of cooperation among members of society.

If the primary subject of justice is the basic structure, then the primary problem of justice is to formulate and justify a set of principles which a just basic structure must satisfy. These principles will specify how the basic structure is to distribute prospects of what Rawls calls *primary goods*. They include the basic liberties, as well as powers, authority, opportunities, income, and wealth. Rawls says that primary goods are things that every rational person is presumed to want, because they normally have a use, whatever a person's rational plan of life ([6], p. 62). Principle (1) regulates the distribution of prospects of basic liberties; (2) regulates the distribution of prospects of powers and authority, so far as these are attached to institutional offices and positions, and (3) regulates the distribution of prospects of the other primary goods, including wealth and income. Though the first and second principles require equality, the difference principle allows inequalities so long as the total system of institutions of which they are a part maximizes the prospects of the worst off to the primary goods in question.

Rawls advances three distinct types of justification for his principles of justice. Two appeal to our considered judgments, while the third is based on what he calls the Kantian interpretation of his theory.

The first type of justification rests on the idea, mentioned earlier, that if a set of principles provides the best account of our considered judgments about what is just or unjust, then that is a reason for accepting those principles. A set of principles accounts for our judgments only if those judgments can be derived from the principles, granted the relevant facts for their application.

Rawls's second type of justification maintains that if a set of principles would be chosen under conditions which, according to our considered judgments, are appropriate conditions for choosing principles of justice, then this is a reason for accepting those principles. The second type of justification includes three parts: (1) A set of conditions for choosing principles of justice must be specified. Rawls labels the complete set of conditions the 'original position.' (2) It must be shown that the conditions specified are (according to our considered judgments) the appropriate conditions of choice. (3) It must be shown that Rawls's principles are indeed the principles which would be chosen under those conditions.

Rawls construes the choice of principles of justice as an ideal social contract. "The principles of justice for the basic structure of society are the principles that free and rational persons . . . would accept in an initial situation of equality as defining the fundamental terms of their association" ([6], p. 11). The idea of a social contract has several advantages. First, it allows us to view principles of justice as the object of a *rational collective choice*. Second, the idea of *contractual obligation* is used to emphasize that the choice expresses a basic commitment and that the principles agreed on may be rightly enforced. Third, the idea of a contract as a *voluntary agreement* which set terms for mutual advantage suggests that the principles of justice should be "such as to draw forth the willing cooperation" ([6], p. 15) of all members of society, including those who are worse off.

The most important elements of the original position for our purposes are a) the characterization of the parties to the contract as individuals who desire to pursue their own life plans effectively and who "have a highest-order interest in how . . . their interests . . . are shaped and regulated by social institutions" ([8], p. 64); b) the 'veil of ignorance,' which is a constraint on the information the parties are able to utilize in choosing principles of justice; and c) the requirement that the principles are to be chosen on the assumption that they will be complied with by all (the universalizability condition) ([6], p. 132).

The parties are characterized as desiring to maximize their shares of primary goods, because these goods enable one to implement effectively the widest range of life plans and because at least some of them, such as freedom of speech and of conscience, facilitate one's freedom to choose and revise one's life plan or conception of the good. The parties are to choose "from behind a veil of ignorance" so that information about their own particular characteristics or social positions will not lead to bias in the choice of principles. Thus they are described as not knowing their race, sex, socioeconomic, or political status, or even the nature of their particular conceptions of the good. The informational restriction also helps to insure that the principles chosen will not place avoidable restrictions on the individual's freedom to choose and revise his or her life plan.[4]

Though Rawls offers several arguments to show that his principles would be chosen in the original position, the most striking is the maximin argument. According to this argument, the rational strategy in the original position is to choose that set of principles whose implementation will maximize the minimum share of primary goods which one can receive as a member of society, and principles (1), (2), and (3) will insure the greatest minimal share. Rawls's claim is that because these principles protect one's basic liberties and opportunities and insure an adequate minimum of goods such as wealth and income (even if one should turn out to be among the worst off), the rational thing is to choose them, rather than to gamble with one's life prospects by opting for alternative principles. In particular, Rawls contends that it would be irrational to reject his principles and allow one's life prospect to be determined by what would maximize utility, since utility maximization might allow severe deprivation or even slavery for some, so long as this contributed sufficiently to the welfare of others.

Rawls raises an important question about this second mode of justification when he notes that this original position is purely hypothetical. Granted that the agreement is never actually entered into, why should we regard the principles as binding? The answer, according to Rawls, is that we do in fact accept the conditions embodied in the original position ([6], p. 21). The following qualification, which Rawls adds immediately after claiming that the conditions which constitute the original position are appropriate for the choice of principles of justice according to our considered judgments, introduces his third type of justification: "Or if we do not [accept the conditions of the original position as appropriate for choosing principles of justice] *then perhaps we can be persuaded to do so by the philosophical reflections*" (emphasis added [6], p. 21). In the Kantian interpretation section of *A Theory of Justice*, Rawls sketches a certain kind of philosophical justification for the conditions which make up the original position (based on Kant's conception of the 'noumenal self' or autonomous agent).

For Kant an autonomous agent's will is determined by rational principles and rational principles are those which can serve as principles for all rational beings, not just for this or that agent, depending upon whether or not he has some particular desire which other rational beings may not have. Rawls invites us to think of the original position as the perspective from which autonomous agents see the world. The original position provides a "procedural interpretation" of Kant's idea of a Realm of Ends or community of "free and equal rational beings." We express our nature as autonomous agents when we act from principles that would be chosen in conditions which reflect that nature ([6], p. 252).

Rawls concludes that, when persons such as you and I accept those principles that would be chosen in the original position, we express our nature as autonomous agents, i.e., we act autonomously. There are three main grounds for this thesis, corresponding to the three features of the original position cited earlier. First, since the veil of ignorance excludes information about any particular desires which a rational agent may or may not have, the choice of principles is not determined by any particular desire. Second, since the parties strive to maximize their share of primary goods, and since primary goods are attractive to them because they facilitate freedom in choosing and revising life plans and because they are flexible means not tied to any particular ends, this is another respect in which their choice is not determined by particular desires. Third, the original position includes the requirement that they will be principles of rational agents in general and not just for agents who happen to have this or that particular desire.

In the *Foundations of the Metaphysics of Morals* Kant advances a moral philosophy which identifies autonomy with rationality [4]. Hence for Kant the question "Why should one express our nature as autonomous agents?" is answered by the thesis that rationality requires it. Thus *if* Rawls's third type of justification succeeds in showing that we best express our autonomy when we accept those principles in the belief that they would be chosen from the original position, and *if* Kant's identification of autonomy with rationality is successful, the result will be a justification of Rawls's principles which is distinct from both the first and second modes of justification. So far as this third type of justification does not make the acceptance of Rawls's principles hinge on whether the principles themselves or the conditions from which they would be chosen match our considered judgments, it is not directly vulnerable either to the charge that Rawls has misconstrued our considered judgments or that congruence with considered judgments, like the appeal to mere consensus, has no justificatory force.

It is important to see that Rawls understands his principles of justice as principles which generate *rights* in what I have called the strict sense. Claims based upon the three principles are to take precedence over considerations of utility and the principles themselves are not justified on the grounds that a basic structure which satisfies them will maximize utility. Moreover, Rawls's theory is not a teleological theory of any kind because it does not define the right as that which maximizes the good, where the good is defined independently of the right. Instead it is perhaps the most influential current instance of a deontological theory.

Nozick's Libertarian Theory There are many versions of libertarian theory, but their characteristic doctrine is that coercion may only be used to prevent or punish physical harm, theft, and fraud, and to enforce contracts. Perhaps the most influential and systematic recent instance of Libertarianism is the theory presented by Robert Nozick in *Anarchy, State, and Utopia* [5]. In Nozick's theory of justice,

as in libertarian theories generally, the right to private property is fundamental and determines both the legitimate role of the state and the most basic principles of individual conduct.

Nozick contends that individuals have a property right in their persons and in whatever 'holdings' they come to have through actions which conform to (1) "the principle of justice in [initial] acquisition" and (2) "the principle of justice in transfer" ([5], p. 151). The first principle specifies the ways in which an individual may come to own hitherto unowned things without violating anyone else's rights. Here Nozick largely follows John Locke's famous account of how one makes natural objects one's own by "mixing one's labor" with them or improving them through one's labor. Though Nozick does not actually formulate a principle of justice in (initial) acquisition, he does argue that whatever the appropriate formulation is it must include a 'Lockean Proviso,' which places a constraint on the holdings which one may acquire through one's labor. Nozick maintains that one may appropriate as much of an unowned item as one desires so long as (a) one's appropriation does not worsen the conditions of others in a special way, namely, by creating a situation in which others are "no longer . . . able to use freely [without exclusively appropriating] what [they] . . . previously could" or (b) one properly compensates those whose condition is worsened by one's appropriation in the way specified in (a) ([5], pp. 178–179). Nozick emphasizes that the Proviso only picks out one way in which one's appropriation may worsen the condition of others; it does not forbid appropriation or require compensation in cases in which one's appropriation of an unowned thing worsens another's condition merely by limiting his opportunities to appropriate (rather than merely use) that thing, i.e., to make it his property.

The second principle states that one may justly transfer one's legitimate holdings to another through sale, trade, gift or bequest and that one is entitled to whatever one receives in any of these ways, so long as the person from whom one receives it was entitled to that which he transferred to you. The right to property which Nozick advances is the right to exclusive control over anything one can get through initial appropriation (subject to the Lockean Proviso) or through voluntary exchanges with others entitled to what they transfer. Nozick concludes that a distribution is just if and only if it arose from another just distribution by legitimate means. The principle of justice in initial acquisition specifies the legitimate 'first moves,' while the principle of justice in transfers specifies the legitimate ways of moving from one distribution to another: "Whatever arises from a just situation by just steps is itself just" ([5], p. 151).

Since not all existing holdings arose through the 'just steps' specified by the principles of justice in acquisition and transfer, there will be a need for a *principle of rectification* of past injustices. Though Nozick does not attempt to formulate such a principle he thinks that it might well require significant redistribution of holdings.

Apart from the case of rectifying past violations of the principles of acquisition and transfer, however, Nozick's theory is strikingly anti-redistributive. Nozick contends that attempts to force anyone to contribute any part of his legitimate holdings to the welfare of others is a violation of that person's property rights, whether it is undertaken by private individuals or the state. On this view, coercively backed taxation to raise funds for welfare programs of any kind is literally theft. Thus, a large proportion of the activities now engaged in by the government involve gross injustices.

After stating his theory of rights, Nozick tries to show that the state is legitimate so long as it limits its activities to the enforcement of these rights and eschews redistributive functions. To do this he employs an 'invisible hand explanation,' which purports to show how the minimal state could arise as an unintended consequence of a series of voluntary transactions which violate no one's rights. The phrase 'invisible hand explanation' is chosen to stress that the process by which the minimal state could emerge fits Adam Smith's famous account of how individuals freely pursuing their own private ends in the market collectively produce benefits which are not the aim of anyone.

The process by which the minimal state could arise without violating anyone's rights is said to include four main steps ([5], pp. 10–25).[5] First, individuals in a 'state of nature' in which (Libertarian) moral principles are generally respected would form a plurality of 'protective agencies' to enforce their libertarian rights, since individual efforts at enforcement would be inefficient and liable to abuse. Second, through competition for clients, a 'dominant protective agency' would eventually emerge in a given geographical area. Third, such an agency would eventually become a 'minimal state' by asserting a claim of monopoly over protective services in order to prevent less reliable efforts at enforcement which might endanger its clients: it would forbid 'independents' (those who refused to purchase its services) from seeking other forms of enforcement. Fourth, again assuming that correct moral principles are generally followed, those belonging to the dominant protective agency would compensate the 'independents,' presumably by providing them with free or partially subsidized protection services. With the exception of taxing its clients to provide compensation for the independents, the minimal state would act only to protect persons against physical injury, theft, fraud, and violations of contracts.

It is striking that Nozick does not attempt to provide any systematic *justification* for the Lockean rights principles he advocates. In this respect he departs radically from Rawls. Instead, Nozick assumes the correctness of the Lockean principles and then, on the basis of that assumption, argues that the minimal state and only the minimal state is compatible with the rights those principles specify.

He does, however, offer some arguments against the more-than-minimal state which purport to be independent of that particular theory of property rights which he assumes. These arguments may provide indirect support for his principles insofar as they are designed to make alternative principles, such as Rawls's, unattractive. Perhaps most important of these is an argument designed to show that any principle of justice which demands a certain distributive end state or pattern of holdings will require frequent and gross disruptions of individuals' holdings for the sake of maintaining that end state or pattern. Nozick supports this general conclusion by a vivid example. He asks us to suppose that there is some distribution of holdings 'D_1' which is required by some end-state or patterned theory of justice and that 'D_1'is achieved at time 'T.' Now suppose that Wilt Chamberlain, the renowned basketball player, signs a contract stipulating that he is to receive twenty-five cents from the price of each ticket to the home games in which he performs, and suppose that he nets $250,000, from this arrangement. We now have a new distribution 'D$_2$.' Is 'D$_2$' unjust? Notice that by hypothesis those who paid the price of admission were entitled to control over the resources they held in 'D$_1$' (as were Chamberlain and the team's owners). The new distribution arose through *voluntary exchanges of legitimate holdings,* so it is difficult to see how it could be unjust, even if it does diverge from 'D$_1$.' From this and like examples, Nozick concludes that attempts to maintain any end-state or patterned distributive principle would require continuous interference in peoples' lives ([5], pp. 161–163).

As in the cases of Utilitarianism and Rawls's theory, Nozick and libertarians generally do not limit morality to justice. Thus, Nozick and others emphasize that a libertarian theory of individual rights is to be supplemented by a libertarian theory of virtues which recognizes that not all moral principles are suitable objects of enforcement and that moral life includes more than the nonviolation of rights. Libertarians invoke the distinction between justice and charity to reply to those who complain that a Lockean theory of property rights legitimizes crushing poverty for millions. They stress that while justice demands that we not be *forced* to contribute to the well-being of others, charity requires that we help even those who have no *right* to our aid.[6]

IMPLICATIONS FOR HEALTH CARE

Now that we have a grasp of the main ideas of three major theories of justice, we can explore briefly some of their implications for health care. To do this we may confront the theories with four questions:

1. Is there a right to health care? (If so, what is its basis and what is its content?)

2. How, in order of priority, is health care related to other goods, or how are health care needs related to other needs? (If there is a right to health care, how is it related to other rights?)

3. How, in order of priority, are various forms of health care related to one another?

4. What can we conclude about the justice or injustice of the current health care system?

In some cases, as we shall see, the theories will provide opposing answers to the same question; in others, the theories may be unhelpfully silent.

We have already seen that the Utilitarian position on rights in general is complex. If by a right we mean a right in the strict sense, i.e., a claim which takes precedence over mere appeals to utility at all levels, including the most basic institutional level, then Utilitarianism denies the existence of rights in general, including the right to health care. If, on the other hand, we mean by right a claim that takes precedence over mere appeals to utility at the level of particular actions or at some institutional level short of the most basic, but which is justified ultimately by appeal to the utility of the total set of institutions, then Utilitarianism does not exclude, and indeed may even require rights, including a right to health care. Whether or not the total institutional array which maximizes utility will include a right to health care will depend upon a wealth of *empirical facts* not deducible from the principle of utility itself. The nature and complexity of the relevant facts can best be appreciated by considering briefly the bearing of Utilitarianism on questions (2) and (3). A utilitarian system of (derivative) rights will pick out certain goods as those which make an especially large contribution to the maximization of utility. It is reasonable to assume, on the basis of empirical data, that health care, or at least certain forms of health care, is among them. Consider, for example, prenatal care, broadly conceived as including genetic screening and counseling (at least for special risk groups), prenatal nutritional care and medical examinations for expectant mothers, medical care during delivery, and basic pediatric services in the crucial months after birth. If empirical research indicates (1) that a system of institutional arrangements which maximizes utility would include such services and (2) that such services can best be assured if they are accorded the status of a right, with all that this implies, including the use of coercive sanctions where necessary, then according to Utilitarianism there is such a (derivative) right. The strength and content of this right relative to other (derivative) rights will be determined by the utility of health care as compared with other kinds of goods.

It is crucial to note that, for the utilitarian, empirical research must determine not only whether certain health-care services are to be provided as a matter of right, but also whether the right in question is to be an equal right enjoyed by all persons. No commitment to equality of rights is included in the utilitarian principle itself, nor is there any commitment to equal distribution of any kind. Utilitarianism is egalitarian only in the sense that in calculating what will maximize utility each person's welfare is to be included.

Utilitarian arguments, sometimes based on empirical data, have been advanced to show that providing health care free of charge as a matter of right would encourage wasteful use of scarce and costly resources because the individual would have no incentive to restrain his 'consumption' of health care. The cumulative result, it is said, would be quite disutilitarian: a breakdown of the health-care system or a disastrous curtailment of other basic services to cover the spiraling costs of health care. In contrast (proponents of this argument continue) a *market* in health care encourages 'consumers' to use resources wisely because the costs of the services an individual receives are borne by that individual.

On the other side of the utilitarian ledger, empirical evidence may be marshalled to show that the benefits of a right to health care outweigh the costs, including the costs of possible over-use, and that a market in health care would not maximize utility because those who need health care the most may not be able to afford it.

Similarly, even if there is a utilitarian justification for a right to health care, empirical evidence must again be presented to show that it should be an equal right. For it is certainly conceivable that, under certain circumstances at least, utility could be maximized by providing extensive health care only for some groups, perhaps even a minority, rather than for all persons.

Utilitarians who advocate a right to health care often argue that this right, like other basic rights, should be equal, on the basis of the assumption of diminishing marginal utility. The idea, roughly, is that with respect to many goods, including health care,

there is a finite upper bound to the satisfaction a person can gain from being provided with additional amounts of the goods in question. Hence, if in general we are all subject to the phenomenon of diminishing marginal utility in the case of health care and if the threshold of diminishing marginal utility is in general sufficiently low, then there are sound utilitarian reasons for distributing health care equally.

Finally, it should be clear that for the utilitarian the issue of priorities within health care, as well as that of priorities between health care and other goods, must again be settled by empirical research. If, as seems likely, utility maximization requires more resources for prevention and health maintenance rather than for curative intervention after pathology has already developed, then this will be reflected in the content of the utilitarian right to health care. If, as many writers have contended, the current emphasis in the U.S. on high technology intervention produces less utility than would a system which stresses prevention and health maintenance (for example, through stricter control of pollution and other environmental determinants of disease), then the utilitarian may conclude that the current system is unjust in this respect. Empirical data would also be needed to ascertain whether more social resources should be devoted to high- or low-technology intervention: for example, neonatal intensive care units versus 'well-baby clinics.' These examples are intended merely to illustrate the breadth and complexity of the empirical research needed to apply Utilitarianism to crucial issues in health care.

Libertarian theories such as Nozick's rely much less heavily upon empirical premises for answers to questions (1)–(4). Since the libertarian is interested only in preventing violations of libertarian rights, and since the latter are rights against certain sorts of interferences rather than rights to be provided with anything, the question of what will maximize utility is irrelevant. Further, any effort to implement any right to health care whatsoever is an injustice, according to the libertarian.

There are only two points at which empirical data are relevant for Nozick. First, whether or not any current case of appropriation of hitherto unheld things satisfies the Lockean Proviso is a matter of fact to be ascertained by empirical methods. Second, empirical historical research is needed to determine what sort of redistribution for the sake of rectifying past injustices is necessary. If, for example, physicians' higher incomes are due in part to government policies which violate libertarian rights, then rectificatory redistribution may be required. And indeed libertarians have argued that two basic features of the current health-care system do involve gross violations of libertarian rights. First, compulsory taxation to provide equipment, hospital facilities, research funds, and educational subsidies for medical personnel is literally theft. Second, some argue that government-enforced occupational licensing laws which prohibit all but the established forms of medical practice violate the right to freedom of contract [3]. Those who raise this second objection also usually argue that the function of such laws is to secure a monopoly for the medical establishment while sharply limiting the supply of doctors so as to keep medical fees artificially high. Whether or not such arguments are sound, it is important to note that Libertarianism is not to be confused with Conservatism. A theory which would institute a free market in medical services, abolish government subsidies, and reduce government regulation of medical practice to the prevention of injury and fraud and the enforcement of contracts has radical implications for changing the current system.

Libertarianism offers straightforward answers to questions (2) and (3). Even if it can be shown that health care in general, and certain forms of health care more than others, are especially important for the happiness or even the freedom of most persons, this fact is quite irrelevant from the perspective of a libertarian theory of justice, though it is no doubt significant for the libertarian concerned with charity or other virtues which exceed the requirements of justice. Nozick and other libertarians recognize that a free market in medical services may in fact produce severe inequalities and that there is no assurance that all or even most will be able to afford adequate medical care. Though the humane libertarian will find this condition unfortunate and will aid those in need and encourage others to do likewise voluntarily, he remains adamant that no one has a right to health care and that hence none may rightly be forced to aid another.

According to Rawls, the most basic questions about health care are not to be decided either by consideration of utility or by market processes. Instead they are to be settled ultimately by appeal to those principles of justice which would be chosen in the original position. As we shall see, however, the implications of Rawls's principles for health care are far from clear.[7]

No principle explicitly specifying a right to health care is included among Rawls's principles of justice. Further, since those principles are intended to regulate the basic structure of society as a whole, they are not themselves intended to guide the decisions individuals make in particular health-care situations, nor are they themselves to be applied directly to health-care institutions. We are not to assume that either individual physicians or administrators of particular policies or programs are to attempt to allocate health care so as to maximize the prospects of the worst off. In Rawls's theory, as in Utilitarianism, the rightness or wrongness of particular actions or policies depends ultimately upon the nature of the entire institutional structure within which they exist. Hence, Rawls's theory can provide us with fruitful answers at the micro level only if its implications at the macro level are adequately developed.

If Rawls's theory includes a right to health care, it must be a right which is in some way derivative upon the basic rights laid down by the Principle of Greatest Equal Liberty, the Principle of Equality of Fair Opportunity, and the Difference Principle. And if there is to be such a derivative right to health care, then health care must either be among the primary goods covered by the three principles or it must be importantly connected with some of those goods. Now at least some forms of health care (such as broad services for prevention and health maintenance, including mental health) seem to share the earmarks of Rawlsian primary goods: they facilitate the effective pursuit of ends in general and may also enhance our ability to criticize and revise our conceptions of the good. Nonetheless, Rawls does not explicitly list health care among the social primary goods included under the three principles. However, he does include wealth under the Difference Principle and defines it so broadly that it might be thought to include access to health-care services. In "Fairness to Goodness" Rawls defines wealth as virtually any legally exchangeable social asset; this would cover health-care 'vouchers' if they could be cashed or exchanged for other goods ([7], p. 540).

Let us suppose that health care is either itself a primary good covered by the Difference Principle or that health care may be purchased with income or some other form of wealth which is included under the Difference Principle. In the former case, depending upon various empirical conditions, it might turn out that the best way to insure that the basic structure satisfies the Difference Principle is to establish a state-enforced right to health care. But whether maximizing the prospects of the worst off will require such a right, and what the content of the right will be, will depend upon what weight is to be assigned to health care relative to other primary goods included under the Difference Principle. Similarly, a weighting must also be assigned if we are to determine whether the share of wealth one receives under the Difference Principle would be sufficient both for health-care needs and for other ends. Unfortunately, though Rawls acknowledges that a weighted index of primary goods is needed if we are to be able to determine what would maximize the prospects of the worst off, he offers no account of how the weighting is to be achieved.

The problem is especially acute in the case of health care, because some forms of health care are so costly that an unrestrained commitment to them would undercut any serious commitment to providing other important goods. Thus, it appears that until we have some solution to the weighting problem, Rawls's theory can shed only a limited light upon the question of priority relations between health care and other goods and among various forms of health care. Rawls's conception of primary goods may explain what distinguishes health care from those things that are not primary goods, but this is clearly not sufficient.

Perhaps because he is aware of the exorbitant demands which certain health-care needs may place upon social resources, Rawls stipulates that the parties in the original position are to choose principles of justice on the assumption that their needs fall within the 'normal range' ([9], pp. 9–10). His ideal may be that the satisfaction of extremely costly special needs for health care may not be a matter of justice but rather of *charity*. If some reasonable way of drawing the line between 'normal' needs which fall within the gambit of principles of justice and 'special' needs which are the proper object of the virtue of charity could be developed, then this would be a step toward solving the priority problems mentioned above.

It has been suggested that the Principle of Equality of Fair Opportunity, rather than the Difference Principle, might provide the basis for a Rawlsian right to health care ([2], pp. 16–18). While I cannot accord this proposal the consideration it deserves here, I wish to point out that there are four difficulties which make it problematic. First, priority problems still remain. For now we are faced with the task of assigning a weight to health care relative to those other factors (such as education) which are also determinants of opportunity. Further, since the Principle of Equality of Fair Opportunity is lexically prior to the Difference Principle, we must again face the prospect that commitment to the former principle might swallow up social resources needed for providing important goods included under the latter.

Second, because it refers only to opportunities for occupying social *positions* and *offices,* rather than to opportunities in general, the Principle of Equality of Fair Opportunity might be thought too narrow to provide an adequate foundation for a right to health care. Rawls might respond either by defining 'position' rather broadly or by arguing that opportunities for attaining positions and offices are related to opportunities in general in such a way that equality in the former insures equality in the latter.

Third, and more importantly, Rawls's Principle of Equality of Fair Opportunity takes 'abilities' and 'skills' as given, requiring only that persons with equal or similar abilities and skills are to have equal prospects of attaining social positions and offices. Yet clearly inequalities in health care can produce severe inequalities in abilities and skills. For example, poor nutrition and medical care during gestation can result in mental retardation, and many health problems hinder the development of skills and abilities. Hence it might be argued that if the Principle of Opportunity is to provide an adequate basis for a right to health care it must be reformulated to capture the crucial influence of health care or the lack of it upon individual development.

Each of the theories of justice under consideration offers a theoretical basis for answering some basic questions concerning justice in health care. We have seen, however, that none of them provides unambiguous answers to all of the questions and that each depends for its application upon a wealth of empirical premises, many of which may not now be available. Each theory does at least rule out some answers and each supplies us with a perspective from which to pursue issues which we cannot ignore. Nonetheless, almost all of the work in developing an account of justice in health care remains to be done.[8]

NOTES

1 In this essay I shall be concerned for the most part with utilitarianism at the institutional level, and I shall proceed on the assumption that a set of institutions which maximizes utility will include rules which bar other direct applications of the principle of utility itself. Consequently, I will mainly be concerned with Rule Utilitarianism, rather than Act Utilitarianism (the latter being the view that the rightness or wrongness of a given act depends solely upon whether it maximizes utility). For an original and interesting attempt to show that Act Utilitarianism is compatible with social norms that bar direct appeals to utility, see [10].

2 Rawls sometimes refers to the "Principle of Equality of Fair Opportunity" and sometimes to the "Principle of Fair Equality of Opportunity." For convenience I will stay with the former label.

3 The phrase "worst off" refers to those who are worst off with respect to prospects of the social primary goods regulated by the Difference Principle.

4 For a detailed elaboration of this point, see [1].

5 For a fundamental objection to Nozick's invisible hand explanation, see [11].

6 P. Singer [12], expanding an argument developed earlier by R. Titmuss, argues that the existence of markets for certain goods may in fact undermine the motivation for charity.

7 See [2].

8 I would like to thank Earl Shelp and William Hanson for their very helpful comments on an earlier draft of this paper.

REFERENCES

1 Buchanan, A. "Revisability and Rational Choice." *Canadian Journal of Philosophy* 5:395–408, 1975.

2 Daniels, N. "Rights to Health Care and Distributive Justice: Programmatic Worries." *Journal of Medicine and Philosophy* 4:174–191, 1979.

3 Friedman, M. *Capitalism and Freedom.* Chicago: University of Chicago Press, 1962, pp. 137–160.

4 Kant, I *Foundations of the Metaphysics of Morals* (transl. by L. W. Beck), New York: Bobbs-Merrill, 1959, Part III.

5 Nozick, R. *Anarchy, State and Utopia.* New York: Basic Books, 1974.

6 Rawls, J. *A Theory of Justice.* Cambridge, Mass.: Harvard University Press, 1971.

7 Rawls, J. "Fairness to Goodness." *Philosophical Review* 84:536–554, 1975.

8 Rawls, J. "Reply to Alexander and Musgrave." *Quarterly Journal of Economics* 88:633–655, November 1974.

9 Rawls, J. "Responsibility for Ends." Stanford University, Unpublished Lecture, 1979.

10 Sartorius, R. *Individual Conduct and Social Norms.* Encino, Calif.: Dickenson Publishing, 1975.

11 Sartorius, R. "The Limits of Libertarianism." In *Liberty and the Rule of Law,* edited by R. L. Cunningham, 87–131. College Station, Texas: Texas A and M University Press, 1979.

12 Singer, P. "Rights and the Market." In *Justice and Economic Distribution,* edited by J. Arthur and W. Shaw, pp. 207–221. Englewood Cliffs, N.J.: Prentice-Hall, 1978.

AUTONOMY, EQUALITY AND A JUST HEALTH CARE SYSTEM
Kai Nielsen

According to Nielsen, justice requires social institutions that work on the premise of moral equality—the life of everyone matters and matters equally. Beginning with this premise and an analysis of basic needs, Nielsen argues that individuals have a moral right to have their health-care needs met. Furthermore, on his account, a commitment to egalitarianism is incompatible with a two- or three-tier system of medical care. Moral equality requires the open and free provision of medical treatment of the same extent and quality to everyone in society. In his view, a system intended to achieve this end would have to take medicine out of the private sector altogether and place both the ownership and control of medicine in the public sector.

I

Autonomy and equality are both fundamental values in our firmament of values, and they are frequently thought to be in conflict. Indeed, the standard liberal view is that we must make difficult and often morally ambiguous trade-offs between them.[1] I shall argue that this common view is mistaken and that autonomy cannot be widespread or secure in a society which is not egalitarian: where, that is, equality is not also a very fundamental value which has an operative role within the society.[2] I shall further argue that, given human needs and a commitment to an autonomy respecting egalitarianism, a very different health-care system would come into being than that which exists at present in the United States.

I shall first turn to a discussion of autonomy and equality and then, in terms of those conceptions, to a conception of justice. In modernizing societies of Western Europe, a perfectly just society will be a society of equals and in such societies there will be a belief held across the political spectrum in what has been called *moral* equality. That is to say, when viewed with the impartiality required by morality, the life of everyone matters and matters equally.[3] Individuals will, of course, and rightly so, have their local attachments, but they will acknowledge that justice requires that the social institutions of the society should be such that they work on the premise that the life of everyone matters and matters equally. Some privileged elite or other group cannot be given special treatment simply because they are that group. Moreover, for there to be a society of equals there must be a rough equality of condition in the society. Power must be sufficiently equally shared for it to be securely the case that no group or class or gender can dominate others through the social structures either by means of their frequently thoroughly unacknowledged latent functions or more explicitly

and manifestly by institutional arrangements sanctioned by law or custom. Roughly equal material resources or power are not things which are desirable in themselves, but they are essential instrumentalities for the very possibility of equal well-being and for as many people as possible having as thorough and as complete a control over their own lives as is compatible with this being true for everyone alike. Liberty cannot flourish without something approaching this equality of condition, and people without autonomous lives will surely live impoverished lives. These are mere commonplaces. In fine, a commitment to achieving equality of condition, far from undermining liberty and autonomy, is essential for their extensive flourishing.

If we genuinely believe in moral equality, we will want to see come into existence a world in which all people capable of self-direction have, and have as nearly as is feasible equally, control over their own lives and can, as far as the institutional arrangements for it obtaining are concerned, all live flourishing lives where their needs and desires as individuals are met as fully as possible and as fully and extensively as is compatible with that possibility being open to everyone alike. The thing is to provide institutional arrangements that are conducive to that.

People, we need to remind ourselves, plainly have different capacities and sensibilities. However, even in the extreme case of people for whom little in the way of human flourishing is possible, their needs and desires, as far as possible, should still also be satisfied in the way I have just described. Everyone in this respect at least has equal moral standing. No preference or pride of place should be given to those capable, in varying degrees, of rational self-direction. The more rational, or, for that matter, the more loveable, among us should not be given preference. No one should. Our needs should determine what is to be done.

People committed to achieving and sustaining a society of equals will seek to bring into stable

Reprinted with permission of the publisher from *The International Journal of Applied Philosophy,* vol. 4 (Spring 1989), pp. 39–44.

existence conditions such that it would be possible for everyone, if they were personally capable of it, to enjoy an equally worthwhile and satisfying life or at least a life in which, for all of them, their needs, starting with and giving priority to their more urgent needs, were met and met as equally and as fully as possible, even where their needs are not entirely the same needs. This, at least, is the heuristic, though we might, to gain something more nearly feasible, have to scale down talk of meeting needs to providing conditions propitious for the equal satisfaction for everyone of their *basic* needs. Believers in equality want to see a world in which everyone, as far as this is possible, have equal whole life prospects. This requires an equal consideration of their needs and interests and a refusal to just override anyone's interests: to just regard anyone's interests as something which comes to naught, which can simply be set aside as expendable. Minimally, an egalitarian must believe that taking the moral point of view requires that each person's good is afforded equal consideration. Moreover, this is not just a bit of egalitarian ideology but is a deeply embedded considered judgment in modern Western culture capable of being put into wide reflective equilibrium.[4]

II

What is a need, how do we identify needs and what are our really basic needs, needs that are presumptively universal? Do these basic needs in most circumstances at least trump our other needs and our reflective considered preferences?

Let us start this examination by asking if we can come up with a list of universal needs correctly ascribable to all human beings in all cultures. In doing this we should, as David Braybrooke has, distinguish *adventitious* and *course-of-life* needs.[5] Moreover, it is the latter that it is essential to focus on. Adventitious needs, like the need for a really good fly rod or computer, come and go with particular projects. Course-of-life needs, such as the need for exercise, sleep or food, are such that every human being may be expected to have them all at least at some stage of life.

Still, we need to step back a bit and ask: how do we determine what is a need, course-of-life need or otherwise? We need a relational formula to spot

needs. We say, where we are speaking of needs, B needs x in order to y, as in Janet needs milk or some other form of calcium in order to protect her bone structure. With course-of-life needs the relation comes our platitudinously as in 'People need food and water in order to live' or 'People need exercise in order to function normally or well.' This, in the very identification of the need, refers to human flourishing or to human well-being, thereby giving to understand that they are basic needs. Perhaps it is better to say instead that this is to specify in part what it is for something to be a basic need. Be that as it may, there are these basic needs we *must* have to live well. If this is really so, then, where they are things we as individuals can have without jeopardy to others, no further question arises, or can arise, about the desirability of satisfying them. They are just things that in such circumstances ought to be met in our lives if they can. The satisfying of such needs is an unequivocally good thing. The questions 'Does Janet need to live?' and 'Does Sven need to function well?' are at best otiose.

In this context David Braybrooke has quite properly remarked that being "essential to living or to functioning normally may be taken as a criterion for being a basic need. Questions about whether needs are genuine, or well-founded, come to an end of the line when the needs have been connected with life or health."[6] Certainly to flourish we must have these things and in some instances they must be met at least to a certain extent even to survive. This being so, we can quite properly call them basic needs. Where these needs do not clash or the satisfying of them by one person does not conflict with the satisfying of the equally basic needs of another no question about justifying the meeting of them arises.

By linking the identification of needs with what we must have to function well and linking course-of-life and basic needs with what all people, or at least almost all people, must have to function well, a list of basic needs can readily be set out. I shall give such a list, though surely the list is incomplete. However, what will be added is the same sort of thing similarly identified. First there are needs connected closely to our physical functioning, namely the need for food and water, the need for excretion, for exercise, for rest (including sleep), for a life supporting relation to the environment, and the need for whatever is indispensable to preserve the body intact. Similarly there are basic needs connected with our function as social beings. We have needs for companionship, education, social acceptance and recognition, for sexual activity, freedom from harassment, freedom from domination, for some meaningful work, for recreation and relaxation and the like.[7]

The list, as I remarked initially, is surely incomplete. But it does catch many of the basic things which are in fact necessary for us to live or to function well. Now, an autonomy-respecting egalitarian society with an interest in the well-being of its citizens—something moral beings could hardly be without—would (trivially) be a society of equals, and as a society of equals it would be committed to (a) *moral* equality and (b) an equality of *condition* which would, under conditions of moderate abundance, in turn expect the equality of condition to be rough and to be principally understood (cashed in) in terms of providing the conditions (as far as that is possible) for meeting the needs (including most centrally the basic needs) of everyone and meeting them equally, as far as either of these things is feasible.

III

What kind of health-care system would such an autonomy-respecting egalitarian society have under conditions of moderate abundance such as we find in Canada and the United States?

The following are health-care needs which are also basic needs: being healthy and having conditions treated which impede one's functioning well or which adversely affect one's well-being or cause suffering. These are plainly things we need. Where societies have the economic and technical capacity to do so, as these societies plainly do, without undermining other equally urgent or more urgent needs, these health needs, as basic needs, must be met, and the right to have such medical care is a right for everyone in the society regardless of her capacity to pay. This just follows from a commitment to *moral* equality and to an equality of condition. Where we have the belief, a belief which is very basic in nonfascistic modernizing societies, that each person's good is to be given equal consideration, it

is hard not to go in that way, given a plausible conception of needs and reasonable list of needs based on that conception.[8] If there is the need for some particular regime of care and the society has the resources to meet that need, without undermining structures protecting other at least equally urgent needs, then, *ceteris paribus*, the society, if it is a decent society, must do so. The commitment to more equality—the commitment to the belief that the life of each person matters and matters equally—entails, given a few plausible empirical premises, that each person's health needs will be the object of an equal regard. Each has an equal claim *prima facie*, to have her needs satisfied where this is possible. That does not, of course, mean that people should all be treated alike in the sense of their all getting the same thing. Not everyone needs flu shots, braces, a dialysis machine, a psychiatrist, or a triple bypass. What should be equal is that each person's health needs should be the object of equal societal concern since each person's good should be given equal consideration.[9] This does not mean that equal energy should be directed to Hans's rash as to Frank's cancer. Here one person's need for a cure is much greater than the other, and the greater need clearly takes precedence. Both should be met where possible, but where they both cannot then the greater need has pride of place. But what should not count in the treatment of Hans and Frank is that Hans is wealthy or prestigious or creative and Frank is not. Everyone should have their health needs met where possible. Moreover, where the need is the same, they should have (where possible), and where other at least equally urgent needs are not thereby undermined, the same quality treatment. No differentiation should be made between them on the basis of their ability to pay or on the basis of their being (one more so than the other) important people. There should, in short, where this is possible, be open and free medical treatment of the same quality and extent available to everyone in the society. And no two- or three-tier system should be allowed to obtain, and treatment should only vary (subject to the above qualification) on the basis of variable needs and unavoidable differences in different places in supply and personnel, e.g., differences between town and country. Furthermore, these latter differences should be remedied where technically and economically feasible. The underlying aim should be to meet the health-care needs of everyone and meet them, in the sense explicated, equally: everybody's needs here should be met as fully as possible; different treatment is only justified where the need is different or where both needs cannot be met. Special treatment for one person rather than another is only justified where, as I remarked, both needs cannot be met or cannot as adequately be met. Constrained by ought implies can, where these circumstances obtain, priority should be given to the greater need that can feasibly be met. A moral system or a social policy, plainly, cannot be reasonably asked to do the impossible. But my account does not ask that.

To have such a health-care system would, I think, involve taking medicine out of the private sector altogether including, of course, out of private entrepreneurship where the governing rationale has to be profit and where supply and demand rules the roost. Instead there must be a health-care system firmly in the public sector (publicly owned and controlled) where the rationale of the system is to meet as efficiently and as fully as possible the health-care needs of everyone in the society in question. The health-care system should not be viewed as a business any more than a university should be viewed as a business—compare a university and a large hospital—but as a set of institutions and practices designed to meet urgent human needs.

I do not mean that we should ignore costs or efficiency. The state-run railroad system in Switzerland, to argue by analogy, is very efficient. The state cannot, of course, ignore costs in running it. But the aim is not to make a profit. The aim is to produce the most rapid, safe, efficient and comfortable service meeting travellers' needs within the parameters of the overall socioeconomic priorities of the state and the society. Moreover, since the state in question is a democracy, if its citizens do not like the policies of the government here (or elsewhere) they can replace it with a government with different priorities and policies. Indeed the option is there (probably never to be exercised) to shift the railroad into the private sector.

Governments, understandably, worry with aging populations about mounting health-care costs. This is slightly ludicrous in the United States, given its military and space exploration budgets, but is also a reality in Canada and even in Iceland where there is no military or space budget at all. There should, of course, be concern about containing health costs, but this can be done effectively with a state-run system. Modern societies need systems of socialized medicine, something that obtains in almost all civilized modernizing societies. The United States and South Africa are, I believe, the only exceptions. But, as is evident from my own country (Canada), socialized health-care systems often need altering, and their costs need monitoring. As a cost-cutting and as an efficiency measure that would at the same time improve health care, doctors, like university professors and government bureaucrats, should be put on salaries and they should work in medical units. They should, I hasten to add, have good salaries but salaries all the same; the last vestiges of petty entrepreneurship should be taken from the medical profession. This measure would save the state-run health-care system a considerable amount of money, would improve the quality of medical care with greater cooperation and consultation resulting from economies of scale and a more extensive division of labor with larger and better equipped medical units. (There would also be less duplication of equipment.) The overall quality of care would also improve with a better balance between health care in the country and in the large cities, with doctors being systematically and rationally deployed throughout the society. In such a system doctors, no more than university professors or state bureaucrats, could not just set up a practice anywhere. They would no more be free to do this than university professors or state bureaucrats. In the altered system there would be no cultural space for it. Placing doctors on salary, though not at a piece work rate, would also result in its being the case that the financial need to see as many patients as possible as quickly as possible would be removed. This would plainly enhance the quality of medical care. It would also be the case that a different sort of person would go into the medical profession. People would go into it more frequently because they were actually interested in medicine and less frequently because this is a rather good way (though hardly the best way) of building a stock portfolio.

There should also be a rethinking of the respective roles of nurses (in all their variety), paramedics and doctors. Much more of the routine work done in medicine—taking the trout fly out of my ear for example—can be done by nurses or paramedics. Doctors, with their more extensive training, could be freed up for other more demanding tasks worthy of their expertise. This would require somewhat different training for all of these different medical personnel and a rethinking of the authority structure in the health-care system. But doing this in a reasonable way would improve the teamwork in hospitals, make morale all around a lot better, improve medical treatment and save a very considerable amount of money. (It is no secret that the relations between doctors and nurses are not good.) Finally, a far greater emphasis should be placed on preventive medicine than is done now. This, if really extensively done, utilizing the considerable educational and fiscal powers of the state, would result in very considerable health-care savings and a very much healthier and perhaps even happier population. (Whether with the states we actually have we are likely to get anything like that is—to understate it—questionable. I wouldn't hold my breath in the United States. Still, Finland and Sweden are very different places from the United States and South Africa.)

IV

It is moves of this *general* sort that an egalitarian and autonomy-loving society under conditions of moderate scarcity should implement. (I say 'general sort' for I am more likely to be wrong about some of the specifics than about the general thrust of my argument.) It would, if in place, limit the freedom of some people, including some doctors and some patients, to do what they want to do. That is obvious enough. But any society, any society at all, as long as it had norms (legal and otherwise) will limit freedom in some way.[10] There is no living in society without some limitation on the freedom to do some things. Indeed, a society without norms and thus without any limitation on freedom is a contradiction in terms. Such a mass of people wouldn't be a society. They, without norms, would just be a mass of people. (If these are 'grammatical remarks,' make

the most of them.) In our societies I am not free to go for a spin in your car without your permission, to practice law or medicine without a license, to marry your wife while she is still your wife and the like. Many restrictions on our liberties, because they are so common, so widely accepted and thought by most of us to be so reasonable, hardly *seem* like restrictions on our liberty. But they are all the same. No doubt some members of the medical profession would feel quite reined in if the measures I propose were adopted. (These measures are not part of conventional wisdom.) But the restrictions on the freedom of the medical profession and on patients I am proposing would make for both a greater liberty all around, everything considered, and, as well, for greater well-being in the society. Sometimes we have to restrict certain liberties in order to enhance the overall system of liberty. Not speaking out of turn in parliamentary debate is a familiar example. Many people who now have a rather limited access to medical treatment would come to have it and have it in a more adequate way with such a socialized system in place. Often we have to choose between a greater or lesser liberty in a society, and, at least under conditions of abundance, the answer almost always should be 'Choose the greater liberty.' If we really prize human autonomy, if, that is, we want a world in which as many people as possible have as full as is possible control over their own lives, then we will be egalitarians. Our very egalitarianism will commit us to something like the health care system I described, but so will the realization that, without reasonable health on the part of the population, autonomy can hardly flourish or be very extensive. Without the kind of equitability and increased coverage in health care that goes with a properly administered socialized medicine, the number of healthy people will be far less than could otherwise feasibly be the case. With that being the case, autonomy and well-being as well will be neither as extensive nor so thorough as it could otherwise be. Autonomy, like everything else, has its material conditions. And to will the end is to will the necessary means to the end.

To take—to sum up—what since the Enlightenment has come to be seen as the moral point of view, and to take morality seriously, is to take it as axiomatic that each person's good be given equal consideration.[11] I have argued that (a) where that is accepted, and (b) where we are tolerably clear about the facts (including facts about human needs), and (c) where we live under conditions of moderate abundance, a health-care system bearing at least a family resemblance to the one I have gestured at will be put in place. It is a health-care system befitting an autonomy respecting democracy committed to the democratic and egalitarian belief that the life of everyone matters and matters equally.

NOTES

1 Isaiah Berlin, "On the Pursuit of the Ideal," *The New York Review of Books* XXXV (March 1987), pp. 11–18. See also his "Equality" in his *Concepts and Categories* (Oxford, England: Oxford University Press, 1980), pp. 81–102. I have criticized that latter paper in my "Formulating Egalitarianism: Animadversions on Berlin," *Philosophia* 13:3–4 (October 1983), pp. 299–315.

2 For three defenses of such a view see Kai Nielsen, *Equality and Liberty* (Totowa, New Jersey: Rowman and Allanheld, 1985), Richard Norman, *Free and Equal* (Oxford, England:

Oxford University Press, 1987), and John Baker, *Arguing for Equality* (London: Verso Press, 1987).

3 Will Kymlicka, "Rawls on Teleology and Deontology," *Philosophy and Public Affairs* 17:3 (Summer 1988), pp. 173–190 and John Rawls, "The Priority of Right and Ideas of the Good," *Philosophy and Public Affairs* 17:4 (Fall 1988), pp. 251–276.

4 Kai Nielsen, "Searching for an Emancipatory Perspective: Wide Reflective Equilibrium and the Hermeneutical Circle" in Evan Simpson (ed.), *Anti-Foundationalism and Practical Reasoning* (Edmonton, Alberta: Academic Printing and Publishing, 1987), pp. 143–164 and Kai Nielsen, "In Defense of Wide Reflective Equilibrium" in Douglas Odegard (ed.) *Ethics and Justification* (Edmonton, Alberta: Academic Printing and Publishing, 1988), pp. 19–37.

5 David Braybrooke, *Meeting Needs* (Princeton, New Jersey: Princeton University Press, 1987), p. 29.

6 *Ibid.*, p. 31.

7 *Ibid.*, p. 37.

8 Will Kymlicka, *op cit.*, p. 190.

9 *Ibid.*

10 Ralf Dahrendorf, *Essays in the Theory of Society* (Stanford, California: Stanford University Press, 1968), pp. 151–78 and G. A. Cohen, "The Structure of Proletarian Unfreedom," *Philosophy and Public Affairs* 12 (1983), pp. 2–33.

11 Will Kymlicka, *op cit.*, p. 190.

INTERNATIONAL MODELS AND PERSPECTIVES

HEALTH CARE REFORM: LESSONS FROM CANADA

Raisa Berlin Deber

In this excerpt from a longer article, Deber provides a descriptive overview of Canada's health-care system while drawing several lessons for the United States as it considers reform. As Deber explains, Canada has in each of its provinces a single-payer system of health-care finance: Everyone is covered by law in a tax-funded system that ensures a relatively comprehensive set of benefits. More specifically, each province covers all "medically necessary" physician and hospital care—most of which is privately delivered—while provinces differ in the extent to which they cover further services such as dental care and prescription drugs. Although the Canadian health-care system always seems to be in crisis, Deber notes, it achieves universal access at relatively low cost with high quality of care and good (if declining) satisfaction among the populace. Lessons for the United States, according to the author, include the following: single-payer systems need not involve cumbersome bureaucracies; they can attain universal coverage less expensively than pluralistic funding approaches; and one major advantage they offer is "the avoidance of risk selection: no one is uninsurable."

To Americans, Canada resembles the girl next door—familiar but often taken for granted. Despite flurries of interest in the Canadian health-care system whenever the United States contemplates implementing universal health insurance, misunderstandings about its nature abound. Indeed, there is no Canadian system; instead, there are a set of publicly financed, provincially run insurance plans covering all legal residents for specified service categories, primarily "medically necessary" physician and hospital care. Neither does Canada have socialized medicine; these services are delivered by private providers. In all industrialized nations, health care seems to be perennially in crisis; however, access and quality in Canada are relatively high, spending relatively well controlled, and satisfaction high, although declining. Canadians remain devoted to their system, but they are increasingly worried that it may not survive.

Recently, several provincial commissions investigated health care and weighed in with their recommendations,[1-3] while the Kirby Senate Committee[4] and the national Romanow Royal Commission[5] are completing extensive research and consultation activities and readying their final reports. What will emerge is unclear, but Canadians have loudly indicated their hopes and fears for the future. Although the Canadian model per se is unlikely to be adopted in the United States, it can provide clear lessons for its neighbor—both positive and negative.

. . .

FEDERALISM AND HEALTH CARE

Because Canada's 1867 constitution assigned most health care responsibilities to provincial jurisdiction,[6] Canadian health policy is inextricably intertwined with federal–provincial relationships. Canada is a federation of 10 provinces plus 3 sparsely populated northern territories. These provinces vary enormously in both size and fiscal capacity, ranging from the Atlantic province of Prince Edward Island, with a 2001 population of 135,000, to the industrial heartland of Ontario, with 11.4 million. The history of the often contentious evolution of the system (and the re-

actions by physicians) has been told elsewhere.[7-10] From the outset, it represented an attempt to balance the desire of Canadians for national standards of service against the differing fiscal capacities of the various provinces and provincial insistence that their jurisdiction be respected.

Financing the Canadian health-care system accordingly evolved incrementally within individual provinces, as they responded to market failure, with national government involvement through a series of programs to share costs with the provinces. Initially, Ottawa provided funding for particular programs, such as public health, hospital construction, and training health personnel. In 1957, the Hospital Insurance and Diagnostic Services Act (HIDS)[11] was passed with all-party approval; it paid approximately half the cost of provincial insurance plans for hospital-based care, as long as the plans complied with specified national conditions. The 1966 Medical Care Act[12] cost-shared provincial insurance plans for physician services under similar provisions. By 1971, all provinces had complying plans insuring their populations for hospital and physician services. Because provinces have jurisdiction, one size does not fit all; there are considerable variations within Canada. In addition, although the financing arrangements were changed in 1977 to a mixture of cash and tax points (reducing the federal tax rates to allow the provinces to take up the resulting "tax room"), the same national terms and conditions initially introduced in HIDS were reinforced in the 1984 Canada Health Act.[13] The system accordingly reflects a hospital/doctor-centered view of health care as practiced in 1957, which is becoming increasingly inadequate.

In order to receive federal money, the provincial insurance plans had only to comply with the following national terms and conditions:

1. Public administration. This frequently misunderstood condition does not mandate public delivery of health services; most care is privately delivered. It represents a reaction to the high overheads associated with private insurance when the system was introduced,[14] and it requires that the health-care insurance plan of a province "be administered and

From *American Journal of Public Health,* vol. 93, no. 1 (2003), pp. 20–24. Copyright 2003 by the American Public Health Association.

operated on a non-profit basis by a public authority appointed or designated by the government of the province"[13] and its activities subject to audit. This administration can be delegated, as long as accountability arrangements are in place.

2. Comprehensiveness. Coverage must include "all insured health services provided by hospitals, medical practitioners or dentists, and where the law of the province so permits, similar or additional services rendered by other health-care practitioners."[13] (Insured dental services are defined as those that must be performed within hospitals; practically, less than 1 percent of dental services so qualify.)

3. Universality. The plan must entitle "one hundred per cent of the insured persons of the province to the insured health services provided for by the plan on uniform terms and conditions."[13]

4. Portability. Provisions must be in place to cover insured people when they move between provinces, and to ensure orderly (and uniform) provisions as to when coverage is deemed to have switched. The details are worked out by interprovincial agreements. Although there are some irritants, in general, out-of-province care incurred during short visits (less than 3 months) remains the responsibility of the home province, which can set limitations (e.g., refuse to cover elective procedures). Out-of-country care is reimbursed at the rates payable in the home province. Since these rates are considerably less than what would be charged in the United States, Canadians leaving the country are strongly advised to have supplementary travel health insurance.

5. Accessibility. Provincial plans must "provide for insured health services on uniform terms and conditions and on a basis that does not impede or preclude, either directly or indirectly, whether by charges made to insured persons or otherwise, reasonable access to those services by insured persons."[13] Other provisions require that hos-

pitals and health providers (usually physicians) receive "reasonable compensation," although the mechanisms are not defined.

In practice, this balancing act means that the federal government cannot act as decision-maker, although it may occasionally attempt to influence policy directions through providing money or attempting to suggest guidelines. However, the comprehensiveness definition gives Ottawa a major influence on what services must be insured by provincial governments. The Canadian Institute for Health Information estimates that approximately 99 percent of expenditures for physician services, and 90 percent of expenditures for hospital care, come from public sector sources. Insurance coverage for such services is not tied to employment. However, other sectors (especially pharmaceuticals, chronic care, and dental care) are much more heavily funded from the private sector, including reliance on employment-based benefits.[15] Overall, about 70 percent of Canadian health expenditures comes from public sources, putting it among the *least* publicly financed of industrialized countries.[16]

For decades, delivery was largely unaffected by public financing. Most hospitals were private, not-for-profit organizations with independent boards. Recently, all provinces except Ontario subsumed hospitals into independent (or quasi-independent) regional health authorities, which were given responsibility for delivering an assortment of services.[17,18] (Ontario retains private not-for-profit hospitals, although the provincial government has become increasingly obtrusive, especially for those hospitals running deficits.) Physicians are private small businessmen, largely working fee-for-service, and moving only slowly (and voluntarily) from solo practice into various forms of groups. In some provinces, provincial governments have been attempting to encourage the move toward rostered group practice paid on a capitated basis, with remarkably little success to date.[19] Individual patients have free choice of physicians. Bills are usually submitted directly to the single payer, which means a decided lack of paperwork for either patient or provider. Indeed, in 1991, the US General Accounting Office estimated that, if the United States could get its administrative costs to the Canadian level, it could afford to cover the entire uninsured population.[20]

ISSUES ARISING

Financing the System In the mid-1980s, Canada faced a deficit trap. To avoid it, they squeezed supply. The federal government unilaterally changed the formula for transfers to the provincial governments, which led to a significant reduction in the cash portion of the transfer. In turn, provincial governments chopped budgets to hospitals, which in turn led to considerable growth in day surgery, reduction in hospital bed numbers, and instability in the nursing employment market.[21] They also attempted to squeeze physician fees. The result was that provincial expenditures per capita for health care, inflation adjusted, were lower in 1997 than they had been in 1989.[22] The search for efficiency proceeded apace, to the point where most hospitals were running at 95 percent occupancy or greater, and most providers felt that they were overworked and underpaid.[23]

Under the rubric of "sustainability," the pent-up demand for restoring funding (and incomes) to previous levels has dominated recent health policy discussions. Advocates of privatization claim that this increased spending cannot be met from public sources, while health reformers argue that if the issue is the ability to meet total costs (rather than the more political question of who will bear them), a single payer should be retained. Some business leaders, recognizing that the search for alternative sources of revenue may represent a greater burden on payroll, support a single payer. Others retain an ideological objection to government involvement. Providers voice support in theory for public payment, but only if it guarantees that they will receive the resources they require to provide the level of services they feel is necessary. The public agrees; they are highly supportive of a single payer, but not if this means they would be denied care. Although it is not clear the extent to which waiting lists are an actual problem (this varying considerably by procedure and geographic area), they remain a highly potent and symbolic issue.

Another key dilemma is comprehensiveness, spoken of in terms of "defining the basket of services." Although provinces are free to go beyond the federal conditions—which establish a floor rather than a ceiling—in practice, many prefer to cut taxes. As care shifts from hospitals, it can shift beyond the boundaries of public insurance. Patients being treated in a hospital have full coverage for such necessities as pharmaceuticals, physiotherapy, and nursing. Once they are discharged, these costs need no longer be paid for from public funds.[24] Some provinces still pay for such care; others do not. The ongoing debate as to what should be "in" or "out" of the publicly financed services, and the role (if any) for user charges, has focused largely but not exclusively on "pharmacare" (coverage for outpatient prescription drugs) and home care.

The "first law of cost containment" states that the easiest way to control costs is to shift them to someone else. These issues have flowed over to massive disputes between levels of government (particularly the federal and provincial governments) and between provincial governments and providers, including some work stoppages by physicians and nurses in certain provinces. These disputes in turn are often resolved by sizeable reimbursement increases, which in turn increases pressure on other provinces to match the enriched contracts.

Delivery There has been strong pressure to modernize delivery and eliminate "silos," which are seen as impeding smooth delivery and efficient use of resources. The US experience with managed care and the UK experience with general practitioner fundholders are frequently cited examples of what should or should not be achieved, depending on the political and managerial preferences of the observer. The push for integration has been expressed in many ways, including establishing regional health authorities and the ongoing attempt to achieve primary care reform. Physicians within the Canadian clinical workforce are unusual in the degree of autonomy they have enjoyed with respect to where they will work and in the volume and mix of services they choose to deliver.[10] Most other clinicians must be hired by a provider organization and are accordingly subject to labor market forces in determining whether (and where) employment is available. The question of whether this state of affairs should be continued or not is an ongoing source of dispute. . . .

LESSONS FOR THE UNITED STATES

Size A common fear about universal health insurance is that it requires a large and cumbersome bureaucracy. In that connection, it is important to recognize both that single-payer systems yield administrative efficiencies and that Canada's model is organized at the provincial (state) level. Canada's 2001 population was 30 million (vs 284.8 million in the United States); the largest provincial plan (Ontario's) served 11.4 million. In contrast, the largest US insurance plan, Aetna, served 17.2 million health care members, 13.5 million dental members, and 11.5 million group insurance customers. A US model organized at the state (or even substate) level would allow for flexibility to account for local circumstances and would probably result in a less bureaucratic system than at present.

Another feature of size is the recognition that most Canadian communities are not large enough to support competition (particularly for specialized services), even should this be considered desirable.[25] Small size also leads to problems in risk pooling, since one expensive case may place the entire plan at fiscal risk. Single-payer models encouraging cooperation are likely to be particularly applicable to the more rural portions of the United States.

Universal Coverage A major advantage of a single-payer system is that one can attain universal coverage at a lower cost than is attained by pluralistic funding approaches. Canada has universal coverage, excellent health outcomes, minimal paperwork, and high public satisfaction, although coverage or reimbursement decisions do tend to become political. One key advantage is the avoidance of risk selection; no one is uninsurable. In a pluralistic system, government often ends up with the worst risks, and the high costs associated with them. A single payer allows these costs to be spread more equitably. Canadian health policy largely accepts the limitations of markets in health care, at least for the portions deemed medically necessary.

It is striking that there are more people in the United States without health insurance than the entire population of Canada, with many more in the United States underinsured. Even in 1998, the United States was spending more per capita from public funds for health care than was Canada, in addition to the considerable spending from private sources.[16] Hospitals, physicians, and patients are faced with considerably less administrative costs than in the United States, although this savings may also translate into considerably less administrative data. The one component in Canada that does use a US mix of public and private financing—outpatient pharmaceuticals—is the one part of the system where costs have been rising most quickly, and access is seen as most problematic.

Jurisdiction Another lesson is that federalism imposes difficulties. Health policy has been damaged by the pitched battles between the national and provincial governments, which have also undermined public confidence in the system. The balance between imposing national standards (and accountability for money spent) and respecting provincial jurisdiction and allowing flexibility is a tricky one, and it would be hard to argue that the present mix is optimal.

CONCLUSION

Despite the angst, the objective evidence suggests that the Canadian model has much to recommend it. Ironically, it is most threatened by proximity to the United States, and the concerted attacks from those favoring for-profit, market-oriented care on both sides of the border.[26,27] The success of earlier reforms may also have produced an excess of "efficiency" at the expense of health-care workers and clients alike.[28] Nonetheless, the Romanow Commission has elicited a national, and heartfelt, public reaction. Canadians prize their system of universal coverage. Various changes at the margin are likely. The shape of the overall system, however, will probably remain relatively stable. The major lesson of the Canadian model is precisely the reluctance of Canadians to lose it.

ACKNOWLEDGMENTS

I thank the organizers and participants in the Rekindling Reform conference, particularly Drs. O. Fein and W. Glazer, and the anonymous reviewers of this report.

REFERENCES

1 *Report and Recommendations: Emerging Solutions.* Québec, Québec: Commission d'étude sur les services de santé et les services sociaux (CESSSS); December 18, 2000. Available at: http://www.cessss.gouv.qc.ca/pdf/en/ 01-109-01a.pdf. Accessed October 11, 2002.

2 *Report of the Premier's Advisory Council on Health. A Framework for Reform.* Edmonton, Alberta: Premier's Advisory Council on Health for Alberta; December 2001. Available at: http://www.gov.ab.ca/home/health_first/ documents_maz_report.cfm. Accessed October 11, 2002.

3 *Caring for Medicare: Sustaining a Quality System.* Regina, Saskatchewan: Saskatchewan Commission on Medicare; April 6, 2001. Available at: http://www.health.gov.sk.ca/ info_center_pub_ commission_on_medicare_bw.pdf. Accessed October 11, 2002.

4 *The Health of Canadians: The Federal Role.* 6 vol. Ottawa, Ontario: Standing Senate Committee on Social Affairs Science and Technology; 2001–2002. Available at: http://www.parl.gc.ca/37/2/parlbus/commbus/sentate/ com-e/soci-e/rep-e/repoct02vol6-e.htm. Accessed November 22, 2002.

5 Commission on the Future of Health Care in Canada. Shape the future of health care: interim report. Available at: http://www.healthcarecommission.ca.gov. Accessed October 11, 2002.

6 *The Constitution Acts, 1867 to 1982.* Ottawa, Ontario: Government of Canada; 1982.

7 Taylor MG. *Health Insurance and Canadian Public Policy. The Seven Decisions That Created the Canadian Health Insurance System and Their Outcomes.* 2nd ed. Kingston, Ontario: McGill–Queen's University Press; 1987.

8 Maioni A. Parting at the crossroads: the development of health insurance in Canada and the United States. *Comp Polit.* 1997; 29:411–432.

9 Naylor CD. *Private Practice, Public Payment: Canadian Medicine and the Politics of Health Insurance 1911–1966.* Kingston, Ontario: McGill–Queen's University Press; 1986.

10 Tuohy CH. *Accidental Logics: The Dynamics of Change in the Health Care Arena in the United States, Britain, and Canada.* New York, NY: Oxford University Press; 1999.

11 Government of Canada. *Hospital Insurance and Diagnostic Services Act.* Statutes of Canada, 5–6 Elizabeth II (c 28, S1 1957), 1957.

12 Government of Canada. *Medical Care Act.* Statutes of Canada (c 64, s 1), 1966–1967.

13 Government of Canada. *Canada Health Act, Bill C-3.* Statutes of Canada, 32–33 Elizabeth II (RSC 1985, c 6; RSC 1989, c C-6), 1984.

14 *Canada Royal Commission on Health Services.* Vol 1. Ottawa, Ontario: Canada Royal Commission on Health Services; 1964.

15 *Preliminary Provincial and Territorial Government Health Expenditure Estimates 1974/1975 to 2001/2002.* Ottawa, Ontario: Canadian Institute for Health Information; October 2001.

16 *OECD Health Data 2001: A Comparative Analysis of 30 OECD Countries* [CD-ROM]. Paris, France: Organization for Economic Cooperation and Development.

17 Church J, Barker P. Regionalization of health services in Canada: a critical perspective. *Int J Health Serv.* 1998; 28:467–486.

18 Lomas J, Woods J, Veenstra G. Devolving authority for health care in Canada's provinces, I: an introduction to the issues. *Can Med Assoc J.* 1997; 156:371–377.

19 Hutchison B, Abelson J, Lavis J. Primary care in Canada: so much innovation, so little change. *Health Aff (Millwood).* 2001; 20(3):116–131.

20 *Canadian Health Insurance: Lessons for the United States. Report to the Chairman, Committee on Government Operations, House of Representatives.* Washington, DC: US General Accounting Office; 1991.

21 Naylor CD. Health care in Canada: incrementalism under fiscal duress. *Health Aff (Millwood).* 1999; 18(3):9–26.

22 Deber RB. Getting what we pay for: myths and realities about financing Canada's health care system. *Health Law Can.* 2000; 21(2):9–56. Available at: http://www.utoronto.ca/ hpme/dhr/pdf/atrevised3.pdf. Accessed November 22, 2002.

23 Armstrong P, Armstrong H, Coburn D, eds. *Unhealthy Times: Political Economy Perspectives on Health and Care in Canada.* Don Mills, Ontario: Oxford University Press; 2001.

24 Williams AP, Deber RB, Baranek P, Gildiner A. From Medicare to home care: globalization, state retrenchment and the profitization of Canada's health care system. In: Armstrong P, Armstrong H, Coburn D, eds. *Unhealthy Times: Political Economy Perspectives on Health and Care in Canada.* Don Mills, Ontario: Oxford University Press; 2001:7–30.

25 Griffin P, Cockerill R, Deber RB. Potential impact of population-based funding on delivery of pediatric services. *Ann R Coll Physicians Surg Can.* 2001; 34:272–279.

26 Evans RG. Going for the gold: the redistributive agenda behind market-based health care reform. *J Health Polit Policy Law.* 1997; 22:427–466.

27 Evans RG, Roos NP. What is right about the Canadian health care system? *Milbank Q.* 1999; 77:393–399.

28 Stein JG. *The Cult of Efficiency.* Toronto, Ontario: House of Anansi Press Ltd; 2001.

UNIVERSAL HEALTH CARE: LESSONS FROM THE BRITISH EXPERIENCE

Donald W. Light

Light discusses the history of the British National Health Service (NHS), its experiment with managed competition late in the twentieth century, and its current structure and trends, before drawing lessons for the United States. Creation of the NHS, he explains, required tremendous British solidarity in the aftermath of mass bombing by the Nazis in World War II; it also required a willingness to make important concessions to the medical profession. A tax-funded single-payer system, the NHS provides universal access to a comprehensive array of benefits at about one-third the per capita cost of American health care. Physicians, meanwhile, enjoy a prerogative not enjoyed by their Canadian counterparts: they may work within the NHS while also maintaining private practices for those British residents (11–12 percent of the population) who opt to pay for private insurance or health services. Lessons for the United States, according to Light, include the following: Health care should be "free at the point of service" because copayments and deductibles create inequities and barriers to care without being cost-effective; universal health care should be funded through income taxes; primary care should be emphasized and supported; specialists should be paid at the same rates; and prescription drug prices should be controlled while genuine breakthroughs in drug development are rewarded.

. . .

BACKGROUND OF THE NHS

The history and development of the NHS—as documented in several highly readable books[1-4]—suggest a number of aspects relevant to achieving universal health care in the United States. In 1911, Parliament passed a very limited national health insurance act that covered workers (but not dependents) for primary care, pharmaceutical drugs, and cash benefits during sickness and disability. Provident societies, doctors' "clubs," and fraternal organizations offered varying degrees of voluntary insurance coverage. Otherwise, health care was financed by private fees, charity, or through public hospitals. Public hospitals tended to be larger, more comprehensive, and better funded than voluntary hospitals, many of which faced mounting debts during the depression of the 1930s. The two hospital systems were poorly coordinated. Access to specialists was uneven, largely owing to specialists gravitating to areas with more private patients. General practitioners (GPs) and members of specialty royal colleges feuded over who was qualified to do what and who could work in hospitals.[5]

Two basic approaches to reform characterized proposals in the 1920s and 1930s. One proposal was to extend the limited 1911 act into comprehensive national health insurance, analogous to universalizing an improved, more comprehensive Medicare in the United States today. Another was to build up and universalize existing, locally funded and run public health services.[1] The first is based on *individuals* having a right to health care, the second on the idea that *society* has an obligation to look after the health of its *people*. This profound difference in the purpose of health care needs to become part of debates in the United States.

The NHS historian Charles Webster believes it took Hitler and mass bombing to break down the petty rivalries, the protective yet often shabby fiefdoms, and factional politics to allow an actual plan to emerge. The terrorist attacks of September 11 pale in comparison. During World War II, more than two million homes in Britain were damaged or destroyed by

From *American Journal of Public Health*, vol. 93, no. 1 (2003), pp. 26–30. Copyright © 2003 by the American Public Health Association.

the Luftwaffe.[2 (chap1)] More than 100,000 people were killed. An Emergency Medical Service was formed that took charge of all medical services in the nation and created a coordinated hospital service, national and regional services for laboratory work and blood transfusions, and national services for surgery, neurology, psychiatry, and rehabilitation. As Webster notes, "The Luftwaffe achieved in months what had defeated politicians and planners for at least two decades." Still, "The bitter jealousies that wrecked the pathetically limited pre-war efforts at reform resurfaced. . . ." They were "deeply damaging and cast a long shadow over the future of the NHS."[2(p8)]

CREATING THE NHS

Leadership matters. In June 1941, Sir William Beveridge, a well-known civil servant, educator, and radio personality, was asked to plan social reconstruction after the war. Beveridge had served as a social worker among the poor in the East End of London. He had witnessed the many contradictory, partial programs for unemployment, child support, medical services, public health, and housing, run by different departments under different rules, not unlike those we have in the United States today. Beveridge decided that the only approach was to address them all at once, in ways that would create partnerships between the individual and the state.[1(chap1–3)]

The Beveridge report, *Social Insurance and Allied Services,* called for comprehensive health care as part of a postwar government master plan promoting education, employment, housing, and social security. Although the report provided only a preliminary and tentative sketch, it captured an essential vision and sold more than 400,000 copies worldwide. The Beveridge plan for a tax-based national health service as a public good offered a basic alternative to the older Bismarck design of national insurance to provide access as an individual right; even today, international reports use "Beveridge" or "Bismarck" to classify these 2 types of universal health-care systems.

Rudolf Klein and others believe that the NHS would have happened even if Beveridge had not written his report because of the shared perspective that had arisen between the world wars on how to solve Britain's health care problems.[1,4] But it might not have happened without Aneurin Bevan, who was appointed minister of health in 1944. He quickly displayed his skill for constructive action, an ability to establish control, and a capacity to steer through the shoals of medical politics. His bold proposal to nationalize all hospitals drew on the wartime Emergency Medical Service. Financing through national taxes addressed the widely differing abilities of local governments to raise funds. At the same time, Bevan concluded that bringing all services under one administration was impractical because local authorities defended their control over public health, and GPs fiercely defended their independent-contractor status. (Independence is a relative term; GPs have had only one contract with one contractor—the government. Nevertheless, defending this "independence" has dominated GP politics for decades.)

Bevan and other leaders had the advantage of a parliamentary system of government that gives the winning party control over the legislative and executive branches. This makes any reform much easier to pass than in the fractured US political structure, designed from the start to impede and frustrate popular reform, even before powerful lobbying groups arise to block or co-opt popular reforms. Still, Bevan found negotiations difficult, filled with broken promises and betrayals, sudden unilateral shifts in positions and threats.[1,2] Getting a specific plan for universal health care passed was difficult and almost did not happen.

One principal obstacle was the doctors. To silence their vociferous opposition, Bevan "filled their mouths with gold."[2(p28)] Senior specialists (consultants) received a lifetime salary and indexed pension as well as the right to continue their private practices. Other inducements included specialist control of private beds in the NHS hospitals, the right to operate independent "firms," power over a separate authority for teaching hospitals, and control over substantial lifetime merit increases to their salaries and pensions. The final result was a tripartite structure: hospitals and specialists under 14 regional boards, general practice under a national contract, and community health services—such as home nurses, midwives, health visitors, maternal and child care, and prevention—under the control of local governments. Eventually, this control was moved to regional health authorities. All units reported to the minister of health and his staff. Yet the NHS was basically a hospital-dominated system in which specialists were a law unto themselves while GPs ran their own practices and undergirded the system.

Even today, the basic design has much to admire. It features largely tax-based financing to fund universal health-care services that are usually free at the point of service. About 60 percent of all institutional long-term care, pharmaceuticals, and vision care are also provided in the NHS.[6(Table2.2)] This universal and relatively comprehensive health service costs about one-third what the United States spends per capita.[7] At this level of funding, everyone can choose a primary care physician and be seen promptly and all urgent cases are treated fully; but elective referrals for specialty care are put on the infamous British "waiting lists" for assessment or treatment.

Waiting lists are a common pressure valve in many systems, a brake on spending far more equitable than the American approach of access by ability to pay and its large number of formal and de facto waiting lists for the working and lower classes. In the NHS, the average waiting time for elective hospital-based care is 46 days, although some patients wait over a year. Differences by social class in funding, services, and access are minimal by international standards, although more affluent people are always more skilled at manipulating any public service.

The British system has always had a private sector for those who want quicker or more luxurious elective care. This sector's clinical quality is no better and may be worse.[6] The proportion of adults who take out private health insurance policies, or get them as a managerial perk, has been flat for several years at about 11.5 percent of the population.[6(Table2.6–7)] These policies provide duplicative coverage for elective procedures for which specialists charge very high fees. Private care is concentrated in the greater London region and a few other cities. Currently, all private admissions and day cases total 2.2 percent of all NHS admissions and day cases.[6(Table2.3,2.10)]

LESSONS FROM MANAGED COMPETITION

Managed competition is one of a series of policy and management imperatives that spread from the United States to Western Europe and other Organization for Economic Cooperation and Development (OECD) countries and then to Eastern Europe and developing countries. International agencies such as the World Bank, the International Monetary Fund, and the World Trade Organization play key roles in such reforms.[8,9] Most European countries joined the competition policy bandwagon but then pulled back as they realized the risks of dislocation, bankruptcy, and the high transaction costs that competition in health care might bring.[10,11]

Margaret Thatcher and many other heads of state joined the international policy movement of competition as a way to challenge entrenched, inefficient, and unresponsive public services in education, municipal services, and health care.[12] Health authorities were changed from being administrative offices to being purchasers. Hospitals, community health services, and specialists became semi-autonomous "trusts" that had to sell their services, although most just continued as before under contracts with their health authorities. Switching from global budgets to unit prices and setting up markets was very costly. Mrs. Thatcher also reconceptualized patients as consumers and encouraged them to be demanding. She then transformed the NHS from a public service for sick patients to a public system of purchasers and providers trying to please patients-turned-consumers. The government aimed to provide greater choice and greater rewards to providers who responded to local preferences. Who could possibly disagree? "Almost everyone." As Klein explains, "Nothing like it had been seen in the NHS policy arena since the opposition provoked by Nye Bevan 40-odd years before."[1(p192–193)]

By 1996, the conservatives concluded that these competition policies were not working well.[13] Even in its perfect form, managed competition has been shown to have deep flaws, and of course it undermines public health and a population-based healhcare system.[12,14,15] Competition required more regulation and government monitoring, because health care has so many kinds of market failure.[9] The costs of setting up and running a market became apparent and large. The salaries of top managers escalated, and the number of managers at least tripled. Overall costs rose, not shrank. A thorough review of US managed care and managed competition by British researchers found little evidence for their alleged benefits.[16] (Perhaps out of bias, few Americans read this major study.)

As a wild card, GPs were offered the opportunity to control funds for a limited number of elective services. "GP fundholding" became the star of the reforms, but evidence showed that only about 15 percent of GP fundholders actually used the power of the purse to wrest better prices or services from specialists and hospitals.[17] Still, the impact on specialists and specialty services was historic. By 1996, most GP fundholders said they did not want the job, and most had neither the taste nor skill for becoming purchasing agents for complex services.[18] Fundholding also disrupted the mandate of health authorities to purchase for the entire population and produced some two-tier access. Morale declined. Sick leaves, days off, and other evidence of despondency increased.[19] In 1997, the Labour Party promised an end to competition and a new era of partnership. It won by a landslide.

THE NEW NHS

The plan for the new NHS by the present government is even more ambitious than the transformation wrought by Margaret Thatcher.[20] The NHS was widely discussed as no longer sustainable, as a quaint utopia no longer affordable. Limiting it to an emergency and welfare service would have been politically feasible and would have fit in with the public–private partnership themes of New Labour. Instead, Tony Blair and his ministers, notably the minister for health, Alan Milburn, have moved toward the far more difficult position of admitting that the NHS has been starved of funds for years and raising the national health insurance tax to fund the largest increases in its history.

The government's new plan also aims to bring GPs from the organizational periphery to the center of the NHS; to organize them into geographic units called primary care trusts; to combine them with community services and with a public health agenda for improving the health status of the population; to develop coordinated programs with housing, employment, education, and the voluntary sector; to devolve most of the centrally held budget to them; and to have them develop new integrated relations with specialists and hospitals. This new master plan addresses most of the segmenting compromises Bevan had to make at the founding of the NHS.[21] A similar vision in the United States was the community-oriented primary care movement of the 1970s.

The Blair government has come to recognize, as its predecessors did not, that waiting lists need to be reduced and restructured. The existing system of each specialist managing his or her waiting list in an uncoordinated way has created a conflict of interest: specialists are rewarded for building up private practices, which only lengthens waiting times for everyone else on the waiting list.[22] The new NHS calls for replacing waiting lists with appointments, removing waiting list management from specialists, rewriting the specialists' contract to reward full-time commitment and productivity, and substantially increasing the number of subspecialists and nurse specialists.

The government is also addressing the historic absence of quality standards by establishing new institutions that set standards for the nation and monitor them in rigorous ways. These measures draw on US models, but the NHS can implement them far more systematically and vigorously than comparable efforts in the United States. The government as payer has set up an entire system for inspecting the quality of medicine delivered at its hospitals and clinics, and quality standards are becoming part of every contract. Chief executives can be—and already have been—replaced for poor performance. Senior specialists whose services are found inferior are the object of formal rehabilitation. Academic medicine is now subject to a commission to oversee the coordination of training for all the health professions. Both of these changes represent a considerable weakening of power by professional associations and the royal colleges in the face of widely publicized evidence of their failing to uphold standards. The unified vision behind these reforms consists of strong national standards together with devolved purchasing and empowering patients and clinicians.

Besides addressing the historic flaws of the NHS, the government plans to unite specialty care

Transferable Policy Lessons From the United Kingdom

The British have made a number of good decisions that are transferable to other systems. Some of these are mentioned in the text and others come from a more comprehensive list.[24]

1. *Health care should be "free at the point of service," a founding principle of the NHS.* Although this is precisely opposite the principle of American employers and politicians as they increase co-payments, the evidence from the United States and abroad supports the British position. Co-payments create inequities, raise barriers to access, and usually do not achieve their goals.[25, 26] They are not very effective in containing costs, because patients have discretion over just a small percentage of ambulatory and elective choices. Most "cost containment" efforts focus on minor, front-end costs rather than addressing major, back-end costs.[27] Moreover, co-payments undermine the goals of appropriate and effective care and discriminate against the working and lower classes. Such evidence seems ignored by advocates of co-payments in Congress and the business community.

2. *Fund health care from income taxes.* Whenever the British have reviewed the option of using health insurance instead of income tax financing, they have found evidence that an insurance-based health-care system costs more to operate, is more inequitable, controls costs less effectively, and provides no basis for population-oriented prevention or public health gains. By sharp contrast, US employers are moving the other way, from large group insurance toward individuals buying their own policies on a voluntary basis, long known as the most costly and inequitable way to structure health insurance, with few means to contain costs, raise quality, or improve the health status of the population.

3. *Establish a strong primary care base for a health-care system.* Every UK resident chooses a personal physician or practice. The system provides incentives to practice in underserved areas and prevents new GPs from setting up in saturated, affluent areas. The primary care base of the NHS is widely celebrated[28] and has been consistently strengthened over the decades. For example, as recruitment into general practice and morale waned and subspecialty medicine grew in the postwar years, the British raised GP lifetime incomes to equal those of subspecialists. Other changes were made to strengthen primary care by providing more practice staff and nurses in order to encourage solo practitioners to come together into teams. More recently, these teams have been further enlarged by bringing together geographic clusters of GP practices into large Primary Care Trusts that include all community health-care services and many social services as well.

4. *Pay GPs extra for treating patients with deprivations and from deprived areas.* Almost 20 years ago, Brian Jarman developed a deprivation scale based on factors that affect clinical care, so that living alone is a factor as well as low income.[29] The British have long paid GPs considerably more for taking care of patients who are more likely to have more problems and whose care is more demanding. American health policy researchers are still debating whether it can be done.

5. *Reduce inequalities in historic funding that usually favor the affluent.* Regional inequities in the United Kingdom are much smaller now than twenty to thirty years ago, and all major budgets are risk adjusted, in sharp contrast to the United States. Reductions have been achieved through national planning, building up hospitals and resources in underserved areas, and giving disproportionately more new funds to less well-funded areas.

6. *Devise a set of bonuses for GP practices that reach population-based targets for prevention.* Starting in 1990, the government added a new element to the GP contract—lump sums or bonuses for carrying out preventive measures on a high percentage of the patient panel (enrollees). For example, a practice could receive about $1250 if it completed the childhood immunization series for 70 percent to 89 percent of all eligible children registered and $3700 if it completed the series for 90 percent or more. The result has been high levels of immunizations and other preventive measures. Another incentive rewards GPs for using generic drugs for 70 percent of their prescriptions. Why don't US health plans follow suit?

7. *Pay all subspecialists on the same salary scale.* This policy conveys the sense that psychiatry is as important and complicated as cardiology and pediatrics as challenging as orthopedics. On what defensible grounds should one specialty (cardiology) be paid more than another (psychiatry)? Equal pay signals to young doctors that they should specialize in what they do best and enjoy. Yet in many systems pay differs greatly by specialty. This decision has many cultural, organizational, and clinical benefits, even though some subspecialties have more opportunities to supplement their incomes than others.

8. *Control prescription drug prices while rewarding basic research for breakthrough drugs.* Like most other countries, the British have a national board that negotiates with the industry. Pharmaceutical companies like to portray this approach, which is nearly universal outside the United States, as "price controls" that can "never work." In fact, nationally negotiated price schedules have worked well for years and saved billions. The British approach goes further, by rewarding breakthrough research and discouraging "me too" research or patent manipulation. It regulates profits, not prices, by having companies submit financial records and by determining set proportions for expenditures (e.g., a limit of 7 percent of sales for spending on marketing) on in patent branded drugs.[30,31] If prices result in higher profits than allowed, the excess profits are paid back. The British approach both ensures and limits profits.[4,5] Meanwhile, providers are given drug budgets within which they have to live. Any other nation or large buyer can learn from this system.

with primary care, primary care with community health care, and all three with social services, so that one ends up with comprehensive, integrated services that are community based. While the government eliminated Community Health Councils, it requires laymen to be appointed to the new governing boards, and it has institutionalized patient power in a number of ways. A nationwide telephone call-in service to trained nurses who answer patients' questions and provide advice has been established. Web-based information on a wide range of health issues and problems has been developed by clinical teams so that citizens are not at the mercy of the bewildering array of unreliable commercial information on the Internet.

In short, what Bevan found he could not achieve in 1948 is now being attempted. Similar efforts are taking place in other European systems that have also been plagued by hospital dominance and protective specialty fiefdoms. These efforts toward population-based health gain and integrated services represent the next generation of health reform, building on the last generation's creation of universal health-care systems. The United States is now more than a generation behind, unable to reduce health disparities in a system characterized by ever-shifting market shares among competing managed care plans that change insurance coverage from year to year and policy to policy for "populations" of employees. The real chasm in US health policy is between the rhetoric to reduce health disparities and the realities of organization and finance.

Given how much US policymakers admire markets and disparage governments, it is interesting that the British are using government power to achieve all the benefits of markets without markets. However, the reality falls short in several ways. Many of the changes are only beginning, although the speed of implementation is remarkable. Specialists and hospitals are resisting, as they have since the NHS was founded. And Blair is pushing to bring in private "partners" (a high-fashion term), especially large corporations. Of course, he thinks he will do so on his terms for the public interest, but one wonders if he knows how persistent and successful large corporations are at reworking the public interest for their business interests. What would happen to the gov-

ernment if it faced highly trained corporate advocates with large expense accounts, who never have to stand for election and never go away?[23] For them, the purpose of health care is to make money, of course in the name of saving money.

Still, governmental leaders in the United Kingdom have achieved much more in the last 3 years than governmental or corporate leaders in the United States have over the past decade. One could do worse than to emulate the new NHS, especially in the United States, where policy leaders do not know how to repair the distrust, backlash, and rising medical costs that resulted from turning over clinical services to for-profit corporations (box). A strong quality movement is building, but it has to improve margins to succeed. The US credo, "No margin, no mission," is stated as a self-evident law of nature, but actually it is contradicted by most health-care systems. The credo in the NHS and in many health care systems is "Mission, not margin," and their mission does not falter when they are in the red, as often they are.

ACKNOWLEDGMENTS

I thank Oliver Fein, William Glaser, Lou Levitt, Aaron Beckerman, and the organizers of Rekindling Reform for inviting me to participate and write this report. I am indebted to helpful comments on earlier drafts by Anne-Emanuelle Birn, Marilyn DeLuca, William Glaser, and astute reviewers.

REFERENCES

1 Klein R. *The New Politics of the NHS*. 3rd ed. New York, NY: Longman; 1995.

2 Webster C. *The National Health Service: A Political History*. New York, NY: Oxford University Press; 1998.

3 Rivett G. *From Cradle to Grave: Fifty Years of the NHS*. London, England: The King's Fund; 1998.

4 Eckstein H. *The English Health Service: Its Origins, Structure and Achievements*. Cambridge, Mass: Harvard University Press; 1958:chap 5.

5 Honigsbaum F. *The Division in British Medicine*. London, England: Kogan Page; 1979.

6 Keen J. Light D, Mays N. *Public–Private Relations in Health Care*. London, England: The King's Fund; 2001.

7 Appleby J. Funding UK health care from general taxes—time for a change? Presented at: The Changing Health Care System: A British-American Dialogue [symposium

organized by the New York Academy of Medicine and the Royal Society of Medicine]; April 25, 2002; New York, NY.

8 Iriart C, Merhy E, Waitzkin H. Managed care in Latin America: the new common sense in health policy reform. *Soc Sci Med.* 2001; 52:1243–1253.

9 Light DW. The sociological character of markets in health care. In: Albrecht GL, Fitzpatrick R, Scrimshaw SC, eds. *Handbook of Social Studies in Health and Medicine.* London, England: Sage; 2000:394–408.

10 [Special issue on comparative institutional responses to competition policy.] *Soc Sci Med.* 2001; 52(8).

11 [Special comparative issue on competition in health care markets.] *J Health Polit Policy Law.* 2000; 25(5).

12 Glaser WA. The competition vogue and its outcomes. *Lancet.* 1993; 341:805–812.

13 Light DW. From managed competition to managed cooperation: theory and lessons from the British experience. *Milbank Q.* 1997; 75:297–341.

14 Light DW. Equity and efficiency in health care. *Soc Sci Med.* 1992; 35:465–469.

15 Light DW. *Homo Economicus.* escaping the traps of managed competition. *Eur J Public Health.* 1995; 5:145–154.

16 Robinson R, Steiner A. *Managed Health Care.* Philadelphia, Pa: Open University Press; 1998.

17 Audit Commission. *What the Doctor Ordered: A Study of GP Fundholding in England.* London, England: Her Majesty's Stationery Office; 1996.

18 Light DW. *Effective Commissioning.* London, England: Office of Health Economics; 1998:chap 3, 5.

19 Williams S, Michie S, Pattani S. *Improving the Health of the NHS Workforce.* London, England: The Nuffield Trust; 1998.

20 Department of Health (UK). *The NHS Plan. A Plan for Investment. A Plan for Reform.* London, England: Stationary Office; 2000.

21 Milburn A. The new NHS—developing the NHS national plan. Department of Health Key Speech delivered at: Royal College of Surgeons; May 18, 2000; London, England.

22 Light DW. How waiting lists work and their hidden agenda. *Consumer Policy Rev* [UK]. 2000; 10: 126–132.

23 *The Other Drug War: Big Pharma's 625 Washington Lobbyists.* Washington, DC: Public Citizen Congress Watch; July 2001.

24 Light DW. Policy lesson from the British Health Care system. In: Powell FD, Wessen AP, eds. *Health Care Systems in Transition: An International Perspective.* Thousand Oaks, Calif: Sage; 1999: 327–365.

25 Evans RG, ML Barer, GL Stoddart. *User Charges, Snares and Delusions: Another Look at the Literature.* Toronto: Ontario Premier's Council on Health, Well-being and Social Justice; 1993.

26 Rasell ME. Cost sharing in health insurance—a reexamination. *N Engl J Med.* 1995; 332:1164–1168.

27 Berk ML, Monheit AC. The concentration of health expenditures, revisited. *Health Aff.* 2001; 20(2):9–18.

28 Starfield B. *Primary Care: Concept, Evaluation and Policy.* 2nd ed. New York, NY: Oxford University Press; 2000.

29 Jarman B. Identification of underprivileged areas. *Br J Med.* 1983; 286:1705–1709.

30 *The Pharmaceutical Price Regulation Scheme.* London, England: Department of Health (UK); 1999.

31 *Pharmaceutical Price Regulation Scheme: Fourth Report to Parliament.* London, England: Department of Health; December 2000.

INSIGHTS FROM HEALTH CARE IN GERMANY

Christa Altenstetter

Altenstetter provides an overview of the history and current structure of German health insurance before offering several insights for the United States. The German system of health insurance, which has been in place for over a century, was the result of several political compromises and the implementation of communitarian values. The basic structure involves these features: universal coverage (92 percent by national health insurance, the rest by private insurance, some individuals opting for both); managed competition and patient choice among sickness funds (for persons covered by national health insurance); and financing by a combination of employer and employee contributions. Benefits offered by sickness funds are very extensive, exceeding even what the Canadian and British public systems offer, while rationing in Germany is essentially a non-issue. Although the system's costs are great by European standards, per capita spending is considerably less in Germany than in the

United States—despite the fact that the German system achieves universal coverage, comparable quality, and more comprehensive benefits. Altenstetter concludes by drawing several lessons for the United States, which she believes can retain its commitment to market forces so long as the health-care market is well regulated within a system of guaranteed universal coverage.

. . .

HISTORICAL COMPROMISES

Several political compromises from the last quarter of the 19th century go a long way toward explaining the success, performance, and durability of German national health insurance. These compromises have had long-lasting effects, determining who has power over national health insurance, the role of government, and the effect of national health insurance on the health-care delivery system (inpatient, outpatient, and office-based care).

The first compromise was the product of industrialization and urbanization, both of which came late in Germany compared with France or the United Kingdom, coinciding with the establishment of German national unity in 1871. Workers began to organize labor unions, fighting both industrial employers and the Prussian State. Under these pressures, business leaders realized it was in their own self-interest to develop "sickness funds" even before Bismarck pioneered a national plan.

The second compromise emerged as a conflict between regional and national forces. Regional elites felt threatened by what they saw as an overwhelming authoritarian state, particularly Bismarck's original plan to control health insurance from a central imperial office. The iron chancellor, known for his militarism, use of coercive powers, and exercise of repressive measures, lost out to these regional forces when national health insurance was created in 1883. Sickness funds, although mandated nationally, were organized on a regional basis.

A third compromise resulted in joint management of sickness funds by employers and employees in the last quarter of the 19th century and then adapted to the conditions of the 20th century. The model of labor and business mediation through nonprofit, self-governing bodies developed in three stages. First, between the 1860s and the 1920s, labor controlled two-thirds and business controlled one-third of the seats on the board of individual sickness funds. During the second period, from around the mid-1920s to 1933, each side had an equal representation. Under the Nazi regime, development was interrupted from 1933 to 1945 because health insurance became subject to total control by Berlin. After 1945, control over sickness funds in West Germany reverted back to business and labor. East Germany kept a state-run delivery system until the West German model was imported in 1989. Since the 1993 reforms, the minister of health has asserted more regulatory authority over the nonprofit, self-governing sickness funds. Based on history, however, it is doubtful that the German state will take on a larger role as in Canada, Britain, or even the United States with Medicare and Medicaid.

The basic structure and principles for securing access to health care—mandatory sickness fund membership, employer- and employee-funded coverage, defined benefits based on the state of medical knowledge, with portability of benefits—thus became embedded in German economic and political institutions (Table 1). As a consequence, German policymakers aimed at extending eligibility, improving benefits, defining quality services, and spreading geographic access to medical services. Efforts to reform health-care delivery were minimal. The medical profession alone defined health-care quality until the 1990s.

Because of solidarity among workers, eligibility also was extended to guest workers (*Gastarbeiter*). In the 1960s, trade unions made their inclusion under social insurance a prerequisite for accepting "importation" of "foreign" workers. Thus, both full- and part-time *Gastarbeiter* have the same rights and obligations under national health insurance and, since 1995, long-term care insurance; they and their families are entitled to the same benefits as other

From *American Journal of Public Health*, vol. 93, no. 1 (2003), pp. 38–40, 42–44. Copyright © 2003 by the American Public Health Association.

TABLE 1   National Health Insurance at a Glance

Scope

No citizen is without insurance—92 percent are covered by National Health Insurance; the rest are insured privately or are wealthy

Mandatory contributions into National Health Insurance

Choice of generalist physicians and specialists, dentists, hospitals, and long-term nursing care

Portability of coverage across all hospitals, doctors' offices, regions, and communities

Chip card (previously uniform forms) serves as membership identification; medical and dental offices, hospitals, and specialized facilities must honor it

Choice of sickness fund (since 1993)

About 7 percent of the population carries commercial insurance (civil servants and the self-employed—about 7.1 million in 2001)

7–10 percent of those covered by National Health Insurance take out private insurance for amenities while hospitalized

Private health insurance is offered by about 50 companies, although the private insurance sector is very restricted given National Health Insurance

Providers

Professional autonomy

Peer review and self-regulation through self-governing bodies

Advice, assistance, and care are mandated; right to representation is institutionalized

Accountability to peers, the public, elected governments, and payers

Income miserable from 19th century through 1960s, when fee-for-service reimbursement was introduced; bonanza lasted until mid-1980s, when income began to decline 2–3 times previous income

Mandatory membership (generalists or specialists) in regional chapters of 2 medical organizations as precondition for practicing medicine and reimbursement under National Health Insurance

- For reimbursement, Federal Association of Panel Doctors
- For actual practice, Medical Chamber controlling medical education, continuing education, and specialty training; setting standards of care for each specialty and subspecialty
- Dentists, pharmacists, and other health professionals share a similar history and guildlike organization

Coverage

Working individuals, their spouses, and their children

Retired persons

Unemployed

All students, whether at community colleges, senior colleges, or universities

In principle, children are covered until age 18 (but, depending on whether a child works or is a student, can continue until age 23 or 25, respectively)

Age limit can be waived for disabled children

Benefits, prevention, and early detection

Any type of medical services delivered by an office-based generalist or specialist

Unlimited hospital care, with copayment limited to 14 days per year regardless of repeat admissions

Prescription drug coverage, subject to copayments

Full salaries for mothers from 6 weeks before childbirth to 8 weeks afterward, including neonatal care for mother (10 visits) and child

Home help

Preventive checkups for children (9 visits from birth to age 6 years, +1 at the beginning of adolescence), plus for adults after age 35

Yearly cancer screening for women starting at age 20 and men at 45

Dental care

Patient-assisting devices (e.g., wheelchair, walker, hearing aid)

Financing (2-Tiered Organization of Sickness Funds)

Mandated employer and employee-financed contributions (payroll tax averaging about 7 percent of salaries and wages for each)

Individuals can be a member of any one of these funds (competing for members since 1993)

First tier

- 7 general regional funds (*Allgemeine Ortskrankenkassen* or AOK)
- 318 company-based funds (*Betriebskrankenkassen*)
- 28 guild funds (*Innungskrankenkassen* or IKK)
- 5 farmers' funds (*Landwirtschaftliche Krankenkassen* or LKK)
- 1 miners' fund (*Bundesknappschaft*)
- 1 sailors' fund (*See-Krankenkasse*)

Second tier: 12 "substitute" funds (*Ersatzkassen*)—originally catered to workers with above-average earnings

German workers. Health insurance also remains unchanged for all workers during unemployment. Their contributions to national health insurance are paid by federally administered statutory unemployment insurance, which is financed on the same basis as national health insurance.

The significance of the historical-political compromises outlined above cannot be underestimated. After 1883, a few policy options were no longer seriously considered. A single-payer system of financing like Canada's was never a real option; nor was a system like the United Kingdom's National Health Service. Instead, given the historical mix of public and nonprofit and faithbased and secular hospitals and specialized facilities, service delivery was based on pluralism.

The central state, however, has retained several important functions within national health insurance. The national government operates as supervisor, enabler, facilitator, and monitor. National professional and management standards became the law of the land, contrary to a strong regional tradition in Germany before 1871 and after 1949. Universal, employer- and employee-funded insurance made it imperative that a line be drawn between regional rights and securing universal quality in health care; it was drawn for national standards. Thus, regional definitions of coverage, entitlements, and eligibility were never allowed to develop. Over time, national standards were to be phased in, setting the conditions for receiving medical services, long-term care, and mental and public health services and for engaging in medical practice. In tandem with these health-care standards, national standards for industrial affairs, social security programs, and other welfare state programs became the rule.

In contrast to centralized policymaking, implementation was reserved for regional governments. Similarly, the provision of medical services and nursing care was left to private, nonprofit, and public providers. The provision of medical and nursing care requires a high degree of cooperation between providers and faith-based and secular welfare organizations. The *Länder* (regions) are also powerful in shaping federal legislation and, to a lesser degree, national standards. Federal legislation of standards that have implications for regional interests can be enacted only with the support of regional governments.

LESSONS FOR THE UNITED STATES

The German experience does have lessons for the United States (Table 2). First, solidarity-based (employer and employee) financing, rather than funding from general taxes, has served health protection and industrial relations in Germany well, even with constant grumbling from employers. German employers have had the unenviable position of enduring the highest nonwage costs in the Organization for Economic Cooperation and Development for twelve years in a row.[1] Yet, despite complaints notably in recent years from employers and physicians, employer- and employee-funded national health insurance remains intact.

Second, universal health care comes with a price; it has never been free for German consumers. Although Germany ranks second among Organization for Economic Cooperation and Development countries (after the United States) in terms of public-mandated spending on health care, it spends 3 percent of gross domestic product less than the United States.[2] Mandated coverage and employer and employee contributions in Germany buy substantially more comprehensive medical services than under any US health maintenance organization or commercial insurance plan.

Endorsing universal health and accepting the conditions that make it work in the United States would mean dramatic power shifts for which neither most of the American public nor stakeholders appear to be ready. However, the price for relying on employer-provided benefits for most of the American labor force is abdication of control and total dependence on employer goodwill. When pinched, employers will offer less coverage, which translates into higher deductibles, co-payments, and benefits exclusions for employees. It also means total dependence on the powerful insurance and pharmaceutical industries. As the historical record has shown repeatedly, elected representatives in the United States cannot be relied on to vote for universal health but tend to be captive to special interest lobbies. The loser is the American patient and consumer.

Third, long-term care has arrived in Germany, although with a time lag of some 120 years when compared with earlier social insurance programs.

TABLE 2   Benefits of Communitarian Health Care for Employers and Employees

Comprehensive, portable benefits and access to quality care

Independent of employers' largesse

No uninsured

No differentiation between high-risk and low-risk employees

Benefit plans do not depend on size of the employer

Employers have the same insurance costs regardless of size

Affordability of offering health insurance to employees less an issue in Germany than in the United States

Same cost-sharing requirements by patients are used under National Health Insurance

No deductibles and maximum annual out-of-pocket costs for employees before benefits kick in

Modest co-payments for all on an equal basis

No variations in health plans and cost sharing

Low administrative costs for sickness funds; although increasing, only 5–6 percent (compared with the United States, with 10 percent of premiums for large employers and 20–25 percent for small employers)

Employer-based human resources departments implement the same national rules

No expenses for advertisement, marketing, and billing

No need to discuss the issue of employees' access to health insurance

All employers and employees get the same value for their contribution

No need to screen any employer for potential risks of their employees

Federal health care reform applies equally to all parties involved

No need to use health characteristics in setting premiums

Source. Adapted from US General Accounting Office.[3]

Mandatory long-term care insurance has provided access to nursing home care and other forms of nonmedical care since 1995, thus keeping the elderly in the mainstream rather than marginalizing them. The employer- and employee-funded contribution into long-term care insurance is set at 1.7 percent, or 0.85 percent for each side. The income ceiling for health and long-term care protection on which the payroll tax is calculated is 3375€ per month starting in January 2002; likewise, the annual income ceiling now is 40500€.

Obviously, coordination at the macro policy level across national health insurance and long-term care insurance is a high priority. An ever-greater need exists for offering integrated services at the community and family level. This seems to work best when home visits are offered by networks of different kinds of providers. In this way, medication can be changed; a referral to a hospital or a specialist can be obtained; and patient-assisting devices, which require a physician's prescription, can be ordered when needed.

Finally, business and labor leaders, federal and regional policymakers, and most segments of the German public remain convinced that solidarity is a better mechanism to resolve conflicts and secure access to health care than fierce competition and adversarial politics. However, there is also agreement that solidarity, subsidiarity, and self-governance can blossom only under 5 conditions: (1) the profit motive (especially investor-owned insurance companies) must be kept out of health care or at least kept to a minimum to save substantial sums, which otherwise pay for advertisements, billing, and marketing; (2) a communitarian and inclusive culture surrounding the delivery of care must be emphasized; (3) countervailing forces (federal vs regional, payer vs provider) should be used and relied on for problem solving[4]; (4) federal or regional offices should act as facilitators, enablers, and monitors of last resort; and (5) the link between the voting public and elected officials must not be severed through special interest politics, which can lose sight of the "woman on the street"

Health policies are the product of politics and a particular institutional and ideological context. Irrespective of ideological differences, US stakeholders and the American public share similar convictions, have similar antigovernment attitudes, endorse a firm belief in "rugged individualism," and, deep down, have in common the strong belief that money has a legitimate place in society. All of these factors mitigate against collective solutions for universal health, whether tax financed or employer and employee funded. However, the situation would be different if we could just get to the point where Americans, like Germans, can say: "Don't take my health insurance away." This works for Medicare; why should it not work for universal health care?

ACKNOWLEDGMENT

The author would like to thank Richard J. Meagher of the CUNY Graduate Center for his assistance in editing and formatting this article.

REFERENCES

1 European Union Delegation of the European Commission to the United States (EURECOM). Institut der Deutschen Wirtschaft. Monthly Bulletin of European Union Economic and Financial News; October 2001.

2 Saalfeld TH. Germany: stable parties, chancellor democracy, and the of informal settlement. In: Müller WC, Strøm K, eds. *Coalition Governments in Western Europe.* New York, NY: Oxford University Press: 2000:32–85.

3 *Private Health Insurance: Small Employers Continue to Face Challenges in Providing Coverage* Washington, DC: US General Accounting Office; October 2001. GAO-02-8.

4 Stone DA. *The Limits of Professional Power.* Chicago, Ill: University of Chicago Press; 1980.

HEALTH CARE REFORM IN FRANCE—THE BIRTH OF STATE-LED MANAGED CARE

Victor G. Rodwin and Claude Le Pen

Noting that the World Health Organization ranked the French health-care system the best in the world, Rodwin and Le Pen describe the system's basic structure as well as recent reforms and challenges. According to the authors, the French generally view their national health insurance as representing an attractive compromise between Britain's National Health Service—associated with excessive rationing and inadequate choice for patients—and the American approach—which focuses on choice but leaves many people uninsured. The French system, which affords universal coverage to an extensive array of benefits, is funded mostly by payroll taxes and government general-revenue funds. A 2004 law, the authors explain, raised taxes and instituted a state-led managed care approach with such developments as computerized record-keeping, practice guidelines, and more use of primary care physicians as gatekeepers; the goal of this recent reform was to modernize the health sector and improve quality while controlling costs. Given the traditional French emphasis on patient choice of providers and on clinical autonomy, Rodwin and Le Pen ask, does the movement toward state-led managed care risk a rebellion among French physicians?

The World Health Organization recently ranked the French health-care system the best in the world.[1] Although the methods and data on which this assessment was based have been criticized, there are good grounds for being impressed by the French system. Yet in August 2004, with the national health insurance (NHI) system facing a severe financial crisis,

France enacted Minister of Health Philippe Douste-Blazy's reform plan. Like previous efforts at health-care reform, this one seeks to preserve a system of comprehensive benefits, which is supported by the major stakeholders.

French policymakers typically view their NHI system as a realistic compromise between Britain's National Health Service, which they believe requires too much rationing and offers insufficient choice, and the mosaic of subsystems in the United States, which they consider socially irresponsible

From *New England Journal of Medicine,* vol. 351, no. 22 (November 25, 2004), pp. 2259–2262. Copyright © 2004 by the Massachusetts Medical Society. All rights reserved.

because 15 percent of the population younger than 65 years of age has no health insurance. Whether reform measures in France have come from the political left or right, French politicians have defended their health-care system as an ideal synthesis of solidarity, liberalism, and pluralism.

Beyond a range of tax increases to finance health care, the recent law seeks to implement what the French call *la maîtrise médicalisée*—a kind of state-led managed care. Like the 1996 reform enacted by then Prime Minister Alain Juppé, it proposes to apply techniques that were designed for managed care organizations in the United States (e.g., computerized medical records, practice guidelines, and incentives to encourage the use of primary care physicians as gatekeepers) to a unitary state system.

The idea of state-led managed care in France has gained momentum over the past decade, but its implementation poses enormous challenges. The idea is compelling for two reasons: it seeks to modernize the health-care sector and increase the quality of care, and it promises to control costs by increasing the efficiency of resource allocation within targeted expenditure limits. In these respects, the reform will reinforce the powerful role of the central state, which will oversee vast institutional renovation, apply administrative and information technology to health care, and design incentives and regulations to improve quality. The limitations of state-led managed care, however, are rooted in the centralization of policymaking in France and the successful resistance of the medical profession to all efforts at micromanaging medical practice and second-guessing physicians' authority.[2]

In contrast to many European nations—such as Britain, the Netherlands, and Germany—France has eschewed two popular ideas in health-care reform: consumer choice and price competition among local health insurance funds and selective contracting between these funds and health-care providers. The avoidance of these approaches reflects France's commitment to the freedom of beneficiaries to choose among all willing providers, as well as the belief that competition would lead to privatization—an unacceptable departure from the "solidarity" principle, which requires mutual aid and cooperation among the sick and the well, the inactive and the

active, and the poor and the wealthy and insists on financing health insurance on the basis of ability to pay, not actuarial risk.

But like the U.S. health-care system, the French system is also structured according to principles of liberalism and pluralism, as a market-based economic system with extensive organizational diversity and individual choice. Most physicians in private practice tenaciously support the present arrangements, embracing the principles enshrined in *"la médecine libérale"*: selection of physicians by patients, freedom for physicians to practice wherever they choose, clinical autonomy, doctor–patient confidentiality, and direct payment to physicians by patients who are reimbursed a good share of their expenditures. With limited and experimental exceptions, France does not use primary care physicians as gatekeepers in the way managed-care organizations do in the United States. Although the hospital system is dominated by public hospitals managed by the Ministry of Health and its regional agencies, private practice remains largely unmanaged.[3]

The NHI system is financed by a mix of mandatory payroll taxes, government general-revenue funds, and a small share of consumer coinsurance. In contrast to Medicare, French NHI coverage increases when a patient's costs increase; there are no deductibles; and pharmaceutical benefits are extensive. Patients with debilitating or chronic illness are exempted from paying coinsurance if they consult physicians who accept NHI reimbursement as payment in full. When patients consult any of the 26.5 percent of physicians who do not do so, a portion of their coinsurance is reimbursed by complementary health insurers, through a system that resembles Medigap coverage for U.S. Medicare beneficiaries. Thus, despite widespread use of coinsurance, patients remain well covered under NHI and enjoy a broad array of choices by European and American standards.

Although French policymakers claim to have a health-care system that reconciles solidarity, liberalism, and pluralism, the system has changed decisively. One change is unique to France. The Juppé reform increased fiscal taxes (on income, capital, cigarettes, and alcohol), reducing the share of employer-based payroll-tax financing from 95 percent of total health-care expenditures to roughly one-half. Since

Basic Indicators, France and the United States, 2002.[*]

Indicator	France	United States
Demographic and Economic Characteristics		
Total population	59,486,000	288,369,000
Population >65 yr of age—%	16.3	12.3
GDP per capita—$	28,094	36,006
Health Care System		
Health care expenditures—% of GDP	9.7	14.6
Per capita health expenditures—$	2736	5267
Public expenditures on health—% of GDP	7.4	6.6
No. of practicing physicians per 10,000 population	33	30
No. of physician consultations per capita	7.9 (1999)	4.2 (1999)
No. of acute care bed-days per 1000 population	1100 (2001)	700 (2001)
No. of acute care beds per 1000 population	4.0 (2001)	2.9
Population satisfied with health system—%	65.0 (1998)	40.0 (2000)
Health Status		
No. of infant deaths per 1000 live births	4.2	6.8 (2001)
Life expectancy at birth—yr	79.3	77.1 (2001)
Life expectancy at 65 yr of age—yr	19.1 (2001)	17.9 (2001)
Life expectancy at 80 yr of age—yr	8.7 (2001)	8.6 (2001)
Disability-adjusted life expectancy at birth—yr	73.1 (1999)	70.0 (1999)
Years of life lost per 100,000 population due to death before 70 yr of age	4182 (1999)	5120 (2000)

*Data on physician consultations in the United States are from the Department of Health and Human Services, National Center for Health Statistics, National Ambulatory Medical Care Survey. Data on the number of physicians in the United States are from the American Medical Association. Data on patient satisfaction are from Eurobarometer Survey Series no. 49 (1998) and the Harvard School of Public Health (2000). Data on disability-adjusted life expectancy at birth are from the World Health Report 2000. All other data are from the Organization for Economic Cooperation and Development (OECD) Health Data, 2004. When data were not available for 2002, the year of the latest available data is indicated in parentheses. GDP denotes gross domestic product; per capita expenditure values are U.S. dollars, adjusted for OECD purchasing-power parities.

the health system is more heavily dependent on central-government financing, the central state's legitimacy in implementing health-care reform has been strengthened. The second change has been driven by the global evolution of medical technology, proliferation of medical specialties, and explosion of medical knowledge—which make most principles of *la médecine libérale* seem anachronistic and render solo private practice quaint at best.[4]

There is emerging consensus on some of the conclusions of a recent task force.[5] First, the secular growth of health-care expenditures will continue. Second, health policy should aim to achieve value for money in the allocation of health-care resources and equity in the distribution of services. Third, when expenditures meet these goals, they must be financed collectively. The first and third propositions do not provoke controversy in France. The second proposition, however, forces recognition of two problems that threaten the sustainability of the health-care system.

First, it is difficult to control expenditures in a system deeply committed to liberalism and pluralism. Although the French health-care system is not expensive compared with that of the United States (see table), France is one of the biggest spenders in

Europe. Second, access to care is no longer a sufficient objective, given that the quality of health services is unevenly distributed among both geographic regions and social classes. This problem is exacerbated by patients' freedom of navigation within the system and the increasing consciousness of possibilities offered by state-of-the-art treatments.

The French health-care system has reached a turning point that should interest clinicians and policymakers in the United States, for the current reform represents the French response to a fundamental question: Can the balance among solidarity, liberalism, and pluralism be maintained while health-care costs are kept under control and the cherished features of the present system are sustained? The birth of state-led managed care in France has clarified the challenge ahead: Can France adapt the NHI system to the exigencies of technological and economic change without provoking insurmountable opposition from the medical profession? In other words, can

the Douste-Blazy reform actually be implemented, or will it provide support for that well-worn aphorism— *plus ça change, plus c'est la même chose?* [the more things change, the more they stay the same]?

From the Wagner School, New York University, and the World Cities Project, International Longevity Center–USA, New York (V.G.R.); and the University of Paris–Dauphine, Paris (C.L.P.).

NOTES

1 World Health Report 2000. Health systems: improving performance. (Accessed November 4, 2004 at http://www.who.int/whr/previous/en/.)

2 De Kervasdoué J. Pour une révolution sans réforme. Pris: Gallimard, 1999.

3 Rodwin VG. The health care system under French national health insurance: lessons for health reform in the United States. Am J Public Health 2003; 93:31–7.

4 Le Pen C. Les habits neufs d'Hippocrate. Paris: Calmann-Levy, 1999.

5 Fragonard B. Rapport du haut conseil pour l'avenir de l'assurance maladie. Paris: Ministry of Health, January 2003.

REFORM PROPOSALS FOR THE UNITED STATES

EXPANDING INSURANCE COVERAGE THROUGH TAX CREDITS, CONSUMER CHOICE, AND MARKET ENHANCEMENTS: THE AMERICAN MEDICAL ASSOCIATION PROPOSAL FOR HEALTH INSURANCE REFORM

Donald J. Palmisano, David W. Emmons, and Gregory D. Wozniak

Representing the position of the American Medical Association, the authors defend a reform proposal that focuses on transforming the health-care market as a means to fostering the development of more high-quality, affordable insurance plans than are currently available. Their proposal recommends three main reforms. First, while employers could continue to offer insurance benefits, employees would be free to purchase group coverage independently of their employment. Second, the current tax exclusion of employer-based health insurance would be replaced by a system of refundable tax credits—inversely related to income—for the purchase of insurance. Third, various enhancements to health insurance markets (e.g., basing premiums on age and sex but not health status, guaranteed renewability of enrollment) would enable more individuals to afford health insurance. A larger health insurance pool would permit lower administrative costs. The predictable result, according to the authors, is that health insurers would become more responsive to consumers' preferences for lower premiums, better benefit packages, and superior care.

A recent editorial[1] in the journal invited a broad discussion of proposals to expand health coverage in the United States. The nature and the extent of the uninsured problem are well documented.[2-9] According to the US Census Bureau,[10] the estimated number of US individuals who did not have health insurance coverage rose from 41.2 million in 2001 to 43.6 million in 2002, involving 15.2 percent of the population. Finding a way to reduce the number of uninsured Americans is imperative.

Since 1998, American Medical Association (AMA) policy has called for reform of the US healthcare financing system according to the principles of tax credits for the purchase of insurance, individuals' choice and ownership of health insurance, and facilitation of new health insurance markets and regulations that are more responsive to variation across individuals and families in their preferences for health insurance.[11-13] The tax credits would be independent of work status, employer-offered health benefits, or the type of plan chosen, whether indemnity insurance, a health maintenance organization (HMO), a preferred provider organization (PPO), or a medical savings account (MSA). AMA policy does not include specific recommendations about a tax credit schedule; rather, it is structured to serve as a broad guide for shaping federal legislation that would expand coverage.

EXPANDING HEALTH INSURANCE COVERAGE

The AMA proposal targets all nonelderly individuals, not only the uninsured or a subgroup of the uninsured. It preserves and enhances the primacy of the patient-physician relationship and continuity of care. It uses tax credits as financial incentives for obtaining and maintaining coverage.

There are 3 key components of the AMA health system reform proposal. The first is to replace the tax exclusion of employer-based health insurance with tax credits that are inversely related to income, refundable and advanceable. With advanceable credits, individuals need not wait until their federal income

taxes are filed to use the credits to purchase insurance. Making the credits contingent on coverage for all family members would ensure maximum enrollment gains. The second is to enable individuals to select and own health insurance. Under the AMA proposal, an employer's offering of health plans will no longer be the only group coverage option for most individuals. More coverage options will enable better matching of insurance benefits with the values and preferences of individuals. The third is to facilitate the formation of new health insurance markets to enhance health insurance offerings. To increase choice in the individual and group health insurance markets, we propose insurance market reforms and incentives to offer a wider range of new, affordable, and permanent insurance options.

TAX CREDITS

The economic benefits of the current federal income tax exclusion of employer health insurance benefits are weighted toward relatively wealthy employed individuals and their families. Those who do not have employer-based coverage and those in the lowest federal income tax brackets receive little or no tax benefit. The total federal income tax subsidy from employer health benefits is estimated to be $188.5 billion in 2004.[14] The tax subsidy from the health benefit exclusion alone is estimated to be $101 billion. Of the total subsidy, 26.5 percent ($50 billion) will go to families with $100,000 or more in income. Families with incomes less than $30,000 will receive 9.8 percent ($18.5 billion) of the subsidy. In 2004, the subsidy will average $1492 overall per family, $2780 for families with income of $100,000 or more, and only $102 for families with less than $10,000 in income.[14]

Tax credits would replace the current federal income tax exclusion of employer-based health benefits with a system of income-related, refundable, and advanceable credits contingent on health coverage for the entire family. Employer spending on employee health insurance benefits would remain fully deductible as a business expense. In developing a tax credit proposal, one must assess tradeoffs among the many combinations of proposal design elements.[15] To achieve near-universal coverage cost-effectively, the credits should be inversely related

From *JAMA*, vol. 291, no. 18 (May 12, 2004), pp. 2237–2239, 2241–2242. Copyright © 2004 by the American Medical Association.

to income and be large enough to ensure that health insurance is affordable for most people.[16] By providing the largest subsidies to those in the lowest income levels, policy makers can target those who, without the tax credit, would be the most likely to be uninsured. Targeting subsidies to low-income individuals also reduces the amount of uncompensated care that currently exists in the health care system.[17]

The tax credit should be refundable to those who purchase health insurance, so those who have tax liability less than the value of the tax credit would receive a refund for the difference. The tax credit could be administered as an advanceable voucher or through some other mechanism. Vouchers are used to provide a variety of services, including food and nutrition, child care, housing, and education. Such vouchers could use existing mechanisms for distribution, such as the federal or state tax system, or state or local agencies. For example, the recent increase in the federal child tax credit was distributed as an advanced credit.[18]

INDIVIDUALLY SELECTED AND OWNED HEALTH INSURANCE

Tax credits large enough to make health insurance affordable would enable individuals to choose coverage that reflects their health insurance and health-care preferences and values. In the current employer-based system, an insured employee cannot change plans if he or she experiences bad service and the employer offers only one plan. In that case, there is little value in "report card" information that compares quality of plans, even if a better-performing plan is available nearby. Comparative information is in high demand when workers are offered multiple plans. A good example is the Federal Employees Health Benefits Program (FEHBP),[19] in which the "individualized group insurance"[20] has given rise to publications of health plan ratings, changes in the plan benefits and premiums, and information on plan patient safety programs.[19] Several other characteristics of the FEHBP are worth noting. Just 5 percent of FEHBP enrollees switch in any year, and many remain for decades with the same choice of plans and providers.[21] Ratings of FEHBP plans are high,[22] and FEHBP is well known for controlling cost increases.[23] Finally, throughout

the years, plans participating in FEHBP have added services of interest to patients.

With more choices, individuals would be more likely to procure coverage and be satisfied with their care.[24-26] Having a choice of plans also increases access to care.[25,27] Insurers and health plans would have incentives to respond to enrollee preferences for information on plan quality, easier access, higher quality, and lower costs.[28,29] Information on quality or other plan characteristics to help individuals make informed choices in health care is becoming increasingly available.[30,31] A well-known economic principle is that a relatively small number of consumers who are willing and able to change their purchase patterns can keep prices down and quality in line with expectations.[32] These market-based mechanisms would lead to improved quality and restraints on cost increases.[33,34] Responsive plans would increase their enrollments and unresponsive plans would fail.

Switching employer health benefits from a defined benefit approach to a defined contribution approach would contribute to the evolution of individually selected and owned health insurance. Defined contribution health benefits clarify the economic cost of the health plan choices to workers.[35,36] When workers choose plans, they become more price conscious and thus select plans with less first-dollar coverage and somewhat higher deductibles.[37,38] Creating incentives for consumers in selecting plans also serves as a cost control.[33] The switch to defined contribution plans also changes insurer incentives. Individuals whose money is part of the transaction expect measurable and demonstrated value from plans. Defined contributions would also make employers' financial obligations for health benefits compensation more predictable in the short run.[36]

NEW HEALTH INSURANCE MARKETS

Prior to the early 1990s, most coverage was through indemnity or fee-for-service plans.[39,40] With indemnity coverage, patients had considerable choice among physicians and other providers. Later, with the expansion of managed care, insurers competed for employers, primarily by offering lower premiums and controlling the delivery of care.[41,42] One approach was to restrict the network of physicians, particularly specialists.[43] Cost increases were reduced, but the patient-physician relationship was seriously challenged. Breaks in the continuity of patient-physician relationships result in patients deferring care and increases in health-care spending.[44,45]

A large proportion of employers offer little or no choice of health plan.[46] Larger firms tend to offer more choices of type of plans, offering an HMO and a PPO, for example, but often from a single insurer.[46] Few small firms, however, offer their employees a choice of plans.[47] For most firms, the overhead of running a multiple-plan health benefits program would be prohibitive. What is needed are ways to expand access to current insurance products and create new group and individual markets that would offer greater continuity of coverage to individuals who work in smaller firms, change employers, or move in and out of employment.[7]

States could allow private-sector employees and other individuals to use their tax credit to purchase coverage in state employee health benefits systems. States could enable the creation or expansion of small group purchasing arrangements, association health plans, and health markets that offer choices to consumers for redeeming their tax credits. To expand coverage in the nonemployer group markets, these alternative insurance risk-pool arrangements could be granted exemptions similar to Employee Retirement Income Security Act exemptions, such as exemption from state insurance regulations of mandated benefits, premium taxes, purchasing pool minimum size restrictions, and small-group rating laws while safeguarding state and federal patient protection laws.[48]

The Achilles heel of individual insurance markets has been adverse selection. Guaranteed issue and strict community rating with extensive benefit mandates have been used as a proposed fix for the problem but with negative effects on costs and number of insured.[49,50] The AMA proposes important insurance market regulations including modified community rating and guaranteed renewability. The resulting modified community rating, based on age and sex, would have risk rating and premium variation but in narrower ranges than with individual risk-rating. The influx of average-risk, current group market enrollees into these new health insurance markets would provide insurers with economies of scale, thereby reducing administrative expenses and the incentives to risk rate.[15,20,51,52]

Even before the Health Insurance Portability and Accountability Act, 75 percent of policies in the individual market were guaranteed renewable.[53] Guaranteed renewability provides incentives for individuals to obtain coverage before they become ill.[54] Once insured, individuals are likely to maintain coverage with the same insurer because switching costs outweigh gains from potentially lower premiums of a different insurer. Less switching reduces insurers' underwriting and policy-issue costs, allowing them to limit premium increases.[55]

With adverse selection, insurers also must have financial incentives to accept and cover individuals who have above-average expected medical expenses. To stabilize the new risk arrangements and avoid channeling them into high-risk pools, high-risk individuals may need subsidies in addition to the tax credit amount. To minimize the effect on the average-risk members of the population, those subsidies should be funded from general tax revenues. An alternative stabilizing mechanism is to provide insurers risk-related subsidies, paid to plans with higher-than-average-risk enrollees by other plans in the market. Another option is a reinsurance pool for insurers, which protects them against expenses of known "high spenders."[55,56]

A combination of reforms and incentives is needed to enable the formation and operation of purchasing arrangements and market innovation such as MSAs, consumer-driven health plans, and other forms of coverage now being developed.[35,57] Internet-based health insurance vendors and small-group purchasing arrangements would expand choice and increase the availability of affordable coverage.[33,58–60] Internet-based vendors also would reduce the administrative costs of offering multiple plans. Web sites now exist that allow consumers to download and compare plan information. Small-group purchasing arrangements already enable employers, particularly small ones, to negotiate with several health plans, expanding the choices beyond what any single employer could offer.

Although employer-based coverage would remain, the improved individual and nonemployer group markets would become good alternatives to traditional coverage. As the size and the extent of new markets increased, they would become more representative of the overall market, and competition for individuals' premium dollars would become intense. Coverage would become more affordable, particularly for those with preexisting or chronic conditions. . . .

ACKNOWLEDGMENT

We acknowledge the helpful suggestions of Robert Otten, MS; James Rodgers, PhD; and Carla Willis, PhD. We also thank Peter McMenamin, PhD, for his contribution on an earlier version of the article.

REFERENCES

1 Fein R. Universal health insurance: let the debate resume. *JAMA.* 2003;290:818–819.

2 Ayanian JZ. Unmet health needs of uninsured adults in the United States. *JAMA.* 2000; 284:2061–2069.

3 American College of Physicians/American Society of Internal Medicine. *No Health Insurance? It's Enough to Make You Sick: Scientific Research Linking the Lack of Health Coverage to Poor Health.* Washington, DC: American College of Physicians; 1999.

4 Hadley J. *Sicker and Poorer: The Consequences of Being Uninsured.* Washington, DC: Kaiser Commission on Medicaid and the Uninsured, The Henry J. Kaiser Family Foundation; 2002.

5 Institute of Medicine. *Care Without Coverage: Too Little, Too Late.* Washington, DC: National Academies Press; 2002.

6 Glied S, Lambrew J, Little S. *The Growing Share of Uninsured Workers Employed by Large Firms.* New York, NY. The Commonwealth Fund; 2003.

7 Short P, Graefe D. Battery-powered health insurance? stability in coverage of the uninsured. *Health Aff (Millwood).* 2003; 22:244–255.

8 Institute of Medicine. *Hidden Costs, Value Lost: Uninsurance in America.* Washington, DC: National Academies Press; 2003.

9 O'Brien E, Feder J, *How Well Does the Employment-Based Health Insurance System Work for Low-Income Families?* Washington, DC: Kaiser Commission on Medicaid and the Uninsured, The Henry J. Kaiser Family Foundation; 1998.

10 Mills R, Bhandan S. *Health Insurance Coverage in the United States: 2002.* Washington, DC: US Dept of Commerce; 2003. Current Population Reports P60–223.

11 American Medical Association, Council on Medical Service. *Empowering Our Patients: Individually Selected, Purchased and Owned Health Insurance.* Chicago, Ill: American Medical Association; 1998. CMS Report 9.

12 American Medical Association, Council on Medical Service. *Health Insurance Market Regulation.* Chicago, Ill: American Medical Association; 2003. CMS Report 7.

13 American Medical Association. *Expanding Health Insurance: AMA Proposal for Reform.* Available at: http://www.ama-assn.org/ama1/pub/upload/mm/363/expandinghealthinsur.pdf. Accessed March 16, 2004.

14 Sheils J, Haught R. The cost of tax-exempt health benefits in 2004. *Health Aff (Millwood).* February 2004:W4-106-W4-112. Available at: http://content.healthaffairs.org/cgi/content/abstract/hlthaff.w4.106. Accessed March 19, 2004.

15 Pauly M, Herring B. Expanding insurance coverage via tax credits: trade-offs and outcomes. *Health Aff (Millwood).* 2001; 20:9–26.

16 American Medical Association, Council on Medical Service. *Principles of Restructuring Health Insurance Tax Credits.* Chicago, Ill: American Medical Association; 2000. CMS Report 4.

17 Hadley J, Holohan J. How much medical care do the uninsured use, and who pays for it? *Health Aff (Millwood).* February 2003:W3-66-W3-80. Available at: http://content.healthaffairs.org/cgi/reprint/hlthaff.w3.66v1.pdf?ck=nck. Accessed March 23, 2004.

18 Internal Revenue Service. Your 2003 advance child tax credit. Available at: http://www.irs.gov/individuals/article/0,,id=111546,00.html. Accessed April 7, 2004.

19 Federal Employees Health Benefits Program. *2003 Plan Guides.* 2003. Available at: http://www.opm.gov/insure/03/guides/index.asp. Accessed March 21, 2004.

20 Pauly M, Percy A, Herring B. Individual versus job-based health insurance: weighing the pros and cons. *Health Aff (Millwood).* 1999; 18:28–44.

21 Francis W. The FEHBP as a model for Medicare reform: separating fact from fiction [Senate Finance Committee Testimony, June 6, 2003]. Available at: http://finance.senate.gov/hearings/testimony/2003test/060603wftest.pdf. Accessed March 16, 2004.

22 Hunter D. *Health Care Choice and Patient Satisfaction.* Washington, DC: Heritage Foundation; 2003.

23 LeMieux J. Bipartisan Commission on the Future of Medicare: memo to the commission, February 17, 1999. Available at: http://medicare.commission.gov/medicare/jeff.html. Accessed November 10, 2003.

24 Schone B, Cooper P. Assessing the impact of health plan choice. *Health Aff (Millwood).* 2001; 20:267–275.

25 Davis K, Schoen C. *Managed Care, Choice, and Patient Satisfaction.* New York, NY: The Commonwealth Fund; 1997.

26 Ullman R, Hill J, Scheye E, Spoeri R. Satisfaction and choice: a view from the plans. *Health Aff (Millwood).* 1997; 16:209–217.

27 Schur C, Berk M. Choice of health plan: implications for access and satisfaction. *Health Care Financ Rev.* 1998; 20:29–43.

28 Ellwood P, Enthoven A, Etheredge L. The Jackson Hole initiatives for a twenty-first century American health care system. *Health Econ.* 1992; 1:149–168.

29 Mays G. *Health Plans' Use of Quality Incentives and Information: Findings From the 2002–03 Community Tracking Study Site Visits* [testimony before Federal Trade Commission and Department of Justice Hearings on Health Care and Competition Law and Policy]. Available at: http://www.ftc.gov/ogc/healthcarehearings/docs/030530may sglen.pdf. Accessed March 18, 2004.

30 National Committee on Quality Assurance. NCQA's health plan report card. Available at: http://hprc.ncqa.org/index.asp. Accessed March 17, 2004.

31 Thompson J, Bost J, Ahmed F, Ingalls C, Sennett C. The NCQA's quality compass: evaluating managed care in the United States. *Health Aff (Millwood)*. 1998; 17:152–158.

32 Baumol W, Willig R. Panzar J. *Contestable Markets and the Theory of Industry Structure.* New York, NY: Harcourt Brace Jovanovich; 1982.

33 Meyer J, Silow-Carroll S. Building on the job-based health care system; what would it take? *Health Aff (Millwood)*. August 2003:W3-415-W3-425. Available at: http://content. healthaffairs.org/cgi/reprint/hlthaff.w3.415v1.pdf?ck=nck. Accessed March 23, 2004.

34 Sheils J, Haught R. *Covering America: Cost and Coverage: Analysis of Ten Proposals to Expand Health Insurance Coverage.* Falls Church, Va: Lewin Group; 2003.

35 Christianson J, Parente S, Taylor R. Defined-contribution health insurance products: development and prospects. *Health Aff (Millwood)*. 2002; 21:49–64.

36 Fronstin P. *Defined Contribution Health Benefits?* Washington, DC: Employee Benefit Research Institute; 2001. EBRI Issue Brief 231.

37 Nichols L. *Can Defined Contribution Health Insurance Reduce Cost Growth?* Washington, DC: Employee Benefit Research Institute; 2002. EBRI Issue Brief 246.

38 Glied S, Remler D, Zivin J. Inside the sausage factory: improving estimates of the effects of health insurance expansion proposals. *Milbank* Q. 2002; 80:603–636.

39 Wholey D, Feldman R, Christianson J. The effect of market structure on HMO premiums. *J Health Econ.* 1995; 14:81–105.

40 InterStudy. *Competitive Edge: HMO Industry Report.* Minneapolis, Minn: InterStudy Publications; 1986–1994.

41 Gold M, Hurley R, Lakem T, Berenson R. A national survey of the arrangements managed-care plans make with physicians. *N Engl J Med.* 1995; 333:1678–1683.

42 Remler D, Donelan K, Blendon R, et al. What do managed care plans do to affect care? *Inquiry.* 1997; 34:196–204.

43 Miller R, Luft H. Managed care plan performance since 1980: a literature analysis. *JAMA.* 1994; 271:1512–1519.

44 Franks P. Cameron C, Bertakis K. On being new to an insurance plan: health care use associated with the first years in a health insurance plan. *Ann Farn Med.* 2003; 1:156–161.

45 Weiss L, Blustein J. Faithful patients: the effect of long-term physician-patient relationships on the costs and use of health care by older Americans. *Am J Public Health.* 1996; 86:1742–1747.

46 The Kaiser Family Foundation and the Health Research and Educational Trust. *Employer Health Benefits 2003 Annual Survey.* Available at: http://www.kff.org/insurance/ ehbs2003-6-set.cfm. Accessed March 16, 2004.

47 Rice T. Gabel J, Levitt L, Hawkins S. Workers and their health plans: free to choose? *Health Aff (Millwood)*. 2002; 21:182–187.

48 Pauly M, Percy A. Cost and performance: a comparion of the individual and group health insurance markets *J Health Polit Policy Law.* 2000; 25:9–26.

49 Zukerman S, Rajan S. An alternative approach for measuring the effects of insurance market reforms. *Inquiry.* 1999; 36:44–55.

50 Sloan F, Conover C. Effects of state reforms on insurance coverage of adults. *Inquiry.* 1998; 35:280–293.

51 Hall M. Of magic wands and kaleidoscopes: fixing problems in the individual market. *Health Aff (Millwood)*. October 2002: W353-W358. Available at: http://content.healthaffairs. org/cgi/content/full/hlthaff.w2.353v1/DC1. Accessed March 16, 2004.

52 Pauly M, Herring B, Song D. Tax credits, the distribution of subsidized health insurance premiums, and the uninsured. *Frontiers Health Policy Res.* 2002; 5:102–122.

53 Harrington S, Niehaus G. *Risk Management and Insurance.* 2nd ed. Burr Ridge, Ill: Irwin McGraw-Hill; 2003.

54 Patel V, Pauly M. Guaranteed renewability and the problem of risk variation in individual health insurance market. *Health Aff (Millwood)*. August 2002:W280–W289. Available at: http://content.healthaffairs.org/cgi/content/ full/hlthaff.w2.280v1/DC1. Accessed March 22, 2004.

55 Harrington S, Miller T. Competitive markets for individual health insurance. *Health Aff (Millwood)*. October 2002: W359–W362. Available at: http://content.healthaffairs.org/ cgi/reprint/hlthaff.w2.359v1.pdf. Accessed March 22, 2004.

56 Swartz K. Government as reinsurer for very-high-cost persons in nongroup health insurance markets. *Health Aff (Millwood)*. October 2002: W380–W382. Available at: http://content.healthaffairs.org/cgi/reprint/hlthaff.w2.380v1. pdf. Accessed March 22, 2004.

57 Gabel J. Lo Sasso A, Rice T. Consumer-driven health plans: are they more than talk now? *Health Aff (Millwood)*. November 2002: W395–W407. Available at: http://content. healthaffairs.org/cgi/reprint/hlthaff.w2.395v1.pdf. Accessed March 17, 2004.

58 Long S, Marquis M. Have small-group health insurance purchasing ailliances increased coverage? *Health Aff (Millwood)*. 2001; 20:154–163.

59 Patel V. Raising awareness of consumers' options in the individual health insurance market. *Health Aff (Millwood)*. October 2002; W367–W371. Available at: http://images. ehealthinsurance.com/ehealthinsurance/expertcenter/Health Affairs_published_awareness.pdf. Accessed March 22, 2004.

60 Long S, Marquis M. Pooled purchasing: who are the players? *Health Aff (Millwood)*. 1999; 18: 105–111.

NATIONAL HEALTH INSURANCE OR INCREMENTAL REFORM: AIM HIGH, OR AT OUR FEET?

David U. Himmelstein and Steffie Woolhandler

Himmelstein and Woolhandler contend that adopting single-payer national health insurance is the only possible reform of American health care that can simultaneously achieve the goals of universal access, affordability, and broad choice of providers. According to the authors, savings on insurance overhead and other bureaucracy along with the elimination of profiteering would offset the costs of achieving universal access to a comprehensive array of benefits. Less drastic, piecemeal reforms, they argue, are insufficient to address the profound structural problems that plague the health-care status quo, as suggested both by previous reforms within the American system and by the experience of other developed nations. While champions of incremental reform claim the advantage of pragmatism, they have proven incapable of advancing meaningful reform through the political system; moreover, according to Himmelstein and Woolhandler, a far greater proportion of Americans favor national health insurance than is generally appreciated.

We advocate single-payer national health insurance (NHI) (Table 3) because it would work and lesser reforms would not. The policy establishment often portrays NHI as an impossible dream: an ultra-left, utopian vision. Yet, most other wealthy capitalist nations have implemented NHI, and it enjoys wide, even majority, public support in the United States.

Most would agree that our health-care system is deeply troubled. At least 41 million people residing in the United States have no health insurance, and millions more have inadequate coverage. Medical care costs are soaring, and job-based coverage is eroding. Public resources of enormous worth—hospitals, visiting nurse agencies, even hospices—built over decades by taxes, charity, and devoted volunteers, are being taken over by companies attentive to profits but indifferent to suffering.

Since the defeat of the Clintons' Rube Goldberg scheme for universal coverage, reform debate has been muted. But the fast developing medical care crisis—business grappling with soaring premiums, workers and unions fighting cutbacks in coverage, governments confronting deficits, and a sharp upturn in the number of individuals who are unemployed and uninsured—ensures a reopening of health policy debate.

From *American Journal of Public Health,* vol. 93, no. 1 (2003), pp. 102–105. Copyright © 2003 by the American Public Health Association.

THE LIMITS OF INCREMENTALISM

Since the passage of Medicare and Medicaid, a welter of incremental reforms have been attempted—and have failed. Health maintenance organizations (HMOs) and diagnosis-related groups promised to contain costs and free up funds to expand coverage. Billions have been allocated to expanding Medicaid, the State Children's Health Insurance Program, and similar state-based insurance programs for poor and near-poor citizens. Medicare and Medicaid have pushed managed care. Oregon essayed rationing; Massachusetts and Hawaii passed laws requiring all employers to cover their workers; Tennessee promised nearly universal coverage; and several states implemented risk pools to insure highcost individuals and insurance regulations to protect consumers.[1] Senators Kennedy and Kassebaum lent their names to insurance market reform legislation. And for-profit firms pledged that market discipline and businesslike efficiency would fix health care.

Fans of incrementalism dismiss NHI as a hopeless home run swing when a bunt—small steps toward universal coverage—would do. Despite incrementalists' claims of pragmatism, however, they have proven unable to shepherd meaningful reform through our political system. Over the past quarter century, incrementalists have trumpeted victories such as those detailed above. Meanwhile, the number

TABLE 3   Key Features of Single-Payer National Health Insurance

1. *Universal, comprehensive coverage:* Only such coverage ensures access, avoids a "two-class" system, and minimizes administrative expense

2. *No out-of-pocket payments:* Copayments and deductibles are barriers to access, administratively unwieldy, and unnecessary for cost containment

3. *A single insurance plan in each region, administered by a public or quasi-public agency:* A fragmentary payment system that entrusts private firms with administration ensures the waste of billions of dollars on useless paper-pushing and profits. Private insurance duplicating public coverage fosters two-class care and drives up costs; such duplication should be prohibited

4. *Global operating budgets for hospitals, nursing homes, HMOs, and other providers, with separate allocation of capital funds:* Billing on a per-patient basis creates unnecessary administrative complexity and expense. Allowing diversion of operating funds for capital investments or profits undermines health planning and intensifies incentives for unnecessary care (under fee for service) or undertreatment (in HMOs)

5. *Free choice of providers:* Patients should be free to seek care from any licensed health care provider, without financial incentives or penalties

6. *Public accountability, not corporate dictates:* The public has an absolute right to democratically set overall health policies and priorities, but medical decisions must be made by patients and providers rather than dictated from afar. Market mechanisms principally empower employers and insurance bureaucrats pursuing narrow financial interests

7. *Ban on for-profit health-care providers:* Profit-seeking inevitably distorts care and diverts resources from patients to investors

8. *Protection of the rights of health care and insurance workers:* A single-payer reform would eliminate the jobs of hundreds of thousands of people who currently perform billing, advertising, eligibility determination, and other superfluous tasks. These workers must be guaranteed retraining and placement in meaningful jobs

of uninsured individuals has increased by 18 million, health care's share of the gross domestic product has risen from 7.9 percent to 13.2 percent, and more and more seniors have been forced to choose between food and medicine. How many more strikes before incrementalism is out?

Incrementalism founders on a simple problem: expansion of coverage must increase costs unless resources are diverted from elsewhere in the system. US health costs are already nearly double those of any other nation and are rising rapidly.[2] The economic climate is cool. Yet, an incrementalist strategy implausibly posits massive infusions of new money, funds that would go mostly to the poor and near poor, who wield little political power. For instance, proposals to offer tax credits for the purchase of coverage would cost about $3000 annually per newly insured person.[3] Employer mandate proposals in California would boost public spending by between $4000 and $10,000 per newly insured person while also increasing employers' costs.[4]

Absent new money, patchwork reforms can expand coverage only by siphoning resources from existing clinical care. Advocates of managed care and market competition once argued that their strategy could accomplish this end by trimming clinical fat. Unfortunately, new layers of corporate bureaucrats have invariably overseen the managed care "diet" prescribed for clinicians and patients. Such cost management bureaucracies have devoured virtually all of the existing clinical savings and antagonized huge swaths of middle-class patients as well as the medical profession.

THE FISCAL CASE FOR NHI

The fiscal case for NHI arises from the observation that bureaucracy now consumes nearly 30 percent of our health-care budget,[5–7] as well as the fact that this enormous bureaucratic burden is a peculiarly American phenomenon. Our biggest HMOs keep 20 percent, even 25 percent, of premiums for their overhead and profit[8]; Canada's NHI has 1 percent overhead,[2] and even US Medicare takes less than 4 percent.[9] HMOs also inflict mountains of paperwork on clinicians and institutional providers. The average US hospital spends one-quarter of its budget on billing and administration, nearly twice the average in Canada.[7] American physicians spend far more time and money on paperwork and billing than their Canadian colleagues.[5] Administration consumes 35 percent of home care agency budgets in the United States, as opposed to 15.8 percent in Ontario (S. Woolhandler, T. Campbell, D.U. Himmelstein, unpublished data, 1999–2000).

Reducing our bureaucratic spending to Canadian levels would save at least $140 billion annually, enough to fully cover the uninsured and upgrade coverage among those now underinsured. Proponents of NHI,[10] disinterested civil servants,[11,12] and even skeptics[13] all agree on this point. NHI would require new taxes, but these taxes would be fully offset by a fall in insurance premiums and out-of-pocket costs. Moreover, the additional tax burden would be smaller than is usually appreciated, because nearly 60 percent of health spending is already tax supported[14] (vs roughly 70 percent in Canada).

Unfortunately, incremental tinkering cannot achieve significant bureaucratic savings. The key to administrative simplicity in Canada (and other nations) is singlesource payment through a public insurer. Canadian hospitals have a global annual budget to cover all costs—much as a health department is funded in the United States—virtually eliminating billing. Physicians bill a single insurer using a simple form, and fee schedules are negotiated annually between provincial medical associations and governments. In contrast, US providers face a welter of plans—at least 755 in Seattle alone[15]—each with its own rules and paperwork.

Even a step from one to two insurers raises providers' administrative costs. Fragmented coverage necessitates eligibility determination and internal cost accounting to attribute costs to individual patients and insurers and undermines global budgeting and health planning efforts. Although many assumed that computerization of billing would cut administrative costs, savings have not materialized.[16] While all nations with NHI have lower health administration costs than the United States, multipayer systems

sacrifice part of this advantage. Thus, Germany's health-care providers employ far more administrators and clerks than Canada's.[17] In the United Kingdom, the implementation of "internal markets" (in effect, a multipayer structure superimposed on the National Health Service) doubled administrative costs.[18]

For insurers, a multipayer structure requires duplication of claims processing facilities and reduces the size of the group that is insured, which increases overhead;[19,20] insurance overhead in the multipayer NHI systems of Germany and the Netherlands is at least double that in Canada.[2] Any degree of participation by private insurers also raises administrative costs.[21] Private insurers in Australia, Germany, and the Netherlands all have high overheads: 15.8 percent, 20.4 percent, and 10.4 percent, respectively.[2] Functions essential to private insurance but absent in public programs (e.g., underwriting and marketing) account for about two-thirds of private insurers' overhead.[22]

THE POLITICAL CASE FOR NHI

The political case for NHI arises from the fact that it would improve care for most Americans, not just the poor: solidarity is stronger than charity, a formulation we first heard from Vicente Navarro. NHI would not just expand current insurance arrangements; it would upgrade coverage for many in the middle class, assuage clinicians' and communities' concerns over the growing corporate dominance of care, and provide a framework for addressing the myriad problems exacerbated by our current irrational financing structure. These problems include the overuse of technology and neglect of caring, the extortionate profits of our drug industry, the imbalance between curative and preventive resources, the mismatch between health investments and need, and the multitude of quality problems that plague us (why is it that virtually every hospital in the United States has a complex computer billing system yet almost none have computerized order-entry systems that would prevent millions of medication errors?).

Among those who already have coverage, NHI would eliminate the fear that today's coverage will subsequently become unaffordable or disappear as a result of a strike, layoff, disabling illness, or college graduation. It would afford them a free choice of providers, a top priority for many Americans according to polls (hence the right-wing appropriation of terms such as "consumer choice health reform") but rare in today's managed care environment. It would encompass many services that are excluded from current coverage—notably long-term care, as well as prescription drugs for the elderly.

Among health workers, NHI can reduce the aggravation of bureaucratic hassles, dampen market-induced gyrations in the financial health of institutions and practices, and refocus the attention of health leaders from profits to health improvement. NHI offers reassurance for health workers and communities now fearful that a distant corporate board may discontinue vital but unprofitable services.

In contrast, incremental reforms divide our potential supporters, proposing fixes for the problems of the uninsured, seniors, disgruntled HMO members, and unhappy physicians and nurses in separate pieces of legislation that compete for resources. And the fundamental problem of corporate control of our health-care system remains unaddressed.

Paradoxically, despite the shift from a Democratic to a Republican administration and the recent assault on social spending and civil liberties, the political climate may be favorable to NHI. The recent spate of corporate scandals has spread appreciation of the corruption and inefficiency of private firms.

Moreover, the corporate class is confused and divided over what should be done about health care, opening space for debate. Between 2000 and 2002, the percentage of employers who thought the health-care system was working "pretty well" declined by 37 percent.[23] Some within business are drawn to voucher schemes (e.g., the defined-contribution program that our own university recently implemented and President Bush's "premium support" proposal for Medicare) that are thinly veiled mechanisms to cut care. Others, however, recognize that such schemes cannot stabilize the health-care system or provide sufficient care to ensure workers' productivity and labor peace. NHI is attractive to some corporate leaders because it would socialize the costs of employee benefits (improving their competitive position vis-à-vis firms in other countries), although this would deprive employers of some of their bar-

gaining leverage. Forty percent of small business owners now favor single-payer NHI.[24]

Predictably, these corporate divisions will soon be reflected in an uptick in media attention to NHI. For a decade the virtual media blackout on NHI has been broken only for occasional assaults on Canada's program. Many of these stories trumpeted the lunatic assertions of rightwing fringe groups (e.g., a recent claim that Canada's health-care system was comparable to Turkey's[25]). Others dramatized the real problems that emerged in Canada during the early 1990s, a period during which health care was starved of funds by governments responsive to pressure from the wealthy, who sought to avoid cross-subsidizing care for the sick and poor.

Whereas once Canadian and US health spending were comparable, today Canada spends barely half (per capita) what we do.[2] Shortages of expensive, high-technology care have resulted. Yet, Canada's health outcomes remain better than ours (e.g., life expectancy in Canada is two years longer[2]), and most quality comparisons indicate that Canadians enjoy care equivalent to that for insured Americans; few Canadians cross the border seeking care.[26] Few if any reporters have noted that a system structured in a manner similar to Canada's, but with double the funding, could deliver high-quality care without the waits or shortages that Canadians have experienced.

The media and policy wonks' dismissal of NHI is remarkable in the face of polls that have consistently shown wide popular support for such reform. While NHI may seem ultra left in the policy milieu, it is dead center in public opinion and even in the opinion of physicians. Even the most negatively phrased surveys reveal that 40 percent of Americans are in favor of single-payer NHI; more sympathetic phrasing elicits support from about 60 percent,[27] polling numbers that have not changed since Richard Nixon was advocating policies that have since become Ted Kennedy's. The Democrats' abandonment of NHI reflects an ideological shift in the party, not in the populace. Indeed, today 62 percent of Massachusetts physicians favor singlepayer NHI.[28] Is any other policy position that enjoys so much support treated so dismissively? Only 17 percent of Americans want to see abortion outlawed![29]

In the name of pragmatism, some public health leaders and many politicians counsel us to abandon, or indefinitely delay, the fight for NHI. To them, corporate power appears unchallengeable and politics so polluted that decent public policy is unthinkable. From this perspective, one would advise Rosa Parks to forgo her futile gesture given the dismal political milieu of 1955.

Rosa Parks understood that even apparently stable systems can change dramatically and unexpectedly, a point also made repeatedly by evolutionary biologist Stephen Jay Gould. The months ahead will see rising pressure for change in our medical care system. Predictably, employers will attempt to shift costs to workers, and governments will attempt to balance budgets on the backs of the poor and the sick. Our tottering medical care system need not veer in that direction, however; a lurch toward NHI is also possible.

In the coming months, our task is to break the iron curtain of media and political silence on NHI. We urge colleagues to publicly endorse NHI (see http://www.physiciansproposal.org) and to enlist other individuals and organizations in the fight for NHI. We are convinced that a striking show of support for NHI among health professionals would uniquely capture public attention, setting in motion vital public discussion of health care's future. For generations, the moral stance of the public health community has helped spark social movements, often against dauntingly powerful foes: the crusade against tobacco and fights for clean water, a sustainable environment, workplace safety, and reproductive rights. Our professions' voices gain extraordinary resonance when we speak courageously in the public interest. A time to raise our cry is again at hand.

CONTRIBUTORS

D. U. Himmelstein and S. Woolhandler participated equally in the writing of this article.

REFERENCES

1 Marquis MS, Long SH. Effects of "second generation" small group health insurance market reforms, 1993 to 1997. *Inquiry.* 2001; 38:365–380.

2 *OECD Health Data 2001* [computer database]. Paris, France: Organization for Economic Cooperation and Development; 2001.

3 Glied SA. Challenges and options for increasing the number of Americans with health insurance. *Inquiry.* 2001; 38:90–105.

4 Lewin Group. Cost and coverage analysis of nine proposals to expand health insurance coverage in California. Available at: http://www.healthcareoptions.ca.gov/final/CA%20 Report%20%20MediCal.pdf. Accessed September 6, 2002.

5 Woolhandler S, Himmelstein DU. The deteriorating administrative efficiency of U.S. health care. *N Engl J Med.* 1991; 324:1253–1258.

6 Himmelstein DU, Lewontin JP, Woolhandler S. Who administers? Who cares? Medical administrative and clinical employment in the United States and Canada. *Am J Public Health.* 1996; 86:172–178.

7 Woolhandler S, Himmelstein DU. Costs of care and administration at forprofit and other hospitals in the United States. *N Engl J Med.* 1997; 336:769–774.

8 Special report. *BestWeek Life/ Health.* April 12, 1999.

9 Heffler S, Levit K, Smith S, et al. Health spending growth up in 1999; faster growth expected in the future. *Health Aff.* 2001; 20(2):193–203.

10 Grumbach K, Bodenheimer T, Woolhandler S, Himmelstein DU. Liberal benefits, conservative spending: the Physicians for a National Health Program proposal. *JAMA.* 1991; 265: 2549–2554.

11 *Canadian Health Insurance: Lessons for the United States.* Washington, DC: US General Accounting Office; 1991. GAO publication HRD-91-90.

12 *Universal Health Insurance Coverage Using Medicare's Payment Rates.* Washington, DC: Congressional Budget Office; 1991.

13 Sheils JF, Haught RA. *Analysis of the Costs and Impact of Universal Health Care Coverage Under a Single Payer Model for the State of Vermont.* Falls Church, Va: Lewin Group Inc; 2001.

14 Woolhandler S, Himmelstein DU. Paying for national health insurance and not getting it. *Health Aff.* 2002; 21(4):88–98.

15 Grembowski DE, Diehr P, Novak LC, et al. Measuring the "managedness" and covered benefits of health plans. *Health Serv Res.* 2000; 35:707–734.

16 Kleinke JD. Vaporware.com: the failed promise of the health care Internet. *Health Aff.* 2000; 19(6):57–71.

17 Himmelstein DU, Lewontin JP, Woolhandler S. *The Health Care Labor Force in the U.S., Canada and Germany—An Analysis Based on Census Data.* Washington, DC: US Office of Technology Assessment; 1993.

18 Rowland D, Pollock AM, Vickers N. The British Labour government's reform of the National Health Service. *J Public Health Policy.* 2001; 22:403–413.

19 *Cost and Effects of Extending Health Insurance Coverage.* Washington, DC: Congressional Research Service, Library of Congress; 1988.

20 Pauly M, Percy A, Herring B. Individual versus jobbased health insurance: weighing the pros and cons. *Health Aff.* 1999; 18(6):28–44.

21 Leigh JP, Bernstein J. Public and private workers' compensation insurance. *J Occup Environ Med.* 1997; 39:119–121.

22 Sherlock Co. Administrative expense benchmarks by health plans. Available at: http://www.sherlockco.com/seerbackground.htm. Accessed June 26, 2002.

23 HarrisInteractive. Attitudes toward the United States' health care system: long term trends. Available at: http://www.harrisinteractive.com/news/newsletters/healthnews/HI_HealthCare-News2002Vol2_Iss17.pdf. Accessed September 8, 2002.

24 *National Survey of Small Businesses*. Menlo Park, Calif: Kaiser Family Foundation; 2002.

25 Beaudan E. Canadian model of healthcare ails. *Christian Science Monitor*. August 28, 2002.

26 Katz SJ, Cardiff K, Pascali M, Barer ML, Evans RG. Phantoms in the snow: Canadians' use of health care services in the United States. *Health Aff.* 2002; 21(3):19–31.

27 Blendon RJ, Benson JM. Americans' views on health policy: a 50-year historical perspective. *Health Aff.* 2001; 20(2):33–46.

28 McCormick D, Woolhandler S, Himmelstein DU, Bor DH. View of single payer national health insurance: a survey of Massachusetts physicians. *J Gen Intern Med.* 2002; 17(suppl):204.

29 Saad L. Public opinion about abortion—an indepth review. Available at: http://www.gallup.com/poll/specialReports/pollSummaries/sr020122.asp. Accessed September 6, 2002.

THE PROBLEM WITH SINGLE-PAYER PLANS

Ezekiel J. Emanuel

Emanuel argues that while single-payer plans (such as that defended by Himmelstein and Woolhandler) are popular among liberals, they represent a fundamentally flawed approach to health-care reform. It is true, he concedes, that single-payer plans can easily achieve universal coverage while eliminating various administrative costs such as insurance underwriting, sales, and marketing. It is also true, he allows, that American health care is in urgent need of overhaul. But the single-payer approach, according to Emanuel, has these substantial disadvantages: (1) It would preserve our dysfunctional, fee-for-service system of delivering health care without reliable instruments for assessing and improving quality of care; (2) While saving impressively on administrative costs, the *total* costs of this approach—including those of unchecked fraud and abuse—are likely to be great; (3) It lacks a credible plan for stemming health-care inflation over time; and (4) It is vulnerable to politicized decision-making regarding funding and coverage.

Many liberals in America dream about single-payer plans. Even if they acknowledge that a single-payer plan cannot be enacted, they still think it the best reform. Another proposal may be politically necessary to achieve universal coverage, but it would be a compromise, a fall-back. Single payer is the ideal.

This is wrong. Even in theory, single payer is not the best reform option. Here's the problem: while it proposes the most radical reform of the health-care financing system, it is conservative, even nostalgic, when it comes to the broken delivery system. It retains and solidifies the nineteenth century,

fragmented, fee-for-service delivery system that provides profligate and bad quality care.

. . .

Reform of the American health-care system needs to address problems with both the financing and the delivery systems. As proponents of single-payer systems note, the financing system is inequitable, inefficient, and unsustainable. There are now forty-seven million uninsured Americans, about 70 percent of whom are in families with full-time workers. Wealthy individuals receive much higher tax breaks than the poor, and insurance premiums are a larger percent of wages for those working at low wages and in small businesses. Many working poor and lower middle class Americans pay taxes to support

Medicaid and SCHIP, yet are excluded from these programs. The employer-based and individual market parts of the financing system are inefficient because they have huge administrative costs, especially related to insurance underwriting, sales, and marketing. The government part of the finance system is inefficient because it fails to address key policy issues, fraud, and—for Medicaid—complex determinations of eligibility. Over the last three decades, health-care costs have risen 2–4 percent over growth in the overall economy. Medicaid is now the largest part of state budgets, forcing states to cut other programs.

But the delivery system is also fraught with problems. First, it is badly fragmented. Currently, 75 percent of physicians practice in groups of eight or less. Of the one billion office visits each year, one-third are to solo practitioners, and one-third are to groups of four or fewer physicians. On average, each year Medicare beneficiaries see seven different physicians, who are financially, clinically, and administratively uncoordinated.

A second problem is that the delivery system is structured for acute care, but the contemporary need is for chronic care. Over 133 million Americans have chronic conditions, and among Americans sixty-five and older, 75 percent have two or more chronic conditions, and 20 percent have five chronic conditions. Consequently, 70 percent of health-care costs are devoted to patients with chronic conditions.

Also, the care that the system delivers is of much poorer quality than Americans realize. Use of unproven, nonbeneficial, marginal, or harmful services is common. The list of offending interventions that are paid for and widely used but either unproven or of marginal benefit to patients is vast—IMRT and proton beam for early prostate cancer, CT and MRI angiograms, Epogen for chemotherapy induced anemia, Erbitux and Avastin for colorectal cancer, and drug-eluting stents for coronary artery disease. Stanford researchers recently showed that between 15 and 20 percent of prescriptions are written for indications for which there is absolutely no published data supporting their use.[1] The Dartmouth studies on variation in practices demonstrate that for many interventions, more services are not better. For instance, heart attack patients in Miami receive vastly more care than similar patients in Minnesota at 2.45 times the cost, yet have slightly worse outcomes.[2]

. . .

In the context of reforming the American health-care system, "single payer" has come to be associated with three key reforms: *a single national plan* for all Americans, *reduced administrative costs*, and *negotiated prices* for hospitals and physicians and perhaps for health-care goods and services, such as drugs. Single-payer plans have two huge advantages.

First, single-payer plans clearly provide for universal health-care coverage. Unlike Massachusetts-style individual mandate reform proposals, single-payer plans do not achieve 95 percent or 97 percent coverage, but true 100 percent coverage for all Americans.

Second, single-payer plans enhance the efficiency of the health-care financing system by eliminating the wasteful costs of insurance underwriting, sales, and marketing. This could save between $60 and $100 billion. Similarly, a single-payer plan with a formulary and negotiated prices would be able to reduce drug costs. McKinsey Global Institute has estimated that bringing drug costs in the United States down to those of other developed countries would save the U.S. system $57 billion.[3] This is a huge and real savings, enough to cover all the uninsured and probably expand the range of covered services to include dental care and other items.

The problem with single-payer plans is that they have an assortment of serious structural problems. To wit:

Institutionalized Fee-for-Service Single-payer plans would preserve the dysfunctional delivery system. We know two things about how to reform the delivery system. First, because no one yet has the secret formula for delivering the best quality health care, a real reform of the financing system needs to foster innovation in delivery and then measure the delivery system to find out what changes improve quality. Second, while the overall contours of reform are unknown, there is a clear need for better integration and coordination of care. Integration requires three *I*'s—infrastructure, information, and incentives. Better delivery of care needs an infrastructure that coordinates doctors, hospitals, home health care agencies, and other providers administratively, fiscally, and clinically. They need to share information easily. And there have to be incentives for this coordination. It will not happen spontaneously.

The problem is that a single-payer approach uses fee-for-service reimbursement to entrench the existing delivery system. Retaining and institutionalizing the fee-for-service payment model would quash the ability to integrate care. Solo practitioners or small groups would have no incentive—financial or otherwise—for integration and coordination of care across providers.

Also, single-payer reform is hostile to the very organizations that have the financial and administrative capacity to build the infrastructure and information systems for the coordinated care delivery systems: insurance companies and health plans. If there is to be an infrastructure for integration of services, information-sharing, and incentives for collaboration, some organization has to develop and implement it. Call it what you will, that organization would look a lot like a health insurance company. (Some might argue that the Veterans Affair's health system is a single-payer system that does a great job of coordinating and integrating care. True, but it covers only thirteen million people. In essence, the VA is a big health plan, like Kaiser. There is no way a single administrative body can efficiently coordinate care for three hundred million people.) In the current system, the financial incentives for health insurance companies lead to perverse behaviors, such as avoiding sick patients. But single-payer plans eliminate not only their problems, but also their potential benefits.

Deceptive Administrative Savings There is no doubt that a single-payer system would produce huge administrative savings, but low administrative costs should not be confused with low total health care costs.

Very low administrative costs in Medicare create an opening for fraud and abuse. The last assessment by the Inspector General of the Department of Health and Human Services occurred in 1996. At that time, the IG estimated that Medicare made about $23.2 billion in improper payments due to insufficient or absent documentation, incorrect billing,

billing for excluded services, and other problems. In 1996, Medicare spent about $200 billion. Thus, fraud was over 10 percent of total Medicare costs. (I leave it to you to imagine why the government has not repeated this assessment in the last decade.) True, the Canadian single-payer system does not report high levels of fraud and abuse, but Canada is not the United States. Canada's population is about one-tenth that of the United States, and Canadians believe in good government.

Furthermore, a plan covering all Americans would be much larger than Medicare. It would have to process more than one billion physician visits, forty million hospitalizations, and 3.7 billion prescriptions each year. This would require sophisticated information technology, but that technology would be a major administrative cost, and keeping it updated could be politically difficult. As we have seen in the IRS and the FBI, there is great aversion to spending money on major IT upgrades.

Finally, monitoring the quality of care delivered to patients also constitutes an administrative expense. It is an administrative burden to systematically assess whether new technologies like cancer genetic fingerprints are in fact beneficial, whether new surgical procedures really lead to longer life, and whether new ways of preparing patients for surgery and handling intravenous lines reduce infections and hospital days.

Nothing would absolutely prohibit single-payer plans from spending more money on administration to detect fraud, improve computerization, address payment issues, and assess quality. Nothing, that is, but a strong ideological commitment to keeping administrative expenses very, very low. The war cry for single-payer plans is very low administrative costs, but repeatedly touting this advantage creates a line in the sand. Indeed, it may exacerbate the inflexibility of a single-payer plan. Because of its size, any agency administering a single-payer plan would have a built-in tendency toward inertia. Further, striving to keep administrative costs low would translate into hiring fewer people to manage the system. Fewer people would mean less expertise for addressing problems and less time to search for creative solutions. This is a prescription for inflexibility and lack of innovation.

Ineffective Cost-Control Strategies Efficiency savings from reduced administrative costs or cheaper drug prices should not be confused with controlling costs overall. Efficiencies, such as reducing administrative waste, are one-time savings. *Controlling costs* means reducing the increase in medical spending year after year. Single-payer plans use the savings from efficiencies to extend coverage to the uninsured and expand covered services without raising the total amount spent on health care. But these one-time savings do not attack the fundamental forces that drive health-care cost inflation. Unless there is some mechanism to control those pressures, the one-time savings would be used up in a few years, and overall health-care spending would go higher and higher. How can single-payer plans respond to this health-care inflation?

There are three possible approaches. One is to "constrain the supply": use the national health plan's control to constrain the introduction and deployment of technology. A single-payer plan could decide to limit the number of MRI scanners, for example. Indeed, in the Physicians' Working Group proposal, the national health plan would negotiate with hospitals on capital expansion and could easily limit how many hospitals can build facilities for MRI scanners or new specialized surgical suites.[4] This strategy creates queuing for access to the technology. As every major country trying this has learned, queuing creates huge public resentment. People on the waiting list get furious at the central administration. Americans, especially the upper middle class, are unlikely to tolerate it.

Constraining supply also promotes gaming of the system and inequality. When technology is limited, patients—and physicians—try to jump the queue. Physicians are not great at creating priority lists based on medical need. Particularly when they have their own practices, their obligation is to their individual patients, not to ensuring that other physicians' patients get care and not to promoting the overall health of the population.

Countries that have tried this approach have found, not surprisingly, that such gaming tends to favor well-off patients. In many facets of life, well-off people have learned how to come out on top in situations where there are limits. Limits on health-care technology gives them one more setting in which their greater gaming skills can be deployed. A study in Winnipeg, Canada, showed that although all Canadians were legally entitled to the same services, the well-off had substantially better access to high technology services that were constrained.[5]

A second approach, a variant of "constrain the supply," is a "low prices and fees" approach. As the only organization paying physicians, hospitals, drug companies, and other health providers, a national health plan would have a huge incentive to squeeze down on fees. This would keep costs down, and since providers would have no one else to turn to, they would have limited recourse.

The United States government uses this low-price approach in Medicaid and Medicare. To save money, every so often Congress or the Medicare administrators roll back the fees paid to hospitals, physicians, and others. Then, just as predictably, those groups scream that they are going broke and lobby Congress to increase the fees. And so the see-saw goes on—prices rolled back and then increased after lobbying. This does not end up saving much, in part because how much is paid out depends not only on the fee or price but also on the volume—on how much is done. So one way physicians respond to lower fees is to ramp up volume; they see a lot of patients for shorter and shorter times. This is easily done because for many diseases there are no data on how often patients should be seen in the physician's office. And it is exactly how Canadian health insurance administrators kept fees low.

The British National Health Service used to do exactly what the Physicians' Working Group wants to do: It paid hospitals a fixed price for operating expenses and controlled capital expenditures to limit expansion and the purchase of new technologies. The result: the hospitals put off maintenance and began falling apart. They put off cleaning and became filthy. They could not buy new equipment or adapt quickly to changes in medical practice. Eventually, even the stiff-upper-lip British rebelled. The British National Health Service reversed course and recently gave hospitals the ability to make their own decisions, including decisions to raise funds or float bonds to expand or buy new technologies.

Both "constrain the supply" and "low prices and fees" are centralized, micromanaging cost control techniques. You do not have to be a die-hard capitalist to think they are bad techniques. Most left-leaning economists agree that it is better to develop incentives and let the market control costs than to have government set prices or supply.

The third approach to cost control in a single-payer system is that adopted by Medicare in the United States: do nothing, and just pay whatever bill comes in. Let the costs go through the roof. The crisis will come later—after the current administrators and politicians are long gone. This is probably why a *New York Times* editorial said, "Even in fantasy, no one has yet come up with a way to pay for Medicare."[6]

These three options are what most single-payer systems in the world have done. None works, and all have long-term consequences.

Politicized Decision-Making As Michael Millenson, a health policy consultant, remarks, when single-payer advocates think about who would run the national health plan, they think of Ted Kennedy. But, he asks, what if the head were Dick Cheney? Medicare reveals what is likely to happen if we have a single-payer plan. Every Medicare decision is subject to political pressure from somewhere. When Medicare tries to lower hospital fees or equalize payments, hospitals pressure their representatives and senators for increases in payments. Patient advocacy groups lobby to have Medicare pay for their favorite technology or treatment. Drug companies use campaign contributions—and patient advocacy groups—to prevent a Medicare formulary and forbid price negotiations that might limit their profits. The

result is that Medicare decisions are made slowly, and rarely on their merits. No federal administrative agency can be completely free of political influence. But single-payer reform plans tend to ignore the importance of administrative independence.

The ideal reform must address not only the inequitable, inefficient, and unsustainable financing system, but also the fragmented delivery system. And it must develop a plan that creates an accountable and innovative delivery system overseen by a (relatively) independent agency that can make hard administrative choices.

REFERENCES

1 D.C. Radley, S.N. Finkelstein, and R.S. Stafford, "Off-Label Prescribing among Office-Based Physicians," *Archives of Internal Medicine* 166, no. 9 (2006): 1021–26.

2 E.S. Fisher, D.E. Wennberg, T.A. Stukel, and D.J. Gottlieb, "Variations in the Longitudinal Efficiency of Academic Medical Centers." *Health Affairs* Web exclusive, October 7, 2004, http://content.healthaffairs.org/cgi/content/full/hlthaff. var.19/DC3.

3 C. Angrisano, D. Farrell, B. Kocher, M. Laboissiere, and S. Parker, "Accounting for the Cost of Health Care in the United States" (The McKinsey Global Institute, 2004), http://www.mckinsey.com/mgi/reports/pdfs/healthcare/ MGI_US_HC_fullreport.pdf.

4 "Proposal of the Physicians' Working Group for Single-Payer National Health Insurance" (Physicians for a National Health Program, 2006), http://www.pnhp.org/publications/proposal_ of_the_ physicians_working_group_for_single-payer_ national_health_ insurance.php.

5 D.A. Alter, A.S. Basinski, E.A. Cohen, and C.D. Naylor, "Fairness in the Coronary Angiography Queue," *Canadian Medical Association Journal* 161, no. 7 (1999): 813–17.

6 "Talking Deficits," *New York Times* opinion, May 23, 2004.

VOUCHSAFE
Ezekiel J. Emanuel and Victor R. Fuchs

After criticizing the "individual mandate" approach to health-care reform, Emanuel and Fuchs sketch their own proposal: a form of managed competition in which all American citizens (or their families) would receive vouchers entitling them to their choice of qualifying health plans. Under this proposal, each year every individual or family representative would have the opportunity to select among five to eight competing plans. All would be free and no plan could turn away applicants. Individuals would also be free to purchase health-care services beyond what is covered by their plan. Regional boards would pay each plan based on the number of enrollees for that year, adjusting payments so that plans attracting sicker enrollees would be compensated more for them. In order to generate funds to pay the plans, the federal government would repeal the tax exemption of employer-sponsored health insurance, raising $200 billion per year, and would institute a value-added tax dedicated exclusively to health care. Addressing the politically sensitive issue of creating a new tax, Emanuel and Fuchs contend that the latter would be offset by various savings: Medicaid would be eliminated; Medicare would be phased out over time (accepting no new enrollees); wages would increase as employers were freed from the need to pay for health insurance; and individuals would no longer have to pay premiums. Finally, the authors argue, costs would be controlled over time by (1) competition of health plans in a well-structured market and (2) the tethering of any increase in federal health-care spending to a proportionate increase in the value-added tax.

Requiring People to buy health insurance as if it were a driver's license has become the health-care policy initiative *du jour.* This "individual mandate" model got its first official embrace when former Massachusetts Governor Mitt Romney, working with his Democratic state legislature, used such a scheme to cover all state residents. In January, California Governor Arnold Schwarzenegger proposed to implement a similar program. And, within the last few days, former Senator John Edwards, a leading Democratic presidential candidate, proposed using the same basic structure on a national scale.

It's great that so many prominent public officials are embracing universal health care, an idea whose time has clearly come. But it's not great to see these public officials embracing such a flawed model of reform. These reforms don't envision a wholesale reinvention of U.S. health care. Instead, they attempt to graft universal coverage onto existing arrangements. That's a mistake, because only comprehensive reforms will eliminate the inefficiencies and perverse incentives of the existing system—a series of flaws that leaves Americans with the worst of all worlds. In the United States, life expectancy is lower and infant mortality is higher than it is in other developed countries. Even so, the United States spends $7,000 per person per year on health care—almost twice as much as is spent on citizens of other high-income countries.

Proponents of individual mandates and other, more incremental reforms insist they are merely being practical—that, if you try to give everybody insurance *and* make it more efficient, the political system will reject it. But there may be a politically realistic way to establish universal coverage while addressing the more fundamental flaws in U.S. health care. It's an idea we first introduced two years ago: universal health vouchers.

Ideally, health-care reform ought to accomplish several goals, starting with universality: All Americans should be covered by a high-quality basic plan, which they can keep whether they change jobs or marital status. But there are other critical goals, too. Americans want to be able to choose their hospital and physicians; they want the ability to change health plans and to buy extra services. Quality is obviously essential; care should be clinically sound and safe. And then there is efficiency. Over time, expenditures should not rise faster than can be justified by higher national income and advances in health care.

Even the most thoughtfully constructed individual mandate reform can make only partial progress on these fronts. An individual mandate would prop up employment-based insurance, which is inefficient and inequitable. It would also increase the number of Americans dependent on income-tested subsidies for programs like Medicaid, which runs up administrative costs (government has to sort out who's eligible for assistance) while providing many of these people with substandard insurance (since the programs' low reimbursements frequently limit access to doctors).

An individual mandate would not address major problems in the organization and delivery of care, nor would it end the squandering of money on lavish executive salaries and perks. And, precisely because an individual mandate would leave the present system for financing medical care fundamentally intact, it's hard to see how it would do much to reduce current overall costs—or future inflation.

A voucher scheme, by contrast, seems far more likely to accomplish these goals. Here's how it would work: Once a year, all Americans would choose a health plan from among five to eight alternatives. All the plans would be free. All the plans would also meet certain criteria—minimal co-payments and deductibles, plus benefits modeled (initially) on those in the Federal Employee Health Benefit Plan. By law, the plans could not discriminate among customers. They would have to accept anybody and promise unconditional renewal, regardless of preexisting medical conditions or other factors that might put people at higher risk of getting sick.

Who would make the decisions about which plans people could buy? Regional health boards would screen the plans and then monitor their performance over time, using criteria set by a federal health board—with the whole system operating like the Federal Reserve system now does. The health boards would also be responsible for paying the plans. Money would come down from the federal health board, which would decide how to divide health-care funds geographically. At that point, the regional boards would pay each plan, based on the number of enrollees in any given year—but with one key adjustment. The regional boards would adjust payments so that plans attracting sicker beneficiaries would get more money. This, along with the prohibitions on denying coverage to people with preexisting conditions, would prevent insurers from profiting by cherry-picking the healthiest subscribers.

So that's how the money would get from the health boards to the health plans. But how would the health boards get their money in the first place? Under the scheme we have in mind, the money would come from the federal government, which would, in turn, draw upon two revenue sources. First, the government would repeal the existing tax exemption on employer-sponsored health insurance— an exemption that would become obsolete once employers stopped providing their workers with basic insurance. That change would raise $200 billion a year. To cover the remaining cost—some $750 billion a year initially—the government would then impose a value-added tax (VAT). Businesses pay VAT at every step of the production and distribution process, adding the cost as they go, so that at the end of the line—when a consumer pays for a good—the consumer ends up picking up the tab at higher prices. The new VAT would be "dedicated," generating money only for health care. A tax of between 10 and 12 percent should be enough to pay for our scheme.

That may sound like a lot—imposing, in effect, a 10 to 12 percent national sales tax—but average Americans would come out ahead. As employers stopped spending money on employee health benefits, wages would go up by 10 to 13 percent. Meanwhile, Americans would no longer have to pay any premiums whatsoever for basic medical coverage. The voucher program would phase out Medicaid and, eventually, Medicare; and, as the programs disappeared, the taxes that support them would disappear, too, leaving the average American even better off. (Medicare would not enroll new members, but it would continue to serve current enrollees until they died or decided—as some might—to opt for the voucher system instead.)

Admittedly, using a VAT would be controversial, because some people believe VATs are too regressive. But the program as a whole would be highly progressive. Indeed, all countries that provide universal health care have a VAT—including the Scandinavian countries, the Netherlands, and Germany. Many liberal analysts, such as Robert H. Frank in *Luxury Fever* and Ed McCaffery in *Fair Not Flat: How to Make the Tax System Better and Simpler,* have recommended a VAT because it taxes spending, not work or saving.

Overall, a voucher system would certainly cost no more than the present system. And, over time, it would actually cost less, as it would hold down health-care inflation. Since the VAT money would be "dedicated," the amount collected from the VAT would set a hard limit on the cost of the basic benefits package—and, ultimately, the services that insurance coverage could purchase. The amount collected would rise as the economy grew. But, if Americans wanted health care spending to grow even more rapidly, they would have to agree to a higher VAT rate. In other words, there would be no open-ended entitlement leading to open-ended inflation, as there is today.

The voucher system would also foster competition among health plans. Because health plans would get a fixed payment per enrollee in exchange for providing a defined set of benefits, they would have to compete for enrollees based on quality and service. They would have a strong incentive to be efficient and to collaborate with their doctors and hospitals to cut down on waste and marginal medical services. Americans who wanted additional services could still get them. But, to do so, they'd have to spend their own after-tax dollars—giving them an incentive to spend judiciously and get value for their money.

To further cut down on costs, we propose using a small portion of the VAT to fund a new, independent Institute of Technology and Outcomes Assessment that would evaluate the effectiveness, cost, and value of new technologies and new applications of existing technologies. The data developed by the Institute would ensure that technologies added to the basic benefit package by the federal health board would be cost-effective. These reports, in turn, would send a signal to drug and device companies to focus their research and development on cost-effective interventions.

These steps would amount to an ambitious overhaul of U.S. health care. But an ambitious overhaul is exactly what U.S. health care needs. Pushing for lesser solutions is the policy equivalent of prescribing aspirin and Band-Aids for cancer—in other words, a form of malpractice.

SINGLE PAYER MEETS MANAGED COMPETITION: THE CASE FOR PUBLIC FUNDING AND PRIVATE DELIVERY

David DeGrazia

After arguing that health-care reform is urgently needed and criticizing various reform proposals, DeGrazia develops the case for merging single-payer finance with managed competition in the delivery of health care. His critique cites various features of multiple-payer systems (e.g., bloated administrative costs, adverse selection) that makes them unlikely to achieve basic goals of health-care reform. The defense of single-payer finance cites extensive empirical evidence that single-payer systems are the most cost-effective way of achieving universal access while protecting patient freedom and maintaining quality of care. An extended reply to objections against the single-payer approach (including some advanced by Emanuel), he argues, neutralizes most objections while leaving intact a few concerns regarding the need for proper incentives in the delivery system. DeGrazia then argues that permitting carefully regulated competition among health plans—in addition to a public system with fee-for-service reimbursement—provides a satisfactory response to the residual concerns. Ultimately, he defends a structural and political compromise between traditional single-payer plans (as represented by Himmelstein and Woolhandler) and managed competition (as represented by Emanuel and Fuchs).

Reprinted, with minor adaptations, by permission of the publisher and author from *Hastings Center Report,* vol. 38, no. 1 (2008), pp. 23–33. Copyright © 2008 by The Hastings Center.

American health care is a terrible mess. Over forty-six million Americans—about 16 percent of the population—lack health insurance; millions more are underinsured.[1] Those lacking health insurance face serious consequences. The Institute of Medicine puts it bluntly: "Uninsured children and adults suffer worse health and die sooner than those with insurance."[2] Moreover, an estimated eighteen thousand unnecessary deaths occur every year in the United States due to lack of insurance.[3] A further consequence for many families is threatened financial security. Meanwhile, the cost of forgoing needed medical services is enormous: an estimated $65–$130 billion per year,[4] exceeding what some leading experts consider necessary to cover all the uninsured.[5] Lack of reliable, continuous access to health care is an intolerable feature of our health-care system.

Other features are also dispiriting. Despite not covering nearly one of every six Americans, we spend *far* more on health care per capita (including the uninsured), and as a fraction of gross domestic product, than do citizens of any other country.[6] Since 2000, overall health-care expenditures have risen at roughly 10 percent per year.[7] American car companies buckle under the strain of paying health insurance premiums. Meanwhile, insured patients frequently complain that insurance companies restrict their choice of doctors and impose bureaucratic hassles. And for years there has been a widespread perception—whether accurate or not—that managed care has damaged quality of care.[8] On the whole, the public is increasingly dissatisfied with American health care.[9] Considering this widespread dissatisfaction, and with Democrats reclaiming power in Congress, it's no surprise that health care reform is back as a leading issue of domestic policy. . . .

At this point, we need to identify the goals of health-care reform. Although perfect unanimity on this matter is impossible, the following four goals enjoy widespread support among Americans and will serve as benchmarks for evaluating proposals for reform: (1) achieving universal coverage; (2) establishing cost controls; (3) enhancing—or at least not diminishing—patients' freedom of choice while minimizing bureaucratic hassle; and (4) sustaining the quality of care.[10]

But are these goals simultaneously achievable? Are they compatible? The best evidence that they are compatible and achievable is the fact that numerous countries have achieved them fairly well. The health-care systems of these countries—including the United Kingdom, Germany, the Netherlands, France, Italy, Sweden, and Canada—all face difficulties, often because of meager funding. But looking at the big picture, all of these countries have universal coverage *while spending far less on health care than we do.* Meanwhile, patients in these countries enjoy considerable freedom of choice, seem less hassled by paperwork and other bureaucracy than we are, and enjoy a quality of care that appears comparable to that enjoyed by well-insured Americans.[11] The basic goals of health care, though in tension with each other, are compatible and achievable—not to utopian levels, but satisfactorily. The urgency of reform must not be obscured by overly pessimistic assumptions.

My thesis is that a single-payer system of national health insurance appears to be the most cost-effective way of achieving the major goals of health care, and is therefore the most morally defensible reform model. As we will see, the single-payer approach offers the most advantages and the fewest disadvantages *when integrated with managed competition in delivery.*

. . .

THE PROPOSALS

The reforms currently on the table fall into six types, which can also be combined in various ways.

Market Reforms The American Medical Association has proposed insurance market regulations, including modified community rating (in which only age and gender would affect premium rates) and guaranteed insurance renewability. These features, the AMA contends, would encourage "consumers" to remain longer with the same insurers, lowering the latter's administrative costs and thereby leading to lower premiums.[12]

Tax Credits A tax credit for the purchase of health insurance is an amount that can be subtracted from the tax one owes. A refundable tax credit permits those who owe no income tax to receive a government payment that can be spent to purchase insurance. One way to ensure funds for tax credits would be to end the federal income tax exclusion of employer-provided insurance. This system deprives the government annually of well over $100 billion of tax revenue. It is also a regressive tax structure: it exempts those fortunate enough to have insurance through their work from paying progressively income-graduated taxes on the employer-paid premiums.[13]

Individual Mandates These would legally require adults who lack health insurance to purchase it for themselves and their dependents. In April 2006, Massachusetts passed such a law,[14] though without the income-related subsidies necessary to achieve universal coverage.[15]

Employer Mandates This measure would require employers to "play or pay": either provide health insurance for their workers or pay into a fund that would cover those not otherwise insured.

Incremental Expansion of Existing Public Sector Programs This strategy would enlarge Medicare, Medicaid, and/or SCHIP until universal coverage is achieved. For example, Medicare might be extended to those fifty-five and older, and SCHIP could be modified to expand enrollment of children. In principle, after two or three such extensions, universal coverage is achievable. Although a proponent of this approach might favor demoting the private insurance industry from prominence—which would clear the way for expanded public programs to merge and cover all Americans, effectively creating a single-payer system—most prefer to leave private insurance largely in place.[16]

Managed Competition This strategy, familiar from Bill Clinton's reform proposal, might naturally combine with individual and employer mandates. A leading option is to adopt the Federal Employees Health Benefits (FEHB) model.[17] While the federal government organizes and manages the system that insures nine million workers and their families, competing insurance companies provide the insurance. Private fee-for-service insurers and more integrated delivery systems (such as HMOs) offer packages of benefits at various premiums. If approved, these plans then compete for enrollees among federal workers, who are free to enroll in any competing plan. In the present proposal, all Americans could en-roll in any of these plans. Two leading proponents suggest a national, quasi-governmental, nonpartisan commission to administer the system and recommend levels of funding and insurance benefits to Congress.[18]

One specific version of this model is a health-care voucher system.[19] In this approach every American under sixty-five would obtain a voucher that would guarantee and pay for the health benefits offered by a qualified, competing insurance plan. Individuals would be able to select any qualified plans while remaining free to purchase services beyond those provided by the plan selected. Funding for the vouchers could flow from an ear-marked value-added tax, tying benefit levels to tax rates so as to motivate fiscally prudent decisions about the extent of services vouchers would cover. According to leading proponents of this approach, employer-based insurance would likely fade away over time, and means-based programs such as Medicaid and SCHIP would be eliminated. Once the voucher plan is inaugurated, no one would be added to Medicare, so that program would phase out, too.

DIFFICULTIES FOR MULTIPLE PAYERS

Despite their various advantages, these proposals share certain difficulties inherited from the private, mostly for-profit insurance industry that they would permit to remain largely in place: massive expenditure on administration, the siphoning off of health-care dollars to profit-making, and probably adverse selection.

First, the administrative costs of private insurance—especially for-profit, private insurance—are much higher than those associated with public insurance. (I will provide evidence for this claim in the next section.) If these very high administrative costs are necessary to gain the alleged comparative benefits of private insurance, the onus is on proponents of private insurance to explain why.

Second, for-profit insurers, which constitute a majority of private insurance companies today, necessarily seek profits, which require that earnings exceed expenditures. This money could instead go to patients in the form of expanded coverage or better care. Nothing intrinsic to health care demands for-profit financing, so siphoning off health-care dollars for profiteering looks from the standpoint of health care's major goals like wasteful discretionary spending. (More on this later, however.)

Perhaps the most serious disadvantage of leaving the private insurance industry largely in place is that it preserves *adverse selection,* which leads insurers to avoid insurance risks and limit their coverage. Adverse selection in health care occurs when a disproportionate number of people in poor health select a particularly generous insurance plan.[20] Where insurance companies compete as payers, they typically differ in the services they cover and in reimbursement rates. Suppose plan A covers outpatient psychiatric services while plan B does not, or A reimburses more generously for such services. Patients with psychiatric problems may gravitate to A, which results in A enrolling many people who need extensive services. This is very costly for the company that administers A. Given variations in different plans' terms, and given that patients may choose from among these plans, the threat of adverse selection encourages health plans to offer less generous benefits and to advertise to wealthier, healthier groups, or to find other ways of avoiding those who most need health care.

Now, a system could address the threat of adverse selection by requiring that each plan cover the same services and charge the same premiums, deductibles, and so on, and by guaranteeing that anyone can enroll in any plan. Standardization of the basic terms of each plan in a system of truly open enrollment tends to level the playing field. But if the terms of each plan are to be uniform, why have different plans at all?

A champion of competing plans might reply that each is to *deliver* health care, never merely provide insurance (as Blue Cross and Blue Shield do). Competition in delivery, the argument goes, will promote quality, thereby justifying higher administrative costs. This may be correct. Note, though, that each move identified for avoiding adverse selection—standardizing prices and covered services, maintaining open enrollment, and requiring competing plans to deliver services—steps in the direction of a single-payer system. Later we will re-

turn to the prospect of merging single-payer financing with competition among private delivery plans.

COST-EFFECTIVENESS

Considerable evidence shows that the single-payer approach is the most cost-effective way to achieve basic health-care goals. Note that cost-effectiveness is not simply a matter of finances. It involves a relation between controlling costs—one of the four goals I identified above—and other goals or values. My claim is that, given appropriate standards for the achievement of the other major goals (universal coverage, patient freedom, and quality), a single-payer system is probably the most affordable way to achieve them. While a precise statement of the appropriate standards lies beyond the purposes of this paper, I suggest roughly the following: universal coverage for all citizens and residents with reasonable access to care even in the least populated areas; broad choice of providers and far less bureaucratic hassle than Americans now face; and quality of care—however measured—no less good than insured patients typically enjoy today.

Why emphasize costs in relation to the other goals? Because doing so counters two popular misconceptions: (1) that covering the currently uninsured (without unacceptable sacrifices in patient freedom and quality) would necessarily cost much more than status quo spending, and (2) that public insurance cannot control costs (without unacceptable rationing).

Before considering the evidence for cost-effectiveness, let us note that it *makes good sense* to expect it of the single-payer approach. What a system of multiple insurers has to do is quite different from what we would require of a single payer. In a pluralistic financing system, most of the payers will have to advertise, elaborate their unique restrictions of coverage, determine patient eligibility, bill patients, try to collect on bad debts—all while paying massive executive salaries and trying to maximize profits. Meanwhile, physicians, group practices, and hospitals have to spend much time and money wading through the bureaucratic complexities of multiple payers with different rules, rates, enrollees, and so on.

A single payer, by contrast, can concentrate on reimbursing providers for patient care. Profit-making is not a goal of the enterprise; breaking even is just fine. There is no need for competitive advertising because there is only one system. Everyone is permanently eligible for services, eliminating in one stroke much unnecessary bureaucracy. Patients need never have medical debts for services covered in the public program because the government will finance the care. There is no need for experts to decipher the rules and regulations of different payers because the single payer will apply the same rules to all enrollees. Billing patients—which requires armies of administrators in competing payers and burdens providers who have to deal with them—is unnecessary. (Patients would receive bills only for services not covered by the universal plan.) Physicians and other professionals have the fee-for-service option of submitting standardized forms recording services rendered, which will then be reimbursed by the public insurer. Alternatively, professionals can receive salaries or other forms of remuneration in group practices or health plans that are paid a lump sum per year to assume full responsibility for a particular person's care (a capitation approach). A third option is to work on a salaried basis for institutions such as hospitals that receive a monthly global budget for all necessary activities. None of these payment schemes requires billing patients.

Global budgeting and other planning are also crucial to controlling costs. A single-payer system will have standardized fees for those professionals who choose the fee-for-service option, and the fees will be based on annual negotiations between the public insurer and professional representatives. Hospitals' global budgets will encourage fiscal discipline. Drug prices, as explained below, will be reasonable and negotiated annually. Careful budgeting will encourage sensible limiting of the supply of high-technology equipment, helping to avoid situations in which equipment that has been purchased but is underutilized motivates providers to artificially create demand (encouraging questionable fee-for-service use of MRIs, for example). In general, global budgeting forces priority setting in an explicit, comprehensive way, which encourages sensible spending.

In addition to savings from streamlined administration and responsible budgeting, the single-payer approach avoids economic incentives that discourage high-quality care and segregate the health care market, making it harder for those who most need insurance to get it. As we have seen, private insurers have reason to seek enrollees who are relatively healthy and wealthy. The profit-making imperative of for-profit insurers motivates "experience rating"—the practice of basing premiums on an individual's particular health profile—rather than the "community rating" that enables wide pooling of risk (which is the traditional idea behind insurance). Fear of adverse selection motivates skimping on benefits, so as not to attract too many expensive patients. Moreover, there are free-rider problems with multiple payers.[21] If plan A wants to improve a doctor's efficiency, it may consider providing her some useful but expensive new technology. But if she has contracts with several insurance companies, the other plans besides A would benefit from the new technology for free. So A has a reason not to seek quality improvement. Another difficulty is that plans are economically discouraged from promoting long-term health with short-term costs if enrollees are unlikely to remain with a given plan long enough for it to realize the savings. All of these problems are avoided if there is only one payer, which will insure the whole population and realize the savings and benefits of efficient delivery and long-term health promotion.

Might these problems also be avoided by the best possible multiplepayer, managed competition approach? Perhaps. The problems associated with adverse selection and experience rating can be avoided if competing plans are required to offer the same benefits with the same premiums and deductibles, if enrollment in any plan is truly open to all, and if insurance is portable. The free-rider problem is avoided if each doctor is limited to working with a single plan. And the problem of discouraging long-term health promotion with short-term costs is avoidable if plans are sufficiently good to encourage enrollees to remain with the same plan for a long time. But the requirements needed to ensure these favorable conditions are far more likely in a single-payer system, which generally permits more regulation than pluralistic financing systems. Finally, the single-payer financing system is the simplest and, as the evidence of the next subsection demonstrates, the least costly way to achieve and maintain universal coverage.

Two further reasons to expect costeffectiveness: First, a single-payer system features *monopsony*—that is, concentrated purchasing power—enabling the negotiation of lower prices. This is crucial, for example, in negotiating with the formidable pharmaceutical industry in order to secure more reasonable prices for medications in this country. Second, a single-payer system could more easily implement a universal information technology system, whose many advantages would include easy and efficient retrieval of any patient's medical records.

Having considered several theoretical reasons to expect a single-payer system to be more cost-effective than pluralistic financing systems, let's turn to the evidence.

THE EVIDENCE

Consider, first, two U.S. government studies. Examining various reform plans, the Congressional Budget Office (CBO) found that only the single-payer plan was likely to achieve universal coverage while saving money (in comparison with then-current spending).[22] A General Accounting Office (GAO) study reached the same conclusion.[23]

Second, Medicare—essentially a single payer providing universal coverage for the elderly—has lower administrative and overall costs per patient than any other approach to health insurance we have tried. It is well known, for example, that the overhead for Medicare is much lower than that for private insurance companies.[24] As explained earlier, Medicare's overhead is also cheaper than that of Medicaid, a means-tested program requiring more complex administration. Further, the funneling of some Medicare recipients through private insurers has resulted in higher expenditures than those associated with traditional, fee-for-service Medicare[25]—exactly as one would expect given independent evidence for the higher administrative costs of private insurance.

Third, to take just one international example, Canada's single-payer system has much lower administrative costs than those of the U.S. system

and much lower total health care costs per capita.[26] Meanwhile, studies consistently suggest that the quality of care in Canada is, on average, no lower than in the United States.[27] As for costs, a debate over administrative savings is noteworthy. One detailed analysis estimated that U.S. spending on health-care administration in 1999 was $1,059 per capita, but only $307 per capita in Canada, suggesting a total excess of administrative spending in the United States of $209 billion.[28] A critical reply contended that the United States' excess administrative costs in 1999, as compared with Canada's, were only $159 billion.[29] Note: a conservative estimate of the annual administrative savings of single-payer financing is *only $159 billion!*

One finds further support for the assertion of cost-effectiveness in the detailed studies of leading scholars. In the mid-1990s, Norman Daniels studied four health-care reform plans proposed by members of Congress, including a single-payer proposal, as well as the American health-care status quo. On every measure Daniels considered—extent of coverage, comprehensiveness of benefits, patient choice, cost controls, and efficiency—the single-payer proposal outperformed competitors.[30] Jack Hadley and John Holahan's 2003 study estimated that covering the American uninsured in public programs would cost about half as much as covering them with private insurance.[31] In a 2004 report, the Institute of Medicine commented that "[s]ingle-payer models, much like Medicare, are generally considered to have substantially lower administrative costs than private insurance plans, since the need for advertising, underwriting, and much eligibility and billing work disappears."[32] In their 2005 book, Julius Richmond and Rashi Fein contended that the single payer offers "the most effective, efficient, and equitable health-care insurance system"—although concerns about political feasibility ultimately led them to favor a different approach.[33] I have found no scholarly studies that cast significant doubt on the cost-effectiveness of the single-payer plan.

FILLING IN OUR SKETCH

Our sketch so far indicates that the publicly financed system would provide universal coverage. There would be no billing of patients for services provided within the system. Hospitals, clinics, and nursing homes would have global budgets to cover all expenses (or perhaps some of these institutions, most feasibly nursing homes, could be paid on a capitation basis). Physicians and other professionals could either work fee-for-service with fees standardized annually, draw a salary from an institution with a global budget, or work for a capitated health plan. Now for further detail.

A key feature is the elimination of out-of-pocket payments for services provided within the tax-funded system. Premiums and deductibles create barriers to access and add substantially to administration. Their value is primarily symbolic: they promote an image of cost-sharing. Even copayments may be unwise for the same reasons. Some single-payer advocates may favor copayments, believing that what they save by inhibiting frivolous seeking of services will be more than copayments cost to administer. Then again, copayments may sometimes inhibit needed care until medical problems worsen—at which time treatment is more costly and possibly less effective. But whatever we decide about modest copayments, generally speaking, the most efficient way to pay for medical services is through taxation, which minimizes monetary transactions and associated administration.

Another feature of the single-payer approach is broad choice of providers, in the sense that patients may seek the services of any health professional working fee-for-service or join any qualifying health plan. (A health plan, however, is likely to have its own restrictions.) On the whole, I suggest, such freedom would improve on the American status quo, with its many economic and institutional restrictions and barriers to access. Moreover, the elimination of billing would *greatly* reduce the hassle confronting patients. The single-payer approach, then, seems likely to achieve the goal of patient freedom.

Will there be any role for private insurance outside the public program? There certainly will be if important categories of services, such as dental or optometric services, are excluded from the public package. Moreover, within the covered categories, there will be some demand for services beyond what is covered, such as cosmetic surgery or psychotherapy for persons who lack any relevant diagnosis.

Such services could be provided for a fee or via ancillary private insurance.

Should American health care preserve more of a role for this industry, as the United Kingdom does, by permitting coverage that *duplicates* what the public plan covers? Drawbacks of this option include possibly fragmenting the market if too high a percentage of the public opts for redundant private insurance; less political support for robust coverage in the public plan; and incentives for physicians to cater to those with private insurance if its reimbursement rates are higher. Then again, allowing duplicative private insurance would be less disruptive to the health-care status quo in this country, for whatever that's worth, than switching to a single-payer plan without this prerogative, and would increase options for providers and the rest of us. If we are to favor this approach—an issue I leave open— then the public program must be good enough that relatively few will be tempted to purchase the redundant private insurance.

Another feature that has only been touched upon is tax-based financing. What tax scheme is optimal is open for discussion. I suggest an earmarked health-care tax both to protect the funds from being appropriated for other purposes and to permit public awareness of health-care spending. Perhaps a progressive income tax would be simplest and fairest. The crucial point, though, is this: Although overall taxes will rise to fund single-payer financing, the elimination of out-of-pocket expenses, employer premiums, and so on—combined with the savings on administration, absence of profit-making within the system, and the like—can be expected roughly to offset the tax increases. That is, we can expect to spend no more on health care *per person on average* than we would in our current system, yet we would better achieve health-care goals. Although medical utilization will rise—appropriately, since everyone will be able to get care when they need it—the savings will roughly offset the increased expenditure needed for universal coverage.[34]

Any honest detailing of the single-payer approach must acknowledge its major disadvantages. These will emerge when I discuss objections. Once they are apparent, I will propose a way of addressing most of them that harnesses the power of market competition without abandoning the advantages of single-payer financing.

RESPONSES TO OBJECTIONS

The Single-Payer Approach Equals Socialized Medicine This is false. Socialist institutions involve not only public funding but also government employment. Although in a single-payer system health care is publicly funded, it is mostly privately delivered. Anyway, the charge of socialism is lame. Were it compelling, we should oppose public libraries, public schools, and the military's medical system.

Patients Do Not Like Severe Restrictions on Their Freedom Yes, so they should like a system that, as the American College of Surgeons noted, appears to be the best way of preserving patients' choice of physicians[35] and generally affords greater freedom from hassle than they currently face. As suggested earlier, the single-payer approach is likely to promote patient freedom.

What about freedom to choose among delivery plans offering different levels of care? Earlier we found that the threat of adverse selection motivated standardizing the range of services covered by plans funded by a single payer. This is a price worth paying to avoid adverse selection. Remember, though, that patients will remain free to purchase services or insurance beyond the public package. Indeed, the value of such freedom of choice—and considerations of political feasibility—may exert some downward pressure on the range of services publicly covered, keeping it more modest than might be justified if these considerations were not acknowledged.

Doctors Will Oppose It They will have relatively little reason to oppose it. The system will greatly reduce their administrative burden—a major savings of time, energy, and expense. It will trust them to deliver medicine appropriately without micromanaging middlemen from remote insurance plans. Doctors will have the option of working independently and for fees or under the terms of a qualifying health plan or hospital. In a recent poll, 63.5 percent of doctors who were asked to identify the health-care system that would provide the best care for the most

people selected the single-payer system.[36] While it does not follow that these doctors preferred the single-payer system overall, they evidently appreciated its ability to deliver high-quality care to the most people.

Doubtless some doctors will resent having fees standardized. But the special interest of maximizing physicians' income is surely less important than the widely accepted goals of health care. Doctors will always earn a good living—especially in a country spending at American levels on health care. And good doctors will take satisfaction in practicing medicine well within a system that serves the interests of patients and society as a whole. Reduced administrative burden and expense should be icing on the cake.

Of course, in saying that doctors have little good reason to oppose the single-payer approach, I am not denying that many doctors may oppose it nevertheless. Any proposal for significant health-care reform faces that possibility.

A Single-Payer System Will Require Rationing All health-care systems have to ration—at the very least they must limit access to exorbitant care of dubious benefit, such as "last chance therapies" available only in clinical trials.[37] Our present system rations by restricting access on the basis of economic and insurance status, restricting care through managed care, and limiting covered services in public programs. Yes, a single-payer system will ration, but it will do so more intelligently and fairly than we do now.

A Publicly Financed System Will Cause Long Waits for Services Like Canadians Have This charge is distorted. Generally speaking and as a matter of policy, Canadians who urgently need care are prioritized, so that only those who *can* wait do. (There have been tragic exceptions, however, just as there are exceptions to the American policy that all who need emergency room care will receive it.) Moreover, while Canadians sometimes come to the United States for medical services—a fact cited to support the claim of intolerable waits—a couple of reality checks are in order. First, a careful analysis suggests that the frequency of Canadians coming to the United States *specifically for medical services*—as opposed to coming for some other reason and then needing medical services during their stay—is tiny.[38] Moreover, Canadian waits occur within a system that is spending much less per person than we spend. Spending at current American levels with the cost-effectiveness of public financing could do much to address the problem.

If Services Are Free, Patients Will Overutilize Them

Copayments, which I have left on the table for further discussion, would discourage unnecessary care-seeking. This problem can also be addressed in other ways. Any genuine threat of overutilization must exist in countries like the United Kingdom and Canada where services are free at point of entry. But these countries spend much less than we do while achieving health-care goals fairly well. Possibly the mechanisms these countries have developed for discouraging overutilization can be put to use in the United States. Part of the solution, no doubt, is for providers to take responsibility for discouraging and even turning away patients who do not genuinely need medical attention. This should be easier in health plans that are paid on a capitated basis, which eliminates financial incentives for unnecessary care.

Quality Will Suffer

As far as I know, there is no hard evidence to support this claim. Indeed, it is contradicted by some of the empirical evidence cited earlier. A single-payer system will reform the way we finance health care but need not change the way we deliver it. Quality is an issue of delivery. With a mixture of fee-for-service financing, capitated payment, and global budgets, delivery can remain much the same.

Would standardized fee schedules and salaries discourage "the best and brightest" from entering medicine? I doubt it, for two reasons. First, the incentives of earning a good living while being able to practice medicine well in a system that's doing its job seem likely to attract better doctors than the incentive of maximizing income in a dysfunctional system. ("Best and brightest" does not mean "greediest and most shallow.") Second, other countries with single payers do not seem to have major problems with quality of care despite spending much less on health care than we do.[39] And spending at current American levels would permit better remuneration.

On the other hand, even if there is no empirical evidence suggesting that quality would suffer under a single-payer system, there may still be cause for concern. Suppose the entire system consisted of professionals working either for fees outside of any health plan or on a salaried basis within a plan. There might not be enough economic incentives to promote the high-quality care that we want—especially for those receiving salaries (and no bonuses or the like to encourage excellence and efficiency). Promoting competition among the plans, and permitting plans to motivate their professionals with a variety of payment schemes, seems more likely to discourage lackluster delivery and encourage excellence. I will return to this idea.

Biomedical Research Will Languish

Why? Nothing inherent to the single-payer approach prevents adequate public investment in research, and private sector research will continue. Take pharmaceutical research. Like the British, we can reward innovation and discourage both "me, too" drug research and patent manipulation (both of which waste many millions of dollars in our current system).[40] We can also spend much more than the British and still save money. Will drug companies refuse to take the financial risks of drug development unless current American-level prices are maintained? Even with these risks, American drug companies have among the highest profit margins in the business world. The proposition that somewhat lower profit margins—a consequence of annual negotiations between industry and the public insurer—would destroy their incentive seems exaggerated. The challenge will be to find sufficient incentives for pharmaceutical companies within a system that annually standardizes drug prices.

Fee-for-Service Payment Discourages Innovation in How Patients Are Treated And How Quality of Treatment Is Monitored

There is some truth to this objection. But it applies only to the independent, fee-for-service segment of a single-payer system. Professionals employed in hospitals, health plans, or other institutions working within global budgets or on a capitated basis have at the very least an incentive to break even, motivating discovery of more cost-effective methods. Insofar as the system will promote competition among health plans and among hospitals, there will be the further incentive to compete successfully for patients, who can choose among providers on the basis of satisfaction. None of this, by the way, is to trivialize the intrinsic incentives of practicing medicine well and enjoying the esteem of colleagues and patients; these incentives drive many professionals. But extrinsic, economic incentives are helpful to most professionals and essential to some.

Fee-for-Service Payment Reduces Efficiency by Encouraging the Provision of Individual Rather than Integrated Services Fair enough, but as with the previous objection, this applies only to the independent, fee-for-service portion of the delivery system. On the whole, this difficulty can be satisfactorily addressed through competition among health plans and other institutions.

HARNESSING COMPETITION

Let's take stock. The most significant objections to the single-payer approach, especially when envisioned as a fee-for-service system, are concerns about inadequate incentives for high-quality, innovative, and integrated care. The solution, I suggest, is to harness some of the power of economic competition without permitting the sort of market that leads to adverse selection, excessive diversion of funds away from patient care, and millions of people without insurance. Thus we return to the idea of managed competition. Competition encourages excellence and efficiency in delivery. Managing the competition can prevent market fragmentation while reducing waste. My proposal, therefore, is single-payer financing and managed-competition delivery.

How different is this proposal from other approaches? It differs from other single-payer proposals[41] in forthrightly acknowledging concerns about this general approach in its paradigmatic fee-for-service form, and in addressing those concerns primarily by harnessing market forces; it also makes no promise to cover "all medically necessary services" and is likely to preserve more of a market open to individual choice. It differs from some single-payer proposals by not making private insurance illegal, as explained earlier.

Will competing health plans include any that are for-profit? Single-payer proposals typically exclude for-profit plans, citing excessive overhead, problems associated with adverse selection, and distortions of clinical decision-making cultivated by the profit motive. I am sympathetic to these charges. Can we trust for-profit plans to serve patients adequately and not subordinate their interests to those of providers and stock-holders? I find it naïve to trust Big Business any more than Big Government. But since the present approach would permit any individual to join any health plan—so that, by law, financial status would not impede enrollment—we could, once insurance is mandated and adverse selection blocked, allow for-profits to join the competition. If we did, that would further distinguish this approach from other single-payer proposals. For-profit plans would receive the same capitation payments from the public insurer that nonprofit plans would receive. If the for-profits waste too much money, or provide low-quality care, they should lose out in the even playing field that includes nonprofit plans.

The approach recommended here also differs from any standard managed competition proposal. Consider the specification of this approach that embraces vouchers as a mechanism. My proposal differs from the voucher proposal, as typically developed, in granting the government (or quasigovernmental body overseeing the health-care system) a greater role in regulation. More specifically, my proposal (1) empowers the public insurer to negotiate annually with industry and professional groups to set drug prices and fees for services delivered by independent professionals, not just capitation rates for health plans; (2) forbids premiums, deductibles, and possibly copayments, so that no one is de facto excluded from any plan by finances; (3) forbids billing of patients for services covered in the public program, massively reducing overhead costs; (4) standardizes the benefits package in the public program to prevent adverse selection, so all plans offer the same benefits, and all independent professionals can be reimbursed for providing those same benefits; and (5) gives doctors a choice between working for a single health plan and working independently on a fee-for-service basis. This proposal offers, I submit, the best of both worlds: public financing and private delivery. Further, while this paper has focused on moral defensibility rather than political feasibility, in American culture it is politically advantageous to integrate market competition into any proposal featuring public financing.

. . .

ACKNOWLEDGMENTS

This paper was written with the support of a visiting scholar fellowship at the Department of Clinical Bioethics, National Institutes of Health, in 2006–2007. The views expressed here are the author's own and do not necessarily reflect those of the NIH. Drafts were presented at Georgetown University, George Washington University, the NIH, the University of Maryland, and the President's Council on Bioethics. I thank attendees of those presentations for invaluable feedback. Special thanks for written feedback to Greg Kaebnick, Joyce Griffin, Paul Menzel, Zeke Emanuel, Steve Pearson, Carrie Thiesen, Maggie Little, David Heyd, Arnon Keren, Joe Millum, and Eric Chwang.

REFERENCES

1 U.S. Census Bureau, *Income, Poverty, and Health Insurance Coverage in the United States: 2005* (Washington, D.C.: Government Printing Office, 2006), 20.

2 Institute of Medicine, "Insuring America's Health: Principles and Recommendations" (Washington, D.C.: National Academies of Science, 2004), http://www.iom.edu/Object.File/Master/17/732/Uninsured6-EnglishFINAL.pdf.

3 Institute of Medicine, "Insuring America's Health: Principles and Recommendations," January 14, 2004, press release.

4 Institute of Medicine, *Hidden Costs, Value Lost* (Washington, D.C.: National Academies Press, 2003), 112.

5 J. Hadley and J. Holahan, "The Cost of Care for the Uninsured," Kaiser Commission on Medicaid and the Uninsured (May 10, 2004): 1–14; J. Richmond and R. Fein, *The Health Care Mess* (Cambridge, Mass.: Harvard University Press, 2005), 233.

6 See G. Anderson et al., "Health Spending in the United States and the Rest of the Industrialized World," *Health Affairs* 24, no. 4 (2005): 903–914. We have far outspent other countries for a long time. See G. Schieber, J.-P. Poullier, and L. Greenwald, "Health System Performance in OECD Countries: 1980–1992," *Health Affairs* 13, no. 4 (1994): 100–112; and G. Anderson et al., "Health Spending and Outcomes: Trends in OECD Countries, 1960–1998," *Health Affairs* 19, no. 3 (2000):150–57.

7 Alliance for Health Reform, "Health Care Coverage in America," updated March 2006; www.CoverTheUninsured.org.

8 See D. Cutler, *Your Money or Your Life* (New York: Oxford University Press, 2004), chapter 8; and K. Donelan et al., "The Cost of Health System Change: Public Discontent in Five Nations," *Health Affairs* 18, no. 3 (1999): 206–216.

9 See Employee Benefit Research Institute, "2006 Health Confidence Survey: Dissatisfaction with Health Care System Doubles since 1998," *EBRI Notes* 27, no. 11 (2006) www.ebri.org, and ABC News/ USA Today/Kaiser Family Foundation Health Care Poll, www.usatoday.com/news/health/2006-10-15-health-poll1.htm.

10 It is difficult to imagine genuine doubt that Americans care greatly about cost controls, patient freedom, and quality, but that they consider universal coverage a high priority might seem less obvious. On this point, see Washington Post-ABC Poll, *The Washington Post,* October 20, 2003; American Hospital Association, "AHA National and Selected Statewide Surveys," www.hospitalconnect.com/aha/campaign2004/index.html; and Kaiser Family Foundation, "Kaiser Health Poll Report: The Public Is Concerned about the Problem," December 2005, www.kff.org/spotlight/uninsured/1.cfm. On the importance to Americans of costs and quality, see Employee Benefit Research Institute, "2006 Health Confidence Survey."

11 See Schieber et al., "Health System Performance in OECD Countries"; K. Donelan et al., "All Payer, Single Payer, Managed Care, No Payer: Patients' Perspectives in Three Nations," *Health Affairs* 15, no. 2 (1996): 254–65; K. Donelan et al., "The Cost of Health System Change"; Anderson et al., "Health Spending and Outcomes"; L. Brown, "Comparing Health Systems in Four Countries: Lessons for the United States," *American Journal of Public Health* 93 (2003): 52–56; R. Blendon et al., "Common Concerns Amid Diverse Systems: Health Care Experiences in Five Countries," *Health Affairs* 22, no. 3 (2003):106–121; and K. Lasser et al., "Access to Care, Health Status, and Health Disparities in the United States and Canada," *American Journal of Public Health* 96 (2006):1300–1307.

12 D. Palmisano, D. Emmons, and G. Wozniak, "Expanding Insurance Coverage through Tax Credits, Consumer Choice, and Market Enhancements," *Journal of the American Medical Association* 291 (2004):2237–42.

13 Alliance for Health Reform, "Health Care Coverage in America."

14 J. Gruber, "The Massachusetts Health Care Resolution: A Local Start for Universal Access," *Hastings Center Report* 36, no. 5 (2006):14–19.

15 Another reason this initiative will not achieve universal coverage is that the mandate is binding only for those who can afford insurance (ibid., p. 17). For other difficulties, see S. Woolhandler and D. Himmelstein, "The New Massachusetts Health Reform: Half a Step Forward and Three Steps Back," *Hastings Center Report* 36, no. 5 (2006):19–21.

16 See Richmond and Fein, *The Health Care Mess,* chapter 8.

17 Ibid., 252–57; and Cutler, *Your Money or Your Life,* chapter 10.

18 Richmond and Fein, *The Health Care Mess,* 258.

19 E. Emanuel and V. Fuchs, "Health Care Vouchers—A Proposal for Universal Coverage," *New England Journal of Medicine* 352 (2005):1255–60.

20 See D. Cutler and S. Reber, "Paying for Health Insurance: The Trade-Off Between Competition and Adverse Selection," *Quarterly Journal of Economics* 113 (1998): 433–66.

21 Cutler, *Your Money or Your Life,* 96–97.

22 Congressional Budget Office, *Universal Health Insurance Coverage Using Medicare's Payment Rates,* December 1991, http://www.cbo.gov/ftpdocs/76xx/doc7652 /91-CBO-039.pdf.

23 United States Government Accountability Office, *Canadian Health Insurance: Lessons for the United States,* June 1991, http://archive.gao.gov/d38t12/144048.pdf.

24 See M. Angell, "Dr. Frist to the Rescue: How Not to Fix Medicare," *The American Prospect,* online article issued February 1, 2003, www.prospect.org/print/V14/2/ angell-m.html; and Physicians' Working Group for Single-Payer National Health Insurance, "Proposal of the Physicians' Working Group for Single-Payer National Health Insurance," *Journal of the American Medical Association* 290 (2003), 799.

25 See Physicians' Working Group for Single-Payer National Health Insurance, "Proposal of the Physicians' Working Group for Single-Payer National Health Insurance," 804.

26 See M. Barer et al., "Reminding Our Ps and Qs: Medical Cost Controls in Canada," *Health Affairs* 15, no. 2 (1996): 217–35; Anderson et al., "Health Spending and Outcomes"; Brown, "Comparing Health Systems in Four Countries"; R. Deber, "Health Care Reform: Lessons from Canada," *American Journal of Public Health* 93, no. 1 (2003):20–24; Anderson et al., "Health Spending in the United States and the Rest of the Industrialized World."

27 See Blendon et al., "Common Concern Amid Diverse Systems"; P. Hussey et al., "How Does the Quality of Care Compare in Five Countries?" *Health Affairs* 23, no. 3 (2004):89–99; and Lasser et al., "Access to Care, Health Status, and Health Disparities in the United States and Canada."

28 S. Woolhandler, T. Campbell, and D. Himmelstein, "Costs of Health Care Administration in the United States and Canada," *New England Journal of Medicine* 349 (2003): 768–73.

29 H. Aaron, "The Costs of Health Care Administration in the United States and Canada—Questionable Answers to a Questionable Question," *New England Journal of Medicine* 349 (2003):801–803.

30 N. Daniels, *Seeking Fair Treatment* (New York: Oxford University Press, 1995), chapter 8.

31 J. Hadley and J. Holahan, "Covering the Uninsured: How Much Would It Cost?" (Web exclusive) *Health Affairs* 22, no. 4 (2003):W3/250–W3/265.

32 Institute of Medicine, "Insuring America's Health," 6.

33 Richmond and Fein, *The Health Care Mess,* 243.

34 See Physicians' Working Group for Single-Payer National Health Insurance, "Proposal of the Physicians' Working Group for Single-Payer National Health Insurance," and Hadley and Holahan, "Covering the Uninsured."

35 P. Cotton, "Single-Payer Plan Gets Cautious Support," *Journal of the American Medical Association* 271 (1994): 731.

36 D. McCormick et al., "Single-Payer National Health Insurance: Physicians' Views," *Archives of Internal Medicine* 164 (2004):300–304.

37 L. Fleck, "Rationing: Don't Give Up," *Hastings Center Report* 32, no. 2 (2002):35–36.

38 S. Katz et al., "Phantoms in the Snow: Canadians' Use of Health Care Services in the United States," *Health Affairs* 21, no. 3 (2002):19–31.

39 For a discussion citing many useful sources, see D. Callahan and A. Wasunna, *Medicine and the Market* (Baltimore, Md.: Johns Hopkins University Press, 2006), 236–46. See also the works cited in notes 12 and 29.

40 D. Light, "Universal Health Care: Lessons from the British Experience," *American Journal of Public Health* 93 (2003), 29.

41 See especially the many fine articles by Steffie Woolhandler and David Himmelstein, including "Proposal of the Physicians' Working Group for Single-Payer National Health Insurance."

ANNOTATED BIBLIOGRAPHY

Bodenheimer, Thomas: "The Oregon Health Plan—Lessons for the Nation (First of Two Parts)," *New England Journal of Medicine* 337 (August 28, 1997), pp. 651–655. Bodenheimer provides a helpful description of the Oregon rationing plan, including changes in the system since its federal approval in 1994.

Cohen, G. A.: *Why Not Socialism?* (Princeton: Princeton University Press, 2009). Cohen presents the fundamental socialist critique of market society in this accessible volume.

Cochrane, John H.: "Health-Status Insurance: How Markets Can Provide Health Security," *Cato Institute* 633 (February 18, 2009), pp. 1–12. In this article, Cochrane argues that the combination of what he calls "health-status insurance" and a competitive market of freely-priced medical insurance solves the central problem in American health care: the lack of long-term, portable health security.

Daniels, Norman: *Justice and Justification: Reflective Equilibrium in Theory and Practice* (Cambridge: Cambridge University Press, 1996). In this collection of essays, Daniels explores the idea that ethical justification involves the achievement of coherence or "reflective equilibrium" in a system of beliefs. Among the practical topics explored are the design of health-care systems as well as aged-based and other forms of rationing.

——: *Am I My Parents' Keeper?* (New York: Oxford University Press, 1988). Daniels seeks a principled approach to allocating health care, income support, and other types of resources to members of different age groups in society. Because we all age, he argues, each of us passes through different life stages. Thus, if we can determine how we would prudently allocate our fair share of social goods to ourselves over different life stages, we can discover what justice demands in the way of allocation between age groups.

Emanuel, Ezekiel J.: "The Cost-Coverage Trade-Off: 'It's Health Care Costs, Stupid'," *JAMA* 299 (February 27, 2008), pp. 947–949. Emanuel argues that the greatest problem facing American health care is not the millions of people who lack insurance, as is commonly supposed, but uncontrolled health-care inflation. Failure to deal with the latter problem, he argues, will cause any solution to the former problem to be transient.

Fleck, Leonard M.: "Just Caring: Oregon, Health Care Rationing, and Informed Democratic Deliberation," *Journal of Medicine and Philosophy* 19 (August 1994), pp. 367–388. Fleck contends that American efforts at health-care reform should be informed by lessons that can be extracted from Oregon's rationing experiment. Most generally, we must learn that the need for rationing is inescapable, that any rationing process must be public, and that fair rationing plans must develop through rational democratic deliberation.

Journal of Medicine and Philosophy 26 (April 2001). This special issue is entitled "Do Children Get Their Fair Share of Health and Dental Care?" Several leading contributors to the bioethics literature address the question contained in the title of the special issue.

Menzel, Paul and Donald W. Light: "A Conservative Case for Universal Access to Health Care," *Hastings Center Report* 36 (July–August 2006), pp. 36–45. The authors argue, contrary to a popular assumption, that conservative values support the case for universal access to health care.

Moreno, Jonathan D.: "Recapturing Justice in the Managed Care Era," *Cambridge Quarterly of Healthcare Ethics* 5 (1996), pp. 493-499. Moreno examines and critically evaluates the managed care movement of the first half of the 1990s, noting with concern the near disappearance of discussions of social justice in the bioethics community. Because managed care is headed in a direction that is ethically unsound and politically unsustainable, he maintains, bioethics needs to ensure that justice recaptures its place in the public mind.

Nelson, James Lindemann: "Measuring Fairness, Situated Justice: Feminist Reflections on Health Care Rationing," *Kennedy Institute of Ethics Journal* 6 (March 1996), pp. 53–68. In this article, Nelson attempts to demonstrate the fruitfulness of an interchange between mainstream discussions of justice in health care and feminist reflections on power, privilege, and justice.

Nozick, Robert: *Anarchy, State, and Utopia* (New York: Basic Books, 1974). In this classic work, Nozick presents his highly influential arguments for libertarianism while addressing other topics of interest such as the nature of rights and the moral status of animals.

Nord, Erik: *Cost-Value Analysis in Health Care: Making Sense Out of QALYs* (New York: Cambridge University Press, 1999). This book provides an in-depth exploration of quality-adjusted life years, a type of outcomes measure frequently used in discussions of health care.

Physicians' Working Group for Single-Payer National Health Insurance: "Proposal of the Physicians' Working Group for Single-Payer National Health Insurance," *JAMA* 290 (August 13, 2003), pp. 798–805. In this article, the physicians' group presents a comprehensive case for their thesis that the United States should make a radical change to single-payer national health insurance.

Powers, Madison and Ruth Faden: "Inequalities in Health, Inequalities in Health Care: Four Generations of Discussion about Justice and Cost-Effectiveness Analysis," *Kennedy Institute of Ethics Journal* 10 (June 2000), pp. 109–127. This article examines how trends in ethical discussions of health-care allocation over the previous two decades transformed the philosophical landscape while encouraging bioethicists to seek normative guidance from outside traditional philosophical discussions about justice.

President's Commission for the Study of Ethical Problems in Medicine and Biomedical and Behavioral Research: *Securing Access to Health Care,* Vol. 1: *Report* (Washington, DC: Government Printing Office, 1983). This influential report presents the commission's conclusions about (1) an ethical framework grounding a societal obligation to provide an adequate level of health care to all citizens, (2) the state of American health care, and (3) changes in health-care delivery that can move the United States in the direction of meeting its societal obligation.

Steinbrook, Robert: "Health Care Reform in Massachusetts—Expanding Coverage, Escalating Costs," *New England Journal of Medicine* 358 (June 26, 2008), pp. 2757–2760. The author reviews data in Massachusetts two years after the state adopted a health-care reform plan that included an individual mandate. He argues that several trends, especially the expansion of coverage, are favorable while other trends, such as escalating costs to the state, are cause for concern.

CASE STUDIES

This appendix contains a set of case studies for analysis and discussion. Some of the cases are essentially records of actual situations. Others, however, are only loosely based on actual happenings, and a few have been constructed simply for their perceived pedagogical value. Most of the cases have been developed only up to a crucial "decision point." Although retrospective case review—concerned with the appropriateness of decisions actually made in any given case—is called for in a few of the cases presented here, most of the cases ask for a prospective rather than a retrospective analysis. Thus, the more common task is to provide an analysis of what should be done within the context of a developing case rather than an analysis of what has actually been done in a case that has already run its course.

When case descriptions feature a richness of factual detail and nuance, they are sometimes characterized as "thick." By way of contrast, case studies of the type presented here may be characterized as relatively "thin," and their somewhat schematic character may cause discomfort. Individuals involved in analyzing such cases often feel that it would be desirable to have more factual details, especially clinical ones. This recurrent desire reflects the well-based axiom that good decision making must be based on "good facts." However, a perceived lack of factual detail should not be allowed to paralyze analysis and discussion. If the proper decision in a certain case is thought to be dependent upon information not provided in the case description, and if it is reasonable to believe that the desired information would or could be available to those confronted with the decision, a discussion of the case can include an examination of the precise way in which the desired information is relevant to the decision.

Two final points are worth noting. First, the last paragraph of each case study identifies some questions raised by the case. These questions are not the only ones worthy of consideration, but they can be used to facilitate analysis and discussion. Second, the title of each case study is followed by a number or numbers within brackets. These numbers refer to the various chapters in this book. Thus, the chapter or chapters most directly relevant to each case are identified.

CASE 1
WITHHOLDING INFORMATION ABOUT RISKS [2]

Marcia W is a 40-year-old female with multiple myeloma, who upon diagnosis shows great interest in having all the information that is necessary to make a decision about further treatment. Dr. C tells her that the response rates to chemotherapy with this disease are very good and that recent research has shown that 50 percent of patients can hope for long-term survival rates, which are tantamount to cure. The other 50 percent of patients die within a year or two. What Dr. C neglects to tell her is that preliminary studies are showing that, over a twenty-year period subsequent to chemotherapy, 10 percent of those who survive the myeloma will contract a form of leukemia that is highly resistant to treatment. When her treatment is discussed in a staff meeting, Dr. C says that he does not want to tell Marcia W about the 10 percent because he is afraid that it might unduly alarm her and cause her not to take treatment, thereby spoiling her chances for long-term survival. Moreover, he states (1) that the research is not conclusive enough to suit him and (2) that 10 percent is such a low figure that he is not morally required to communicate the risk. After all, he suggests, one cannot inform a patient of *every* risk.

(1) Does Marcia W have a right to the information about the possible risk of leukemia? (2) Is this 10 percent chance of contracting leukemia significant for her decision making? (3) Will this information harm her by making it impossible for her to make an autonomous decision? (4) Is the refusal to disclose justified by the low 10 percent figure and the serious consequences of refusing treatment?

CASE 2
A PATIENT'S REQUEST FOR A POSSIBLY USELESS TREATMENT [3]

After arriving at his doctor's office, Jeff R complains of the flu and requests an antibiotic. His description of symptoms convinces Dr. T that he has the flu. Dr. T explains to Jeff R that antibiotics are physiologically useless against the flu and other conditions caused by viruses (as opposed to bacteria). In dealing with patients who have the flu, she ordinarily recommends rest and fluids and sometimes recommends over-the-counter drugs. But Jeff R insists on an antibiotic, so she considers writing a prescription. On the one hand, she figures that an antibiotic will cause Jeff R no harm and might even help psychologically by making him feel that something is being done for his condition. On the other hand, she is aware that overuse of antibiotics makes it more likely that bacteria in the environment will become resistant to available antibiotics.

(1) Should Dr. T honor Jeff R's request for antibiotics? (2) Is it appropriate for physicians to offer treatments whose sole purpose is to provide psychological comfort when that comfort is based on a false belief or misunderstanding?

CASE 3
VOLUNTARY STERILIZATION AND A YOUNG, UNMARRIED MAN [3]

Gregory X, who is 25 years old, unmarried, and childless, wants a vasectomy. (Vasectomy is a sterilization procedure that, until recently, had been considered irreversible but at present can sometimes be surgically reversed.) He goes to Dr. H, a urologist in a clinic in a large city hospital, because he cannot afford the surgery elsewhere. He tells Dr. H that he has decided, after several years of thought, never to be a parent. The vasectomy will now ensure that and make it unnecessary for any woman he loves to run the various risks associated with the available means of contraception. Dr. H has doubts about performing the surgery on a young, unmarried man. He asks Gregory X to consider the feelings of a possible future wife who will not have any say about the sterilization decision. Gregory X insists on the surgery.

(1) Should Dr. H accede to Gregory X's request despite his reservations, since Gregory X cannot afford the vasectomy elsewhere? (2) Is there anything morally problematic about Gregory X's request?

CASE 4
THE DENTIST AND PATIENT AUTONOMY [2, 3]

A 36-year-old man, Patrick M, contacts the office of an endodontist. (Endodontics is a specialized field of dentistry.) Patrick M wants to arrange for a procedure commonly called a "root canal" to be performed on each of his teeth. A root canal is a common (somewhat involved) procedure used as an alternative to extracting a diseased tooth. It consists of removing the damaged or diseased blood vessels and nerves contained within the tooth. The tooth is thus "devital" but functions normally. If this procedure is not done on a diseased tooth or if the tooth is not extracted, infection will very likely develop in the necrotic tissue and spread into the jaw bone and surrounding tissues.

The endodontist is startled by the idea of performing a root canal on all of Patrick M's teeth. Further discussion makes Patrick M's motivation clear. He is a fervent survivalist, dedicated to planning for every contingency in the expectation that some conflagration is about to destroy society. Patrick M is attempting to ensure—by having all of his teeth desensitized—that he will never suffer a toothache. Although the endodontist cannot escape a sense of amusement over what he considers a bizarre situation, Patrick M seems fully prepared both to undergo a difficult set of procedures and to pay what will be a huge overall bill. Still, the endodontist feels that it would be unethical to remove healthy tissue. He feels that he is being asked to perform a procedure that is not indicated by the existing conditions and may never be indicated, judging by the excellent overall health of the teeth.

(1) Is there any significant difference between the dentist-patient relationship and the physician-patient relationship? (2) Should the endodontist accede to Patrick M's desires?

CASE 5
LIBERTY AND THE ELDERLY PATIENT [2]

Ronald X is 71 years old. A widower, he lives alone in an apartment, but he receives some assistance from a cleaning woman and a friendly neighbor. Ronald X is presently in a hospital because of a broken leg, but he is ready to be discharged. Ronald X also suffers from arteriosclerosis, a condition that results in his experiencing periods of confusion during which he sometimes wanders purposelessly around the city, running some risks to himself. Ronald X's children do not want him to return to his home. They believe that he needs the supervised care provided in a nursing home. Ronald X, when not in a confused state, repeatedly expresses his awareness of the problems he faces stemming from his arteriosclerosis and of the resultant risks he runs. Nonetheless, he would rather run those risks than be confined to institutional care. The health-care professionals and Ronald X's children decide that he will not be discharged from the hospital until an appropriate nursing home is found. At that time, he will be sent to the nursing home. When Ronald X insists on being discharged from the hospital, the medical professionals sedate him to a level sufficient to gain his compliance.

(1) Are the health-care professionals and Ronald X's children making an unjustified leap from his occasional risk-running behavior to the conclusion that he lacks sufficient competence to determine the shape of his own life? (2) Is this paternalistic limitation on Ronald X's liberty morally obligatory? morally permissible? morally reprehensible?

CASE 6
RITALIN FOR A NORMAL BOY [3]

Teresa T and George L, two highly educated and successful professionals, bring their son, Mike, into the office of his pediatrician, Dr. S, with some concerns about Mike's behavior. In school the boy has had difficulties sitting still and following directions, and sometimes has trouble concentrating on his studies both in school and at home. After an extensive discussion with Mike and his parents, Dr. S is convinced that the boy does not have Attention Deficit/Hyperactivity Disorder or any other condition meriting a diagnosis. Mike appears to be a normal, energetic boy who faces many of the behavioral challenges that normal, energetic boys commonly face in school and other highly structured environments.

Despite this reassurance, Teresa T and George L ask Dr. S to write a prescription for Ritalin for Mike. As they explain, they have read that Ritalin can help children (and adults) to improve their concentration regardless of whether they have a medical diagnosis. "Besides," Teresa T asks, "who can draw a bright line between illness and normalcy these days?" Although Dr. S is aware that Ritalin and other stimulants are sometimes prescribed to children like Mike, he expresses reservations about prescribing cognition-affecting medications for children who are basically well. His reservations persist when further discussion reveals that Teresa T and George L are thinking of administering Ritalin to Mike only occasionally, when he needs to prepare for and take a test or complete a difficult assignment.

(1) Do physicians have a responsibility to restrict prescriptions to those patients who have a diagnosable illness or disorder? Does it matter whether the medication in question affects cognition? Does it matter whether the patient is a child? (2) Is there a meaningful boundary between illness, dysfunction, and other medical conditions on the one hand and medical normalcy on the other? If so, does this boundary determine the limits of appropriate medical practice? (3) Does the provision of medications to children who lack a diagnosable condition—in order to enhance their performance in competitive contexts—pose a social threat that merits our serious attention? If so, what is the nature of this threat and how might the medical profession or society address it?

CASE 7
AGGRESSIVE ADVERTISING FOR COSMETIC SURGERY [3]

"Shape Up for Summer!" the advertisement advises. "Don't Be Ashamed to Hit the Beach." Appearing in a variety of magazines for teenage girls and women, the ad offers several types of cosmetic surgery, including breast augmentation and liposuction. Although the five versions of the ad feature different models, each model is a Caucasian woman of college age who is slim, large breasted, and dressed in a bikini. The ad provides contact information for a team of physicians who specialize in cosmetic surgery.

(1) Is it ethically acceptable for physicians to provide services that employ their medical skills for ends other than treating a medical illness, dysfunction, or other diagnosable condition? (2) Is it ethically acceptable for physicians to stimulate demand for such services with attention-grabbing advertisements that may take advantage of some people's insecurities (e.g., about their physical attractiveness)? (3) Is medicine best understood as a business or as a profession with stricter moral norms than those governing business?

CASE 8
THE NURSE AND INFORMED CONSENT [2]

Michael G, who is dying of leukemia, is in a hospital, where he is receiving chemotherapy. A registered nurse involved in his care, Nurse L, learns that he has never received information about alternative natural therapies. She gives Michael G the information and discusses the advantages and disadvantages of the various alternatives. After extensive reflection and consultation with his family, Michael G decides to leave the hospital and to make arrangements to try one of the alternative therapies. He informs the attending oncologist of his decision. When the oncologist learns about the source of Michael G's information, he charges Nurse L with unprofessional conduct and asks that her nursing license be revoked. Nurse L argues that the patient has the right to know about the alternatives and that a failure to inform him vitiates his "informed consent" to the chemotherapy.

(1) Was Nurse L acting in a morally correct way when she gave Michael G the information? (2) Should the physician in charge have the final word about the information a patient receives? (3) If Michael G did not know about the alternative therapies, was his agreement to the chemotherapy *informed* consent?

CASE 9
THE OFFICE NURSE AND INFORMED CONSENT [2]

Joan R is going through menopause. Her physician, Dr. W, wants her to begin estrogen therapy. After talking with the physician, Joan R agrees to the therapy. She stops at the nurse's desk in Dr. W's office to pick up her prescription. In the course of the conversation, Nurse M realizes that Dr. W has not informed Joan R that other options are available to her and that there is wide disagreement about which option is preferable. Instead of taking only estrogen, Nurse M reasons, Joan R could choose to take estrogen together with a progestin, or she could choose to take no hormones at all. Each of these options is thought to carry different potential benefits and risks.

(1) Should Nurse M provide Joan R with that information? (2) Should Nurse M suggest to Joan R that she initiate an additional discussion with Dr. W in order to obtain more information? (3) Should Nurse M express her concern in this matter to Dr. W? If so, how should she approach him?

CASE 10
PAIN RELIEF, CULTURAL BELIEFS, AND THE ROLE OF A FAMILY MEMBER [2]

Marie F, a 40-year-old Haitian immigrant, is hospitalized with terminal lung cancer. Initially, the nurse responsible for Marie's care complied with her (competent) request for pain medication. Then Marie's brother, Jean, arrived from another city and found his sister delirious and mumbling incomprehensibly (as patients often do under a heavy dose of pain medication). In accordance with the voodoo religion of his family's culture, Jean took Marie's behavior to suggest the presence of evil spirits in her body; if not exorcised, he thought, the spirits would bring harm to their entire family. Upon learning that Marie's delirious mumbling occurred after she was given pain medication, Jean demanded that the medication be discontinued, explaining, "The medicine brought the spirits into her, so we need to stop the medicine to get the spirits out!" At this point, the nurse feels conflicted between honoring Marie's request for pain control measures and respecting her family's religion. (She also wonders whether this religion assumes that an adult male should make medical decisions on behalf of female family members—as some traditional belief systems assume—but she is reluctant to broach this issue with Jean.)

(1) How should the nurse responsible for Marie's care handle this predicament? (2) Does the principle of self-determination apply to competent adults regardless of cultural context? (3) Would continuing to administer pain medication to Marie entail a failure to respect the religious beliefs expressed by Jean?

CASE 11
CONFLICT BETWEEN THE INTERESTS OF A PATIENT AND HIS WIFE [2]

An elderly man, Bill S, has been paralyzed by a stroke but apparently retains decision-making capacity. There is no significant chance that the paralysis can be reversed. The patient's physician, Dr. Z, believes the patient should enter a nursing home when he is ready to be discharged from the hospital. Bill S, however, insists on returning home, although the only available caretaker is his rather frail, elderly wife, Amy S, who has a heart ailment. Amy S knows that she is incapable of the physical demands required to care for her husband, and she knows that he will refuse nursing care at home. She explains to her husband that, if her health fails, he will have to enter a nursing home anyway and she may become bedridden or die. Amy S pleads with Dr. Z to intercede when her husband remains adamant. Because Bill S is very attached to his physician, Dr. Z believes that by threatening to withdraw from the case he might be able to get Bill S to change his mind.

(1) How should Dr. Z deal with this situation? (2) Should the interests of family members, when they conflict with a patient's interests, have any bearing on medical decision making? (3) Is it ever appropriate for a physician to pressure a patient to do what is morally right?

CASE 12
AN HIV-INFECTED SURGEON AND A DUTY TO DISCLOSE [2]

Dr. M, a surgeon, has learned that he has been infected with the human immunodeficiency virus (HIV). A prominent study estimates that surgeons cut themselves, on average, 2.5 times for every 100 surgical procedures and that, in approximately one-third of those cases, the patient is touched with the instrument carrying the surgeon's blood. According to the study, for every 1,000 cases in which an HIV-infected surgeon's blood mixes with that of a patient, a patient will become infected in at most 3 cases. Thus, there is *some* risk that a patient operated on by Dr. M will be infected.

(1) Does Dr. M have an obligation to refrain from performing surgery? (2) If not, does Dr. M have an obligation to inform those on whom he plans to operate that he is infected with the virus? (3) Suppose the positions were reversed and a patient, Dorothea L, is the one infected. Is Dorothea L obligated to inform Dr. M of her infection?

CASE 13
"WOULD A COCHLEAR IMPLANT BE BEST FOR OUR CHILD?" [3]

Having become parents one year ago, Sean and Mary McG are considering cochlear implant surgery for their infant child, Gregory, who, like his parents, was born deaf. Cochlear implants are surgically implanted devices that often, but not always, enable partial hearing and speech comprehension in deaf individuals. Neither Sean nor Mary McG has had cochlear implant surgery, which was unavailable when they were young; both speak and read English, their first language, but now rely mostly on American Sign Language (ASL) in each other's company. When they first learned about cochlear implant surgery, the parents were enthusiastic about the possibility of reducing the effects of deafness, which they consider a serious disability, in their child. But some deaf friends of theirs have expressed strong opposition to cochlear implants, stressing their limited efficacy and criticizing efforts to assimilate deaf people into mainstream hearing culture. "Take more pride in being deaf," they say to Sean and Mary McG. "Take pride in our shared language, ASL, and Deaf culture. The whole attitude that says deafness is a disability reflects the majority's prejudice against deafness and the preference that everyone adjust to hearing culture and lifestyle." The McGs feel conflicted. Although they might allow their son to decide for himself when he is older—say, ten or even fifteen—they understand that success rates for cochlear implants are much higher when the surgery is performed in the first few years of life.

(1) Is being deaf objectively disadvantageous, notwithstanding the many achievements of deaf individuals and the deaf community? Or does the classification of deafness as a disability largely reflect the hearing majority's prejudices? (2) What decision regarding cochlear implant surgery would best promote Gregory's long-term interests?

CASE 14
AN INTERSEX INFANT AND DECISIONS ABOUT "NORMALIZATION" [3]

Accompanied by her husband, Fred, Jenny D has just given birth to a boy. The infant's penis is extremely small, creating an appearance of sexual ambiguity ("Is that a boy or a girl?"). In confronting cases involving "intersex" or ambiguous genitalia, many physicians have assumed that healthy psychosexual development requires early social assignment to one gender and a corresponding genital appearance. Accordingly, the attending physician—in consultation with colleagues including a sexologist—ask Jenny and Fred D to consider surgical removal of their infant's testicles, additional surgery, and hormonal treatment to make the child more female in appearance, and a plan to raise their infant as a girl. The parents consider this option along with an alternative approach: avoiding surgery and hormone treatment, raising their child as a boy, providing any psychological counseling he may need, and allowing him to make any major decisions about his sexuality when he is older.

(1) What decision for the present would seem most conducive to the child's long-term interests? (2) What should the medical team do to facilitate the parents' decision making?

CASE 15
PREVENTING PHYSICAL MATURATION IN A BRAIN-DAMAGED GIRL [3]

On January 3, 2007, the news media broke the controversial story of Ashley, a severely retarded, nine-year-old girl whose parents authorized medical interventions designed to impede her physical development. Ashley was born with static encephalopathy, a brain impairment that resulted in her cognitive development being arrested at that of a normal three-month-old. She is unable to talk, walk, sit up, turn over, or eat without assistance. In view of her severe incapacity, her parents authorized the Children's Hospital in Seattle to provide what they called "the Ashley treatment": powerful estrogen therapy to stunt the girl's growth, removal of her breast buds to prevent breast maturation, and hysterectomy (removal of her uterus) to prevent the discomfort of menstruation and eliminate any possibility of pregnancy.

According to Ashley's parents, the medical interventions were motivated by the girl's best interests. Remaining small—at under 80 pounds and four feet five inches tall—means that Ashley can be held in their arms, moved more easily, taken outside the house and out of town more often, and bathed in a standard bathtub. These possibilities, they maintain, are good for her physically (e.g., for her circulation) and psychologically (since more outings entail more stimulation). In sum, the Ashley Treatment was designed "to improve our daughter's quality of life and not to convenience her caregivers."

(1) Did Ashley's parents and doctors judge correctly that the Ashley treatment was in her best interests? (2) Does it seem likely that some of the motivation behind the unorthodox interventions was to convenience her caregivers? If so, how does that affect the appropriate moral evaluation of their choice? (3) Are medical interventions designed to arrest a patient's physical development contrary to human dignity? (4) Do such interventions fall within the bounds of appropriate medical practice?

CASE 16
UNPROTECTED SEX AND PATIENT CONFIDENTIALITY [2]

For two months, Brian P, who suffers from depression, has been seeing Dr. A in weekly psychotherapy sessions. Brian P, who is gay, has long struggled with feelings of social rejection and with insecurity about his attractiveness; in the past year, he has also experienced the trauma of learning that he is HIV-positive. Shortly after Dr. A feels that he and Brian P have established a strong rapport, Brian P explains that he and a man he has been dating, George S, have begun to have unprotected sex. Even more startling to Dr. A is Brian P's stated intention not to tell George S that he (Brian) is HIV-positive. Careful to avoid a judgmental tone, Dr. A presents the advantages of safe sex and recommends that Brian P inform George S. But Brian P fears that either of those options would lead to his being rejected. While he does not want to harm his partner, Brian P—apparently in denial—claims that unsafe sex is not very likely to transmit HIV (despite Dr. A's assertions to the contrary). Moreover, Brian P reasons, HIV infection is not as bad as it used to be, since a combination of drug therapies now makes long-term survival possible for many HIV-infected individuals.

Dr. A is deeply disturbed by Brian P's intention to continue to have unsafe sex with George S without disclosing his HIV-positive status to him. While Dr. A is sure he would breach confidentiality (as a last resort) if a patient intended to kill an identified third party, Brian P does not intend to kill his partner. Moreover, Dr. A and Brian P have achieved a trust that makes psychotherapy more likely to succeed, a trust that would be put at risk if Brian P's confidentiality were breached. Still, Dr. A feels some obligation to protect George S by warning him if Brian P continues on the present course.

(1) Do health professionals have a "duty to warn" that can override their obligation to maintain patient confidentiality? (2) If so, does this duty extend to cases like the present one? (3) What should Dr. A do?

CASE 17
A RANDOMIZED CLINICAL TRIAL AND A PHYSICIAN'S RESPONSIBILITY TO A PATIENT [2, 4]

Dr. L has agreed to request the participation of his patients in an RCT designed to test a new drug whose purpose is to treat and cure a disease that is about 70 percent fatal. One of the participants in the trial, Bruce W, has been a patient of Dr. L's for 11 years. There are

90 participants in the RCT. Placebos have been given to 36. The other 54 have been given the new drug. None of the patients is told which treatment he or she is receiving, although all know they are taking part in an RCT. After 24 of the 36 patients on placebos and 15 of those receiving the new drug die, Bruce W asks Dr. L whether he is a placebo recipient and whether there is any good reason to think the new drug is effective. Dr. L knows that Bruce W is a placebo recipient and that the data so far tend to support the view that the experimental drug is effective and prevents death. Dr. L and other physicians involved in the trial prefer not to end it at this time because of concerns about the validity of the study if it is terminated prematurely.

(1) Should the experiment be ended and the remaining patients put on the new therapy immediately? (2) Should Dr. L decline at this point to provide Bruce W with the requested information? (3) Does Dr. L have an obligation to his patient, Bruce W, which should take precedence over concerns about establishing the validity of the RCT's results?

CASE 18
ANTI-AGING RESEARCH [3, 4]

Aging in one sense simply means getting older. Aging in a second sense involves the usual physiological changes that accompany getting older—for example, cells are increasingly subject to chromosomal aberrations; the immune system weakens, making one more susceptible to infections; nerve cells become damaged by chromatin; and collagen fibers become rigid, causing skin to wrinkle. Aging in both senses is now the topic of controversial research, which aims to gain insight into the physiology of aging with a possible eventual payoff of being able to extend the human lifespan. Some enthusiasts of anti-aging research consider it a prejudice to regard aging—in the sense of the characteristic forms of physical deterioration—as anything other than a disease, or set of diseases, that should be resisted through medical means no less than cancer is. Critics suggest that aging is a natural part of the human life cycle and that the current life expectancy in developed nations is all that human beings should aspire for.

(1) Is physiological aging natural in a sense that implies that it should be accepted rather than resisted? Or can it be regarded as a medical condition worthy of treatment? (2) Is there a natural human lifespan beyond which it is morally problematic to try to go? (3) Should the scientific community pursue anti-aging research?

CASE 19
ENROLLING INELIGIBLE PATIENTS IN A CLINICAL TRIAL [2, 4]

Participation in the clinical trial of a drug intended to benefit cancer patients is contingent upon the fulfillment of certain requirements. These include having only a certain type of cancer; having at least an eight-week life expectancy; having normal kidney, liver, and heart functioning; and having the ability to perform everyday functions. The validity of the trial depends upon the enforcement of these requirements. The trial is being conducted by colleagues of Dr. T who have asked him to enroll eligible patients in the trial, with the latter's consent, of course. Dr. Y, who is Dr. T's patient, has exhausted the therapies available for his form of cancer. Dr. Y hears about the clinical trial. Although he knows that he cannot meet all the requirements for participation, he tells Dr. T that he wants to be enrolled and asks that Dr. T fudge the data, if necessary, since otherwise he has no chance for survival.

(1) Should Dr. T fudge the data to give Dr. Y one last chance? (2) Since Dr. Y is also a physician and understands that his participation will compromise the validity of the trial, is his insistence on participation incompatible with his professional commitment?

CASE 20
BRAIN-DAMAGED GIBBONS AND THE MARCH OF SCIENCE [4]

In 2017, the United States Air Force commences a study to learn about "the basic mechanisms responsible for brain damage in head-injured fighter pilots." In this study, which involves the use of gibbons (one of the "lesser ape" species), a subject's head is cemented tightly in a helmet and subjected to a sudden jerking movement, generating an extremely strong impact. While the gibbon's skull is not fractured, neurological damage is caused by the impact of the brain against the hard skull. Anesthesia is carefully used so that the gibbons are completely unconscious during the procedure. The head trauma causes some subjects to become permanently comatose; others become conscious after anesthesia wears off (and are then given standard pain medications as needed). All become irreversibly brain-damaged and too disabled to feed themselves. Each lives alone in a small cage for approximately one month—during which time various tests are conducted—before they are killed and their brains analyzed.

(1) Can nonhuman animals be harmed by loss of freedom, disability, or death (as distinct from pain, distress, and suffering)? Does social isolation constitute a harm for highly sociable animals, such as primates? (2) Are some harms so great that no animal subjects should ever be forced to incur them? (3) Does the species of animal subjects matter in considering whether a study is justified? If so, how? (4) Does the importance of the research objective justify the study? Thousands of head-injured humans are hospitalized every year. Should they be considered as possible subjects for studies that cause no additional harm to them? Could more use be made of autopsy studies?

CASE 21
PHYSICIAN DISAGREEMENT REGARDING A PATIENT'S WISHES [2, 5]

John H, a 59-year-old male, has been diagnosed as having cancer, the primary site of which is the pancreas. His condition is rapidly deteriorating. John H has requested that he not be resuscitated if he should go into cardiac arrest. He has also stated that he wishes no further treatment. Dr. W, who is John H's personal physician, and Dr. R, the oncologist in the case, agree that he should not be resuscitated, and "Do not resuscitate" is written on his chart. However, when John H begins to experience severe internal bleeding, he asks his physicians if they can do something. Whether John H is competent at this point is unclear. Dr. W does not want to take measures to stop the bleeding, in keeping with John H's original request for no further treatment. Dr. R sees the request "to do something" as taking precedence over the earlier request for no additional treatment. If they do not act quickly to stop the internal bleeding, John H will die as a result of blood loss.

(1) What is the most appropriate response in this situation? (2) When a patient who is in a great deal of pain, weak, and close to death makes a request that seems at odds with a decision he made when he may have been more fully autonomous, which request should guide those caring for him?

CASE 22
HONORING A LIVING WILL [2, 5]

Esther K, a 65-year-old woman with a long history of diabetes, has been diagnosed as having pancreatic cancer. At the time of diagnosis, she refused all aggressive therapies and later wrote a living will, in which she stated clearly that she did not want any "extraordinary means" used to prolong her life. She specified the "extraordinary means" as chemotherapy, respirators, or resuscitation efforts. Three months after diagnosis, Esther K was admitted to the hospital in a confused state with discoloration on her foot and some evidence of necrotic tissue on the top of her foot. Observation over the next couple of days revealed that the necrosis had spread, and the surgeon, Dr. P, diagnosed gangrene. Dr. P wanted to remove the foot before the gangrene spread. Esther K was somewhat confused but nonetheless agreed to the surgery. The family was very upset with Dr. P for suggesting the surgery and for considering her competent to give consent. The family thinks that in the spirit of the living will she would not want the surgery, which would fall into the class of "extraordinary means." Furthermore, the family thinks that Esther K is too confused to give reflective consent, and this may be borne out by the fact that the patient whispered to the nurse that she consented only because she was afraid Dr. P would no longer take care of her and might order her out of the hospital.

(1) How specific must a living will be in order for it to be morally decisive? (2) Is there a danger of assuming that a consent is valid merely because it coincides with what the physician wishes to do? (3) What weight should be given to the family's judgment in this case?

CASE 23
REFUSAL OF LIFE-SUSTAINING TREATMENT BY A MINOR [2, 5]

Jimmy T is an 11-year-old boy who suffers from lymphoma. The oncologist has indicated that without chemotherapy Jimmy is likely to die within six months. She has also indicated that chemotherapy provides an effective cure in only 20 percent of cases like Jimmy's; in most of the cases, chemotherapy produces at best an additional three-month to six-month extension of life. Jimmy is also compromised by an incurable neurological disease. This disease will eventually make it impossible for him to walk, talk, use his hands effectively, or control his excretory functions. Already his speech is slurred, and he cannot hold a pencil. Even without the lymphoma, the prognosis for him because of the neurological disease is death by the age of 18. Jimmy has been raised in a strong religious environment, and his belief in God has been an important comforting factor for him. After having the facts fully explained to him, he has accepted his situation and the inevitability of his death at a young age. He says that he does not want the chemotherapy and that he is ready to "go to God." His parents, however, cannot reconcile themselves to losing Jimmy. They override Jimmy's decision and tell the oncologist to proceed with the chemotherapy.

(1) Should minors of Jimmy's age be permitted to participate in decisions of this magnitude? (2) Whose decision, the parents' or the child's, should be decisive? (3) How should the oncologist deal with this situation?

CASE 24
A POSSIBLE CONFLICT OF INTEREST FOR A PROXY DECISION MAKER [5]

Joe and Liz C married fifteen years ago. (Before that, he was a widower and she was divorced.) For the past seven years the marriage has been relatively unhappy, due to the revelation of Liz C's affair with one of her husband's colleagues. Two weeks ago Liz C had a stroke. It is clear that some of her capacities will be damaged by the stroke, but the extent of incapacitation is currently unknown. Right now she cannot speak and has incurred respiratory difficulties and an acute infection. Joe C has requested that her conditions not be treated. "Make her as comfortable as possible and let her die in peace," he urged the medical team. "After all, she always said she didn't want to be an invalid. I'm sure she wouldn't want to live." But the attending physician, Dr. H, remembers Joe C's remarking a couple of times that he could not imagine taking care of an invalid wife. Moreover, Dr. H, who has known the couple for years, is aware of the affair that took place long ago, and he has often sensed a deep bitterness on the part of Joe C toward his wife. Dr. H therefore wonders about Joe C's motives and about whose interests would be served if Liz C were allowed to die. Without being quite sure how to proceed, he decides he cannot simply take for granted Joe C's testimony about his wife's preferences.

(1) If the medical team is unable to uncover more information regarding Liz C's wishes regarding treatment in her present circumstances, how should her best interests be determined? (2) If her best interests favor treatment of her infection and breathing difficulties as well as rehabilitative therapy—in apparent conflict with Joe C's wishes— should these interventions be initiated? Should Joe C's interests be given any significant consideration?

CASE 25
ANENCEPHALIC NEWBORNS, ORGAN DONATION, AND SOCIAL POLICY [5, 6]

It is estimated that 1,000 to 2,000 babies are born in the United States each year with anencephaly, the total or almost total absence of the cerebral hemispheres. Many of these infants are stillborn; the prognosis for those born alive is that they will live for only a few hours, days, or weeks. Although the organ systems of some anencephalic infants are underdeveloped, there are many cases in which organs (e.g., a heart or kidneys) could be transplanted to other infants whose lives might thereby be saved. Some parents of anencephalic infants would undoubtedly consent to organ donation as a way of creating some redeeming value out of a tragic situation. Still, numerous reservations have been expressed about the idea of transplanting the organs of anencephalic infants. In particular, for transplants to have a reasonable prospect of success, the vital organs must be taken from an anencephalic infant before it meets the criteria of (whole) brain death; thus, harvesting its vital organs is tantamount to killing the infant. At present, there is no legal mechanism through which this sort of organ donation can be accomplished.

(1) Is it disrespectful, unfair, or otherwise immoral to transplant the organs of an anencephalic infant? (2) Should we adopt a social policy that would permit (with parental consent) harvesting the organs of an anencephalic infant? (3) If an anencephalic infant is stillborn, would it be justifiable to attempt resuscitation purely for the purpose of keeping organs intact until they can be harvested? (4) If it is justifiable to harvest the organs of an anencephalic infant, would it be justifiable to harvest the organs of someone in a permanent vegetative state?

CASE 26
NEONATAL CARE AND THE PROBLEM OF UNCERTAINTY [5]

Bobbie C is now 6 months old. He was born prematurely with a birth weight of 800 grams and had multiple problems from the beginning. Bobbie developed hyaline membrane disease due to his undeveloped lungs and the need for a respirator. He also developed rickets. A CAT scan revealed some calcium deposits in the brain, which might or might not compromise his mental functions. Within the first month, Bobbie developed thrombocytopenia (low platelet count), for which he was given transfusions. He now suffers from a depression of his immunological system, perhaps related to the transfusions. He shows little interest in eating, and all attempts to bottle-feed him have failed after a couple of days. His health-care costs are being supported by Medicaid, and they are estimated to be in the neighborhood of $550,000 for his six months of hospitalization. Now the health-care staff and the attending physician are considering the possibility of a bone marrow transplant to deal with the thrombocytopenia and the immunosuppression. The chances of success in an infant this small are minimal, and the procedure is largely experimental in infants having this condition. If the transplant is successful, it will alleviate only one of his many problems.

(1) In view of the many uncertainties in this case, what is the proper treatment decision? (2) Should society be expected to shoulder such an expense for an infant who is so physiologically and, perhaps, mentally compromised? (3) Do the parents have a right to reject further aggressive therapies? to insist on them?

CASE 27
IS NUTRITION EXPENDABLE? [5]

Mildred D, a 78-year-old woman, suffers from diabetes, which has been controlled largely by diet. She has a history of heart disease and has suffered two heart attacks. She has now had a stroke, which has rendered her semicomatose and paralyzed. She must be fed through an NG (nasogastric) tube, and the sustenance that she receives in this way is the only thing that keeps her going. Mildred D has previously indicated to her family that in such a circumstance she would not want to be resuscitated. Her condition is slowly deteriorating, but it looks as though the dying process will be a long one. It seems that she will never return from the twilight zone in which she now resides. Angiography indicates that a substantial portion of the brain has been destroyed by the stroke. Her three children want to stop the tube feedings, but the physician objects that it is unethical to "starve" a patient so that she will die sooner.

(1) Is it morally legitimate to withhold nutrition in this case? (2) Does the family have the right to make such a decision for the patient? (3) Should the refusal of resuscitation be considered an indicator that the patient would also refuse nutrition?

CASE 28
DEATH BY DEHYDRATION [5, 6]

Roberta W is a 67-year-old unmarried female. A retired teacher, she is cared for by her brother and his wife in their home. Roberta W suffers from severe emphysema and related heart problems. She also suffers from a collection of nagging medical problems, including bloatedness, hemorrhoids, and a hernia. She is largely confined to her bed. Occasionally she feels well enough to sit up for an hour or so, but eating, going to the bathroom, and personal grooming are experienced as exhausting and burdensome. Roberta W is weary of the circumstances of her life, and she regrets being a burden to her brother and his wife, although they do not seem to resent the demands placed upon them by her care. Roberta W's prognosis is somewhat unclear, and she may well live for several years in her present state, but she continually says that she would rather be dead. At one point, when her hernia was especially bothersome to her, she had a conversation with her physician, Dr. R. He said that the hernia could easily be corrected by surgery but that it was very unlikely that she would survive the surgery because of her emphysema and heart problems. She said that she wanted the surgery anyway. "If I die, fine; if I survive, at least I have one less problem." Dr. R responded that no responsible surgeon would perform an operation in such circumstances.

Roberta W now asks Dr. R to admit her to the hospital. Her plan is to stop drinking and to refuse any form of medical hydration, but she wants to be in the hospital so that any discomfort can be controlled through medication. She has read that patients who refuse all hydration will usually die within a week or so.

(1) If Roberta W refuses all hydration, is she committing suicide? (2) Should Dr. R accept Roberta W's plan and cooperate with her in executing it? Should his cooperation be understood as physician assistance in suicide? (3) Would it have been morally justified for a surgeon to have provided the hernia surgery that she had wanted at an earlier time?

CASE 29
A BRAIN-DEAD MOTHER GIVES BIRTH [5, 7]

Rosa J suffered a fatal seizure while she was 23 weeks pregnant. Although Rosa J was declared brain-dead the day after the seizure, cardiopulmonary function was maintained by means of a respirator and allied technology for nine weeks, until she gave birth to a healthy baby girl by cesarean section. During this time, the physicians used steroids to help the lungs of the fetus mature and monitored fetal growth with ultrasound examinations. Rosa J was fed intravenously and given antibiotics for infections when necessary. After the birth, the respirator was disconnected. The baby was given an excellent chance to survive, although she weighed only three pounds. From the time of the seizure, all decisions about Rosa J and the fetus she was carrying were made by physicians in consultation with Rosa J's family.

(1) Should Rosa J have been maintained on a respirator for nine weeks after being declared brain-dead simply in order to give the child she was carrying a better chance to survive? (2) Was Rosa J being used merely as a means to others' ends? (3) Is someone who is brain-dead a "person" and, therefore, on a Kantian account an individual who cannot be used merely as a means to others' ends?

CASE 30
EMBRYONIC STEM CELLS AND A PRESIDENTIAL DECISION [7, 8]

In a short speech delivered to the nation August 9, 2001, President George W. Bush offered some general reflections on the ethics of research on embryonic stem cells and also announced a decision he had made about the use of federal funding to support such research.

"As a result of private research, more than sixty genetically diverse stem cell lines already exist. They were created from embryos that have already been destroyed, and they have the ability to regenerate themselves indefinitely, creating ongoing opportunities for research. I have concluded that we should allow federal funds to be used for research on these existing stem cell lines, where the life and death decision has already been made.

"Leading scientists tell me research on these sixty lines has great promise that could lead to breakthrough therapies and cures. This allows us to explore the promise and potential of stem cell research without crossing a fundamental moral line, by providing taxpayer funding that would sanction or encourage further destruction of human embryos that have at least the potential for life."

The President's decision was widely viewed as an effort to craft a political compromise on a volatile policy issue. The essence of the decision was this: Research on preexisting stem cell lines—that is, those already in existence as a result of the prior destruction of embryos—would be eligible for federal funding, but research on stem cell lines derived from embryos destroyed after August 9, 2001, would not be eligible for federal funding.

In March 2009, President Barack Obama fulfilled a campaign promise by signing an executive order lifting the Bush restrictions on embryonic stem-cell research (ESCR) and directing the National Institutes of Health to develop guidelines to decide which stem cell lines it would be ethical to use. (In addition to the lines that were eligible for federal funding under the Bush policy, there are many additional lines that have been funded through private sources.) Representing a political compromise, the NIH guidelines that were finalized in July 2009 limited federal funding to lines created from excess fertility clinic embryos, provided they were obtained in a way that met certain criteria—such as ensuring that couples were not offered financial incentives to donate embryos that might later be used for research. In December of the same year, NIH authorized the first lines of embryonic stem cells for research under the Obama policy.

(1) Was the Bush federal funding policy too restrictive, too permissive, or fully justified? (2) Is the Obama policy more or less morally defensible than the Bush policy? (3) What would be an optimal policy regarding federal funding for ESCR if neither the Bush approach nor that of Obama is optimal?

CASE 31
MATERNAL PKU AND FETAL WELFARE [7]

Martha J, a 23-year-old female, was born with PKU (phenylketonuria), an enzyme deficiency that prevents the metabolization of phenylalanine. Children born with PKU are ordinarily placed on a special low-phenylalanine diet for at least the first five years of their life. Although the diet is necessary to prevent severe retardation, it is very burdensome, not only because normal foods are very limited but also because the main source of protein is a bad-tasting "medical food." Because Martha J was placed on this special diet in her childhood, she does not suffer from retardation.

Martha J is four months pregnant. Although her inability to metabolize phenylalanine is no longer a problem for her own well-being, there is a problem for the fetus she is carrying. Unless Martha J maintains the same low-phenylalanine diet throughout the course of her pregnancy, her fetus is at grave risk for severe retardation, microcephaly, congenital heart disease, and other disorders. Martha J's religious beliefs have motivated her to decide against abortion. Nevertheless, she is ambivalent about her pregnancy, because she is unmarried and depressed by the breakdown of her relationship with the child's father. She is also finding it very difficult to adhere to the same dietary restrictions that she found so oppressive in her childhood. Dr. R, the obstetrician who is caring for Martha J, has repeatedly emphasized the importance of adhering to the prescribed diet, but Martha J acknowledges that she has been inconstant in doing so.

(1) Should Dr. R encourage Martha J to reconsider the possibility of abortion? (2) If Martha J is resolved to carry her fetus to term, how should Dr. R deal with the fact that she is not maintaining the prescribed diet? (3) If all else fails, should Dr. R seek a court order that would place Martha J in a supervised setting where dietary restrictions could be enforced?

CASE 32
A FETUS WITH TURNER'S SYNDROME [7, 8]

Barbara J is a 37-year-old woman who is pregnant and in her 20th week. She is married and has one child, a 4-year-old girl. At the advice of her obstetrician, Barbara J has undergone amniocentesis, so that tests could be performed for chromosomal abnormalities and neural-tube defects. The tests have just come in, and Barbara J is told that the fetus has been diagnosed with a chromosomal abnormality known as Turner's syndrome.

A normal female has two X chromosomes. In Turner's syndrome, one of the two X chromosomes is missing; there is a total of only 45 chromosomes. Females who have Turner's syndrome have a characteristic appearance: short stature, webbing of the neck, sagging eyelids, low hairline on the back of the neck, and multiple moles. The syndrome is also characterized by narrowing of the aorta, the failure of menstruation and breast development, and infertility. Although many patients with Turner's syndrome have difficulty performing tasks that require spatial orientation, they can otherwise function normally in society.

(1) How serious are the appearance and developmental problems associated with Turner's syndrome? (2) Would abortion be morally justified in this case? Does it make a difference that the fetus is already at 20 weeks?

CASE 33
PRENATAL DIAGNOSIS AND SEX SELECTION [7, 8]

A 32-year-old woman, Lisa B, goes to the prenatal diagnostic center of a major hospital. She is intent on arranging for chorionic villi sampling (CVS) in order to determine the sex of the fetus she is carrying. A genetic counselor explains to her that the center has an established policy against making prenatal diagnosis (whether CVS or amniocentesis) available for purposes of sex selection. The genetic counselor, in defending the policy, tells her that there is a collective sense at the center that abortion purely on grounds of sex selection is both morally and socially problematic.

Lisa B proceeds to explain her situation. She and her husband already have three children, all of whom are girls. They want very much to have a male child but, for economic reasons, are determined to have no more than one more child. Indeed, if they had a boy among their three children, they would not even consider having a fourth. They feel so strongly about this fourth child's being a boy that, if they cannot gain assurance that it is a male, they will elect abortion. Lisa B insists that it is unfair for the center to deny her access to prenatal diagnosis.

(1) Should the center consider this case an exceptional one and make CVS available? (2) Would the center be well advised to develop a different policy regarding the availability of prenatal diagnosis for purposes of sex selection?

CASE 34
PREIMPLANTATION GENETIC DIAGNOSIS AND HUNTINGTON'S DISEASE [7, 8]

Heather D is a 24-year-old female whose father suffers from Huntington's disease, an autosomal dominant genetic disease whose symptoms first emerge (ordinarily) between the ages of 30 and 50. Huntington's disease is characterized by a progressive physical and mental deterioration leading to death in ten to fifteen years. Heather D knows that there is a

50 percent chance that she has inherited the defective gene from her father, but she has decided not to undergo testing to determine whether she has inherited the gene, because she would rather not know. Heather D and her husband want to have a child, but both of them have a strong desire that their child not be at risk for Huntington's disease. They have rejected the possibility of prenatal diagnosis and selective abortion, in part because Heather D realizes that diagnosis of her fetus as carrying the defective gene would entail the knowledge that she also carries the gene, and because Heather D's husband is morally opposed to abortion. A genetic counselor has suggested an alternative involving preimplantation genetic diagnosis. Several embryos could be formed in vitro using Heather D's eggs and her husband's sperm. These embryos could be tested for the presence of the Hungtington's gene, with only embryos free of the gene being transferred to Heather's uterus. If any embryos were found to carry the defective gene, they would be quietly discarded.

(1) Is Heather D's decision not to be tested for the Huntington's gene a wise one? (2) Does the genetic counselor's suggestion provide a satisfactory solution to the problem? (3) Is preimplantation genetic diagnosis and the discarding of affected embryos morally equivalent to prenatal diagnosis and selective abortion?

CASE 35
CYSTIC FIBROSIS AND A FINDING OF NONPATERNITY [8]

At the age of 19 months, Jennifer C was diagnosed with cystic fibrosis (CF), an autosomal recessive genetic disease. The characteristic pattern is that a child inherits the CF gene from both parents, each of whom is a carrier. Jennifer C's parents, who have been married about three years, are anxious to clarify their risk for having another child with this disorder. They are referred to a genetic counselor, who arranges for DNA testing to confirm their carrier status. The results from the laboratory indicate that Jennifer's mother is a carrier but her husband is not. In fact, DNA analysis shows clearly that he is not the biological father of the child. The genetic counselor is unsure how to proceed.

(1) Should the genetic counselor communicate the finding of nonpaternity to the couple, perhaps jeopardizing their young marriage? Should the genetic counselor first speak privately with the woman? (2) If the woman is willing to identify the biological father, should the genetic counselor notify him that he is almost certainly a carrier of the CF gene?

CASE 36
IVF AND A POSTMENOPAUSAL WOMAN [8]

Emily L is a 59-year-old woman who plans to retire at the age of 60 from her job as a financial executive. She has been married for ten years to a man who also plans to retire within the next year. He is presently 64 years of age. Both Emily L and her husband are in good health and look forward to carving out a new life in retirement. In fact, they have decided that this would be a good time for them to raise a child, so they want to arrange for Emily L to become pregnant. They are aware that it is now possible for postmenopausal women to bear children by employing egg donation, in vitro fertilization (IVF), and embryo transfer to the womb of the postmenopausal woman, who would receive hormonal treatments. The idea is that Emily L's husband would provide the sperm for IVF, making him the biological father of the child. When Emily L and her husband explain their plan to Dr. T at the Metropolitan Fertility Clinic, Dr. T is uncertain whether the clinic should support Emily's attempt to become pregnant. Dr. T has successfully produced pregnancies in women who have experienced early menopause, but she is not comfortable with the age of the prospective parents in this particular case.

(1) Is the plan formulated by Emily L and her husband morally sound? If not, what is problematic about it? (2) Should Dr. T and the clinic support Emily L's attempt to become pregnant?

CASE 37
BABY M [8]

In February 1985, Mary Beth Whitehead entered into a commercial surrogacy agreement with a married couple, Elizabeth and William Stern. Mary Beth Whitehead agreed, for a fee of $10,000, to be artificially inseminated with William Stern's semen and to bear a child that upon birth would be given over to the couple and adopted by Elizabeth Stern. Elizabeth Stern was living under a possible diagnosis of multiple sclerosis and was reluctant to bear the risks associated with pregnancy. Mary Beth Whitehead was married and had two children at the time she entered into the surrogacy contract.

Mary Beth Whitehead eventually became pregnant and Baby M was born March 27, 1986. (The baby was named Sara by Mary Beth Whitehead and Melissa by the Sterns.) Upon giving birth, Mary Beth Whitehead realized that she did not want to part with the child, but she did give the child over to the Sterns on March 30. The next day, clearly in emotional turmoil, she implored the Sterns to let her keep the baby for another week. The Sterns reluctantly agreed. When Mary Beth Whitehead subsequently refused to return Baby M to the Sterns, William Stern filed a complaint seeking legal enforcement of the surrogacy contract. In response, Mary Beth Whitehead and her husband fled with Baby M from New Jersey to Florida. The Whiteheads continually changed their location in Florida in an effort to escape detection, but Florida authorities eventually located Baby M when she was about four months old. The child was returned to New Jersey and placed in the temporary custody of the Sterns while the trial court considered how the matter was to be resolved.

Eight months later, when Baby M was about one year old, the trial court announced its judgment. The trial court (a) found the surrogacy contract to be valid, (b) ordered the termination of Mary Beth Whitehead's parental rights, (c) awarded sole custody of Baby M to William Stern, and (d) authorized adoption by Elizabeth Stern.

The New Jersey Supreme Court ultimately took a very different position. The court concluded that commercial surrogacy contracts are invalid and unenforceable in New Jersey. Four principal concerns were expressed. First, a surrogate mother cannot be forced by a prebirth contract to surrender her child because she is in no position to make an *informed* choice prior to birth. Second, commercial surrogacy contracts are tantamount to baby selling. Third, commercial surrogacy contracts would allow the rich to exploit the poor. Fourth, there is a risk of psychosocial harm to the resultant child. Although consideration of Baby M's best interests led the court to award primary custody to the Sterns, the court found no basis for the termination of Mary Beth Whitehead's parental rights and therefore concluded that she (as the child's legal mother) was entitled to visitation.

(1) Is it the trial court or the New Jersey Supreme Court that provided the best overall resolution of the issues involved in this case? (2) Should commercial surrogacy contracts be recognized as valid and legally enforceable? (3) Who should be recognized as the legal mother of Baby M? Would it make a difference if Mary Beth Whitehead, instead of being both the genetic and gestational mother of Baby M, had been only the gestational mother

of Baby M, that is, if an egg provided by Elizabeth Stern had been fertilized with her husband's sperm and then transferred to the uterus of Mary Beth Whitehead?

CASE 38
IVF, EMBRYO SPLITTING, AND DELAYED TWINNING [8]

Karen T and Roger T, a married couple in their late 30s, have been trying for several years to start a family. After consulting with Dr. M at the University Reproductive Center, the couple decided to try IVF, even though their expenses for this procedure would amount to at least $8,000. Karen T expressed worries about the possible hazards of the fertility drugs commonly used to enhance the production of mature eggs, but she ultimately agreed to undergo drug treatment, and several eggs were recovered via a minor but uncomfortable surgical procedure. The eggs were subsequently fertilized with Roger T's sperm. Of the seven embryos ultimately produced by this process, four were frozen at the four-cell stage, and the other three were transferred to Karen T's uterus, but without success. Later, three of the remaining embryos were thawed and transferred to Karen T's uterus, again without success.

Concerned about the risks of fertility drugs, the risks and discomfort of the egg-recovery process, and the overall expense of the procedure, the couple is now reluctant to start another course of IVF. They propose the following plan to Dr. M. The one remaining embryo should be thawed and split into four cells, so that each can begin the process of division and growth. Implantation should be attempted with two of the newly formed embryos; the other two should be frozen. Further, they suggest, if Karen T becomes pregnant and gives birth to a healthy child, the couple can wait two or three years and then attempt to achieve pregnancy with the remaining embryos. This plan could result in genetically identical children of different ages.

(1) Should Dr. T act in accordance with the wishes of the couple? (2) Is embryo splitting morally defensible as an adjunct to IVF and embryo transfer? (3) Is embryo splitting and delayed twinning less morally problematic than cloning via somatic cell nuclear transfer?

CASE 39
JUSTICE AND ABORTION FUNDING [7, 9]

Sara G is a 35-year-old mother of four children whose husband deserted her about a month after she became pregnant with her fifth child. The ages of her four children range from 1 to 6 years. She knows nothing about her husband's whereabouts and is currently being supported by public assistance. Sara G is less than three months pregnant and wants an abortion. Her reasons are as follows: (1) She does not have the skills to get a job whose earnings will even come close to the public assistance she receives. If she has to pay for child care from whatever meager wages she could earn, the money left could not support her family at even the subsistence level, so, at least until the children are older, she will be dependent upon public assistance. The sums she receives are barely adequate to take care of her present family. Adding another member would mean even further deprivation for her present family. (2) Her caseworker has agreed that, when the four children are a bit older, Sara G will go into a job-training program that will enable her to get a job paying enough to get the family off public assistance and to give her children a better start in life. Sara G has undergone a battery of psychological tests to help determine what kind of work she should be capable of doing with the right education and training. The social worker and psychological counselor are both confident that Sara G can do the work necessary to make a good living for herself and her family. Having another child would only postpone the time when Sara G will be self-supporting, and in the meantime her family would be living at a very inadequate level.

Because Sara G is on public assistance, she must get an authorization from the social work agency to secure funding for any medical procedure that is not necessitated by an emergency. In cases involving abortion, the final decision is made by a social worker.

(1) Should the social worker authorize funding for the abortion? (2) What moral justification could be advanced to support an authorization? a refusal to authorize? (3) What restrictions, if any, should there be on the Medicaid funding of abortion?

CASE 40
JUSTICE, MENTAL DISABILITY, AND PUBLIC POLICY [9]

State representative Jeremy H has introduced a state bill that would establish homes for the care and education of children with major learning disabilities, such as severe retardation and autism. The bill would provide one home for every twelve children presently institutionalized in five state institutions for children with such disabilities. The present annual cost of maintaining the five institutions is $100 million. Providing the new form of care for the present institutionalized population of 8,000 is expected to cost about $130 million annually.

Jeremy H argues that the currently institutionalized children live in antiquated buildings lacking basic human necessities and amenities. The children frequently spend whole days in their cheerless rooms; many are not even properly clothed. Supervised by an overworked, largely untrained staff, they receive almost nothing in the way of education, entertainment, or structured activities. Jeremy H argues that justice requires removing these individuals from such subhuman conditions and offering them an opportunity for a more "normal" life.

A physician, Dr. M, is opposed to the bill and testifies at a legislative hearing. He argues that the money required to make the change could be used more efficiently to provide health care for three groups: normal children, women lacking access to gynecological and prenatal services, and working adults whose employers do not provide health insurance. He also argues that the occurrence of retardation and other mental disabilities can be greatly reduced through prenatal diagnosis.

(1) Should the proposed bill be enacted into law? (2) Do the mentally retarded have a right to lead a life as "normal" as possible, given their limitations?

CASE 41
JUSTICE, HEALTH CARE, AND POVERTY [9]

Amanda R is 25 years old. Although she holds both a full-time and a part-time job, she has a very low income and does not have any health-care insurance. At the same time, Amanda R's income is just high enough to prevent her from qualifying for any government-funded health care such as that provided by Medicaid. While experiencing severe chest pain and difficulty in breathing, Amanda R goes to the emergency room of a local for-profit hospital. Before she receives any care, clerical personnel in the hospital determine her financial status and the fact that she is uninsured. By the time she is examined, Amanda R's chest pains stop, and her breathing difficulties disappear. A medical staff member gives her a cursory examination, which does not include an electrocardiogram, and sends her home, suggesting that she go to her own physician the next day for a more thorough examination.

(1) If the medical staff member's decision not to give Amanda R a more thorough examination and not to admit her for further observation was based on her lack of health-care insurance, can that decision be morally justified? (2) Suppose that Amanda R's symptoms had not eased while she was in the emergency room and that the medical staff member had decided that Amanda R did need hospital admittance, observation, and testing. However, suppose that, instead of admitting her to the for-profit hospital, Amanda R had been sent by ambulance to a community (not-for-profit) hospital. Would that behavior have been morally acceptable?

CASE 42
HEALTH CARE REFORM IN MASSACHUSETTS [9]

In April 2006, under the leadership of Governor Mitt Romney, Massachusetts passed significant health-care legislation. The new law had several key elements. First, eligibility for Medicaid was somewhat expanded. Second, it required individuals with income levels above the poverty line to purchase a private insurance policy for themselves or their families, with the state offering partial subsidies to families within 300 percent of the poverty line. Third, a new state agency called "the Connector" was designed to connect people with private health insurance plans and to help design affordable plans. In addition, citizens were permitted to use pre-tax dollars to buy health insurance, and businesses employing more than ten people were required to pay a small fee if they declined to provide health insurance to their employees.

The results of this Massachusetts legislation (as of 2009) have both favorable and unfavorable aspects. The percentage of uninsured persons fell from 6.4 percent in 2006 to 2.6 percent in 2008, a sizeable improvement in coverage. At the same time, the state is struggling to control rapidly rising health-care costs and the legislature voted to cut back on benefits for thousands of legal immigrants. Moreover, Boston Medical Center has sued the state on the grounds that the new law has driven the hospital into deficit. According to critics, Massachusetts-style health-care reform is doomed to failure because, rather than addressing the structural inefficiencies of the American health care status quo, it essentially just requires people to buy health insurance without enabling (through adequate subsidies) enough of the poor to do so. In a word, neither universal coverage nor cost controls is possible with this approach. On the other hand, a strong majority of Massachusetts residents express support for the reform in polls. Some even take the state experiment as a model for health-care reform on a national level. MIT economics professor Jonathan Gruber expressed this opinion: "I think the Massachusetts model is an excellent one for what it tried to accomplish: moving to universal coverage by building on the existing insurance infrastructure."

(1) Is health-care reform along the line of the Massachusetts approach—featuring an "individual mandate" to purchase insurance—likely to achieve universal coverage, cost controls, and other important health-care goals? (2) Would health-care reform that more drastically restructured the health insurance market or massively expanded public insurance be more likely to achieve major health-care goals? (3) Which sort of reform is preferable, all things considered: Massachusetts-style reform or more fundamental reform? What role should considerations of political feasibility play in this discussion?

ABOUT THE CONTRIBUTORS

TERRENCE F. ACKERMAN is Professor and Chair of the Department of Human Values and Ethics at the College of Medicine, University of Tennessee, Memphis.

CHRISTA ALTENSTETTER is Professor of Political Science at Queens College (Flushing, New York).

MARCIA ANGELL is Senior Lecturer, Department of Social Medicine, Harvard University.

GEORGE J. ANNAS is Edward R. Utley Professor and Chair of the Department of Health Law, Bioethics, and Human Rights at the Boston University School of Public Health.

JOHN D. ARRAS is Porterfield Professor of Biomedical Ethics, Professor of Philosophy, and UVA Alumni Association Distinguished Professor at the University of Virginia.

JAMES L. BERNAT is Professor in the Department of Medicine, Section of Neurology, Dartmouth Medical School.

R. B. BRANDT was Professor of Philosophy at the University of Michigan.

DAN W. BROCK is Frances Glessner Lee Professor of Medical Ethics in the Department of Social Medicine and Director of the Division of Medical Ethics, Harvard University.

BARUCH BRODY is Leon Jaworski Professor of Biomedical Ethics and Director of the Center for Medical Ethics and Health Policy at Baylor College of Medicine, and Professor of Philosophy at Rice University.

HOWARD BRODY is Director, Institute for the Medical Humanities, Professor of Family Medicine, and John P. McGovern Centennial Chair at the University of Texas Medical Branch.

ALLEN E. BUCHANAN is James B. Duke Professor of Philosophy and Public Policy Studies at Duke University.

DANIEL CALLAHAN is a cofounder of the Hastings Center (Garrison, New York), where he is Director of International Programs.

CHRISTINE K. CASSEL is President and Chief Executive Officer of the American Board of Internal Medicine and the ABIM Foundation.

JAMES F. CHILDRESS is John Allen Hollingsworth Professor of Ethics in the Department of Religious Studies and Professor of Medical Education at the University of Virginia.

KEVIN C. CHUNG is Professor of Plastic Surgery at the University of Michigan Medical School.

CARL COHEN is Professor of Philosophy in the Residential College, University of Michigan.

ROBERT A. CROUCH is Research Assistant at the Poynter Center for the Study of Ethics and American Institutions, Indiana University.

RAISA BERLIN DEBER is Professor of Health Policy, Management, and Evaluation on the Faculty of Medicine, University of Toronto.

REBECCA DRESSER is Daniel Noyes Kirby Professor of Law and Professor of Ethics at Washington University in St. Louis.

CARL ELLIOTT is Professor in the Center for Bioethics and in the Departments of Pediatrics and Philosophy at the University of Minnesota.

EZEKIEL J. EMANUEL is Chair of the Department of Clinical Bioethics, National Institutes of Health and Special Advisor for Health Policy to the Director of the Office of Management and Budget.

DAVID W. EMMONS is Director of Economics and Health Policy Research at the American Medical Association.

MARTHA J. FARAH is Walter H. Annenberg Professor of Natural Sciences, Professor of Psychology, and Director of the Center for Cognitive Neuroscience at the University of Pennsylvania.

LEONARD M. FLECK is Professor of Philosophy and Medical Ethics at Michigan State University.

JOHN C. FLETCHER was Emily Davie and Joseph S. Kornfield Professor of Biomedical Ethics at the School of Medicine, University of Virginia.

CAROL FREEDMAN is a psychotherapist and philosopher, currently working in the Professionals' Program at the Institute of Living (Hartford, Connecticut).

VICTOR R. FUCHS is Henry J. Kaiser, Jr., Professor of Economics and of Health Research and Policy, Emeritus, at Stanford University.

BERNARD GERT is Stone Professor of Intellectual and Moral Philosophy, Emeritus, at Dartmouth College, Adjunct Professor of Psychiatry at Dartmouth Medical School, and Research Professor in the Department of Social Medicine at the School of Medicine, University of North Carolina, Chapel Hill.

LEONARD H. GLANTZ is Associate Dean for Academic Affairs, Emeritus, and Professor of Health Law, Bioethics and Human Rights at the School of Public Health, Boston University.

LAWRENCE O. GOSTIN is Associate Dean for Research and Academic Programs and Linda D. and Timothy J. O'Neill Professor of Global Health Law at the Georgetown University Law Center and Professor of Public Health at Johns Hopkins University.

MICHAEL A. GRODIN is Professor of Health Law, Bioethics and Human Rights at the Boston University School of Public Health, Professor of Socio-Medical Sciences and Community Medicine and Psychiatry at the Boston University School of Medicine, and Professor of Philosophy at Boston University.

LISA ABELOW HEDLEY is a lawyer, film producer, director, and screenwriter.

DEBORAH S. HELLMAN is Jacob France Research Professor of Law at the University of Maryland.

SAMUEL HELLMAN is A. N. Pritzker Distinguished Service Professor in the Department of Radiation and Cellular Oncology, University of Chicago.

EDWIN CONVERSE HETTINGER is Professor of Philosophy at the College of Charleston (South Carolina).

ROGER HIGGS is Professor of General Practice and Primary Care at the School of Medicine and Dentistry, King's College, London.

DAVID U. HIMMELSTEIN is Associate Professor of Medicine at Harvard Medical School and Chief of the Division of Social and Community Medicine, Cambridge Hospital.

JOSEPHINE JOHNSTON is Research Scholar at the Hastings Center (Garrison, New York).

LEON R. KASS is former Chair of the President's Council on Bioethics and Addie Clark Harding Professor, the Committee on Social Thought and the College, University of Chicago.

SOPHIA KOLEHMAINEN is Deputy Director of the Cedar Tree Foundation (Boston).

ALEXANDER A. KON is Associate Professor of Pediatrics and Bioethics at the Medical Center, University of California, Davis.

PETER D. KRAMER is Clinical Professor of Psychiatry and Human Behavior at Brown University.

HELGA KUHSE is Honorary Senior Research Fellow at the Centre for Human Bioethics, Monash University (Melbourne).

CLAUDE LE PEN is Professor of Economics at the University of Paris-Dauphine.

DONALD W. LIGHT is Professor of Comparative Health Care Systems and Director of the Division of Social and Behavioral Medicine at the University of Medicine and Dentistry of New Jersey, School of Osteopathic Medicine.

MARGARET OLIVIA LITTLE is Associate Professor of Philosophy as well Director and Senior Research Scholar, Kennedy Institute of Ethics, Georgetown University.

PAUL LITTON is Associate Professor of Law at the University of Missouri, St. Louis.

BRUCE LOWENSTEIN has a private practice in psychotherapy and provides outpatient services for Helen Hayes Hospital (West Haverstraw, New York).

RUTH MACKLIN is Professor of Bioethics at the Albert Einstein College of Medicine (New York).

WENDY K. MARINER is Professor of Law, Professor of Socio-Medical Sciences and Community Medicine, and Director of the Patient Rights Program at Boston University.

DON MARQUIS is Professor of Philosophy at the University of Kansas.

JEFF MCMAHAN is Professor of Philosophy at Rutgers University (New Jersey).

DIANE E. MEIER is Director of the Center to Advance Palliative Care, Director of the Lilian and Benjamin Hertzberg Palliative Care Institute, Professor of Geriatrics and Internal Medicine, and Catherine Gaisman Professor of Medical Ethics at Mount Sinai School of Medicine in New York City.

VICKI MICHEL was Associate Director of the Pacific Center for Health Policy and Ethics at the University of Southern California.

FRANKLIN G. MILLER is Special Expert, Intramural Research Program, National Institute of Mental Health, and Bioethicist, Department of Clinical Bioethics, National Institutes of Health.

CLAUDIA MILLS is Professor of Philosophy at the University of Colorado, Boulder.

R. PETER MOGIELNICKI is Professor of Medicine (General Internal Medicine) at Dartmouth Medical School.

SHERRI GROVEMAN MORRIS is an attorney and intersex activist who founded the U.S. branch of the Androgen Insensitivity Syndrome Support Group and has served on the Board of Directors of the Intersex Society of North America.

THOMAS H. MURRAY is President and Chief Executive Officer of the Hastings Center (Garrison, New York).

LISA H. NEWTON is Professor of Philosophy and Director of the Program in Applied Ethics at Fairfield University (Connecticut).

KAI NIELSEN is Professor Emeritus of Philosophy at the University of Calgary (Alberta, Canada) and Adjunct Professor of Philosophy at Concordia University (Montreal, Quebec).

DAVID ORENTLICHER is Samuel R. Rosen Professor of Law and Co-Director of the Center for Law and Health at Indiana University School of Law–Indianapolis.

JULIE GAGE PALMER is Lecturer in Law, University of Chicago Law School.

DONALD J. PALMISANO is former President of the American Medical Association, Clinical Professor of Surgery, and Clinical Professor of Medical Jurisprudence at Tulane University School of Medicine (New Orleans).

EDMUND D. PELLEGRINO is former Chair of the President's Council on Bioethics, former President of the Catholic University of America, and John Carroll Professor Emeritus of Medicine at Georgetown University Medical Center.

TIA POWELL is Director of the Montefiore-Einstein Center for Bioethics (New York).

LAURA M. PURDY is Professor of Philosophy at Wells College (Aurora, New York).

TIMOTHY E. QUILL is Professor of Medicine, Psychiatry, and Medical Humanities at the University of Rochester School of Medicine and Dentistry, and Director of the Center for Ethics, Humanities and Palliative Care.

JAMES RACHELS was Professor of Philosophy at the University of Alabama at Birmingham.

JOHN A. ROBERTSON holds the Vinson & Elkins Chair of Law at the University of Texas Law School.

VICTOR G. RODWIN is Professor of Health Policy and Management at the Robert F. Wagner School of Public Service, New York University.

MICHAEL J. SANDEL is the Anne T. and Robert M. Bass Professor of Government at Harvard University.

PIETER J. J. SAUER is Professor of Pediatrics at the University Medical Center Groningen (Netherlands).

SUSAN SHERWIN is Professor of Philosophy, Emerita, at Dalhousie University (Fairfax, Nova Scotia).

MARK SIEGLER is Professor of Medicine, the Lindy Bergman Distinguished Service Professor, and Director of the Maclean Center for Clinical Medical Ethics at the University of Chicago.

PETER SINGER is Ira W. DeCamp Professor of Bioethics, Center for Human Values, Princeton University, and Laureate Professor, Centre for Applied Philosophy and Public Ethics, University of Melbourne.

BONNIE STEINBOCK is Professor of Philosophy at the University at Albany, State University of New York.

JUDITH JARVIS THOMSON is Professor of Philosophy, Emerita, at the Massachusetts Institute of Technology.

TOM TOMLINSON is Professor in the Department of Philosophy and Director of the Center for Ethics and Humanities in the Life Sciences at Michigan State University.

ROBERT D. TRUOG is Professor of Medical Ethics, Anesthesiology, and Pediatrics at Harvard Medical School and Senior Associate in Critical Care Medicine at Children's Hospital Boston.

BONNIE POITRAS TUCKER is Professor of Law, Emerita, at Arizona State University.

EDUARD VERHAGEN is Medical Director of the Department of Pediatrics at the University Medical Center Groningen (Netherlands).

ROBERT WACHBROIT is Research Scholar at the Institute for Philosophy and Public Policy, University of Maryland.

LEROY WALTERS is Joseph P. Kennedy Professor of Christian Ethics, Kennedy Institute of Ethics, and Professor of Philosophy at Georgetown University.

MARY ANNE WARREN is Professor of Philosophy, Emerita, at San Francisco State University.

MARK R. WICCLAIR is Professor of Philosophy and Adjunct Professor of Community Medicine at West Virginia University and is Adjunct Professor of Medicine at the University of Pittsburgh, where he is also affiliated with the Center for Bioethics and Health Law.

PAUL ROOT WOLPE is the Griggs Candler Professor of Bioethics and Director of the Center for Ethics at Emory University (Atlanta).

STEFFIE WOOLHANDLER is Associate Professor of Medicine at Harvard Medical School.

GREGORY D. WOZNIAK is Senior Economist at the American Medical Association.

The Business of Fashion

DESIGNING, MANUFACTURING, AND MARKETING

FOURTH EDITION

Leslie Davis Burns
Kathy K. Mullet
Nancy O. Bryant

OREGON STATE UNIVERSITY

Fairchild Books
New York

Executive Editor: Olga T. Kontzias

Senior Associate Acquiring Editor: Jaclyn Bergeron

Assistant Acquisitions Editor: Amanda Breccia

Editorial Development Director: Jennifer Crane

Associate Development Editor: Abigail Wilentz

Creative Director: Carolyn Eckert

Assistant Art Director: Sarah Silberg

Production Director: Ginger Hillman

Associate Production Editor: Linda Feldman

Copyeditor: Nancy Reinhardt

Ancillaries Editor: Noah Schwartzberg

Executive Director & General Manager: Michael Schluter

Associate Director of Sales: Melanie Sankel

Cover Design: Erin Fitzsimmons

Cover Art: Shoes: Richard Boll/Getty Images; Thread: Tamara Staples/Getty Images;
Gucci Fall 2001: Courtesy of WWD/Davide Maestri; Yarn: Kristin Duvall/Getty Images

Back Cover Art: Courtesy of WWD/George Chinsee

Text Design: Kyle Gell

Page Layout: Precision Graphics

Photo Research: Alexandra Rossomando

Illustrations: Mike Miranda

Library of Congress Catalog Card Number: 2011922455

ISBN: 978-1-60901-110-9

GST R 133004424

Printed in the United States of America

CH16 TP09

Contents

Extended Contents

Preface

Since the publication of the third edition of *The Business of Fashion: Designing, Manufacturing, and Marketing*, the textile, apparel, accessories, home fashions, and retailing industries have continued to undergo tremendous change. Supply chain management, product lifecycle management, and fast fashion have evolved into strategies for globalization, sustainability, and corporate social responsibility. Web-based communications and commerce are the norm, mass customization in a variety of applications has expanded, international trade agreements continue to affect sourcing options, and retailing venues continue to expand. As such, the fourth edition of this book attempts to capture the dynamics of the fashion industry by emphasizing the technological changes, organizational changes, and changes in the global dimensions of its various components.

The Business of Fashion focuses on the organization and operation of the U.S. fashion industry—how fashion apparel and accessories and home fashions are designed, manufactured, marketed, and distributed—within the global economy. As we investigate this ever-changing industry, it is important to set current strategies within their historical context. Thus, Chapter 1 begins with a history of the U.S. textile and apparel industry—from its inception in the late 1700s to the development and implementation of supply chain management strategies, globalization, e-commerce, and corporate social responsibility strategies. Once this historical context is set, we turn to current organizational structures and forms of competition among companies within the fashion industry.

Chapter 2 discusses types of company ownership within the fashion business, including sole proprietorships, partnerships, and corporations. Because of the prevalence of licensing, licensing contracts and the advantages and disadvantages of licensing are discussed. Marketing channels within the industry (i.e., direct, limited, and extended), as well as marketing channel integration, are outlined and explained. The chapter ends with an overview of the laws affecting the textile, apparel, accessory, and home fashions industries, including international trade agreements, laws protecting inventions and designs, and laws related to business practices.

Chapter 3 outlines the organization and operation of the U.S. textile industry—that is, the designing, manufacturing, and marketing of fabrics used in the production of apparel and home fashions. Leathers and fur are materials that are used for apparel and accessories and follow much of the same processing and marketing as other fabrics. We follow textile production from color forecasting and fiber processing through the marketing of seasonal lines of fabrics. Recent developments and issues within the industry such as technological advancements and environmental issues provide a basis for our understanding of future trends in the textile industry.

Chapter 4 focuses on the general classifications and organizational structures of apparel companies that produce men's, women's, and children's apparel and accessories. Comparisons between ready-to-wear and couture, and among types of producers, classifications of brand names, and price zones, reinforce an appreciation of the complexities of the apparel and accessory industries. The major divisions within ready-to-wear organizations are introduced (research and merchandising, design and product development, operations, sales/marketing, advertising/sales promotion, and finance and information technology). Trade associations and trade publications also are introduced in this chapter.

Chapter 5 begins a four-chapter sequence on the creation and marketing of fashion apparel. This sequence follows an apparel line/collection through the various stages of research, design, style selection, and marketing. Chapter 5 focuses on the various forms of research conducted prior to the development of the line/collection: consumer research, product research, market analysis, and fashion research. The chapter explains the importance of accurately profiling the company's target customer. Chapter 6 highlights the design stage—design inspiration, designing for the market niche, planning the line, designing sketches, and writing garment specification sheets. The creation of an apparel line continues in Chapter 7, which discusses design development and style selection, including the development of first patterns, sewing of prototypes, initial cost estimates, and selection of styles for the final line. The discussion concludes at the stage when the final line is marketed to retail buyers.

Chapter 8 describes locations of and roles played by marts and trade shows in facilitating the marketing of apparel, accessories, and home fashions. Next, it discusses how merchandise is sold through corporate selling and sales representatives. The chapter ends with an overview of marketing strategies used by apparel and home fashions companies in the distribution and promotion of their lines. Throughout this sequence of events in the creation and marketing of apparel, accessories, and home fashions lines, the chapters highlight new technological developments, including product lifecycle management, Web-based communications including social media, global perspectives, and organizational changes within the industry.

Chapter 9 begins a four-chapter sequence on the production and distribution of apparel and home fashions. Preproduction processes, including determining production orders, factoring, ordering production fabrics, pattern finalization, pattern grading, making the production marker, and production cutting are described. Chapter 10 outlines the sourcing options for apparel and home fashions production and the criteria used by companies in making sourcing decisions. Applications of corporate social responsibility in assessing the advantages and disadvantages of domestic and foreign production of apparel, accessories, and home fashions are also discussed. Chapter 11 explores the various methods by which apparel is produced. Production sewing systems and technological developments in production equipment are described. The chapter ends with a summary of product finishing and the creation of floor-ready merchandise. Once produced, the merchandise is distributed to retailers, often through distribution centers. Chapter 12 summarizes distribution strategies and processes used by apparel, accessory, and home fashions companies. A description of the various types of store and nonstore retailers ends this chapter.

Our focus turns to accessories and home fashions in Chapters 13 and 14. A strong relationship exists between these industries and the textile and apparel industries. Thus, an overview of the organization and operation of the primary accessories industries is included in Chapter 13. Chapter 14 introduces the various facets of the home fashions industry, with specific focus on the use of textiles in the production of home fashions such as sheets, towels, and draperies.

In introducing students to this dynamic, multifaceted business, the book incorporates real-world examples from its component industries. Career profiles are also included near the end of each chapter to give readers a sampling of the many career opportunities throughout the fashion industry. Other end-of-chapter features that help students prepare for their own entry into the fashion business include chapter summaries, lists of key terms, discussion questions, class activities, and references.

Acknowledgments

Many people have assisted with the development of this book, and we would like to thank them for their time, effort, and support. Leslie Burns would like to thank her students, former students, and colleagues at Oregon State University, who shared their ideas and resources in the development of the book. Leslie particularly thanks her coauthor, Nancy Bryant, who collaborated with her on the first three editions. Nancy brought extensive technical expertise and knowledge of the apparel industry to this work. She greatly appreciates her new coauthor, Kathy Mullet, whose expertise in design, production, and industry trends is highlighted in this fourth edition. Kathy Mullet would like to express her appreciation to Leslie Burns and Nancy Bryant for allowing her to work with them on the fourth edition of this book. Kathy would like to thank her former students for their continual sharing of information about the apparel industry. Many other professional contacts in the apparel industry also most willingly shared their expertise. The support of her colleagues at Oregon State University is deeply appreciated.

We wish to thank the many readers and reviewers of the current and previous editions of this book. Their excellent input is reflected throughout. We owe our deepest appreciation to Jaclyn Bergeron, Jennifer Crane, Linda Feldman, Sarah Silberg, Elizabeth Marotta, and Noah Schwartzberg at Fairchild Books and to Pamela Crews at Precision Graphics for their patience, professional attention to details, and invaluable assistance with this book. Thank you!

Leslie Davis Burns
Kathy K. Mullet
Nancy O. Bryant
Oregon State University

PART 1

Organization
of the U.S. Textile, Apparel, and Home Fashions Industries

CHAPTER 1

From Spinning Machine to Globalization

In this chapter, you will learn the following:

- the history of the transition of the apparel industry from a craft industry to a factory-based industry to an information-based global industry

- the technological developments in the textile, apparel, and home fashions industries

- the historical basis for the emergence of supply chain management, corporate responsibility, technological applications, and consumer focus

- the forms of interindustry cooperation and technologies needed for the success of global supply chain management

- current strategies in the textile, apparel, home fashions, and retailing industries, including e-commerce, fast fashion, and pop-up retail

- the role of corporate social responsibility throughout the supply chain

The U.S. textile, apparel, and home fashions industries consist of large and small companies that design, produce, and market fibers, textiles, apparel, and home fashions for consumers in the United States as well as around the world. U.S. textile and apparel manufacturing companies employ approximately 500,000 people with employment in the states of California, Georgia, and North Carolina, accounting for about 44 percent of all workers (Bureau of Labor Statistics, 2010). When apparel and home fashions distribution through retailers is included, these industries contribute to the economy of virtually every community in the nation. Whereas the U.S. textile and apparel industries contribute less than 1 percent to the U.S. gross domestic product, contributions in research and development, design, and marketing have supplementary benefits to the U.S. economy. Indeed, U.S. apparel brands are some of the best known in the world. How did it all begin? How did these industries develop and grow into the dynamic industries they are today? To fully understand the modern textile, apparel, and home fashions industries, a brief review of how they began, grew, and changed over the past 220-plus years is important.

1789–1890: Mechanization of Spinning, Weaving, and Sewing

For thousands of years, the spinning and weaving of fabrics were labor-intensive hand processes. Then, in England, in the mid-1700s, the spinning of yarn and weaving of cloth began to be mechanized. At that time, England's cotton and wool textile industries were the most technologically developed in the western world. In response to a growing demand for textiles both in England and abroad, a series of advances in the spinning and weaving of fabrics by English inventors brought the British industry to world prominence. These inventions included the following:

- the flying shuttle loom invented by John Kay in 1733
- the spinning machine or "jenny" invented by James Hargreaves in 1764
- the water-powered spinning machine invented by Sir Richard Arkwright in 1769
- the mechanized power loom invented by Reverend Edmund Cartwright in 1785–1787

In addition, the process for printing fabrics was also being mechanized. England was protective of its technological developments, and severe penalties existed for attempting to take blueprints and/or machines or their parts out of the country. Even the mechanics themselves were restricted from leaving the country. At the time, the textile factory system in England was not only one of the most productive but also one of the most dehumanizing and unhealthy for the workers subjected to it. England's labor reform movement in the mid-1800s was a call for reform in the textile industry (Yafa, 2005).

In the United States, a fledgling cotton industry was taking root, but America lacked England's advanced technology for spinning and weaving cotton fibers. Then, in 1789, Samuel Slater, a skilled mechanic, brought English textile technology to the United States by memorizing the blueprints of the Arkwright water-powered spinning machine. Farmers were permitted to leave England, so he declared himself a farmer and came to the United States. He settled in New England where a ready supply of water existed. Hired by Moses Brown, a merchant, Slater set up a spinning mill similar to the one shown in Figure 1.1. Who would have thought that this small spinning mill in Pawtucket, Rhode Island, would prove that cotton yarn could be spun profitably in the United States? This mill, which opened in 1791, sparked the textile industry in the United States. Within a few years, spinning mills had sprung up all over New

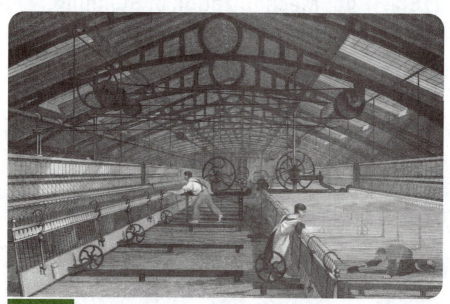

Figure 1.1 Early spinning mills, as introduced by Samuel Slater, included carding, drawing, roving, and spinning.

England. By the mid-1800s, towns such as Waltham, Lowell, Lawrence, and New Bedford, Massachusetts, and Biddeford, Maine, became centers of the newly emerging textile industry. A reliance on British inventions still existed; any technological changes were based on reproducing and improving textile machinery used in England.

Although the spinning process was becoming mechanized, the weaving process continued to be contracted out to individual handweavers. In 1813, Francis Cabot Lowell originated a functional power loom. He set the stage for vertical integration within the industry; his factory was the first in the United States to perform mechanically all processes from spinning yarn to producing finished cloth under one roof. As early as 1817, power looms were being installed in textile mills all over New England. Despite the technological developments in weaving, however, the contracting out of the weaving process to handweavers for complex fabrics continued until the late 1800s.

The mechanization of spinning and weaving made these processes so much faster that fiber producers were pressured to supply a greater amount of cotton and wool. However, cotton growers in the South were limited by the time needed to handpick seeds from cotton. In 1794, Eli Whitney patented the **cotton gin** (gin for engine), which could clean as much cotton in one day as 50 men (see Figure 1.2). As a result of this invention, the cotton growers soon were able to supply New England's spinning and weaving mills' increased demand for fiber.

To be closer to this very important source of cotton, manufacturers built textile mills in the southern states. The Northeast continued to be a primary producer of wool fabrics. By 1847, more people were employed in textile mills than in any other industry in the United States. Unfortunately, the squalor of the textile factory towns in England was also found in textile factory towns in the northeastern and southeastern United States. It took many years for unions and

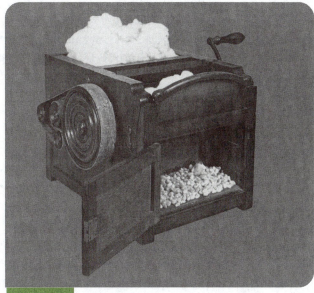

Figure 1.2 The Whitney Cotton Gin, patented by Eli Whitney, increased the speed and quality of the cotton cleaning process.

labor reforms to improve the pay and factory working conditions for those in the textile industry. In the meantime, consumer demand for cotton increased, and, by the late 1890s, three-quarters of the clothing in Europe and the United States was made from cotton (Yafa, 2005).

The **ready-to-wear (RTW)** industry had its beginnings in the early eighteenth century. To meet the demand for ready-made clothing, tailors would make less expensive clothes from scrap material left over from sewing custom-made suits. Sailors, miners, and slaves were the primary target market for these early ready-made clothes, which were cut in "slop shops" and sewn by women at home. The term **slops** later became a standard term for cheap, ready-made clothing.

In the early nineteenth century, the demand for ready-to-wear clothing grew. The expanding number of middle-class consumers wanted good-quality apparel but did not want to pay the high prices associated with custom-made clothing. However, it was not until the sewing process of apparel production became mechanized that ready-to-wear apparel became available to the majority of consumers. Sewing machine inventions by Walter Hunt (1832), Elias Howe (1845), and Isaac Singer (1846) made it possible for apparel to be produced by machine, thereby speeding the process by which it could be made. From 1842 to 1895, 7,339 patents for sewing machines and accessories were issued in the United States. The advertisement in Figure 1.3 shows how competitive the business had become. The sewing machine allowed relatively unskilled immigrant workers to sew garments in their homes. In addition, sewing factories were established, with some of the first men's clothing factories appearing as early as 1831. In fact, Singer's sewing machine, patented in 1851, was designed for factory use.

In the United States, men's RTW developed first. Children's RTW followed, with boys' apparel developing before that for girls. The last to develop was RTW apparel for women. Men's RTW developed first because men's size standards existed for apparel producers to use. In addition, in the late nineteenth century, the styling of men's apparel was less complicated than that of women's. The term **size standards** refers to the proportional increase or decrease in garment measurements for each size produced. Patterns could be made for a range of men's sizes. Thus, multiple sizes could be cut and sewn using mass-production methods. One of the first large-scale applications of menswear size standards was in the sewing of uniforms during the Civil War.

By 1860, a variety of ready-made men's clothing was available. Indeed, between 1822 and 1860, the ready-to-wear segment of the menswear tailoring industry grew larger than the custom-made segment. Because of this increased demand, the number of sewing factories also grew. A number of other advances contributed to the growth of the industry at this time. During the late 1800s,

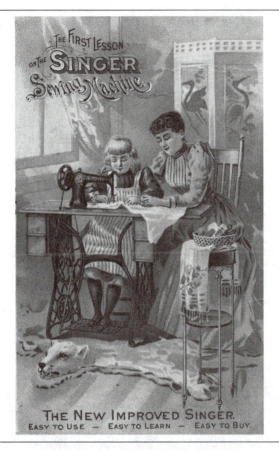

Figure 1.3 Sewing machine inventions provided increased speed in the production of apparel.

motorized cutting knives and pressing equipment were developed. Mass production of apparel was also facilitated by the invention of paper patterns. Ebenezer Butterick started a pattern business in 1863; James McCall started a similar one in 1870. Thus, by the end of the nineteenth century, mechanization of the textile and apparel production processes resulted in a growing number of companies.

With the availability of ready-made clothing, distribution outlets to consumers in cities increased. Brooks Brothers, one of the first well-known men's apparel stores, opened in New York City in 1818 and catered primarily to sailors and working-class men who could not afford custom-tailored clothing. The mid-1800s saw the development of dry goods stores in cities, which later became department stores:

- In New York City's Greenwich Village, Lord & Taylor opened in 1826; in 1903, it was moved to Fifth Avenue.

- In Haverhill, Massachusetts, Macy's Wholesale and Retail Dry Goods House (see Figure 1.4) opened in 1857.

- In Chicago, Marshall Field's opened in 1852, and Carson Pirie Scott & Co. opened in 1854.

- In Philadelphia, John Wanamaker and Co. opened in 1869.

Although these stores initially offered a limited range of products, by the end of the Civil War, the range of merchandise expanded and included apparel.

To those consumers unable to shop in the cities, illustrated catalogs offered a wide variety of goods by the latter part of the nineteenth century. With the expansion of the U.S. postal service due to the introduction of parcel post in 1913, the continued development of railroads, and the introduction of rural free delivery (RFD) in 1893, a growing mail-order business for ready-made clothing was created by such companies as Montgomery Ward (established in 1872) and Sears, Roebuck & Co. (established in 1886). Table 1.1 summarizes these supply and demand needs for the emergence and growth of the textile and apparel industries in the United States. See Table 1.2 for a listing of other significant historical events during this time period.

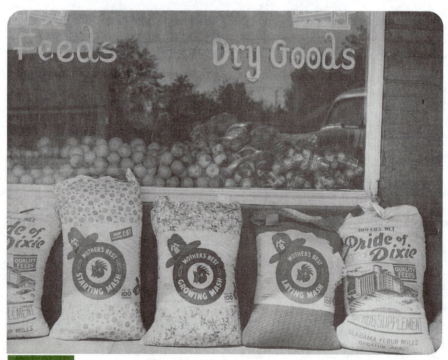

Figure 1.4 Early general stores sold "dry goods," including fabrics and ready-to-wear apparel in addition to hardware and food.

Table 1.1	Supply and Demand Needs for the Emergence and Growth of Textile, Apparel, and Home Fashion Industries in the United States

SUPPLY

- The need for plenty of fabric that could be produced quickly and the means to sew it quickly was achieved by the following:
  - spinning machine (1764)
  - power loom (1785–87)
  - cotton gin (1794)
  - sewing machine (1832, 1845, 1846)
- The need for a ready supply of labor was achieved by immigrant workers who
  - began production sewing in their homes
  - were employed by sewing factories

DEMAND

- The need for customers and consumer demand for mass-produced apparel was achieved by the following:
  - sailors, miners, and slaves who needed inexpensive, ready-made clothing (slops)
  - an expanding number of middle-class consumers who wanted good-quality apparel at reasonable prices
- The need for a distribution system for mass-produced apparel, accessories, and home fashions was achieved by the following:
  - mail-order catalogs
  - general stores in rural areas
  - department stores (mid-1800s) in cities

1890–1950: Growth of the Ready-to-Wear Industry

Although most men's apparel was available ready-made by the mid-nineteenth century, the women's RTW industry did not expand until the late nineteenth century (see Figures 1.5, 1.6, and 1.7). The first types of RTW apparel produced for women were outerwear capes, cloaks, and coats. Because these garments fit more loosely than fashionable dresses, sizing was not a critical problem. Manufactured corsets, petticoats, and other underwear items were also accepted by consumers, perhaps because these clothing items were hidden from public view. By the beginning of the twentieth century, RTW skirts and shirtwaists (blouses) were offered for sale. The popularity of the shirtwaist, made fashionable by Charles Dana Gibson's "Gibson girl," shifted women's apparel

Table 1.2	Historical Events 1789–1890: Mechanization of Spinning, Weaving, and Sewing
1791	Samuel Slater, who came to the United States in 1788, opens the first U.S. spinning mill.
1793	Hannah Slater, Samuel's wife, invents the 2-ply cotton sewing thread.
1794	Eli Whitney's cotton gin is patented.
1818	Brooks Brothers opens in New York City.
1851	Isaac Singer patents the sewing machine for factory use.
1853	Levi Strauss joins the family business founded by his brother-in-law, David Stern, which will come to be known as Levi Strauss & Co.

Mid-1800s to late 1890s: Dry goods stores (forerunners of today's department stores) are opened:

    1826–Lord & Taylor

    1841–Jordan Marsh

    1842–Gimbels

    1849–Famous-Barr

    1852–Marshall Field's

    1854–Carson Pirie Scott & Co.

    1857–R.H. Macy & Co.

    1862–Stewart's

    1867–Rich's

    1869–John Wanamaker and Co.

    1872–Bloomingdale Brothers, Inc.

    1898–Burdines

1854	The first U.S. trade association, Hampden County Cotton Manufacturers Association, starts in Hampden County, Massachusetts.
1860	Census data on the women's clothing industry indicates 96 manufacturers producing apparel worth $2,261,546 annually.
1865	William Carter begins knitting cardigan jackets in the kitchen of his house in Needham Heights, Massachusetts. The William Carter Co. will grow to be one of the nation's largest children's companies.

production away from a craft industry to a factory-based industry. It was the shirtwaist and the popularity of separates—that is, coat, blouse (shirtwaist), and skirt worn by young working women in the cities—that provided the basis for the development of the women's RTW industry.

The production of RTW apparel was labor intensive. A ready supply of immigrant workers spurred the growth of the mass production of apparel. By 1900, approximately 500 shops in New York City were producing shirtwaists. The contracting system of production grew in popularity, as it was estimated that a $50 investment was all that was necessary to start a business with a few workers and a bundle of cut garments obtained from a manufacturer or wholesaler. Production was divided into two segments:

1. a large number of sewing operations located in the homes of immigrants producing lower-priced garments

2. a relatively small number of large, modern sewing factories engaged in the production of better-quality garments

These sewing factories, primarily on the Lower East Side of New York City, were notorious for their poor working conditions. The term **sweatshop** originally referred to the system of contractors and subcontractors whereby work was "sweated off." Later, the term became associated with the long hours, unclean and unsafe working conditions, and low pay of contract sewing factories, as well as with the dismal conditions of home factories, where contract workers sewed clothing.

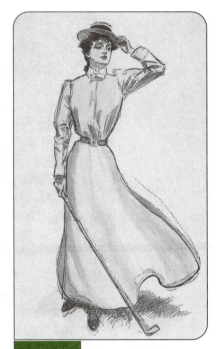

Figure 1.5 Gibson Girl, illustration by Charles Dana Gibson, 1899.

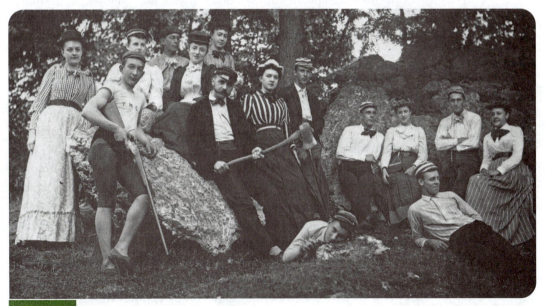

Figure 1.6 By the 1890s, most men's apparel and some women's apparel were available ready-to-wear.

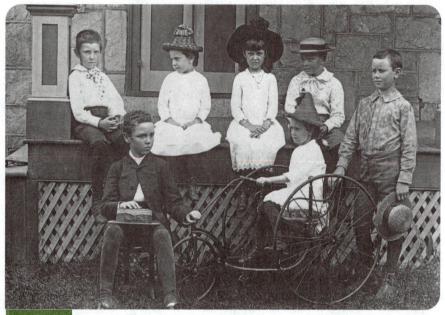

Figure 1.7   Ready-to-wear children's apparel was available for purchase by the 1890s.

In an effort to improve working conditions for the employees in the industry, most of whom were young immigrant women, the International Ladies' Garment Workers' Union (ILGWU) was formed in 1900 at a convention in New York City. The tragic fire in the Triangle Shirtwaist Co. factory on March 25, 1911, in which 146 young women died, brought public attention to the horrid working conditions and increased support for the ILGWU. It is now the Textile, Manufacturing, and Distribution Division of the union UNITE HERE, which represents workers in the hospitality, food service, textile, apparel, and retailing industries.

In the 1920s, the women's fashion industry in New York moved from the Lower East Side to Seventh Avenue. This area of midtown Manhattan became known as New York's garment district, and it has remained the hub of women's fashion. The manufacturing of menswear was less centralized, with Chicago, Baltimore, and New York emerging as manufacturing centers.

At the beginning of the twentieth century, the majority of RTW clothing was made from cotton and wool. Silk fabric, imported from France and Italy, was highly desired for its luxurious qualities. However, it was very expensive, and the supply was limited. Therefore, when synthetic substitutes for natural fibers were initially explored, "artificial silk" (rayon, made from wood pulp) was the first to be developed and patented in the United States. The first American rayon plant was opened in 1910. Synthetic dyestuffs for textile dyeing were developed and available by the beginning of the twentieth century.

Other inventions made during this time became staples in the RTW industry. An invention called *the locker* was demonstrated at the Chicago World's Fair in 1893. Named *the zipper* in 1926, it was to have a major impact on the apparel industry. First used to fasten boots, the zipper was not generally used in fashion apparel until the 1930s.

Fashion magazines, beginning with *Vogue*, were first published in 1892. These magazines provided consumers with up-to-date fashion information and helped spur the desire for new fashions. Between 1910 and 1920, a variety of communication channels helped unite the fledgling RTW industry. Trade publications, such as the *Daily Trade Record* (menswear), established in 1892, and *Women's Wear Daily*, established in 1910, provided a great impetus to the RTW industry (see Figure 1.8)

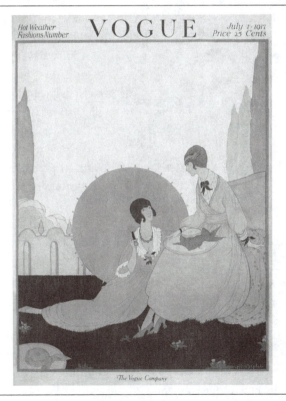

Figure 1.8 1917 *Vogue* magazine cover illustrates the simpler designs of women's fashions of the age.

Another step in the developmental progress of the RTW industry was the result of wartime manufacturing. World War I spurred the need for the manufacture of military uniforms, and, in turn, helped streamline apparel production methods. Also important to the U.S. textile and apparel industries was the closing of French and British fashion houses during the war, which allowed American fashion to develop from 1914 to 1918.

Although most items of women's clothing were available ready-made by the early 1900s, growth in the garment industry came about with the simplification of garment styles in the 1920s (see Figure 1.9). Who knows which came first? The simpler styles may have spurred the growth of the industry, but industry methods also affected the styles of apparel that could be produced for, and thus adopted by, consumers. By the 1920s, mass-produced clothing was available to the majority of individuals. The era of inexpensive fashion had begun. New styles and variety became more valued than costly one-of-a-kind apparel by the majority of consumers. Retail stores increased their inventory ratio of moderately priced clothing in proportion to more expensive goods.

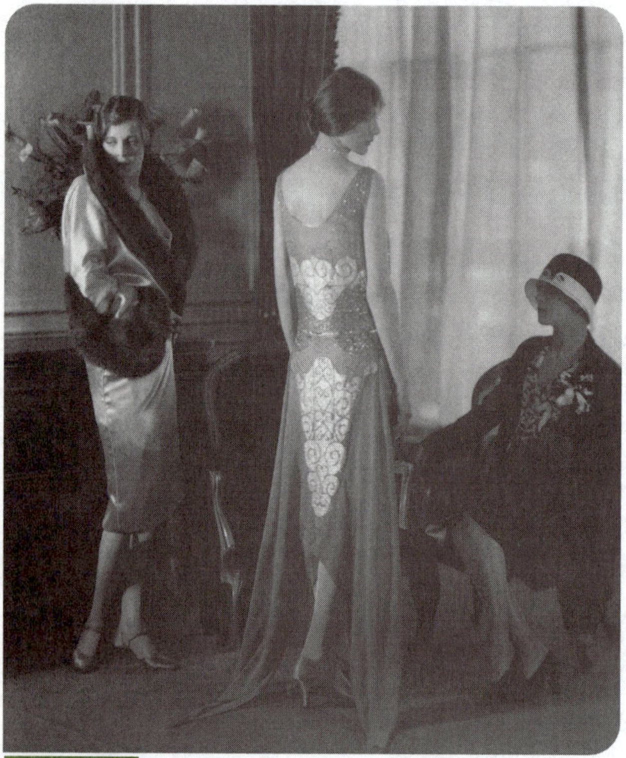

A new development in retailing during this decade was the country's first outdoor shopping mall. The Country Club Plaza was built in 1922 in Kansas City, Kansas. It remains a gem among shopping malls, with its Spanish-style architecture and fountains reminiscent of Seville, Spain.

The boyish chemise-style dresses of the 1920s were easy to manufacture because there were few contours to shape and fit. This loose, boxy style also fit a wider variety of figures than did previous styles. However, this style was not favored by the textile manufacturers because it utilized approximately one-third less yardage per garment than the styles of the previous decade. With the growing popularity of movies,

Figure 1.9 Fashions with simplified designs and the "feeling of Paris couture" are sold at Bergdorf Goodman and highlighted in a 1928 issue of *Vogue* magazine.

movie stars began to influence the fashion preferences of consumers. Fashion news also became available over a new invention—the radio. Fortunately for textile manufacturers, the women's garment styles of the 1930s used more fabric than those of the 1920s.

New York City remained the center of the women's fashion industry, and Seventh Avenue was becoming synonymous with women's fashion. By 1923, New York City was producing nearly 80 percent of U.S. women's apparel in the city's growing garment district. Also during the 1920s, specialized sewing machines were developed, such as overlockers (sergers) and power-driven cutting equipment.

As mass communications expanded in the 1920s, so did the flow of fashion information. France dominated the fashion scene, where a new generation of high-fashion designers, including Patou, Chanel, Vionnet, and Schiaparelli, was rising. Covering the fashion shows in Paris and bringing this news to American consumers was a huge undertaking. In 1926, more than 100 reporters covered the Paris couture openings for newspapers and magazines.

When the stock market crashed in 1929, it devastated all aspects of the American economy. Repercussions were felt in Paris, as retail stores and private clients canceled orders overnight. The Great Depression of the 1930s, which resulted from the 1929 stock market crash, caused a severe blow to the textile and apparel industries. These and other industries did not recover until the start of World War II. In 1929, it was estimated that New York had 3,500 dress companies; by 1933, there were only 2,300.

However, the 1930s brought about the development of the first "synthetic" fibers synthesized entirely from chemicals. Because most manufactured fibers were developed as substitutes for natural fibers, their properties were intended to emulate those of silk, wool, and cotton. Nylon, the first synthetic fiber, was conceptualized by E. I. du Pont de Nemours and Company in 1928, successfully synthesized in 1935, marketed in 1938, and introduced in nylon stockings in 1939. However, nylon production for consumer use was interrupted by World War II, so its widespread use for consumer products did not come until after the war.

It also became more common for manufacturers to contract and subcontract some of the sewing operations to other companies, known as **contractors** and **subcontractors**. Some contractors specialized in specific processes, such as fabric pleating. For example, the manufacturer would ship the needed quantity of yard goods to the contractor for pleating. The contractor would return the pleated goods to the apparel manufacturer. Then the manufacturer would proceed with cutting and sewing operations.

During the 1930s, a large number of dress and sportswear companies emerged and grew in New York. In addition, the sportswear industry in California and other western states began to expand. The California sportswear industry actually began in the 1850s, when Levi Strauss & Co. began production of work trousers. It was not until the 1930s that sportswear made by other companies, such as White Stag, Jantzen, Cole of California, Pendleton Woolen Mills, and Catalina, became popular (see Figure 1.10). The sportswear trend was further legitimized by American designers, such as Claire McCardell and Vera Maxwell. These designers introduced informal, casual "designer" clothing in the late 1930s.

A number of fashion magazines also debuted in the 1930s, each catering to a particular segment of consumers. *Mademoiselle*, established in 1935, and *Glamour*, first published in 1939 as *Glamour of Hollywood*, catered to fashionable college coeds and young working women (see Figure 1.11). *Esquire*, first published in 1933, was designed to enlighten men about the world of fashion and elegance. Movies of the era also served as a source of fashion information for consumers, and movie stars became the fashion leaders of the day.

Brand names of manufacturers gained strong consumer recognition during the 1930s. One of the first to gain national recognition was the Arrow shirt. Launched in 1905, the Arrow shirt advertising campaign continued for many

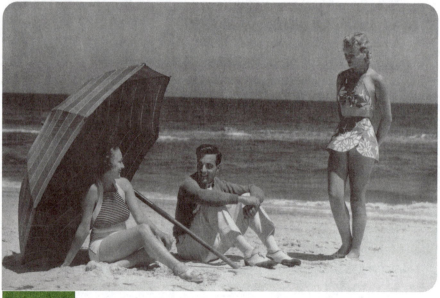

Figure 1.10 The 1930s brought a growth in the sportswear industry and the influence of sports on fashion.

years. The ads featured color fashion illustrations of a very sophisticated male, wearing an Arrow shirt, engaged in a variety of activities suitable to a man of taste and leisure. These ads remain classic examples of lifestyle advertising.

By the 1930s, the college student and young working woman were clearly identified as target customers for the fashion industry; special markets included junior and large-size customers. Size standards were widely adopted by the industry after the U.S. Department of Agriculture published size measurements in 1941. The demand for good-quality RTW was strong, and fashion news spread quickly.

A number of changes in the 1940s had profound influences on the U.S. apparel industry. Although World War II devastated the fashion industry in France, Paris emerged once again after the war as a prominent player in the international fashion industry. However, the war did allow American designers such as Claire McCardell to become

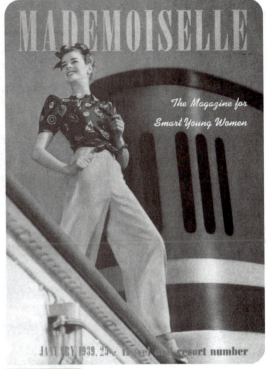

Figure 1.11 *Mademoiselle*: The magazine for smart young women; 1939.

well-known among consumers. The United States became known as the sportswear capital, and it held on to this title even after the Paris fashion houses reopened.

The U.S. fashion industry founded several organizations during the 1930s and 1940s to strengthen and promote the industry. These organizations included The Fashion Group International, the New York Couture Group, and the California Fashion Creators. The Coty American Fashion Critics Award was founded in 1942 to recognize outstanding American fashion designers.

By the 1940s, the production of ready-to-wear clothing was located primarily in modern factories. Because of rising costs in New York City, factories had been built in New Jersey, Connecticut, and upstate New York. Apparel manufacturing factories also were springing up in other parts of the country. The apparel industry in California, centered in Los Angeles, emerged as the hub for the growing active and casual sportswear industry in the West. Dallas, Texas, also gained prominence in apparel manufacturing. See Table 1.3 for a listing of other significant historical events during this time period.

Table 1.3   Historical Events 1890–1950: Growth of the Ready-to-Wear Industry

1892	American *Vogue* magazine begins publication.
1892	*Daily Trade Record*, the trade newspaper for the RTW men's wear industry, begins publication; became *Daily News Record* in 1916.
1900	The International Ladies' Garment Workers' Union (ILGWU) is founded.
1901	Walin & Nordstrom Shoe Store opens in downtown Seattle.
1902	James Cash Penney, age 26, opens a dry goods and clothing store in Kemmerer, Wyoming. Opening day receipts totaled $466.59.
1904	New York seamstress Lena Bryant introduces ready-to-wear maternity wear. Her company, named Lane Bryant, becomes the first plus-size ready-to-wear producer.
1907	Herbert Marcus, Sr., his sister Carrie, and brother-in-law, A.L. Neiman, start Neiman Marcus department store in Dallas.
1908	Filene's opens its "automatic bargain basement" in Boston. Merchandise in the upstairs store is automatically marked down 25 percent every week for three weeks, then sent to the basement. This practice marks the beginnings of the off-price store.
1909	Pendleton Woolen Mills begins producing woolen blankets and robes.
1909	In November, 20,000 New York shirtwaist makers stage the largest strike by American women to that time.
1910	*Women's Wear Daily*, trade newspaper for the women's wear industry, begins publication.
1911	146 garment workers die in a fire at the Triangle Shirtwaist Co. factory in New York's garment district. The tragedy stimulates a movement to end sweatshop conditions.
1914	The Amalgamated Clothing Workers of America Union is formed as the primary union for the men's wear industry.
1920	Membership in the ILGWU grows to 200,000.
1922	Country Club Plaza, the country's first outdoor shopping mall, opens in Kansas City, Kansas.
1923	Pushed by the growing demand among women for ready-to-wear clothing, New York leads the growing industry, manufacturing 80 percent of all women's apparel.
1925	The first Sears Roebuck & Co. store opens in Chicago.
1926	J. M. Haggar starts his own men's wear company in Dallas, Texas, using assembly lines to manufacture men's trousers.
1927	The average price for women's full-fashioned silk stockings is $11.50 per dozen; by 1933 the price plummets to a low of $5.10 per dozen.
1928	Sanford Cluett develops a process to compress fabric under tension to reduce shrinkage, and the "Sanforized" trademark is licensed to cotton finishers.
1932	Sales at Sears, Roebuck & Co. retail stores surpass catalog sales.
1934	Membership in the ILGWU grows to 217,000.
1939	Textile Workers Union is founded.
1939	Nylon stockings are introduced.

Table 1.3	Historical Events 1890–1950: Growth of the Ready-to-Wear Industry *(continued)*
1941	Congress fixes Thanksgiving, which previously had been a floating holiday in November, as the fourth Thursday in November. Fred Lazarus Jr. is credited with the idea as a way to expand the Christmas shopping season.
1941	Employment in the textile industry peaks at approximately 1.4 million.
1944	The Fashion Institute of Technology is founded to support New York's fashion industry.
1947	Leslie Fay is established—and becomes one of the largest women's apparel companies.
1949	Bloomingdale's opens its first branch store in Fresh Meadows, New York.

1950–1980: Diversification and Incorporation

The 1950s saw not only a general growth in consumer demand for apparel, but also a shift in the product mix demanded by consumers. Because of lifestyle changes, casual clothing and sportswear were an expanding segment of the fashion industry. In fact, between 1947 and 1961, wholesale shipments of casual apparel and sportswear increased approximately 160 percent. During the same period, suit sales decreased by approximately 40 percent.

Teenage fashion developed as a special category during the 1950s (see Figure 1.12). It reached its peak during the youth explosion of the 1960s, when **mass fashion** became affordable to the majority of the population. Mass fashion focused on simplified styling and sizing, mass production sewing in large factories, with distribution through retail chain stores. In 1965, half the U.S. population was under 25, and teenagers spent $3.5 million annually on apparel.

Spurred by increased orders from the military in the early 1950s, the textile industry also grew. In 1950, Burlington ranked as the largest Fortune 500 textile manufacturer, with annual sales just over $1 billion. Developed in the 1940s, acrylic and polyester were available to the U.S. market by the early 1950s. Triacetate was introduced in 1954, and it provided a less heat-sensitive alternative to acetate, a previously developed synthetic fiber. The use of synthetic fibers in apparel provided consumers with easy-care, wrinkle-free, and "drip-dry" clothing that freed them from the high demands of caring for cotton and woolen clothing. These new fibers provided lower-cost and lighter-weight alternatives. Fashion trends and technological developments in textiles became intertwined. Textile mills developed new texturizing processes that made possible such innovations as stretch yarn. Nylon stretch socks became available in 1952. Later in the decade, nylon stretch pants became a fashion sensation.

In the 1960s, synthetic fibers began to overtake natural fibers in popularity. Apparel designers, such as Pierre Cardin, experimented with space-age

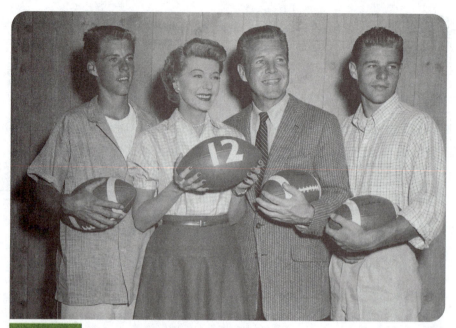

Figure 1.12 Ozzie and Harriet Nelson, with sons Ricky (left) and David (right). Spurred by the popularity of television and pop music, teenage fashion became a separate category in the 1950s.

materials. Plastic was used extensively, and heat-fusing techniques were developed. The natural fiber industry fought back with strong organizations such as the Cotton Council and the International Wool Secretariat. Eventually, natural fibers would again gain public favor, but not until after the 1970s—the decade of America's love affair with polyester.

After World War II came Christian Dior's New Look, and consumer attention turned again to Paris. During the 1950s and 1960s, Parisian haute couture continued to set fashion trends worldwide. However, increased productivity in mass-produced clothing made it possible for designer fashions to be copied and reproduced at a fraction of the cost of haute couture (see Figure 1.13). During this period, ready-to-wear fashions became the standard worldwide, and "Chanel" suits, which were less expensive copies of the originals, were available to everyone. Since the 1970s, haute couture has been overshadowed by mass-market apparel. In fact, currently all haute couture designers also create ready-to-wear collections.

One of the most apparent changes in the apparel industry during the late 1950s and throughout the 1960s was the increase in large, publicly owned apparel corporations. In 1959, only 22 public apparel companies existed, but, by the end of the 1960s, more than 100 apparel companies had become publicly owned corporations. Some companies that "went public" early on were Jonathan Logan, Bobbie Brooks, and Leslie Fay.

Because of the growth of suburbia in the United States, fewer people lived in cities, and consumers wanted shopping outlets closer to their new homes. Thus, the shopping mall emerged. In 1956, Southdale Center, the first enclosed shopping mall, was built in a suburb of Minneapolis. During the 1960s, shopping malls appeared in virtually every suburb. Typically, regional or national department stores served as anchors.

During the 1960s and 1970s, American designer names saw increased prominence. Although American designers were first promoted by the Lord & Taylor department store in New York in the 1930s, it was not until the late 1960s that stores such as Saks Fifth Avenue featured specific American designers. During this time, fashion designers became celebrities. Aware of the broad appeal of their names, designers such as Halston and Bill Blass ventured into licensing their names for apparel and accessories.

However, rising labor costs in the United States led to increased prices of apparel for consumers. In an attempt to keep costs down, retailers explored the idea of low overhead, self-service, and high-volume stores for apparel and other products. The strategy was successful, and retailers such as Kmart (see Figure 1.14), Target, Walmart, and Woolco, known as discounters, flourished. In addition, as labor costs continued to rise, apparel manufacturing companies

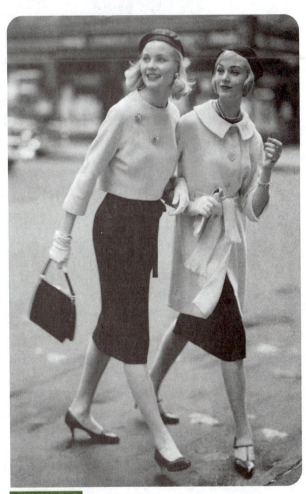

Figure 1.13 Ready-to-wear apparel of the 1950s, such as these Sportwhirl fashions, copied the haute couture designs of the time.

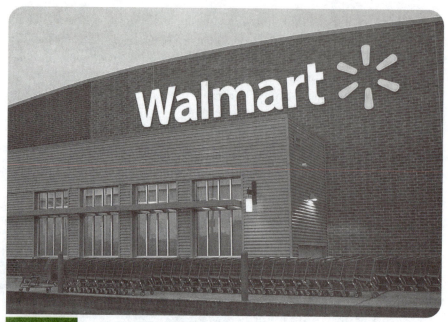

Figure 1.14 Discount retailers such as Walmart grew from retail strategies to keep merchandise costs to consumers as low as possible.

searched for a cheaper workforce. Their search began within the United States, particularly in the Southeast. Then, it was expanded outside the United States, particularly in Hong Kong and Southeast Asia. Textile technology, once the domain of American companies, was increasingly imported from abroad. In 1967, for the first time in its history, the United States ran a trade deficit in textile machinery.

The 1970s saw the beginning of trends in which companies became vertically integrated, and large, publicly owned conglomerates bought apparel companies. For example, during this time, General Mills acquired Izod, David Crystal, and Monet jewelers; Consolidated Foods purchased Hanes hosiery and Aris gloves; and Gulf & Western bought Kayser-Roth.

Technological advances in the textile industry included a new generation of photographic printing and dyeing processes. Computer technology entered the textile and apparel manufacturing areas. The popularity of polyester double knit and denim fabrics sparked sales in the textile industry. However, increased competition from textile companies outside the United States cut into profits, and textile imports rose 581 percent between 1961 and 1976. See Table 1.4 for a listing of other significant historical events during this time period.

Table 1.4	Historical Events 1950–1980: Diversification and Incorporation
1951	Employment in the apparel and knitwear industries in New York City peaks at 380,000.
1952	Stiletto heels are introduced by Christian Dior.
1952	Orlon® acrylic is introduced; by 1956, over 70 million Orlon sweaters are sold.
1955	Mary Quant opens her boutique, Bazaar, in London.
1956	Southdale Center, the first enclosed shopping mall, is built in a Minneapolis suburb to serve shoppers. Dayton's serves as an anchor department store.
1957	*Gentlemen's Quarterly* is first published and distributed through men's wear stores.
1957	Christian Dior dies, and Yves Saint Laurent takes over as head designer of the House of Dior.
1958	Supp-hose, a 100 percent nylon stocking designed for women suffering from leg fatigue, is patented by the Chester H. Roth Co.
1958–59	To the benefit of intimate apparel, hosiery, and swimwear companies, DuPont introduces its first spandex fiber.
1960	Hanes-Millis Sales Corp. becomes the first national sock manufacturer to distribute its products through wholesalers.
1960	The first Bobbin Show takes place in Columbia, South Carolina, with 12 exhibitors.
1960	American Apparel Manufacturers Association (AAMA) is founded.
1962	Dayton's opens their discount store chain, Target.
1962	Sam Walton opened the first Walmart discount store; the company incorporates as Wal-Mart Stores Inc. in 1969.
1964	John Weitz becomes the first American designer to put his name on a menswear collection.
1967	Pierre Cardin and Bill Blass boutiques open in Bonwit Teller's New York store.
1968	Calvin Klein Ltd. is established.
1968	Polo Ralph Lauren is created.
1968	Minimum wage is increased to $1.60 per hour.
1969	The Gap opens in San Francisco, selling records, cassettes, and Levi's. The store draws its name from the "generation gap."
1969	Target opens its first distribution center in Fridley, Minnesota.
1969	Dayton Corporation and J.L. Hudson Company merge to create Dayton-Hudson Corporation.
1970	L'eggs Products introduces egg-shaped packaging and self-service distribution for hosiery.
1970	Walmart opens its first distribution center and its home office in Bentonville, Arkansas
1971	Diane Von Furstenberg introduces her jersey wrap dress, which is an immediate success.
1972	The Care Labeling of Textile Wearing Apparel and Certain Piece Goods Act goes into effect.
1972	Nike brand footwear debuts.
1973	No nonsense hosiery is first distributed by Kayser Roth.
1975	Giorgio Armani Co. is founded, and Armani launches his first menswear line.
1975	Geoffrey Beene becomes the first American designer to show his collections during fashion openings in Milan, Italy.

Table 1.4	Historical Events 1950–1980: Diversification and Incorporation *(continued)*
1975	*John T. Molloy's Dress for Success* is published.
1975	The first Zara store opens in Coruña, Spain.
1976	Liz Claiborne, Inc. is created and later grows to be one of the largest U.S. women's apparel companies.
1976	The nation's first major warehouse retailer, Price Club, opens in San Diego.
1976	The Amalgamated Clothing Workers of America Union merges with the Textile Workers of America and the United Shoe Workers of America unions to form the Amalgamated Clothing and Textile Workers Union (ACTWU).
1977	Ralph Lauren is the stylist for the Annie Hall character for the movie *Annie Hall*.
1978	Calvin Klein introduces his first menswear collection.

1980–1995: Imports and Quick Response

In the 1970s and early 1980s, the U.S. textile and apparel industries saw a decline in consumer demand for their products and an increase in labor, energy, and materials costs. Consumer demands for lower prices, quality merchandise, and better service were reflected in business strategies. During the 1980s, several of the largest department store groups were leveraged by management or as part of acquisitions and takeovers. Among the largest of these deals were the following:

- May Department Stores' acquisition of Associated Dry Goods in 1986
- Robert Campeau's purchase of Allied Stores in 1986 and Federated in 1988
- Macy's purchase of Bullock's and I. Magnin in 1988

Store acquisitions continued through the 1990s and early 2000s as:

- Federated Department Stores acquired Macy's in 1994 and Broadway Stores in 1995.
- Profitt purchased Saks Fifth Avenue and smaller regional stores in 1998.
- In 2005, Federated Department Stores acquired May Department Stores and realigned the retailers under two names: Bloomingdales and Macy's. With this acquisition, retailers such as Abraham & Straus, Bon Marché, Burdines, Filene's, L.S. Ayres, Marshall Field's, Meier & Frank, and Robinsons-May were converted to the Macy's moniker.

However, not all retailers were able to adapt to the changing retailing environment. By the late 1990s, many well-known retailers were out of business, including B. Altman & Co., Bonwit Teller, Gimbels, E. J. Korvette, I. Magnin, Peck & Peck, and The Broadway. At the same time, stores such as Nordstrom, The Limited, Gap, Target, and Walmart were thriving.

The 1980s and 1990s also saw an increase in vertical integration among manufacturing and retailers. **Vertical integration** is a business strategy whereby companies control several steps of the design, production, marketing, and/or distribution of products. Strategies included the following:

- manufacturers (e.g., Nike, Tommy Hilfiger, Liz Claiborne) opening or expanding retail store operations

- department and specialty stores entering into partnerships with manufacturers and contractors to produce private-label merchandise for their stores

- retail stores (e.g., The Limited, Gap, Banana Republic, Old Navy, Victoria's Secret, Eddie Bauer) adopting a **store brand** concept, whereby the store offers only merchandise with the store name as its brand

During the early 1980s, certain segments of the industry were affected by the continued growth of textile and apparel imports. Companies such as Liz Claiborne, founded in 1976, and Nike, Inc. founded in 1972, were producing apparel worldwide in order to obtain the best labor price for production. Concern about rising labor costs in the United States and the continued surge of imports led industry executives to join forces in examining ways to improve the productivity of the U.S. textile and apparel industries. Analyses indicated that apparel manufacturers and retailers were working with a 66-week cycle to go from raw fiber to a garment on the retail selling floor. It was estimated that for 55 weeks—83 percent of this cycle—products were in inventory. Thus, products were actually being processed for only 11 weeks (*Quick Response*, 1988). Industry executives recognized that this represented a huge inefficiency.

In 1984–1985, the Crafted with Pride in U.S.A. Council engaged Kurt Salmon Associates, textile and apparel industry analysts, to analyze industry inefficiencies. This project developed the idea of **Quick Response (QR)** to describe a philosophy that promoted potential ways to increase efficiencies. The following year, the Crafted with Pride in U.S.A. Council sponsored pilot projects linking fabric producers, apparel manufacturers, and retailers to determine if QR was feasible and to identify obstacles and difficulties in implementing QR strategies. Results from these pilot projects, in terms of increases in sales, stock turnover (the number of times during a specific period that the average inventory on hand has been sold), and return on investment (relationship between company profits and investment in capital items), were positive.

A few mass merchants and department stores, as well as top name-branded manufacturers, ventured to implement new technologies (Hasty, 1994). Because investments in technology led to higher productivity, companies found that their investments paid off quickly. Pioneers in QR included textile companies such as Milliken and Burlington; apparel manufacturers such as Haggar, Levi Strauss, and Arrow; and retailers such as Dillard's, J.C. Penney Company Inc., and Belk, among others.

What Is Quick Response?

The phrase *Quick Response* is an umbrella term used to identify various management systems and business strategies in the textile and apparel industries that reduce the time between fiber production and sale to the ultimate consumer. Specific definitions of QR varied, depending on the industry division:

- For textile producers, QR focused on connections among fiber producers, fabric producers, and apparel manufacturers.
- For apparel manufacturers, QR focused on increased use of technology and connections among fabric producers, apparel producers, and retailers.

In general, these strategies included the following:

- increased speed of design and production through the use of computers
- increased efficiency with which companies communicate and conduct business with one another
- reduced amount of time goods are in warehouses or in transit
- decreased amount of time needed to replenish stock on the retail floor

Quick Response was a change from the **push system** of the past, in which supply-side strategies were used to push the products produced on the consumer. In contrast, QR was a **pull system** of demand-side strategies based on the flow of timely and accurate information about consumers' wants and needs from consumers to the manufacturers.

During this time, Quick Response strategies were implemented at all stages of the textile and apparel manufacturing and distribution processes, generally referred to as the marketing channel or marketing pipeline, from fiber production to retail sale to the ultimate consumer. Business strategies that fell under the QR umbrella included the following:

- use of computer-aided design and manufacturing systems
- use of the most efficient fabric and apparel production systems

- use of UPC bar codes on merchandise and shipping cartons
- receiving and sharing of product information
- sending of orders and other forms electronically

In other words, any business strategy that improved accuracy and/or quality and reduced the amount of time spent in the production and distribution of fabric and apparel was considered part of QR.

It soon became apparent that the key barrier in the implementation of QR was the use of a variety of computer systems by manufacturers and retailers and the lack of standards within the industry. Thus, in the mid-1980s, inter-industry councils were formed to establish voluntary communications standards. Once these standards were instituted and adopted, companies that had embraced QR saw growth in sales and market share. By the late 1990s, virtually all successful firms had implemented some QR strategies. Even though the phrase Quick Response was used in conjunction with the slogans Made in U.S.A. and Crafted with Pride in U.S.A., QR strategies were also adopted by overseas apparel manufacturers, especially those manufacturers that worked with large retailers in the United States (Douglas-David, 1989).

Industry Cooperation and Partnerships

For Quick Response strategies to be successful, cooperation among the various components of the textile, apparel, and retailing industries was essential. A level of trust between companies was also a must for the strategies to be effective. For example, with QR, because fabric is inspected for flaws at the mill, apparel producers do not have to reinspect it at the apparel plant. However, the apparel producers must trust that the fabric producers have adequately inspected the fabric. A number of partnerships were formalized to focus on ways in which companies within the various industries could best cooperate to increase productivity. These partnerships included **Textile/Clothing Technology Corporation** ([TC]^2), industry linkage councils, the Crafted with Pride in U.S.A. Council, and the American Textile Partnership.

In the late 1970s, Harvard professors John T. Dunlop and Frederick H. Abernathy assessed the productivity of the U.S. apparel industry within the global economy. They argued that new approaches were needed to reduce labor costs if the apparel industry was to maintain its market share. This study led to a two-day conference of industry, union, government, and university representatives to plan a joint research and development program. Thus, in 1980, the Tailored Clothing Technology Corporation ([TC]^2) was established

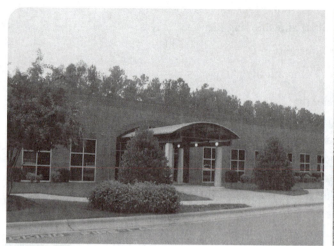
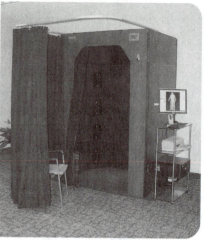

Figure 1.15 Established in 1980, [TC]² (left) conducts research and development for the apparel industry such as the 3-D body scanning technologies (right).

by the Amalgamated Clothing and Textile Workers Union (ACTWU), three men's suits manufacturers (Hartmarx, Palm Beach, and Greif), and the menswear division of fabric producer Burlington Industries (Kazis, 1989). In 1985, the name was changed to the Textile/Clothing Technology Corporation to better reflect its broader focus (see Figure 1.15, left). Currently, [TC]² remains a nonprofit consortium of over 200 textile, apparel, retail, labor, and government organizations, which "provides a range of solutions for the global soft goods industry specializing in technology development and supply chain improvement" ([TC]², 2010).

Since its beginning, [TC]² has focused on developing, testing, and teaching advanced apparel technology that could contribute to the reduction of direct labor costs involved in the production of apparel made in the United States. Initially, its work focused on automating the men's tailored clothing industry, but the group's current work is much broader in nature and represents needs throughout the entire fiber-textile-apparel industry. The work of [TC]² includes 3-D body scanning (see Figure 1.15, right), sizing (SizeUSA), and ink-drop printing. [TC]² also provides numerous educational programs and seminars for the sewn products industries.

In the mid-1980s, a number of councils were formed to develop and encourage the use of voluntary standards to facilitate faster, more accurate information flow between producers and suppliers. The Voluntary Interindustry Communications Standards (VICS) Committee was formed in 1986 by a group of industry executives who wanted to "take a global leadership role in the ongoing improvement of the flow of product and information about the product throughout the entire supply chain in the retail industry" (VICS Mission Statement). Their initial efforts focused on establishing agreement among retailers and producers regarding the use of the **Universal Product Code (UPC)** system (**bar codes**) to identify products and to acquire accurate information on consumers' purchases on an individual stock-keeping unit (SKU) basis; in addition, they sought to gain agreement on a single set of communication formats and **electronic data interchange** (EDI).

VICS was very successful in meeting these objectives. In 1987, the UPC-A bar code was recommended for branded general merchandise, including apparel. This voluntary standard was later endorsed by the National Retail Merchants Association (now called the National Retail Federation) and the International Mass Retailer Association. Shipping container marking (SCM) standards were also established. These marking standards support the flow of merchandise through distribution centers and are still used today.

In terms of EDI, a retail-specific version of the ANSI X.12 standard was published and made available through the Uniform Code Council. This standard was developed by the American National Standards Institute (ANSI), a national voluntary organization of companies and individuals who develop standardized business practices. The retail-specific version of the ANSI X.12 standard focused on electronic transmission of data for business transactions, such as purchase orders and invoices, and is currently used across the industry.

Once these standards were put in place, the VICS committee focused on conducting cost/benefit analyses of using VICS for UPC marking, EDI, and shipping container marking. Under a new name, the Voluntary Interindustry Commerce Solutions (VICS) Association, this organization now focuses on improving supply chain processes through recommendations for floor-ready merchandise standards, logistics standards, item-level tagging, and technologies for Internet commerce.

The Crafted with Pride in U.S.A. Council was a "one-industry" approach to marketing textiles and apparel made in the United States. From its conception in 1984, the Crafted with Pride in U.S.A. Council played an important role in coordinating unified efforts among the various segments of the industry to communicate to consumers that "buying American" matters for them and for the U.S. economy. This was accomplished by the use of TV spots, magazine supplements, syndicated columns and newsletters, labels and hangtags, in-store displays, and other promotions (see Figure 1.16).

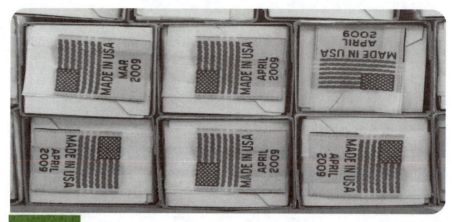

Figure 1.16 Beginning in the 1980s, many companies promoted Made in the USA production, such as L. Gambert, producer of the shirts shown here.

During the 1990s, a number of other partnership groups were formed to build cooperative efforts. The American Textile Partnership (AMTEX) was created to "enhance the competitiveness of the U.S. Textile Industry, from fibers through fabricated products and retail, by implementing technologies developed in collaborative R&D programs that link the scientific and engineering resources of government, universities, and industry" (AMTEX Mission Statement). AMTEX linked Department of Energy laboratories operated by the U.S. government with nonprofit technical organizations such as [TC]². See Table 1.5 for a listing of other significant historical events during this time period.

1995–Present: Supply Chain Management, Globalization, and Corporate Responsibility

Beyond QR: Supply Chain Management and RFID

By the late 1990s, QR strategies had been adopted by large and small companies alike. Three types of apparel companies made up the supply chain for soft goods (Parnell, 1998):

- Companies that performed almost all of their own manufacturing, from yarn or fabric to finished garments or other textile products
- Companies that had a particular niche within the industry, performing specific manufacturing operations such as manufacturing yarns or fabrics, finishing fabrics, or performing sewing operations

Table 1.5	Historical Events 1980–1995: Imports and Quick Response
1980	[TC]² begins operation to research and demonstrate new computer technology in the textile and apparel industries.
1984	Giorgio Armani launches a second, lower-priced line, called Emporio Armani.
1984	Donna Karan New York is founded by Donna Karan and her husband Stephan Weiss.
1984	Crafted with Pride in U.S.A. Council is formed.
1986	The Voluntary Interindustry Communications Standards (VICS) Committee is formed.
1986	May Department Stores acquires Associated Dry Goods.
1987	Christian Lacroix opens a new couture house in Paris.
1987	Nike introduces Air Max, the first Nike footwear to feature Nike Air bags.
1988	Target becomes the first mass merchandiser to introduce UPC scanning in all Target stores and Distribution Centers.
1990	Tom Ford joins Gucci and becomes creative director in 1994; he later becomes creative director for Yves Saint Laurent.
1990	Dayton-Hudson Corporation purchases Marshall Field's.
1990	Nike introduces "Reuse-A-Shoe" program whereby consumers can drop off worn athletic shows which Nike grinds up and uses for new sports surfaces.
1990	Walmart becomes the nation's number one retailer.
1992	Allied Stores Corporation and Federated emerge from bankruptcy as Federated Department Stores, Inc. with 220 department stores in 26 states.
1992	Macy's files for protection under Chapter 11.
1991	Donna Karan launches her menswear line.
1992	Levi Strauss & Co. establishes a code of conduct for hired contractors worldwide.
1994	The North American Free Trade Agreement (NAFTA) goes into effect.
1994	Federated Department Stores acquires Macy's.

- Companies that were involved in the design, marketing, and distribution of apparel but contracted sewing operations to other companies, either domestically or in other countries

For each type of company, QR highlighted the importance of and need for additional partnerships among companies throughout the soft goods pipeline. With advances in information technology, the ways companies designed, manufactured, and distributed soft goods were affected. This philosophy of sharing and coordinating information across all segments of the soft goods industry was termed **supply chain management** (SCM). Supply chain management comprises the "collection of actions required to coordinate and manage all activities necessary to bring a product to market, including procuring raw materials, producing goods, transporting and distributing those goods, and managing the selling process" (Abend, 1998, p. 48).

Similar to QR, the goals of SCM are to reduce inventory, shorten the time for raw material to become a finished product in the hands of a consumer, and provide better service to the consumer. Collaboration, trust, and dependability are the cornerstones to making both the QR and the SCM processes effective. However, SCM goes beyond QR in that SCM companies share forecasting, point-of-sale data, inventory information, and information about unforeseen changes in supply or demand for materials or products.

By 2002, large companies such as VF Corporation invested in the information technology infrastructure to make SCM a reality. As **business-to-business (B2B)** Web-based technologies emerged, both smaller and larger companies have implemented effective supply chain management strategies for information sharing. Through the use of password-protected websites, businesses can share information and conduct business transactions effectively and efficiently (Figure 1.17).

As supply chain management strategies brought increased efficiencies to companies, new technologies continued to provide companies with tools for communication and integration. One such tool was **Radio Frequency Identification (RFID)** (see Figure 1.18). RFID is sometimes referred to as the next generation bar code since its primary functions are to increase supply chain

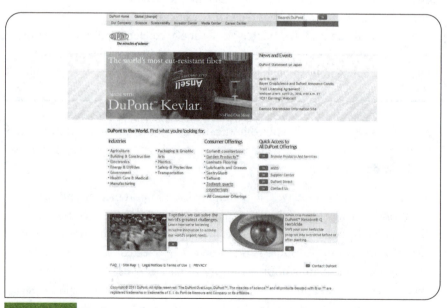

Figure 1.17 Businesses rely on Web technologies for communications to clients and consumers.

management through the tagging of containers, pallets, and individual items so that they can be accurately tracked as they move through the supply chain. However, unlike bar codes, RFID tags do not rely on line-of-sight readability. In fact, multiple RFID tags can be read simultaneously; they have memory and therefore can store and update data, and they provide fully automated data collection. Large global retailers, such as Walmart and Target, have pushed the adoption of

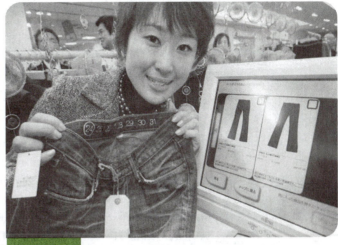

Figure 1.18 Sales associate demonstrating RFID technology to improve supply chain management.

RFID by requiring all their suppliers to apply RFID tags to pallets and cases.

Although RFID tags are significant in increasing efficiencies along the supply chain, concerns have been raised about item-level tagging. For example, because RFID tags are always "on," are there privacy issues when tags are placed on individual items? Pilot projects in 2005–2006 by companies such as Mitsukoshi, a Japanese department store, and Marks & Spencer, a U.K. retailer, found that using RFID tags on certain individual apparel items could improve their inventory management. In 2008, Indexport S.A., the licensed manufacturer of Hush Puppies in Spain, integrated RFID technology into their distribution, allowing them to identify and track each pair of shoes distributed (Hush Puppies, 2008). By 2009, American Apparel had fully integrated RFID technology at the store level, resulting in increased sales based on better inventory management and allowing employees to spend more time with customers (Roberti, 2009). RFID tags are also being used as a means to identify authentic products from counterfeit products. With retailers such as Walmart and Target requiring RFID technologies of their suppliers, RFID equipment, tags, and accessories are becoming more affordable and available to a broader spectrum of companies.

Globalization

Globalization is the process whereby nations' economies become intertwined and interdependent. Although the textile, apparel, home fashions, and retailing industries have been an integral part of the process of globalization for decades, the end of the twentieth century and the beginning of the twenty-first century brought increased attention to how the industries would adapt to and reflect the evolving global economy. Trade among countries for fibers, fabrics, apparel, home fashions, and the machinery needed to produce textiles and apparel has contributed to globalization. From its inception, the textile and apparel industries have offered countries opportunities for increased employment and economic growth. Regulation of international trade has evolved over the centuries, with countries setting up trade incentives and barriers as mechanisms for improving their economies or protecting domestic industries.

In 1995, the World Trade Organization (WTO) was created as a vehicle by which member countries (153 as of 2010) would negotiate trade agreements with an overall goal of enhancing international trade. As compared to **bilateral trade agreements** between two countries, the WTO contributes to the creation of **multilateral trade agreements** or trade agreements among multiple countries. With regard to textiles and apparel, many of the barriers to trading these were removed over a 10-year period (1995–2004). Thus, countries such as the United States that protected their domestic production of textiles and apparel through the use of quotas (numerical limits on imports) and tariffs (taxes on imports) were required to lower or eliminate these barriers to trade. The work of the World Trade Organization to increase opportunities for trade among member countries brought about dramatic shifts in the design, marketing, and production of apparel worldwide. These new rules resulted in countries redefining their roles in order to maximize their competitive advantages within the global economy:

- Countries such as the United States and France are focusing primarily on design and marketing.
- Countries such as China and India are focusing primarily on production.
- Other countries have found appropriate niches for their expertise and infrastructure. For example, Japan and Taiwan are producers of high-tech textiles.

Globalization and the opportunities and challenges for the textile, apparel, home fashions, and retailing industries are discussed throughout the book. Trade laws, free trade agreements, the WTO, and implications for the global textile, apparel, home fashions, and retailing industries are discussed in greater detail in Chapter 10.

Fast Fashion and Pop-Up Retail

Within this context of globalization and supply chain management, international companies have expanded their capabilities of vertical integration across countries. At the same time, consumers are demanding high-quality and fashion-forward products at reasonable prices. Creating this ultra-fast supply chain that focuses on consumer demand is known as **fast fashion**. Fast-fashion companies introduce new products in small quantities on a continuous basis with little or no replenishment. One of the most successful fast-fashion companies is Zara (see Figure 1.19), a member of The Inditex Group, a vertically integrated group of more than 100 companies. Zara is headquartered in Spain, with over 1,400 stores in 76 countries and more than 400 cities in Europe, the Americas, Asia, and Africa. Its success has been dependent upon the following:

- vertical integration (controlling many stages of the supply chain)
- designers working alongside production planners and market specialists
- making design and production decisions based on consumer demand
- offering consumers limited quantities of multiple styles of merchandise
- the ability to produce merchandise in weeks instead of months

Indeed, Zara can design and produce a garment and distribute it to a retailer in just 15 days. Swedish company H&M, and U.S. companies such as Bebe, Forever 21, and Charlotte Russe have also implemented fast-fashion philosophies.

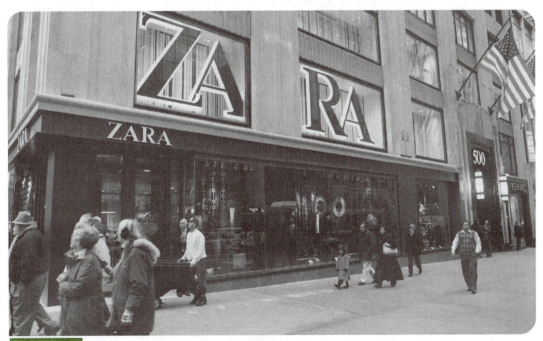

Figure 1.19 Zara is an example of a successful global fast-fashion company.

Fast fashion relies on constant communication among all elements of a company's supply chain—from customers to store personnel, from store managers to designers and merchandisers, from designers to buyers and sourcing agents, from buyers to contractors, from contractors to warehouse managers and distributors. Fast fashion has created an expectation among consumers of always seeing something new in stores and on the Internet. Although not all companies may be able to or even want to focus on all elements of fast fashion, aspects such as producing merchandise closer to the time the ultimate customer buys it are being copied by large and small companies worldwide.

If apparel and accessories can come and go quickly, then why can't retail stores do the same? Starting in the late 1990s, **pop-up retail** has emerged as an important trend. In 2002, Target opened its first pop-up store, a store with holiday merchandise that floated on the Hudson River. In 2003, Target opened a temporary 1500-square-foot store in Rockefeller Center, Manhattan, for its Mizrahi exclusive licensing collection of women's apparel. The store was open for only six weeks, from early September through the middle of October. In Spring 2004, Target opened a temporary (5 weeks only) store in the Hamptons with a focus on summer merchandise. Since then, Target has created a number of other pop-up stores. The retailer, Vacant, only operates pop-up stores with a series of traveling temporary (1 month only) retail establishments in empty spaces in cities around the world, selling limited collections of merchandise from new designers as well as established brands ("Pop-up Stores," 2007).

When the U.S. recession hit in 2008, pop-up stores created opportunities for landlords to fill space on a temporary basis and allowed retailers to test new locations and merchandise (Misonzhinik, 2009). In 2009, Gap Inc. used pop-ups in Los Angeles and New York to sell their new 1969 Premium Jeans. Pop-up stores are also being used for seasonal sales such as holiday, back-to-school, and Halloween. Pop-up retailers often use social media websites such as Facebook and Twitter to create excitement around the merchandise and store. See Table 1.6 on p.40 for other significant historical events during this time period.

Intraindustry and Interindustry Partnerships

In order to create competitive advantages, companies have sought ways of differentiating themselves within the marketplace. One strategy that has been successful across industry sectors has been **intraindustry** and **interindustry partnerships**; that is, partnering with companies that are in the same sector of the industry but have different target customers (intraindustry), or with companies in a different industry that share common target customers (interindustry).

As an example of intraindustry partnerships, retailers such as H&M and Target created exclusive limited licensing agreements with name designers. H&M has partnered with prestigious designers such as Karl Lagerfeld (2004), Viktor and Rolf (2006), and Roberto Cavalli (2007), with short-term exclusive licensing agreements. Since its inception in 2006, Target's GO International fashion program has provided limited-time collections of over a dozen designers including Luella Bartley (2006), Proenza Schouler (2006), Richard Chai (2008), and Zac Posen (2010). Target's Designer Collaborations program has included special collections for Target by designers such as Anna Sui (2008), Alexander McQueen (2009), and Jean Paul Gaultier (2010). Other intraindustry partnerships include Stella McCartney and Adidas who in 2004 joined forces on a collection called Adidas by Stella McCartney. In 2009, Pendleton Woolen Mills and Opening Ceremony created a collection of trendy apparel using traditional Pendleton fabrics and motifs called Pendleton Meets Opening Ceremony (see Figure 1.20). As an example of an interindustry partnership, from 2006 to the present, Nike has partnered

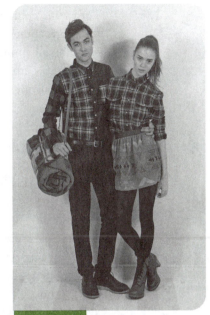

Figure 1.20 Partnerships, such as Pendleton Meets Opening Ceremony, create unique fashions and expand the lines of both companies.

with Apple to create iPod and iPhone compatible footwear. When inserted into the sole of a Nike running shoe, the sensor allows runners to choose Nike-created Sport Music as well as track and store workout information on their iPods, iPhones, and/or online. These types of intraindustry and interindustry partnerships have allowed companies to create unique product lines and thus differentiate themselves from competitors.

E-Commerce

With the introduction of **e-commerce** in the mid-1990s, many companies began experimenting with online business. At this time, the idea of multichannel retailing meant that a brick-and-mortar store might also have a seasonal catalog. A number of issues needed to be resolved before online retailing would become readily accepted by consumers, and retailers struggled with the relationship between traditional stores and online extensions. Both retailers and consumers were skeptical about the security of ordering merchandise online.

For example, in 1998, Liz Claiborne launched its website lizclaiborne.com as an information/branding website only; not until 2000 did they relaunch the site as an e-commerce destination.

By the beginning of the twenty-first century, online retailing had become an important component of many retailers' multichannel approach. Across categories, online retail sales have grown every year since 2000 with $155 billion in U.S. sales in 2009. The apparel, accessories, and footwear category accounted for $27 billion in sales in 2009 with a prediction of at least 10 percent annual growth for the next few years (Stambor, 2010). Top business-to-consumer online retailers in the apparel and accessory category include J.C. Penney Co. Inc., Victoria's Secret, Macy's, Target Corp., Gap Inc. Direct, L.L. Bean, and Nordstrom ("Top 500," 2010). New technological developments in website design include online tools that mimic the tactile experiences consumers have in bricks-and-mortar apparel and accessories stores. In addition, today consumers expect true **multichannel retailing** that seamlessly integrates brick-and-mortar and online operations so that they can, for example, check merchandise availability on mobile devices while sitting in the parking lot of the retailer ("E-commerce," 2010). Pop-up retail and e-commerce within the textile, apparel, and home fashions industries is discussed in greater detail in Chapter 12.

Corporate Social Responsibility

As the twentieth century came to a close, reflections of the industries 100 years earlier revealed that the same inhumane conditions of the early textile factory towns in England and the United States were found again in factories around the world. A combination of public outcry, student activists, and media attention brought these issues to forefront of government Therefore, in 1996, President Clinton created the Apparel Industry Partnership, a voluntary partnership of apparel and shoe manufacturers, trade unions, and consumer and human rights organizations, to create a standardized code of conduct for apparel companies. The Fair Labor Association was formed in 1998 and the Workers' Rights Consortium was formed in 1999. Over the past 15 years, most companies have implemented codes of conduct, and they routinely monitor factories.

By 2011, companies have incorporated socially responsible business practices throughout the supply chain. What does this mean for the current business of fashion? In general, **corporate social responsibility (CSR)** refers to business practices that contribute positively to society. Companies that engage in corporate social responsibility ask the question: how do we design, produce, and distribute the highest quality and environmentally sustainable products under the best factory and business conditions in a profitable manner? Indeed, in today's business environment, manufacturers, marketers, and retailers must provide consumers with competitively priced merchandise that is designed, manufactured, and distributed in responsible ways that foster sustainability from both environmental and business perspectives (see Figure 1.21).

Corporate social responsibility in the textile, apparel, and home fashions industries is evidenced throughout the supply chain. **Socially responsible supply chain management** is achieved through design, sourcing, and distribution decisions that positively affect social, environmental, and economic systems:

- **Socially responsible design** includes practices that enable designers to influence the social, environmental, and economic systems through design solutions. This is achieved through inclusive design, environmentally responsible design, health-related design, and design that promotes fair trade.

- **Socially responsible production** is achieved through safe and healthy working conditions, environmentally responsible production, fair wages, and production that promotes fair trade.

- **Socially responsible marketing** considers consumers' desire to purchase goods and services that have been produced and distributed with sustainability in mind and in safe and humane conditions by individuals who are paid a fair or living wage.

- **Socially responsible distribution** is achieved through safe and sustainable practices for getting products to the ultimate consumer.

As a framework for the business of fashion, corporate social responsibility is discussed throughout the book in relation to the policies, practices, and business decisions described in each chapter. To be sustainable into the next decade, the business of fashion must reflect a global value system of social responsibility.

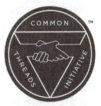

Figure 1.21 Patagonia's Common Threads campaign highlights trends in apparel production focusing on environmental responsibility.

Table 1.6	Historical Events 1995–Present: Globalization, Internet, and Fast Fashion
1995	The two primary labor unions in the textile and apparel industries—the Amalgamated Clothing and Textile Workers Union and the International Ladies Garment Workers Union—merge to become the Union of Needletrades, Industrial and Textile Employees (UNITE).
1995	Federated Department Stores acquires Broadway Stores.
1995	The World Trade Organization (WTO) begins as an international organization for negotiating trade agreements.
1996	The Kathie Lee Gifford sweatshop scandal: merchandise she endorsed is found to have been made in South American sweatshops.
1996	President Clinton creates the Apparel Industry Partnership to develop a plan to eliminate sweatshops.
1996	www.macys.com is launched.
1996	Patagonia uses only 100% organic cotton for all its cotton garments.
1997	Designer superstar Gianni Versace is murdered.
1997	Nike begins using organic cotton in its jersey t-shirts.
1997	Walmart becomes the largest private employer in the United States, with 680,000 U.S. associates and another 115,000 international associates.
1998	[TC]^2 makes a 3D body measurement system commercially available.
1998	Liz Claiborne, Inc. launches lizclaiborne.com as a branding/information Web site. It is relaunched in 2000 as an e-commerce Web site.
1998	Dayton Hudson Corporation purchases Associated Merchandising Corporation.
1998	Activists found the United Students Against Sweatshops (USAS).
1998	The Fair Labor Association is formed through the efforts of the Apparel Industry Partnership.
1999	The Workers Rights Consortium (WRC) is created as an alternative monitoring system to the Fair Labor Association.
1999	Walmart becomes the largest private employer in the world, with 1,140,000 associates.
2000	Dayton Hudson Corporation is renamed Target Corporation; 2004 Associated Merchandising Corporation is renamed Target Sourcing Services.
2000–06	Liz Claiborne expands to 40 brands, with $4.85 billion in sales; acquisitions include Monet (2000), Mexx (2001), Ellen Tracy (2002), Juicy Couture (2003), Enyce (2003), and Mac & Jac (2006).
2001	When terrorists fly commercial airplanes into the World Trade Center and the Pentagon, how business is conducted changes forever.
2002	José Mariá Castellano Rios, CEO of Inditex/Zara, is named International Retailer of the Year by the National Retail Federation.
2002	Target creates its first pop-up retail outlet: a boat on Chelsea Pier featuring holiday merchandise.
2003	Target launches its exclusive licensing agreement with Isaac Mizrahi.

Table 1.6	Historical Events 1995–Present: Globalization, Internet, and Fast Fashion *(continued)*
2004	Tom Ford leaves Gucci and YSL to start his own line of luxury men's wear.
2004	UNITE and HERE (Hotel Employees and Restaurant Employees International Union) merge to create the union, UNITE HERE; it re-affiliates with AFL-CIO in 2009.
2004	Facebook is launched from a dorm room at Harvard University.
2005	Quotas on textiles and apparel imported from World Trade Organization (WTO) members are phased out.
2005	Federated Department Stores acquires May Department Stores, realigning stores into eight operating divisions: one Bloomingdale's and seven Macy's.
2005	Nike's Considered Boot, its first sustainable product, debuts.
2006	Target introduces GO International, featuring British designer, Luella Bartley.
2006	Twitter is launched, allowing users to post "micro-blogs".
2007	Kohl's launches its exclusive licensing agreement with Vera Wang, introducing Very Vera by Vera Wang.
2007	Federated Department Stores changes its name to Macy's, Inc.
2007	Facebook reaches over 50 million active users.
2008	Nike launches its Nike Considered Design, a collection of footwear that combines sustainability principles with sport innovations.
2008	Swimmers wearing Speedo's LZR Racer suits break multiple world records while wearing the suit; the suit is banned by FINA, the governing body of swimming starting in 2010.
2009	Macy's and Bloomingdale's launch social media programs to reach customers.
2010	Two Bloomingdale's stores open in Dubai.
2010	Facebook reaches over 400 million active users with more than 70 translations.

Summary

Since their beginnings in the Industrial Revolution of the eighteenth and nineteenth centuries, the textile and apparel industries have maintained an important place in the American economy. Spurred by the mechanization of spinning, weaving, and sewing processes, the textile and apparel industries moved from craft industries to factory-based industries. Immigrants provided the necessary labor force for these growing industries.

By the 1920s, ready-made apparel was available to most consumers. Two types of apparel production were developed—modern, large factories, and small contractors who sewed piecework at home. The textile and apparel industries emerged from the Great Depression of the 1930s with the need to address growing and changing demands from consumers. Technological advancements in synthetic fibers provided a new source of materials for apparel. However, it was not until after World War II that these easy-care fibers hit the American market.

The 1950s saw growth and expansion of apparel companies, many becoming large, publicly owned corporations. This growth continued through the 1960s. However, as labor costs in the United States increased and consumer demand for lower-cost clothing also increased, companies began moving production outside the United States.

As imports of textiles and apparel surged, the American industry examined how it could increase productivity and global competitiveness. The result of this analysis was the development of the Quick Response system, an industry-wide program made up of a number of strategies to shorten the production time from raw fiber to the sale of a finished product to the ultimate consumer. Quick Response strategies are seen in all segments of the textile, apparel, and retailing industries. Interindustry cooperation through joint research ventures, [TC]^2, interindustry linkage councils, the Crafted with Pride in U.S.A. Council, and the American Textile Partnership increased the effectiveness of Quick Response strategies.

Enhanced information technology has allowed for increased partnerships throughout the soft goods pipeline. Supply chain management (SCM) encompasses these information-sharing processes to improve the efficiency and effectiveness of the textile and apparel industries. RFID tagging has evolved as an important tool for companies wanting to increase their efficiencies in SCM.

Since the beginning of the twenty-first century, the textile and apparel industries have been adapting to new rules associated with international trade and consumer demand for high-quality, fashionable, and reasonably priced goods. Strategies such as fast fashion, pop-up retail, and e-commerce will tap the industries' capabilities for effective integration and communication. The textile and apparel industries will continue to be integral industries for globalization and economic growth. With globalization comes the integration of corporate social responsibility throughout the textile and apparel supply chain including socially responsible design, production, marketing, and distribution.

Key Terms

bar codes	cotton gin
bilateral trade agreement	e-commerce
business-to-business (B2B)	electronic data interchange (EDI)
contractor	fast fashion
corporate social responsibility (CSR)	globalization

interindustry partnership

intraindustry partnership

mass fashion

multichannel retailing

multilateral trade agreement

pop-up retail

pull system

push system

Quick Response (QR)

Radio Frequency Identification (RFID)

ready-to-wear (RTW)

size standards

slops

socially responsible design

socially responsible distribution

socially responsible marketing

socially responsible production

socially responsible supply chain management

store brand

subcontractor

supply chain management

sweatshop

Textile/clothing Technology Corporation ([TC]^2)

Universal Product Code (UPC)

vertical integration

Discussion Questions and Activities

1. What technological developments were imperative for the development and growth of the textile and apparel industries in the United States and in global markets?

2. Look in a historic costume book, and select a fashion from at least 15 years ago. What social and technological developments were necessary for the production and distribution of the fashion?

3. In your own words, define supply chain management. Why would a textile or apparel manufacturer want to adopt SCM strategies? What technological developments have led to supply chain management?

4. What are the disadvantages and advantages of fast fashion for textile, apparel, and home fashions companies? What are the advantages and disadvantages of fast fashion for consumers?

5. Go to your favorite apparel and/or accessory website. What are the characteristics of the website that assist you in making selections and purchases? How might the website be improved?

6. In your own words, define coporate social responsibility in the textile, apparel, home fashions, and retailing industries. What business practices and decisions are instrumental for effective corporate social responsibility?

References

Abend, Jules. (1995, October). Textiles making all the right moves. *Bobbin*, pp. 40–45.

Abend, Jules. (1998, May). SCM is putting a buzz in industry ears. *Bobbin*, pp. 48–54.

American Textile Manufacturers Institute. (1978). *Textiles: Our First Great Industry*. Charlotte, NC: American Textile Manufacturers Institute.

Bedell, Thomas. (1994, March). Innocents lost: The great Triangle fire. *Destination Discovery*, pp. 24–31.

Bicentennial of U.S. textiles. (1990, October). *Textile World*.

Brill, Eileen B. (1985). From immigrants to imports. In *WWD/75 Years in Fashion, 1910–1985*. Supplement to *Women's Wear Daily*, pp. 10–14. New York: Fairchild Publications.

Bureau of Labor Statistics (2010). *Textile, Textile Product, and Apparel Manufacturing. Career Guide to Industries*, 2010–2011 Edition. United States Department of Labor, http://www.bls.gov

Butenhoff, Peter. (1999, May). Future perfect: Will past tensions dissolve with SCM? *Apparel Industry Magazine*, pp. SCM-2–SCM-4.

Davis-Meyers, Mary L. (1992). The development of American menswear pattern drafting technology, 1822 to 1860. *Clothing and Textiles Research Journal*, 10 (3), pp. 12–20.

Douglas-David, Lynn. (1989, October). EDI: Fiction or reality? *Bobbin*, pp. 86–90.

E-commerce: More than just an e-Store. (2010, June). Whitepaper of Jesta I.S. Inc. [online] Available: http://www.jestais.com [June 29, 2010].

Ewing, Elizabeth. (1992). *History of Twentieth Century Fashion* (3rd ed.). Lanham, MD: Barnes & Noble Books.

Ferdows, Kasra, Lewis, Michael A., and Machuca, Jose A.D. (2004). Rapid-Fire Fulfillment. *Harvard Business Review*, Vol. 82, No. 11.

Fraser, Steven. (1983). Combined and uneven development in the men's clothing industry. *Business History Review*, 57, pp. 522–547.

Hasty, Susan E. (Ed.). (1994, March). *The Quick Response Handbook*. Supplement to *Apparel Industry Magazine*.

Hohanty, Gail F. (1990). From craft to industry: Textile production in the United States. *Material History Bulletin*, 31, pp. 23–31.

Hosiery and Underwear. (1976, July). Issue devoted to the history of hosiery and underwear. NY: Harcourt Brace Jovanovich.

Hush Puppies (2008). RFID Projects, *RFID Magazine*, pp. 32-29.

Kazis, Richard. (1989, August/September). Rags to riches? *Technology Review*, pp. 42–53.

Kidwell, Claudia B., and Christman, Margaret C. (1974). *Suiting Everyone: The Democratization of Clothing in America*. Washington, DC: Smithsonian Institution.

Kramer, William M., and Stern, Norton B. (1987). Levi Strauss: The man behind the myth. *Western States Jewish Historical Quarterly*, 19 (3), pp. 257–263.

Melinkoff, Ellen. (1984). *What We Wore*. New York: Quill.

Misonzhnik, Elaine. (2009). Pop-up stores fill vacant space, create a win/win model in a down market. *Retail Traffic*. [online] Available: http://retailtrafficmag.com/retailing/operations/0818-pop-up-stores/ [June 27, 2010].

Parnell, Clay. (1998, June). Supply chain management in the soft goods industry.

Apparel Industry Magazine, pp. 60–61.

Pop-up Stores a Fresh Approach for the Savvy Retailer (February 10, 2007). *Retail Times*. [online] Available: http://www.retailtimes.com.au/index.php/page/Pop-up_Stores_a_fresh_approach_for_the_savvy_retailer [June 27, 2010].

Quick Response: America's Competitve Advantage [slide set program guide] (1988). Washington, DC: American Textile Manufacturer's Institute

Richards, Florence S. (1951). *The Ready-to-Wear Industry 1900–1950*. New York: Fairchild Publications.

Roberti, Mark (2009, July 2). American Apparel RFID Project. *RFID Journal Blog*. [online] Available http://www.rfidjournal.com/blog/entry/5015/ [June 27, 2010]

Stambor, Zak. (2010, March 8). E-retail will influence 53% of purchases by 2014, Forrester says. *Internet Retailer*. [online] Available: http://www.internetretailer.com/2010/03/08/e-retail-will-influence-53-of-purchases-by-2014-forrester-says [June 27, 2010].

Steele, Valerie. (1988). Paris Fashion: A Cultural History. New York: Oxford University Press.

Stegemeyer, Anne. (1996). *Who's Who in Fashion* (3rd ed.). New York: Fairchild Publications.

Symbol Technologies, Inc. (2006). *Synchronize Your Supply Chain with RFID*. Holtsville, New York: Author.

[TC]² Coporate Headquarters (2010). [TC]² Home Page [online]. Available: http://www.tc2.com [June 27, 2010].

Top 500 Guide (2010). *Internet Retailer*. [online]. Available: http://www.internetretailer.com/top500/list/ [June 27, 2010].

Yafa, Stephen. (2005). *Big Cotton*. New York: Viking/Penguin Books.

CHAPTER 2

Business and Legal Framework of Textile, Apparel, and Home Fashions Companies

In this chapter, you will learn the following:

- the ways in which a business can be owned and operated—sole proprietorships, partnerships, and corporations

- terminology related to business organization

- the ways in which businesses within the textile, apparel, home fashions, and retailing industries compete

- the definition of licensing and how textile, apparel, and home fashions companies use licensing agreements

- the primary marketing channels used by textile, apparel, and home fashions companies

- the federal laws that can affect textile, apparel, and home fashions companies

Business Organization and Company Ownership

*T*extile, apparel, and home fashions companies come in all sizes and types. Some are large corporations that employ thousands of people; others are small companies with one or two employees. Regardless of size and organizational structure, every company in the textile, apparel, and home fashions supply chain is in business to make a profit by providing customers with the products and services they desire and need. Because many people planning careers in the textile, apparel, and home fashions industries hope to own their own businesses someday, an understanding of the various types of business organizations is an important starting point before our further examination of the operation of these companies. In addition, information about business organizations is important for planning careers and assessing companies in terms of employment and advancement opportunities. Depending on their objectives, needs, and size, textile, apparel, and home fashions companies can be owned and organized in a number of ways. The three most common legal forms of business ownership are sole proprietorships, partnerships, and corporations. They are compared in Table 2.1. Each of these forms of business can be found among textile, apparel, and home fashions companies.

Sole Proprietorships

The **sole proprietorship** is a very common form of business ownership in which an individual, the "sole proprietor," owns the business and its property. Indeed, from a legal perspective, the sole proprietor or owner is indistinguishable from the company itself. The sole proprietor typically runs the overall day-to-day operations of the company but may have employees to help with specific aspects of the business. Employees may be full-time, part-time, or hired to conduct certain tasks. Any profit from the business is considered personal income of the sole proprietor and taxed accordingly; the owner is personally liable for any debt the business may incur.

When starting a company, sole proprietors are often referred to as **entrepreneurs**. According to Entrepreneur.com, entrepreneurs "assume the financial risk of the initiation, operation and management of a business." As such, entrepreneurs often create a new business as either a sole proprietorship, partnership, or a limited liability company, depending on the number of people involved in the creation of the business.

Table 2.1 Comparisons among Sole Proprietorships, Partnerships, and Corporations

Business Organization Form	Sole Proprietorship	Partnership	Corporation
Ease of formation	Easy to form Business licenses required	Easy to form Business licenses required Written contract advisable	Difficult to form Charter required Registration with the SEC required for publicly held corporations
Operational strategies	Owner also runs the business	Partners can bring range of expertise to running the business	Board hires individuals with specific expertise to run the business
Liability	Unlimited personal liability	Unlimited personal liability for each partner	Limited liability; stockholders not personally liable for corporate debt
Tax considerations	Sole proprietor's income taxed as personal income	Partners' income taxed as personal income	Double taxation (corporation's income taxed, and dividends taxed as personal income)
Potential for employee advancement	Limited, depending upon size of company	Some incentive for employees to become partners	Employees can move up through the ranks
Examples	Small companies Freelance designer Independent sales representative	Small or medium-size companies Designer and marketer who join forces to form an apparel company	Large companies May be private or publicly held (e.g., Celanese Corporation, Liz Claiborne, VF Corporation, Macy's Inc.) Some may be multinational

ADVANTAGES OF SOLE PROPRIETORSHIPS

This type of business ownership has a number of advantages. For one thing, only a few business licenses are needed. For example, in Los Angeles, the following licenses are needed to open an apparel manufacturing business:

- City of Los Angeles business license
- garment license
- resale license
- public health license
- federal employer identification number (if there are employees)
- state employer identification number (if there are employees)
- registration number (for labeling purposes, in lieu of putting the company name on labels)

Sole proprietorships are also easy to dissolve. When the sole proprietor decides to stop doing business, the sole proprietorship is essentially ended. Another advantage of a sole proprietorship is the control and flexibility given the sole proprietor, who often finds personal satisfaction in being the boss and making the decisions regarding the direction the business will take. This personal satisfaction is the characteristic of this form of business ownership that individuals most often desire.

DISADVANTAGES OF SOLE PROPRIETORSHIPS

This type of business ownership also has a number of disadvantages. The biggest disadvantage is that sole proprietors are personally liable for any business debts. This means that if the business owes money, creditors can take all business and personal assets (such as the owner's home) to pay the debts of the business. This **unlimited liability** is one of the largest risks a sole proprietor takes in starting the business.

Another disadvantage of sole proprietorships is that because there are no partners, the sole proprietor needs to have expertise in all areas of running the business. For example, an apparel designer who wants to start his or her own business must do the following:

- handle the design aspect of the business
- work with fabric suppliers, contractors, and retailers
- deal with accounting
- manage personnel
- market the product

The difficulty in running all aspects of the business is often overwhelming for new sole proprietors. In some cases, sole proprietors will hire employees who have expertise in specific areas in which the owner is not familiar. For example, a designer may hire an accountant to manage the financial aspects of the business.

In a sole proprietorship, raising **capital** (funds or resources) for business initiation or expansion can be difficult. Capital needed to start or expand the business may be obtained in the following ways:

- tapping the owner's personal funds
- purchasing goods and services on credit
- borrowing money from banks, friends, family members, or other investors

A well-written business plan is essential for a sole proprietor to garner funds from banks and other investors. As with other forms of business ownership, sole proprietorships must keep books of account for federal, state, and municipal income tax and other regulatory purposes. Profits are taxed as personal income.

EXAMPLES OF SOLE PROPRIETORSHIPS

Sole proprietorships tend to be small companies, the resources and complexities of which can be handled by one owner. Individuals may start companies as sole proprietorships and then, as the company grows, change the form of ownership to a partnership or corporation. Examples of sole proprietorships within textile, apparel, and home fashions industries might include the following:

- a freelance textile or apparel designer who sells his or her work to larger textile or apparel companies
- an independent sales representative who sells apparel lines to retailers
- an apparel retailer who owns a small specialty store

The Bureau of Labor Statistics estimates that more than one out of every four fashion designers is self-employed (U.S. Department of Labor, 2010).

Partnerships

There are times when two or more people want to join forces in owning a business. In these cases, a **partnership** may be formed. According to the Uniform Partnership Act (UPA), a partnership is an "association of two or more persons to carry on as co-owners of a business for profit." A partnership may be formed between two individuals or among three or more individuals through written contracts called **articles of partnership**. Although contracts will vary, they typically include the following:

- the partnership's name
- the partners' and officers' names
- the intentions or purposes of the partnership
- the amount and form of contributions (e.g., money and real estate) from each partner
- the length of the partnership
- procedures to add and eliminate partners
- the way profits or losses will be divided among the partners
- the degree of management authority each partner will have
- the designation of which partners, if any, are entitled to salaries
- how partnership affairs will be handled if a partner dies or is disabled

Profits are shared among the partners, known as **general partners**, according to the conditions laid out in the partnership contract. Profit from a partnership is taxed as part of each partner's personal income. Similar to sole proprietors, partners have unlimited liability. This means that, together, they are liable for the entire debt of the partnership as outlined in the partnership contract. Dissolution of a partnership can result from the following:

- a partner's withdrawal
- the entry of new partners
- a partner's death
- a partner's bankruptcy
- a partner's incapacity or misconduct
- the goals of the business becoming obsolete

LIMITED PARTNERSHIPS

Sometimes individuals want to join or invest in a partnership, but they do not want to have the unlimited liability for partnership debt that may be larger than their investment. This can be achieved through a **limited partnership**. In this type of partnership, a limited partner has **limited liability**, that is, he or she is liable only for the amount of capital that he or she invested in the business. Any profits are shared according to the conditions of the limited partnership contract. Establishing limited partnerships can be an attractive way for general partners to raise capital to initiate or expand their business. Typically, the limited partner does not take an active role in managing the business, which is handled by the general partners.

ADVANTAGES OF PARTNERSHIPS

Partnerships have some advantages over sole proprietorships. Similar to sole proprietorships, partnerships are relatively easy to establish; the same business licenses are required to start a partnership as a sole proprietorship. Unlike sole proprietorships, where only one person owns the business, partners can pool their range of expertise and resources to run the company. For example, one partner in an apparel company may have expertise in design, and another partner may have expertise in business and accounting.

Raising capital for partnerships is also somewhat easier than for sole proprietors because the resources of more than one person can be tapped, and the combined resources of partners can be used as collateral when borrowing money. Through the use of limited partnerships, resources can also be raised for business initiation or expansion. As with sole proprietorships, a quality business plan is needed for partnerships to secure funding from investors.

Another advantage of partnerships over sole proprietorships is that advancement opportunities for employees are greater: employees may be given the opportunity to become partners in the business. This can be a valuable incentive when recruiting and hiring employees.

DISADVANTAGES OF PARTNERSHIPS

Partnerships also have a number of disadvantages. As with sole proprietorships, the primary disadvantage of partnerships is liability exposure. This means that each partner is personally liable for any debt of the partnership, regardless of which partner was responsible for incurring the debt. In addition to books of account, the UPA also requires that partnerships keep minutes of meetings and business records.

Another disadvantage of a partnership is the potential for disagreement among partners in running the business or setting the future direction of the business. Partnerships often dissolve because of such disagreements. As with sole proprietorships, a partnership is dependent on its owners, and dissolution is presumed when a partner leaves the partnership. Although ease of dissolution of a partnership can be viewed as an advantage, it can also lead to a lack of continuity in the business operations.

EXAMPLES OF PARTNERSHIPS

Partnerships are typically small to medium-size companies that require a combination of specialized skills to be successful. For example, two or more individuals may start an apparel company, each bringing unique skills (e.g., design, marketing, operations, and so on) to the business. A number of large apparel manufacturers, such as Calvin Klein, Esprit de Corp., and Liz Claiborne, started as partnerships.

- Calvin Klein borrowed money from his friend Barry Schwartz to start his design company, and the two remained partners in the business until it was sold to Phillips-Van Heusen in 2003.

- In the 1960s and 1970s, Doug Tompkins, Susie Tompkins, and Jane Tise owned an apparel company called Plain Jane. In 1979, the Tompkins bought out Tise and renamed the company Esprit de Corp. The Tompkins divorced in the early 1990s and the company is now a private corporation.

- Elisabeth "Liz" Claiborne started her business in 1976 with her husband, Arthur Ortenberg, and a manufacturing expert, Leonard Boxer, as partners. Later, Jerome Chazen joined as a partner. Within a year, the company was making a profit, and in 1981, it became a publicly traded corporation.

Corporations

The **corporation** is the most complex form of business ownership because corporations are considered legal entities that exist regardless of who owns them. Corporations are created through the filing of **articles of incorporation** (sometimes referred to as articles of organization or articles of association) with the state or federal government. General requirements of articles of incorporation include the following:

- name of corporation
- purpose and power of the corporation
- time frame or period of existence
- authorized number of shares/owners
- types of shares
- other conditions of operation

Typically, corporations are designated by the words Corporation, Corp., or Inc. Although assets owned by the corporation, such as buildings or equipment, are tangible, the corporation itself is considered intangible.

Unlike a sole proprietorship or partnership, ownership of a corporation is held by **stockholders** (or shareholders), who own shares of stock in the corporation. Each share of stock represents a percentage of the company, so that if someone owns 50 percent of the stock in a company, he or she owns 50 percent of the company. Stockholders in a corporation are liable only for the amount they paid for their stock. Thus, if the company fails, stockholders are not liable for the corporation's debts beyond their investments in the company's stock.

The **board of directors** of the corporation is elected by the stockholders. Each stockholder has a percentage of votes in electing the board that reflects the percentage of stock he or she owns. The board of directors is the chief governing body of the corporation. It plans the direction the company will take and sets policy for the corporation. The board also hires the officers of the corporation (e.g., the president, chief executive officer, chief financial officer, and so on), who run the business. Stockholders may participate in the management of the business, but many stockholders in corporations have very little or no participation in day-to-day operations.

Profit is paid out to stockholders in the form of **dividends**, which are taxed as personal income. Stockholders may also receive dividends in the form of additional stock in the company. Figure 2.1 shows some examples of corporations in the textile, apparel, and home fashions industries.

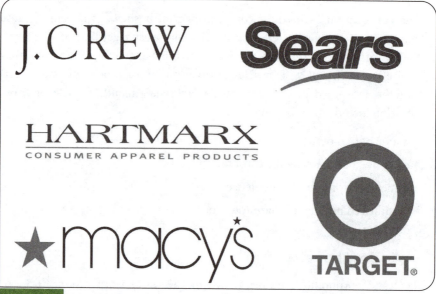

Figure 2.1 Trademarked logos of apparel, accessory, and home fashions corporations.

TYPES OF CORPORATIONS

C Corporations and S Corporations

The most common type of corporation is the **C corporation**, or **regular corporation**. This type of corporation distributes profits to shareholders through dividends. Therefore, earnings of the corporation are taxed twice—once at the corporate level, and again at the individual level. This is known as **double taxation**. For small domestic corporations with a limited number of domestic individual shareholders, **S corporations** are becoming more common. S corporations are given special status by the Internal Revenue Service whereby earnings are taxed only at the individual level, thus eliminating double taxation.

Publicly Traded and Privately Held Corporations

Differences between publicly traded and privately held corporations are primarily in terms of the ownership and transferability of shares of stock. In publicly traded corporations, (or **publicly held corporations**), at least some of the shares of stock are owned by the general public. **Publicly traded corporations** usually have a large number of stockholders who buy and sell their stock on the public market, either through an exchange (New York Stock Exchange, American Stock Exchange, or National Association of Securities Dealers Automatic Quotation System [NASDAQ]), or through brokers "over the counter." Publicly traded corporations must submit financial information to the Securities and Exchange Commission (SEC), which regulates the securities markets. Table 2.2 lists selected publicly traded corporations in the textile and home fashions industries. Table 2.3 lists selected publicly traded corporations in the apparel industry.

  Privately held corporations (also called **private corporations, closely held corporations**, or **close corporations**) are those in which the shares are owned

Table 2.2 Examples of U.S. Publicly Held Fiber and Textile Corporations

Celanese Corporation	(NYSE: CE)
Culp, Inc.	(NYSE: CFI)
DuPont	(NYSE: DD)
International Textile Group	(OTC US: ITXN)
The Dixie Group	(NASDAQ GM: DXYN)
Unifi, Inc.	(NYSE: UFI)

Table 2.3   Examples of U.S. Publicly Held Apparel, Footwear, and Home Fashions

Carter's, Inc.	(NYSE: CRI)
Cherokee, Inc.	(NASDAQ GS: CHKE)
Coach, Inc.	(NYSE: COH)
Columbia Sportswear Company	(NASDAQ GS: COLM)
Decker's Outdoor Corp.	(NASDAQ GS: DECK)
Ethan Allen Interiors, Inc.	(NYSE: ETH)
Fossil Inc.	(NASDAQ GS: FOSL)
G-III Apparel Group Ltd.	(NASDAQ GS: GIII)
Hanesbrands, Inc.	(NYSE: HBI)
K-Swiss Inc.	(NASDAQ GS: KSWS)
Kenneth Cole Productions, Inc.	(NYSE: KCP)
La-Z-Boy Inc.	(NYSE: LZB)
Liz Claiborne, Inc.	(NYSE: LIZ)
Maidenform Brands	(NYSE: MFB)
Mohawk Industries Inc.	(NYSE: MHK)
Nike, Inc.	(NYSE: NKE)
Oxford Industries, Inc.	(NYSE: OXM)
Perry Ellis International	(NASDAQ GS: PERY)
Phillips-Van Heusen Corporation	(NYSE: PVH)
Polo Ralph Lauren Corporation	(NYSE: RL)
Quiksilver Inc.	(NYSE: ZQK)
Sealy Corporation	(NYSE: ZZ)
Sketchers USA Inc.	(NYSE: SKX)
The Jones Group	(NYSE: JNY)
Timberland Company	(NYSE: TBL)
True Religion Apparel Inc.	(NASDAQ GS: TRLG)
Under Armour, Inc.	(NYSE: UA)
VF Corporation	(NYSE: VFC)
Warnaco Group, Inc.	(NYSE: WRC)
Wolverine World Wide Inc.	(NYSE: WWW)

by a small number of individuals; that is, the stock is not available in public markets and has not been issued for public purchase. Typically, the stockholders of a private corporation are highly involved in the operations of the company. Vera Wang Bridal House, L.L.Bean, Patagonia, Pendleton Woolen Mills, KEEN Inc., HMX LLC (owner of brands such as Hickey Freeman, Hart Schaffner Marx, and Bobby Jones), Maidenform Brands, Inc., and Retail Brand Alliance (owner of Brooks Brothers and Carolee jewelry) are examples of private corporations in the apparel and retailing industries.

Multinational corporations are either private or publicly traded corporations that operate in several countries. In today's global economy—with increased world production and trade of apparel, accessories, and home fashions—multinational corporations have grown in number and importance. Multinational corporations can be set up in the following ways:

- in horizontally integrated corporations, operations throughout the world are involved in producing the same or similar products

- in vertically integrated corporations, operations throughout the world are involved in specific aspects of the production across the supply chain

- diversified corporations include some aspects of both horizontal and vertical integration

Examples of multinational corporations include Nike, Inc. and Walmart.

Limited Liability Companies

Authorized in 1977 and expanded in 1988, **Limited Liability Companies (LLC)** provide business owners with tax advantages (as with partnerships) along with limited liability (as with corporations). These companies are owned by a few members who all participate in management of the company.

Although LLCs are more complex to form than partnerships, they are easier to form than corporations. Examples include small companies, such as PFW Productions, LLC, the production company for Portland (Oregon) Fashion Week, and Sweetface Fashion Company LLC, a joint venture with Jennifer Lopez that designs and markets women's comtemporary fashions.

ADVANTAGES OF CORPORATIONS

Corporations have a number of advantages over other forms of business ownership. The main advantage of incorporation is the limited liability of the owners (stockholders). If the corporation fails, creditors cannot seize the personal assets of the stockholders to pay the corporate debt. This is the primary reason why two or more individuals may decide to create a private corporation rather than a partnership when beginning a business.

Another advantage corporations have is the flexibility and ease with which ownership can be transferred. Unlike a sole proprietorship or partnership, a corporation does not cease to exist if one of its owners withdraws or dies. Shares are simply transferred to heirs or sold. In most cases, stockholders are free to sell their stock at any time. Because of this ease of transferring ownership, corporations seldom dissolve because of ownership issues.

Unlike the management of a sole proprietorship or partnership, management of a corporation is not dependent on ownership. The management group runs the day-to-day operations of the company regardless of who owns the business that day. This allows the board of directors to hire the best-qualified individuals to manage the specialized areas of the company.

In addition, in large corporations, there is great potential for employee advancement within the organization. Employees may work in specialized areas of the company and advance through the ranks—such potential for advancement can serve as employee incentive.

For publicly traded corporations, the act of "going public," or becoming a publicly traded corporation, can be a benefit to businesses in raising capital to expand or diversify. When a corporation goes public, investors buy shares of stock based upon how well they believe the company will perform in the future. These investments can then be used to expand or improve the company.

DISADVANTAGES OF CORPORATIONS

With all of these advantages, why are not all businesses corporations? Despite the apparent advantages, a number of disadvantages exist. It is much more complicated to establish a corporation than a sole proprietorship or partnership. As previously noted, a corporation is organized around a legal charter or articles of incorporation that outline its scope and activity. Because of this, legal fees and other costs involved in incorporation are higher than for other forms of business ownership. This is especially true if a company wants to become a publicly traded corporation or "go public" through the selling of shares to public investors. It is estimated that the costs of an **initial public offering (IPO)** can be up to 25 percent of the company's equity (the difference between the company's assets and its liabilities).

The corporation's articles of incorporation also restrict the type of business performed by the corporation. In other words, the board of directors or officers of a publicly traded apparel company cannot shift from producing apparel to producing automobiles without filing new articles of incorporation.

Corporations are organized under the laws of specific states, and each state has statutes that govern corporations. There are also federal laws (i.e., Securities Act of 1933, Securities Exchange Act of 1934) that regulate publicly held corporations in the issuing and selling of their shares of stock. Other federal laws that govern businesses, including corporations, are described later in this chapter.

Another disadvantage to corporations are corporate taxes. Because they are legal entities, corporations are taxed on their income at a tax rate higher than that on personal income. In addition, for C corporations, dividends paid to stockholders are considered personal income, and, therefore, they are subject to personal income tax.

Corporations are often large companies that can have thousands of employees. Because of this, employees sometimes view corporations as impersonal and bureaucratic. In addition, unlike other forms of business ownership, owners of corporations, especially publicly traded corporations, might not be involved in the day-to-day operations of the business. Employees who are not stockholders may not have the same commitment to the corporation that owners of sole proprietorships or partnerships may have.

Despite these disadvantages, the limited liability associated with corporations and ease of transferring ownership make them very attractive for investors who want to own part of specific companies. Thus, privately held and publicly traded corporations are the most powerful forms of business in the textile and apparel industries. In fact, some categories within the industry, such as intimate apparel, are dominated by large corporations. Within the intimate apparel category, corporations control most of the production and distribution:

- Maidenform Brands, Inc. with brands including Maidenform®, Flexees®, Control It®, and Lilyette®

- Warnaco with brands including Calvin Klein® underwear, Warner's®, and Olga®

- HanesBrands, Inc. with brands including Playtex®, Bali®, L'eggs®, Just My Size®, Barely There®, and Wonderbra®

- Kayser-Roth Corporation with brands including No nonsense® and HUE®

- Fruit of the Loom, Inc. with brands including BVD®, Fruit of the Loom®, and Underoos®

- Vanity Fair Brands, LP (subsidiary of Fruit of the Loom) with brands including Vanity Fair®, Lily of France®, Vassarette®, Curvation®, and Bestform®

Terms Associated with Company Expansion and Diversification

As you read trade and consumer literature about companies' organizations and operations, you will come across a number of terms (e.g., merger, consolidation, takeover, and conglomerate) related to the company's organization. In order to interpret the literature, it is important to have a basic understanding of these terms.

A **merger** is the blending of one company into another company. If company A and company B merge, the result will be a larger company A, which will assume ownership of company B's assets and liability for all of company B's debts. For example, in 2010, Tommy Hilfiger Corporation was acquired through a merger agreement by Phillips-Van Heusen Corporation, whose other investments include Calvin Klein, Arrow, Izod, Bass, and VanHeusen.

A **consolidation** is the combining of two companies, with the result being a new company. If company A and company B consolidate, the result is company C.

A **takeover** results when one company or individual gains control of another company by buying a large enough portion of its shares. For example, in 2005, adidas Group, a German company, completed a takeover of its North American-based rival Reebok. Similarly, in 2008, Nike acquired Umbro (UK football brand) through a takeover. Takeovers can be either mergers or consolidations; friendly, in that the company that is taken over agrees to the association; or hostile, in that the company that is taken over does not agree to the association. Being informed about possible mergers and consolidations within the industry is important for management-level textile and apparel executives in their strategic decision making.

Conglomerates are diversified companies (typically corporations) that are involved with significantly different lines of business. The biggest advantage for conglomerates is their ability to realign assets among companies to increase efficiencies, support expansions, and minimize the impact of losses. For example, LVMH Group is a conglomerate including companies focusing on wine and spirits (e.g., Moët & Chandon champagne), fashion and leather goods (e.g., Louis Vuitton, Céline, Givenchy, Marc Jacobs), perfumes and cosmetics (e.g., Parfum Dior, Benefit cosmetics,), watches and jewelry (e.g., TAG Heuer, Zenith, De Beers), and retailing (e.g., DFS Galleria, Sephora).

Forms of Competition

The goal of every sole proprietorship, partnership, and corporation in the textile, apparel, and home fashions industries is to earn a profit by providing products and/or services that are desired by the ultimate consumer. However, many companies are vying for the consumer's dollar. Thus, companies, whether they are sole proprietorships, partnerships, or corporations, compete with one another. Companies that successfully compete will make a profit that will either be reinvested in the company or paid to the company's owners or stockholders.

Competitive Strategies

Companies compete in a number of ways that, in part, determine their business strategies. Companies typically compete on any of the following bases:

- the *price* of the merchandise to the retailer or consumer
- the *quality* of the design, fabrics, and construction
- *innovation*—how unique or fashionable the merchandise is
- *services* offered to the business customer or ultimate consumer
- a combination of these factors

One company that produces children's wear may have lower prices than its competition; another may provide better-quality merchandise; another may produce children's wear that is more innovative; and still another may provide consumers with catalogs or other services. Thus, a company's business practices are based on competitive strategies.

For example, Hanna Andersson, a children's apparel manufacturer and multichannel retailer headquartered in Portland, Oregon, is known for its socially responsible business practices (see Figure 2.2). As their mission statement states:

> To share our passion for outstanding quality and our care for children by providing uniquely styled, long lasting, and comfortable clothing that lets kids be kids and is inspired by our Swedish heritage and socially responsible business practices.

This corporate philosophy is demonstrated in a number of ways. Organically grown cotton is used for sleepers, long johns, and T-shirts; garments are also tested for harmful substances. The Hanna Helps program gives grants to nonprofit organizations that focus on children's lives. Through their Cash for Kids program, the company gives $100 checks each year made out to the schools of children of Hanna Andersson employees. The children present the checks to the school

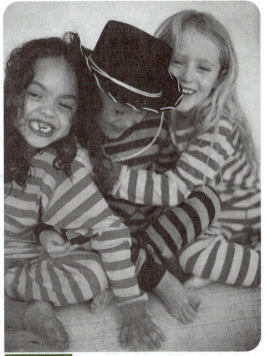

Figure 2.2 One of Hanna Andersson's competitive advantages is to focus on quality, functionality, durability, and environmental responsibility of their designs.

principal, and they help to decide how the funds should be used. Donations are made to programs that support home-schooled children, as well as to schools of children mentored by Hanna Andersson employees. Such corporate practices are one way Hanna Andersson separates itself from its competition and appeals to the company's customers.

Competitive Situations or Market Forms

Five primary competitive situations or market forms exist among U.S. companies:

1. monopoly
2. oligopoly
3. oligopsony
4. pure or perfect competition
5. monopolistic competition

In a **monopoly**, one company typically dominates the market and, thus, can price its goods and/or services at whatever level it wishes. Because a monopoly essentially eliminates or drastically reduces competition, federal laws prohibit companies from buying out their competition and, in effect, becoming a monopoly. Only essential services, such as utilities, can legally operate as monopolies in today's market, and the prices they charge are heavily regulated by the government.

In an **oligopoly**, a few companies dominate and essentially have control of the market, thereby making it very difficult for other companies to enter. The dominant companies compete among themselves through product and service differentiation and advertising. Although oligopolies are not illegal, the dominant companies are not permitted to set artificial prices among themselves. In many ways, the athletic footwear industry can be considered an oligopoly because it is dominated by a few companies. For example, Nike (including Converse) and adidas Group (including Reebok), account for the largest share of athletic footwear worldwide. Thus, these companies have some control over the price they charge for their goods.

Oligopsony exists when there is a small number of buyers for goods and services offered by a large number of sellers. This type of competition is most often found in agricultural products (e.g., cocoa) whereby numerous growers sell to a limited number of buyers worldwide.

In **pure competition**, or **perfect competition**, there are many producers and consumers of similar products, so price is determined by market demand. The market for agricultural commodities, such as cotton or wool, is the closest to pure competition that can be found in the textile and apparel industries. In these cases, the price for the product—raw cotton or wool—is determined by supply and demand of the commodity. For example, supply and demand for cotton are estimated two years in advance. Cotton supplies can be affected by weather conditions, production yield, trade negotiations, legislation, and other factors that impact how many bales of cotton are produced. When supplies are high and demand stable or low, prices of cotton can decrease. When supplies are low and demand high, prices of cotton can increase.

The most common form of competition in the textile, apparel, and home fashions industries is **monopolistic competition**, in which many companies compete in terms of product type, but the specific products of any one company are perceived as unique by consumers. For example, many companies produce denim jeans, including Levi Strauss & Co., Lee, Wrangler, Guess?, 7 for All Mankind, Marc by Marc Jacobs, Joe's, Gap, True Religion, and Calvin Klein. However, through product differentiation, advertising, distribution strategy, and pricing, each company has created a unique image. By creating this unique image in consumers' minds, each has, in some respect, a monopoly in terms of its specific product and, therefore, has some control over price. A consumer who wants only 7 for All Mankind jeans and seeks out that particular brand may be willing to pay a premium for that brand.

Within monopolistic competition, each company must create a perceived difference between its product and the competition's products. This can be achieved in the following ways:

- The product is differentiated by design characteristics.
- The company uses advertising to create public awareness of its brand name or trademark (see Figure 2.3).
- The company buys the use of a well-established brand name, trademark, or other image through licensing programs.
- A retailer creates **private-label brand** or **store brand** merchandise that is unique to its store or catalog. Examples of private-label brands are Arizona (JCPenney), Classiques Entier and Halogen (Nordstrom), and Charter Club and INC International (Macy's). Examples of store brands are Abercrombie and Fitch, Gap, Banana Republic, and Ann Taylor.
- A manufacturer may expand its services to consumers, as when it opens retail stores (e.g., Polo Ralph Lauren, Liz Claiborne, Tommy Hilfiger) or offers goods through catalogs, websites, and other nonstore venues.

In these ways, consumers associate a company's goods with a particular unique image.

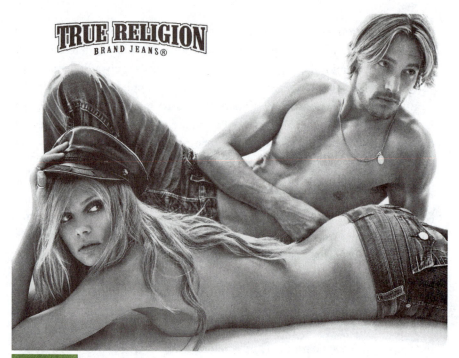

Figure 2.3 Apparel and accessory companies strive to create unique images to gain competitive advantage.

Licensing

One of the methods used by textile and apparel companies to create a perceived difference in their product is **licensing**. Because of the widespread use of licensing within the textile, apparel, and home fashions industries, an understanding of the role it plays in textile and apparel production is important. Licensing is the selling by the owner (*licensor*) of the right to use a particular name, image, or design to another party (*licensee*), typically a manufacturer, for payment of royalties. The licensee buys the right to use the name, image, or design, referred to as the *property*, on merchandise to add value to the merchandise. Licensing has grown dramatically as companies recognize the value of established brand names, characters, and **brand extensions**. Examples of licensed products include the following:

- loungewear and performance underwear produced by Exquisite Apparel with the brand name Dickies

- men's dress shirts produced by Phillips-Van Heusen with the Ike Behar brand name

- hosiery manufactured by Kayser-Roth Corporation under the brand name Calvin Klein hosiery
- children's apparel produced by Franco Apparel Group under the brands Starter Baby, Starter Kids, Eddie Bauer, New Balance, Laura Ashley Collection, Baby Inc., and professional sports teams
- Andrew Marc and Marc New York brands owned by Jones Apparel Group manufactured by G-III Apparel Group
- sheets and pillowcases under the Lauren Ralph Lauren label manufactured by WestPoint Stevens

Some companies' products are entirely licensed (e.g., Hang Ten); other companies license only certain product lines (e.g., Vera Wang fragrances, Donna Karan sunglasses, Polo by Ralph Lauren boys' wear). Many name brands use licensing agreements to expand their production and distribution in other countries; for example, Liz Claiborne apparel, handbags, and related accessories are produced by Trimera Group for distribution in Canada.

Types of Licensed Names, Images, and Designs

The types of names, images, and designs that are licensed vary widely, although the majority falls into the following categories:

- *Character and entertainment licensing:* Such images as cartoon characters, movie or television characters, and fictional characters are often licensed to appear on a range of merchandise, from sleepwear to backpacks to sheets and towels. Examples include the following:
  – Disney characters
  – *Peanuts* or *South Park* cartoon characters
  – *Toy Story* characters
  – likenesses of Spiderman or Superman
  – *Alice in Wonderland* characters

  In recent years, licensed merchandise relating to movies and movie characters has been extremely popular, particularly for infant and children's clothing and other children's merchandise.

- *Corporate licensing:* The licensing of brand names and trademarks of corporations such as IBM, Harley-Davidson, or Coca-Cola is also common. This type of brand extension licensing extends a brand that is well known in a particular product area to a different product area. Examples include Porsche sunglasses, Coca-Cola stuffed-toy polar bears, Pillsbury Doughboy potholders, and Harley-Davidson armchairs.

- *Designer name licensing:* Designers, including Pierre Cardin, Chanel, Yves Saint Laurent, Ralph Lauren, Calvin Klein, Giorgio Armani, Vera Wang, Donna Karan, and many others, license their names as brand names for products including scarves, jewelry, fragrances, cosmetics, home fashions, and shoes.

- *Celebrity name licensing:* Celebrities also license their names to create immediately recognized brands of merchandise. Examples include the following:
  - Jennifer Lopez, and Sarah Jessica Parker, who have licensed their names and images to perfumes
  - Ashley and Mary-Kate Olsen (Dualstar Entertainment Group), who have an exclusive licensing agreement with Steven Madden, Ltd. for a line of footwear and with Absolute Black for a line of sunglasses both under their brand, Elizabeth and James
  - Eminem, who partnered with Nike on a limited collection of footwear
  - Kathy Ireland's collection of home furniture, rugs, ceiling fans, home accessories, and bedding that bears her name through licensing agreements with a number of home fashions companies

- *Exclusive licensing for a retailer:* In recent years, retailers have teamed up with celebrities and designers to create merchandise sold exclusively at a particular retailer, creating a unique form of private-label merchandise. Examples include the following:
  - Jaclyn Smith's line of apparel licensed to Kmart
  - Vera Wang's Simply Vera exclusive brand for Kohl's
  - Target's GO International program that has featured exclusive licenses with designers including Luella Bartley, Tracy Feith, and Zac Posen
  - Shaun White shoes and clothing available through an exclusive license with Target

- *Nostalgia licensing:* Manufacturers license the names and images of legends, such as Marilyn Monroe, James Dean, and Babe Ruth, as well as old-time movies and radio and TV shows, such as *The Lone Ranger*, *Superman*, and *King Kong*.

- *Sports and collegiate licensing:* Professional sports team and university logos are licensed to appear on sport-related merchandise, such as sweatshirts with the Green Bay Packers logo, jackets with the Boston Red Sox logo, and caps with the Oregon State University logo.

- *Event and festival licensing:* The names or logos of such events as the Kentucky Derby, the Indianapolis 500, Wimbledon, the Olympics, the World Cup, and the Masters golf tournament are also licensed for use on products.

- *Art licensing:* Manufacturers license great works of art to be reproduced on their merchandise.

The success of licensing depends on consumers' desire for goods with a perceived difference based on brand name, trademark, or image. The diversity of types of licensed goods attests to its effectiveness in creating a favorable perceived difference in the eyes of consumers.

The Development of Licensed Products

A well-established image-oriented property is a must for the success of any licensed product. When such a property exists, the development of licensed products based on it involves a number of steps. The stages of development of licensed products are as follows:

1. The image or design, commonly referred to as the *property*, is created. For example, the red, white, and blue logo of Tommy Hilfiger is established.

2. Consumers are exposed to the property through the media. The Tommy Hilfiger name and trademark are used in advertising, hangtags, publications, and so on.

3. The property is marketed by the licensor to build name or image recognition. Tommy Hilfiger builds a reputation among consumers for trendy fashion, quality, and value. The name and trademark are associated with these characteristics in consumers' minds.

4. Merchandise with the property added is produced by a variety of manufacturers. Tommy Hilfiger licenses the name and trademark to several manufacturers of apparel, accessories, and fragrances.

5. Merchandise is distributed by retailers. Retailers who have been successful with Tommy Hilfiger sportswear will also want to carry licensed Tommy Hilfiger merchandise, such as accessories and fragrances.

6. Merchandise is demanded by consumers. Consumers identify with the Tommy Hilfiger name and perceive the licensed products as having an added value because the Tommy Hilfiger name and trademark are attached to the merchandise.

The Licensing Contract

The terms of the agreement between the licensee and licensor are outlined in a contract. Typically, a licensing agreement will include the following elements:

- *Time limit:* For many licensed products, timing is everything. For example, the contract for the image of a currently popular movie character may be for a shorter time than for a classic designer name.

- *Royalty payment:* Typically, royalties of 7 to 14 percent of the wholesale price of the goods sold are paid by the licensee to the licensor.

- *Image:* Contract clauses specify how the image will appear, giving the licensor control over graphics, colors, and other design details. For example, Ocean Pacific (OP) controls the design of all graphics on its licensed merchandise.

- *Marketing and distribution:* Licensors often want to control the consistency of the marketing of their licensed merchandise. Also, many designers do not want their licensed merchandise distributed through discount or off-price retailers, and they put clauses in their contracts to prevent it.

- *Quality:* Clauses about the materials and manufacture of merchandise and the submission of samples of merchandise for approval by the licensor give the licensor control over the quality of the product.

- *Advances:* Contract clauses set the amount of the advance money that will be paid up front and then deducted from the royalty payments.

- *Guarantees:* Contracts often guarantee that a minimum dollar amount will be paid to the licensee, even if royalties fall below this amount.

- *Notification of agreements to customs department:* If goods are being manufactured offshore, or outside the United States, this notification is needed so the goods will clear customs and not be confiscated as counterfeit goods. Contract clauses assure licensees that the licensor will provide notification if it is needed.

Advantages of Licensing

Licensing agreements have a number of advantages for both the licensee and licensor. For the licensee, the value added to the merchandise by a licensed name, image, or design comes in many interrelated forms. The licensee gets automatic brand identification (see Figure 2.4). For example, a youth T-shirt with a picture of characters from the 2009 movie *Avatar* received automatic recognition from children and parent-consumers.

In many instances, the licensed product is trusted for qualities that stem from the licensor—a designer name attached to a handbag adds fashion credibility to the handbag. For manufacturers, a licensed product can also be a marketing shortcut for launching new products. By purchasing the rights to a designer or celebrity name, a fragrance company can launch a new fragrance with immediate brand name recognition.

The licensor also gains from licensing agreements. Licensing allows for brand extension into other categories of merchandise without revealing to consumers that the licensor is not manufacturing the merchandise. Such arrangements allow companies to expand their product lines by taking advantage of the manufacturing and distribution expertise and facilities of other companies.

For example, when Nike decided to expand its product line into women's swimwear, rather than spending the resources to develop the expertise in this area, it licensed its name to Jantzen, one of the world's largest women's swimwear manufacturers. With such an agreement, Nike was able to take advantage of the expertise at Jantzen, and Jantzen had the opportunity to expand its business by producing a new line of women's swimwear for a new target market.

As another example of this cooperation between corporations in licensing,

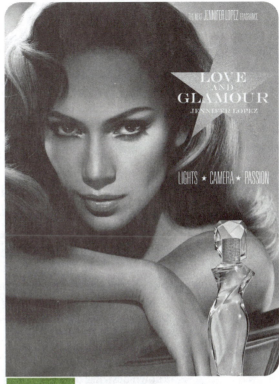

Figure 2.4 Celebrity name licensing of products adds immediate image and name recognition to the products.

Hartmarx, a well-known and well-respected producer of men's tailored clothing, is one of Tommy Hilfiger's licensees, handling both tailored and business-casual clothing and slacks for Tommy Hilfiger (owned by Phillips Van-Heusen). Hilfiger controls the design, distribution, and visual presentation of the products, and Hartmarx handles the production.

Designer–manufacturer licensing collaborations are common in intimate apparel and legwear, as shown in the following examples:

- Tommy Hilfiger Group has a licensing agreement with Israel-based Delta Galil Industries Ltd. to produce and market women's intimate apparel with the Tommy Hilfiger label.

- HanesBrands, Inc. licenses legwear under the Donna Karan and DKNY labels.

- Kayser-Roth produces Calvin Klein hosiery.

For well-established names or images, licensing arrangements can also be very lucrative. It is estimated that designers such as Calvin Klein and Ralph Lauren make millions of dollars each year in royalties from licensed merchandise.

Disadvantages of Licensing

There are also a number of disadvantages for the licensor and licensee. For the licensor, overuse of licensing arrangements may result in a saturation of the property in the marketplace. This can lead to consumers who do not perceive a distinct image with the property. For example, with hundreds of licensing agreements, Pierre Cardin's name can be seen on everything from luggage to cookware to children's apparel. Because of this, the name has lost some of its prestige.

When a licensed product sells well, the licensor must rely on the licensee's ability to react by producing goods quickly. Depending on the licensing contract, licensors also risk a loss of control over quality or distribution of licensed merchandise. To assure consistent quality, the licensor must provide constant monitoring of production quality by inspecting samples or production facilities.

A tragic example of the risk involved with losing control of a licensed name is that of the designer Halston. In the 1960s and 1970s, Halston became a well-known designer of expensive apparel worn by celebrities. In 1973, Halston sold the exclusive rights to his name to Norton Simon Industries (NSI). In 1982, NSI asked Halston to design a line of affordable mass-merchandised clothing for JCPenney. The introduction of this line resulted in high-end retailers dropping his designer-priced collection. Although Halston received some royalties until his death in 1990, he never regained control over the use of the Halston name, which changed ownership at least eight times during its almost 40-year history. Today the Halston name continues to regain prestige with its current owners the Weinstein Company and Hilco Consumer Capital LLC hiring Sarah Jessica Parker as its creative consultant and designer Marios Schwab, who created his first collection in 2010.

The major disadvantage of licensing for the licensee is the risk associated with predicting the popularity of the licensed name or image. Timing is extremely important for the success of many licensed products, and licensees must be experts in understanding and predicting consumer demand. Sometimes, however, the license does not turn out as anticipated. This often happens when big-budget movies flop.

Licensees also incur the expense of controlling channels of distribution and trying to prevent the counterfeiting of the licensed goods. They are also responsible for additional costs related to the manufacture of the licensed products according to the licensor's rules and regulations. For example, many licensors have rules governing where a product may be manufactured, which may make production more expensive than it otherwise might be. However, despite these disadvantages, licensing will continue to be an important business strategy for many companies.

Marketing Channels

In addition to understanding the different forms of business ownership and competitive strategies of companies in the textile and apparel industries, it is important to differentiate among the various marketing channels within the industry. **Marketing channels** are routes that products follow to get to the ultimate user. They consist of businesses that perform manufacturing, wholesaling, and retailing functions in order to get merchandise to the consumer. Marketing channels have several structural systems, including the following (see also Table 2.4):

- direct marketing channel
- limited marketing channel
- extended marketing channel

With the **direct marketing channel**, apparel manufacturers sell directly to consumers. For example, consumers may purchase goods directly from the manufacturer through catalogs or over the Internet. Although some apparel products are available to consumers through this channel, consumers do not have the resources to deal directly with manufacturers for all of their apparel

Table 2.4 Marketing Channels

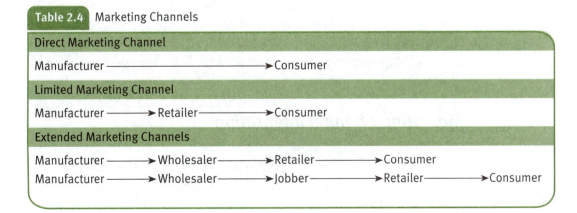

| Direct Marketing Channel |
| Manufacturer ⟶ Consumer |
| Limited Marketing Channel |
| Manufacturer ⟶ Retailer ⟶ Consumer |
| Extended Marketing Channels |
| Manufacturer ⟶ Wholesaler ⟶ Retailer ⟶ Consumer |
| Manufacturer ⟶ Wholesaler ⟶ Jobber ⟶ Retailer ⟶ Consumer |

purchases, nor do manufacturers have the resources to deal directly with individual consumers. Therefore, consumers must rely on retailers to search for and screen manufacturers and products for them.

In a **limited marketing channel**, retailers survey the various manufacturers and select (i.e., buy) merchandise that they believe their customers will want. Retailers also serve as gatekeepers by narrowing the choices for consumers and providing them with access (through retail outlets) to the merchandise, thus performing an important service to consumers. Retailers may also arrange for the production of specific goods (private-label merchandise) that they then make available to their customers. In some cases, apparel manufacturers sell merchandise through their own retail stores (e.g., Ralph Lauren, Nike, Guess?, Juicy Couture, Diesel). Because of the use of a retail store in the process, this form of distribution is considered a limited marketing channel rather than a direct marketing channel, even though the product is sold by the manufacturer. The limited marketing channel is the most typical marketing channel for apparel and home fashions products.

Extended marketing channels involve one of the following:

- Wholesalers acquire products from manufacturers and make them readily available to buyers, usually retailers.
- Intermediaries buy products from wholesalers at special rates and make them available to retailers. Intermediaries are sometimes referred to as jobbers in this segment of the industry.

Extended marketing channels are used in the distribution of many basic items, such as T-shirts, underwear, and hosiery. For example, a company may produce white T-shirt "blanks" and sell them to wholesalers. The wholesalers will sell the T-shirts to manufacturers that will have designs screen-printed on the shirts, using a textile converter for the screen printing process. The shirts are then sold to retailers. However, because of the increased time involved, this type of marketing channel is seldom used for fashion goods that companies want to get to the consumer as quickly as possible.

Marketing Channel Integration

Marketing channel integration is the process of connecting the various levels of marketing channels so that they work together to provide the right products to consumers in the right quantities, in the right place, and at the right time. Integration can be created through conventional marketing channels or through vertical marketing channels.

Conventional marketing channels consist of independent companies that separately perform the designing, manufacturing, and retailing functions. For example, KEEN Inc. with headquarters in Portland, Oregon, designs outdoor footwear that is manufactured by contractors and sold through a variety of brick-and mortar and online retailers. Each of these segments represents separate companies. **Vertical marketing channels** (also called **vertical integration**) consist of companies that work as a united group to design, produce, market, and distribute merchandise. Examples of vertical marketing channels include the following:

- An apparel manufacturer sells merchandise only through its own (or franchised) retail stores.

- A textile producer also manufactures and distributes finished textile products (e.g., hosiery, sheets, towels) to retail stores.

- Private-label (e.g., JCPenney's Arizona brand, Nordstrom's Caslon and Pure Stuff brands) and store brand merchandise (e.g., Crate and Barrel, The Limited, Gap, Old Navy) are produced specifically for a retailer.

In some cases, manufacturers will sell their merchandise through their own stores as well as through other retailers. This distribution strategy is known as **dual distribution**. Many manufacturers, such as Tommy Hilfiger, Liz Claiborne, Ralph Lauren, Pendleton, and Nike, distribute merchandise through both their own brick-and-mortar stores and through other brick-and-mortar retailers. Thus, they are engaged in dual distribution.

A growing distribution strategy for companies is a **multichannel distribution** approach. In multichannel distribution, companies offer merchandise through varying retail venues: brick-and-mortar stores, catalogs, and/or websites. For example, J. Jill offers merchandise through brick-and-mortar stores, catalogs, and a website. Multichannel retailing is discussed more in Chapter 12.

Marketing Channel Flows

A **marketing channel** connects the companies within it in several streams, including ones for physical flow, ownership flow (or title flow), information flow, payment flow, and promotion flow. Each stream relates to specific functions that companies perform throughout the marketing channel.

- *Physical flow:* This is the tracking of merchandise from the manufacturer to the retailer or ultimate consumer. It includes warehousing (or storing), handling, and transporting merchandise so that it is available to consumers at the right time, at the right place, and in the right quantity.

- *Ownership flow* or *title flow:* This is the transfer of ownership or title from one company to the next. For example, does the retailer own the merchandise when it leaves the manufacturer's distribution center or when the retailer actually receives the merchandise? The point at which the title is transferred is negotiated between the manufacturer and retailer.

- *Information flow:* This is communication among companies within the marketing channel pipeline. Increased information flow between manufacturers and retailers has resulted from many supply chain management strategies.

- *Payment flow:* This is the transfer of monies among companies as payment for merchandise or services rendered. This includes both the methods used for payment and to whom payments are made.

- *Promotion flow:* This is the flow of communications designed to promote the merchandise either to other companies (trade promotions) or to consumers (consumer promotions) in order to influence sales.

Laws Affecting the Textile, Apparel, and Home Fashions Industries

This section briefly reviews a number of federal laws and international treaties that affect the textile, apparel, and home fashions industries. Obviously, not all of these laws will affect all companies, but it is important to note the variety of areas that are covered by federal laws and international treaties—everything from protecting personal property to protecting consumers to protecting fair trade. In addition to these federal laws, a number of state and municipal laws may apply to companies. Professionals in the industries must be aware of and abide by these laws, the details of which can be found in federal, state, and municipal government documents.

Laws Protecting Textile, Apparel, and Home Fashions Inventions and Designs

Many companies in the textile, apparel, and home fashions industries are involved in creating, inventing, or designing new processes and products. Laws related to patents, trademarks, and copyrights were established to protect such inventions and creations.

Laws protecting original garment designs vary from one country to another. Unlike designs created in European countries, in the United States, apparel designs, in and of themselves, are not protected. The United States has generally held a philosophy that laws protecting industrial design (including apparel) would impede design innovation. Inventions, textile print designs, and logos are protected under patent, trademark, and copyright laws, respectively; however, apparel designs are not protected by U.S. law. Some believe this lack of design protection in the United States inhibits apparel design innovation in the United States and has resulted in many U.S. designers working instead in Europe (Keyder, 1999). The laws in Europe do provide more design protection than do current U.S. laws. As noted by Virginia Brown Keyder (1999), an attorney who specializes in design law:

> European design law, though widely divergent in terms of detail at the national level, continues to afford stronger protection to the designer and is fast becoming harmonized across Europe. In addition, EU [European Union] design law is increasingly being used as a model of legal reform throughout the world.

An example of how a designer in France used French laws to protect his work occurred in 1994 when French designer Yves Saint Laurent took Ralph Lauren to court in a dispute over the copying of a tuxedo dress ("Tuxedo Junction," 1994).

PATENTS

According to the U.S. Patent and Trademark Office, a **patent** grants property rights to an inventor, which includes "the right to exclude others from making, using, offering for sale, or selling the invention in the United States or importing the invention into the United States." A patent allows the inventor or producer the exclusive right to use, make, or sell a product for a period of 20 years. From a legal perspective, products must be new inventions or technological advancements in product design. In the textile, apparel, and home fashions industries, patents can be acquired for technological advancements in textile processing, apparel production, or in products themselves.

For example, Nike acquired a patent (#5,396,675) for a "method of manufacturing a midsole for a shoe and construction therefore." Patents cannot be acquired for garment designs per se. If someone else uses a patented product or process, the owner of the patent has the right to sue the party for patent infringement. For example, in 2007, Reebok sued Nike for patent infringement. Reebok claimed that Nike's flexible sole athletic shoes infringed on Reebok's patent for "collapsible shoe" technology.

TRADEMARKS AND SERVICEMARKS

A **trademark** or **trade name** is a "word, phrase, symbol, or design, or a combination of words, phrases, symbols, or designs, that identifies and distinguishes the source of the goods of one party from those of others" (U.S. Patent and Trademark Office). **Servicemarks** are similar to trademarks but refer to identifications for services rather than for products. The Lanham Act (Federal Trademark Act) provides for federal registration and protection of trademarks. Although any company can claim rights to a trademark or servicemark by using the TM or SM designators, trademarks can be registered through the U.S. Patent and Trademark Office or through the Secretary of State in a state for products that are not in interstate commerce. Federal trademarks are effective for as long as they are used and registrations are updated. Once it has been registered, the ® symbol is used, and others cannot use the trademark without permission. If they do, they can be sued for trademark infringement. Trademark and patent searches are conducted by attorneys who specialize in ensuring that a trademark, trade name, patent, or business name is available for use.

Trademarks and trade names may not be generic terms such as *wonderful* or *exciting*, or, in the apparel industry, such generic terms as *trouser* or *dress*. In the early 1990s, Fruit of the Loom claimed to have ownership of the word *fruit* and sued another company for trademark infringement for using the word *fruit* as a trademark on apparel goods. Fruit of the Loom did not win the case. On the other hand, in 2006, Pendleton Woolen Mills filed a trademark infringement suit against Kmart Corporation for a line of flannel sheets sold at Kmart stores with packaging that indicated "Pendleton flannel sheet set" and featured an Indian trade blanket design similar to designs used by Pendleton Woolen Mills. Pendleton did not have a licensing agreement with Kmart or the company that manufactured the sheets and had not authorized the use of the Pendleton name. The lawsuit was resolved with Kmart pulling the sheets from their stores and donating them to charity. Kmart also recognized Pendleton's trademark rights by paying Pendleton an undisclosed amount of money.

In the textile, apparel, and home fashions industries, registered trademarks and trade names are widespread and include the following:

- trade names of manufactured fibers used for apparel and home fashions (e.g., Dacron® polyester, Lycra® spandex)

- trade names of natural fiber associations and companies (e.g., Cotton Incorporated's cotton symbol, Wool Company's Woolmark symbol)

- apparel and home fashions manufacturers' trade names (e.g., Levi's Dockers®, WestPoint Steven's Vellux®)

- trademarks of apparel and footwear manufacturers (e.g., Nike's swoosh, the stitching on the back pocket of Levi's jeans)

Well-known and well-respected trade names and trademarks take years to establish through concentrated efforts in designing goods that meet the needs of consumers, quality control, and advertising. Consumers become confident

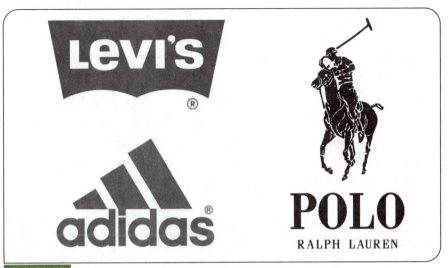

Figure 2.5 Tradenames and trademarks provide immediate consumer recognition and are protected against illegal copying.

that goods with a well-known trade name or trademark will meet certain standards in terms of quality and/or image. Thus, they desire these goods. Figure 2.5 shows some well-known trademarks and trade names.

Consumers' desire for apparel with well-known and visible trade names and trademarks has led to numerous **trademark infringements** and a proliferation of **counterfeit goods** (goods bearing unauthorized registered trade names or trademarks). Typically, counterfeit goods are of much lower quality than the authentic merchandise and are sold at a fraction of the genuine merchandise's price. Counterfeiters exploit consumer awareness and trust of a brand image by producing low-quality merchandise, and they do not pay royalties to the companies that may have spent millions creating that awareness and trust.

To establish trademark infringement in court, the plaintiff must prove the following:

1. Its trademark has achieved a secondary meaning (that is, the consumer associates the trademark with the company or product).

2. The trademark is nonfunctional (that is, the trademark is ornamental or does not contribute to the function of the product).

3. There is likelihood of confusion by the consumer for "famous" trademarks, or the trademark has been weakened by the association with the infringing product.

The International AntiCounterfeiting Coalition estimates that more than $600 billion worth of counterfeit goods are sold every year to knowing or unknowing consumers. A number of laws are in place to protect businesses against counterfeits:

- The Trademark Counterfeiting Act of 1984 created criminal sanctions against the domestic manufacture of counterfeit goods. Retailers who knowingly sell counterfeit goods can also be criminally liable

- The Anticounterfeiting Consumer Protection Act of 1996 allowed increased law enforcement by federal, state, and local law officials to seize counterfeit goods.

- The Stop Counterfeiting in Manufacturerd Goods Act of 2006 made shipment of falsified labels and packaging illegal and strengthened the penalties against counterfeiters.

Companies also discourage trademark infringement by doing the following:

- monitoring the production of their goods.

- using fabric codes and coded labels to distinguish authentic goods from imitations.

- working with the U.S. Customs and Border Protection to stop the flow of imported counterfeit goods into the United States. In 2008, over 80 percent (in dollar value) of the counterfeit goods seized by the U.S. Customs and Border Protection originated in China.

Trade dress is a subset of trademark law, only instead of protecting the identifying words or logos, the law of trade dress protects the overall look or image of a product itself or the packaging of a product, provided that the overall look or combination of features has come to identify the manufacturer of the product. Classic examples of trade dress are the distinctive shape of a Coca-Cola bottle and the turquoise packaging of merchandise purchased at Tiffany & Co.

Although it is more difficult to prove trade dress infringement than trademark infringement, and courts generally do not want to interfere with competition, trade dress infringement has been tested in the courts with mixed rulings. For example, Columbia Sportswear Company settled a trade dress infringement against the Orvis Company, which agreed to remove from its product line a pullover windbreaker that Columbia described as a "substantial copy" of Columbia's Gizzmo parka. In another example, jewelry manufacturer Denny Wong Designs won a trade dress lawsuit against Po Sun Hon jewelry company. Rulings indicated that Hon had illegally copied Wong's registered

Tropical Memories Plumeria flower jewelry. In this case, it was ruled that the consumer was confused by the copied merchandise.

COPYRIGHTS

Copyrights protect a number of written, pictorial, and performed works, including literature, music, films, television shows, artworks, dramatic works, and advertisements. Under the Copyright Act of 1976 (with periodic amendments through 2009), the copyright holder has the exclusive right to use, perform, or reproduce the material for life of the author plus 70 years, or if the work is of corporate authorship (e.g., Disney characters) for 95 years from publication or 120 years from creation, whichever expires first. All works published before 1923 are considered to be in the public domain. Under the *fair use* doctrine, works protected by copyright can be used on a limited basis for educational or research purposes. Reproduction of material protected by copyright without permission is considered infringement.

In the U.S. textile, apparel, and home fashions industries, although garment or product style is not protected by copyright, original textile prints and graphic designs are protected, even when incorporated into a garment or home fashions item. In order to be able to collect damages when a copyright is infringed, the copyright must be registered with the Copyright Office of the U.S. Library of Congress. A textile designer may also put a copyright notice (©) in the selvage of the fabric, although this notice is not necessary. A designer owns the copyright unless the designer is a salaried employee of a company; then the copyright is held by the employer. Any unauthorized reproduction of the textile print or design protected by copyright is considered copyright infringement, and once the copyright is registered, the copyright holder can take the infringer to court. Examples of copyright infringement in the textile industry include the following:

- dishonest textile converters who buy apparel or home fashions at retail in order to copy the textile print

- unscrupulous apparel or home fashions manufacturers that work with one converter to develop new prints, and then take the samples to another converter to have them reproduced more cheaply

- fraudulent retailers that copy textile prints for use in their private-label merchandise

U.S. copyrights are partially protected in the international market under the Berne Convention, an international treaty designed to help fight infringement across national borders.

Federal Laws Related to Business Practices and International Trade

Many federal laws relate to how a company must run its business, including requirements concerning fair competition, international trade, environmental practices, consumer protection, and employment practices.

FAIR COMPETITION

A number of federal laws have been established to assure fair competition. Table 2.5 reviews the primary laws that prohibit monopolies and unfair or deceptive practices in interstate commerce. Any textile and apparel company that distributes products or services across state lines is governed by these laws. These laws are all administered by the Federal Trade Commission (FTC).

INTERNATIONAL TRADE

Federal regulations and international treaties also exist concerning the international trade of products, including textiles, apparel, and home fashions (see Table 2.6). The primary objective of these laws and treaties is to establish fair

Table 2.5 Federal Laws Related to Competition

- Sherman Antitrust Act (1890): outlawed monopolies and attempts to form monopolies.
- Clayton Act (1914): amended the Sherman Antitrust Act by
  - forbidding a seller from discriminating in price between and among different purchases of the same commodity
  - outlawing exclusive dealing and tie-in arrangements
  - forbidding corporate asset or stock mergers where the effect may be to create a monopoly
  - forbidding persons from serving on boards of directors of competing corporations
- Federal Trade Commission Act (1914): declared unlawful unfair methods of competition in or affecting commerce and unfair or deceptive acts or practices in interstate commerce. The FTC's Bureau of Competition investigates potential law violations and serves as a resource for policy makers regarding competition (http://www.ftc.gov).
- Robinson-Patman Act (1936): amended the Clayton Act by preventing large firms from exerting excessive economic power to drive out small competitors in local markets.
- Cellar-Kefauver Act (1950): made it illegal to create a monopoly by eliminating competition through company mergers and acquisitions.
- Wheeler-Lea Act (1938): amended the Federal Trade Commission Act by allowing the FTC to stop unfair competition, even if a competitor is not shown to be harmed by a business practice when a consumer is injured by deceptive acts or practices.

Table 2.6 Laws, Agreements, and Organizations Related to International Trade Practices

- General Agreement on Tariffs and Trade (GATT, 1947): a multinational agreement regarding global trade policies. In international trade of textiles and apparel, GATT allowed for the use of tariffs (taxes on imports) to protect domestic industries and for quantitative limits (quotas) on certain textile and apparel merchandise entering the United States from specified countries during a specified period of time.
- Multifiber Arrangement (MFA I: 1947–1977, MFA II: 1977–1981, MFA III: 1981–1986, MFA IV: 1986–1991, extensions to MFA IV: 1991, 1992, 1993): a general framework for international textile trade that operated under the authority of GATT and allowed for the establishment of bilateral agreements between trading partners. The MFA was phased out in 2005 when international trade for textile, apparel, and home fashions industries came under the jurisdiction of the World Trade Organization.
- World Trade Organization (WTO, 1995): the World Trade Organization (WTO) Agreement on Textiles and Clothing (ATC) provided for the reduction and phasing out of quotas on textiles and apparel imported from WTO member countries in three stages between 1995 and 2005. The ATC was approved as part of the Uruguay Round Agreements Act by the U.S. Congress in December 1994 and went into effect on January 1, 1995. In 2011, the WTO had 153 member countries. Most quotas had been phased out for member countries.
- U.S. Free Trade Agreements and implementation dates:
  - Australia (2005)
  - Bahrain (2006)
  - Central America–Dominican Republic–United States Free Trade Agreement (CAFTA-DR, 2005): Costa Rica, El Salvador, Guatemala, Honduras, Nicaragua, the Dominican Republic, and the United States
  - Chile (2004)
  - Israel (1985)
  - Jordan (2001)
  - Morocco (2006)
  - North American Free Trade Agreement (NAFTA, 1994)United States, Canada, and Mexico:
  - Oman (1985)
  - Peru (2009)
  - Singapore (2004)
- U.S. Trade Preference Programs
  - African Growth and Opportunity Act (AGOA)
  - Andean Trade Promotion and Drug Eradication Act (ATPDEA)
  - Caribbean Basin Trade Partnership Act (CBTPA)
  - Haitian Hemispheric Opportunity Through Partnership for Encouragement Act (HOPE Act)

trade among countries. Because of shifts in international relations, these laws and treaties are reviewed and amended regularly. Any textile, apparel, or home fashions company that imports goods into or exports goods from the United States is affected by these laws and treaties. In the United States, trade policy is set by the executive branch of the government and carried out by the U.S. Trade Representative. The implementation and administration of trade laws are conducted by several departments, including the following:

- The Export Trade Act is administered by the Federal Trade Commission.

- The Department of Commerce oversees the Committee for the Implementation of Textile Agreements (CITA) and the Office of Textiles (OTEXA).

- The U.S. Customs and Border Protection oversees the physical control of imports and the collection of tariffs (taxes on imports), and prevents counterfeit goods from entering the country.

ENVIRONMENTAL PRACTICES

Federal environmental laws regulate business practices related to environmental pollution. The goal of these laws is to protect the environment from toxic pollutants. In the fashion industries, these laws particularly affect chemical companies that manufacture fibers. These companies' processes often produce or require the use of toxic substances, and their factories may emit toxic substances considered pollutants. Table 2.7 lists the primary environmental laws, which are administered by the Environmental Protection Agency (EPA).

Table 2.7   Federal Laws Related to Practices to Protect the Environment

- National Environmental Policy Act of 1969: established the national charter for the protection of the environment
- Clean Air Act (1970): controls air pollution through air quality standards to protect public health
- Endangered Species Act (1973): provides for the conservation of threatened or endangered plants and animals and the habitats in which they are found
- Resource Conservation and Recovery Act of 1976: controls the management of solid waste products and encourages resource conservation and recovery
- Toxic Substances Control Act (1976): allows regulation of the manufacturing, use, and disposal of toxic substances
- Clean Water Act (1977): controls water pollution by keeping pollutants out of lakes, rivers, and streams
- Pollution Prevention Act (1990): focused on reducing pollution through cost-effective changes in production, operations, and use of raw materials

CONSUMER PROTECTION

Beginning in the 1930s and 1940s, a number of laws were enacted to protect the health and safety of consumers (see Table 2.8). Over the years since then, many additional protections have been added. These laws require companies to label truthfully the fiber content and care procedures of products and prohibit companies from selling flammable products. They are administered by either the Federal Trade Commission or the Consumer Product Safety Commission.

EMPLOYMENT PRACTICES

To assure fair hiring and employment practices among companies, a number of laws have been enacted to regulate child labor and homework (piecework contracted to individuals who do the work in their homes) and to prohibit discrimination based on such characteristics as race, sex, age, or physical disability. Any company with employees is regulated by these laws (see Table 2.9).

Table 2.8   Federal Laws Associated with Practices for Consumer Protection

- Wool Products Labeling Act (1939), Fur Products Labeling Act (1952), the Textile Fiber Products Identification Act (1958, effective 1960, last amended 2006): require specified information to be on textile and fur product labels; require the advertising of country of origin in mail-order catalogs and promotional materials. Administered by the FTC.
- Enforcement Policy Statement on U.S. Origins Claims (1997): provides guidelines for labeling products as *Made in the U.S.* to be "all or virtually all" made in the United States.
- Flammable Fabrics Act (1953, last amended 1990): regulates the manufacturing of wearing apparel and fabrics (including carpets, rugs, and mattresses) that are so highly flammable as to be dangerous when worn. Sets standards of flammability and test methods. Sets standards for flammability of children's sleepwear. Originally administered by the FTC; administration transferred to the CPSC in 1972.
- Consumer Products Safety Act (1972): established the Consumer Products Safety Commission (CPSC) to reduce or eliminate risk of injury associated with selected consumer products.
- Care Labeling of Textile Wearing Apparel and Certain Piece Goods Act (1971, last amended 2000): requires that care labels be affixed to most apparel and be attached to retail piece goods. Administered by the FTC.
- Federal Hazardous Substance Act (1960; last amended 1995): addresses issue of choking, ingestion, aspiration of small items by children, and hazards from sharp points and edges on articles intended for use by children by requiring that decorative buttons or other decorative items on children's clothing pass use and abuse testing procedures. Prohibits the use of lead paint on children's articles, including clothing. Administered by the CPSC.

| Table 2.9 | Federal Laws Related to Employment Practices |

- Fair Labor Standards Act of 1938 (last amended 2004): guarantees fair employment status by establishing minimum wage standards, child labor restrictions, and other employment regulations.
- Equal Pay Act of 1963: amends the Fair Labor Standards Act by requiring employers to provide equal pay to men and women for doing equal work.
- Age Discrimination in Employment Act (1967): prohibits an employer from discriminating in hiring or other aspects of employment because of age. Administered by the Equal Employment Opportunity Commission (EEOC).
- Occupational Safety and Health Act of 1970 (last amended 2004): created the Occupational Safety and Health Administration (OSHA); assures safe and healthful working conditions for employees by setting general occupational safety and health standards, and requiring that employers prepare and maintain records of occupational injuries and illnesses. Administered by the Department of Labor/OSHA.
- Equal Employment Opportunity Act of 1972: prohibits discrimination by employers in hiring, promotions, discharge, and conditions of employment if such discrimination is based on race, color, religion, sex, or national origin.
- Americans with Disabilities Act (ADA) of 1990: prohibits discrimination against qualified individuals with disabilities in all aspects of employment; prohibits discrimination on the basis of disability by requiring that public accommodations and commercial facilities be designed, constructed, and altered in compliance with accessibility standards. Administered by the Office of the ADA, Department of Justice.
- Family and Medical Leave Act of 1993: grants eligible employees up to a total of 12 work weeks of unpaid leave for one or more family and medical reasons (e.g., birth of a child, care of an immediate family member).
- Immigration and Nationality Act (last amended 2000): establishes conditions for temporary employment in the United States by non-U.S. citizens.
- Trade Adjustment Assistance Reform Act of 2002 (last amended 2006): reauthorized the Trade Adjustment Assistance Program (first established in 1974), which provides aid to workers whose employment is negatively affected by increased imports.

Summary

Depending on the objectives, needs, and size of textile, apparel, and home fashions companies, they are owned as sole proprietorships, partnerships, or corporations. The advantages and disadvantages of each form of business ownership are related to the ease of formation and dissolution (advantage of sole proprietorship and partnership and disadvantage of corporations), the degree of liability that owners have for business debts (advantage of corporations and disadvantage for sole proprietorship and partnerships), and operational strategies (some advantages and disadvantages for each form of ownership).

Each company—whether a sole proprietorship, partnership, or corporation—competes with other companies on the basis of price, quality, innovation, service, or a combination of these factors. Within the textile, apparel, and home fashions industries, the competitive strategies include monopolies, oligopolies (e.g., athletic shoe industry), oligopsonies, pure competition (e.g., textile commodities), and monopolistic competition, the most common of the five. In monopolistic competition, although companies compete in terms of product type (denim jeans), the specific product attributes of any one company (7 for All Mankind jeans) are perceived as different from the product attributes of other companies (Guess? jeans, Calvin Klein jeans).

Companies create this perceived difference through product differentiation, advertising, licensing programs, private-label merchandise, or services offered. In licensing programs, the owner (licensor) of a particular name, image, or design (property) sells the right to use the name, image, or design to another party, typically a manufacturer (licensee), for payment of royalties. For example, Hartmarx pays Tommy Hilfiger royalties for the use of the Tommy Hilfiger name on a line of men's tailored clothing. Tommy Hilfiger controls the design, distribution, and presentation of the products; Hartmarx controls the production. A licensing contract outlines the terms of the licensing agreement. Licensing programs can be advantageous to both licensors and licensees in terms of expanding product lines and exposure. Possible disadvantages include market saturation and problems in timing of the release of the product.

To get merchandise to the consumer, direct, limited, and extended marketing channels are used by businesses that perform manufacturing, wholesaling, and retailing functions. In conventional marketing channels, separate companies perform these functions; in vertical marketing channels, a single company performs multiple functions.

A number of federal laws affect businesses in the textile, apparel, and home fashions industries. Laws related to patents, trademarks, and copyrights protect the identity, inventions, and designs of designers and companies. For example, a textile designer's fabric design is protected by the copyright law so that others cannot legally copy it. Laws have also been established that relate to how companies must run their businesses, including requirements regarding competition, international trade, protecting consumers, protecting the environment, and employment practices.

CAREER PROFILES

Individuals who have careers in the apparel, accessories, and home fashions industries may be part of companies that are sole proprietorships, partnerships, or corporations.

Owner, Sole Proprietor
Women's Specialty Store

Position Description:
Responsible for all of the purchasing (buying), advertising, supervising of personnel, special events (in-store and community), in-store selling, and visual merchandising.

Typical Tasks and Responsibilities:

- Write orders for merchandise.
- Handle special orders.
- Organize and implement store promotions.
- Determine pricing policies.
- Determine policies regarding merchandise returns.
- Handle in-store customer service.
- Oversee ongoing merchandising of the store to create a "fresh" look.
- Hire, train, schedule, and motivate sales associates.

Corporate Executive Officer, Chairman of the Board
Privately Owned Children's Apparel Manufacturer and Retailer

Position Description:
Ultimately responsible for everything from financial decisions to store maintenance. Conceive and create all new products sold wholesale by the company. Run the retail stores. Work with all management personnel, including those who report directly to the chairman, along with the 300 company employees. Motivate and supervise employees at all levels. Sell all products to customers at wholesale and retail.

Typical Tasks and Responsibilities:

- Set the vision of the organization.
- Model the values of the company with regard to professionalism, integrity, and community involvement.
- Apply knowledge of the latest trends and ideas in the market to the design and sale of new products.
- Oversee the overall management of the organization.
- Make sure everyone remembers that the customer is always right.

Key Terms

articles of incorporation
articles of partnership
board of directors
brand extension
C corporation
capital
close corporation
closely held corporation
conglomerate
consolidation
conventional marketing channel
copyright
corporation
counterfeit goods
direct marketing channel
dividend
double taxation
dual distribution
entrepreneur
extended marketing channel
general partner
information flow

initial public offering (IPO)
licensing
limited liability
Limited Liability Company (LLC)
limited marketing channel
limited partnership
marketing channel
marketing channel integration
merger
monopolistic competition
monopoly
multichannel distribution
multinational corporation
oligopoly
oligopsony
ownership flow
partnership
patent
payment flow
perfect competition
physical flow
private corporation

Key Terms *(continued)*

private-label brand	store brand
privately held corporation	takeover
promotion flow	title flow
publicly held corporation	trade dress
publicly traded corporation	trademark
pure competition	trade name
regular corporation	trademark infringement
S corporation	unlimited liability
servicemark	vertical marketing channel
sole proprietorship	vertical integration
stockholder	

Discussion Questions and Activities

1. Interview a small-business owner in your community. Find out whether the business is a sole proprietorship, partnership, LLC, or corporation. Ask the owner why this form of business ownership was chosen and what he or she views as the primary advantages and disadvantages to the ownership form. Find out what business licenses were required of the owner to start the company. Compare this information with information others in class receive.

2. Suppose you wanted to invest (buy stock) in a publicly traded corporation. Where can you find information about the corporation? Select a publicly traded corporation in the textile, apparel, and home fashions industries, and find information about the company.

3. What are some examples of licensed textile, apparel, and home fashions products that you own? Which category of licensed goods does each fall into? What characteristic of the property or product was appealing to you as a consumer? Why?

4. Currently, textile designs and prints are protected by copyright from illegal copying, but apparel designs (designs of the garment itself) are not protected in the United States. Do you think that apparel designs should also be covered under copyright law? Why or why not? Justify your response.

References

American Apparel Manufacturers Association. (1992). *Federal Standards and Regulations for the Apparel Industry*. Arlington, VA: Author.

Bosworth, Mike. (1999, April). Gavels pound on knockoff vendors. *Apparel Industry Magazine*, pp. 86–90.

Committee for the Implementation of Textile Agreements, U.S. Department of Commerce. (2010). Retrieved July 14, 2010, from http://otexa.ita.doc.gov/cita.htm

Entrepreneur.com (2010). Definition of Entrepreneur. Retrieved June 27, 2010, from http://www.entrepreneur.com/encyclopedia/term/159078.html

Fisher, Bruce D., and Jennings, Marianne M. (1991). *Law for Business* (2nd ed.). St. Paul, MN: West Publishing Co.

Gerber, David A. (1984, September 14). Protecting apparel designs: Tough, but there are ways. *California Apparel News*, p. 24.

Hirtle, Peter B. (2010, January 4). Copyright Term and Public Domain in the United States. [online]. Available: http://copyright.cornell.edu/resources/publicdomain.cfm [July 14, 2010].

Hughes, John. (1991, January 4–10). Getting it in writing. *California Apparel News*, pp. 16–17.

International AntiCounterfeiting Coalition (2010). About Counterfeiting. Retrieved July 14, 2010, from http://www.iacc.org/

Keyder, Virginia Brown. (November 12, 1999). *Design Law in Europe and the U.S.* Presentation at the Annual Meeting of the International Textile and Apparel Association, Santa Fe, NM.

Office of Textiles and Apparel, U.S. Department of Commerce. (2010). Trade Agreements. Retrieved July 14, 2010, from http://otexa.ita.doc.gov/

Tuxedo Junction: YSL, Ralph square off. (1994, April 28). *Women's Wear Daily*, pp. 1, 15.

U.S. Department of Labor (2010-11). Bureau of Labor Statistics, Occupational Outlook Handbook. Retrived June 27, 2010, from http://www.bls.gov/oco/home.htm

U.S. Patent and Trademark Office (2010). U.S. Department of Commerce. Retrieved June 27, 2010, from http://www.uspto.gov/

World Trade Organization (2010). WTO Structure. Retrieved July 14, 2010, from http://www.wto.org/

CHAPTER 3

Structure of the U.S. Textile Industry

In this chapter, you will learn the following:

- the importance of textile knowledge for the successful design, production, and marketing of apparel and home fashions

- terms used in describing textiles and textile manufacturing

- the organization and operation of the textile industry

- procedures followed in the processing and marketing of natural and manufactured fibers, yarns, and fabrics

- current developments in the textile industry, including international trade, supply chain management strategies, and responses to environmental issues

onsider the following scenarios: an apparel designer is starting a new line of apparel, but before she begins, she examines the newest fabrics shown by textile companies in their showrooms; or, a buyer for a home fashions retailer decides to attend a textile trade show in order to become familiar with the newest trends in colors and fabrics. These scenarios highlight the integrated nature of the textile, apparel, home fashions, and retailing industries. As textiles are the foundation of the soft-goods industries, an understanding of the organization and operation of the textile industry is important for all professionals. Therefore, this chapter describes such organization and operation as well as the marketing of fibers and fabrics. It also gives an overview of new developments in the field.

What Are Textiles?

Before we review the organization and operation of the U.S. textile industry, let us first reexamine the basic terminology used to describe textiles. This terminology forms the basis for an understanding of the fabrics used in apparel and home fashions. First, what are **textiles**? The term *textile* is used to describe any product made from fibers. There are four basic components of textile production:

- fiber processing
- yarn spinning
- fabric production or fabrication
- fabric finishing

Fibers comprise the basic unit used in making textile yarns and fabrics. Fibers are classified into **generic families** according to their chemical composition and can be divided into two primary divisions:

- natural fibers
- manufactured (man-made) fibers

Natural fibers include those made from natural protein fibers of animal origin (e.g., wool, cashmere, camel, mohair, angora, and silk) and natural cellulose fibers of plant origin (e.g., cotton, flax, jute, bamboo, and sisal). Leather and fur are considered natural-fiber products created from the **pelts**, **skins**, and **hides** of various animals. Leather and fur are unique textiles in that the fibers are not spun into yarns and then constructed into fabrics. Instead, the pelts are tanned to create supple and durable "fabrics."

Whereas natural fibers have been used in making textiles for thousands of years, manufactured fibers have been around for about 120 years. In the mid-1800s, scientists became interested in duplicating natural fibers.

- In 1891, "artificial silk," made from a solution of cellulose, was commercially produced in France.
- In 1924, the name of this fiber was changed to rayon.
- In 1939, nylon, the first fiber to be synthesized entirely from chemicals (synthetic), was introduced by E. I. du Pont de Nemours and Company.

Since then, many more manufactured fibers have been developed, including the following:

- cellulose-based fibers (e.g., lyocell, acetate)
- synthetic fibers (e.g., acrylic, aramid, modacrylic, olefin, polyester, and spandex)
- mineral-based fibers (e.g., glass, gold)

Until the 1930s, fiber production in the United States focused entirely on natural fibers. By the end of the 1940s, natural-fiber production accounted for 85 percent of the nation's textile mill fiber consumption, and manufactured-fiber production accounted for only 15 percent. By 1965, manufactured fibers accounted for more than 42 percent of total fiber consumption by U.S. textile mills. Today, manufactured fibers account for approximately 75 percent of total fiber consumption and 25 percent is accounted for by natural fibers.

Yarns refer to the collection of fibers or filaments laid or twisted together to form a continuous strand strong enough for use in fabrics. Yarns are classified as **spun yarns** made from shorter staple fibers, or **filament yarns** made from long continuous fibers. Filament yarns can be either plain or textured. The type of yarn selected will affect the performance, tactile qualities, and appearance of the fabric.

Fabric construction or **fabrication** processes include the following methods used to make fabrics:

- from solutions (e.g., films, foam)
- directly from fibers (e.g., felt, nonwoven fabrics)
- from yarns (e.g., braid, knitted fabrics, woven fabrics, and lace)

The fabric construction process used often determines the name of the fabric (e.g., satin, jersey, lace, felt). It should be noted that the fiber name is not interchangeable with the fabric name.

Dyeing and finishing the fabric complete the textile production process. **Finishing** refers to "any process that is done to fiber, yarn, or fabric either before or after fabrication to change the *appearance* (what is seen), the *hand* (what is felt), or the *performance* (what the fabric does)" (Kadolph & Langford, 2002, p. 270). **Greige goods** (also referred to as *grey*, *gray*, or *loom state goods*) are fabrics that have not received finishing treatments, such as bleaching, shearing, brushing, embossing, or dyeing. Once finished, the fabrics are then referred to as **converted goods**, or **finished goods**. Finishes can be classified in the following ways:

- *general* or *functional*
- *mechanical* or *chemical*
- *durable* (permanent) or *renewable* (impermanent)

Both greige goods and finished fabrics are used in a variety of end uses: apparel, home fashions, other sewn products such as sleeping bags and flags, and industrial uses such as liners for highways and hoses.

Organization of the Textile Industry

Overview of the Industry

The textile industry is one of the oldest manufacturing industries in the United States. With its beginnings during the Industrial Revolution, the textile industry has been an important part of the U.S. manufacturing base for over 200 years.

Over the past 20 years, the U.S. textile industry has seen a dramatic decline. This decline can be attributed to the following factors:

- increase in the technologies and capabilities of textile industries worldwide
- the loss of trade protection from less expensive imports (particularly those being imported from Asian countries) that came with the phase-out of quotas by WTO members
- the growth of vertical integration by retailers (e.g., Walmart, Target, JCPenney) and their decision to purchase fabrics closer to where the apparel or home fashions are being produced

Some segments of the textile mill products sector, like industrial fabrics, carpets, and specialty yarns, are highly automated, innovative, and competitive on a global scale, so they will be able to expand exports. According to the U.S. Department of Commerce, the one area of the U.S. textile industry that has seen growth over the past few years is the carpet and rug industry. Corporations producing carpets in the United States include Milliken Carpet, The Dixie Group, and Mohawk Industries, Inc. Chapter 14 discusses home fashions in greater detail.

Structure of the Industry

Companies within the textile industry take part in one or more of the four basic components of textile production: fiber processing, yarn spinning, fabric production, and fabric finishing. The structure of the textile industry is illustrated in Figure 3.1. Some companies specialize in certain aspects of textile production, as shown in the following examples:

- **Throwsters** modify filament yarns for specific end uses, such as increasing luster or texture through altering the yarn.
- **Textile mills** concentrate on the fabric construction stage of production (e.g., weaving, knitting, nonwoven fabric, lace).
- Companies that specialize in finishing fabrics are called **textile converters**.
- Finished fabrics are sold to apparel and home fashions manufacturers, retailers that sell fabrics, or jobbers that sell surplus goods.
- Retailers that sell private-label merchandise may also work directly with converters and/or textile mills.

Within the textile industry are a number of large corporations that operate through a vertically integrated marketing channel. Each corporation handles all four steps—from processing the fiber to finishing the fabric—within its own organization. Some vertically integrated companies are also involved in the production of end-use products, such as towels, sheets, or hosiery. Vertically integrated companies include companies that produce textile products made from both natural and manufactured fibers. Although vertically integrated companies may process fibers, they might not actually produce their own fibers. For example, a vertically integrated company that produces cotton knit fabrics might not be involved in growing the cotton. Instead, raw cotton might be purchased from cotton growers. Some companies are partially integrated, in that they focus on several steps of production. For example, some knitting operations (e.g., hosiery, sweaters) not only knit, dye, and cut the fabrics, but they also construct the knitted garments to be sold to retailers.

One of the oldest vertically integrated textile companies in the United States is Pendleton Woolen Mills, headquartered in Portland, Oregon. Pendleton was

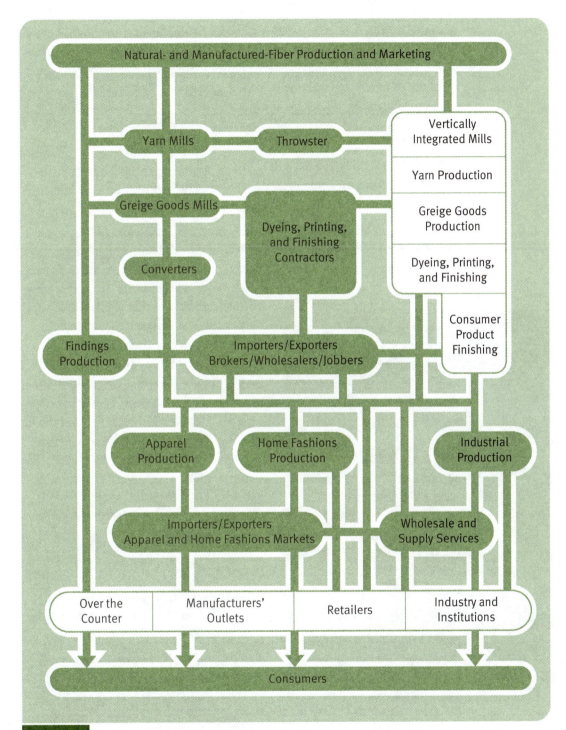

Figure 3.1 This flowchart depicts the structure of the textile industry.

started by Clarence and Roy Bishop in Pendleton, Oregon, in 1909. Led by a fourth generation of Bishops, the company now manufactures woolen menswear, women's wear, and blankets; nonwoolen apparel; and over-the-counter fabrics. It is involved with the following:

- the selection and processing of wool
- the designing and weaving of fabrics
- the development of garments
- the shipment and sale of garments, over-the-counter piece goods, and blankets

Such vertical integration allows for coordination among all production steps and increased control of quality throughout the production of the textiles and end-use products. For example, Pendleton textile designers work closely with the apparel designers in engineering the plaid fabrics that will work best for pleated skirt designs.

A number of trade publications cater to the textile industry by providing timely information about trends in the industry, new products, company success stories, and technological advancements. Table 3.1 lists selected trade publications in the textile industry.

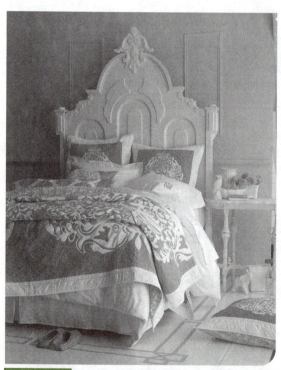

Figure 3.2 Textiles are used for a variety of end-use products, including apparel, hosiery, and home fashions.

End Uses of Textiles

Although apparel and home fashions are the primary end uses for textiles, it is important to note the variety of other goods made from natural and manufactured fibers. End uses for U.S. textiles vary widely (see Figure 3.2), as shown in the following estimates:

- Thirty-six percent of the total pounds of textiles produced in the United States goes into fabrics for men's,

Table 3.1	Selected Trade Publications in the Textile Industry

EmergingTextiles.com (www.emergingtextiles.com): online statistical reports on textiles and apparel trade including prices, country reports, and tariff and quota updates

Fiber Economics Bureau Publications (www.fibersource.com):

- ***Fiber Organon*** (www.fibersource.com): published monthly; statistical journal summarizing producer information on the natural and manufactured-fiber markets including monthly production and shipments, quarterly trends and analyses, and trade information

- ***Manufactured Fiber Handbook*** (www.fibersource.com): the official data source on the U.S. manufactured-fiber industry

- ***Manufactured Fiber Review*** (www.fibersource.com): monthly newsletter review of the latest U.S. data on manufactured fibers

Nonwovens Industry (www.nonwovens-industry.com): published monthly; for manufacturers, converters, distributors, and suppliers of nonwoven soft goods; covers manufacturing processes, distribution, and end-use applications of nonwoven textile products

Southern Textile News (www.textilenews.com): published bi-weekly; offers textile news, including trade matters; new advancements in textile equipment; developments in yarn, thread, knits, wovens, nonwovens, cotton, dyeing and finishing, and apparel; updates on mill news

Textile World (www.textileworld.com): published monthly; for textile executives in their dual role as technologists and managers; leading resource for textile news and information; covers technical developments in the textile industry

Women's Wear Daily (WWD) (www.wwd.com): published daily, Monday through Friday (except holidays); covers all aspects of the business of fashion and beauty including textile, apparel, and home fashions designers, manufacturers, marketers, and retailers

women's, and children's apparel and hosiery; over-the-counter retail piece goods; and craft fabric.

- Twenty-five percent goes into floor coverings, such as carpets, rugs, and paddings.

- Twenty-three percent goes into industrial and other products, such as tires, ropes and cordage, tents, belting, bags, shoes and slippers, and medical and surgical supplies.

- Sixteen percent goes into home fashions products, such as drapery and upholstery fabrics; sheets, pillowcases, and mattresses; blankets; bedspreads; tablecloths; and towels.

Fiber Processing and Yarn Spinning

The development and marketing of natural versus manufactured fibers vary greatly. In general, natural fibers, as part of the larger agricultural industry, are the product of a crop that is grown and harvested or of an animal that is raised. Manufactured fibers, on the other hand, are created by large nonagricultural corporations through research and development efforts.

Natural-Fiber Processing

Of the natural fibers produced in the United States, cotton has the largest production and wool the second largest production. Worldwide, China, the United States, India, and Pakistan are the four largest producers of cotton, accounting for approximately two-thirds of the production.

Cotton is obtained from the fibers surrounding the seeds of the cotton plant. The plant is grown most satisfactorily in warm climates where irrigation water is available. Cotton is grown in 17 states, with the combined production of Texas (the leading cotton-producing state), Arkansas, Mississippi, Georgia, California, North Carolina, Tennessee, and Louisiana accounting for 85 percent of U.S. production (National Cotton Council of America, 2010). According to the National Cotton Council of America, 64 percent of cotton produced in the United States each year goes into apparel, 28 percent is used for home furnishings, and 8 percent is used for industrial products.

In conventionally grown cotton, synthetic fertilizers, insecticides, herbicides, fungicides, and defoliants are used. The significant amounts of chemical pesticides and fertilizers—as well as water—used in production have led to criticism of the industry. Organic cotton has emerged as an environmentally responsible approach to growing cotton. Rather than using synthetic chemical fertilizers and pesticides, the following organic techniques are used:

- Natural fertilizers, such as manure, are used. These fertilizers biodegrade.
- Fields are weeded by hand, or cover crops are planted to control weeds.
- Crops are rotated for disease control.
- Beneficial insects that consume destructive insects are introduced.
- Once harvested, certified organic cotton is stored without the use of chemical rodenticides and fungicides.

According to the Organic Trade Association (2010), organic cotton was grown in 22 countries worldwide with the top ten producer countries led by India and including (in order of rank) Turkey, Syria, Tanzania, China, United States, Uganda, Peru, Egypt, and Burkina Faso. Although production of organic cotton represents only .76 percent of total worldwide cotton production, this is an increase over the .03 percent of 2005.

As a result of consumer interest, many apparel and home fashions producers and retailers (e.g., Nike, Patagonia) have organic cotton programs, thus increasing the demand for certified organic cotton. The United States Department of Agriculture (USDA) sets standards and certifies cotton (and other organic agricultural products). The USDA Organic Certification is used in advertising end-use products to the consumer. In 1994, Mission Valley Textiles was the first woven apparel and home furnishings fabrics mill in the United States to receive the government's organic fiber processing certification (Rudie, 1994). Since then, numerous companies have adopted organic cotton programs. Organic cotton and naturally colored cotton programs are discussed later in this chapter.

In traditional cotton production, after the cotton is picked, a cotton gin is used to separate the fiber, called "cotton lint," from the seeds. (The seeds, a valuable by-product of the cotton industry, are used to produce cattle feed and cottonseed oil.) The cotton lint is then packed into large bales and shipped to yarn and textile mills. The spinning process of cotton yarns is highly automated; cotton fibers are cleaned, carded, combed, and drawn and spun to create yarns. For blended yarns, other fibers, such as polyester, nylon, or wool, are blended with the cotton during the spinning process. Figure 3.3 shows a cotton processing plant.

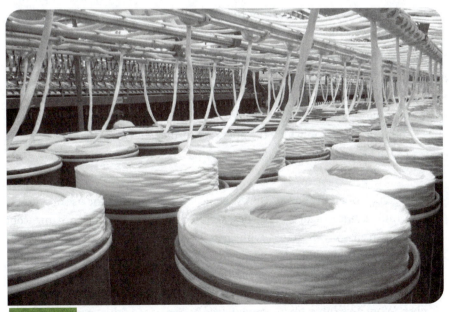

Figure 3.3   Cotton yarn production includes multiple steps, from carding and combing cotton fibers to drawing and spinning yarns.

Wool fibers are derived from the fleece of sheep, goats, alpacas, and llamas. Worldwide, the largest producers of wool are Australia, New Zealand, and the United Kingdom. China and Italy are the world's largest wool buyers. Although wool production occurs in every state and has a long history in the United States, currently it plays a minor role in U.S. textile production.

Most wool comes from a number of specific breeds of sheep, including Delaine-Merino, Rambouillet, Hampshire, and Suffolk. Some breeds of sheep can graze in areas of the country with extreme climates that are unsuitable for other livestock. Farm flock production (animals raised in a more confined area) is best suited for other breeds of sheep. Because wool growers often produce small amounts of wool, the use of wool co-ops or pools and warehousing operations is common.

The steps in wool processing are as follows:

1. The first step is shearing the sheep. Shearing usually takes place once a year in the spring, just before lambing. Using electric clippers, a skilled shearer can remove the fleece from a sheep in five minutes. Some shearers can shear more than 100 sheep per day. A chemical shearing process is also used on a limited basis.

2. Bags of wool fleece are inspected, graded, and sorted according to the diameter and length of the wool fibers.

3. Fibers are scoured to remove grease (unrefined lanolin) and impurities. The lanolin is separated from the wash water, purified, and used in soaps, creams, cosmetics, and other products.

4. Clean wool fibers from different batches are blended to achieve uniform color and quality.

5. Fibers are carded, a process that straightens the fibers and removes any remaining vegetable matter. Wool to be used in worsted fabrics undergoes a combing process in which the fibers are further straightened.

6. The fibers are drawn and spun into yarns.

Organic wool is produced using organic feed and without the use of synthetic hormones, insecticides, pesticides, and feed additives. In 2010, organic wool was grown in six U.S. states, with over 80 percent of certified organic wool grown in the United States coming from New Mexico, followed by Montana and Maine (Organic Trade Association, 2010).

Wool fabrics are often processed by the same company that processes the fiber. Wool, like other fibers, can be dyed at one of the following stages in the production process:

- immediately after it is washed and blended (stock dyed or vat dyed)
- after it has been spun into yarns (yarn dyed)
- after it has been woven or knitted into fabric (piece dyed)

Wool absorbs many different dyes uniformly. Some wool producers market wools that, rather than being dyed, are sorted and sold in natural sheep colors, ranging from cream to a broad spectrum of browns, blacks, and grays.

Mohair comes from the wool of the Angora goat. In the United States, mohair production has steadily decreased over the past 20 years, with production found primarily in Texas, Arizona, and New Mexico. Almost all of the raw mohair fiber produced in the United States is exported for processing, primarily to China. This is because most U.S. textile mills have equipment designed to process cotton and wool—which are much larger industries in the United States than is mohair. Cotton and wool fibers measure two inches or less, whereas mohair fibers are often four to six inches long. Therefore, machinery designed to process cotton and wool cannot be used for mohair. Worldwide production has also declined as other luxury fibers have gained favor.

Cashmere comes from the undercoat wool of the Cashmere or Kashmir goat. Most of the world's cashmere comes from China, Mongolia, and Tibet. China, Italy, and the United Kingdom are the world's largest buyers of cashmere. Cashmere is considered a luxury fiber because of its cost and is often blended with other, less-expensive wools. However, demand for cashmere has grown in recent years as high-end designers (e.g., Burberry, Gucci, Armani) have included cashmere products in their collections and consumer desire for the soft fibers has increased.

Leather Production

Leather is obtained from the skins and hides of cattle, goats, and sheep, as well as from a variety of reptiles, fish, and birds. Most skins and hides are by-products of animals raised primarily for their meat or fiber. Thus, the leather industry is a bridge between the meat industry from which the hide is a by-product and the manufacture of basic raw material into nondurable goods, such as shoes and wearing apparel. Pelts are categorized according to the following weights:

- The term **skins** refers to pelts weighing 15 pounds or less when shipped to the tannery.
- The term **kips** refers to pelts weighing from 15 to 25 pounds.
- The term **hides** refers to pelts weighing more than 25 pounds.

Animal pelts go through a number of processes that transform them into leather. They are first cleaned to remove hair. Then, they are tanned, colored or dyed, and finished (e.g., glazed, embossed, napped, or buffed).

Tanning is the process used to make skins and hides pliable and water resistant. The tanning process can use a number of agents, including vegetable materials, oils, chemicals, and minerals, or a combination of more than one type of agent. With vegetable tanning, natural tannic acids found in extracts from tree bark are used. Because vegetable tanning is extremely slow and labor intensive, it is seldom used in commercial tanning. Oil tanning uses fish oil (usually codfish) as a tanning agent. Oil tanning is used to make chamois, doeskin, and buckskin. One of the quickest tanning methods is through the use of chemicals, typically formaldehyde.

Two tanning methods use minerals—alum tanning and chrome tanning. Alum tanning is rarely used today. Chrome tanning, the least expensive and most commonly used method, requires the use of heavy metals and acids, which are toxic. The chrome tanning process also produces acidic waste water with a pH of 4.5 to 5.0 (acidic). Thus, this industry is heavily regulated by the Environmental Protection Agency (EPA) and must meet their waste standards for air, liquid, and solid wastes. This explains why there are few leather tanneries and finishers in the United States and a growth of tanneries in developing countries where labor costs are less and environmental standards are not as strict. However, tanning systems that include recycling chromium have been developed and have allowed U.S. companies to reduce the amount of chromium found in waste.

The few U.S. tanneries remaining are typically small privately held companies. Approximately 3,000 individuals are employed in the U.S. leather and hide tanning and finishing industry with the majority working in production (U.S. Bureau of Labor Statistics, 2010). This is down from the approximately 7,000 individuals in 2005. **Regular tanneries**, the most common type of tannery, buy skins, kips, and hides and sell finished leather. Leather **converters** buy skins, kips, and hides, contract with a tannery to tan them according to specifications, and then sell the finished leather. Most of the U.S. companies tan and finish cattle hides. As costs increase, raw hides are typically being shipped overseas for finishing.

Compared to other textiles, leather production is a relatively slow process. Because of the longer lead time needed in the production from hide to finished product, leather producers often must make styling and color decisions before other textile producers. Therefore, they are keenly involved with trend forecasting and market research. Casual footwear and automobile upholstery account for most of the leather market in the U.S. Leather is also used for such products as apparel (e.g., jackets, coats) and handbags (see Figure 3.4).

Fur Production

Fur fibers are considered luxury products that come from animals valued for their pelts, such as mink, rabbit, beaver, and muskrat. Pelts are the unshorn skins of these and other animals. Fur is divided into two categories: farm-raised and wild fur. Farm-raised fur is derived from reproducing, rearing, and harvesting

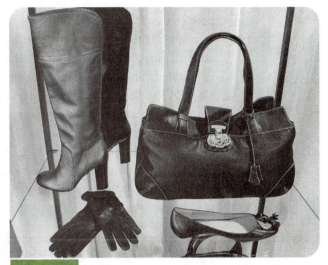

Figure 3.4 End uses for leather include footwear, apparel, handbags, and other accessories.

domestic fur-bearing animals in captivity. Mink and fox are the most popular pelts produced on fur farms. In addition, chinchilla, fitch, nutria, and other furbearers are raised in smaller numbers, while some countries produce large quantities of pelts from sheep, goats, and rabbits as a valuable by-product of meat production. Wild fur is derived from the selective and regulated harvesting of surplus fur-bearing animals that are not endangered or threatened species and that do not live in captivity. Fur pelts are sold at fur auctions to fur processors. Major fur auction houses are located in Copenhagen, Frankfurt, Helsinki, Hong Kong, Leipzig, New York, Seattle, St. Petersburg, Toronto, and Vancouver.

The tanning process for fur, known as **tawning**, differs from the tanning of hides for leather. To tan fur pelts, salt, water, alum, soda ash, sawdust, cornstarch, and lanolin are used. Each ingredient is natural and nontoxic, and the tawning process produces neutral waste water with a pH of 7 (neutral—neither acidic nor alkaline). Many furs are also bleached or dyed to improve their natural color or to give them a nonnatural color (e.g., blue, green). Pelts are also glazed to add beauty and luster to the fur.

Fur production and the wearing of fur have been politically charged topics for many years. In the 1970s, efforts of animal rights and other organizations (e.g., World Wildlife Fund, Fur Conservation Institute of America) pushed for the enactment of the Endangered Species Conservation Act of 1973, which protected endangered animal species in 80 countries worldwide. More recently, animal rights groups have organized anti-fur campaigns, creating an intense and widespread debate over the humane treatment of animals used for fur production and environmental claims of the fur industry. The Fur Commission USA (2010) Animal Welfare Committee certifies fur farmers who are committed to humane treatment in all aspects of fur farming, including "attention to nutritional needs; clean, safe and appropriate housing; prompt veterinary care; consideration for the animals' disposition and reproductive needs; and elimination of outside stress." However, even with such assurances, anti-fur activists continue to campaign against the killing of animals for the production of luxury goods.

Manufactured-Fiber Processing

Since the first synthetic fiber (nylon) was introduced in 1939, the demand for synthetics has steadily increased. The Asia-Pacific region, particularly China and India, will continue to be the largest producer of manufactured fibers. By 2012, China is expected to manufacture over 70 percent of all polyester output.

The largest synthetic textile company in the United States is INVISTA, a multinational company and the world's largest producer of nylon and spandex. Originally the textiles and interiors division of DuPont, it was renamed INVISTA in 2004. INVISTA produces and markets fiber brand names such as Lycra spandex and Antron nylon carpet fiber. Table 3.2 lists selected U.S. manufactured-fiber producers. Many of these companies are said to be **horizontally integrated**, in that they produce several fibers or variations of fibers that are at the same stage in the process (i.e., fiber processing). For example, INVISTA produces several types of nylon.

New manufactured fibers are developed through research efforts that take up to five years before the fiber is available on the market. According to the Textile Products Identification Act, when a fiber belonging to a new generic family is invented, the U.S. Federal Trade Commission assigns it a new generic name. Currently, more than 25 generic fibers are recognized by the FTC; see Table 3.3 for a listing of these fibers.

The steps in producing manufactured fibers are as follows:

1. The raw material is converted into a group of related chemical compounds that are treated with intense steam heat, chemicals, and pressure. During this process, which is called *polymerization*, the molecules become long-chain synthetic polymers. The molten resin is then converted into flakes or chips.

Table 3.2   Selected Manufactured-Fiber Producers and Fiber Trade Names

American Fibers and Yarns Co.
- Impressa Olefin
- Innova Olefin

Celanese Corporation
- Celanese Acetate
- Celstar Acetate

DAK Americas
- Dacron Plus Polyester

DuPont Performance Materials
- Kevlar Aramid
- Nomex Aramid
- Tyvek Olefin

FiberVisions, Inc.
- Herculon Olefin

Honeywell Nylon, Inc.
- Anso Nylon 6
- Caprolan Nylon 6
- Zeftron Nylon 6

Honeywell International
- Spectra Olefin

INVISTA, Inc.
- Antron Nylon 6.6
- Cordura Nylon 6.6
- TACTEL Nylon 6.6
- Lycra Spandex

Lenzing Group
- Tencel Lyocell

Nylstar, Inc.
- Meryl Nylon

Solutia, Inc.
- Acrilan Acrylic
- Duraspun Acrylic
- SEF Modacrylic
- Ultron Nylon 6.6

Sterling Fibers, Inc.
- Creslan Acrylic
- Creslite Acrylic
- Cresloft Acrylic

Wellman, Inc.
- Wellon Nylon
- Fortrel Polyester
- ComFortrel Polyester
- Ultra Polyester

2. The flakes or chips are melted and extruded to form filaments. Variations in the appearance of the filaments may be obtained at this stage by changing the shape of the fiber or adding chemicals to modify the fiber characteristics.

3. The cold-drawing process winds and stretches the filaments from one rotating wheel to a second faster-rotating one. This straightens the molecules and permanently introduces strength, elasticity, flexibility, and pliability to the yarn.

Table 3.3	Names of Generic Fibers

acetate	olefin (polypropylene)
acrylic	PBI (polybenzimidazole)
anidex	PBO (polyphenylenebenzobisozazole)
aramid	PEN (polyethylene naphthalate)
azlon	PLA (polylactic acid fiber)
elastoester	polyester
glass	rayon
lyocell (subcategory of rayon)	saran
melamine	spandex
metallic	sulfar or PPS (polyphenylene sulfide)
modacrylic	triacetate
nylon	vinal
nytril	vinyon

Manufactured fibers can be modified in terms of shape (cross-section), molecular structure, chemical additives, or spinning procedures to create better-quality or more versatile fibers and yarns. Generic fibers are also combined within a single fiber or yarn to take advantage of specific fiber characteristics. Yarn variations include monofilament and multifilament yarns, stretch yarns, textured yarns, and spun yarns. Companies continue to invest in research to create fiber and yarn innovations to meet consumer demand. Innovations such as microfiber yarns (introduced in 1986) and TENCEL Lyocell (introduced in 1992) have met with favorable consumer response. Many of the same companies in the United States that produce manufactured fibers also produce yarns (e.g., INVISTA, Solutia, and Wellman). In addition, many textile mills focus on producing yarns with natural, manufactured, and blended fibers (e.g., Carolina Mills, Frontier Spinning Mills, Patrick Yarns, Richmond Yarns, Unifi, and Waverly Mills).

Fiber Marketing and Distribution

Marketing Natural Fibers

Natural fibers are considered commodities; they are bought and sold on global markets, with prices based upon market demand. For example, in the mid-1990s, cotton prices soared as consumer demand went up and cotton supplies dwindled because of devastating weather and insect-related crop failures in China (the world's largest producer of cotton) and other major producing countries, such as India and Pakistan. The largest commodity markets for cotton in the United States are Dallas, Houston, Memphis, and New Orleans; for wool, Boston; and for mohair, a warehouse system throughout Texas. These natural fibers are sold to mills for yarn spinning and fabric production. Furs are sold at public auction.

Not until the late 1940s and early 1950s, when the popularity of manufactured fibers was growing, were marketing efforts for natural fibers initiated by each trade association that represents a specific fiber. These trade associations—such as Cotton Incorporated, the American Wool Council, the Mohair Council of America, and the Cashmere and Camel Hair Manufacturers Institute (CCMI)—are supported by natural-fiber producers and promote the use of the natural fibers through activities such as research, educational programs, and advertising on television and in trade and consumer publications. Through these activities, natural-fiber trade associations have become an important support arm for the apparel and home fashions industries, and strong relationships have developed between the trade associations and the apparel and home fashions companies that use natural fibers.

Founded in 1961, Cotton Incorporated is a research and promotional organization supported by U.S. cotton growers and importers of cotton products. Cotton Incorporated's members receive technical services, color and trend forecasting services, and promotional services. In 2000, Cotton Incorporated opened a new research and development headquarters in Cary, North Carolina. The research facility includes **textile testing**, product care, and color labs. Cotton Incorporated's Seal of Cotton trademark (see Figure 3.5) is used on hangtags and in advertisements, along with the association's slogan "The Fabric of Our Lives." In recent years, Cotton Incorporated has sponsored collections of new designers during the spring fashion shows in New York City. Cotton Incorporated is also involved in market research. Research results are published as print and Web reports in the *Lifestyle Monitor*. It includes consumer segment profiles, retail patronage profiles, summaries of consumers' attitudes, and forecasts.

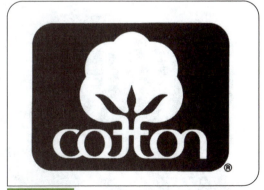

Figure 3.5   Cotton Incorporated's trademark for products made of 100 percent (upland) cotton.

Trade associations focusing on wool fall into the following two categories:

- those that focus on wool production (e.g., California Wool Growers Association, Montana Wool Growers Association)

- those that focus on product development, marketing, and education (e.g., American Wool Council and Australian Wool Innovation Limited)

Established in 1955, the American Wool Council is a division of the American Sheep Industry Association. Its programs are involved in all aspects of wool marketing, from raw wool marketing and product development to registered trademark programs, advertising, and publicity. The American Wool Council has been involved in standardizing quality levels of wool and promoting wool applications with spinners, weavers, knitters, designers, manufacturers, and retailers.

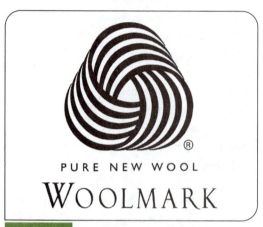

Figure 3.6 The Woolmark, a registered trademark of The Woolmark Company, is used on hangtags and in advertising.

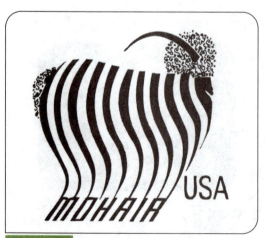

Figure 3.7 Registered trademark of the Mohair Council of America.

The Woolmark Company was established in 1937 as the International Wool Secretariat (IWS) and is now a subsidiary of Australian Wool Innovation Limited. In 1964, the Woolmark program, with its well-known Woolmark symbol (see Figure 3.6), was created to identify quality products made from new wool. The Woolmark Blend symbol was introduced in 1971 to identify products made from at least 50 percent new wool. Its services include trend and color forecasting, textile testing, licensing the Woolmark symbols, and global market analyses.

Established in 1966, the Mohair Council of America is "dedicated to promoting the general welfare of the mohair industry" (Mohair Council of America). The council's programs focus on market surveys, research, and development activities, including advertising, workshops, and seminars. Because most of the mohair produced in the United States is exported, the council conducts foreign as well as domestic market research and promotion. The council's trademark is shown in Figure 3.7. Other trade associations focusing on natural fibers include the Cashmere and Camel Hair Manufacturers Institute, International Linen Promotion Commission, National Cotton Council, and International Silk Association.

Trade associations also play an important part in marketing leather and fur. Associations such as the Leather Industries of America and the Fur Information Council of America are involved with promotion, including advertising and consumer education programs. The mink industry also has a number of breeder associations, such as the Fur Commission USA and the Canada Mink Breeders Association, that are involved in promotion efforts.

The trade associations discussed above concentrate their efforts on specific segments of the natural-fiber industry (see Figure 3.8). The National Council of Textile Organizations (NCTO) has a broader mission, as it represents the entire spectrum of the textile sector, including fiber producers, textile mills, and other textile suppliers. The NCTO is highly involved with lobbying efforts in Washington, D.C., on the behalf of the U.S. textile industry. As its website states: "NCTO is also mobilizing global resources in its efforts to preserve the U.S. textile industry. Through new powerful international alliances, our voice is heard and has an impact from Washington, DC, to Geneva, to Beijing." (National Council of Textile Organizations, 2010). Table 3.4 lists selected trade associations in the textile industry.

Marketing Manufactured Fibers

Manufactured fibers are most often produced by **vertically integrated** companies. Prices are set primarily by the cost of developing and producing the fibers. Manufactured fibers are sold either as commodity fibers or brand name fibers.

- *Commodity fibers* are generic manufactured fibers (parent fibers) sold without a brand name attached.

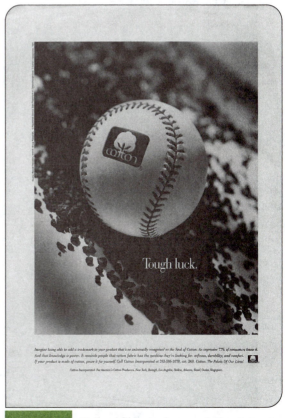

Figure 3.8 Natural fiber trade associations promote the use of natural fibers through **advertising**.

Table 3.4   Selected Textile Trade Associations

American Association of Textile Chemists and Colorists (AATCC)
P.O. Box 12215
Research Triangle Park, NC 27709
Tel: (919) 549-8141
Fax: (919) 549-8933
www.aatcc.org

American Fiber Manufacturers Association (AFMA)
1530 Wilson Blvd.
Suite 690
Arlington, VA 22209
Tel: (703) 875-0432
Fax: (703) 875-0907
www.afma.org

American Wool Council
c/o American Sheep Industry Association
9785 Maroon Circle
Suite 360
Centennial, CO 80112
Tel: (303) 771-3500
Fax: (303) 771-8200
www.sheepusa.org

Association of Nonwoven Fabrics Industry
1100 Crescent Green, Suite 115
Cary, NC 27518
Tel: (919) 233-1210
Fax: (919) 233-1282
www.inda.org

Australian Wool Innovation Limited (Wool-mark Company)
1120 Avenue of the Americas, Suite 4107
New York, NY 10036 USA
Tel: (212) 626- 6744
www.wool.com

Carpet and Rug Institute
730 College Drive
Dalton, Georgia 30720
Tel: (706) 278-3176
Fax: (706) 278-8835
www.carpet-rug.com

Cotton Incorporated
6399 Weston Parkway
Cary, NC 27513
Tel: (919) 678-2220
Fax: (919) 678-2230
www.cottoninc.com

Fur Information Council of America (FICA)
8424 A Santa Monica Blvd. #860
West Hollywood, CA 90069
Tel: (323) 848-7940
Fax: (323) 848-2931
www.fur.org

Industrial Fabrics Association International
1801 County Road B W
Roseville, MN 55113-4061
Tel: (651) 222-2508
Fax: (651) 631- 9334
www.ifai.com

Leather Industries of America
3050 K Street, NW, Suite 400
Washington, DC 20007
Tel: (202) 342-8086
Fax: (202) 342-8583
www.leatherusa.com

Mohair Council of America
233 W. Twohig Ave.
San Angelo, TX 76903
Tel: (800) 583-3161
www. mohairusa.com

Table 3.4 Selected Textile Trade Associations *(continued)*	
National Council of Textile Organizations 910 17th Street NW, Suite 1020 Washington, DC 20006 Tel: (202) 822-8028 Fax: (202) 822-8029 www.ncto.org	**Synthetic Yarn and Fiber Association** 737 Park Trail Lane Clover, SC 29710 Tel: (704)-589-5895 Fax: (803)746-5566 www.thesyfa.org

For example, a carpet labeled "100 percent" nylon is probably manufactured with commodity nylon fibers.

- Manufactured fibers are also sold under **brand names** (or **trade names**) given to the fibers by manufacturers. Brand names distinguish one fiber from another in the same generic family. Modified manufactured fibers with special characteristics are typically sold under brand names (See Table 3.3). Examples include the following:
  - Lycra spandex (INVISTA)
  - TENCEL Lyocell (Lenzing Fibers)
  - Dacron polyester (INVISTA)
  - Fortrel polyester (Wellman, Inc.)
  - Ascend nylon (Solutia, Inc.)
  - Antron nylon carpet fiber (INVISTA)

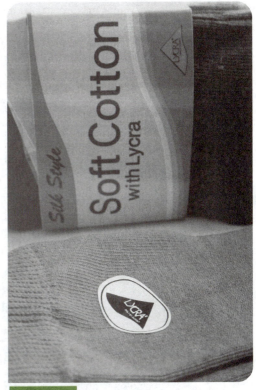

To establish consumer recognition of brand name fibers, promotion activities focus on the company, the brand name, and the specific qualities of the fiber (see Figure 3.9). Companies spend a great deal of money establishing brand name identification among consumers, and brand name fibers are generally higher in price than commodity fibers. Advertisements also connect brand name fibers with specific end uses. Therefore, cooperative advertising between manufactured fiber companies and apparel and home fashions manufacturers is common.

Licensed brand name programs, or **controlled brand name programs**, set minimum

Figure 3.9 Brand name manufactured fibers are advertised to increase name recognition among customers.

standards of fabric performance for the trademarked fibers. Determined through regular textile testing, these standards are established as a form of quality assurance and relate to a specific end use. The following examples illustrate minimum standards for trademarked fibers:

- The Wear-Dated brand of nylon carpet fibers produced by Solutia, Inc. has minimum standards for wear and soil resistance, stain resistance, color and light fastness, and tuft bind (adhesion to carpet backing).

- The Trevira polyester program (Trevira is a company in the Reliance Group) establishes minimum standards for fabric quality for specific end uses.

- Coolmax is a registered trademark of INVISTA. It certifies high-performance fabrics that include INVISTA and, in some cases, other companies' fibers.

The standards set through these programs can be especially beneficial to apparel and home fashions manufacturers in quality assurance and marketing end-use products.

Fiber producers also design and create **concept garments** to promote their new fibers to textile mills. For example, when Solutia, Inc. has a new product to show textile mills, it will often show the new product in garment form. When creating concept garments, fiber companies will either create fabrics and the garment on their own machinery, or work with a textile mill and manufacturer that will produce small runs of the concept garment. For example, INVISTA shows samples of Coolmax fabrics made into actual performance garments as part of their marketing program.

As with natural fibers, **trade associations** are also important to the manufactured-fiber industry. The American Fiber Manufacturers Association (AFMA) began in 1933, first as the Rayon Institute, and then as the Man-Made Fiber Producers Association. The current name was adopted in 1988. The AFMA focuses on domestic production of synthetic and cellulosic manufactured fibers. Programs include government relations, international trade policy, the environment, technical issues, and education services. AFMA's statistics division, the Fiber Economics Bureau, collects and publishes data on production and trade of manufactured fibers.

Color Forecasting in the Textile Industry

Color is an important criterion used by consumers in the selection of textile products, including apparel and home fashions. Therefore, an understanding of consumers' color preferences is crucial to successfully marketing a particular textile product. Whereas some classic colors remain popular over many years, fashion colors have a shorter fashion lifecycle. Because color is typically applied at the textile production stage, textile companies are often involved in determining which colors are to be used in the end-use products. Through the process of **color forecasting**, color palettes or color stories are selected and translated into fabrics produced by a company for a specific fashion season. Color forecasting is also conducted by apparel and home fashions manufacturers (see Chapter 5).

The Color Association of the United States (CAUS) is a nonprofit service organization that has been involved in color forecasting since 1915. More than 700 companies, including fiber producers, textile companies, apparel manufacturers, and home fashions producers, belong to CAUS. A committee of volunteers from these companies determines general color palettes for the coming 18 to 24 months. Twice a year (in March and September), swatch cards (see Figure 3.10) are sent to member companies for their use in determining color palettes for their own products.

The International Colour Authority (ICA) is an international **color forecasting service**. Teams of representatives from member companies and color experts meet biannually to determine general color palettes approximately 22 to 24 months before the products they produce will be available to the consumer. ICA services provide some of the earliest predictions in the industry. Separate palettes are created for menswear, women's wear, leather, home fashions, and paints. Forecasts are then sent to member companies for their use.

A number of other color forecasting services also sell color forecasts to companies. These forecasts may be specific to a particular target market and product (e.g., women's apparel, children's apparel). Often the services will also include style and fabrication forecasting. "The color box" provides subscribers with four-color and design forecasts per year for menswear, children's wear, and women's wear. Color forecasting services include the following:

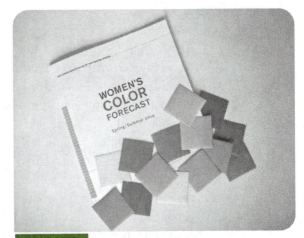

- Trendstop.com is a highly regarded online global color and trend forecasting service that provides subscribers with current research on a variety of international fashion trends.

- Headquartered in Paris, Promostyl is an international color, fabric, and

Figure 3.10 Swatch cards from color forecasting services assist textile companies in their color decisions.

style forecasting service that provides trend analyses for men's, women's, and children's apparel 12 to 18 months ahead of the fashion season.

- Peclers Paris also offers color and trend forecasts for fashion, industrial design, and home fashions.

- Color forecasts may also be conducted by trade associations for their member companies. For example, Cotton Incorporated provides color forecasting services to its members.

Textile, apparel, and home fashions companies also conduct their own color forecasting, which is more specific to their product and target market than the information provided by color forecasting services. This type of color forecasting is accomplished through the following steps:

- reviewing color predictions from color forecasting services

- tracking color trends by examining the colors that were the best and worst selling from previous seasons

- observing general trends that may affect color preferences of the target market

- looking at what colors have been missing from the color palettes in order to select colors that may be viewed as "new"

Fabric Production

Textile Mills

Textile mills focus on the fabric construction or fabrication stage of textiles. According to North American Industry Classification System (NAICS, 2010) definitions, Sector 313 Textile Mills are companies "that transform a basic fiber (natural or synthetic) into a product, such as yarn or fabric, that is further manufactured into usable items, such as apparel, sheets, towels, and textile bags for individual or industrial consumption." The two most common fabric construction methods are weaving and knitting. Except for vertically integrated companies that produce both woven and knitted goods, textile mills typically specialize in the production of one type of fabric. In addition to fabric production, woven textile mills often spin their own yarn (see Figure 3.11), whereas knitters typically purchase their yarn. All textile mills sell greige goods. Greige goods may be used "as is" or bought by converters who finish the goods. In addition to selling greige goods, vertically integrated companies also finish the goods themselves and may produce end-use products, such as home textiles (e.g., sheets and towels).

Mills sell staple and/or specialty (novelty) fabrics. Staple fabrics, such as denim or tricot, are produced continually each year with little change in construction or finish. Novelty fabrics have special design features (e.g., surface texture, specialty weave) that are fashion-based and, therefore, change with fashion cycles. Because of this, fashion fabrics require shorter production runs and greater flexibility.

The knitting industry has two main divisions:

- the knitted products industry, which manufactures end-use products, such as T-shirts, hosiery, and sweaters

- the knitted fabrics industry, which manufactures knitted yard goods sold to apparel and home fashions manufacturers and retailers

Textile mills are found throughout the world, with eastern Asian countries (China, Taiwan, Japan) and India accounting for most of the world's textiles. Many multinational companies have textile mills in a variety of countries. For example, headquartered in Greensboro, North Carolina, International Textile Group (ITG) comprises six companies: Cone Denim, Burlington Worldwide Apparel, Cone Decorative Fabrics, Narricot, Saftey Components, and Carlisle Finishing. ITG has global operations in China, Hong Kong, Vietnam, Mexico, and Nicaragua. Similarly, Springs

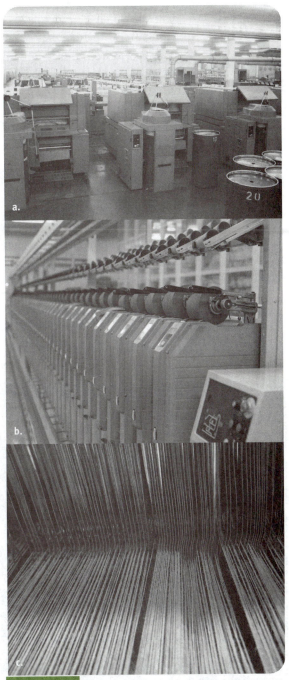

Figure 3.11 Fabric production is highly automated. These machines are used for carding fibers (a), spinning them into yarn (b), and weaving fabric (c).

Global, which is a merger of Springs Industries of the United States and Coteminas of Brazil, has operations in Argentina, Brazil, Canada, Mexico, Turkey, India, China, Vietnam, and the United States.

Textile Design

Textile design involves the interrelationships among the following:

- color (e.g., dyeing, printing)
- fabric structure (e.g., woven or knitted fabric)
- finishes (e.g., napping, embossing)

In addition to knowing about color and fabric structure, textile designers must have expertise in computer-aided design or graphics software and an understanding of the technology used in producing textiles. The use of computer-aided design or graphics software allows the textile designer to experiment with color and fabric construction, and then to print and prepare exact instructions to replicate the fabric design (see Figure 3.12).

Textile designers specialize according to printing method and fabric structure; they may be freelance designers or work for textile design studios, textile

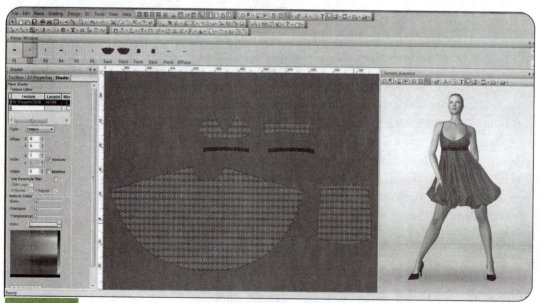

Figure 3.12 Computer-aided design helps a designer see how a new fabric or design will look in a garment.

mills, or converters. For example, one textile designer may work for a textile mill and specialize in direct roller-printing processes; another may be a freelance designer of graphics for T-shirts and specialize in screen printing processes. The term **textile stylist** is currently used to designate individuals who have expertise in the design and manufacturing of textiles, as well as an understanding of the textile market. The stylist's combination of design, technical, and consumer/business expertise is particularly important in reflecting consumer preferences in the textiles being designed. Designers and stylists may work directly with apparel and home fashions manufacturers to create special prints, or with retailers to create prints to be used for private-label merchandise.

Textile Converters

Textile converters buy greige goods from mills; have the fabrics dyed, printed, or finished; and then sell the finished fabrics. Textile converters focus on the following:

- aesthetic finishes (e.g., glazing, crinkling)
- performance finishes (e.g., colorfast, stain resistant, water resistant, durable pressed)
- dyeing or printing fabrics

Textile converters are experts in color forecasting and understand consumer preferences in fiber content, fabric construction, and various aesthetic and performance fabric finishes. Often textile converters will contract with dyers, printers, and finishers to create fabrics that they market to apparel and home fashions manufacturers, jobbers, and retailers. Some converters specialize in a certain type of fabric; others may design several types of fabrics. Most converters that print fabrics use rotary printing presses. **Digital printing** with ink jet printers is becoming more widespread (see Chapter 11). Because the fabric is finished close to the time when consumers will be purchasing the end-use product, converters play an important role in analyzing and responding to changing consumer preferences.

Although most fabric finishing is done by converters, not all finishing operations are handled by them. For example, apparel and home fashions manufacturers and retailers fulfill the converter's functions to some extent when they specify to a textile mill the color they want a fabric dyed. Woolen and worsted wool fabrics are seldom sold through converters, but rather are generally sold finished by mills. In addition, industrial fabrics are typically sold directly from mills because they are made to meet buyer specifications and may require special performance tests. Also, converters are seldom used in the manufacturing of sweaters and other knitwear, which are typically knitted and then constructed into garments by the same company.

Other Fabric Resources

Textile jobbers and fabric retail stores buy and sell fabric without any involvement in producing or finishing the fabric. Textile jobbers buy from textile mills, converters, and large manufacturers, and then sell to smaller manufacturers and retailers. Typically, jobbers will buy mill overruns (fabrics the textile mill produces beyond what was ordered) or discontinued fabric colors or prints. For example, a textile jobber may buy extra or discontinued fabric from a textile mill and sell it to a small apparel manufacturer who does not need a large volume of fabric. Retail fabric stores sell over-the-counter piece goods primarily to home sewers. Fabric stores may purchase their bolt yardage from fabric wholesalers that have purchased large rolls from textile mills.

Textile brokers serve as liaisons between textile sellers and textile buyers. For example, a broker may connect a small textile mill wanting to sell greige goods to a small converter that wants to buy them. Textile brokers differ from jobbers in that brokers never own the fabric.

Textile Testing and Quality Assurance

The textile industry is highly involved in quality assurance programs and textile testing. Textile testing involves inspection and measurement of textile characteristics (e.g., strength, flammability, abrasion resistance, colorfastness) throughout the production and finishing of the textile. Standard test methods developed by the American Society for Testing and Materials (ASTM) and the American Association of Textile Chemists and Colorists (AATCC) are used by companies in testing the quality and specific performance requirements of the textile materials they use.

Although the terms **quality control** and **quality assurance** are sometimes used interchangeably, they have different meanings:

- *Quality control* involves inspecting finished textiles to make sure they adhere to specific quality standards as measured by a variety of textile testing methods (see Figure 3.13).

- *Quality assurance* is a broader concept, covering not only the fabric's general functional performance (quality), but also how well it satisfies consumer needs for a specific end use. For example, a textile to be used in children's ap-

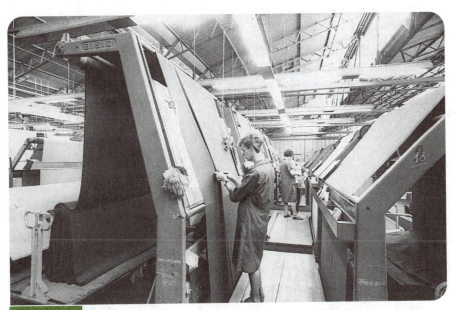

Figure 3.13 Fabrics are inspected by trained experts to ensure that they meet quality standards.

parel must not only meet minimum standards of functional performance but also specifications such as colorfastness that are important to the consumer of children's apparel. Whereas a textile mill may test for general functional performance of the fabric, often the apparel or home fashions manufacturer or retailer must determine if the fabric meets the specifications of importance to its consumers. This is why the testing of fabrics is often conducted by the following:

– apparel and home fashions manufacturers (e.g., Nike, Pendleton Woolen Mills)
– retailers (e.g., JCPenney, Target) of these goods
– independent textile testing companies contracted by manufacturers or retailers

Marketing and Distribution of Fabrics

Marketing Seasonal Lines

Fiber producers, textile mills, and converters take part in the marketing of textile fabrics. Most manufactured-fiber producers have showrooms that exhibit fabrics and end-use products made from their fibers. Textile showrooms are located in most major U.S. cities (e.g., Los Angeles, Dallas, Atlanta, Chicago), although New York is the primary market center for textile mills, converters, and textile product manufacturers. Internationally, textile showrooms are prevalent in the major cities of countries with large numbers of textile mills, as well as large marketing headquarters (e.g., Paris, Milan, Taipei, Hong Kong, Shanghai, Tokyo). Showrooms house the fabric samples to be marketed by textile mills or converters to designers and apparel or home fashions manufacturers.

Textile mills and converters market their textile fabrics as Fall/Winter and Spring/Summer seasonal lines. Each fabric line includes a grouping of fabrics with a similar theme or **color story**. It is the responsibility of the merchandising or marketing staff of textile companies to show fabric samples to prospective buyers in their showrooms or at textile trade shows. Samples of Fall/Winter lines of fabrics are shown to prospective fabric buyers in October or November, approximately nine to twelve months before the end-use product (e.g., apparel) hits the stores. Spring/Summer lines of fabrics are shown in March or April. During these shows, apparel and home fashions companies will purchase yardage for their samples. Some large manufacturers may order their end-use fabrics at this time, but most will wait until their own orders from retailers are known. For large accounts, fabric samples can be "confined," which means that the textile company will not sell the fabric to other end-use companies.

Fabric companies also promote their lines through sites on the Internet and through other online services. Such online marketing of fabrics offers an efficient method for companies to advertise their products to prospective fabric buyers. A number of Internet companies focus on connecting fabric/textile sellers with fabric/textile buyers in the apparel industry.

Textile Trade Shows

Textile **trade shows** exhibit textile mills' newest fabrics for the coming fashion seasons. Typically held twice per year, in spring (March) and fall (October/ November), textile trade shows offer visitors a look at general trends in color, textures, prints, and fabrications (see Figure 3.14). For example, a textile trade show held in March 2010 would exhibit Spring/Summer 2011 fabrics.

Because every apparel line or collection begins with fabrics, textile shows provide designers and manufacturers with inspirations for their next line or collection. "A designer's creativity is limited by what a fabric can be made to do, so, in a sense, a collection doesn't really start with the [apparel] designer but with the fabric mill" (Schiro, 1995, p. L16). Below is a listing of selected textile trade shows:

- Direction, an international textile design show held in New York City, focuses on trendsetting textiles from around the world.

- Sourcing at MAGIC, held in Las Vegas in association with MAGIC Marketplace, connects apparel and accessory manufacturers with fabric and trim suppliers from around the world.

- Interstoff, managed by Messe Frankfurt, is one of the largest textile trade show organizations in the world. Interstoff includes the following:
  - Interstoff Asia (Hong Kong)
  - Interstoff Rossija (Moscow)
  - Intertextile Beijing
  - Intertextile Shanghai
  - Source It (Hong Kong)
  - Texworld (Paris)
  - Texworld India (Mumbai)
  - Texworld USA (New York City)
  - Yarn Expo

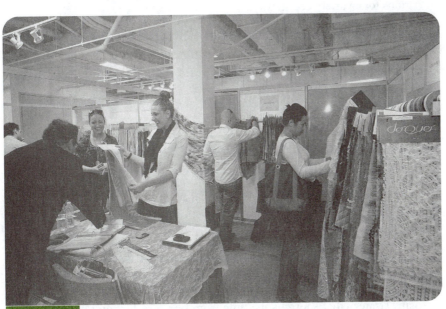

Figure 3.14 Textile trade shows provide opportunities for textile companies to promote their lines to manufacturers.

- Première Vision, held in Villepinte, near Paris, focuses on high-quality and innovative fabrics. Designers often get inspirations for apparel designs from the textiles shown at Première Vision. Première Vision has expanded worldwide to include the following:
  - Première Vision Shanghai
  - Première Vision New York
  - Première Vision Moscow
  - Première Vision Tokyo
- Material World New York, sponsored by the American Apparel and Footwear Association, is a growing textile trade show in the United States.
- Ideacomo, held in Como, Italy (near Milan), was created in 1975 by silk apparel producers near Como. It now focuses on medium- to high-market luxury and innovative fabric collections of member companies.
- L.A. International Textile Show, held at the California Market Center and sponsored by the Textile Association of L.A., is one of the largest textile trade shows in the United States. It focuses on creative domestic and European designer fabric and trim collections and other textile resources.
- Taipei Innovative Textile Application Show (TITAS) focuses on high-tech and innovative textiles (primarily from Asian countries) and their applications for a variety of end uses.

Leather producers also use biannual trade shows to market their products. Some of the best known are LE CUIR A PARIS, China International Leather Fair, Moscow International Fur Trade Fair, and Fur and Fashion Frankfurt Fair.

Developments in the Textile Industry
Technological Advances

In order to compete successfully in a global economy, the U.S. textile industry has invested in new technology to increase productivity in textile mills and improve communication among textile mills, their suppliers, and their customers. These investments in technology are part of Quick Response, supply chain management, and product lifecycle management.

As discussed in Chapter 1, *Quick Response* is an umbrella term that refers to any strategy that shortens the time from fiber production to sale to the ultimate consumer. Supply chain management takes QR further by enhancing the communications and partnerships among industry sectors. In the textile industry, Quick Response and supply chain management strategies include computer-aided textile design, computerized knitting machines, and computer-controlled robots (see Figure 3.15). Enhanced communication links between textile companies, their suppliers, and their customers have also contributed to effective supply chain management strategies.

The textile industry has also played an important role in the research, development, and implementation of new strategies to increase productivity and competitiveness. According to the National Council of Textile Organizations, the U.S. textile industry has increased productivity by 50 percent over the last 10 years and ranks second among all industrial sectors in productivity increases. Examples of investment in technologically advanced equipment and processes include digital textile printing (see Figure 3.16) which has reshaped the way in which fabric designs are created. Digital textile printing is "the process of creating printable designs for fabric on a computer, which can be sent directly from the computer to fabric printing machinery without the use of screens and color separation" (Campbell & Kim, 1999, p. 113).

Another technological advancement that has affected the textile industry is **nanotechnology**. Nanotechnology is the "manufacturing technology that operates in the range of nanometers, one-billionth of a meter" ("Nanotechnology's new potential," 2006). Nanotechnology applications in textile manufacturing have been used to create faster and more precise textile-processing machinery, and have improved the quality and speed of textile surface coatings/finishes. It is expected that new nanotechnology applications will provide competitive advantages for companies incorporating this technology into the manufacturing processes. Optical fibers with integrated electronics have also been developed, allowing fibers that can sense, process, and store data to be woven into fabric. Initial applications for these **"smart" fibers** and materials include military uniforms, medical devices, protective garments for extreme environments, and performance athletic wear.

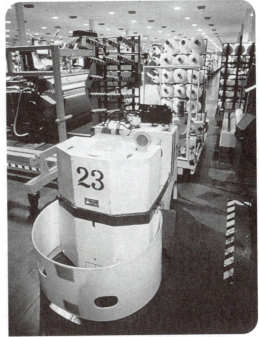

Figure 3.15 Computer-controlled robots are used to transport packages in textile mills. Such investments in technology have increased the textile industry's productivity.

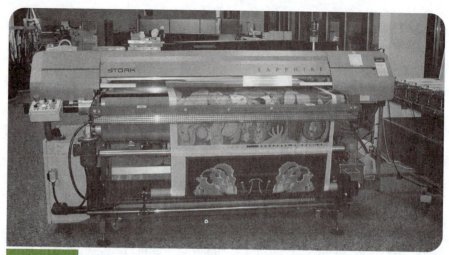

Figure 3.16 Digital printing allows companies to send fabric designs from computers directly to fabric-printing machinery.

Environmental Issues

Demand for environmentally responsible products, once limited to younger consumers and consumers who had a sense of social responsibility, has become mainstream. Companies, including textile producers, are working to improve environmental conditions and to show they are environmentally conscious. They are incorporating environmentally responsible processes (see Figure 3.17), such as the following:

- manufacturing products that include organic or recycled materials
- using less toxic materials, such as low-impact dyes
- using less water in production

Apparel manufacturers are also pressuring textile producers to supply environmentally responsible textiles. Therefore, a number of environmentally responsible textile manufacturing processes have been implemented, including organically grown cotton, cleaner dyeing and finishing processes, and waste reduction (see discussion of organic cotton earlier in this chapter).

Each year, textile companies spend billions of dollars to ensure that their processes are environmentally responsible through efforts in conserving water, energy, and electricity and in recycling products (e.g., paper and plastic) and natural resources (e.g., water and energy). Plants are built or adapted with environmental impact in mind. For example, Malden Mills' (producer of Polartec and Polarfleece fleece fabric) plant in Lawrence, Massachusetts, has built-in environmental systems that reduce water use, reuse heat, and treat wastewater.

Trade associations and other organizations have played an important role in research, implementation, and promotion of environmentally safe processes. The Sustainable Style Foundation (SSF), headquartered in Seattle, Washington, "is an international, member-supported nonprofit organization created to provide information, resources, and innovative programs that promote sustainable living and sustainable design" (SSF, 2010). Founded in 2003, SSF provides the most current information about sustainable style to designers, producers, and consumers; promotes sustainable style in the media; and uses "popular culture to influence consumer choices."

A number of "environmentally cleaner" processes have been implemented in the cotton industry. These include naturally colored cotton, organic cotton, "cleaner" dyeing methods, and reduced water use. For example, one cotton producer, Sally Fox, developed naturally colored cotton in various shades of green, brown, and red. Natural colors had been bred out of modern cotton because the colored fibers were too short and weak for automated textile manufacturing. Fox began crossing the longer, stronger white cotton fibers with colored cotton

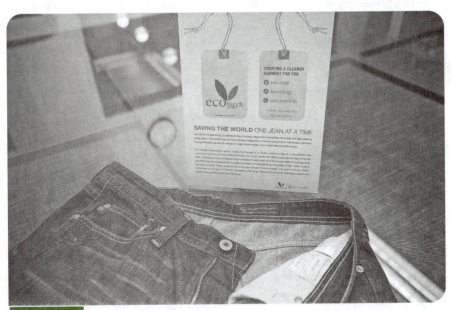

Figure 3.17 EDUN is a socially and environmentally conscious clothing company that seeks to foster sustainable employment in developing nations and to use organic materials in their clothing collections.

to create Foxfibre cotton, the first naturally colored cotton that could be processed with modern textile equipment (Vreseis, 2007). The natural colors did more than eliminate the need for dyeing the cotton; instead of fading, naturally colored cotton actually deepens in color when washed. In addition, Foxfibre cotton has a silky feel and a wool-like elasticity. Foxfibre, Colour-by-Nature, and Colorganic are all registered trademarks for naturally colored cottons.

Fox is also committed to organic cotton production, in which synthetic chemical fertilizers and pesticides are used minimally or not used at all. Fox is not the only cotton producer interested in organic cotton. According to the Organic Trade Association, sales of organic cotton have been steadily rising over the past five years, with estimates that it will continue to grow 15 percent per year over the next few years. Organic cotton fibers are now used in end-use products, ranging from cotton puffs and ear swabs to sheets and blankets to diapers to fashion apparel. The challenge for companies is finding enough quality organic cotton. Some companies use only organic cotton (e.g., Patagonia), whereas others use a blend of organic and regular cotton.

Because the majority of textiles are colored using chemical dyes to create bright, colorfast characteristics, some manufacturers are attempting to lessen the environmental impact of cotton production through the use of "cleaner" dyeing processes, including synthetic "low-impact" dyes, natural dyes, and undyed, unbleached cottons. Natural dyes are extracted from a variety of leaves, barks, flowers, berries, lichens, mushrooms, roots, wood, peels, nutshells, minerals, shellfish, and insects. However, many of these sources do not produce stable dyes for textiles.

A number of manufactured-fiber companies developed more environmentally responsible production processes, including the use of recycling. For example, in 1988, Courtalds Fibres UK developed lyocell, a cellulosic fiber made from harvested wood pulp (and, therefore, a subcategory of rayon) that is processed with recycled nontoxic solvents. In its production, virtually all the dissolving agent is recycled. In addition, waste emissions (air and wastewater) are lower than for other manufactured-fiber production. The resulting fiber is machine washable and is stronger than cotton or wool—as well as having a silkier touch. Currently, the only company manufacturing lyocell in the United States is Lenzing, Inc. (headquartered in Austria) under the TENCEL trade name. Fabrics made from 100 percent lyocell or in a variety of blends are used for apparel, accessories, and home fashions.

In addition to lyocell, some companies are making rayon from bamboo fibers. Because of its fast growth rate, renewability, and ability to take in greenhouse gases, the use of bamboo is being promoted by environmentalists. Rayon made from bamboo fibers has a silk-like hand, making it popular for apparel and home fashions. Linda Loudermilk's Luxury eco collection combines fabrics made from bamboo and other renewable plants in high-fashion collections shown on New York City runways.

Polyester staple fibers are also being recycled from plastic soda bottles, which are made of polyethylene teraphthalate, or PET. The process of making recycled polyester fibers includes the following steps:

1. All caps, labels, and bases made of other materials are removed from the bottles.

2. The bottles are sorted by color (clear and green).

3. The bottles are chopped.

4. The pieces are washed and dried.

5. The pieces are heated, purified, and formed into pellets.

6. The purified polyester is extruded as fine fibers that can be spun into thread, yarn, or other materials.

It takes an average of 25 plastic soda bottles to make one garment. Foss Manufacturing LLC produces Fortrel Ecospun®, a polyester that contains 100 percent recycled fiber used by dozens of apparel companies (see Figure 3.18). It is estimated that 2.4 billion bottles are kept out of landfills per year through the manufacturing of Fortrel Ecospun® fibers.

Several companies are also recycling scrap yarns and fabric as a means of reducing the amount of scrap materials ending up in landfill. Recycled scrap denim is being used in a variety of products, including fabrics, pencils, and paper. Milliken Floor Covering promises to recover all carpets returned to them through renewing the product, donating them to charities, recycling them, or using them in energy cogeneration (an environmentally responsible means of producing power). According to Milliken's Web site, since 1999, the company's carpet manufacturing plants have not sent any waste to landfill.

As Martin Bide stated in his article *Fiber Sustainability: Green is not Black + White*, the development or use of sustainable fibers is not clear cut (AATCC Review 2009). Everything comes with some environmental advantage or disadvantage. What he does foresee is that the consumer of the future will be more of a realist, and will have a longer view of sustainability. This consumer will buy fewer clothes, avoid cotton/polyester blends, wash in cold water with less water, line dry the clothes, and recycle the fabric at the end of the garment's wearing cycle.

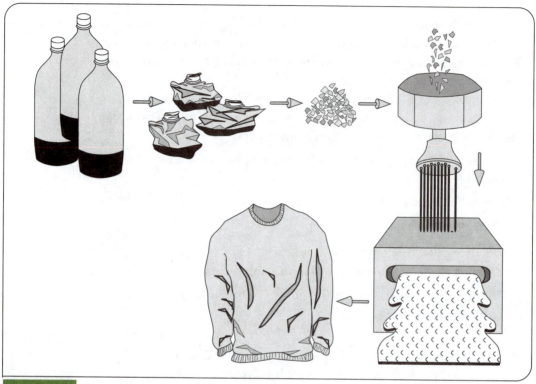

Figure 3.18 Fortrel Ecospun® is made of 100 percent recycled plastic bottles and is used in a variety of end products.

Summary

The textile industry includes companies that contribute to the four basic stages of textile production: fiber processing, yarn spinning, fabric production or fabrication, and fabric finishing. Some companies specialize in one or more of the production processes; vertically integrated companies handle all four. Both natural and manufactured fibers are processed in the United States.

Natural fibers produced in the United States include cotton, wool, mohair, and other specialty fibers. Leather and fur, also produced in the United States, are considered natural-fiber products. Natural fibers are commodities bought and sold on international markets and are generally promoted by trade associations that focus on specific fibers. These trade associations encourage the use of the various natural fibers through such activities as market research, advertising, and consumer education programs.

Manufactured fibers are typically produced by large vertically integrated companies. They are marketed either as commodity fibers or brand name (trademarked) fibers, such as Lycra spandex fiber or Dacron polyester fiber. Brand name fibers are advertised by companies in order to create consumer awareness and preference for the specific fibers. Trade associations are also involved in promoting manufactured fibers.

Textile companies are often involved in determining the colors to be used in end-use products. Through the process of color forecasting, color palettes are selected and translated into fabrics produced by a company for a specific fashion season. Color forecasts are available from nonprofit service organizations, such as the Color Association of the United States, or from color forecasting services. Companies may also conduct their own color forecasting.

Textile mills focus on fabric production and sell greige goods; some textile mills will finish the fabric as well. Textile design involves the interrelationships among color (e.g., dyeing, printing), fabric structure (e.g., woven, knitted), and finishes (e.g., napping, embossing). Textile converters specialize in fabric finishing. They buy greige goods and finish the fabric according to textile mills', apparel manufacturers', or retailers' specifications. Other fabric resources include textile jobbers, textile brokers, and fabric retail stores. Through quality assurance programs, textile mills, apparel manufacturers, and retailers test textiles according to standards for end-use products. Textile mills and converters market their textile fabrics as Fall/Winter and Spring/Summer seasonal lines in showrooms and at textile trade shows held throughout the world.

In order to compete successfully in a global economy, the U.S. textile industry continues to invest in new technology to increase the productivity of textile mills and improve communication among textile mills, their suppliers, and their customers. These investments in technology are part of Quick Response and supply chain management strategies, designed to shorten the time from fiber to finished product. Nanotechnology and "smart" fibers and materials are paving the way for high-tech fabrics for a variety of specialized end uses.

The textile industry is addressing environmental concerns through manufacturing and by making available to consumers products that include organic or recycled materials, are produced with less-toxic materials such as low-impact dyes, use less water in production, or have incorporated other environmentally responsible processes.

CAREER PROFILES

Careers in the textile industry are as varied as the industry itself. Textile chemist, textile designer, textile production supervisor, and textile marketer are just a few of the many careers available in this industry.

Textile Designer
Product Development Department, Publicly Held Retailer

Position Description:

Part of a dynamic product development team responsible for creating private-label merchandise for a major publicly held retail corporation. Work with textile mills in designing fabrics to be used in private-label merchandise.

Typical Tasks and Responsibilities:

- Create color artwork for prints, stripes, and yarn dyes using CAD.
- Approve lab dips for production use.
- Track lab dip status.
- Prepare presentation boards.
- Travel overseas.

Independent Sales Representative
Fabrics and Trims

Position Description:

Show lines of fabrics and trims to designers and merchandisers, send samples, help design products, follow up with vendors to see that goods are delivered through production, negotiate prices, and make presentation books and boards.

Typical Tasks and Responsibilities;

- Drive to accounts in several states and Canada—traveling two to three days per week minimum.
- Show lines to designers and merchandisers.
- Pack and unpack sample bags.
- Keep price lists organized.
- Manage the office and finances; purchase supplies and office equipment.
- Work with purchasing agents.
- Write orders, follow-up letters, and price quotes.
- File, update files and materials, and keep the office clean.

Key Terms

brand name

cashmere

color forecasting

color forecasting service

color story

concept garment

controlled brand name program

converted goods

converter

cotton

digital printing

fabric construction

fabrication

fiber

filament yarn

finished goods

finishing

generic family

greige goods

hide

horizontally integrated

kip

licensed brand name program

mohair

nanotechnology

pelt

quality assurance

quality control

regular tannery

skin

"smart" fiber

spun yarn

tanning

tawning

textile

textile converter

textile jobber

textile mill

textile stylist

textile testing

throwster

trade association

trade name

trade show

vertically integrated

wool

yarn

Discussion Questions and Activities

1. What are the advantages and disadvantages to a textile company being horizontally integrated? Vertically integrated? How are the advantages and disadvantages of each type of integration related to the types of textile companies that are horizontally and vertically integrated?

2. Follow a cotton/polyester blend woven fabric from the fiber production to the marketing of the fabric to apparel manufacturers. What are the primary stages of production and marketing? Give the approximate time frame for this process.

3. What are the differences between the production and marketing of natural fibers and manufactured fibers? Why do these differences exist?

4. What roles do trade associations play in the promotion of natural and manufactured fibers? Give examples of the activities performed by trade associations. Bring in examples of cooperative advertising between trade associations and end-use producers.

5. What are greige goods? Why are converters important in creating the end-use products that can best meet the needs of consumers?

6. Select an item of clothing, such as a jacket or coat. How many different textiles and fibers are used to make the garment?

7. Form debate groups to debate whether cotton is enviromentally more or less harmful to the ecosystem than polyester; or whether disposible or cloth diapers are better when balancing production costs, water and energy use, and disposal.

References

Bide, M (2009, July) Fiber sustainablity: green is not black + white. *AATCC* Review. Vol 9 (7) p34–37.

Bureau of Labor Statistics (2010). U.S. Department of Labor, Textile, Textile Product, and Apparel Manufacturing. Retrieved December 10, 2010, from http://www.bls.gov/oco/cg/cgs015.htm

Campbell, J.R. and Kim, Eundeok. (1999, November). Concepts in digital textile printing that affect the approach to textile design. Proceedings Annual Meeting of the Textile and Apparel Association. Santa Fe, NM, pp. 113–114.

Fur Commission USA (2010). Fur farming in North America. Retrieved December 10, 2010, from http://www.furcommission.com/farming/index.html

Kadolph, Sara J., and Langford, Anna L. (2002). *Textiles* (9th ed.). NY: Fairchild Publications.

Mohair Council of America www.mohairusa.com

Nanotechnology's new potential in apparel machinery (2006, September 8). Just-style.com. Retrived September 8, 2006 from http://www.just-style.com

National Cotton Council of America (2010). World of Cotton. Retrieved December 10, 2010, from http://www.cotton.org/econ/world/detail.cfm

National Council of Textile Organizations (2010). About NCTO. Retrieved December 10, 2010, from http://www.ncto.org

North American Industry Classification System (2010). Definitions: 313 textile mills. Retrieved December 10, 2010, from http://www.census.gov/epcd/naics02/def/NDEF313.HTM#N313

Organic Trade Association (2010). Organic Wool Fact Sheet. Retrieved December 10, 2010, from http://www.ota.com/organic/environment/wool.html

Rudie, Raye. (1994, February). How green is the future? *Bobbin*, pp. 16–20.

Schiro, Anne-Marie. (1995, May 7). Mills weave trends in fabric of fashion. *The Oregonian*, p. L16.

Sustainable Style Foundation (2010). About us. Retrieved December 10, 2010, from http://www.sustainablestyle.org

Vreseis, Ltd. (2007). Sally Fox: Innovation in the field. [online]. Retrieved April 15, 2007, from http://www.vreseis.com

CHAPTER 4

Ready-to-Wear:
Company Organization

In this chapter, you will learn the following:

- the difference between the ready-to-wear industry and haute couture

- the various types of ready-to-wear companies

- the organizational structure of apparel and accessory companies

- the merchandising philosophies of apparel and accessory companies

- the primary trade associations and trade publications in the apparel industry

*The majority of apparel and accessories produced and sold is called **ready-to-wear (RTW)**. As the term implies, the apparel is completely made and ready to be worn (except for finishing details, such as pants hemming in tailored clothing) at the time it is purchased. In the United Kingdom, this merchandise is called* off-the-peg; *in France, it is called **prêt-à-porter**; and in Italy, it is called* moda pronto. *RTW apparel is made in large quantities using mass-manufacturing processes that require little or no hand sewing.*

Ready-to-Wear: What Does It Mean?

Many apparel and accessory companies produce seasonal lines or collections of merchandise. Lines or collections are groups of styles designed for a particular **fashion season**. The primary difference between a line and a collection is the cost of the merchandise—the term **collection** typically refers to more expensive merchandise. Often name designers will create and offer collections; other apparel companies will offer **lines**.

Apparel and accessory companies typically produce four to six new collections or lines per year, corresponding to the fashion seasons: Spring, Summer, Fall I, Fall II, Holiday, and Resort or Cruise. These fashion seasons coincide with the times consumers would most likely wear the merchandise, not to when companies design or manufacture the merchandise or when the merchandise is delivered to stores. For example, a company may start to design a Fall season line in September, market the line in March, actually manufacture it from March through April, and deliver the merchandise to the stores in June.

Not all companies produce lines for all six fashion seasons. The number of lines a company will produce depends on both the product category and the target market (the group of customers for whom the line is designed). For example, a company that produces men's tailored suits may create only two lines per year (Fall and Spring), whereas a men's sportswear company may create five lines per year (Fall I, Fall II, Holiday, Spring, and Summer). Some companies produce more than six lines per year. A number of apparel and accessory companies produce smaller lines that are shipped to retailers more frequently; the frequent infusion of new merchandise appeals to customers. Fast fashion companies such as Zara, H&M, and Forever 21 create lines that are delivered to stores every few weeks. Many companies that produce store brands (e.g., Victoria's Secret, Ann Taylor, Express) or other forms of private label merchandise (e.g., Worthington for JCPenney) also ship goods to their retail stores frequently. Chapters 5 and 6 discuss in more detail the development of collections and lines.

As discussed in Chapter 1, the standardization of sizing was necessary for the development of the ready-to-wear industry. Sizes in RTW are based on a combination of standardized body dimensions, company size standards, and wearing and design ease. Clothing sizes were developed by grouping computed average circumference measurements of a large group of people (of average height) into specific size categories. For example, the men's size 42 relates to an "average height" (5 feet 10 inches to 6 feet) male with a chest circumference of 42 inches and waist of 36 inches. These body measurements or dimensions are what are referred to as the standardized size. Standardized tables of body dimensions are available from the American Society for Testing and Materials (ASTM) for various figure types.

The apparel industry does not adhere strictly to the "set" standardized sizes. A company may develop its "company size" based on a target customer with a smaller waist in comparison to the hip circumference, or a larger chest in comparison to the waist circumference. The term *athletic fit* is used to refer to a men's suit built to fit the male body with a larger chest-to-waist ratio than the standardized size (for example, a size 42 athletic fit might be based on a chest circumference of 42 inches and a waist circumference of 35 inches). Because of the wide variety of body types, companies will focus on the "company size" that is most appropriate for their target customer. This is why many consumers find that one brand of apparel fits them better than other brands.

As nonstore retailing (e.g. catalogs, Internet) of apparel has increased, direct-marketing apparel companies have worked to develop consistent body measurements and related size measurements for all styles that the company produces. A fit that can be determined accurately from a catalog's or website's body measurement chart can reduce returns and thus increase customer satisfaction with the product and the company.

The size chart lists the body measurements for the company's apparel. Wearing ease and design ease allowances are added to the body measurements to create the garment measurements. Each company decides how much wearing ease and design ease to add to create the "look" for the company. Some styles are designed to fit more loosely than other styles. The company sizing will reflect these style aspects. Each company's size range is based on its predetermined body measurements, plus ease. The size measurements increase and decrease in specified increments from the base or sample size to create the size range. The size increments used to create the various sizes are discussed in more detail in Chapter 9.

A national sizing survey was completed in 2003 using 3-D body scanning technology (see Chapter 11). Approved by the U. S. Department of Commerce, the project, called Size USA, set up body scanning sites in more than 12 large cities across the United States and collected body measurement data from thousands of consumers. Part of the funding for this survey was provided by apparel producers, including JCPenney, Sears, Liz Claiborne, VF Corporation, Dillard's, Target, Russell, and Lands' End (for more information, see http://www.sizeusa.com). [TC]² provided the scanning equipment. A similar survey was conducted in the United Kingdom. Apparel companies may access the enormous data bank of body dimensions provided by this survey. With the quantity of new data available, the development of new and adapted size ranges, such as those targeted to specific age or ethnic groups, are possible.

The Difference between Ready-to-Wear and Couture

Designer names, such as Chanel, Christian Dior, and Yves Saint Laurent, first became famous in the realm of French haute couture (high fashion) and later became associated with expensive ready-to-wear. Because of the continued prominence and importance of these designer labels, it is important to understand the distinction and the relationship between couture and ready-to-wear. **Couture** is a French term that literally means "sewing." In general, couture apparel is distinguished by the following characteristics:

- produced in smaller quantities
- utilizes considerable hand-sewing techniques
- sized to fit an individual's body measurements

Generally, more expensive fabrics are used in couture apparel than in RTW.

The term couture is derived from **haute couture** (pronounced oat coo-tur), which literally means "high sewing." As discussed in Chapter 1, the haute couture industry developed in Paris during the nineteenth century. At that time, apparel was produced by dressmakers and tailors who custom-fit each garment to the client. The garment's style and fabric were selected for or by each client, the client's body measurements were taken, and the garment was completed after one or more fittings during the construction process. For persons who did not have personal dressmakers or tailors, apparel was produced in the home by whoever had the necessary skills.

Selecting a fabric and creating a garment prior to an order from a client was a new concept, attributed to Charles Frederick Worth, the founder of the haute couture business during the second half of the nineteenth century. He created several gowns, which were modeled by his wife. Clients came into his shop and selected a style to be copied for them, custom-fit to their body measurements. Soon he had a clientele of wealthy and noble patrons. He used exquisite fabrics and trims and employed a bevy of seamstresses to complete the intricate handwork. In time, other designers followed Worth's lead, and the haute couture business was formed. These designers "created" new fashions, while the rest of the western fashion world followed their lead.

During the early twentieth century, the *Chambre Syndicale de la Couture* was formed by the French Ministry for Industry to provide an organizational structure and to offer protection for designers against their designs being copied. Currently, the *Chambre Syndicale* does the following:

- arranges the calendar for the showings of the collections twice per year
- organizes accreditation for press and buyers who want to attend the showings
- assists the couture houses so each gains the maximum press coverage possible

In Summer 2010, there were 11 official members of the *Chambre Syndicale* and, therefore, they could be called couture houses: Adeline André, Anne Valérie Hash, Carlota Alfaro, Chanel, Christian Dior, Jean Paul Gaultier, Givenchy, Dominique Sirop, Franck Sorbier, Maurizio Galante, and Stéphane Rolland. Foreign correspondent members include Elie Saab, Giorgio Armani, Maison Martin Margiela, and Valentino. To be a member of the Paris haute couture requires specific qualifications, including the following:

- the use of one's own "house" seamstresses
- the presentation of Fall/Winter and Spring/Summer collections each year
- adherence to the dates of showings set by the *Chambre Syndicale*
- registration of the original designs to protect against copying

Each designer's business is called a **couture house**. Thus, there is the House of Dior, the House of Givenchy, and the House of Chanel. The haute couture designer is called the **couturier** (or **couturière** if the designer is a woman) or the "head of the house." Whereas some couturiers control their own businesses, many couture houses are owned by corporations that finance them. In recent years, some financial backers have been known to hire and fire head designers frequently. A Paris haute couture designer typically has a **boutique** (store) located on one of several "fashion avenues" in Paris. The boutique sells the designer's licensed products, such as perfume, scarves, jewelry and other accessories, and home fashions. Some boutiques sell boutique collections of apparel as well as shoes.

The **salon de couture** is the showroom of the couture designer. The salon is typically located on the second floor of the building that houses the designer's boutique. Entry to the second level, the salon, is limited to those with invitations to a collection show. The **atelier** (pronounced ah-tal´-lee-aye) **de couture**, or workrooms, may be on the floors above the salon or in a separate building.

The twice-per-year Paris haute couture collection openings continue to be huge events in the fashion world and are covered in detail by the fashion press (see Figure 4.1). Fall/Winter fashion season haute couture collections are typically shown in July, and Spring/Summer fashion season haute couture collections are typically shown in January. The press, buyers, other designers, celebrities, and wealthy clients are in attendance. While the fashion influence of the couturiers waxes and wanes, the designs presented are considered to represent a laboratory of design creativity.

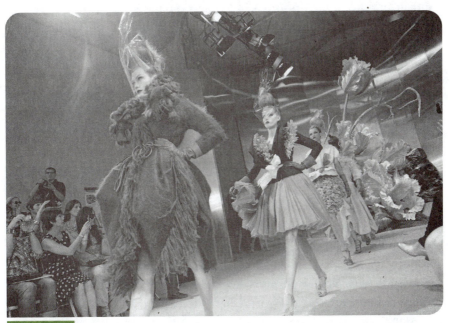

Figure 4.1 Paris haute couture collections, such as Dior Haute Couture, attract extensive press coverage.

Paris haute couture houses also produce RTW (*prêt-à-porter*) collections. These RTW collections may be sold in the house boutique, in freestanding boutiques, or in upscale department or specialty stores. Currently, all haute couture houses offer prêt-à-porter collections.

In addition to the couturiers who are members of the *Chambre Syndicale*, there are other designers who consider themselves to be couture designers. Generally, a couture designer is distinguished by the following:

- uses high-quality fabrics
- creates original designs (as opposed to copying another's designs)
- uses high-quality construction and hand-finishing details
- custom-fits the garment to a client's body measurements

Couture designers may produce all custom work (ordered by a specific client), or they may present a seasonal collection and then take custom orders selected from the collection. There are couture designers in New York, Los Angeles, and other cities around the world.

The term *couture* is sometimes used in the apparel industry to impart an elite ambience to an apparel collection. For example, an apparel company might produce a high-priced RTW collection and call it a couture collection. Indeed, some stores even have what they call couture departments. However, if mass-production techniques are used in producing the apparel, and if garments are not custom-fit to the client, the line should be called RTW and *not* couture.

Types of RTW Apparel and Accessory Producers

From large corporations to small companies, from those that produce innovative, trendy merchandise to those that produce classics, RTW companies come in all types and sizes and vary tremendously in their organization. Because of the diversity found in RTW apparel company organization, any attempt to classify types of apparel producers is difficult. However, according to industry analysts, the major types of apparel suppliers can be grouped into the following categories: manufacturers, jobbers, contractors, and licensors.

Manufacturers perform all functions of creating, marketing, and distributing an apparel line on a continual basis. These companies may make products in their own plant(s) or factories (e.g., American Apparel), but they typically use outside companies, or contractors, to perform the manufacturing function. Manufacturers include the following:

- multidivision companies that produce several product lines of nationally advertised merchandise (e.g., Levi Strauss & Co., VF Corporation)
- companies that specialize in one or more product categories, such as infants' and children's wear (e.g., Carter's) or fleece wear (e.g., Russell Athletic)

Manufacturers may produce brands of merchandise distributed nationally or regionally, licensed products, or private label merchandise for a specific store. Retail distribution of products will vary depending on the manufacturer.

Jobber is the traditional term for a company that buys fabrics and acquires styles from independent designers, or that copies or designs lines itself, but uses contractors to make its products. This type of company became popular in the early 1900s, with New York (Seventh Avenue) men's and women's apparel companies serving as intermediaries. They carried huge inventories of merchandise and could make prompt deliveries to retailers. As retailers started sending their own buyers to New York, and as resident buyers became more popular, the need for jobbers declined.

Today, because so many apparel producers contract out the manufacturing functions, the use of the term *jobber* is not as widespread as it used to be. Instead, most apparel, accessory, and home fashions producers are referred to as manufacturers, regardless of whether or not they use contractors. In fact, this definition of **manufacturer** offered by industry analysts suggests a broader perspective: "Manufacturers in the apparel industry are the main contractors of apparel production. Some have internal production capabilities, but most contract out a substantial portion of actual production to contractors" (Southern California Edison Company, 1995, Appendix A).

Contractors are companies that specialize in the sewing and finishing of goods. Contractors are used by the following:

- manufacturers who do not own any manufacturing factories and contract all sewing and finishing operations
- manufacturers that lack sufficient capacity in their own plants or have specialized needs for a short time and use contractors to address these needs
- retailers for private label and store brand merchandise

According to the industry definition, "contractors in the apparel industry are the many, usually small factories in which most apparel production actually takes place. Several different types of industry entities source apparel goods from contractors, including manufacturers, retailers, buyers, importers, and trading companies" (Southern California Edison Company, 1995, Appendix A). Most contractors specialize in a product category (e.g., knit tops) or have specialized equipment (e.g., embroidery machines) and skilled workers. The term **item house** is used to describe contractors that specialize in the production of one product. For example, item houses are used in the production of baseball caps. Contractors offer their customers fast turnarounds. **Full-package contractors**, in working with retailers, also offer fabric procurement and apparel design services that were traditionally part of the manufacturers' role.

Some manufacturers and contractors produce goods for the sole use of a particular retailer (or retail corporation) as a private label brand or retail store/direct-market brand merchandise. Some retailers offer a combination of national brands and private label merchandise (e.g., Nordstrom, Macy's), whereas other retailers offer only store brand merchandise (e.g., Gap, The Limited, Eddie Bauer, Talbot's). Some manufacturers and contractors will produce merchandise for both national brands and private label or store brands; other manufacturers and contractors will produce merchandise for one national or private label/store brand only.

Licensors are companies that have developed a well-known designer name (e.g., Calvin Klein, Donna Karan, Ralph Lauren), brand name (e.g., Guess?, Hang Ten), or character (e.g., Mickey Mouse, Barbie, Beauty and the Beast) and sell the use of these names or characters to companies to put onto merchandise. As discussed in Chapter 2, successful licensing depends on a well-known name or image (property). It should be noted that these categories are not mutually exclusive. For example, a manufacturer may use a contractor or may license its brand name to a company that produces product categories different from its own. The details of these various types of apparel production will be discussed in later chapters.

Classifications and Categories of Apparel and Accessory Producers

Apparel and accessory producers are classified in the following ways:

- by the type of merchandise they produce
- by the wholesale prices of the products or brands
- by an industry classification system for governmental tracking

An examination of these classification systems is in order to better understand the diversity of apparel organizations.

Gender/Age, Size Range, Product Category

The apparel and accessory industries are divided into the primary categories of men's, women's, and children's apparel and accessory (including footwear) manufacturers. Some companies produce apparel and accessories in only one of these categories; others produce apparel and accessories for more than one. In some cases, companies began as producers of one category of apparel and/or accessory; then they branched out into one or more other categories as the companies grew. For example, Levi Strauss & Co. began as a producer of men's apparel, and later expanded into women's and children's wear. Nike started as a sport footwear company and expanded into apparel and sports equipment.

The separate gender/age categories have their roots in the early history of the U.S. apparel and accessory industries. Apparel and accessory producers specialized in one category because of a variety of factors. The types of machinery used for producing men's apparel were often different from the types needed for women's apparel. The sizing standards developed differently for men's, women's, and children's apparel and footwear. The number of seasonal lines produced per year differs for each category; therefore, the production cycle varies.

The organizational structure of retail stores is related to these categories of apparel, another reason why the apparel and accessory industries remains divided into the three primary categories of men's, women's, and children's apparel and accessories. Retail buyers are often assigned responsibilities in one of the three categories of apparel and accessories. For example, a menswear buyer buys apparel for the retail store from men's apparel producers. This allows the producers and retailer to establish and maintain profitable working relationships.

Within each of the three primary categories, apparel producers are subdivided into additional categories. Apparel producers generally specialize in one or several subcategories. These subcategories relate to the classification of apparel. Apparel classifications are by type of garment produced (product type). Traditional classifications by product type for women's apparel include the following:

- outerwear (coats, jackets, and rainwear)
- dresses
- blouses
- career wear (suits, separates, and career wear dresses)
- sportswear and active sportswear (separates, such as pants, sweaters, and skirts; and active sportswear, such as swimwear and tennis wear)

- evening wear and special occasion
- bridal and bridesmaid dresses
- maternity wear
- uniforms
- furs
- accessories
- intimate apparel, which is further classified into the following categories:
  – foundations (girdles or body shapers, bras, and other shape wear)
  – lingerie (petticoats, slips, panties, camisoles, nightgowns, and pajamas)
  – loungewear (at-home wear, robes, and bed jackets,)

Foundations and lingerie worn under other clothing are sometimes referred to as *innerwear*. In addition, lingerie and loungewear are sometimes divided into daywear and nightwear.

The various subcategories are organized by size category and clothing classification (see Table 4.1). For example, some apparel companies manufacture apparel only in the misses (also referred to as *missy*) or the junior-size category. Some companies produce apparel in misses and women's (large) sizes, while other companies manufacture misses, women's, petite, and tall sizes. Figure 4.2

Table 4.1 Children's, Men's, and Women's Wear Categories and Size Ranges

CHILDREN'S WEAR

Subcategories (organized by gender and size)

Infants	sized by weight/height or sizes 0 to 3 months (or newborn, 3 months), 6 to 9 months (or 6 months, 9 months), 12 months, 18 months, 24 months, or S-M-L-XL
Toddler	sizes 2T, 3T, 4T, 5T
Boys	sizes 4, 5, 6, 7, and 8 to 20 (even numbers only). Also Slim sizes 4S, 5S, 6S, 7S, and 8S to 20S (even numbers only), and Husky sizes 8H to 26H (even numbers only), or S-M-L-XL-XXL
Girls	sizes 4, 5, 6, 6X, and 7, 8, 10, 12, 14, 16, 18. Also Slim sizes 4S, 5S, 6S, 7S, and 8S to 16S (even numbers only), or S-M-L-XL
Girls Plus	sizes 8 1/2 to 20 1/2 (even numbers only), or 7+, 8+, 10+, 12+, 14+, 16+, 18+, 20+, or M-L-XL
Preteen (girls)	sizes 6 to 16 or 8 PT to 16 PT (even numbers only)
Young Junior	sizes 3 to 13 (odd numbers only)

Table 4.1   Children's, Men's, and Women's Wear Categories and Size Ranges *(continued)*

MENSWEAR

Subcategories (organized by classification of apparel)

Tailored clothing	**suits, sport coats, evening wear (tuxedos), overcoats:** sizes: 36, 38, 39, 40, 41, 42, 43, 44, 45, 46, 48, 50, 52, 54, 56, 58, 60 based on chest circumference. lengths: Regular, Short, Long, Extra Long Regular, Athletic, and Portly fit **separate trousers:** sized by waist (29 to 44)/hemmed at retailer
Sportswear	**sport shirts:** sizes S-M-L-XL-XXL-XXXL **pants:** sized by waist/inseam (29 to 44 waist and 28 to 34 inseam), or sizes S-M-L-XL **casual jackets:** sizes 36 to 50 or S-M-L-XL. Also Tall, Extra Regular, Big & Tall sizes
Furnishings	**shirts:** sized by neck/sleeve length (e.g., 16/34), or S-M-L-XL-XXL sizes **sweaters:** sizes S-M-L-XL-XXL **underwear:** sized by waist size **robes and pajamas:** sizes S-M-L-XL-XXL **neckwear:** sizes regular, long, and extra long **socks** (based on shoe size)
Active sportswear, swimwear, athletic wear, windbreakers	sizes S-M-L-XL-XXL-XXXL may include Tall and Big & Tall sizes
Uniforms and work wear	**overalls, work pants:** sized by waist/inseam, or S-M-L-XL-XXL-XXXL **work shirts:** sizes S-M-L-XL-XXL-XXXL Regular, Tall, Big & Tall sizes

WOMEN'S WEAR

Classifications include: outerwear, dresses, career wear, blouses, sportswear and active sportswear, evening, bridal, maternity, uniforms, furs, intimate apparel, accessories

Misses	sizes 0 to 18 (even numbers only: 2, 4, 6, 8, 10, 12, 14, 16, 18), or sizes XS-S-M-L-XL
Women's (large size, queen, plus, custom)	sizes 14W to 26W (even numbers only), or Plus sizes 1X, 2X, 3X
Petite (under 5'4")	sizes 0P to 16P, under 5'4" (even numbers only)
Women's Petite	14WP to 20 WP (even sizes only)
Tall (over 5'9")	sizes 10T to 18T (even numbers only)
Junior	sizes 1 to 15 (odd numbers only)
Junior Petite	sizes 1JP to 15JP (odd numbers only)

Note: Not all companies produce the entire size range in the size categories listed.

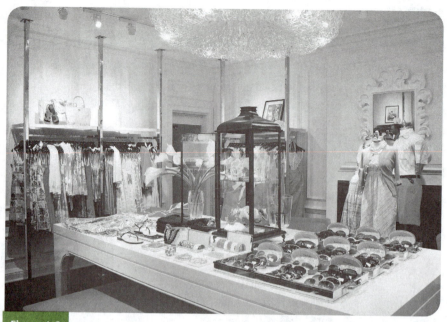

Figure 4.2 Women's apparel includes size categories including misses (missy), junior, and women's.

shows how the measurements in several different size categories vary. Within one size range, an apparel producer may manufacture clothing in one or more of the product classifications previously listed.

In addition to the difference between size categories of misses and junior apparel, there are styling differences as well (see Figure 4.3). The junior size range is designed for a customer who is approximately 16 to 22 years old, whereas the misses size category is designed for a target customer who is approximately 22 years old and upward. The styling, fabrics, and trims of misses apparel have a more mature fashion look than that of junior apparel.

Traditional menswear classifications include the following:

- tailored clothing (structured or semi-structured suits, coats, and separates, such as sport jackets and dress slacks)
- sportswear (casual pants, including jeans)
- furnishings (dress shirts and casual shirts; sweaters; neckties, handkerchiefs, and other accessory items; underwear and night wear; hosiery; and hats and caps)
- active sportswear (athletic clothing, including golf wear, tennis wear, swimwear)
- uniforms and work wear (work shirts and pants, overalls)

Table 4.1 lists these classifications and typical sizes offered. The number of seasonal lines produced per year in menswear varies with the classification of apparel. Tailored-clothing producers tend to develop a large Fall line and a somewhat smaller Spring line, while most sportswear producers develop four to six seasonal lines per year.

In children's wear, the subcategories are organized by age-related size categories and by gender (see Table 4.1). Many children's wear manufacturers produce apparel in both infant and toddler sizes. In the older-size categories, apparel companies usually specialize in either boys' wear or girls' wear. Seasonal lines produced in children's wear typically include Back-to-School (the largest line), Holiday, Spring, and Summer lines.

Price Zones

Ready-to-wear apparel companies typically specialize in one or more **price zones** or **price points**. These categories are based on either the approximate wholesale price of the merchandise or the suggested retail price of the merchandise.

The price zone categories include the following:

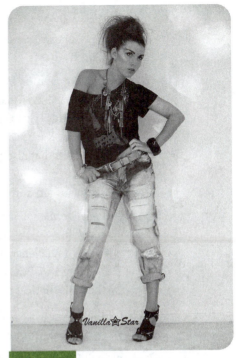

Figure 4.3 Junior apparel is differentiated from misses (missy) apparel through sizing for a younger customer and trendier styling.

- *Designer:* The designer price zone is the most expensive of the price zones. It includes collections of name designers such as Calvin Klein, Donna Karan, Vera Wang, Giorgio Armani, and Chanel, as well as collections of brands such as St. John Knits. Although this category is sometimes referred to as *couture*, it should not be confused with couture apparel that is custom-made to the body measurements of an individual.

- *Bridge:* Bridge lines traditionally fall between designer and better price zones. These may include designers' less expensive lines, sometimes called **diffusion lines** (e.g., Armani Collezioni), or those brands that are situated between designer and better price zones (e.g., Eileen Fisher, Adrienne Vittadini).

- *Better:* Lines in the better price zone are generally nationally known brand names, such as Emporio Armani, DKNY in women's wear, or Nautica in menswear. Many store brands (e.g., Banana Republic) and private label merchandise (goods that carry the retailer's name) are also in this price zone (e.g., Nordstrom's Caslon and Classiques Entier brands).

- *Moderate:* Lines in the moderate price zone include nationally known sportswear brand names (e.g., Dockers, Guess?, Jones New York Sport) or store brands (e.g., Gap, A/X Armani Exchange) and other reasonably priced lines (e.g., Kasper suits). Moderate lines also include less expensive lines of companies that also produce better merchandise (e.g., Mexx). Private label and store brand merchandise may also be in this price zone (e.g., JCPenney's Arizona brand and Macy's INC International Concepts brand).

- *Budget or mass:* Found primarily at mass merchandisers and discount stores, budget lines are the least expensive of the price zones. These may include store brands of retailers with low prices as a competitive strategy (e.g., Old Navy—see Figure 4.4). Private label merchandise for discount stores is also considered to be in the budget price zone category (e.g., Kmart's Jaclyn Smith brand).

It is important to note that the price zones can be considered a continuum for classification purposes. For example, some lines may be considered to be between budget and moderate, while others may be considered between moderate and better. Also, a brand may be offered in the bridge price zone as direct-mail

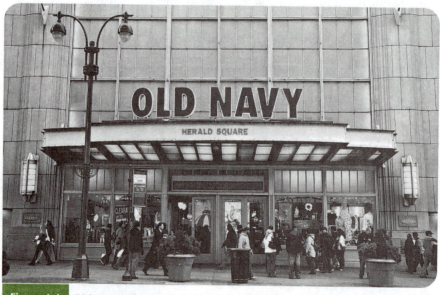

Figure 4.4 Old Navy offers store brands in the budget price zone.

merchandise, while the same brand may be offered in the designer price zone at retail stores. Some companies produce labels in several price zones, or brand tiers. Giorgio Armani includes the Giorgio Armani label, the Emporio label, and the A/X Armani Exchange label, each targeted for a different price zone.

Brand Name Classifications

Apparel and accessory companies also vary in the brands they produce. Brand names fall into one of the following categories:

- *International designer brands:* some designers have international recognition and sell their licensed merchandise through boutiques or other high-end retail venues. Examples include Armani, Chanel, and Calvin Klein.

- *National/local designer brands:* some designers have more local or national recognition and sell their merchandise through boutiques in their community or country (Figure 4.5).

- *International name brands:* Some companies have established international recognition as a brand name. Examples include companies such as Nike and Adidas as well as store brands such as H&M and Zara.

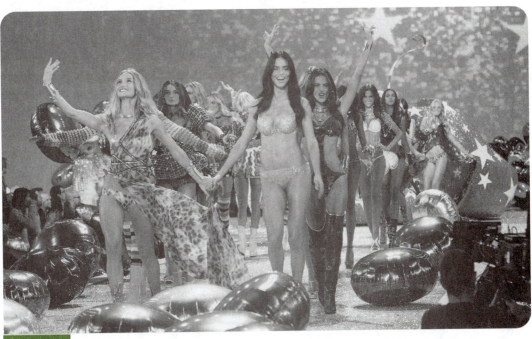

Figure 4.5 Victoria's Secret is an example of a retail store/direct market brand or "store brand."

- *Private label brands:* A **private label brand** is specific to a particular retailer who oversees the design and marketing of the brand. Examples include JCPenney's Worthington label and exclusive licensing agreements, such as Target's Mossimo private label brands.

- *Retail store/direct market brands:* In some cases, the retailer and the brand are one in the same. These are sometimes referred to as **store brands**. Examples include Gap, Banana Republic, A&F, Victoria's Secret, and L.L.Bean.

- *Lifestyle brands:* A **lifestyle brand** is a term used to describe brands that are associated with a particular target customer's activities and way of life. Tommy Bahama is a good example of a lifestyle brand as the merchandise is associated with the lifestyle of individuals who live or vacation in tropical locations.

- *All other brands:* In addition to these brands, licensed merchandise and specialized brands exist. Examples include Wilson, Mickey & Co., and Looney Tunes/Warner Bros.

North American Industry Classification System

The U.S. Department of Commerce categorizes companies based on their chief industrial activity. Industry data is often compiled and reported according to these categories. In the past, Standard Industrial Classification (SIC) numbers were used. With the phasing out of the SIC system, the **North American Industry Classification System (NAICS)** was created. In this classification system, industry sectors in the United States, Mexico, and Canada can be compared. The following are primary NAICS groups for textiles and apparel:

- NAICS 313: Textile Mills
- NAICS 314: Textile Product Mills (produce non-apparel textile products)
- NAICS 315: Apparel Manufacturing
- NAICS 316: Leather and Allied Product Manufacturing

Within these major groups, additional numbers are used to designate more specific products (e.g., 31521 refers to cut-and-sew apparel contractors). Table 4.2 lists the NAICS categories for textiles and apparel.

Table 4.2 North American Industry Classification System (NAICS)

313 Textile Mills

Industries in the Textile Mills subsector are establishments that transform a basic fiber (natural or synthetic) into a product, such as yarn or fabric, that is further manufactured into usable items, such as apparel, sheets, towels, and textile bags for individual or industrial consumption. The further manufacturing may be performed in the same establishment and classified in this subsector, or it may be performed at a separate establishment and be classified elsewhere in manufacturing.

The main processes in this subsector include preparation and spinning of fiber, knitting or weaving of fabric, and the finishing of the textile. The NAICS structure follows and captures this process flow. Major industries in this flow, such as preparation of fibers, weaving of fabric, knitting of fabric, and fiber and fabric finishing, are uniquely identified. Texturizing, throwing, twisting, and winding of yarn contain aspects of both fiber preparation and fiber finishing and are classified with preparation of fibers rather than with finishing of fiber.

314 Textile Product Mills

Industries in the Textile Product Mills subsector are establishments that make textile products (except apparel). With a few exceptions, processes used in these industries are generally cut and sew (i.e., purchasing fabric and cutting and sewing to make nonapparel textile products, such as sheets and towels).

315 Apparel Manufacturing

Industries in the Apparel Manufacturing subsector are establishments with two distinct manufacturing processes: (1) cut and sew (i.e., purchasing fabric and cutting and sewing to make a garment); and (2) the manufacture of garments in establishments that first knit fabric, and then cut and sew the fabric into a garment. The Apparel Manufacturing subsector includes a diverse range of establishments manufacturing full lines of ready-to-wear apparel and custom apparel: apparel contractors, performing cutting or sewing operations on materials owned by others; jobbers, performing entrepreneurial functions involved in apparel manufacture; and tailors, manufacturing custom garments for individual clients are all included. Knitting, when done alone, is classified in the Textile Mills subsector, but when knitting is combined with the production of complete garments, the activity is classified in Apparel Manufacturing.

Table 4.2	North American Industry Classification System (NAICS) *(continued)*

316 Leather and Allied Product Manufacturing

Establishments in the Leather and Allied Product Manufacturing subsector transform hides into leather by tanning or curing and fabricating the leather into products for final consumption. It also includes the manufacture of similar products from other materials, including products (except apparel) made from "leather substitutes," such as rubber, plastics, or textiles. Rubber footwear, textile luggage, and plastic purses or wallets are examples of "leather substitute" products included in this group. The products made from leather substitutes are included in this subsector because they are made in similar ways leather products are made (e.g., luggage). They are made in the same establishments, so it is not practical to separate them.

The inclusion of leather making in this subsector is partly because leather tanning is a relatively small industry that has few close neighbors as a production process, partly because leather is an input to some of the other products classified in this subsector, and partly for historical reasons.

SOURCE: U.S. Census Bureau (http://www.census.gov/epcd/naics02/naicod02.htm).

Organizational Structure of Apparel Companies

The organizational structure of a typical apparel company is shown in Figure 4.6. Although companies will vary in terms of their exact organizational structure, the following activities are often included:

* research and merchandising
* design and product development
* sales and marketing
* operations
* advertising and sales promotion
* finance and information technology

Very large companies may have separate departments or divisions with dozens of employees who handle each of these activities. On the other hand, in very small companies, a few employees may handle several of these activities.

In reviewing Figure 4.6, it is important to note the connections among all of the areas or divisions. Communication among the various activities is imperative for the success of the company. Merchandisers must communicate with designers; designers must communicate with production management and marketers; those in information technology must understand the computer needs of all areas. This can be a challenge for large companies.

Research and Merchandising

The term **merchandising** generally refers to the process of synthesizing information to make decisions regarding the characteristics of merchandise manufactured and/or sold by a company (e.g., product category, price, promotion, retail venue, etc.) This process includes conducting necessary trend and market research and developing strategies to get the right merchandise, at the right

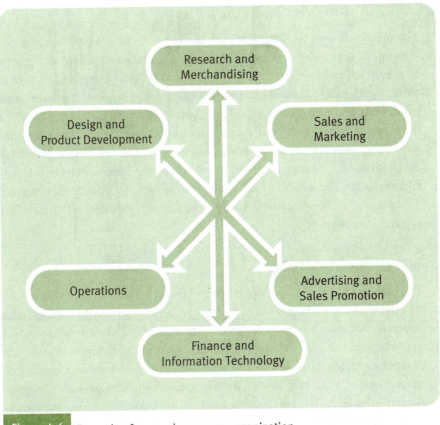

Figure 4.6 Example of apparel company organization

price, at the right time, in the right amount, to the right locations to meet the wants and needs of the target customer.

The merchandising area of apparel and accessory companies may include merchandise managers, merchandise coordinators, and fashion directors. These individuals research and forecast fashion trends and trends in consumer purchasing behavior in order to develop color, fabric, and garment silhouette directions for the company's merchandise. When making these forecasts, merchandisers interpret these trends for the company's target market, which is determined by their customer's age, gender, income, and lifestyle. The role of merchandisers in apparel and accessories companies can vary. In some companies, they facilitate the creation of lines; in other companies, they oversee the fashion direction of the company. The merchandising function of the apparel company is discussed in greater detail later in this chapter and in Chapter 5.

Design and Product Development

The merchandisers work closely with those in the design and product development area, who interpret the trend forecasts and create designs to be manufactured by the company. Generally, merchandisers and designers work together on the seasonal and line planning. Those in the design and product development area include designers, assistant designers, product developers, stylists, pattern makers, and sample sewers. For companies that have their own factories, the design and product development area may also include the management and operation of the company-owned factories, including the employment and training of sewing operators. Chapters 5 through 7 focus on the design and product development activities of an apparel company.

Sales and Marketing

The sales and marketing area of the apparel company works to sell the company's merchandise to the retail buyers. The sales and marketing division includes regional sales managers and sales representatives, as well as those who conduct marketing research for the company. The sales and marketing staff show the company's merchandise to retail buyers in the company's showrooms during market weeks and at trade shows (see Figure 4.7). Some companies will employ their own sales staff; others will contract with independent sales representatives to handle their merchandise. Chapter 8 discusses the marketing and sales activities of an apparel/accessory company.

Operations

The operations area includes the pre-production, material management, quality assurance, sourcing, production, distribution, and logistics functions. The preproduction, production, material management, and quality assurance areas of an apparel/accessory company include those people involved with the material inspection and buying, production (see Figure 4.8), and quality assurance. (Some companies refer to these activities as product engineering.) It also includes those who identify and monitor domestic and foreign contractors to sew the garments, if the company contracts out these services. Once produced, merchandise is shipped and distributed to retailers. Chapters 9 through 11 focus on production, planning, and control. Chapter 12 focuses on distribution strategies of apparel companies.

Advertising and Sales Promotion

Working with the design and product development staff and the sales and marketing staff, those in the advertising and sales promotion area focus on creating promotional and advertising strategies and tools to sell the merchandise to the retail buyers and to the ultimate consumer (see Figure 4.9). Often these services are contracted to an outside advertising agency that specializes in these activities.

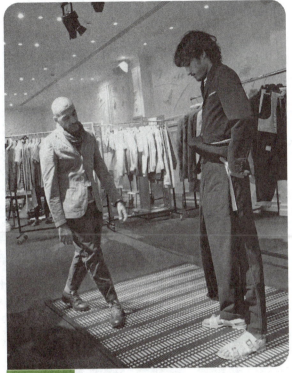

Figure 4.7 Sales and marketing: designer Antonio Marras assists a model at a Kenzo showroom.

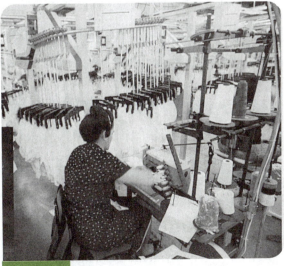

Figure 4.8 Operations: sourcing, production, and quality assurance.

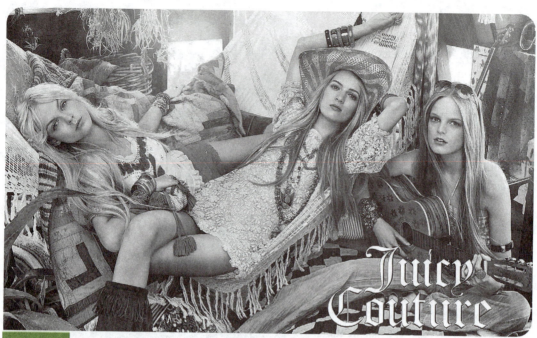

Figure 4.9 Advertising and sales promotion: print advertisement for Juicy Couture.

Finance and Information Technology

Because all companies are in business to make a profit, effective financial management of companies is imperative to their success. More than simply "churning out numbers," those in the finance area of an apparel company are responsible for the overall financial health of companies and work closely with all other areas.

With the increased importance of computer systems in the design and production of products and in the product data management of companies, information technology (IT) areas of companies play important roles in overseeing companies' computer operations. Those who work within IT must have technical expertise, and they must understand the operation of the apparel industry. Some companies have chosen to outsource their information technology area.

Merchandising Philosophies of Apparel and Accessory Companies

With the overall goal of the merchandising area to make a profit by offering merchandise that meets the wants and needs of consumers, merchandisers set the overall direction for the merchandise assortment and work closely with the other areas of the apparel/accessory company that carry out the design, production, marketing, and distribution of the goods. Effective merchandising and product development depend on the following:

- the company's product category (e.g., men's sportswear, women's dresses, children's outerwear)
- the price zone(s) of its merchandise
- its marketing strategy

Companies can be classified according to their merchandising philosophy, based upon where in the product lifecycle their merchandise belongs:

- ***Design innovators:*** Design innovators depend upon their innovative designs to attract their target market, which is generally composed of fashion innovators (see Figure 4.10). Because their target market represents a very small number of customers, competition among design innovators is intense. The odds of a company succeeding are probably less than one in one hundred. Designers for such fashion-forward companies often rely on their skill, reputation, and advertising to attract customers. Examples

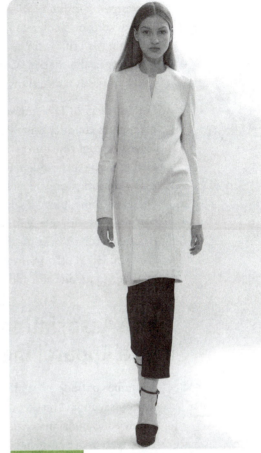

Figure 4.10 A design innovator company, such as Calvin Klein, depends on its innovative designs to attract its target market.

of brands representing design innovator companies include Calvin Klein, Betsey Johnson, Vivienne Westwood, and Anna Sui. Design innovators may also be small companies started by young designers who offer merchandise through boutiques and small specialty stores and who cater to customers who are fashion innovators.

- ***Design or fashion intepreters:*** Rather than creating their own design innovations, a number of companies interpret successful innovative trends of other companies for their own target market. Although design skills and reputation are often key factors in the success of these interpreters, the risk of creating unsuccessful innovations is reduced.

- *Design or fashion imitators:* Imitators are those who produce affordable knockoffs or similar copies of fashions that have received media attention. Timing is crucial for the imitators, who must react immediately to new trends in the market. Companies that quickly reproduce gowns worn by celebrities at award shows (e.g., Academy Awards) are considered imitators.

Regardless of how innovative a company's merchandise is, all successful companies conduct some type of market research and typically obtain direct feedback from consumers on the product line through processes such as style testing. To be successful in today's global economy, companies must accurately assess consumer preferences, based on style testing and analyses of trends in retail sales. Companies get sales information through their own stores or through partnerships with retailers, and they can produce and ship merchandise quickly, often within weeks. As discussed in Chapter 1, fashion companies such as Zara and H&M offer innovative merchandise very quickly by using a variety of methods to predict and address accurately consumers' preferences.

Trade Associations and Trade Publications in the Apparel Industry

A number of trade associations in the apparel industry promote their industry segments, conduct market research, sponsor trade shows, and develop and distribute educational materials related to various segments of the apparel industry. The largest of these associations is the American Apparel & Footwear Association (AAFA), which serves as an umbrella trade association for apparel companies. Representatives of member companies and other professionals in the industry are active in many committees. Activities of the AAFA include the following:

- compilation of statistical information related to apparel manufacturing, industry forecasts, and trend forecasts
- publication of educational materials and information for use by industry analysts and company executives

Other trade associations focus their efforts on specific divisions of the RTW industry, such as intimate apparel, men's sportswear, or knitwear, to name just a few (see Table 4.3).

A number of trade publications focus on the apparel industry and are of use to professionals in the RTW industry. (See Table 4.4 for a listing of selected trade publications in the apparel industry.) These publications range from daily newspapers to monthly magazines (see Figure 4.11).

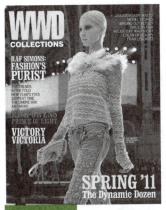 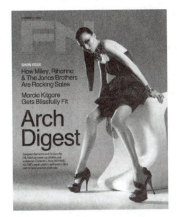 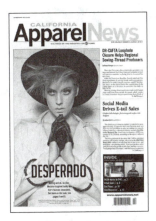

Figure 4.11 Trade publications, such as *WWD* and *FN*, provide fashion industry professionals with industry-related news and information.

Table 4.3	Selected Trade Associations in the Apparel and Accessory Industries
American Apparel and Footwear Association (AAFA)	www.apparelandfootwear.org
American Apparel Producers' Network (AAPN)	www.aapnetwork.net/
American Association of Textile Chemists and Colorists (AATCC)	www.aatcc.org/
American Textile Machinery Association	www.atmanet.org/home.aspx
Canadian Apparel Federation (CAF)	www.apparel.ca
Council of Fashion Designers of America	www.cfda.com
Fashion Footwear Association of New York	www.ffany.org/
Fashion Group International, Inc.	newyork.fgi.org/index.php
The Hosiery Association	hosieryassociation.com/
International Apparel Federation	www.iafnet.com/
International Association of Clothing Designers and Executives	www.iacde.net/en/
International Formalwear Association	www.formalwear.org/
International Swimwear/Activewear Market	www.isamla.com/
MAGIC International	www.magiconline.com/

Table 4.3   Selected Trade Associations in the Apparel and Accessory Industries *(continued)*

Organic Trade Association	www.ota.com/ofc-1.htm
SPESA, Sewn Products Equipment Suppliers of the Americas	www.spesa.org/default.html
Sporting Goods Manufacturers Association	www.sgma.com/
Underfashion Club	www.underfashionclub.org/

Table 4.4   Selected Trade Publications in the Apparel Industry

Apparel Magazine: Targeted to apparel and soft goods businesses. Focus on business and technology. Print and online.

California Apparel News: Covers fashion industry news with an emphasis on regional companies and markets on the West Coast. Weekly print newspaper and online.

Earnshaw's Magazine: Targeted to retailers of fashion and accessories for newborns and young children. Print and online.

FN on WWD.com: Footwear news. Online only.

Just-style.com: General news for the international textile and apparel industries; market research reports and analyses. Online only.

Stores: Provides information of general interest, as well as reports on electronic commerce, loss prevention, and computer software and hardware. Print and online.

Women's Wear Daily (WWD): Covers national and international news in the women's and children's fashion industry for retailers and manufacturers. Covers textiles, accessories, and fragrances, in addition to apparel. Daily print newspaper and online.

Summary

Most of the apparel and accessories produced and sold today is considered ready-to-wear (RTW), that is, it is completely made and ready to be worn at the time of purchase. RTW apparel and accessories are possible because of standardized sizing and mass-production techniques used in the apparel and accessory industries. Apparel and accessory companies typically produce four to six lines or collections corresponding to the fashion seasons: Spring, Summer, Fall I, Fall II, Holiday, and Resort or Cruise. Fast fashion companies can produce more than 12 lines per year.

It is important to note the distinctions between RTW and couture. In couture, garments are made to the specific body measurements of an individual rather than to standardized sizes found in RTW. In addition, couture garments are generally made with some hand-sewing techniques and from more expensive materials than RTW. Haute couture collections are shown twice per year (in July and January) to the media, others in the fashion industry, and wealthy clients.

Based on their organization and operations, RTW apparel and accessory companies fall into the following categories: manufacturers, jobbers, contractors, and licensors. Apparel companies are also classified according to the type of merchandise they produce, the price zones of their products or brands, and by the North American Industry Classification System (NAICS) established by the government.

A typical apparel and accessory company includes areas or divisions that focus on the following activities: research and merchandising; design and product development; sales and marketing; operations including production, planning, control, and distribution; advertising and sales promotion; and finance and information technology. Merchandisers set the overall direction for the merchandise assortment and work closely with the other divisions of the company that carry out the design, production, marketing, and distribution of the goods. Companies vary in their merchandising philosophies and may be innovators, interpreters, or imitators. All successful companies rely on consumer and market research, as well as sales data, for setting their fashion direction.

A number of trade associations in the apparel industry promote, conduct market research, sponsor trade shows, and develop and distribute educational materials related to various segments of the apparel industry. Examples include the American Apparel and Footwear Association (AAFA) and MAGIC International. A number of trade publications focus on the apparel industry and are used by professionals in the RTW industry. Examples include *Women's Wear Daily* and *Apparel.*

Careers within apparel companies include positions in merchandising; product/fashion development; sales and marketing; preproduction; production, control, and quality assurance; and advertising and promotion.

Women's Merchandise Manager
Better Men's and Women's Apparel Company

Position Description:

Manage and control the development of merchandise from color, fabric, and style selection to presentation and sales marketing. Work with the development team, which consists of a designer, pattern maker, sample sewer, and product engineer. The merchandise manager is ultimately responsible for the line.

Typical Tasks and Responsibilities:

- Analyze wholesale and retail performance of the product.
- Read trade and fashion publications to keep current on market direction.
- Communicate with retail accounts to gain sales information.
- Estimate units per style/color for the designated season (design development team produces patterns; merchandising decides in which fabrics each style will be available).
- Write and deliver presentations to sales representatives; attend sales meetings held throughout the year.
- Travel domestically to meet with sales representatives and retail accounts three to four times per year.
- Travel to New York twice per year for major development trips.
- Work with the fabric design department to develop fabrics and patterns for future seasons.
- Work with contractors to develop garments not produced by the company's factories.
- Work with quality control on production problems.
- Work with design to develop a style plan; design follows up with prototype development.
- Attend fitting sessions; sign off on all pieces to be included in the line.

CAREER PROFILES

Key Terms

atelier de couture

boutique

collection

contractor

couture

couture house

couturier, couturière

diffusion line

fashion season

full-package contractor

haute couture

item house

jobber

licensor

lifestyle brand

line

manufacturer

merchandising

North American Industry Classification System (NAICS)

prêt-à-porter

price point

price zone

private label brand

ready-to-wear (RTW)

salon de couture

store brand

Discussion Questions and Activities

1. Name your three favorite apparel brands. What companies manufacture these brands? How would you classify these brands in terms of product category, wholesale price zone, and type of brand name?

2. Examine copies and/or online versions of trade publications in the apparel industry. To whom does each of the trade publications cater (i.e., what are the publications' target markets)? What types of information are included in the trade publications? How might this information be used by professionals in the industry?

3. Discuss the advantages and disadvantages of producing four seasonal lines per year versus six seasonal lines per year versus twelve lines per year. What are some examples of merchandise that is well suited to four, six, and twelve lines per year? Why?

4. What roles do each of the following divisions play in an apparel company: research and merchandising; design and product development; sales and marketing; operations including production, planning, control, and distribution; advertising and sales promotion; and finance and information technology? In which area would you like to have a career? Why?

References

American Society for Testing and Materials. http://www.astm.org/

Fédération Française de la Couture du Prêt-à-Porter des Couturiers et des Créatures de Mode. http://www.modeaparis.com/

North American Industry Classification System. http://www.census.gov/epcd/naics02/naicod02.htm

Size USA. http://www.sizeusa.com

Southern California Edison Company. (1995, February). *Southern California's Apparel Industry: Building a Path to Prosperity*. Rosemead, CA: Author.

Eight Steps in the Design Process

Step 1 Research and Merchandising

Market Research:	Fashion Research:
Consumer Research	Fashion Trend Research
Product Research	Color Research
Market Analysis	Fabric and Trim Research
Target Customer Profile	

Seasonal and Line Planning

Step 2 Design

Design Inspiration

Plan the Line

Sketch Design and Obtain Vendor Samples

Select or Develop Fabrics and Trims

Review and Select Styles to Develop for Line

Write Garment Specifications Sheet and Quick Cost

Step 3 Design Development and Style Selection

Make First Pattern

Cut and Sew Prototype

Approve Prototype Fit, Revise Style, or Drop Style

Estimate Cost (initial cost estimate)

Present and Review Line

Select Styles for Final Line (line adoption)

Determine the Final Cost

Order Fabric, Trims, and Findings for Sales Samples

Order Sales Samples Cut and Sewn

Step 4 Marketing the Apparel Line

Designer and National Brands:
Sales Representatives Show Line at Market and
through Other Promotion Strategies

Retail Buyers Place Orders

Private-Label Brands:
Design Team Shows Line to Merchandisers/Buyers

Buyers Place Orders

Step 5 Preproduction

Order Production of Fabrics, Trims, and Findings

Finalize Production Pattern and Written Documents

Grade Production Pattern into Size Range

Make Production Marker

Inspect Fabric

Spread, Cut, Bundle, and Manage Dye Lots
for Production

Step 6 Sourcing

Select Production Facility

Step 7 Apparel Production Processes, Material Management, and Quality Assurance

Sew Production Order (may include approval
of first size run by contractor)

Finish, Inspect, Press, Tag, and Bag Order

Step 8 Distribution and Retailing

Send Retailer's Order to Manufacturer's
Distribution Center

Pick Orders (may include Quality Assurance Check)

Send to Retail Store Distribution Center
or Directly to Retailer

Review Season's Sales Figures

PART 2

Creating and Marketing an Apparel Line

CHAPTER 5

Creating a Line:

Research

In this chapter you will learn the following:

- the concept of an apparel line

- the various types of market research used to understand the target consumer

- the scope of the job responsibilities of the apparel designer and merchandiser in conducting and interpreting market research

- resources for fashion trends, color trend, and fabric trend forecasting

Step 1: Research and Merchandising

Step 1 Research and Merchandising

Market Research:	Fashion Research:
Consumer Research	Fashion Trend Research
Product Research	Color Research
Market Analysis	Fabric and Trim Research
Target Customer Profile	

Seasonal and Line Planning

↓

Step 2 Design

↓

Step 3 Design Development and Style Selection

↓

Step 4 Marketing the Apparel Line

↓

Step 5 Preproduction

↓

Step 6 Sourcing

↓

Step 7 Apparel Production Processes, Material Management, and Quality Assurance

↓

Step 8 Distribution and Retailing

Creating an Apparel Line

Combining a group of apparel items into a collection or a line involves a series of steps. Each step is closely related to and influenced by all the other steps in the process. The next several chapters will discuss these steps sequentially. The Eight Steps in the Design Process flowchart at the beginning of Part 2 will help acquaint you with the big picture. Each stage in the design process will be explored in greater detail in Parts 2 and 3. Step 1, Research and Merchandising, is discussed in Chapter 5. The Step 1 flowchart at the beginning of this chapter shows the research and merchandising step in detail. It is important to keep in mind that this flowchart is a generic one. Some apparel companies deviate from this sequence for a variety of reasons. The industry is constantly changing in areas such as computer integration, speed of production, geographic location for production, regulations on goods manufactured outside the United States, number of new lines introduced each year, and distribution channels. These changes affect the sequence of steps in the design process. A company may also follow one sequence for some lines and use a modified sequence for other lines. In addition, several activities may occur simultaneously during the progress of a line's development.

The terms *line*, *group*, and *collection* are used to designate a combination of apparel items presented together to the buying public for a particular season. The term **collection** is used generally to refer to the apparel presented through runway shows each fall and spring by the high-fashion designers in Paris, Milan, New York, London, Tokyo, and other locations. The runway shows of designer collections often include a wide range of apparel, including swimwear, dresses, suits, sportswear, evening wear, and, of course, bridal wear as the finale. The designer collections may include approximately 100 to 150 apparel items. Collections are typically inspired by a theme and reflect the design philosophy of the head designer.

An apparel **line** consists of one large group or several small groups of apparel items, or styles, developed around a theme that may be based on such factors as color, fabric, design details, or a purpose (such as golf or tennis) that links the items together (see Figure 5.1). A line is composed of a variety of items or styles within a category of clothing, such as shirts, pants, jackets, vests, and sweaters. Each line is developed for a specific target customer and could consist of as many as 50 or 60 apparel items. A designer, often with a team of several others, such as a design assistant and a product developer, will be assigned responsibilities for the creation of the line. Some designers will have responsibility for several lines. Sometimes, several small **groups** will be developed within a line, each with its own theme. A group might use three to five fabrics in varying combinations and include approximately a dozen apparel items, all carefully coordinated.

Whereas many apparel companies focus on developing seasonal lines (typically four to six seasons per year), some apparel companies develop new groups to ship every four to six weeks throughout the year. This merchandising strategy places new merchandise in retail stores at frequent intervals, an enticement for many customers to shop often. Liz Claiborne is a company known for providing new style groups approximately every six weeks. Another merchandising strategy focuses on providing new merchandise on a continual basis. Zara, based in Spain, exemplifies fast fashion, a quick-cycle approach to design-produce-distribute discussed in Chapter 1. Zara designs the product as well as owns its retail stores; therefore, it can quickly design, produce, and distribute new merchandise. New styles arrive in Zara's retail stores weekly.

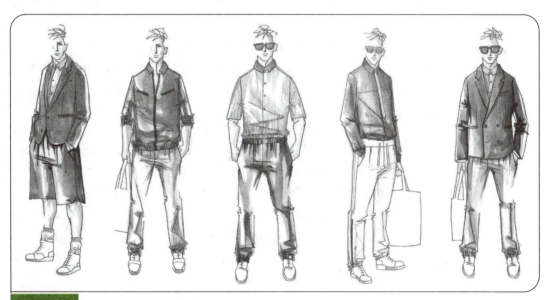

Figure 5.1 A line is a group of products developed around a theme.

Just as fashion, in general, follows an evolutionary pattern, apparel designers who work for companies generally create new seasonal lines in an ongoing, evolutionary manner. New lines tend to develop from previous lines, with some repetition or modification of successful styles. Styles repeated from one seasonal line to the next are called **carryovers**. The target customer, general market trends, fashion trends, color trends, fabric trends, and retailers' needs are all taken into careful consideration in the planning and development of an apparel line.

The stereotypical image of a fashion *designer* is that he or she sits at a drawing table, sketching garment idea after garment idea. The sketches are handed to other employees who turn them into garments. Is this what really happens in the apparel industry? In actuality, the creation of an apparel line is a carefully orchestrated series of processes—a team effort, involving many people. The designer's job includes a variety of responsibilities, such as the following:

- researching the market
- selecting the colors, fabrics, and garment styling for the line based on fashion direction from merchandisers
- consulting with product engineers on costing factors
- preparing the preliminary specification sheets
- presenting technical drawings or sketches of new garment styles
- providing suggestions for linings, interfacings, trims, buttons, and other components
- releasing the approved styles for pattern making
- responding to inquiries about the styles during preproduction and production

A designer typically works with a **merchandiser** to plan the overall look of an apparel line, the color story, the fabrics, the price, and the number of styles for each line (see Chapter 6 for this discussion). The merchandiser's role is to see that all the company's needs for the line are met. This might include seasonal as well as line planning and coordinating several lines presented by the company. The merchandiser is also responsible for the following:

- conducting market research
- developing and maintaining the line estimate and price targets to meet budget objectives
- reviewing the designer's proposed line
- approving the line

Years of experience in design or retailing provide the perspective needed for the apparel company's merchandiser.

The creation and design development stage of one line overlaps with the production stage of the previous line and the selling stage of the line presented prior to that one. A two-year **master calendar** of a company that is developing four seasonal lines a year will shows that at any given time, designers and merchandisers are handling at least three lines, each in a different stage of the product cycle. Developing a line would be much easier if one had the final sales statistics from the previous line before beginning to work on the creation stage of the new line. Unfortunately, this is not possible in the fast-paced world of fashion. Ever-increasing numbers of shopping malls, factory outlet malls, and direct mail and electronic shopping options have provided increased opportunities for purchasing apparel and accessories. To help meet consumers' wishes, the timeline in today's apparel industry calls for creating more lines more quickly than even five years ago.

Market Research: Understanding Consumer Market Trends

The most important concept for success in the apparel industry is that the company needs to know its target market and provide the merchandise assortment desired by its customers—when they want it and where they will purchase it. In other words, consumer demand is the driving force in the apparel industry. The industry expression, "You can make it only if it sells," relates to the concept of the consumer-driven market. Thus, the success of any apparel, textile, or home fashions company depends on determining the needs and wants of the consumer. To determine what customers will need and want, and when and where they will want it, a variety of types of research must be conducted. This process is called **market research**.

Market research can be defined as "the systematic and objective approach to the development and provision of information for the marketing management decision-making process" (Kinnear & Taylor, 1983, p. 16). Market research is divided into two general categories (Kinnear & Taylor, p. 17):

1. basic research that deals with extending knowledge about the marketing system

2. applied research that helps managers make better decisions

Company executives, merchandisers, and designers conduct applied market research as a part of the planning process.

Applied market research includes the following three types of research:

- **consumer research,** which provides information about consumer characteristics and consumer behavior
- **product research,** which provides information about preferred product design and characteristics
- **market analysis**, which provides information about general market trends

All three types of market research will be discussed in this chapter.

Each form of applied market research provides valuable information to company executives, merchandisers, and designers about the wants and needs of their target market customers. Some forms of market research take considerable time to conduct, analyze, and interpret. Because of the fast-paced nature of the fashion business, fashion products require a short research-and-development stage. Timing is crucial to the fashion item's successful sale in the marketplace. Therefore, companies generally conduct market research on an ongoing basis.

Trade associations, such as the American Apparel and Footwear Association and Cotton Incorporated, also conduct market research, providing information that can be very beneficial to apparel manufacturers and retailers. (Selected trade associations are discussed in Chapters 3 and 4.) Examples of other sources of information to assist with conducting research will be discussed in this chapter.

Consumer Research

Consumer research provides information about consumer characteristics and consumer behavior. Some forms of consumer research study broad trends in the marketplace. Research on **demographics** focuses on understanding the following characteristics of consumer groups:

- age
- gender
- marital status
- income
- occupation
- ethnicity
- geographic location

Consumer research may also focus on **psychographics**. Psychographic characteristics of consumer groups include the following:

- buying habits
- attitudes
- values
- motives
- preferences
- personality
- leisure activities

Demographic information helps describe who the customer is, while psychographic information helps explain why the customer makes the choices he or she makes. Some of these demographic and psychographic characteristics will be discussed further in the market analysis section of this chapter.

Numerous companies conduct consumer and market research. The ACNielsen Company was founded in 1928 and is considered the pioneer company in this field. Some market research companies include a fashion division. For example, NPD Fashionworld is the apparel division of the market research firm NPD Group of Cambridge, Massachusetts.

Apparel companies may conduct and interpret their own consumer research. For example, Macy's worked with the consulting firm dunnhumby to gather data through surveys, focus groups, store intercepts and customer purchases diaries to determine their customers' needs and wants. Peter Sachse, chief marketing director for Macy's, stated that the one reassuring outcome of this research was, "We don't need new customers. All we need to do is take care of the ones who already love us." (NRF Retail Innovation and Marketing Conference Highlights, *Stores*, April 2010, p. 22)

Consumer research is also conducted by companies expanding their markets beyond U.S. consumers to better understand the preferences of these new consumer groups. For example, some women's activewear companies in the United States are expanding into the European market. To market a U.S. company's activewear apparel in France, it is important to research the French activewear consumer if the product is to succeed in that marketplace. It is essential to learn, among other things, that the styles of activewear preferred by French women are not the same as those currently most popular in the United States.

Color preferences vary among countries and cultures. These preferences might be related to the country's climate, personal skin tones of the residents, or cultural heritage. When expanding into a new market, consumer research dealing with color preferences of the intended new market would be important for the success of the line.

Conducting consumer research related to fashion items can be a challenge. Apparel purchase decisions are based on a number of factors—including psychological, social, and financial considerations—of which consumers are often not consciously aware. Therefore, results of market research indicate that consumers often do not actually purchase what they indicate they would purchase when queried in advance.

Product Research

Product research provides information about preferred product design and product characteristics. When new products are developed, or existing products are modified, it is advantageous to assess how well a new or revised product will fare in the marketplace. To try to determine customer preferences, one could conduct product research such as the following:

- survey potential consumers orally

- send a questionnaire

- offer a free trial of a product in exchange for feedback

Sometimes an apparel company will conduct substantial market research before introducing a new line, especially if the company is interested in developing a new product type. Some large apparel manufacturers, such as JCPenney (for their private-label merchandise) and VF Corporation, have been testing style preferences for years.

Is it possible to predict how apparel consumers will react to a style? Style testing techniques, refined by some of the most respected names in apparel manufacturing, show that one can predict what consumers will want to buy. Some companies use outlet store sales to gather data on how consumers react to various styles and prices. JCPenney surveys mall shoppers and uses in-house video testing to guide the decisions of its buyers as well as its manufacturing operations.

Listening to comments from sales representatives, retailers, and customers about the success of a line provides another part of the feedback necessary for continued success. Designer John Galliano stated that "he plans to communicate regularly with Bergdorf [Goodman] sales staff to find out what's happening on the floor, including reactions to the cut, fit, and finishing of the clothes, right down to the durability of a button. That kind of information is a gold mine for the designer" (Socha, 1997, p. 12).

One of the newest ways in which companies are collecting data about their customers is through social media, such as Facebook and Twitter. Companies are not only setting up websites to advertise their products, but using social networking to ask customers what they want. Shannon Walton, a spokesperson for Schoeller, states, "The everyday user is available 24/7. We are taking a more social approach to the end user" ("Consumer connections," *Textile Insight*, January/February 2010, p. 18).

Market Analysis

Market analysis provides information about general market trends. Planning ahead to meet the future needs of the consumer is a critical part of continued success in the apparel industry. Market analysis in the apparel, accessories, and home fashions industries can be subdivided into long-range forecasting (or research) and short-range forecasting. **Long-range forecasting** projects market trends one to five years in advance, while **short-range forecasting** focuses on market trends one year or less in advance. Both long-range forecasting and short-range forecasting strategies are used for market analysis. Long-range forecasting includes researching economic trends related to consumer spending patterns and the business climate that affects the apparel industry. Sample research questions include the following:

- Will interest rates be increasing on money borrowed by an apparel manufacturer to purchase fabric?

- Will corporate taxes for the apparel company be increasing?

- Will cost-of-living expenses rise because of inflation, resulting in fewer apparel purchases by consumers?

- Will rising labor costs result in noticeable increases in the purchase price for apparel?

All of these trends can influence the company's plans and the consumer's future purchases (Figure 5.2).

Long-range forecasting also includes sociological, psychological, political, and global trends. For example, changes in international trade policies will affect long-range forecasting. Political fluctuations among countries can affect sourcing options when planning offshore production. Currency devaluation, economic downturn, and financial turmoil around the world have an impact on the U.S. apparel industry.

Other aspects of long-range forecasting deal with ongoing changes in the apparel industry. Sources of information on these changes include the following:

- The *Apparel Strategist* (www.apparelstrategist.com) is a publication that is directed specifically toward market analysis in the apparel industry.

- Npd Group (www.npd.com), publishes online market research for the apparel and footwear industries.

- Kurt Salmon Associates (KSA) is an example of a company that specializes in conducting and publishing soft-goods business expertise and market analysis.

- Cotton Incorporated, a textile trade organization discussed in Chapter 3, conducts product trend analysis and consumer marketing. *Lifestyle Monitor* is published monthly by Cotton Incorporated (see www.cottoninc.com). Cotton Incorporated also publishes *Lifestyle Monitor Trend Magazine* semi-annually.

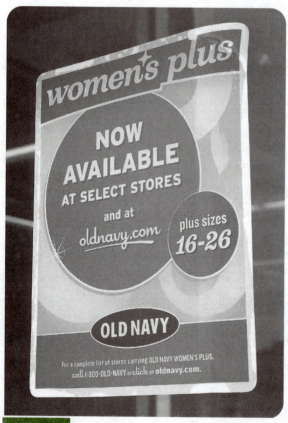

Figure 5.2 Market analysis provides the data needed for apparel companies to expand their markets by offering new size ranges.

The apparel marketplace is in a constant state of flux. Changes in a company's target market, market shifts, or new markets all need to be considered. Two major catalog companies, L.L. Bean and Lands' End, saw the need to engage a younger consumer. "Fashionable designer brands recently have been creating modern versions of the classics that Bean and Lands' End have been selling for years, and the catalog retailers are determined not to be outdone by hipster upstarts" (Smith, 2009, p. D.5). Each introduced new lines, which are geared to consumers in their 20s and 30s. The two companies are using social media to promote their new lines.

Another market currently of interest to the apparel industry is the aging boomers market. Market research on apparel spending patterns suggests consumers over age 55 will spend less on apparel than this group spent before reaching age 55. As the fashion-conscious baby boomers reached age 55, their apparel spending patterns changed. "The aging of America is slowly sneaking up on the apparel indus-

Table 5.1	Average Annual Apparel and Apparel Services Expenditures by Age Group						
Year	Under 25 Years	25–34	35–44	45–54	55–64	65–74	75 and over
2003	1,117	1,849	2,091	1,953	1,562	1,190	611
2004	1,371	2,134	2,142	2,217	1,200	1,200	604
2005	1,577	2,082	2,365	2,318	1,784	1,313	584
2006	1,464	2,152	2,368	2,176	1,892	1,212	639
2007	1,477	2,106	2,335	2,191	1,888	1,323	732
2008	1,351	1,965	2,235	2,228	1,622	1,381	755

SOURCE: Retrieved June 30, 2010 from U. S. Department of Labor, Bureau of Labor Statistics, Consumer Expenditure Survey, Web site: http://www.bls.gov/cex/

try, and the purse strings are beginning to tighten as the boomers age" (Behling, 1999, p. 53). Table 5.1 lists average annual expenditures on apparel and apparel services by age group between the years 2003 and 2008.

Sustainability and environmental concerns are other examples of long-range trends that affect apparel companies. Companies are becoming more sustainable and energy efficient. American & Efrid, a global thread manufacturer, kicked off an eco-driven program in 2009 called 10 Threads of Sustainability, which includes sustainable packaging, recycled polyester thread, and energy efficiency goals (Walzer, 2010, p.22).

Some companies have made the commitment to use fabrics made from recycled products, such as aluminum cans or plastic bottles. For example, Patagonia uses postconsumer recycled (PCR) materials in some of its product line (see Figure 5.3). These fabrics are made using recycled polyester garments and by utilizing other recycled plastics. The use of PCR material in its product line reflects Patagonia's decision to offer products consistent with its company's and customers' values. Patagonia's environmental assessment coordinator Eric Wilmanns stated, "From a lifecycle analysis approach, we look not only at the materials and energy we use, but also what goes into sustaining our products, how they are used, and what eventually happens to them when consumers are finished using them" (Welling, 1999, p. AS26). In 2007, Patagonia introduced a major expansion of its garment recycling program. Customers may return used Polartec fleece garments, Patagonia fleece, Patagonia cotton tees, and Capilene baselayers to Patagonia via mail or to any Patagonia retail store ("Patagonia announces ...," 2007). The fabrics from these used garments are then used to produce new PCR material. Patagonia's company philosophy regarding environmental concerns extends to all aspects of its business.

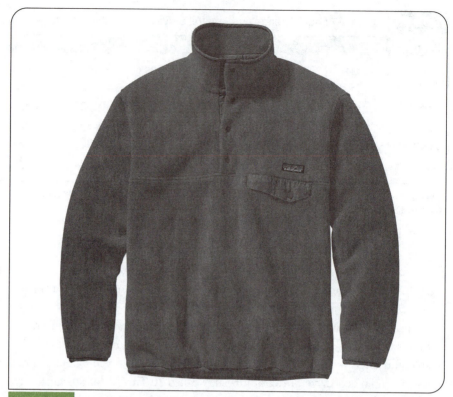

Figure 5.3 Patagonia's Synchilla vest is made from fabric containing postconsumer recycled (PCR) fiber.

What about forecasting long-range fashion trends? Is it possible to forecast fashion trends several years in advance of a season? Long-range forecasting can reap benefits. Many trend forecasting firms provide short-term and long-range trend forecasts. For example, Fiona Jenvey, CEO of Mudpie Ltd., states "Currently there is a trend for longevity and classic as a reaction to both considered consumption and sustainability (buy better less often); this translates in fashion to vintage, design re-issues, or 'vintage inspired'. Retailers and designers should use trend information as a tool for creating an original desirable product, which represents the values of the brand" (fibre2fashion, 2010).

Short-range forecasting is critical to an apparel company's success. Planning meetings are held with designers, merchandisers, planners, and sales personnel to discuss the company's short-range forecasts and strategic planning. This planning includes such components as determining the desired percentage of increased sales growth for a company. For example, perhaps the company managers have determined that a 5 percent growth in sales should be planned.

The designer for each apparel line that the company produces may be asked to increase the line with a 5 percent sales growth factor in mind. Using sales figures from the current selling season, the designer (and merchandiser) may select one or several styles that are selling particularly well and add one or several similar styles to the upcoming line. Seasonal and line planning are discussed in more detail in Chapter 6.

Short-range forecasting also includes the careful study of what the competition is doing. If a competitor seems to be expanding one of its lines, for example, the water sports category of apparel, then perhaps it would be wise to study whether this growth area would be feasible for your company. Apparel, accessories, and home fashions companies constantly observe the marketplace competition.

Short-range forecasting also includes predicting changes in retailing. A retailer may be in the process of expansion, with a number of new stores ready to open in the forthcoming year. If this retailer has been a strong client of an apparel manufacturer in the past, the expansion can signal increased orders for the apparel company. As retailers file for bankruptcy, merge, and divide, it is important for the apparel company to be wary of shipping goods to retailers who may be in the process of disruption.

Target Customer

Each apparel company's goal is to position its apparel lines to be different from the competition and to be enticing to potential customers. The merchandising and design staff's objective is to develop the right product for the company's target customer at the right time in the marketplace. This is called its brand position. Eddie Bauer, headquartered in Seattle, describes its brand position as follows:

> Innovation, quality and an appreciation of the outdoors: The passions of our founder, Eddie Bauer, remain the cornerstone of the Eddie Bauer business today. In conjunction with innovative design and exceptional customer service, Eddie Bauer offers premium-quality clothing, accessories, and gear for men and women that complement today's modern lifestyle. (Eddie Bauer, 2010)

Within a company's position in the marketplace, each apparel line produced by the apparel company requires a clearly defined **target customer** (see Figure 5.4).

The profile, or description, of the target customer usually includes the following demographic and psychographic characteristics determined for the majority of customers:

- gender
- age range

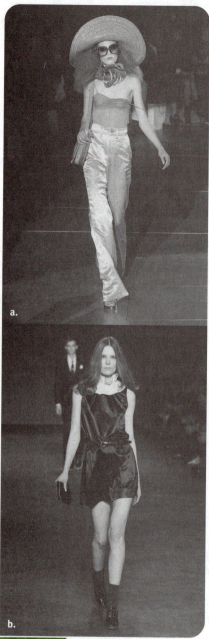

- average income
- lifestyle
- buying habits
- geographic location
- price zone

A swimwear company may produce several lines, each based on a specific target customer profile. One line may be designed for very conservative misses customers, while other lines may range from appealing to conservative customers to updated misses customers to fashion-forward junior customers. Developing a well-defined target customer profile for each line helps the designers and merchandisers focus the line to the specific audience, or market niche. For example, Eddie Bauer outlines its target customer for its classic Eddie Bauer line as follows:

- 42 to 46 years old
- college educated
- average income $70,000
- young families and empty nesters, currently working
- quality and value are a priority
- prefer an active, casual lifestyle

Some companies develop a very detailed target customer profile. A photograph of the "typical" customer might be included with the target customer profile statement to help merchandisers, designers, product developers, and sales representatives visualize the customer. The models used for product advertisements are also selected to portray the image of the target customer. The design team relies on the target customer profile for the following:

- to identify market trends, especially those related to its target customer
- to develop the initial direction for the line
- to develop style sketches (concept sketches) and color concepts

Figure 5.4 The target customer for Marc lines (a) is similar to the target customer for the more expensive Marc Jacobs designer lines for women (b). The main difference between the two markets is the price zone.

VF Corporation, parent company to Wrangler, Lee, The North Face, JanSport, and 7 For All Mankind has used a variety of strategies to develop the products that consumers want and need for specific brands. According to VF Corporation's president and CEO, a company must recognize that it will constantly be changing its business to respond to the continuous changes going on with consumers. It must focus on creating a continuous link between consumer research and new product development. "We focus on specific target consumer segments, defined by differences in key attitudes, lifestyles, and needs. The discovery part is learning everything we can about each brand's specific target consumer—who she is, how she thinks, how her life is changing, and what she really needs" (Hill, 1998, p. AS-5).

GENDER

Whereas some companies produce lines of unisex clothing (for example, a T-shirt company), most lines are focused on men's, women's, or children's apparel. Many companies produce both men's and women's apparel, but they will have separate lines specifically designed for each gender. Other apparel companies produce only men's apparel or only women's apparel.

In the children's wear industry, many companies produce infants' and toddlers' apparel for both boys and girls. While some companies produce children's apparel for both girls and boys, many companies produce only girls' apparel or boys' apparel.

AGE RANGE

Companies tend to focus on a specific age range, as defined in their target customer profile statement for each of their lines. For a line of junior apparel, a company might profile its customers as ages 15 to 25. This does not mean that a woman over the age of 25 would not wear the apparel in this line. Rather, the design team visualizes the majority of customers as falling within the age range of 15 to 25 and keeps this age range firmly in mind while creating the line. A company may decide to adjust the targeted age of its customer. Raising the upper age of the age range of the target customer might be a logical adjustment as the average age of the population increases. Perhaps the company wants to retain an established customer by broadening the age range at the older end, yet continue to include the established target customer in its target market. After acquiring a loyal customer who likes a company's brand, it could be very cost effective to adjust the styling slightly over time to continue to appeal to this customer as he or she ages.

LIFESTYLE AND GEOGRAPHIC LOCATION

A study of the target customer's lifestyle might include information such as the following:

- type of career
- stage in career
- geographic location and its population size
- social or political direction
- education
- attitudes
- values
- interest in fashion (for example, prefers classic looks or is a fashion trendsetter)
- price consciousness

Lifestyle preference descriptions could suggest that the target customer is focused on entertainment or is comfortable with technology. Obtaining such results through lifestyle research can help define the various target groups.

The term **lifestyle merchandising** was coined to recognize the importance of appealing to the target customer's lifestyle choices. The proliferation of popular lifestyle magazines, direct-mail catalogs, and websites indicates the importance of appealing to customers' lifestyles. For example, the fitness market has a myriad of lifestyle magazines. Not surprisingly, some apparel companies design clothing to appeal to a specific lifestyle preference.

Tommy Bahama is an apparel, accessories, and home fashions company that exemplifies lifestyle merchandising. The brand is a "purveyor of island lifestyles" (Tommy Bahama, 2010). Relaxed fashions, some in tropical prints, as well as island-inspired accessories, home fashions, and store decor all contribute to promoting the island lifestyle.

Some companies may focus a line on a specific geographic location. For example, the resort market in Florida might be a location for a targeted customer. There is a special fashion "look" to resort apparel in Florida that may not sell well in other geographic locations. The garment style characteristics, fabric design motifs, and colorations of apparel for Florida resort wear are easily recognized if you are familiar with that market.

PRICE ZONE

The target customer profile also typically includes a targeted price zone, such as moderate, better, or bridge price, as discussed in Chapter 4. Each line will be planned to fall within the specified price zone, based on the target customer profile. Within the line, not every style of shirt will sell for the same price. There will be a range of prices, based on differences in styling and fabric variations. However, the overall prices for the line will fall within expected ranges for the determined price zone. If a company is known to produce goods in the moderate price zone, a jacket style in its line priced in a better price zone will look overpriced in comparison to the rest of the line. A customer would question why the price is higher than expected and might not purchase the jacket due only to its price.

The design team always keeps the target customer profile in mind in order to create a line that will appeal to the customer. It is important for a company to review and update its target customer profile from time to time. The target customer profile is an important component of an apparel line's marketing campaign, both to the retailer and to the ultimate customer.

Fashion Research

In addition to market research, fashion research is also conducted. Fashion research focuses on trends in silhouettes, design details, colors, fabrics, and trims. Similar to market research, fashion research may be conducted and interpreted by fashion research or forecasting firms, or by apparel companies themselves.

Fashion Trend Research

Fashion trend research tends to be a daily activity for the designer and the merchandiser. **Trend research** activities include reading or scanning appropriate **trade publications**. Each segment of the apparel industry has specific trade newspapers and magazines directed toward fashion trends in that industry segment. Examples include the following:

- *Children's Business* and *Earnshaw's Infant, Girls, and Boys Wear Review*, focusing on children's wear industry fashion trends

- *Footwear News* for the footwear industry

- *Sportswear International* for the menswear, women's wear, and children's wear apparel and accessories industries

These trade publications require subscriptions, so they are not available for individual purchase at specialty magazine stores.

Trade newspapers include *Women's Wear Daily* and *California Apparel News*. *Women's Wear Daily* covers fabrics, fashion ready-to-wear, sportswear, furs, and financial news daily. In addition, each day of the week is targeted to specific market segments (for example, accessories, innerwear, and legwear are covered on Mondays). A few newspaper and magazine retailers offer these publications over the counter, but, for the most part, they are available by subscription only. Several trade publications are available online; for example, *Women's Wear Daily* is available at www.wwd.com.

European **fashion magazines**—such as *French Vogue, Italian Vogue, Elegance,* and *Book Moda Alta Moda* (women's wear); *Book Moda Uomo* and *Vogue Homme* (menswear); and *Vogue Bambini* (children's wear)—are important sources for fashion trends. Many of the specific fashion magazines are provided to the design team by the apparel company. Some of these fashion magazines are available for purchase at specialty magazine stores in larger cities. Other specialized publications are available only by subscription from fashion publication subscription services in New York and Los Angeles.

Popular fashion magazines, read by the target customer, are sources for fashion trend information and provide an insight into the preferences of the customer. Designers and merchandisers peruse the appropriate publications, depending on their target market. Examples of popular fashion magazines include *Vogue, Elle, Harper's Bazaar, W, Glamour, Allure, Self, Vanity Fair, Town & Country, Essence, In Style, Lucky, Savvy, YM, Seventeen, Jump, Men's Vogue, Details, Maxim,* and *GQ* (see Figure 5.5). These magazines are readily available to the public at news and magazine stands and bookstores. Some of these magazines, such as *Elle, Glamour, Harper's Bazaar, Seventeen, Teen,* and *Teen People,* have editorial websites on the Internet or have previews of the current issue's contents on the Internet. A convenient and fast way for designers and merchandisers to search for fashion trend information related to a specific target customer is by using online access.

Apparel companies and retailers often subscribe to **fashion forecasting services**. Some of these forecasting services cover a broad range of fashion trends. Some specialize in color trends, while others provide both fashion trend and color trend analysis. Examples of fashion trend forecasting services based in the United States include the following:

• The Doneger Group, based in New York, provides merchandising consulting and fashion trend and color forecasts for the apparel and accessories markets. The Doneger Group publishes the *Tobe Report,* a fashion consulting publication for retailers.

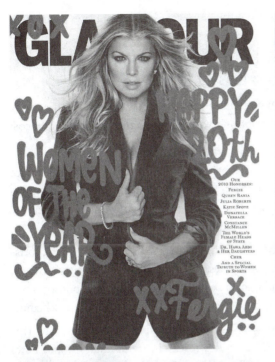
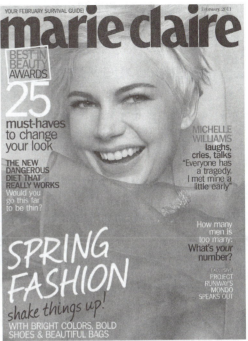
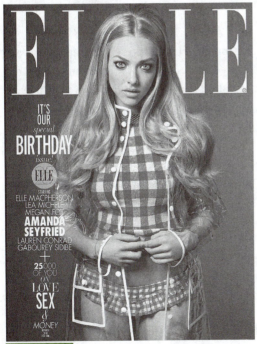
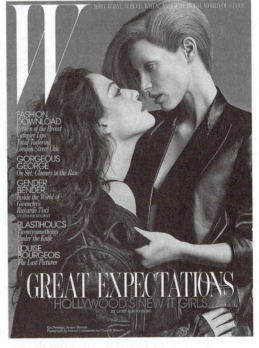

Figure 5.5 Popular fashion magazines are a source of fashion trend information.

- Margit Publications, a division of the Doneger Group, publishes a variety of trend and color forecasts.

- Here & There provides trend and color forecasts as well as collections reports, retail reports, and textile reports.

Publications such as these help merchandisers and designers analyze upcoming fashion trends. An annual subscription to a fashion trend newsletter might cost several hundred dollars.

- Trend Union is a fashion trend, fabric, and color trend forecasting service based in Paris that conducts fashion and fabric trend seminars in locations such as New York, Seattle, San Francisco, and Los Angeles several times a year in addition to its forecasting publications.

- Promostyl provides trend books focusing on menswear, women's wear, sportswear, streetwear, youth, and accessories. The company produces style trends, color trends, and fabric trend books. Based in Paris, Promostyl sponsors conferences in many major cities throughout the world on a continuous schedule.

- Worth Global Style Network (WGSN) is an example of an online subscription fashion resource. WGSN provides research, trend analysis, and news service daily to its online subscribers. (See Chapter 3 for more examples of trend forecasting companies.)

Recent runway shows are another source of fashion trend information. Several resources provide runway images of recent designs shown in Milan, Paris, London, and New York. Fashion information is available online as well. There are many websites that show the latest styles as seen on the runways of Milan, Paris, London, and New York. These sources provide examples of current fashions, rather than forecasting future trends. However, many of the new styles shown are those that set new trends and provide a sense of fashion direction for many moderate- and mass-priced manufacturers. Some sources are accessible without a fee, whereas other sources require an online subscription. Often a free introductory preview is available to assess their usefulness before subscribing. A big advantage of these online sources, like online magazines, is their ease of accessibility.

The design team often attends textile and apparel trade shows geared to a specific segment of the market. Trade shows are held in various locations around the world, from Las Vegas to Beijing. Attendance at trade shows might be for a variety of purposes. Often the attendee's company is represented at the trade show. Some designers and merchandisers attend trade shows specifically to view the latest trends. An added benefit for those attending trade shows is that fashion trend and color forecasting seminars geared to a specific product market are presented. Some of these trade shows, such as MAGIC and The Super Show, sponsored by Sporting Goods Manufacturers Association (SGMA), are discussed in Chapter 8.

Computer software programs have been developed to assist with consumer-driven fashion forecasting. Some software programs provide more than total sales figures. The software enables an apparel company to determine specifically who is buying what, and where, taking into account factors such as weather, special events in the area, and store promotions.

Fashion trend research also involves **shopping the market**. Although this sounds like fun, it actually requires considerable concentration and constant vigilance. Merchandisers and designers look for new trends that may influence the direction of an upcoming line. Bodice design details in evening wear may inspire a design detail in a swimsuit, for example. One aspect of shopping the market involves visiting retail stores that carry the company's line. Talking with retailers about how the line is selling provides helpful information for predicting fashion trends. Watching retail store customers' reactions to the line provides helpful feedback. Studying the competitors' lines in retail stores is also important for predicting trends.

The "fantasy" aspect of trend research involves viewing the high-fashion couture and ready-to-wear collections in Paris, Milan, London, Tokyo, and New York. Designers and merchandisers for some apparel companies are given the assignment to view these twice-yearly collections. The high-fashion collections are often filled with avant-garde styles probably not worn by the target customer. However, important fashion trends can be extracted and then modified for a line in the moderate price zone.

Some designers and merchandisers also study customers "on the street," or, if the line is an active sportswear line, they watch potential customers on the ski slopes or at the beach participating in the specific sport. Fashion is a reflection of the time and the lifestyle of the society from which and for which it is created. Therefore, trend research involves the collection of information from multiple sources on a continuing basis. The design team does not create in a vacuum; instead, it is influenced by everything on a daily basis. It is important to visit art museums, concerts, and movies, and to participate in other activities that expose the design team to fashion-related trends.

Color Research and Resources

When color trends in apparel, accessories, or home fashions are reviewed over time, it becomes clear that certain staple colors appear frequently in the fashion cycle. In apparel, black, navy, white, and beige are considered staple colors and are seen almost continuously season after season. One or more **staple colors** are included in each line. Pendleton Woolen Mills is known for maintaining a group of staple colors in its classic apparel lines. Pendleton's tartan navy and tartan green are examples of colors that are color matched season after season. If a customer has purchased a navy Pendleton jacket from its classic line, a pair of navy slacks purchased several years later will match the color of the jacket (unless it has faded because of improper care or excessive wear). Pendleton tracks the sales, ranked by dollar volume and color, to ensure that long-term, high-selling colors are represented in each line. Talbots is another company that provides color-matched apparel season after season. The Talbots true red, # 25, and cherry red, #26, are examples of colors that are continued season after season.

Some companies vary a staple color slightly from season to season to reflect fashion influences. One season, a navy may be a violet-navy, while another season, the navy may be a black-navy. This lends an updated fashion look to staple colors. If a print fabric in the line contains navy, then it is necessary to match the navy in the print fabric to the solid navy.

Other colors, called **fashion colors**, appear less frequently over time than staple colors. Fashion colors often follow cycles, reappearing in a different shade, value, or intensity from one fashion season to the next. For example, an orange-red may evolve into a blue-red, which may evolve into a blue-magenta. It is interesting to follow the trend of a fashion color over a period of years. A color such as aubergine (eggplant) will recur every few years. It may be slightly redder one season, slightly bluer another. For those who have tried to match the color of an item purchased in a previous season or year, it becomes painfully obvious that the lifecycle of some fashion colors is very short. Some customers have learned to purchase all color-matched pieces of a line at one time to avoid disappointment later, when they might be unable to match the color of a shirt they would like to purchase to wear with the pants purchased a year earlier.

Some fashion colors sell more readily, and, therefore, tend to reappear more frequently than others. In the United States, dark reds and wine tones tend to recur often. Orange is a color that flatters fewer people's personal coloring than some other colors, such as blue. Thus, orange does not occur as frequently in the color cycle as some other colors. Apparel designers and merchandisers keep in mind color preferences of their target customers as they look at color trends.

The color forecasting services used by textile producers (see Chapter 3) are also used by apparel companies. These services study color trends in textiles, apparel, home fashions, and related fields. Some color forecasting services predict color trends 18 months in advance of when the product is available to consumers, while others, for a higher subscription fee, predict farther ahead. An apparel company subscribes to the color forecasting service based on the category, such as men's apparel, as well as the length in advance for which forecasts are provided. Most services publish color forecasts twice a year for men's, women's, and children's apparel (see Figure 5.6). Some color forecasting services include forecasts for the home fashions industry.

Resources for color forecasting services based in the United States include the following:

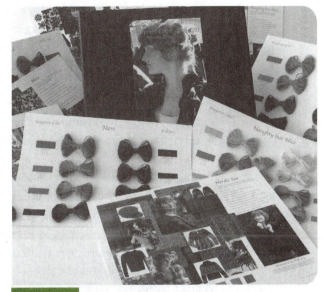

Figure 5.6 Color trend reports are issued by color forecasting services.

- Color Association of the United States (CAUS) produces seasonal predictions with fabric swatches twice a year. Annual memberships range from $650 to $1,350, which includes two seasonal forecasts for one category (women's, men's, youth, interiors/environmental).

- Pantone, based in Carlstadt, New Jersey, publishes the Pantone View Color Planner twice a year, providing seasonal color direction 24 months in advance (see Chapter 6 for more information about color), and offers color consulting services. Pantone View Home is targeted to the home fashions industry.

- Here & There, mentioned earlier in this chapter, provides both fashion trend and color forecasting services.

- Huepoint Color is an American color company dedicated to forecasting the best seasonal colors and color standards on different formats such as cotton yarn, cotton fabric, CMYK, and RGB.

These are a few of the many color resources available. Most apparel, accessories, and home fashions companies subscribe to several color forecasting services to provide a broader view of color trends.

Many people wonder how color trends are determined. Does "someone" predict that ruby red will be the color of the fall season, and that all designers will then include ruby red in their lines? Although this is not the case, color forecasting services do conduct color research to assist the fashion industry in the assessment of the color trends. Some U.S. forecasters rely on the color directions of fabric producers in Europe. They might watch to see whether these colors are adopted by fashion-forward designers and consumer fashion innovators in the United States. Other color forecasting services will focus on analyzing trends in consumer color preferences through sales data.

From the wide variety of possible colors, a palette of certain hues, values, and intensities that reflect upcoming color trends will be identified by the color forecasting service. Many apparel companies subscribe to several color forecasting services. It is interesting and informative to compare the similarities and differences of several color forecasting services' predictions for the same season.

The color trends presented by the color forecasting services are represented by a grouping of paint chips, fabric swatches, or yarn pompons, arranged attractively in a spiral-bound notebook or magazine format. These color palette charts may include up to several dozen colors. The colors selected tend to span a range of darks and lights, neutrals, and fashion colors. Thus, one color service will not predict all dark colors while another service shows all light colors. Designers and merchandisers will be able to identify certain overall trends recurring among the various color forecasting services.

After studying the color trends, designers and merchandisers will select a **color palette**, or color story, for the upcoming season, taking into consideration the many factors important to the success of their line. A designer may note that varying shades of purple have appeared in many of the color forecasts, indicating a purple trend. Some services provide fashion names for the color chips. The various shades of purple might be named violet, plum, dahlia, wisteria, African violet, and lavender. The specific name may be transferred to the color name used by the apparel company for that color, or a new name may be created by the apparel company to identify their company's seasonal color. The theme of a line might be linked to the color names used. For example, color names such as adobe, cactus, sage, and sandstone might be selected to correlate with a southwestern theme for a line.

Fabric and Trim Research and Resources

The designer and merchandiser research the fabric and trim market in addition to studying fashion and color trends. The designer undertakes fabric research, beginning with such broad fabric trends as the trend toward the use of spandex blended with wool for career apparel or the use of microfibers for men's suits and raincoats. This research might include such trends as the use of metallic fibers in fabrics or the use of chenille yarns in suitings. Resources for this type of fabric research include the same trade publications that designers and merchandisers use for fashion trends, as well as textile trade publications.

For more specific fabric trends, textile mills, textile trade associations, and textile manufacturers are eager to acquaint designers with the latest fibers, fabrics, and textures. Fabric manufacturers employ sales representatives who supply designers with fabric swatch cards, usually in response to a phone call by the design team member to the textile sales representative. Sample yardage can also be ordered from the sales representative. Many fabric manufacturers have showrooms in New York and other cities that display the latest fabrics. The textile trade associations' headquarters are excellent resources as well. For example, a designer might visit the New York office of Cotton Incorporated to research a wide range of woven and knit cotton fabrications.

A very effective way to research fabric resources is to visit one of the textile trade shows (see Chapter 3 for a discussion of these trade shows). The shows are usually held twice a year, in the fall and the spring. American fabric manufacturers hold their textile trade shows in New York and Los Angeles. Here, many fabric manufacturers have booths displaying the latest and most enticing fabrics. In addition, smaller shows are held in cities such as Chicago and Seattle.

Some of the international fabric manufacturers bring their fabric lines to New York and Los Angeles to show to the American designers who are not able to travel to Europe. For example, Première Vision Preview New York features Italian, French, Spanish, Austrian, and Portuguese fabrics. The Los Angeles International Textile Show features both imported and domestic fabrics, trims, and findings.

Some designers travel to the European textile trade shows held twice a year to see the latest goods produced by fabric manufacturers in Europe (see Chapter 3 for detailed information). European textile trade shows include the following:

- Première Vision, showcasing Europe's fabric manufacturers, is held in Paris (see Figure 5.7).

- Texworld is also held in Paris twice a year, showcasing fabrics from 42 countries.

- Italian fabrics are featured along with those of many other countries at Ideacomo and Ideabiella near Milan.

- Prato Expo in Florence, Italy, hosts textile companies from Europe, North America, and Asia.

- Interstoff Asia, held in Hong Kong, provides an opportunity to feature Asian-produced textiles.

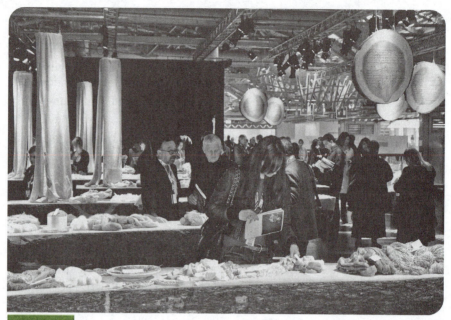

Figure 5.7   Designers attend textile trade shows for fabric research and inspiration.

Designers can place orders for **sample cuts** from the textile producers. Each cut is usually three to five yards long, enough yardage to produce a prototype garment in order to evaluate the possible use of the fabric. The sample cuts are sent to the apparel company after the order is placed at a trade show. Sample cuts can also be ordered directly from the sales representative after the trade show. For many designers, though, these textile shows serve a similar purpose as the couture design shows—as an inspiration and a means to sift through the multitude of ideas for trends appropriate to their company's target customers.

Some types of apparel are especially suited to the use of specialty trims and fasteners. Outdoor activewear is one example. A new design idea might be sparked by a novelty trim or fastener. Trims, as a source of design inspiration, will be discussed in Chapter 6. Research regarding new products is an important aspect for designers and merchandisers. Product trade shows, trade publications, and specialty trim sales representatives are sources of information about such new products.

Armed with information from market research—fashion and color trend research, and fabric and trim research—the designer is ready to bring everything together in the creation of a new line.

Summary

Creating an apparel line begins with research. Sales figures from the current selling season are taken into consideration as the designer and merchandiser plan the upcoming line. However, a fashion apparel company cannot survive long if it only repeats what has sold well in the past. Market research is often conducted to help predict what specific items or general trends will appeal to customers in the upcoming season. The merchandiser's and designer's job responsibilities include long-range forecasting of major social, economic, retail, apparel manufacturing, and customer trends. Short-range forecasting is also tied to the economy, political climate, availability of resources, and customer needs. The target customer profile, describing such aspects as the target customer's age, lifestyle, and intended price zone, requires constant updating and careful consideration in the creation of an apparel line.

The merchandiser and designer conduct fashion trend research on a daily basis by reading fashion publications, attending fashion events, and developing the ability to sense the fashion mood of the times. They translate this information into styles for the target customer. Color forecasting services provide information for color trend research, another important component of the creation stage. The apparel company may subscribe to one or more of these services. Fabric trend research is another aspect of the designer's responsibility. This may include scrutinizing fashion and textile industry publications and attending textile trade shows in New York and European and Asian fashion centers. While research is being conducted on the upcoming line, it is important to remember that the designer may also be working on fabric and style development for a subsequent line, is involved with production of the current line, and is watching the sales figures on the line currently selling in retail stores.

CAREER PROFILES

If you are particularly interested in fashion-related research or the analysis of market trends, color, or fashion trends, additional coursework in consumer behavior, market analysis, statistics, and some related job experience may be helpful.

Fashion Trend Forecaster
Publisher of Trend Forecasting Report

Position Description:

Scan stores in trendsetting locales to identify key fashion trends, analyze shopping behavior, advise retail store buyers, and write trend forecasts.

Typical Tasks and Responsibilities:

- Travel extensively to determine trends.
- Gauge shifting trend patterns and public interest in product innovation.
- Scan merchandise in trendsetting stores.
- Talk with sales associates to discuss trends.
- Confer with retail store buyers about significant trends affecting their businesses.
- Observe and analyze shopping behavior.
- Write trend forecasts for trend reports.

Key Terms

carryover

collection

color palette

consumer research

demographics

fashion color

fashion forecasting service

fashion magazine

group

lifestyle merchandising

line

long-range forecasting

market analysis

market research

master calendar

merchandiser

popular fashion magazine

product research

psychographics

sample cut

shopping the market

short-range forecasting

staple color

target customer

trade publication

trend research

Discussion Questions and Activities

1. What are some examples of trends that can be predicted by long-range forecasting (perhaps five years from now)? How might these trends affect the apparel industry?

2. What are some examples of short-range trend forecasting (perhaps six months from now) in men's apparel, women's apparel, and children's apparel? How might these trends be reflected in an apparel line?

3. Describe what you perceive as the target customer profile for the following national brands: Roxy, Polo Ralph Lauren, DKNY, and Tommy Hilfiger.

4. What are some current color trends in women's wear? In menswear? What color or colors do you predict will be popular next season in women's wear? In menswear? Why do you think these colors will be popular?

5. What are some fabric trends that are on the upswing in the fashion cycle?

6. What are some examples of specific sources of research information for designers and merchandisers? How would you locate examples of these?

References

Behling, Dorothy U. (1999, January). Aging boomers may shift the apparel empire. *Bobbin*, pp. 53–54.

Eddie Bauer (2010). About Eddie Bauer Retrieved June 28, 2010, from http://investors. eddiebauer. com/about

Kinnear, Thomas C., and Taylor, James R. (1983). *Marketing Research: An Applied Approach*. New York: McGraw-Hill Book Company, pp. 16–17.

"NRF Retail Innovation and Marketing Conference Highlights" (2010, April) *Stores*, pp. 22–23.

Patagonia announces major expansion of garment recycling program. (2007, January 28). Patagonia.com Retrieved February 21, 2007 from http://www.patagonia.com/ pdf/en_US/common_threads_pr_expansion.pdf

Smith, Ray (2009, December 31) Style: Two dowdy clothing brands go for vogue— Catalog retailers LL Bean and Lands' End launch lines aimed at younger customers; a relaxed, lived-in style. *The Wall Street Journal,* p. D.5.

Socha, Mike. (1997, December 7). Romancing the store. *Women's Wear Daily*, p. 12.

Tommy Bahama (2007). Tommy Bahama Home Page Retrieved June 28, 2010, from http://tommybahama.com/index.jsp

Walzer, Emily (2010, January/February) Consumer connections. *Textile Insight*, p. 18.

Walzer, Emily (2010, January/February) Insight on what's next. *Textile Insight,* p. 22.

Welling, Holly. (1999, December). Patagonia: small world view of big business. *Apparel Industry Magazine,* pp. AS-26–32.

Interview Ms. Fiona Jenvey, CEO and Founder, Mudpie Ltd. Retrieved June 21, 2010, from http://www.fibre2fashion.com/face2face/mudpie-ltd/ms-fiona-jenvey.asp

CHAPTER 6

Creating a Line:
Design

The discussion of the creation, marketing, production, and distribution of a line in the following seven chapters provides an overview of the processes that occur from the inception of a line until the product reaches the ultimate customer. There are many variations of the specific sequence of processes used by apparel companies. For the most part, a traditional design and manufacturing sequence of processes will be used to avoid confusion. Alternative possible sequences will be discussed where appropriate.

In this chapter, you will learn the following:

- the various sources of design inspiration

- the market forces that direct a company's design focus

- the scope of the job responsibilities of the design and merchandising team in designing a line

- the interrelationship between design and merchandising in developing a new season's line

- the ways computer-aided design and graphic design software systems are used in the design process

- the use of product lifecycle management systems to track each style as it progresses through the design, style selection, marketing, preproduction, production, and distribution processes

Step 2: Design

Step 1 Research and Merchandising

Step 2 Design

| Design Inspiration |
| Plan the Line |
| Sketch Design and Obtain Vendor Samples |
| Select or Develop Fabrics and Trims |
| Review and Select Styles to Develop for Line |
| Write Garment Specifications Sheet and Quick Cost |

Step 3 Design Development and Style Selection

Step 4 Marketing the Apparel Line

Step 5 Preproduction

Step 6 Sourcing

Step 7 Apparel Production Processes, Material Management, and Quality Assurance

Step 8 Distribution and Retailing

Design Inspiration

*T*he design stage of creating a line combines the designer's and merchandiser's interpretations of market and fashion trends, their understanding of the target customer, and new design inspirations appropriately interpreted for the target customer. Where do designers come up with the multitude of new designs each season? Designers' inspirations for a new line can come from a variety of sources that may have been part of the market and fashion research conducted. All the research information discussed in the previous chapter sifts through the designer's mind during this phase of the design process. For example, designers may be inspired by studying pictures of design ideas from fashion trend sources, collecting swatches of interesting fabric textures and trims, developing some innovative design details, conducting research about a historical period or another culture, or searching the marketplace for a "lightning bolt" idea. Designers may visit historical costume and textile collections, such as the Fashion Institute of Technology's collection or the Metropolitan Museum of Art's Costume Institute, both in New York City. Apparel companies located close to such extensive costume and/or textile resources may pay an annual fee so that their designers can have continual access to the collections. These sources of design inspirations are then interpreted for the specific company's target customer. The interrelationships of various types of information needed to create a new line are shown in Figure 6.1.

A Theme for the New Line

Based on market research, design inspirations, and discussions among the designers and merchandisers who are coordinating the various lines for a company, a theme for the line might be developed. Not every group or line will have a theme, but a theme can help sell a group or a line to retailers and consumers. In some cases, an advertising campaign may be developed around a chosen theme. For example, a company producing an outdoor fishing group might use the theme of a popular sport fish (see Figure 6.2). The theme might be carried through in the graphic art used on items in the group.

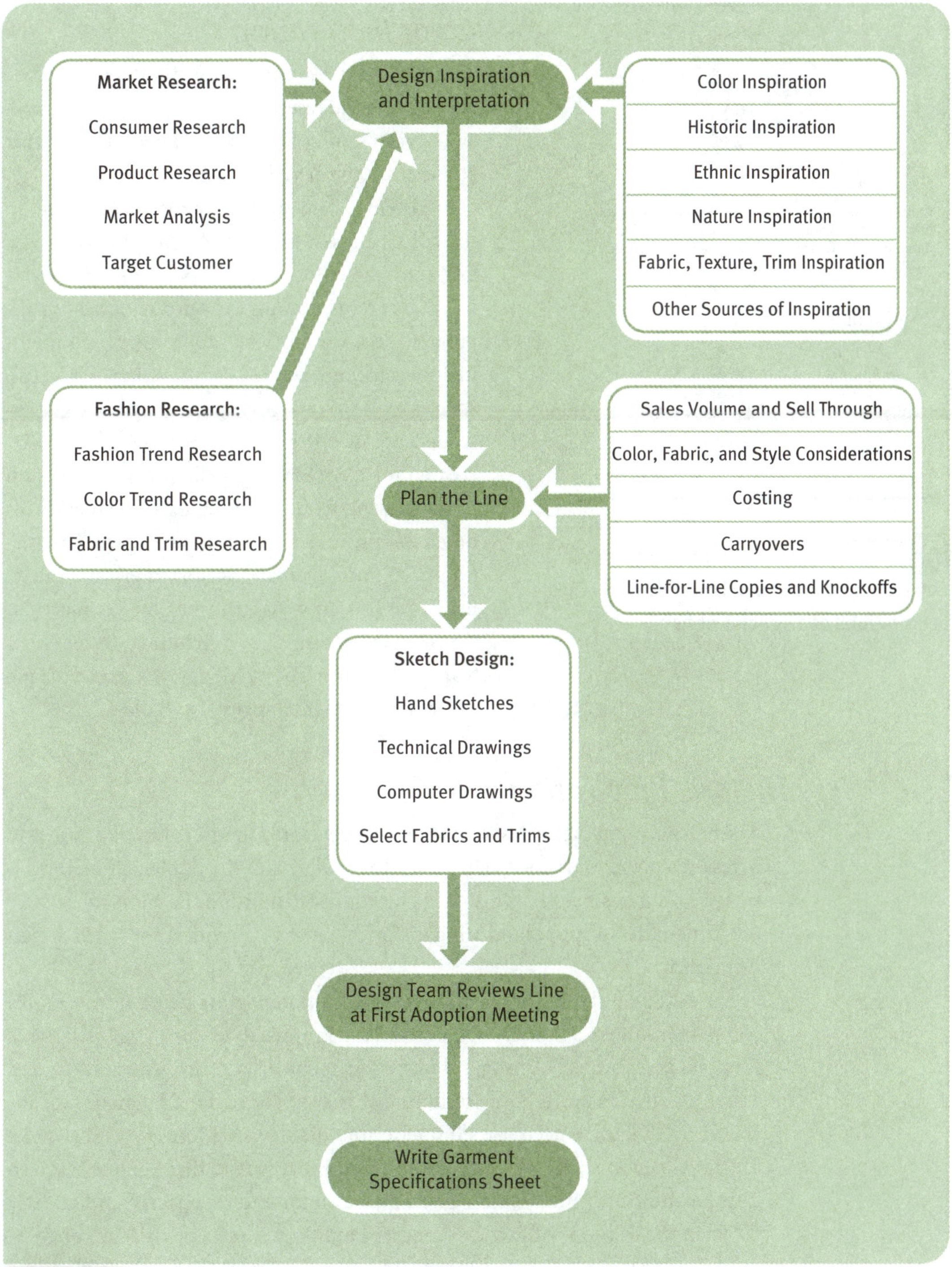

Market Research:

Consumer Research

Product Research

Market Analysis

Target Customer

Design Inspiration and Interpretation

Color Inspiration

Historic Inspiration

Ethnic Inspiration

Nature Inspiration

Fabric, Texture, Trim Inspiration

Other Sources of Inspiration

Fashion Research:

Fashion Trend Research

Color Trend Research

Fabric and Trim Research

Plan the Line

Sales Volume and Sell Through

Color, Fabric, and Style Considerations

Costing

Carryovers

Line-for-Line Copies and Knockoffs

Sketch Design:

Hand Sketches

Technical Drawings

Computer Drawings

Select Fabrics and Trims

Design Team Reviews Line at First Adoption Meeting

Write Garment Specifications Sheet

Figure 6.1 Step 2 Design expanded to show how a new line is created.

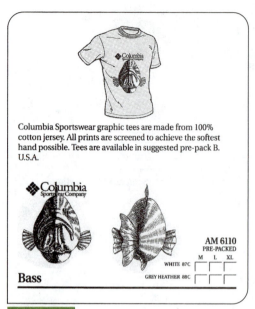

Columbia Sportswear graphic tees are made from 100%
cotton jersey. All prints are screened to achieve the softest
hand possible. Tees are available in suggested pre-pack B.
U.S.A.

Figure 6.2 A group within a line might be designed around a theme, such as the colorations of a species of fish.

Color Inspiration

The design team studies color trend reports gathered during the research phase and discusses possible groups of colors, also referred to as **color stories,** for the new line while thinking about a color theme. The theme might be reflected in the colors chosen for some of the new styles. For example, the colorations seen on a golden trout might be an inspiration for a group of fishing apparel. Colors for fabrics used in the group might include various hues, tones, and values of the fish species' colorations. A graphic design of a golden trout leaping up to catch a fishing fly could be created for a T-shirt in the line. A small version of the leaping trout could be used as an embroidered or printed motif on other pieces in the group. As another example, an Americana theme might be chosen for a group of misses pieces in a Spring collection with a "country flavor" that features fabrics in ruby red, navy blue, and bisque colors in solids, small prints, and plaids.

Historic Inspiration

The high-fashion name designers typically develop a theme for a collection and invest heavily in marketing that theme to retailers and the public. Often the designer's theme is based on historical or ethnic inspiration. Fashion silhouettes or garment details popular during historical periods provide a source of design inspiration.

For example, the Empire silhouette was fashionable during the early 1800s. Named for France's Emperor Napoleon, the Empire style was worn by his wife, Empress Josephine. The long, tubular dress included a raised waistline located just under the bustline. Some fashion historians believe that Napoleon was inspired by the ancient Greek silhouette for this new fashion look. This style, known as *neoclassical,* became a fashion trend that spread throughout Western Europe and the United States. The Empire silhouette reappeared in the early 1900s in the fashions of French designer Paul Poiret, seen in his *Directoire* Revival dress (Mackrell, 1990). Once again, other designers copied this style as the fashion look spread throughout Europe and the United States. In the 1960s, the raised waistline of the Empire silhouette appeared again, this time in an above-the-knee minidress version, as well as a long version. In the early 1990s, and again in the first decade of the twenty-first century, the Empire style made fashion headlines. Figure 6.3 shows how the Empire style was adapted for different eras.

As another example of historical inspiration, both American designer Adrian and French designer Balenciaga were inspired by the bustle silhouette of the 1870s and 1880s for their designs created in the 1940s and 1950s. The bustle has been an important design silhouette from earlier times through to the present (see Figure 6.4).

Garment details of historic eras serve as another source of inspiration for designers. French designer Karl Lagerfeld used Renaissance fashion details as inspiration for a Chanel design in the 1988–1989 collection (Martin & Koda, 1989). The ruff collar popular on Renaissance clothing may inspire a group, a line, or a collection (see Figure 6.5). A sleeve detail from the Renaissance period could be an inspiration for a young girl's party dress. Other examples of often-used sources of historically inspired fashions include the following:

- ancient Greek and Roman costume
- medieval costume
- eighteenth-century fashions
- Victorian fashions
- Flapper dress of the 1920s

Retro Fashion

A return to the fashion look of more recent decades is called a **Retro** fashion or *Retro look*. In the twenty-first century, fashion looks reminiscent of the 1980s were added to the mix of Retro looks from the 1960s and 1970s. Retro fashions tend not to be exact replicas of the previous fashion look; instead, they include a

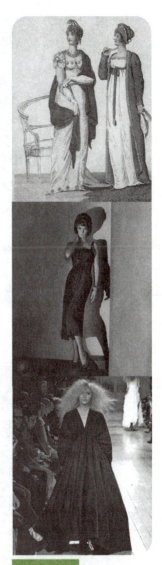

Figure 6.3 The Empire style recurred periodically throughout fashion history. Shown here are examples from the early nineteenth century (1807), the middle twentieth century (1950's), and the early twenty-first century (2011).

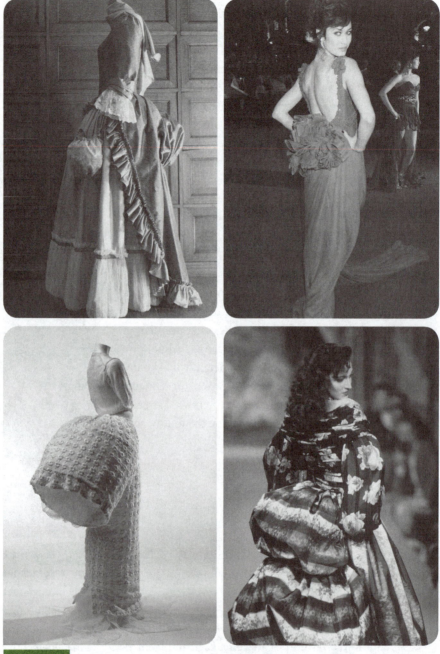

Figure 6.4 Various bustle silhouettes through time: (clockwise from top left) period dress from early 1700s France, a Valentino dress from 2008, a Christian Lacroix dress from 1987, and a Rei Kawakubo for Comme des Garçons dress from 2010.

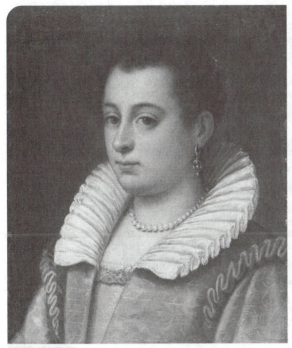 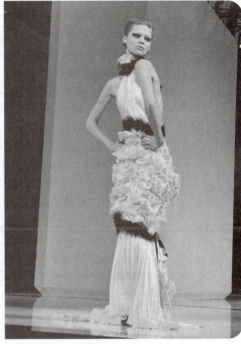

Figure 6.5 Fashion details from one era may inspire new fashion details in another.

"new" fashion twist, for example:

- A Retro look design may have style details of the earlier fashion but be made from a currently popular fabric rather than a fabric similar to that used in the earlier fashion.

- The Retro look might include updated style details that are different from the original, while the fabric might resemble the fabric used for the earlier fashion.

Ethnic Inspiration

Designers may be inspired by the clothing styles of other cultures. The global environment has increased interest in products from the far reaches of the world. Consumers who purchase and wear fashions inspired by other cultures may derive a sense of adventure and vicarious enjoyment of that culture. Designers seek inspiration from exotic cultures with clothing styles, fabrics, and accessories that are unique. Some designers travel to other locales to seek inspiration for a new line.

Asian clothing styles have been a source of inspiration historically, as well as for current fashions. *Chinoiserie* is a French term for a style that incorporates Chinese motifs. The fabrics of China were used to create Western high-fashion apparel during the 1850s. The Chinese influence on Western fashion grew during the last decades of the 1800s. In the United States, Chinese motifs became fashionable in home fashions, chinaware, house style details, and such clothing styles as the kimono sleeve, Mandarin collar, and frog closures. Chinese clothing and fabrics continue to inspire apparel designers today.

In 1995, the Costume Institute of the Metropolitan Museum of Art in New York presented *Orientalism: Visions of the East in Western Dress*. This exhibition and the catalog (Martin & Koda, 1994) featured apparel inspired by Asian cultures from various decades. Included in the exhibit were several examples of Asian-inspired garments from recent collections of American designers Ralph Lauren, Oscar de la Renta, and Todd Oldham. For French designer Karl Lagerfeld's Fall 2006 Chanel collection, he

> was inspired by the tour de force exhibit at London's Royal Academy, *China: The Three Emperors, 1662–1795*. This show revealed that the emperors Kangxi, Yongzheng, and Qianlong, conquering Manchu warriors from the north, were also highly refined artistic patrons and poets. Lagerfeld took the exquisite pale-jade objects that the emperors commissioned and used them as the starting point for his dazzling evening embroideries... (Bowles, 2006, p. 142).

Yves Saint Laurent, a former French couture designer, is renowned for his use of various national and ethnic groups and cultures as inspirations for his collections. He created collections inspired by such regions as Russia, Africa, China, and Spain (Saint Laurent, Vreeland, et al., 1983). In 2010, designer Alberta Ferretti took her cue from a traveler to Marrakech. "Blurry prints in soft shades of the savannah sunset show up in ethereal evening gowns, while tribal motifs appear on hippie-ish bootleg pants paired with soft camisoles "(At Ease, 2010, p 7)."

Nature as a Source of Inspiration

Design inspiration is anywhere and everywhere. Nature is another example of a source of inspiration, from flora to fauna, from sky to wind to water. For New York designer Zac Posen's Spring 2004 collection, he was inspired by images of the Sargasso Sea (out in the blue Atlantic, a vast bed of floating seaweed where mysterious sea creatures swim), and long walks along the sultry beach at sunset. From Botticelli's famous Venus on the half-shell, and from an illustrated science book about seashells, Posen borrowed his soft hues, his muted palette of sea foam and lavender (with jolts of vibrant reds and yellows) (Talley, 2003, pp. 94, 122).

New York designer Gene Meyer's visit to St. Petersburg, Russia, "sparked the theme for his Fall 1999 collection called "In the Shadow of the Winter Palace." "… St. Petersburg was just amazing. It was a combination of the way the city basked in sunlight, the bright pearly sky, and the snow everywhere that inspired me" (Knight, 1999, p. 16). The inspiration might be the designer's impetus for developing the color story for a group or collection, or the designer might be inspired by the shape or texture of the inspirational source.

Fabric, Texture, and Trim Inspiration

Whereas some designers who create apparel for the higher price zones research a specific period or culture for inspiration, many designers often rely on studying new fabric and texture trends. Sources of information and inspiration used for fabric research are discussed in Chapters 3 and 5. An intriguing fabric texture or interesting print might serve as the design inspiration and become the foundation for a group. Several fabrics in prints, plaids, and solid colors, and with smooth as well as textured surfaces, might be combined to create an interesting group. During this design stage of creation, some designers work with specific fabric ideas gathered at textile shows or obtained directly from textile manufacturers as they begin to sketch garment design ideas (see Chapters 3 and 5). Less frequently, designers might develop a design sketch and then seek the perfect fabric for it. Another option for designers at some companies is to develop, or work with others to develop, a new textile fabrication or a textile print for the new line.

Special trims and **findings** (also known as notions or sundries), such as buttons or fasteners, can be important features of some garment designs. A unique trim can transform an ordinary or classic garment into a new look. For children's apparel, special ribbons, trims, and appliqués frequently "make" the design. A unique clasp or closure on a swimsuit design can increase its appeal (see Figure 6.6), or a special button on a classic jacket may create a fresh look. Designers constantly seek interesting trims and findings as sources of inspiration.

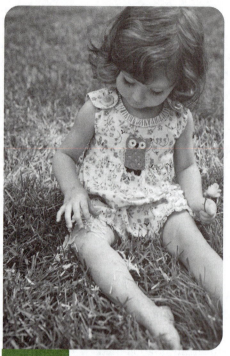

Figure 6.6 Findings such as buttons and trims provide innovative and fun design details.

Other Sources of Inspiration

The inspiration for a garment within a line or for an entire line can come from an infinite variety of sources. Sources of inspiration are often linked to the social spirit of the times, also called the **zeitgeist**. Events and the general spirit of the popular culture might be reflected in new apparel lines. "Tommy Hilfiger, who travels extensively, said he's most inspired by the younger generations in cities across the globe. The most influential factor in every major city are the kids on the streets who set the trends" (Knight, 1999, p. 16). Ask designers what inspired them to create a particular line, and you may be surprised to learn that Japanese kites were the inspiration for a line of swimsuits or that graffiti was the inspiration for a line of sportswear.

The Market Niche

Successful designers and merchandisers are able to interpret their design inspirations appropriately for their target customer. As noted in Chapters 4 and 5, many apparel companies specialize in a certain type of product, such as casual clothes, swimwear, or evening wear. The apparel company's **product type**, or product line, is the basis for the development of its line. For example, Lacoste is known for the company's polo-style knit shirts. If you are familiar with this company, a certain type of product comes to mind when the name of the company is mentioned (see Figure 6.7). Consistency in a company's product type helps the customer develop company brand recognition, build product loyalty, and encourage repeat customers. Thus, the design team, which consists of designers, product developers, and merchandisers, will develop the line for the new season with the product type as its foundation.

The importance of keeping the target customer profile in mind when creating a line was discussed in Chapter 5. A strong connection exists between the type of product included in the line and the company's target customer. The blend of product type with target customer is referred to as the **market niche**. Developing and maintaining a line based on the market niche is important to the success of the apparel line. The line for the new season will include some variation of styles to appeal to the variety of customers' needs and tastes within the market niche. For example, a misses swimwear manufacturer will include some very conservative swimsuit styles as well as some styles that have an updated look (see Figure 6.8). The misses swimwear line might be divided into several groups to appeal to a variety of misses customers. Based on the changing needs and preferences of the target customer, a company's product line may change over time. If the product line does not change at all, customers might become bored with the same look and decide that they do not need to purchase another item so similar to items they already own. Examples of product line changes include the following:

- A company might decide to change the direction of its product from a focus on career suits to a focus on coordinated separates after sensing that women are no longer interested in the look of a matched suit.

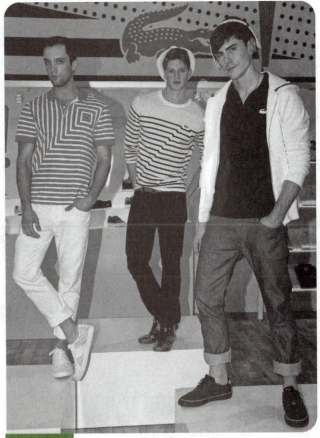

Figure 6.7 Consumers associate the name of a company, such as Lacoste, with a specific fashion image.

- A sportswear company may decide to add a golf apparel group to its product line because of the growth in popularity of golf among its target customers.

Sometimes new designers and/or merchandisers are hired by a company to help revamp the product type. However, if a new look for a product is too radical, or if the product type is changed too quickly, it can cause problems for the retailer and the customer. Retaining the loyal customer is important, just as it is important to attract new customers for company growth. The customer who is familiar with and enjoys wearing the company's product may not understand the new look. Balancing the relationships among the current product look, changes that need to occur in the product to maintain interest and provide fashion change, and keeping the target customer happy is one of the responsibilities of the design team.

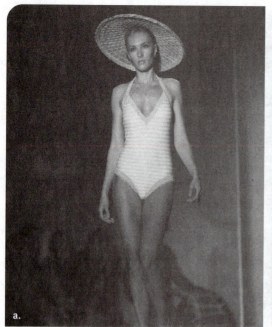
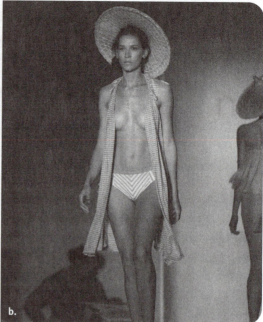

Figure 6.8 A swimwear line includes styles ranging from conservative (a) to fashion forward (b) looks.

Planning the Line

Although the research and design inspiration stages of the design process—consisting of market research, as well as trend, color, and fabric-and-trim research—continues throughout the year, at a specified time in the year, the design team must begin to develop concrete ideas for the new season's line. Based on the number of lines a company produces each year, each apparel company maintains a master calendar with target due dates for completion of the stages of the creation and production of each line (see the Eight Steps in the Design Process flowchart at the beginning of Part 2). The design team looks at the due date for the finalization of a line and then works backward to determine when to move from the research stage to the design stage.

The Design Team's Role

The creation of each line relies on a team of people. Designers typically work with merchandisers and product developers on the creation of each new style in the line (see Figure 6.9, an example of an apparel company's design team organizational chart). As discussed in Chapter 5, many larger apparel companies employ a merchandiser whose responsibility it is to oversee and guide the designer or design team to determine what, when, at what price, and how much apparel to produce.

A merchandiser often works with designers of several lines to oversee the coordination among the lines. In some companies, especially smaller ones, the designer also performs the job responsibilities of the merchandiser. Some companies employ both designers and product developers. A product developer takes the designer's idea and is responsible for developing the product. The product developer does the following:

- researches possible fabrics and trims
- works with vendors in securing all components for the style
- coordinates all aspects of style creation

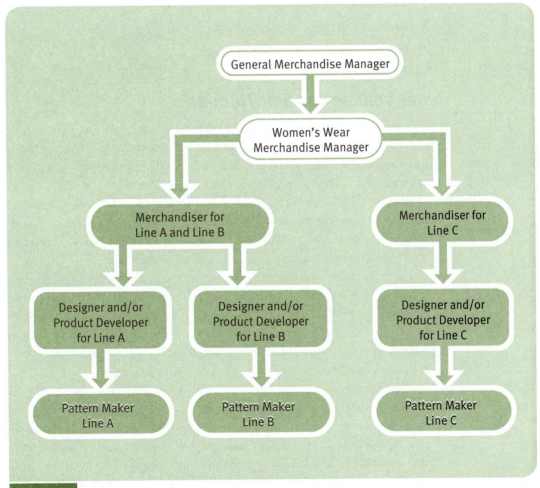

Figure 6.9 Apparel company organization chart.

At some smaller companies, the designer also handles the product development responsibilities.

The designer(s) and merchandiser(s) attend planning meetings during the research and design stages. At planning meetings, the sales figures (including sales volume and sell-through) for the previous season are reviewed, the sales projections for the new season are considered, and the overall plan and schedule for the upcoming season's line are discussed. This might include the following:

- decisions about the target number of styles to include in the line
- the ratio of jackets compared to vests or the ratio of skirts compared to pants
- the styles that will be repeated from the previous season (carryovers)
- the types of silhouettes for various styles
- the decision to try something new to be added to the line
- the colors and fabrics that will be used
- the costs of all components for the line

Sales Volume and Sell-Through

There is an expression in the fashion business—"you're only as good as your last line"—that means a company's success is measured by how well the previous season's line sold. Success of a line is measured by sales volume and also by sell-through at the retail level. **Sales volume** is the actual level of sales in terms of either the total number of units of each style sold or the total number of dollars consumers spent on the style (dollar volume). Manufacturers tend to measure the success of a line by the total number of units sold, while retailers tend to measure the success of a line by the dollar volume.

The designer and merchandiser have to hit the targeted sales volume with a mix of repeated styles, revised styles, and new styles. Because of the number of lines typically produced per year, the sales volume figures are not usually available in time to rely on the number of units sold during the previous season in order to predict accurately the strategy for the line under development. Therefore, one's intuition also becomes a part of planning the line.

A line may sell well at market to the retailer (see Chapter 8), but a delay in delivery to the retailer could reduce the dollar volume at the retail store. This is one reason why another measurement tool, the line's sell-through, is considered a good indicator of the line's success. **Sell-through** denotes the percentage of items sold at retail compared to the number of items in the line that the retailer purchased from the manufacturer. For example, if 300 items in a line were delivered by the apparel manufacturer to the retail store and 250 of the items were sold, the sell-through would be 83 percent. Keep in mind that markdowns—that is, items that were put on sale—enter into the overall success of the line as well. A strong sell-through is the goal for both the manufacturer and the retailer. The sales figures from the current and previous selling seasons are important guidelines in planning how many and what types of apparel items to include in the new line.

Color, Fabric, and Style Considerations

During planning meetings, colors and fabrics for the new season's line are discussed. A color story will be developed based on the color research conducted before the planning meetings. Lines need a balance between some staple colors and some fashion colors (see Chapter 5). The line needs to have a cohesive look, so a great deal of time is spent deciding on the correct balance of colors. The group of colors selected for the line may need to include a color that the design team does not expect to sell well because they know that buyers expect to see a balance of colors in the color group (for example, a light color may be needed to balance the color story of a group of medium and dark colors).

Most garment styles will be produced in more than one color. A specific style may be available in three or four different solid colors, or in three or four color variations of the same print. The varieties of colors available for a style are called **colorways**. Producing the same style in several colorways is efficient in terms of development cost since fewer patterns, spec sheets, prototypes, and cost estimates need to be prepared than if each style were produced in only one colorway. This variety also offers more options to retailers that might want to buy part of a line but not duplicate the same colorways as competing local retailers will offer in their stores. It also allows a retailer to select the colorway choices that the retailer thinks are best suited for its customers.

As discussed in Chapter 5, designers typically attend textile trade shows and are aware of the new colors and fabrics available. Fabric vendors will provide samples of fabrics that the design team is considering for use in the upcoming line. Therefore, decisions regarding the colors and fabrics are frequently made before the garment styles are determined. The new line needs to provide a balance among the colors, styles, and prices offered.

Costing

The production cost of each style in a line is an important factor for designers to consider throughout the design stage. Thus, many companies include cost personnel as a part of the team during the planning meetings for a new line. Their role is to provide cost estimates on the new styles in the line as the styles develop. There are many factors to keep in mind related to costing. Even prior to providing an initial cost estimate, each company has pricing strategies that guide costing. Examples of pricing strategies include the following:

- It is important that two garments in the same line do not compete against each other for sales. Some manufacturers follow a pricing strategy that specifies that the prices of two different shirt styles should not be the same—and style differences in the two styles need to support the price difference. A shirt made from a more expensive fabric might have fewer garment details, while a shirt made from a less expensive fabric could have more details to be sold at similar (but not identical) price.

- Pricing strategies need to make sense to the customer. Comparing two shirts in a line with different prices, it needs to be apparent to the customer that the higher-priced shirt is made from the more expensive fabric or that the higher priced shirt has more complex style details to justify the price.

- With the pricing strategy called **price averaging**, a shirt manufactured from a more expensive fabric is priced to equalize a shirt manufactured from a less expensive fabric. The manufacturer averages the costs of the two shirts to keep the price of both styles similar. Thus, the shirt made from the more expensive fabric is priced slightly low, while the shirt made from the less expensive fabric is priced slightly high. If both styles sell equally, the company breaks even. If more shirts are sold that are made from the less expensive fabric, the company comes out ahead; if more shirts are sold that are made from the more expensive fabric, the company loses some profit.

- **Target costing** is a pricing strategy that developed as a result of a significant change made by the apparel industry in the design-produce-sell cycle. The process had been to create a new style, and then calculate its cost based on materials and labor. Now, price tends to drive the style decisions, especially in the moderate and budget/mass price zones, as well as in private-label and store brand merchandise. The style and fabric components are manipulated by setting a cost first, and then determining how many yards of fabric and at what price, estimating the cost of other components such as a zipper or buttons, and estimating how many minutes of labor are needed to produce the design, based on a per-hour labor price. For example, the design team might determine that they want to produce a jacket to sell at $75 retail ($37.50 wholesale). The team knows from previous seasons' costs that it takes 30 minutes to sew a basic jacket, and that one and one-half yards of fabric are required for a typical style. After estimating a cost per yard of a typical fabric and other components, the design team can calculate the cost. If the estimated total is less than the target cost, more design details (adding labor and materials cost) or more expensive fabrics or trims can be added to enhance the style and still meet the target cost.

The target costing process has been used for some time for certain types of goods, such as styles produced for a specific retail chain (sometimes called *special makeups*) and private-label goods. The design of private-label goods and store brand merchandise will be discussed in more detail later. One of the driving forces behind target costing is that in today's market (with the exception of the couture and some designer price zones), the upper limit of price is based on what the target customer is willing to pay.

Carryovers

A line of apparel typically does not consist of only new styles. In a new line, some styles will be carryovers, some styles will be modifications of good sellers, and some styles will be new designs. A carryover will repeat the same garment style as a successful garment style from a previous season, but often in a new fabric and color. Thus, carryovers provide a less expensive route to add a fresh look to a line. If the new fabric has identical textile characteristics as the previous fabric, the development cost will be minimal because the production patterns made for this style can be reused. However, if the new fabric is different—for example, it has a different shrinkage factor—a new pattern and prototype will need to be made.

Companies vary regarding the number of new items compared with the number of carryovers for each line. For an idea of the approximate ratio for a company that produces apparel in the moderate wholesale price zone, some companies target about one-third of the line to be carryovers, one-third as revisions of previous styles, and one-third as new designs. The percentage of new styles could be as low as 10 percent at some mass to moderate price zone companies, whereas a bridge or designer label might produce mostly new styles. Some styles in a new line might be revisions of a style from a previous season. One or more design details, such as a collar or pocket, might be changed for the new season to revise a style. This process cuts down on the development time, saves some cost, and also provides some degree of confidence that the revised style will sell well in the marketplace.

Line-for-Line Copies and Knockoffs

Rather than starting with a designer's sketch for a new design, a "new" style might be added to a line in another way. Sometimes while shopping the market or looking through fashion magazines, a designer or merchandiser will find a garment that seems ideal for the company's upcoming line. Thus, the designer and merchandiser may decide to create a copy of an existing garment. Copying a garment may be done in several ways. For example, a unique design, such as a shirt with innovative design details, may seem perfect for the upcoming line. The designer might request that a **line-for-line copy** of the shirt be made by the pattern development department and produced in a similar fabric. The new shirt would be an exact replica of the original; thus the term *line-for-line copy* is used.

Another example is taking a garment that exists in a higher price zone and copying it to be sold at a lower price. This can be done by selecting a less expensive fabric, or by eliminating or modifying some of the design details. These methods are used to create **knockoffs**, designs that are similar to the original, but not exact replicas. Moderate price clothing lines often knockoff successful designer looks once the style has become poplar.

Is it legal to copy an existing garment design? The United States has laws to protect against copyright and trademark infringement (see Chapter 2). A specific "invention" in a garment (for example, a unique molding process to create a seamless panty) can be patented in the United States. However, in some countries (including the United States), the actual garment design is considered to be in the public domain. Therefore, it is quite common to see line-for-line copies and knockoffs in the U.S. apparel business. An article in *Women's Wear Daily* stated that creating knockoffs "is a practice so commonplace, and one not clearly prohibited by law, that most designers who have been copied have felt helpless to stop it" (Wilson, 1999, p. 8). Design laws are more strict in some European countries, as evidenced by the 1994 case, in which French designer Yves Saint Laurent took Ralph Lauren to court in France in a dispute over the design copy of a tuxedo dress (see Figure 6.10) ("Tuxedo Junction," 1994).

Several court cases in the United States regarding trade dress law, a part of trademark law (see Chapter 2), have brought the issue of copying into the headlines. As reported by *Women's Wear Daily*, "there have been several recent legal challenges, and now that the Supreme Court has taken up a case with the potential to define what constitutes a violation of existing trade dress law, the practice of knockoffs is under the spotlight, raising questions among manufacturers of what the ramifications of such a decision could be" (Wilson, 1999, p. 8).

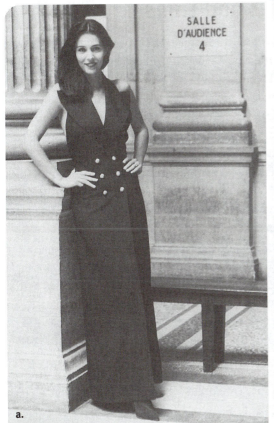 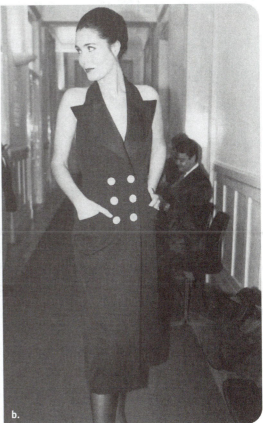

Figure 6.10 The tuxedo dress as presented by Yves Saint Laurent (a), and the tuxedo dress as presented by Ralph Lauren (b).

Many factors need to be considered during the planning of a line. Among them is the overall number of styles to be included in the line. Some of these styles will be carryover styles from the previous line, some styles will be revisions of previous styles, and some styles will be new designs. Decisions are also made about the following:

- the number of top styles in relation to the number of bottom styles
- styling variety (such as single-breasted and double-breasted jackets)
- color and fabric offerings for each style
- cost to produce each style
- overall pricing balance of the line

Selection of Fabrics and Trims

Sourcing for the right fabrics and trims must often be accomplished at the planning stage of the design process. The fabrics and trims are usually selected before a design is approved for inclusion in a line. Each design sketch or tech drawing includes a small sample of the intended fabric, called a **swatch**, which is attached to the sketch or drawing. It is essential that the fabric be chosen before a design is reviewed by the merchandiser, designer, and cost personnel for possible inclusion in the final line. The design sketch or tech drawing will also include any trim swatches that will be used and may indicate specific findings as well. Sometimes the actual fabric intended for the design is not yet available from the textile manufacturer. In these cases, a facsimile fabric will be used temporarily for the design development stage.

Textile mills produce a large quantity of printed textiles each season. Many apparel companies purchase printed fabrics directly from textile mills for their lines. However, sometimes an apparel company prefers to work with a textile converter (see Chapter 3) to develop a printed textile. A new textile design can be created from the following:

- an existing print that is revised into a new colorway
- a new textile print developed by the designers, assistant designers, or product developers (for example, if they cannot find the right print on the market)
- a textile design that is purchased from a company or a freelance textile designer who creates and sells original artwork for the printed textile industry

When an apparel company purchases a piece of textile design artwork, it owns the rights to copy or change the print as it wishes. Thus, the apparel company's staff can reconfigure a textile design's scale, motif, colors, or repeat to suit their needs.

The Design Sketch

At some point in the design stage (usually determined by the master calendar due date), the designer will begin to transform interpretations of design inspirations into garment idea sketches. A designer might develop some garment sketches early in this stage, and then face a pressing deadline for sketching the remaining pieces. Is it difficult to create 20 new sweater or swimsuit designs each season? By constantly seeking inspiration from a variety of sources, most designers have plenty of new ideas.

Hand Sketches

Some designers rely on hand sketches of their garment ideas. The designer's sketches do not look like the finished artwork of a fashion illustration. In fact, some designers state that they are not good at drawing. Partially because of time constraints, some designers use a body silhouette called a **croquis**, or **lay figure**, as a base from which to develop their garment design sketches. A swimwear designer may have numerous copies of a croquis available, onto which the swimsuit design idea will be drawn in pencil or marker. Some designers place lightweight paper over the croquis and create their garment sketches on an overlay sheet. Other designers begin with a sheet of drawing paper and sketch the garment idea portrayed on a body silhouette (see Figure 6.11). Some designers add color to their sketches by using colored pencils or markers. Often a back view sketch is shown as well as the front view.

Technical Drawing

Some garment design sketches do not include the body silhouette. If only the garment design is drawn, without an indication of the body, the sketch is sometimes called a *technical drawing*, or **tech drawing**. The garment is drawn as it would appear lying flat, as on a table, so sometimes the term **flat**, or **flat sketch**, is used to indicate this type of drawing. Tech drawings are used by some companies in place of design sketches, especially in the active-sportswear industry. Activewear garments might have many details. Tech drawings might include a close-up sketch of a detail, such as a

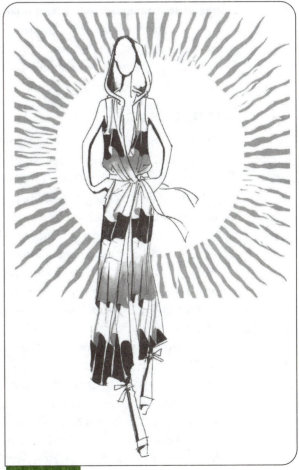

Figure 6.11 Some designers sketch their garment design ideas on a body silhouette.

pocket, cuff, or collar, as well as the back view. Tech drawings are especially useful and often necessary for pattern making and production needs. Sometimes specific dimensions, such as the size and/or placement of a patch pocket, are indicated on the tech drawing.

Computer-Aided Design and Graphics Software

Computer-aided design (**CAD**) software was in use by the 1970s. CAD software developed specifically for the apparel industry was introduced in the early 1980s. Since then, software upgrades have dramatically improved apparel CAD software. Current CAD software used for pattern making (and also for preproduction and production) is much easier to learn than the software used in the 1980s. Graphics software is especially useful for drawing and textile design. Software upgrades have also improved the "user friendliness" of these programs. In the past, the cost of CAD and graphics systems was a hurdle for some companies. The price for computer systems has dropped substantially, making CAD and graphics systems affordable to even small apparel companies.

APPAREL DESIGN

Some designers prefer to draw flats or tech drawings by hand. However, many, if not most, apparel companies expect their designers to create tech drawings using CAD or graphics software programs (see Figure 6.12). CAD systems used for pattern making, pattern grading (sizing), and marker making (developing the master cutting plan) will be discussed in other chapters.

Two major advantages of using a CAD or graphics system to create design sketches are the time-saving potential and the capability to try out numerous design ideas quickly. The designer may select a garment sketch from the previous season's line as a starting point and simply modify design details for the new design for the upcoming line. This procedure greatly speeds up this phase of the design process.

Some designers may think it stifles their creativity to sketch on a computer. They prefer to "think" with pencil in hand. To assist the artist, there are graphics computer programs that allow the designer to use a pencil-like stylus to simulate the act of drawing. After becoming familiar with the process of sketching by CAD or graphics software, most designers find that the speed with which a design can be modified is such an advantage that they have no desire to revert to drawing by hand. However, for the high-end designer price zones, hand sketching design ideas may still be the preferred process. This is due, in part, to the differences in the creation process involved, which will be discussed later.

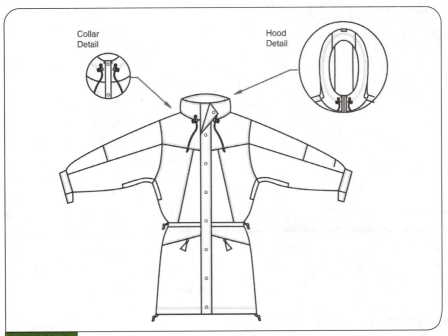

Collar
Detail

Hood
Detail

Figure 6.12   Tech drawings can be used to show design details.

Designs can be created using the following approaches:

- The computer can store a croquis (see Figure 6.13), or a series of croquis, in various poses. The designer selects a desired pose, which then appears on the computer screen. The desired garment sketch can be drawn onto the croquis.

- Some software programs provide a style library of basic garment silhouettes, such as shirts and pants, as well as garment components, such as collar and pocket styles. The designer creates the new style by bringing the desired components together (see Figure 6.14).

- New garment designs are drawn by using true proportions from a croquis stored in the system.

- New garment designs are drawn by specifying exact measurements.

To visualize what the garment style might look like in a specific color or print, the computer-generated garment drawing can be colored in several possible ways. For example, computer graphics programs can be used to simulate the color of a specific fabric swatch by blending colors on the computer monitor to create an accurate color match. The drawing of the new garment

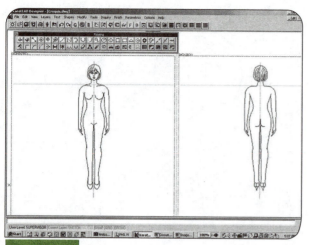

Figure 6.13 A body image called a croquis can be used as the lay figure for drawing the new garment style.

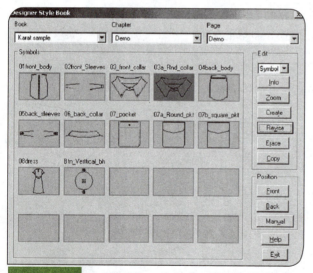

Figure 6.14 A library of garment components stored in the computer can be selected and imported into a tech drawing to develop a new style.

style can then be printed to compare the printed color on paper to the actual color of the fabric swatch.

Some of the graphics software programs are integrated with the same color system used by textile producers so an exact match can be produced very quickly by keying in the color number. The Pantone color system is supported by a number of graphics software programs and is used by textile producers to match the printed visual version of the garment with the actual fabrics. These integrated systems can be used to produce accurate color matching of the line sheet used later to sell the line at market.

A scanner can be used to input an existing fabric print into the computer system. A facsimile of the fabric will appear on the computer screen. The scale of the print or plaid fabric motif can be adjusted to approximate the correct size of the motif for the scale of the drawing. This is much faster than hand drawing and coloring fabric motifs.

Some of the more complex software programs can simulate the drape of the fabric on the designer's computer drawing (see Figure 6.15). The computer technology of simulating the three-dimensional drape of fabric is called **virtual draping**. This is discussed further in Chapter 7.

Using CAD or graphics software at the design stage helps to integrate later steps in the design process. The designer's CAD drawing will be the basis for garment technical drawings used in design development and production. The integration of computers in the entire design process is discussed later in this chapter and at each step in the design process.

It has become increasingly important for designers to be proficient with CAD and graphics software systems, and design students will increase their opportunities for future employment by developing the ability to use a computer system to sketch their design ideas.

TEXTILE DESIGN

Computer-aided design and graphics software programs are also important tools for textile design. Since textile design is such an integral part of the garment design, it is important for apparel designers and merchandisers to know as much as possible about the textile design process. More frequently today than in the past, apparel designers find textile design and/or graphic design assignments a part of their responsibilities. For example, an apparel designer may need to design a graphics logo for a T-shirt to coordinate with a print fabric used in a line, or perhaps the apparel designer will need to redesign or recolor an existing textile print.

At some companies, textile designers work side by side with the apparel design team. For example, at Pendleton Woolen Mills in Portland, Oregon, the design of the woven plaid fabric is integrated with the garment design. The textile designers calculate the spacing of the plaid repeat to coincide with the pleat widths of the skirt pattern, or vice versa, depending on the requirements for the specific style. This is not an easy task, as the designer must keep in mind the size range in which the style will be produced.

Computer software systems provide numerous advantages for textile design. Some of the computer textile design systems can print the newly created print design directly onto fabric. Several repeats of the print design can be joined together to simulate a large piece of the printed textile. Viewing a large section of the print design helps the textile designer visualize the scale, repeat, and color combination (see Figure 6.16). Changes can be made immediately. This is

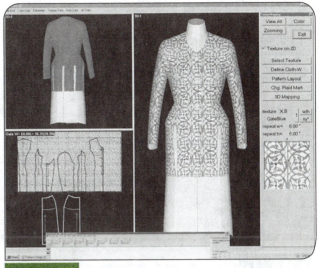

Figure 6.15 Virtual draping software creates a visual image of the scanned fabric shown on the 3-D image of the garment style.

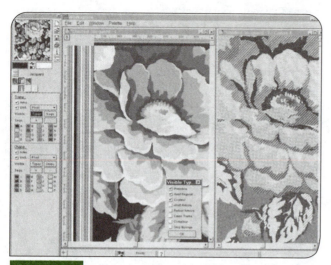

Figure 6.16 Textile designers experiment with various color combinations while designing prints.

much faster and less expensive than sending a printed paper sample to a textile mill to make a length of sample yardage of the print, called a **strike off** (see Chapter 9).

It took years to develop processes to print directly onto fabric without backing the fabric with paper to stabilize it. Now, fabric can be printed digitally in sufficient yardage to create entire garments. This technology opens the field to cost savings, time savings, and totally new customization possibilities. With digital printing, the textile design moves from the designer's computer screen to fabric without the textile producer having to make a strike off and perfect the sample fabric. Not only is there a cost savings, but there is a time savings as well. Sometimes it takes weeks for a textile print developed by traditional processes to reach final approval. The ability to perfect the print design quickly and inexpensively using digital printing adds flexibility to the design process. According to the J.Crew director of CAD, "more work can be shown, in a shorter time, than was possible before. This helps everyone in getting a real sense of what something's going to really look like before we ever get involved with the mill" (Weldon, 1999, p. 40). Additional benefits of digital printing are the capability to produce very small runs for limited production or to create custom prints.

Some companies use computer software programs to develop textile prints that can be electronically communicated to textile mills. The textile print computer file can be delivered electronically to the textile mill. According to Craig Crawford, director of design technology at Liz Claiborne:

> Liz Claiborne also has found that CAD shortens the process of translating a design into a printed piece of fabric. Now that we're giving them a digital file, the mill doesn't have to scan it, they don't have to produce the colors, and they don't have to clean it up. All they have to do is adjust it for production. It used to [take] four to eight weeks for a strike off to come back. Now that we can make all our adjustments with them before we ever let the ink hit the fabric, it's more like two weeks to a month (Swedberg, 2004, p. 40).

Networking of computer systems allows direct communication with textile mills—or direct printing on greige goods. Eliminating the labor spent recreating these designs in strike offs and samples shortens production cycles and significantly reduces miscommunication and simple human errors.

Where will digital printing technology lead the industry next? A designer specializing in digital printing at [TC][2] "is breaking industry paradigms by creating and applying custom prints to individual pattern pieces and producing them on a digital printer" (Weldon, 1999, p. 40). This technology merges the textile print and the fit-and-style options of the pattern to exact customization for the customer. Customization is discussed in more detail in Chapter 11.

Designers Who Create by Draping

Some designers create a design idea three-dimensionally by using actual fabric as a starting point, instead of beginning with a sketch of a garment (see Figure 6.17). For this design process, a mannequin or dress form in the sample size is used. Fabrics vary in their **hand** (tactile qualities) and ability to drape around the body. Working with the actual fabric can be a source of design inspiration, especially for fabrics with special draping qualities, such as charmeuse or permanently pleated fabric. Fabrics that are plaid or striped or that have a large print motif are suited to creating the initial design by the **draping** process. Couture designers and some ready-to-wear designers creating lines in the designer price zone frequently use draping to create the initial design.

Some ready-to-wear designers and some couture designers develop the design from the designer's sketch by draping in **muslin**. Muslin is an inexpensive trial fabric, similar

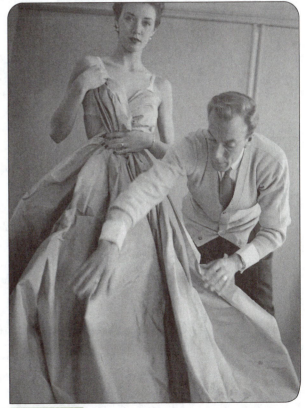

Figure 6.17 Some designers, such as the late Jacques Fath, create three-dimensionally by draping designs in fashion fabric on a live model.

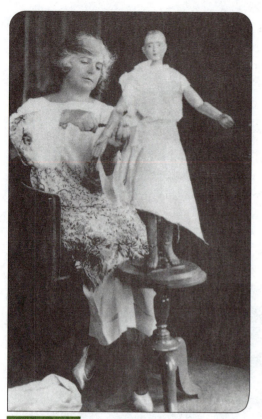

Figure 6.18 French designer Madeleine Vionnet developed her design ideas by draping fabric on a small-scale wooden mannequin and later perfecting the designs on a full-size mannequin.

to cotton broadcloth. It helps the designer determine silhouette, proportion, and design details, but it does not have the drape of many fashion fabrics. For many fabric types and garment styles, muslin serves the purpose adequately.

The muslin trial garment is sometimes referred to as the **toile**, the French word for *cloth*. French designer Madeleine Vionnet created innovative bias cut garments during the 1920s and 1930s. She always draped, rather than sketched, her design ideas. She worked out the design in fabric on a small-size wooden mannequin (see Figure 6.18). Her design team then draped a full-size replica in muslin. A prototype in fashion fabric was then cut using the pattern pieces developed from the muslin toile. Donna Karan is an example of a contemporary designer who creates designs by draping.

There are advantages to developing the design idea by draping, especially if fashion fabric is used. Seeing the design develop, sensing the drape of the fabric, molding the fabric into a three-dimensional shape, and evolving the design during the process bring a great deal of creativity to the design process. However, draping a design may take more time than preparing a design sketch or tech drawing, and draping requires more fabric than if one first makes a pattern and then cuts fabric from the pattern. Therefore, many designers rely on drawings for the design phase of the process.

Product Management Systems

There are increasing demands on apparel, accessories, and home fashions manufacturers to produce new styles quickly. The traditional methods of designing, marketing to retail buyers, producing, and distributing to retailers are no longer effective for many companies. Many forces have affected the need to accelerate the pace of these industries. Several of the most critical factors include the following:

- the length of time a style is in process

- the international scope of sourcing and production

- the need for all partners in the pipeline to communicate accurately and quickly

Following is a typical scenario in today's fashion industry: Imagine that you are a New York-based apparel designer, carefully formulating the next season's color palette, while meticulously developing the Summer line to which it will apply. Here's the catch. Your design partner is based in Los Angeles, your patternmaker and sample maker are 8,000 miles away in India, and your dyeing mill is in China. How do companies handle all the necessary data, in the shortest time possible, across thousands of miles?

Computer technology has provided the means to help meet these requirements. Beginning in the early 1990s, product data management, also known as product information management or product development management systems, were developed to provide a means to track via computer the style's technical information package needed by the preproduction and production facilities. Generally, this management approach began once the new style had been adopted. Often the design team worked through the initial stages of creating a new style using their computer systems or using hand-drawn garment sketches (or tech drawings), along with handwritten or computer-generated style information sheets (spec sheets). Once the style moved to the preproduction department, style information might then be input into that department's computer system. Thus, time delays, errors, and miscommunication of style information between the various departments were constant concerns.

By the late 1990s, it became increasingly important to begin electronic management of product information related to the style at its inception. This led to expanding the style-information tracking process to include style information from the very beginning of its design through its delivery at the retail store. The two technologies that provide electronic management of files are as follows:

- **product data management (PDM)**, also referred to as **product development management (PDM)**

- **product lifecycle management (PLM)**

These technologies differ somewhat. PDM solutions "take a product-centric focus to information management. Unlike image- or document-focused management systems, PDM centers on the product, or style at hand, grouping together everything related to that product, including specifications, sketches, and other information, which can then be reviewed and updated by other parties.

Sometimes referred to as **PDM/PLM** when combining product data (development) management and product lifecycle management, this approach requires all computer systems in the pipeline to be compatible in order to share product data. The designer's sketch is created in a software program that interfaces with the garment spec sheet software, and on down the pipeline. All partners have online access to the style information. Lectra, a leading software and hardware provider for the industry, developed software that integrates the entire product development process. It works with a simple-to-use graphical interface that allows all users to access the full range of data and to visualize each step in the development of a collection: design, technical specifications, bills of materials, size charts and measurements, sewing instructions, costing, planning control, pattern making, marker making, and packaging.

Since all partners have instantaneous access to any change made for a style, the person responsible for inputting the data accurately carries a heavy responsibility. One of the product developers at Nike commented on how nervous she was the first time she logged into the PDM system. She knew that if she input data incorrectly, the error would be transmitted to everyone in the system. In spite of this concern, the advantages of using a PDM/PLM system are tremendous for total work flow management. In summary, product lifecycle management "ties together the whole process from concept development to production" (Kusterbeck, 2005, p. 44).

As mentioned earlier in this chapter, the Liz Claiborne company often designs its own textiles using a CAD system. The company has expanded its computer network to include its offshore partners. According to Craig Crawford, director of design technology at Liz Claiborne, "networking products allow Liz Claiborne to send textile designs to its offshore offices and mills via an internal network. All the company's CAD designers have access to the network, and they can drag-and-drop their production-ready artwork into a file folder for pickup in Asia" (Swedberg, 2004, p. 42).

Design Team Reviews Line

Typically, many more design ideas are sketched than will appear in the final line. At a line review meeting (also called a **first adoption meeting**), the designer presents the design sketches to the review team (for example, the merchandiser, fit or production engineer, and head of sample sewing) according to the timeline on the master calendar (see Figure 6.19). Some designers present the new line as a formal presentation with beautifully rendered drawings, fabric swatches, and perhaps an indication of the design theme or inspiration shown on presentation boards or storyboards. The designer might make an oral presentation to the design team, upper management, or private label managers to "sell" the line.

This first adoption meeting is the first of several review processes that the line must undergo. There will be several subsequent line reviews before the final adoption. The review team discusses and evaluates each of the designs. The team will have determined during previous planning meetings how many of each type of apparel item it will be possible to include in the line. Out of 60 design ideas presented for review, perhaps only 30 or 40 sketches will be selected to continue into the design devel-

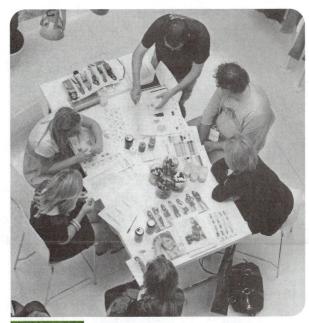

Figure 6.19 At review meetings, the designer, merchandiser, and production engineer discuss the feasibility of each style in the line.

opment stage. Some of these designs will be dropped at later stages as well. At other companies, the merchandisers may request that all or most of the designs be developed as prototypes to better visualize the product.

Guided by the total number of pieces previously determined for the line, other factors enter into the decision to accept or drop designs from the line. The balance of the line is an important factor in deciding which designs should be included. For a misses career line, jacket style variations are considered so that there will be a range of styles to suit a variety of customers. For example, it is important to include a balance of the number of short versus long, boxy versus fitted, single versus double-breasted jackets, and jackets with collars versus collarless jackets. The ratio of solid to plaid or print fabrics is another consideration. Skirt style variations must be balanced—short versus long, fitted versus flared, full versus pleated. The skirts need to coordinate with as many of the jacket styles as possible. The mix of classic and fashion-forward styles needs to be considered.

Anticipated cost is an important factor in the review process. The anticipated prices need to be similar to the previous season's prices, unless a new market niche is sought. Some cost considerations are discussed in the section on planning the line earlier in this chapter. It is important that style features match price. For example, a customer expects to pay less for a short, single-breasted style than for a longer, double-breasted jacket. The team discusses cost estimates and possible style, design details, findings, and fabric changes that might reduce cost.

Other factors to consider include ease of adjusting the style to fit varied body types. For example, elastic added at the sides of the skirt waistband can enhance the adaptability of a garment to fit more figure shapes, especially in the misses and larger-size markets. However, for the junior market, elastic in the waistband may be considered a negative feature and could adversely affect sales. Ease in alterations is another consideration. A wrap skirt with a curved, faced hemline is not easily shortened and cannot be lengthened.

There is a constant struggle among the following personnel:

- production personnel who want new styles to be similar to previous styles and as simple to construct as possible
- merchandisers who want the line to "sell itself" in the marketplace with great prices and high quality
- designers who want highly creative, complex styles

This may explain why some companies call the conference room where design reviews are conducted the *war room*. It is important for the designer to be prolific with design ideas and to develop an impersonal attitude about the designs that need to be modified or are dropped from the line.

In summary, the merits of each style as it fits in the big picture of the overall line will be discussed at the design review meeting. Sometimes design details will need to be modified to lower the expected cost or to coordinate better with other styles. The team is guided in their review process by the following aims:

- to create a cohesive theme
- to include an appropriate number of items and a balance of styles
- to fit the overall merchandising orientation of the company for the season (e.g., fit the price and lifestyle of the target customer)

Writing the Garment Specification Sheet

The designer often has some specific design details in mind that need to be conveyed to the pattern maker and sample sewer in order to create the sample or prototype garment at the next stage of the design process. These details, as well as other vital information, are conveyed on a **garment specification sheet**, also called a *garment spec sheet*, or shortened still more to *spec sheet*. Examples of types of design details that need to be specified include the following:

- the placement and spacing of buttons
- any edge stitching or top stitching
- the spacing between pleats or tucks
- findings, such as the number, size, and style of buttons; zipper length, color, and style; snaps and buckles
- pocketing, lining fabric, and interfacings

Any information not specified will be decided by the patternmaker. Thus, it is the designer's responsibility to specify all garment aspects that are important to the look of the design. A drawing of the garment design is included on the spec sheet along with fabric swatches. The spec sheet may also include the measurement specifications and construction specifications (see Chapter 9).

A **style number** is assigned to each new style in the line. This number (which might include a letter code as well) is coded to indicate the season and year in which the line will be presented to buyers, along with other information desired by the apparel company. The style number may include a category indicator, such as swimwear or sportswear, and the size category of junior, misses petite, or tall. The style number is used as the style's reference throughout development, marketing, and production.

Summary

In creating an apparel line, the design process follows the research process. The design team works with planning and production personnel to plan the calendar of due dates in order to provide garments to the retailer at the season's outset. The line is planned to provide the right product type for the target customer at the right time and at the right price. The sales volume and sell-through of a line at the retail level are important indicators used to plan the upcoming line. Striking the right balance between carryover styles, revisions of popular styles from the previous season, and new styles is critical to the success of the line.

The merchandiser may work with the designer to develop a theme for a new line. A theme for a line can help sell the products. An example of a color theme for a sport fishing group is one based on the colors of a sport fish. This theme can be enhanced by the use of the fish image as a graphic design on a T-shirt in the collection. Historical and ethnic clothing are sources of design inspiration, as are new fabrics, textures, trims, and fasteners.

Some designers hand sketch their garment design ideas, some use a computer-aided design or graphics program, some prepare technical drawings, and some create the design idea three-dimensionally in fabric by draping. The designer is responsible for creating far more design ideas than will be selected for the line. The designer is also responsible for selecting fabrics, trims, and linings for each design and specifying details, such as buttons and top stitching. The garment specification sheet includes all the pertinent information required to complete a pattern and prototype of the design.

Increasing demands for the fast development, production, and delivery of goods has put pressure on the textile and apparel industries. These demands are coupled with the physical distance between various partners in the global marketplace that rely on one another for sourcing. Electronic technologies have provided the means for instant communication and accurate tracking of each style. Product data management and product lifecycle management systems provide electronic connectivity for instantaneous communication among all parties in the creation, design development, style selection, preproduction, marketing, production, and distribution of goods.

If you are considering a career as a designer or merchandiser for an apparel company, you need to have a creative flair, good technical knowledge, and confidence.

Assistant Designer
Privately Owned Sportswear Company

Position Description:
Assist the design director and merchandise manager.

Typical Tasks and Responsibilities:

- Create a catalog of the season's prototype garments, including computer illustrations and colorways of all garments.
- Create and weave yarn dyes on the computer and scan in prints.
- Prepare all of the information necessary for the textile mills to do strike offs and handlooms.
- Update and change data when changes in colors are made.
- Design garments from initial sketches through fit sessions.
- Prepare special computer projects for sales reps—drawing and coloring garments and creating mini catalogs.
- Work with all fit models.
- Work with overseas correspondence in the absence of the designer.

Designer
Publicly Held Sportswear and Athletic Shoe Company

Position Description:
Work with merchandisers and marketers to design lines. Work with the graphic designer and textile designer in creating the line.

Typical Tasks and Responsibilities:

- Provide ideas, direction, images, and concept(s) for the season's line.
- Research fabric vendor resources.
- Select fabrics for the garments in the line.
- Work with pattern makers in creating patterns for the garments in the line.
- Provide follow-through to production of all garments in the line.
- Give presentations of the line to various groups for feedback.

CAREER PROFILES

Key Terms

color story

colorway

computer-aided design (CAD)

croquis

draping

findings

first adoption meeting

flat

flat sketch

garment specification sheet

hand

knockoff

lay figure

line-for-line copy

market niche

muslin

price averaging

PDM/PLM

product data management (PDM)

product development management (PDM)

product lifecycle management (PLM)

product type

Retro

sales volume

sell-through

strike off

style number

swatch

target costing

tech drawing

toile

virtual draping

zeitgeist

Discussion Questions and Activities

1. What are some current societal trends (zeitgeist) that might provide an inspiration for a group or line of apparel?

2. What might be an example of an *unconventional* source of design inspiration? Why might it be considered unconventional?

3. Review current designers' collections, and try to identify their source of inspiration. Do any of the designers share a common inspiration?

4. What are some current styles in the stores that might be considered knockoffs of designers' styles?

5. What are some of the job responsibilities of a merchandiser and a designer in the design stage of the design process? What are some activities that might be helpful for you to complete as students to help prepare you for these job responsibilities? Examples include a target customer collage for a specific company, a trend board for a jacket line for a year in advance, or an inspiration board for a children's wear beach group.

References

At Ease (2010, June 17). *Women's Wear Daily*, p 7.

Bowles, Hammish. (2006, May). Show business. *Vogue*, pp. 142, 144, 146.

Knight, Molly. (1999, September 24). Globetrotting for inspiration. *DNR*, pp. 14–16.

Kusterbeck, Staci. (2005, December). Jones Apparel Group. *Apparel*, p. 44.

Mackrell, Alice. (1990). *Paul Poiret*. New York: Holmes & Meier.

Martin, Richard, and Koda, Harold. (1989). *The Historical Mode*. New York: Rizzoli International Publications.

Martin, Richard, and Koda, Harold. (1994). *Orientalism: Visions of the East in Western Dress*. New York: Metropolitan Museum of Art. Distributed by Harry N. Abrams, Inc.

Saint Laurent, Yves, Vreeland, Diana, et al. (1983). *Yves Saint Laurent*. New York: Metropolitan Museum of Art.

Talley, Andre Leon. (2003, November) Remembrance of things past. *Vogue*, pp.94, 98,122.

Swedberg, Jamie. (2004, May). Designers embrace CAD differently. *Apparel*, pp. 38–42.

Tuxedo Junction: YSL, Ralph square off. (1994, April 28).*Women's Wear Daily*, pp. 1, 15.

Weldon, Kristi. Identifying expert CAD users. (1999, October). *Apparel Industry Magazine*, pp. 38–44.

Wilson, Eric. (1999, November 2). The culture of copycats. *Women's Wear Daily*, pp. 8–9.

Wolcott, James, Luther, Marylou, and Parmal, Pamela. (2005). *Beene by Beene/Geoffrey Beene*. New York: The Vendome Press.

CHAPTER 7

Design Development and Style Selection

In this chapter, you will learn the following:

- the steps required to develop a sketch into a prototype garment and to prepare the garment for design team review

- the use of computers for product life management

- reasons why a style might be eliminated from the line during the review process

- style factors that influence the estimated cost of a new garment style

- the relationships among traditional design development processes and private label and store brand product development.

Step 3: Design Development and Style Selection

Step 1 Research and Merchandising

Step 2 Design

Step 3 Design Development and Style Selection

Make First Pattern

Cut and Sew Prototype

Approve Prototype Fit, Revise Style, or Drop Style

Estimate Cost (initial cost estimate)

Present and Review Line

Select Styles for Final Line (line adoption)

Determine the Final Cost

Order Fabric, Trims, and Findings for Sales Samples

Order Sales Samples Cut and Sewn

Step 4 Marketing the Apparel Line

Step 5 Preproduction

Step 6 Sourcing

Step 7 Apparel Production Processes, Material Management, and Quality Assurance

Step 8 Distribution and Retailing

*A*t this point in the design process, the line for the new season consists of a group of sketches with fabric swatches that have made it through the design team's preliminary selection process. This chapter discusses how the first pattern is developed from the designer's sketch, swatch, and garment specification sheet and how the prototype garment is cut and sewn from the first pattern (see Step 3: Design Development and Style Selection flowchart, at the beginning of this chapter, and Figure 7.1, an expanded view of Step 3). The prototype is then tried on a fit model whose body measurements match the company's size standard.

The designer, merchandiser, patternmaker, and production engineer analyze the fit and design, and discuss cost factors. An initial cost estimate is calculated. This is an important factor in deciding the feasibility of producing the style. Changes may be made to the prototype, or perhaps the pattern will be modified and a new prototype will be cut and sewn. This process continues with all the styles for the line. The styles in the line are reviewed, and final decisions are made to determine which styles will be adopted for the final line. Participating in the development of a new style from its sketch (or the first drape) to a finished prototype is an exciting part of the design process. On the other hand, it can be a difficult decision to cut some styles from the line after seeing the prototypes and liking all of them. After the final styles have been approved and final cost has been determined, sales samples are cut and sewn. Marketing of the line is discussed in Chapter 8.

This chapter focuses on the development process typically used by apparel companies that manufacture brand merchandise. This is apparel whose brand labels are well recognized by the public, including Levi Strauss & Co., Tommy Hilfiger, Calvin Klein, and Nike. Later in the chapter, private label and store brand product development processes are discussed. Increased vertical integration and changes in the design–retail relationship during the 1980s led to the growth and expansion of this alternative product development process. With private label and store brand product development, retailers are a part of the design team and/or are in charge of the manufacturing process. Such changing roles and relationships among design, production, and retail will continue in our complex economic market.

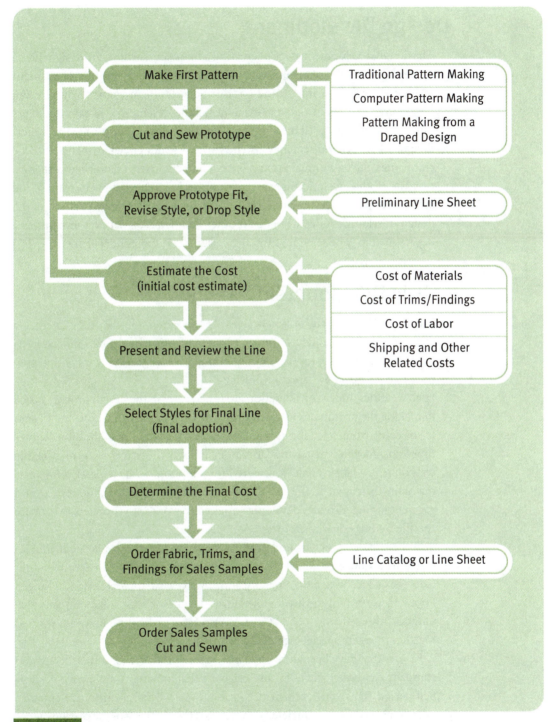

Figure 7.1 Step 3 Expanded: Design Development and Style Selection

Design Development

The design development stage of creating a line occurs within the design development department of an apparel company. Other names for this department include design department and product development department. Design development teams in this department include designers, assistant designers (also called design assistants), and product developers (also called technical designers). Merchandisers may also be part of the design department. At some companies, the patternmakers and production engineers (also called cost engineers or product technicians) are a part of the design development team. If the apparel company also has production patternmakers, they may be a part of the design development department. At other companies, a pattern development department may be separate from the design development department.

Fabric Development

Fabric is a key element of a new style. At the same time that the pattern for the new style is under development, potential fabrics for the new style are under consideration. A product developer might be assigned to work with textile mills to develop a new fabric or finish.

New fabrics under consideration are tested early in the design process (prior to making the prototype) for such properties as colorfastness, crocking (transfer of color from one fabric to another fabric), pilling, and abrasion. Sometimes an independent testing laboratory is used to perform specified textile tests on a new fabric being considered for adoption. Some apparel companies maintain their own testing labs that might conduct both textile testing and garment testing. Product developers might also work with suppliers to procure specific findings or trims for the new style.

Some apparel designers and product developers work with fabric manufacturers to produce custom fabrics to meet specific needs. For example, after Gore-Tex's success as a woven fabrication, activewear apparel designers longed for a knit version of the breathable fabric. The fabric's manufacturer was able to meet this need when W. L. Gore & Associates and Nike employees worked together to create special technical-performance fabrics.

Fabrics that have been developed by a textile producer for a specific apparel company can be restricted for use solely by that apparel company for a specified period. This adds exclusivity to the product, which in turn can enhance sales. Such a fabric is **proprietary**; that is, it is the property of the private owner (the apparel company). Dri-FIT ® is a proprietary fabric for Nike , as is Synchilla® for Patagonia.

As discussed in Chapter 6, textile prints are sometimes developed for the new line by the apparel company. At the same time that the new styles are under development, the designer, assistant designer, or product developer will work with the textile converter to ensure that the prints will be approved and ready for production on schedule.

The designer responsible for the line will have selected a color story, or palette, for the line (see Chapter 6). The colors for the line might be represented by color chips or fabric swatches. **Color management** deals with handling the technical aspects of matching the colors of the fabrics, trims, and findings to ensure that the colors of the finished product match the designer's color swatches. Much work goes into selecting the specific hue, value, and intensity for each color in the color palette. Therefore, it is essential that the fabrics and trim colors of the finished product match the intended color swatch. Color management begins during design development, as the product developer, assistant designer, or designer work with textile mills to procure the exact color match.

For prints, the colors used need to match any solid-colored fabrics intended to coordinate with them. Color matching is challenging, especially when the various fabrics used in a line are composed of a variety of fibers. Different fibers require different types of dyes, so color matching the wide variety of fibers, fabrics, thread, buttons, zippers, and other findings requires constant attention during the design development and preproduction steps. Color management continues in production processes.

Preparation for Pattern Development

As discussed in Chapter 6, the designer sketches an idea for a new style as the preliminary design step by hand or by using a CAD or graphics system (see Figure 7.2). After the design team has approved the style for development, the designer's sketch, fabric swatch, and garment specification sheet are delivered to the design development department to begin the patternmaking process. In the case of apparel manufacturers that use contractors, the first pattern may be developed by the contractor, or the pattern may be developed by the apparel manufacturer. The responsibility for developing the first pattern is fairly common for contractors who provide full-package (FP) contractor services.

Other designers prefer to drape the preliminary design idea using either muslin or a fashion fabric on a mannequin or dress form (see Chapter 6). After careful markings have been made, the fabric pieces of the draped design are removed from the mannequin. The "drape" is then ready for patternmaking.

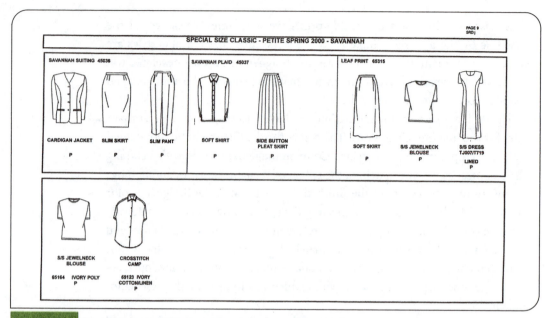

Figure 7.2 The designer's CAD sketches are prepared for the first adoption meeting.

Making the First Pattern

As noted earlier, some apparel manufacturers develop the line, create the design sketches with accompanying fabric swatches, and write the garment specification sheet. Then they use either domestic or offshore contractors to manufacture the garments. These firms are called *CMT contractors* because they cut, make, and trim the garments. The steps between those involving making the pattern and cutting and sewing the **prototype**, or sample, may be performed by either the apparel company or the contractor.

It may be advantageous for those apparel companies that use contractors to retain the capability to develop the pattern and prototype in-house because schedule delays and communication and visual interpretation problems are possible when a contractor develops the pattern and prototype. A number of factors must be considered by each apparel manufacturer regarding the patternmaking, grading, and marker making responsibilities. One of the potential problem areas when using contractors for patternmaking has to do with the base pattern used. A **base pattern** is a non-stylized basic pattern in the sample size from which the stylized pattern is derived. Two contractors producing different styles for the same line might not use identical base patterns for patternmaking. This can cause differences in the fit of the finished stylized garments between a style produced by one contractor and another style produced by another contractor. More offshore contractors now have computer pattern-making systems that eliminate many of the problems that apparel companies previously encountered when they had contractors perform the patternmaking functions.

At some companies, the designer is also the first patternmaker. This tends to be the case in very small companies or in some specialty areas, such as children's wear. Some designers enjoy being involved in the development of their design ideas from sketches into patterns and then prototypes. For designers who also are responsible for making the first pattern and prototype, their design ideas or the construction procedure might evolve during the development process. Thus, they might modify the design during the process of making the pattern and/or sewing the prototype. From the designer's sketch, the assistant designer or patternmaker begins the patternmaking process, called **flat pattern** design. The patternmaker's role is critical to the accurate translation of the designer's idea. It is important that the patternmaker accurately assesses from the sketch the following information:

- the overall silhouette desired
- the amount of ease (from very snug to very oversized)
- the designer's desired proportions for the design details

An existing pattern is used to begin the new design. This pattern could be a base pattern (also called a **block** or a **sloper**) in the company's sample size. For example, a basic shirt block might be used as the base pattern for a new shirt style. The patternmaker creates the new pattern by adding pattern design details such as a collar, pocket, button band, back yoke, and sleeve pleats to the base pattern, as indicated in the designer's sketch or tech drawing.

Another process frequently used by the patternmaker is to select a similar style from a previous season. For example, a shirt style for a new season might be similar to a pattern that has already been made for the previous season. Modifying an existing pattern can be the fastest way to create the pattern for the new style. Selecting the most appropriate previous style for the starting point of a new style may require some discussion between patternmaker (or assistant designer) and the designer. Alternatively, the designer might make a note to the patternmaker on the design sketch or tech drawing suggesting a previous style from which to begin.

The intended fabric for the final garment is an important consideration during patternmaking. For example, the amount of gathers to incorporate into a sleeve depends on the hand, or tactile qualities, of the fabric specified by the designer. The patternmaker may experiment by gathering a section of the intended fabric or a facsimile fabric to better determine the ideal quantity of gathers. To develop patterns for garments made from stretch fabrics, it is necessary to know the exact amount of stretch of the fabric in all directions. The patternmaker selects the base pattern or previous style pattern to correspond to the specific stretch factor of the intended fabric for the new style.

Fabric shrinkage is another patternmaking consideration. After the fabric sample has been wash tested to determine accurately its shrinkage in all directions, the pattern is made sufficiently larger to account for the shrinkage factor. All pattern pieces are expanded, based on accurate length and width shrinkage ratios.

The patternmaker needs expertise/knowledge in the following areas:

- patternmaking, so that a garment illustration can be translated into a pattern

- understanding of fit and the ways in which shape and fullness are incorporated into the design

- textiles, so that fiber and fabric characteristics are accounted for in the design development

- production aspects, such as the sequence of sewing operations used by a production facility that affect how the pattern is built, so the style can be made easily and cost effectively in the factory

- the types of equipment at the production facility, in order to produce a pattern that can be sewn satisfactorily by the factory

The patternmaker may work with traditional paper patterns, or the pattern might be created using a computer-aided design system. There are similarities and differences between these patternmaking methods; both methods are discussed.

TRADITIONAL PATTERNMAKING

The base patterns, as well as stylized patterns, are often made of a heavy paper called **tagboard**, *oak tag*, or *hard paper* (see Figure 7.3). Tagboard is similar in weight to the paper used for file folders. This heavy paper is sturdy, and the edges can be traced rapidly to copy a pattern as the beginning point for the new pattern. Traditional patternmaking procedures require either that the patternmaker trace the base pattern onto pattern paper, called *soft paper*, or that new patterns be made directly onto new tagboard. Style details are developed, col-

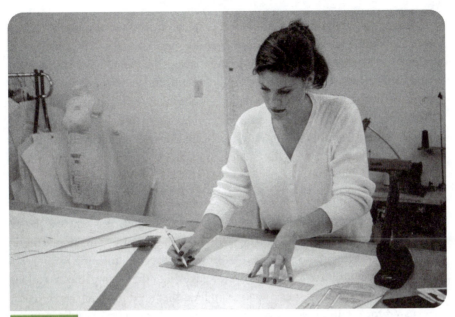

Figure 7.3   Tagboard patterns from previous seasons are used as reference for making patterns for new styles.

lars can be created, new sleeves designed, and pleats or gathers added in order to create the pattern pieces for the new style.

COMPUTER PATTERNMAKING

Computer patternmaking was developed for use in the apparel industry in the early 1980s. The use of computers has become essential in all steps of a design's development. Companies such as Gerber Technology and Lectra, have led much of the industry in developing and providing software to handle almost every step of a garment's production. Today, the computer-aided design has become part of the product lifecycle management (PLM). By using computer pattern design software, the pattern can be communicated electronically among all departments to integrate the business and manufacturing systems seamlessly. This, in turn, speeds the product through production and reduces the possibility of errors (see Chapter 9 for additional discussion).

Many apparel companies use **pattern design systems (PDS)** for some or all of the patternmaking functions (see Figure 7.4). The computer patternmaking process is similar to the flat-pattern process previously discussed. The base patterns and all previous style patterns are stored in the computer's files or on a server. To begin a new style, either a base pattern or the pattern pieces for a similar style from a previous season is pulled from the computer's file and appears on the screen. The patternmaker uses a mouse, or stylus (which looks similar to a pen) to select specific areas to change on the pattern. Patternmaking commands are either selected from a menu shown on the screen or typed on a keyboard. Once the patternmaking is completed, the pattern can be plotted (drawn) in full size (see Figure 7.5).

Computer technology continues to bring remarkable advances in ease of use, adaptability, and cost effectiveness of PDS. Some of the advantages of PDS include the following:

- *Speed:* Since the base patterns and patterns from previous styles are stored in the computer system and used to begin the pattern for a new style, no time is spent tracing an existing pattern to begin patternmaking. To add seam and hem allowances, the patternmaker specifies the amount of seam and hem allowances to add to selected edges, and the cutting lines are added in an instant. The lengths of two seam lines that need to match can be compared for accuracy with a computer command. Markings and labels, such as grainlines and notches, are stored in a library and can be quickly added to the pattern pieces. To add gathers, the patternmaker indicates where and how much the pattern should be enlarged, and the pattern piece is spread to insert gathers instantly. A paper pattern, on the other hand, must be slashed in several places and then spread in order to insert additional width or length for gathers. If the design is modified later in the design process, changes in the pattern can be made more quickly by PDS than they usually can with a paper pattern. Another advantage of using a PDS that enhances the speed of patternmaking is its capability to adjust other pattern pieces automatically. For example, a change made by the patternmaker on the jacket front pattern would generate the same change to be reflected on the facing and lining pattern pieces.

- *Accuracy:* Using PDS eliminates the incremental growth that can occur when hand tracing a pattern due to the thickness of the pencil lead. Seam lengths and seam allowance widths are more exact than is possible by hand. By always using a stored pattern for the base pattern, consistency in pattern design across all styles is assured. When the patternmaker makes a modification in one pattern piece that affects other pattern pieces, some PDS software programs make an automatic change in the corresponding pattern piece(s). For example, if a change is made in the front side seam length, the back side seam length is automatically corrected. This can greatly reduce potential errors, as well as increase the speed of patternmaking.

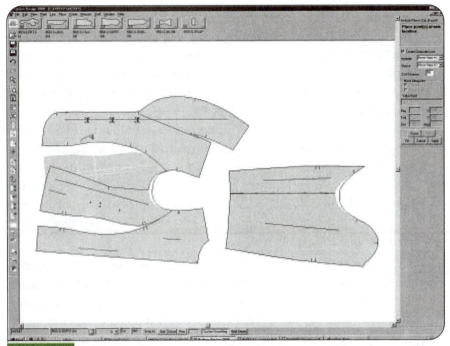

Figure 7.4   Pattern design systems provide speed and accuracy for pattern-making.

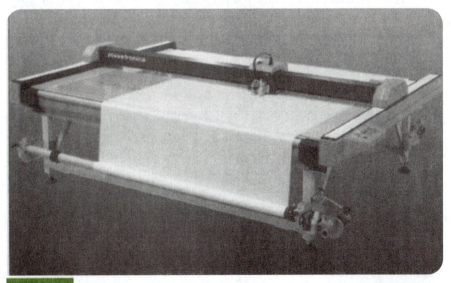

Figure 7.5   After a pattern is completed on a pattern design system, the pattern pieces are drawn full size on a plotter.

- *Integration with spec sheets:* Some computer software programs provide an interface between the patternmaking process and the garment specification sheet (spec sheet). Some PDS programs allow the patternmaker to write parts of the spec sheet as the pattern is being made on PDS. A file of potential sewing steps is retrieved and edited on one screen, while the pattern is being made and viewed on another screen. The measurement specifications can also be written during the patternmaking process. With some PDS software programs, the widths and lengths of the pattern being made in the sample size can be requested at any time during the patternmaking process. This information is the basis for the completion of the measurement specifications (which are discussed in more detail in Chapter 9). The possibility of an error in the spec sheet is reduced when the patternmaker writes the spec sheet simultaneously with making the pattern.

- *Integration with production:* Later in the product development process, production is faster if the pattern pieces have been stored in the computer than if it is necessary to input the pattern pieces for computerized grading and marker making. These processes will be discussed in Chapter 9.

Although the advantages of PDS are many, some patternmakers and company executives note that there are disadvantages. Possible disadvantages of using PDS include the following:

- *Cost:* The initial cost of PDS is high, although some of the new technology systems cost less than earlier versions. Some apparel manufacturers, especially smaller companies, may not see a substantial return on their investment for some years. If a company produces only a limited number of new styles per season, PDS will not be utilized to its maximum.

- *Time:* Another aspect of cost has to do with time involved in training patternmakers. One of the hurdles with learning a computer software system is learning the operating system and memorizing the commands and the various steps needed to complete a process. Typically, patternmakers are sent to the computer software company's headquarters for a week or two of intensive training on the system. In addition to the dollar cost of the training, there is the cost of lost time while training occurs and the greater time required to make patterns while the new system is being mastered.

- *Technical support:* If the system goes down, the delay can cause great problems and affect the subsequent production steps. Any delays can be extremely costly to the manufacturer and retailer. Fortunately, most PDS companies have excellent technical support by phone and online, easing the time loss and stress.

- *Visualization difficulties:* For patternmakers who are used to working with full-size patterns, the use of PDS requires an adjustment because they are looking at reduced-size pattern pieces on the computer screen. When working by hand, the patternmaker slashes the pattern for gathers and spreads the pattern the desired amount. These decisions often are based on what looks correct. When patternmakers use PDS, they select the quantity of gathers to add. The new pattern piece, with the selected quantity of gathers, then appears on the screen. In other words, the patternmaker must choose the quantity before seeing how the pattern looks. However, if the quantity of gathers seems too great or too small, it takes very little time with PDS to undo the maneuver and request a different quantity of gathers. With experience, it becomes easier for patternmakers to visualize scale using PDS.

In the future, an increasing number of apparel companies will use PDS. Costs of PDS programs have been reduced as more price competition among CAD companies has developed and technology costs have decreased. Many CAD systems operate with standard computer industry PCs, providing additional price competition in the huge PC market. Most large apparel manufacturers already rely completely on computer-generated patternmaking. An increasing number of small apparel companies use CAD systems in order to be fully integrated with their manufacturers.

PATTERNMAKING BY DRAFTING

Rather than beginning the patternmaking process with a base pattern, some companies prefer to draft the pattern by using body measurements. The pattern shapes are drawn based on the body dimensions plus ease allowances. Pattern drafting can be done using paper and pencil, or using a CAD program. Pattern drafting to create stylized patterns is used more frequently in Asia than in North America.

PATTERNMAKING FROM A DRAPED DESIGN

As discussed in Chapter 6, some designers, especially in the designer and bridge price zones, create the initial garment by draping the design on a mannequin. The fabric, either fashion fabric or muslin, is draped onto the sample size mannequin. The design is developed by cutting into the fabric, molding the fabric to the desired shape, and then pinning the fabric in place. After finalizing all aspects of the design, the style lines and construction details of the drape are very carefully marked in preparation for removal from the mannequin. The fabric pieces are removed and laid flat over pattern paper. The shapes of the pattern pieces are traced onto paper; then the pattern is perfected, and markings such as grainlines, notches, buttonholes, seam and hem allowances, and facings are added.

Some companies digitize the paper pattern into a computer pattern design system. This allows the remaining stages of the design development process, preproduction, and production processes for the new style to be handled electronically.

Regardless of the procedure by which the pattern is made—by using flat pattern design with paper, by using PDS, by drafting, or from a draped design—the full-scale final pattern of the style is now ready to be cut and sewn into a prototype for style review.

Making the Prototype or Sample Garment

The next step in the design development process is to cut and sew the prototype or sample garment. As mentioned in Chapter 6, some apparel companies use computer software systems to create three-dimensional replicas of the styles in the line that show simulated fabrics draped on the mannequin viewed on the computer screen (see Figure 7.6). Rather than continuing the development process by cutting and sewing the sample, some companies use these computer-generated images to sell the styles to the retail buyers. This marketing process will be discussed later as well.

Most companies produce a sewn prototype. This provides the opportunity for the following:

- to test the design in the selected fabric(s)
- to evaluate the style on a live fit model
- to test the construction sequence
- to use a physical sample to perform a cost analysis for materials and labor costs
- to see all the styles in the line as a whole

The prototype made from the first pattern for the new style may be cut and sewn by an in-house sample or sewing department, or it might be made by a contractor. If the contractor has a compatible computer system, the pattern can be sent electronically to the contractor. Many contractors, especially those located in Asia, realize that their business opportunities expand greatly if they invest in computer systems.

SAMPLE CUTTING AND SEWING

The completed pattern is delivered to the sample sewing department, accompanied by a swatch of the intended fabric for the actual garment and the garment specification sheet. If the intended fabric is available (sometimes as a sample cut ordered from the textile mill), it will be used to make the prototype garment. Sometimes the intended fabric is not yet available, so a substitute or facsimile fabric, as similar as possible to the intended fabric, will be used.

The garment spec sheet will indicate any special cutting instructions. For example, a shirt with back yoke may require that the shirt's striped fabric be cut on the lengthwise grain for the body, sleeves, and collar, and on the crosswise grain for the yoke. Stretch fabrics for swimwear and bodywear may require some pattern pieces to be cut with the greatest stretch in the horizontal direction and other pattern pieces to be cut with the greatest stretch in the vertical direction. The sample cutter will match plaids where specified and make other decisions about how the pattern pieces are laid on the fabric (layout). The sample cutter will cut all pieces needed for the prototype. A sample room may use a cutter that cuts directly from a PDS program from which the pattern was developed (Figure 7.7). The pattern is removed from the fabric after cutting; then the pattern is usually returned to the design development department rather than accompanying the fabric pieces of the prototype through the sample sewing process.

The **sample sewer** is highly skilled in the use of a variety of sewing machines as well as in the production processes used in factories. Without an instruction sheet and rarely consulting the pattern pieces, the sample sewer sews the entire prototype garment. The sample sewer moves from one piece of equipment to

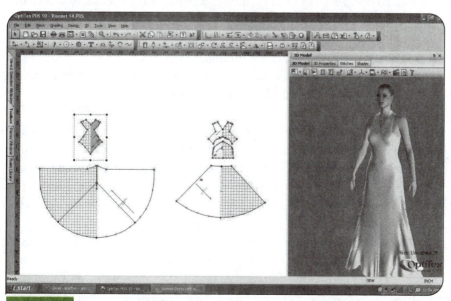

Figure 7.6   Computer generated sample garment.

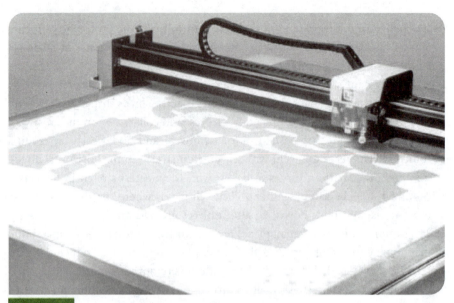

Figure 7.7   The sample cutter is used to cut the garment pieces for the sample or prototype.

the next, until the garment is finished. The sample sewer may need to send a section of a prototype to another area for work. For example, it may be necessary to embroider a logo onto a shirt front after it is cut out and before the shirt is sewn. Keeping the work flowing smoothly is also part of the process. Generally, for companies that produce prototypes in-house, the prototype is completed within a few days after cutting.

If the design development department is located near the sample sewing room, the sample sewer might consult with the patternmaker regarding a specific sewing process or technique, or they may discuss possible alternative solutions to a pattern or construction problem (see Figure 7.8). A team approach among patternmaker, cutter, and sample sewer is an advantage. After the sample sewer finishes making the prototype, it is sent back to the design development department for evaluation. Often the patternmaker reviews the prototype first to assess whether any changes need to be made before the style is reviewed by the designer and merchandiser.

APPROVING THE PROTOTYPE

The fit of the company's products is important in achieving a competitive advantage through product differentiation. Therefore, an assessment of how each

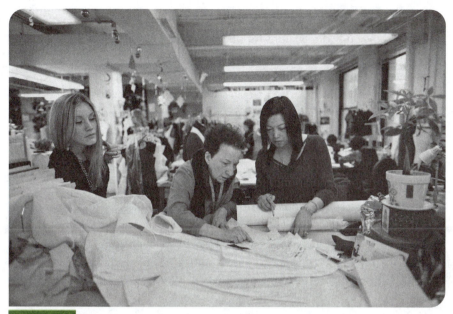

Figure 7.8 The patternmaker and the sample sewer discuss possible alternatives for a design detail.

style fits can be very important to a company. A **fit model** is used to assess the fit, styling, and overall look of the new prototype. The fit model is a person selected to represent the body proportions that the apparel company feels are ideal for its target customer and that correspond to the base pattern size used to make the prototype. Some fit models, called in-house models, may work for the company in another capacity and are asked to try on prototypes as needed as a part of their job duties. Other companies hire a professional fit model who may work for a number of apparel companies. With professional fit models, specific appointments will be made for fit sessions, requiring both lead time to book the appointment and on-time delivery of prototypes for the fit session. Fit models can provide valuable information about the comfort and ease of the garment.

Menswear fit models tend to have well-proportioned bodies and usually are about 5 feet, 10 inches to 6 feet tall. In misses apparel, fit models differ from runway models and photographic models. A misses fit model has body proportions that are "average," with a height of 5 feet, 5 inches to 5 feet, 8 inches, as compared to the tall and svelte runway models. Large-size, tall, and petite fit models are used for their respective size categories. In children's wear, the fit model outgrows the sample size very quickly, requiring the apparel company to search for a new fit model every few months.

In junior and misses apparel, there are wide variations among apparel companies in the body dimensions for one size (Workman, 1991). For a pant created to fit an individual with a 25-inch waist, one company may use a 36-inch hip measurement for its size standard, and another company may use a 37-inch hip measurement. The pattern's crotch depth measurement may also differ among companies. Finding the "perfect" fit model for an apparel company can be a challenge, especially for swimwear and innerwear companies that make garments that fit closely to the body. The model's cup size and bust contour are factors in selecting the fit model. Some fit models are in very high demand, especially in the more populous market centers.

Body forms (such as dress forms, torso forms, and pant forms) can be a valuable tool for assessing the fit and design of a prototype. Body forms based on specified body dimensions are used by many apparel companies. Customized body forms, made to a company's measurement specifications, are also available from a variety of body form companies. New developments in 3-D body scanning allow an apparel company to have their fit model's individual shape duplicated as a body form. Thus, assessing the fit on a true-to-life body form can provide great accuracy when the fit model is not available. Other developments in body forms include the use of more pliable materials that better replicate the malleable characteristics of flesh. Body forms made from these materials are especially valuable for swimwear, underwear, and lingerie companies.

When several prototypes are ready for assessment, a fit session is scheduled with the fit model. While the garment fit is a part of the assessment, much of the discussion among designer, assistant designer, and patternmaker may focus on the prototype's overall style and garment details. Sometimes production engineers are asked to provide feedback about potential difficulties in factory production of the style. If any of these aspects need revision, either the existing prototype will be redone or the pattern will be revised and a new prototype will be cut and sewn. The final design will be approved by the designer and/or the merchandiser. The style might be eliminated from the line at this point if reworking the design does not seem feasible.

After the prototype has been completed, a wash test might be performed on the finished garment using a typical home-laundering-type washer and dryer. The wash test performed on garments to be sold in other countries would use the type of laundering equipment used by the customer in those countries to simulate the conditions under which the garment will be laundered. Occasionally, problems that were not evident when the individual fabrics or trims were tested arise after laundering a garment.

Three-Dimensional Tools

Three-dimensional technology provides the ability to move from the two-dimensional pattern to a three-dimensional image of a garment draped onto a body form. When using 3-D for patternmaking, a designer can construct garments over a digital image, rotate them, zoom in, and visualize how the piece will look. Even different fabric drape can be selected to stimulate how the final garment will hang. Originally developed as a "virtual dressing" tool at the retail level, the customer could envision how a garment might look on them. Lands' End was one of the first retailers to introduce online shoppers to the software My Virtual Model™. The customer inputs personal data such as coloring, body build, and favorite colors. The program shows the virtual model on the computer screen wearing suggested styles in colors from the catalog.

Three-dimensional technology has many applications in the apparel industry in addition to allowing designers and product developers to view a design three-dimensionally before the pattern is made, sample cut, and sewn. The concept of designing entirely on the computer may seem far off, but the reality is that not only can we create the three-dimensional image of the garment style with replica fabric on the computer screen, but retail buyers can write their orders from the garments viewed on the screen. No prototype samples need to be sewn. The cost savings related to design development are substantial.

Advances in computer technology will allow the three-dimensional virtual garment to be transferred into a two-dimensional pattern. Other advances include the technology to compute the cost difference (in material usage and time to sew) between slightly different versions of a design.

Preliminary Line Sheet

A sketch or a tech drawing of each new style in the group or line will be used to develop a preliminary line sheet showing all the styles in the line (see Figure 7.9). Fabric swatches and other pertinent details might also be listed. The line sheet is used within the department to help all the team members keep track of the styles in the group as they are developed. The preliminary line sheet will become the basis for the development of the final line sheet, or line catalog, used later to market the line.

Determining the Initial Cost Estimate

The cost to mass-produce the style is an important consideration in the selection of styles for the final line. Thus, preliminary costing needs to be done prior to the decision to adopt or reject a style. An **initial cost estimate**, also called **precosting**,

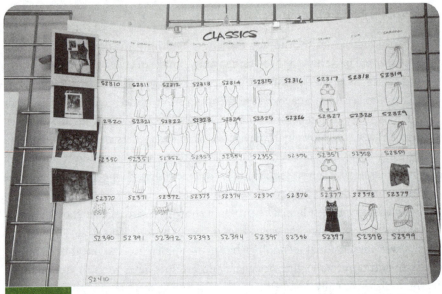

Figure 7.9   The preliminary line sheet is used by the design team during the development process of the line.

for the style is based primarily on material cost and labor cost. A "quick cost" may have been calculated during the design stage; however, until the prototype is constructed, the quick cost serves only as a preliminary estimate. To calculate the cost more accurately, an initial cost estimate is determined based on the components of materials, trims and findings, labor, and other related costs.

MATERIAL COST

The cost of the materials is estimated based on the number of yards of fabric required to make the prototype. Included in the cost of materials are such items as interfacing, pocketing, and lining needed for the prototype. To calculate the quantity of yardage required to make a new style, a layout plan of the pattern pieces, called a **marker**, needs to be made. The term costing marker refers to the layout plan for the pattern pieces that are used to determine the yardage (called **usage**) to produce one garment of the new style (see Figure 7.10). If the pattern for the new style was made using PDS, the pattern pieces for this style have been stored in the computer and can be brought into a computer program that is used to develop the costing marker. The pattern pieces are arranged within a rectangular space representing the width and length of the intended fabric. Various layouts can be analyzed to determine the best arrangement of pattern pieces using the least quantity of fabric. This process is repeated for the lining and other materials required for the new style.

In theory, the quantity of the various fabrics needed to produce one medium-size garment in the new style multiplied by the apparel company's cost for the fabrics would be used to arrive at a total materials cost. If the company produces the same number of small sizes and large sizes as medium sizes, then using the size medium to average the quantity of fabrics needed should provide a good estimate of the yardage required for one garment. How-

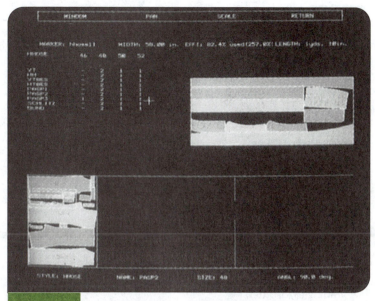

Figure 7.10 A costing marker created from the pattern pieces stored in the pattern design system is used to determine the quantity of material required for one garment.

ever, if the company in fact sells many more size small items than size large items, the average cost of materials would be higher than the actual cost. Conversely, if many more size large items were sold than size small items, then the average cost of materials would be too low. Therefore, some companies may use a size other than size medium to calculate their average usage.

TRIM AND FINDINGS COST

The quantity of all trims and findings used for the new style must be included in the initial cost estimate. Examples of trim items include braid or lace, and findings include items such as elastic, zipper, and buttons. For the initial cost estimate for the cotton pants shown in Table 7.1, one button and one zipper are needed to make this style. Note that the cost of one button is based on the cost when a gross of buttons is purchased. The cost per item is based on a large quantity purchase for other trims and findings as well.

LABOR COST

The other major component of the initial cost estimate is the cost of labor to cut and sew the new style. The labor cost is determined by estimating the number

Table 7.1   Cost to Manufacture a Pair of Cotton Pants in the United States

Style #8074	Quantity	Price/Yard	Amount	Subtotal
1. Materials				
fabric	1.7 yd.	$2.90	$4.93	
interfacing	0.2 yd.	$0.55	$0.11	
ship fabric to company ($0.20 x 1.7)		$0.20	$0.34	
Total Materials Cost				$5.38
2. Trim/Findings				
buttons	1	$2.00/gross	$0.02	
zipper (7")	1	$0.13	$0.13	
Total Trim/Findings Cost				$0.15
3. Labor				
marking ($45/order)		$0.23		
grading ($70/order)		$0.35		
cutting ($75/order)		$0.38		
sewing labor (0.5 hour @$15.00)		$7.50		
Total Labor Cost				$8.46
4. Other				
packaging/hanger, hangtag, labels		$0.15		
freight		$0.35		
duty (none, U.S. production)		$0.00		
shipping agent, consolidator fees (none)		$0.00		
Total Other Costs				$0.50
5. Cost to Manufacture				**$14.49**

WHOLESALE PRICE: The manufacturer determines the wholesale price to include overhead and profit. If keystone markup is used, then the wholesale price paid by the retailer to the manufacturer will be **$28.98.**

of minutes required to cut (and fuse interfacing), sew, and finish the garment multiplied by the cost per minute of labor for a specific sewing factory. To estimate the number of minutes required to cut, sew, and finish a new style, sewing time data from similar styles produced in the previous season can be very useful. For an accurate labor cost estimate, it is necessary to select a possible site for production since labor costs vary considerably around the world. In some countries, the labor cost varies month by month. One approach to estimating the labor cost for a new style is to use the known cost of labor to sew a similar garment from the previous season. However, due to economic and political conditions, it may not be feasible to use the same factory that produced a similar style for the previous season. At this point in the development process, the cost is just an estimate. An exact cost will be calculated later. As production time nears, costs might be researched in several countries to select the source country for the best production cost (see Chapter 10).

OTHER COSTS

When establishing the initial cost estimate, it is necessary to include other items that affect the cost. Table 7.1 details some of these items: packaging and/or hanger, hangtags, labels, and freight charges. If a style is produced offshore, other costs might include duty charges and fees to shipping agents and freight consolidators.

TARGET COSTING

Designing a product based on target costing (also discussed in Chapter 6) works a little differently from the product development sequence discussed previously. The designer's sketch is reviewed by the cost engineer, also called a product technician. The cost is carefully estimated from the designer's sketch. The design team works out fabric choices, garment details, and construction factors to bring the design within the required cost for each style in the line. The design sketch may need to be reworked to meet the target cost and to be approved; then a prototype garment is cut, sewn, and given final approval after a careful cost estimate has been made. Each style that is approved is added to the line. The line might be composed of five groups, with three to four styles in each group.

Target costing is frequently used by retailers as they develop private label goods. The retailer's design department sets a specific cost for each item that will be produced. During the design development process, style features and fabrics are adjusted in order to meet the target cost.

Style Selection

Each style in the new line goes through a similar process of development and costing. When all the styles have received the approval of the designer (and merchandiser), the line is ready for design review. Because of the lag time

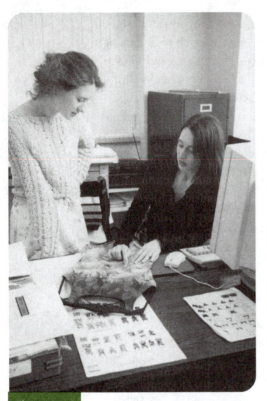

Figure 7.11 The design team carefully reviews each style in the line.

in receiving some fabrics, the review garments may have simulated textile elements in order to visualize the style in the intended fabric. For example, sometimes a print or stripe is painted onto a fabric to simulate the final textile design. Occasionally, these simulated prototypes are even used for promotional photos, since the difference between the mock-up and the actual garment will not be apparent in the photograph.

Presenting and Reviewing the Line at the Line Review Meeting

On the scheduled master calendar date, the new line is presented for review. The merchandiser, designer, assistant designer, production engineer, and any other review team members (such as a selected sales representative) assemble for the line review meeting (see Figure 7.11). Upper management may also be included in the review session. The individual garment styles may be displayed on walls in the conference room (sometimes referred to as the war room), or fit models may try on the garments to present the styles to the review team.

Sometimes the designer or merchandiser begins the review session with a presentation. Design presentation boards or concept boards may be included as a part of the presentation, showing fabrics, various colorways, inspirational pictures, and garment sketches. The presentation might include information about the following:

- the concept or inspiration for the line
- how the styles coordinate or work together
- the target customer profiles for various styles within the line

It may be to the designer's advantage to "sell" the styles in the line to the company review team.

Each style in the line is reviewed, and questions are asked by the review team to determine how well the style works in the areas of cost, production, styling, relationship to the rest of the line, and fabric and trims.

- *Cost:* Will the estimated cost result in a retail price that is within the range of the target customer's expectation? Is its cost in proportion to that of other similar styles? Are there changes in design that might reduce the cost? Could less expensive buttons be substituted? For companies that do cost averaging among several similar items (see Chapter 6), is this approach feasible?

- *Production:* Are there any potential difficulties in production? Are there changes in design that could make production easier or less expensive? Could a seam be eliminated?

- *Styling:* Does the style fit the "look" of the target customer? Does the styling look too fashion forward or too conservative when compared with the rest of the line? Could pockets be added if this is important to the target customer? Does the style look sufficiently different from competitors' styles?

- *Relationship to the rest of the Line:* Does the style work well with other styles in the line? Is there another style so similar that the two will compete with each other? Is the style so different from others that it looks out of place in the line?

- *Fabric and trims:* Are there potential problems with the fabric? If the fabric is new to the line, will it snag, pill, or wrinkle? Has the fabric been adequately tested? Are there potential problems with lengthy lead time required for a fabric or high minimum yardage requirements by the textile mill?

Each of these points, as well as others, is discussed by the review team for each of the styles in the line.

Selecting the Styles for the Line at the Final Adoption Meeting

At the conclusion of the line review meeting, some styles will be eliminated, and some changes may be required in a few styles. For styles in which changes are required, patterns are modified and new prototypes are sewn and approved. The line is thus honed to develop a tight group, line, or collection of styles with the hope that all styles will sell well at market.

Occasionally, one or more styles are included in a line that the review team speculates may not sell well to the retail buyers. A company may want to experiment with a slightly more fashion-forward look. The line may include one or two jackets with more updated styling than has been shown in the past to see how the retail buyers react to these styles.

Thus, the styles that have been approved join to become the new line. It is reviewed and finalized at the final adoption meeting.

Determining the Cost to Manufacture

The cost to manufacture each of the styles to be shown in the new line must be determined before showing the line at market. Establishing as accurate a cost as possible is important to the successful financial outcome of the line. A design that sells well but is underpriced can be a disaster for the apparel company. The amount that the company calculates will be spent to make the garment is called the **cost to manufacture**.

Calculating the cost requires knowledge about production techniques and facilities. Production engineers, or cost engineers, use known costs as well as estimated costs for unknown factors to arrive at the cost to manufacture each of the styles. There is always the possibility that a style will actually cost more than was calculated, or perhaps less. However, it is critical that the cost to manufacture be as accurate a figure as possible. Forgetting to include the cost of a hanger or plastic bag can affect the overall profit when multiplied by thousands of items produced in that style.

If an apparel company uses contractors for production, they can be asked to do one of the following:

- examine a prototype garment of the style to provide a cost figure
- sew a sample garment, and thus provide a cost figure
- review a complete and detailed spec sheet and provide a firm cost

The **wholesale price** is the price quoted to the buyers at market and is the amount the retail store will pay the apparel company for the goods. The wholesale price is the cost to manufacture the style plus the manufacturer's overhead and profit. Some apparel companies double the cost to manufacture (sometimes referred to as "keystone") to arrive at the wholesale price (refer to Table 7.1).

Preline

Some apparel companies invite their key retail accounts (those retail buyers who place large orders with them) to preview the line prior to its introduction at market. The preview is sometimes referred to as **preline**. The line might be composed of actual samples, or virtual samples shown on the computer. These retail buyers provide their opinion to the apparel company about the potential success of the styles they are shown. Retailers might place orders at this time.

Advantages to the apparel company of holding a preline showing include the following:

- knowing in advance which styles will sell well, allowing the apparel company to plan production needs accordingly so it has adequate quantities of anticipated successful products and avoids producing poor-selling styles

- maintaining a strong working relationship with key retail accounts

- receiving feedback from retailers about styles that might sell better if changes were made

A disadvantage is that, since the styles have not yet been produced in the factory, unknown factors may still emerge that will require later changes in a style that buyers have already ordered.

Some companies forecast sales without actual written orders from retailers. For example, black ski pants tend to be constant sellers at market. In advance of orders being placed, the skiwear company may begin production of a certain number of black ski pants to avoid the pressure on production during that industry's very short production season.

Preparation for Market

Now that the new line is ready to be shown to retail buyers, additional **samples** or **duplicates** need to be made (see Chapter 9) so that sales representatives throughout the country or world can sell the line by showing samples to retail store buyers. The marketing process involved in selling the line will be discussed in detail in Chapter 8.

Ordering and Making Sales Samples

Each sales representative and/or each market center showroom will require a representative group of styles from the new line to show to the retail store buyers. Because of cost limitations, not every style in every colorway will be made for sales representatives' samples, or duplicates. However, line catalogs, or line sheets, will show all colorways. As soon as the line is final, the styles that will be made as samples to sell the line at market are selected. The quantity of fabric, as well as linings, buttons, zippers, and other supplies required for the samples, are calculated and ordered. If the textile producer is late in delivering the ordered fabrics, complications in producing the samples on time may occur. Late arrival of fabric could result in the samples not arriving in time for the sales representatives to show at market.

Contractors or the apparel company's sewing factories cut and sew the sample garments. If any production difficulties arise during this small production run, there is an opportunity to make an adjustment to ensure a smooth run later during production of the retailer's goods. Late delivery of samples from the sewing facility could also cause complications at market.

The apparel company may also produce a fashion show and visual presentation of all the company's lines at a special event for the company's sales representatives. This line presentation creates enthusiasm for the new season's goods and helps the sales force sell the line at market. The line's designer (and merchandiser) may be responsible for producing the line presentation. Social events might also be held when the representatives gather for the line presentation. Events such as golf or tennis tournaments, which involve friendly competition among the sales representatives, build company spirit.

Line Catalog or Line Sheet

As soon as the new line has been finalized, a **line catalog** (also called a **line sheet** or line style book) is prepared. This is a catalog, usually with color illustrations, of all the styles available in the line in the various colorways available for each style. Color photographs of featured styles may also be included. Charts show the sizes and colors available for each style and can serve as order sheets as well. Wholesale prices and sometimes suggested retail prices for each style are included. Figure 7.12 shows a typical line catalog page. The line catalog is used by sales representatives and buyers to augment the sample garments shown during presentations. More information about the selling process is presented in Chapter 8.

Most companies use specialized CAD or graphics software to produce the color illustrations of the garments for the line catalog. The technical details about scanning the actual fabric prints into these computer systems for the line catalog are discussed in Chapter 6. Typically, if the first sketch used in the design stage is produced using a computer system, this sketch is revised as needed and then used for the line catalog.

It is important that the line catalog accurately represent the colors of the actual fabrics for each style. Retail buyers expect the finished goods to match the colors depicted in the line catalog. Some apparel companies show actual fabric swatches in their line catalogs, or they send a set of fabric swatches with the line catalogs. Seeing the actual fabric texture, plaid repeat, or variety of print colorways helps sell the line to the retail buyers.

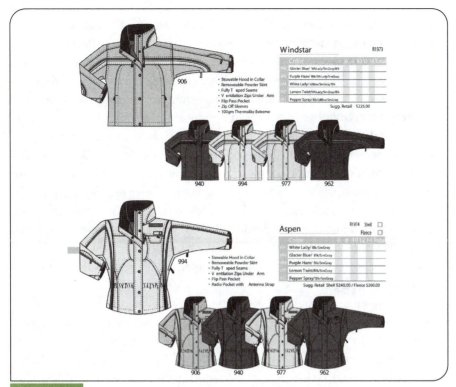

Figure 7.12 Sales representatives use line catalogs in their presentations.

Private Label and Store Brand Product Development

In today's marketplace, there are a variety of ways in which the creation and development of an apparel line occurs. Possible design–retail relationships include the following:

1. traditional design development in which the garment carries the brand name or designer brand of the apparel company

2. private label product development or store brand product development through one of the following arrangements:

  • The retailer provides the garment specifications, and the manufacturer or contractor sources the goods (**specification buying**).

  • The retailer and the manufacturer collaborate in the creation of the retailer's line.

  • The manufacturer or contractor designs the entire program for the retailer.

It is important to understand the differences between traditional design development and private label or store brand development as they affect the design, production, and pricing strategies for apparel, accessories, and home fashions.

We have traced the progress of a style from its creation through its development stages, using a model based on a conventional marketing channel used for **brand merchandise** in the apparel industry. The apparel company conceives the design, controls manufacturing (using their own factories or contractors they select), and then markets the product to the retailer. The retail buyer evaluates the sample garment and decides whether or not to purchase the style in anticipation of the retailer's target customer desiring the product. A profit is expected at each step of the marketing channel. Conventional design development, marketing, and production involve several profit-making steps, including sewing by a contractor and selling by a sales representative. The final price of the product to the ultimate consumer usually reflects the number of profit-making steps.

As the price of apparel at the retail level has escalated in recent years, retailers and apparel companies have sought ways to reduce costs and increase their share of the profit. Using offshore production in countries with lower labor costs is one solution. Another approach is to reduce the number of steps involved in the marketing channel. By reducing the number of profit-making steps, either the cost of the product can be reduced, or the profit to the remaining companies can be increased (or both). If a retailer works directly with an apparel company to co-create a product or a line, the sales representative's position is no longer needed. If a retailer decides to create a product to sell in its retail stores and goes directly to a sewing contractor, the apparel company's services are not needed. These are examples of private label product development or store brand product development.

Private Label and Store Brand Product Development Processes

Creating private label or store brand merchandise can be achieved in several ways. One method for developing private label or store brand goods is for the retailer to work directly with the manufacturer, sewing contractor, or their agents, providing them with garment specifications. Retailers such as Target, JCPenney, and Nordstrom have their own product development departments for developing their store brand merchandise. These companies work directly with contractors to source and produce the goods to their very detailed specifications. Target, JCPenney, and Walmart, among others, have sourcing offices in Asia. Thus, the retailer assumes the responsibility of designing the product as well as overseeing its production. One advantage to the retailer in dealing directly with the contractor for production is that the retailer has no intermediaries to deal with, thus avoiding communication pitfalls and eliminating the need to share the profits. From the contractor's viewpoint, working directly with the retailer has certain risks. The contractor usually carries the financing for the materials during the production process. After delivery of the goods to the retailer, the contractor is paid for both labor and materials. This is different from the conventional market channel discussed earlier, in which the apparel company often carries the financing of the materials. As these new marketing channels expand and are modified, the advantages, disadvantages, and risks to contractor and retailer may vary as well. Some retailers own their production facilities, carrying all the risk while reducing the number of intermediaries in the marketing channel.

Another of the private label or store brand development processes uses an apparel company's design and development staff to create the entire program for the retailer. Nike, an apparel company that produces lines of apparel under its own label, also develops special lines for other sports specialty retail stores carrying the retailer's label. This type of collaborative business is very common in the apparel industry. One advantage to the retailer is that the apparel company handles all the production processes. Often the apparel company has a strong working relationship with vendors, relieving the retailer of developing systems to oversee the production.

The third type of the private label or store brand development process teams a retail partner with a manufacturer in the creation of the retailer's line. In a new development for the retailer, Bloomingdale's has a joint venture with Tahari, a fashion-forward apparel company. This type of venture is called **co-branded apparel**. The company offers complete collections of jackets, skirts, pants, dresses, sweaters, T-shirts, and outerwear ("Private label's new identity," 1999, p. 8) in place of more traditional private label merchandise based on single items.

Development of Private Label and Store Brand Products

The British retailer Marks & Spencer has been a leader in private label apparel since its merchandise development department was established. "The company's low prices were the result of trading direct with manufacturers for cash, a principle which remains unchanged to this day. Marks & Spencer's goods are immediately recognized by their 'St. Michael' trademark, which first appeared on 'pajamas and knitted articles of clothing' back in 1928" (Bressler, Newman & Proctor, 1997, p. 68). Rather than purchasing lingerie items from apparel companies to sell in their retail stores, Marks & Spencer determined the goods they wanted to produce and then went directly to contractors who produced the goods. By eliminating the apparel company's role (and its profit) in the design and manufacturing process, Marks & Spencer could produce and sell its goods at very appealing prices.

Soon, other retailers began to realize the advantages of private label product development. In the 1950s, Hong Kong was well-known for its knitwear manufacturing, especially sweaters. The quality was good, production was dependable, and prices were low. Retailers such as Frederick and Nelson (no longer in business) contracted with knitwear companies in Hong Kong to produce exclusive products such as sweaters for their retail stores. The sweater label read "Made Exclusively for Frederick and Nelson in Hong Kong." This private label product development remained a small part of the specialty and department store retail picture in the United States until the 1980s.

The growth of off-price stores and factory outlet mall stores in the 1980s increased pressure on department and specialty store retailers to offer products at competitive prices. Added to retailers' pressures was the fact that apparel companies such as Liz Claiborne, Tommy Hilfiger, Polo Ralph Lauren, and Nike opened retail stores of their own. One remedy for department store retailers was to increase the percent of private label merchandise they carried. Thus, the private label business continues to expand, both within department store retailers and with specialty retailers.

With private label goods, all the risk in selling is in the retailer's hands. The risk to retailers is lessened by the fact that basic goods (as compared to fashion goods) have long-term sales potential. Thus, as department store retailers built and expanded their private label business in the early 1990s, most chose to produce basic garment styles such as polo shirts, shorts, casual pants, and jeans, well suited for private label manufacturing. Another advantage of producing these types of private label goods is that it makes differentiation between a national brand and a private label item difficult to discern. A customer could purchase a private label polo shirt for several dollars less than the national brand shirt that looked nearly identical. The price-conscious customer would eagerly select the private label polo shirt and be well satisfied with its quality (see Figure 7.13).

Some retailers link their private label lines to celebrities to enhance the stature of the label and the retail store. Kmart offers Jaclyn Smith labels. In an interesting twist, some retailers have signed licensing deals with Seventh Avenue fashion designers. Target signed an exclusive licensing deal with designers Gene Meyer, Issac Mizrahi, and Cynthia Rowley. For these fashion designers, the financial risk of designing under their own business has been transferred to the retailer.

As sales volume of private label merchandise increased, retailers developed more fashion-forward private label merchandise in addition to the basic items that were "safe" choices to begin their private label businesses. To do so, retailers organized product design teams similar to the design teams at apparel companies. Mass retailers such as Target and JCPenney were some of the first retailers to have private label product development departments (see Table 7.2).

Most department and chain stores strive toward a balance between national brands and their private label merchandise. In 2007, private label apparel made up 42 percent,

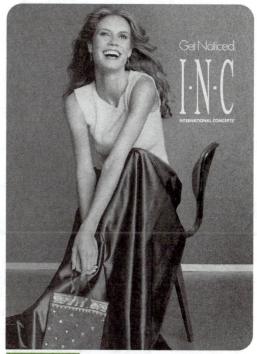

Figure 7.13 Department stores offer a number of private label apparel brands, such as INC International for Macy's.

Table 7.2	Selected Apparel Private Labels
Store	**Labels**
Dillard's	Allison Daley, Investments, Westbound, Copper Key, Aigle, Caribbean, Daniel Cremieux, Murano, Roundtree & Yorke, Class Club, First Wave, Starting Out
Macy's, Inc.	Charter Club, Karen Scott, INC International, Alfani, Greendog, Club Room, Style & Co.
JCPenney	Worthington, St. John's Bay, Arizona/Arizona Kids, Stafford, Okie Dokie
Kmart	Joe Boxer, Jaclyn Smith, Kathy Ireland, Basic Editions, Route 66, Small Wonders
Kohl's	Apt 9, Croft & Barrow, Sonoma, Urban Pipeline
Gottschalks	Shaver Lake
Nordstrom	Caslon, Classiques Entier, Halogen, Baby Nay, Façonnable
Sears	Canyon River Blues, Covington, Classic Elements, Personal Identity, Stacy Adams
Target	Merona, xhilaration
Walmart	Starter, No Boundaries, George, Faded Glory

national brand apparel 34 percent, designer 6 percent, and 18 percent other for most department stores (Cohen, 2009). For example, Macy's offers a variety of private label lines, such as Charter Club and INC International, in addition to the national brands, such as Levi Strauss & Co., Quiksilver, Koret, and Pendleton. However, with the recession during 2009, retailers begin to recognize that private label merchandise isn't necessarily the safest bet in challenging times (Cohen, 2009). Branded merchandise is recognized and the retailer does not assume the risk of selling their private label. By May 2009, national brands had increased to 35.3 percent and private label decreased to 40.8 percent in total apparel sales volume (Cohen, 2009).

Store Is Brand

During the 1980s and early 1990s, a number of specialty retailers opened businesses that sell 100 percent private label merchandise or store brands (see Chapter 4). This strategy, known as **store-is-brand**, results in the retail outlet (i.e., store, catalog, website) and the apparel brand being one and the same in the consumer's mind. Examples of companies that employ this strategy include The Limited, Victoria's Secret, Express, Gap, Banana Republic, Old Navy, Casual Corner, Eddie Bauer, Talbots, and Benetton. As with other retailers that offer private label merchandise, companies that offer only store brands either employ their own designers and/or product developers who turn their designs over to contractors for production, or their buyers seek out full-package contractors who design, develop, and produce specified merchandise exclusively for the store. Exceptions include Benetton and Zara, both vertically integrated companies that control production from fabric to finished garment.

Advantages and Disadvantages of Private Label and Store Brand Product Development

Retailers may decide to offer private label merchandise, expand their private label business, or offer only store brands. As noted earlier, one of the major advantages to private label and store brand product development is the reduction in the number of intermediaries involved, providing an increased profit (gross margin) to the retailer and/or a reduced price for the consumer.

Another advantage of private label and store brand business is that the retailer can fill in voids in some product categories. Also, the customer is looking for value, and private label merchandise can provide that value. Quality private label products offered at a good price can build and maintain store loyalty, as well as private label loyalty among customers. One of the goals for retailers is to make the private label into a well-defined brand in the customer's mind. "More private-brand managers are charged with making sure the brand's message is consistent across categories and seasons, with the goal of creating destination brands" (Ryan, 2003, p. 32).

Store differentiation is another advantage. National-brand merchandise is available at many retail and specialty stores, creating a sameness to these stores' merchandise. Once customers become familiar with retailers' private label brands or store brands, they may choose to shop at that retailer's location because the store merchandise has an appeal and is different from what other stores offer. James Coggin, president of Saks stated, "Our private label initiative is extremely important to Saks Inc. because it provides a way to differentiate ourselves from our competitors and allows us to provide quality merchandise for our customer at a greater gross margin return than normal brands" (Hye, 1999, p. 17). Presenting exclusive merchandise to the customer who wants to associate with the retailer's image is an advantage of private labeling.

Retailers have the closest tie to the customer. They have a finger on the pulse of what the customer really is buying and what she or he wants. Retailers want increasing control over more aspects of the product than branded manufacturers offer them.

The major drawback to private label and store brand business has been mentioned. The retailer takes all the risk. Since the retailer usually owns the merchandise, if it does not sell well, the retailer loses profit.

Summary

The design development stage in the progress of a new line begins with the delivery of the designer's approved sketch. Development of the new style includes making the first pattern using either traditional paper patternmaking techniques or computerized PDS. A prototype is cut from the pattern and sewn by a sample sewer, using the intended fabric (or a substitute facsimile if the actual fabric is not yet available). The new prototype is tried on a fit model for review of the design and fit by a design team and revised if necessary. Sometimes, several prototypes of a new style are sewn in order to perfect the design.

The cost for the final design is estimated. The line is reviewed again, at which time each style is scrutinized carefully by the design team. The final line consists of styles that have been approved at this stage. Additional samples of styles in the line are sewn for sales representatives, and a line catalog and other types of promotional materials are prepared for marketing purposes.

Computer applications in design development continue to expand. Each year, more apparel companies realize the need to utilize this technology in order to survive in today's marketplace. The computer integration of design, patternmaking, and production is another critical step for continued survival in the ever-increasing pace of the apparel industry.

The changing structure of apparel marketing channels will continue to bring changes in the relationship between the apparel company, contractor, sales representative, and retailer. Trends in the apparel industry include continued expansion of private label and store brand product development, the use of product lifecycle management systems, and 3-D tool development.

Career opportunities in the development area include assistant designer/patternmaker, cutter, sample sewer, supervisor, or specification technician.

Pattern Engineer
Publicly Held Sportswear and Athletic Shoe Company

Position Description:

Create fit-approved and manufacturable patterns from design sketches through CAD patterns and flat patterns, ensuring design concepts are correctly interpreted and production capabilities are considered. Manage approximately 90 to 150 styles annually, from inception through distribution. Provide construction, specification, and fabric utilization expertise for the design and development of the line.

Typical Tasks and Responsibilities:

- Draft prototype patterns on CAD.
- Develop preliminary specifications and construction details for sewers and engineers.
- Collaborate with design, development, and engineering departments to interpret sketches into cost-effective production styles.
- Monitor fit sessions, review garments for accuracy of measurements and construction details, and revise patterns.
- Calculate and provide fabric-utilization information throughout the development process.
- Oversee the sample-making process on assigned styles.
- Prepare traced patterns, specifications, construction details, usage, and special grading requirements for contractors' samples.

Specification Buyer
Sportswear Manufacturer and Retailer

Position Description:

Responsible for assisting the product engineer in the documentation of all sample reviews and the follow-up communication to vendors relating to specification development, product evaluation, and control of specification files.

CAREER PROFILES

Typical Tasks and Responsibilities:

- Be responsible for fit reviews.

- Create specification packages (bill of materials, construction, size specifications).

- Sketch front and back details of garments.

- Read electronic mail from product engineer and domestic and overseas vendors.

- Tag, log, and track all incoming samples.

- Perform engineer's tasks when needed.

- Complete counter sample reviews and preproduction reviews.

Key Terms

base pattern	pattern design system (PDS)
block	precosting
brand merchandise	preline
co-branded apparel	proprietary
color management	prototype
cost to manufacture	sample
duplicate	sample sewer
fit model	sloper
flat pattern	specification buying
initial cost estimate	store-is-brand
line catalog	tagboard
line sheet	usage
marker	wholesale price

Discussion Questions and Activities

1. Discuss how an apparel company interested in converting from paper patternmaking to a pattern design system (PDS) might decide what system to purchase.

2. Discuss why a designer might use draping techniques as opposed to patternmaking when developing a garment design. What are advantages and disadvantages to each method?

3. Select a garment, such as a jacket. How might the design and materials be changed to reduce the cost?

4. For a retailer, what are some advantages and disadvantages in producing private label merchandise?

5. For an apparel company, what are some advantages and disadvantages in producing a special private label apparel line for a retailer?

References

Bressler, K., Newman, K., and Proctor, G. (1997). *A Century of Lingerie*. Edison, NJ: Chartwell Books.

Cohen, M. (2009, August 1). The challenges of private label apparel. *License Global*. Retrieved from http://www.licensemag.com

D'Innocenzio, A. (1998, October 7). Punching up private label. *Women's Wear Daily*, pp. 14–15.

Hye, J. (1999, November 17). Saks sources technology for private label. *Women's Wear Daily*, p. 17.

Private label's new identity. (1999, March 11). *Women's Wear Daily*, pp. 1, 8, 20.

Ryan, T. (2003, June). Private labels: Strong, strategic & growing. *Apparel*, pp. 32–37.

Workman, J. (1991). Body measurement specifications for fit models as a factor in clothing size variation. *Clothing and Textiles Research Journal*, 10 (1), pp. 31–36.

CHAPTER 8

Marketing a Line of Apparel or Home Fashions

In this chapter, you will learn the following:

- the marketing process within apparel and home fashions companies

- the histories, functions, and activities of U.S. apparel, accessory, and home fashions market centers, marts, market weeks, and trade shows

- the nature of the selling function of apparel and home fashions companies, specifically the roles of sales representatives and showrooms

- the distribution and sales promotion strategies used by apparel and home fashions companies

Step 4: Marketing the Apparel Line

Step 1 Research and Merchandising

Step 2 Design

Step 3 Design Development and Style Selection

Step 4 Marketing the Apparel Line

Designer and National Brands
Sales Representatives Show Line at Market and through Other Promotion Strategies

Retail Buyers Place Orders

Private-Label Brands
Design Team Shows Line to Merchandisers/Buyers

Buyers Place Orders

Step 5 Preproduction

Step 6 Sourcing

Step 7 Apparel Production Processes, Material Management, and Quality Assurance

Step 8 Distribution and Retailing

*W*ithin the organizational structure of an apparel or home fashions company, the area called research and merchandising *typically focuses on market research and developing sales, promotion, and distribution strategies (see Chapter 4). Marketing divisions or departments in apparel or home fashions companies are organized in a number of ways, depending on the size and goals of the company. Figure 8.1 shows a variety of organizational structures for marketing divisions of apparel companies.*

Although the marketing area of an apparel or home fashions company is most often associated with the promotion and sales of the products, it should be noted that without an accurate understanding of the target customer attained through market research, and without designing and producing goods and services that meet the needs of the target customer, even the best of promotion strategies will undoubtedly fail. Thus, the marketing of apparel and home fashions products connects the research conducted previously with the appropriate strategies for getting the product to the right consumers at the right price and in the right place.

The term **market** can be used in the following ways:

- One may say that a particular product has a *market*, meaning that there is consumer demand for the product. Chapter 5 discusses research used in assessing the consumer demand or market for a product.

- The term *market* can also be used to refer to a location where the buying and selling of merchandise takes place. For example, retail buyers often talk about going to market to purchase merchandise for their stores.

- One can also *market* a product, meaning that the product will be promoted through advertising in the media and public relations efforts.

This chapter examines apparel and home fashions markets as locations where apparel and home fashions companies sell their merchandise to retailers. It also explores the distribution and promotion strategies that apparel companies use in marketing their goods to retailers and consumers.

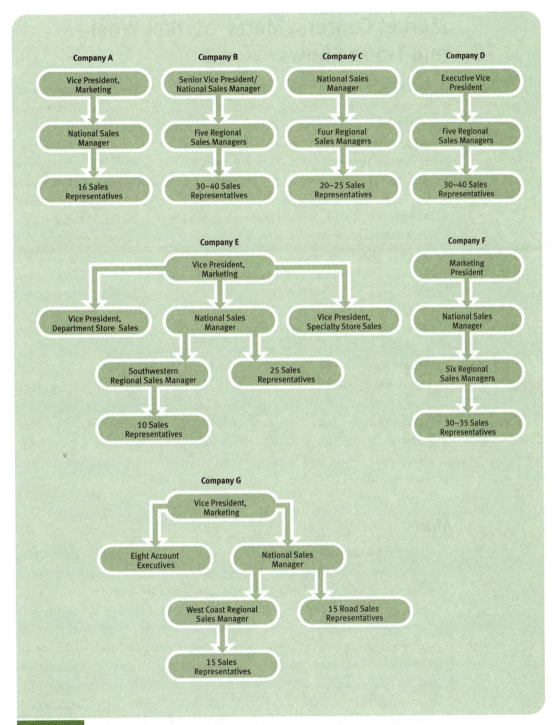

Figure 8.1 Examples of Marketing Division organizational structures.

Market Centers, Marts, Market Weeks, and Trade Shows

Historically, New York City was the first apparel, accessory, and home fashions market center in the United States. Buyers from large, upscale stores traveled to New York City once or twice a year to view the new lines and purchase merchandise for their stores. In addition, manufacturers' salespeople would travel from town to town within a specific region, inviting buyers from local stores to see the lines in a hotel room or in the retailers' stores. With the growth of apparel and home fashions manufacturing and retailing in the 1950s, regional market centers began to be established. In the early 1960s, the first regional apparel and merchandise marts were built. After experiencing growth throughout the 1980s, some regional apparel and home fashion marts saw a decline in the 1990s. This was because of consolidation of companies within the industries, increased competition among marts, the growth of private label merchandising and store brands, the growth of trade shows as an important means for retailer buyers to connect with manufacturers, and the growth of electronic and web-based communications between manufacturers and retailers.

With the decline of the importance of the regional marts, there was a growth in the importance of market centers for the industries. The term **market center** is used to refer to those cities that house marts and showrooms, are home to important trade shows, and also have important manufacturing and retailing industries. In the United States, these cities include New York City, Los Angeles, Dallas, Atlanta, and Chicago. Internationally, these cities include Paris, London, Milan, Tokyo, Hong Kong, Seoul, and Taipei.

Marts

A **mart** is a building or a group of buildings that houses showrooms in which sales representatives show apparel and home fashions lines to retail buyers. Most major cities (except for New York) have marts; some are devoted entirely to textiles, apparel, accessories, home fashions, and related goods (e.g., Los Angeles's California Market Center, a.k.a. the CMC); some also house showrooms for a variety of types of products. For example, the Merchandise Mart in Chicago includes showrooms for apparel, home furnishings, kitchen and bath, contract furnishings, contemporary art, antiques, and fine crafts. Some marts are also part of larger market center complexes (e.g., Dallas Market Center) which include multiple mart buildings for a variety of merchandise. Figure 8.2 shows the locations and names of the major market centers and regional marts in the United States.

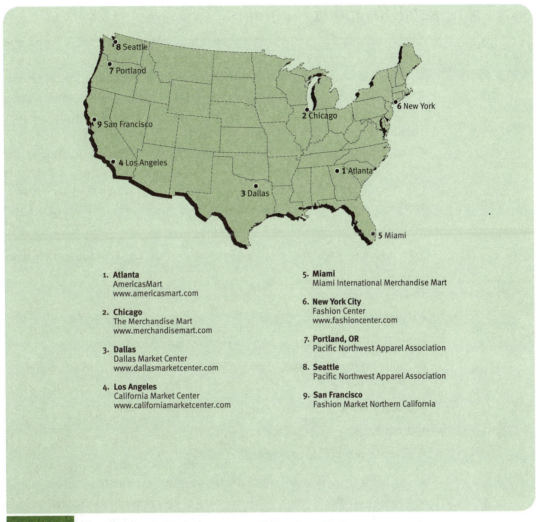

1. **Atlanta**
   AmericasMart
   www.americasmart.com

2. **Chicago**
   The Merchandise Mart
   www.merchandisemart.com

3. **Dallas**
   Dallas Market Center
   www.dallasmarketcenter.com

4. **Los Angeles**
   California Market Center
   www.californiamarketcenter.com

5. **Miami**
   Miami International Merchandise Mart

6. **New York City**
   Fashion Center
   www.fashioncenter.com

7. **Portland, OR**
   Pacific Northwest Apparel Association

8. **Seattle**
   Pacific Northwest Apparel Association

9. **San Francisco**
   Fashion Market Northern California

Figure 8.2 U.S. apparel and home fashions markets and marts.

All marts also include exhibition halls that are filled with temporary showrooms or booths. These are used during **market weeks,** the primary times during the year in which seasonal lines are shown to retail buyers by apparel or home fashions companies or sales representatives without permanent showrooms at that mart. Exhibition halls are also used for trade shows. To facilitate the buyers' trips to market, apparel and merchandise marts publish and/or post on their websites directories for market weeks that list the apparel and home fashions lines being offered, sales representatives, and services available at the mart.

Retail Relations Programs

Marts compete for retailer buyers' attention through a variety of programs and services designed to enhance the buyer's experience and allow them to be more efficient and effective in their jobs. These programs are commonly known as **retail relations programs**. For example, in response to shorter turnaround times and faster delivery of apparel, and because buyers are purchasing less merchandise more often, the larger marts are open year round, typically 5 days a week, 52 weeks a year. This allows buyers to come at any time during the year, not just during market weeks. Most marts currently have ongoing retail relations programs, including a number of services designed to assist retail buyers during market weeks and trade shows. These services include the following:

- educational seminars (e.g., trend reports, visual merchandising, new merchandising strategies)
- seminars for first time or new buyers
- fashion shows
- programs to connect buyers with representatives and vendors
- opportunities for buyers to join together for purchasing, marketing, and advertising purposes
- credit and financing assistance
- discounts on travel expenses
- entertainment (e.g., concerts, food fairs)

A number of marts offer seminars focusing on international markets and sourcing (purchasing goods and services) in other countries. Topics include how to do business in Mexico or China, labeling requirements for exporting goods, and other issues surrounding exporting.

Although the growth of apparel and merchandise marts outside of New York City was primarily due to the need for regional market centers, the larger apparel and merchandise marts (e.g., California Market Center in Los Angeles, Dallas Market Center) are now considered national and international resources; many marts are working to attract international buyers from Mexico, Canada, Central and South America, Asia, and Europe. Services offered to international buyers include travel assistance, office space with free international phones, and translation services.

Marts are sometimes viewed as self-contained in that they generally house consultants' offices, restaurants, banks, hotels, auditoriums, health clubs, dry cleaners, business centers, and other services for retail buyers. Marts may also be involved in many aspects of the apparel and home fashions industries. For example, the California Market Center includes offices of fixture and display companies, employment agencies, buying offices, trade associations, and private label manufacturers. Thus, when buyers come to market, the mart serves as a one-stop location for all of their needs.

Market Weeks and Trade Shows

Market weeks and trade shows are the primary opportunities for designers, manufacturers, and retailers to connect and conduct business.

Market Weeks

Market weeks are the times of the year when retail buyers come to showrooms or exhibit halls to see the seasonal fashion lines. During market weeks, retail buyers do the following:

- set appointments with manufacturers' sales representatives of name brands
- set appointments with contractors for private-label and store-brand merchandise
- discover new lines
- attend fashion shows
- attend trend seminars and other educational sessions
- review manufacturers' lines
- place orders for name brand merchandise for their stores
- place orders for private-label and store-brand merchandise

They typically come to market weeks with a specific amount that they can spend (referred to as their **open-to-buy**) for specific categories of merchandise. Marts generally sponsor a variety of market weeks throughout the year, each focusing on a particular product category (e.g., women's, juniors', men's, children's, bridal, swimwear, and so on) and fashion season (e.g., Fall, Holiday, Resort, Spring, Summer). Market week dates are set years in advance during meetings with representatives from the various marts and New York City fashion councils. In general, market weeks for Fall fashion season are held in March and April, and market weeks for Spring fashion season are held in October and November. Market weeks may also be sponsored in conjunction with an industry trade association. Through these joint efforts, buyers are exposed to a greater variety of apparel manufacturers at a single location than they would be otherwise. Table 8.1 outlines the typical months in which U.S. women's and children's ready-to-wear market weeks are held for each fashion season.

Market weeks provide advantages for both the apparel and home fashions manufacturer and the retailer. The advantages of market weeks for apparel and home fashions manufacturers include the following:

- Sales representatives can show the new lines to a large number of retail buyers in a very short time. Retailers may also place orders during market week shows.

- Sales representatives can talk with the buyers and acquire information regarding consumer and retail trends.

- Based on buyer interest, sales representatives also can determine which pieces in the line will most likely be put into production.

- Through such market week activities as fashion shows and displays, apparel and home fashions companies can receive publicity for their lines with the potential for securing new retail accounts.

- Manufacturers can often view the lines of competing companies (although many exclusive lines are available for viewing to retail buyers only).

Table 8.1   Women's and Children's Ready-to-Wear (RTW) Market Weeks

Fashion Season	Market Weeks
Summer	NYC market: October All other markets: January
Fall I	NYC market: January All other markets: March–April
Fall II	NYC market: February All other markets: June
Holiday and Resort	NYC market: June All other markets: August
Spring	NYC market: August All other markets: October–November

For retail buyers, the advantages of market weeks include the following:

- Market weeks allow them to review a large number of lines of merchandise in a very short time.

- By attending seminars held during market weeks, they are also able to acquire information about fashion trends, advertising, visual merchandising, and a number of other topics.

- Buyers can also become aware of new lines that they may want to purchase for their stores.

Individuals involved with product development often attend market weeks to identify manufacturers that may be able to produce private label or store brand merchandise. Thus, market weeks are important times for the apparel and home fashions companies in determining the success of their lines.

Trade Shows

Trade associations and specialized trade show producers sponsor their own shows for the purpose of promoting lines of apparel, accessories, and home fashions (see Figures 8.3 and 8.4). These trade shows, lasting anywhere from

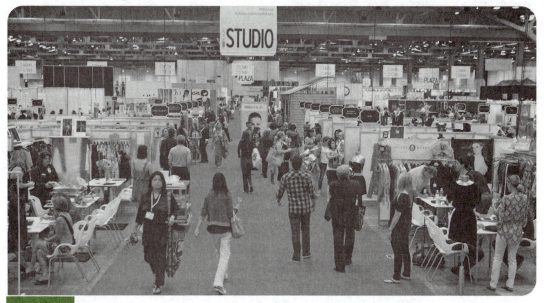

Figure 8.3 Retail buyers attend trade shows such as WWDMAGIC to view lines from a number of companies.

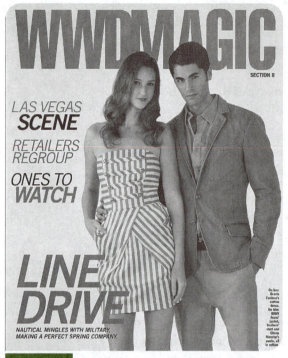

Figure 8.4 The WWD and MAGIC partnership has created one of the largest trade shows in the United States for apparel and accessories.

three to eight days, are typically located in the exhibition halls of marts, at large hotels, or at convention centers. For example, the Javits Center in New York City is the home to many apparel and accessories trade shows each year including AccessoriesTheShow, FFANY, and FAME trade shows. Las Vegas has become a U.S. hub for trade shows including MAGIC, Accessories-TheShow, and Moda. Below are selected examples of trade shows for several categories of merchandise.

SHOES AND ACCESSORIES

- AccessoriesTheShow, New York City and Las Vegas

- WSA (World. Shoes. Accessories) Show, Las Vegas

- Fashion Footwear Association of New York (FFANY), New York City

ACTIVE SPORTSWEAR AND SPORTING GOODS

- Outdoor Retailer, Salt Lake City, UT
- Action Sports Retailer (ASR), San Diego, CA, and Costa Mesa, CA

APPAREL FASHIONS AND ACCESSORIES

- ENK International Trade Events (Accessories Circuit, Fashion Coterie, Children's Club, Sole Commerce), New York City

- Fashion Avenue Market Expo (FAME), New York City and Las Vegas

- Men's Apparel Guild in California (MAGIC) Marketplace, Las Vegas
  – MAGIC—menswear
  – WWDMAGIC—women's wear
  – Project—contemporary fashion
  – Premium at MAGIC—men's contemporary designers

     – S.L.A.T.E.—skate, surf, and street fashion

     – Street Unlimited—young men's

     – KID Show (held in conjunction with MAGIC, Las Vegas)

     – Pool Trade Show (held in conjunction with MAGIC) boutique market

     – Sourcing at MAGIC—global sourcing resources

- Moda Manhattan and Moda Las Vegas, New York City and Las Vegas

- STYLEMAX, Chicago

HOME FASHIONS

- NeoCon World's Trade Fair (design for the built environment), Chicago

- At Home, New York International Gift Fair, New York City

Some companies rely heavily on trade shows for presenting their lines; others present their lines primarily during market weeks in New York City and/or at apparel and merchandise marts and may exhibit at only one or two of the primary trade shows. Retail buyers, product developers, and sourcing agents may attend both market weeks and trade shows to review lines and services for their stores. Websites for trade shows include exhibitor information, buyer information, product search services, show information and registration, and show evaluations.

Trade shows have utilized virtual trade shows through online exhibits of lines and expanding buyers' opportunities to purchase goods online. Virtual trade shows for textiles, home fashions, graphics (e.g., T-shirt graphic designs), and specialized apparel (e.g., protective clothing, uniforms) are quite common. It's important for retail buyers and product developers to examine a line in person so that they can evaluate color, fabric, and quality. Therefore, because of the desire to touch and examine textile, home fashions, and apparel products, face-to-face trade shows will still remain popular for these product categories.

U.S. Market Centers

New York City

New York City (NYC) is considered the preeminent U.S. market center for apparel, accessories, and home fashions. As noted in Chapter 1, NYC has a long history and tradition of being the heart of apparel manufacturing and marketing in the United States. Interestingly, NYC is the only U.S. market center that does not have a designated apparel or merchandise mart. Instead, showrooms are located throughout a portion of Manhattan known as the *garment district,* the *garment center*, the *fashion center,* or the *fashion district*. NYC's fashion center is an area in midtown Manhattan located between Fifth Avenue and Ninth Avenue and between 35th Street and 42nd Street (see Figure 8.5). The central area is between Seventh Avenue (designated *Fashion Avenue* in 1972) and Broadway. The fashion center began as a manufacturing center but as costs of space increased, many of the manufacturing operations were forced to move to locations outside Manhattan where real estate costs are lower. However, the fashion center is now better known as a design, marketing, and sales center rather than as a manufacturing center.

Currently, the NYC garment district or fashion center includes more than 800 fashion companies, including studios, showrooms, or headquarters with yearly revenues of $1.5 trillion. It is estimated that more than 20,000 out-of-town buyers visit the fashion center every year. For companies that also have their design headquarters in NYC, showrooms are often in the same building—if not on the same floor—as the design area. Although NYC is the home of design and marketing efforts for a wide variety of companies, the NYC market is best

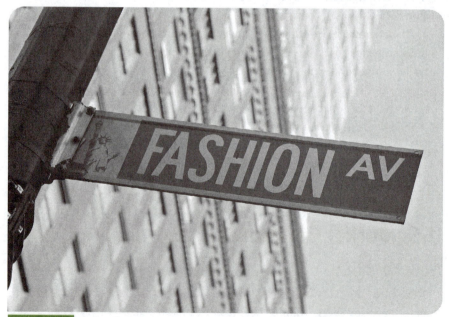

Figure 8.5 New York City's fashion center, located in midtown Manhattan, is the home to studios and design and marketing headquarters of hundreds of companies.

known for women's apparel and for designer and bridge price zones. Virtually all name designers (e.g., Vera Wang, Calvin Klein, Donna Karan, Ralph Lauren, Jill Stuart, Michael Kors, and so forth) have offices in NYC. NYC is also home to Mercedes-Benz Fashion Week, where twice a year nearly 100 U.S. and international designers, including Nicole Miller, BCBG Max Azria, Cynthia Rowley, Derek Lam, Betsey Johnson, Vera Wang, Ralph Lauren, and Badgley Mischka (just to name a few), hold their runway shows at Lincoln Center (see Figure 8.6). In addition to being the home of marketing efforts for a number of companies, New York City is also the location of corporate headquarters for companies such as Jones Apparel Group, Danskin, Phillips-Van Heusen, Polo Ralph Lauren, Donna Karan International, and Vera Wang, just to name a few. And, of course, New York is the headquarters of Fairchild Fashion Group media company (owned by Condé Nast) that publishes *WWD*, *WWDMen's*, *FN*, and WWD.com.

In an effort to facilitate buyers' trips to NYC, certain buildings have tried to specialize in specific apparel categories. However, despite some attempts to specialize buildings, NYC, in general, is not very convenient for retail buyers,

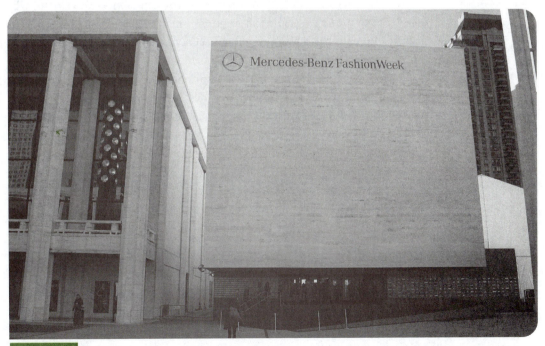

Figure 8.6 Designers present new collections twice per year at Mercedes-Benz Fashion Week in New York City.

who must go from building to building to visit showrooms during their buying trips. Resources for accessories, for example, are spread throughout the garment district, adding to the inconvenience. Thus, in comparing the NYC market with the apparel marts in other cities, NYC is often viewed as less personal and more overwhelming.

To add greater convenience for retail buyers, the Fashion Center Business Improvement District (FCBID), funded by owners of property devoted to the garment industry, was created to provide additional services and capital improvements to enhance the fashion center. FCBID activities include an information kiosk on the corner of Seventh Avenue and 39th Street, a website (www. fashioncenter.com), maps with color-coded industry identifiers, and sanitation and security crews to maintain a safe environment. Other projects and initiatives of the Fashion Center Business Improvement District, the Council of Fashion Designers of America, and the Design Trust for Public Space (i.e., Made in Midtown project) have sought to make the fashion center affordable to fashion businesses. Indeed, since the mid-1980s, NYC has enacted special zoning restrictions in the area to preserve affordable manufacturing space and to encourage multi-use buildings.

Given the fact that the city is expensive, crowded, and inconvenient, why does NYC continue to serve as an important market center? In addition to its historic foundation as a fashion center, NYC offers companies access to buying offices, textile wholesalers, findings and trim wholesalers, consultants, advertising agencies, offices of major trade associations, and publishing companies located in the city. As a cultural center, designers can draw inspiration from the continuous influx of art, theater, dance, opera, and other cultural events. They can also view historic costume and textile collections at the Metropolitan Museum of Art and the Fashion Institute of Technology. In addition, because so many companies have showrooms in NYC, the NYC market remains a "must attend" for many buyers, regardless of whether they attend market weeks elsewhere.

Los Angeles

Whereas NYC is considered the primary market center on the East Coast, Los Angeles is considered the primary market center on the West Coast. Located in Los Angeles' downtown Fashion District, the California Market Center (CMC), which opened in 1964, houses hundreds of showrooms for women's wear, menswear, children's wear, accessories, textiles, and gifts and home decor (see Figure 8.7). In addition to the major markets, the CMC offers a number of category-specific specialty markets, such as the following:

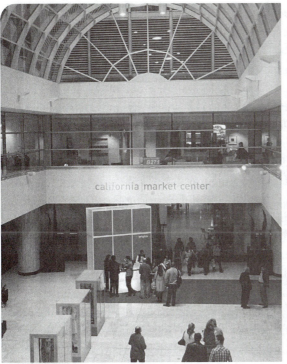

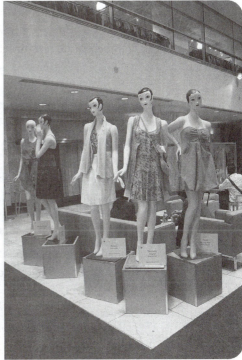

Figure 8.7 The California Market Center in Los Angeles is the largest apparel and accessory market center on the West Coast.

- the L.A. International Textile Show
- Los Angeles Kids Market
- Transit: The LA Show
- CMC Gift and Home Market

The California Market Center has become one of the most technologically advanced of the market centers. This market center caters to retail buyers primarily in the western and southwestern states (e.g., California, Arizona, New Mexico, Nevada, Utah, Oregon, Washington, and Idaho), but it also attracts buyers from across the United States and internationally.

The New Mart, across the street from the California Market Center, provides additional space and has showrooms for many designers and brand name apparel manufacturers (currently 95 showrooms) with hundreds of apparel and accessory resources.

The L.A. Mart® is home to the Design Center (LAMDC) and L.A. Gift and Home Center. The L.A. Mart has approximately 200 showrooms for furnishings, lighting, gifts, and services for interior designers. The LAMDC houses trendsetting furniture and home fashions showrooms for both residential and commercial design projects. The L.A. Gift and Home Center features custom and nationally branded home and lifestyle merchandise.

Similar to New York City, Los Angeles was once one of the nation's largest garment manufacturing centers, but it too has shifted its emphasis to design and marketing. L.A. Fashion District has evolved from being a production center to a design and marketing center. The LA Fashion Business Improvement District was created to vitalize the district through projects to improve business and safety. With the passage of the North American Free Trade Agreement (NAFTA) in 1994 and the Dominican Republic–Central American Free Trade Agreement (CAFTA-DR) in 2004, much of Los Angeles' apparel manufacturing industry has moved to Mexico, Central America, and China. However, despite job losses in manufacturing, in 2008 the LA fashion industry included over 6,800 companies employing 98,000 individuals and drew $36.3 billion in direct sales ("Otis Report," 2009). Designers and producers who have remained in LA find they can monitor production and replenish fashion merchandise faster than if the products were manufactured off-shore (outside the United States).

When we think of California, casual apparel and sportswear come to mind; Los Angeles is best known for sportswear, swimwear, and the "L.A. Style" of casual chic. Companies with headquarters in the Los Angeles area include American Apparel, BCBG Max Azria Group, Inc. (Vernon, CA), Guess? Inc., Hot Cotton, Inc., Joe's Jeans, Inc., Lucky Brand Jeans (Vernon, CA), Quiksilver, Rock & Republic, Sketchers USA, Inc., St. John Knits International, Inc., Tarrant Apparel Group (maker of JCPenney's Arizona jeans and other private labels), and Pacific Sunwear of California (PacSun) (Anaheim, CA), to name a few. Los Angeles and San Francisco areas also include a number of contractors for branded and private label merchandise. California is also home to the headquarters of a number of other large apparel/retailing companies including Ashworth, Inc. (Carlsbad, CA), Bebe Stores, Inc. (Brisbane, CA), Levi Strauss & Co. (San Francisco), Patagonia (Ventura, CA), and Wet Seal (Foothill Ranch, CA).

Chicago

The Chicago Merchandise Mart and the Chicago Apparel Center cater to industry customers from around the world. For apparel and accessories, their clientele comes primarily from the northern and midwestern regions of the United States. The Chicago Merchandise Mart was opened in 1930 by Marshall Field & Company as the largest wholesale center in the United States. Since that time, the Merchandise Mart has remained one of the largest trade centers in the world. As a design center, the Merchandise Mart is the venue for the gift and home markets, as well as for NeoCon.

Built in 1977, the Apparel Center (official name is 350 West Mart Center) is located next to the Chicago Merchandise Mart. During market weeks, the Apparel Center's 140,000-square-foot Expo Center can accommodate 500 booths from temporary vendors (see Figure 8.8). Stylemax trade show offers over 4,000 brands of women's apparel and accessory lines. And some consider the Merchandise Mart's na-

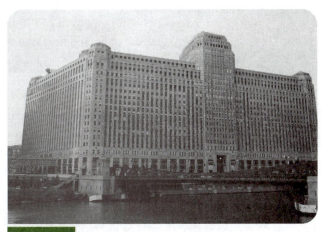

Figure 8.8 The Merchandise Mart in Chicago is the venue for gift and home markets.

tional bridal market to be second only to New York's. Chicago is also home to the headquarters of Hartmarx, a prominent manufacturer of men's and women's wear, and Sears, Roebuck and Co.

Dallas

In the south, Dallas has become the key apparel market center. The Dallas Market Center (DMC) includes four buildings:

- World Trade Center—dedicated in 1974, includes hundreds of showrooms for gifts, decorative accessories, furniture, rugs, fabric, and toys. Fashion-CenterDallas® showcases fashion apparel and accessories.

- Trade Mart—opened in 1959 and expanded in 2007 includes showrooms for gifts, decorative accessories, housewares, tabletop, and stationery.

- International Floral and Gift Center®—opened in 1999, the IFGC is the only U.S. wholesale trade center that includes permanent showrooms for floral and holiday trim industries.

- Market Hall—opened in 1960 and expanded in 1963, includes temporary exhibit space for a variety of trade and consumer shows.

DMC offers more than 50 markets a year for merchandise including textiles; women's, men's, and children's apparel and accessories; and home furnishings and gifts. The DMC offers more that 2,000 showrooms with more than 12,000 apparel lines and more than 25,000 lines of decorative accessories, home furnishings, holiday, gift, and floral items. Buyers from over 75 countries visit the DMC annually.

As with California, the passage of the North American Free Trade Agreement and Texas' proximity to Mexico have resulted in decreased employment in the apparel production industry in Texas. However, increased trade with Mexico has increased employment in sectors of the industry other than production as companies have located operations along the Mexican border. For example, VF, the world's largest manufacturer of jeans, has operations in Texas. Dallas is also home to the corporate headquarters of Haggar Clothing Co, a menswear manufacturer, and Williamson-Dickie Mfg. JCPenney Corporation is headquartered in Plano, Texas, near Dallas.

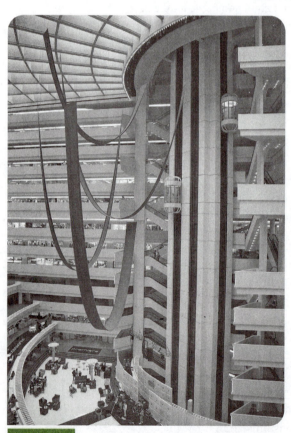

Figure 8.9 The Apparel Mart of AmericasMart 3 in Atlanta includes 15 floors of showrooms and a large fashion theater.

Atlanta

AmericasMart in Atlanta includes:

- AmericasMart 1: the Merchandise Mart (opened in 1961)
- AmericasMart 2: the Gift Mart (opened in 1992)
- AmericasMart 2 West
- AmericasMart 3: the Apparel Mart (opened in 1979 as the Atlanta Apparel Mart)

AmericasMart hosts more than 55 markets per year. The Apparel Mart consists of 15 floors, including a large fashion theater (see Figure 8.9), and it has the capacity to house 2,000 showrooms and 11,000 apparel and accessory lines, including more than 800 children's wear lines. Because NYC does not have a mart, the Atlanta Apparel Mart is the largest mart on the East Coast. Corporate headquarters of Carter's, Inc. and Oxford Industries are also located in Atlanta.

Other Regional Markets

In addition to these market centers, regional markets exist in many U.S. cities. These markets often cater to a more localized clientele or focus on a more concentrated product category. The most prominent of these regional markets are in Miami, San Francisco, and Seattle and Portland, OR.

MIAMI

Known for swimwear, sportswear, and children's wear, Miami's apparel industry grew as a result of Cuban immigration in the 1960s. The Miami International Merchandise Mart opened in 1968 and was the primary wholesale facility in the southeast United States. The mart is now in the middle of legal issues involving its owner. During the 1980s, Miami saw change and increased growth in its apparel industry because of the arrival of offshore production, particularly in Caribbean Basin countries. The United States had trade initiatives with countries in the Caribbean Basin (e.g., Honduras, Guatemala, Dominican Republic), which allowed goods cut in the United States and sewn in one of these countries to be imported into the United States with tariff (taxes on imports) benefits. With the passage of CAFTA-DR in 2004, Miami has attracted a number of apparel manufacturers that produce in these areas of the world, and it has served as a U.S. hub for imports from these areas.

SAN FRANCISCO

In the 1980s and 1990s, San Francisco's apparel industry supported two apparel marts (e.g., the San Francisco Apparel Mart and the Fashion Center) Currently Fashion Market Northern California offers five markets per year with a focus on moderate, better, and contemporary collections for regional buyers. Apparel/home fashions/retailing companies with headquarters in San Francisco include Levi Strauss & Co., Gap, Inc., Jessica McClintock, Gymboree, and Williams-Sonoma, Inc. In addition, a number of apparel companies have headquarters near San Francisco including Bebe (Brisbane, CA), The North Face (San Leandro, CA), JanSport (San Leandro, CA), Restoration Hardware (Corte Madera, CA), Ross Stores (Pleasanton, CA), and Marmot (Santa Rosa, CA).

SEATTLE AND PORTLAND

Since the closure of the Seattle Trade Center apparel mart in 1999, the Pacific Northwest Apparel Association offers NW Trend Shows for five fashion seasons each year. These shows are an important regional format for buyers and exhibitors from Washington, Oregon, Idaho, Montana, Alaska, and British

Columbia. As with other regional shows, exhibitors tend to be independent sales representatives who offer lines from a number of companies. Seattle is famous for its men's and young men's sportswear and outerwear manufacturers. In the late 1970s, Seattle was the home to Brittania Sportswear, then the largest privately owned sportswear manufacturer in the United States. In Brittania's wake came a second generation of sportswear companies that achieved success in the 1980s, including Seattle Pacific Industries (Unionbay, Reunion), Generra (no longer headquartered in the Seattle area), and BUM Equipment (no longer headquartered in Seattle). Proximity to Asian contractors is an advantage for Seattle companies that source in that region of the world. With the inclusion of established sport and outdoor wear companies/retailers, such as Cutter and Buck, Tommy Bahama, Zumiez, Eddie Bauer (Bellevue, WA), and Recreational Equipment Incorporated (R.E.I.) in Kent, Washington, plus successful brick-and-mortar retailers such as Nordstrom, and e-retailers such as Amazon.com, Seattle has gained prominence in the fashion industry.

Over the past 20 years, Portland, Oregon has grown as a market center for activewear and outdoor gear. With the headquarters for Nike, Columbia Sportswear, and Adidas North America, Inc., it has attracted a variety of smaller sportswear and footwear companies including KEEN Footwear and LaCrosse Footwear, Inc. In addition, Portland is the home to the headquarters for other apparel companies including Pendleton Woolen Mills and Hanna Andersson.

OTHER U.S. MARKETS

A number of other U.S. cities, including Boston, Charlotte, Denver, Kansas City, and Minneapolis offer regional markets for apparel, accessories, home fashions, and furnishings. Regional trade associations and general merchandise marts often sponsor apparel market weeks relying on traveling sales representatives who set up temporary showrooms or booths. These markets cater to buyers within a fairly small region—primarily within a 250-mile radius of the mart. For these buyers, attending a regional market is much less costly and time consuming than traveling to a larger apparel mart or to NYC. In addition, even buyers who attend other markets may attend these regional markets to supplement their stock between major market weeks.

International Market Centers

Although the focus on this book is on the U.S. fashion industries, international market centers such as Paris, London, Milan, Rome, Tokyo, Hong Kong, Seoul, Taipei, Rio de Janeiro, Buenos Aires, and Sydney play important roles within the global fashion industries. These large cities are home to thriving fashion industries including design, marketing, production, and distribution/retail. Paris, London, and Milan have long histories as "fashion capitals" in Europe. Hong Kong and Tokyo reign as the fashion capitals of Asia, and Rio de Janeiro and Buenos Aires are important fashion market centers in South America. Trade shows in Europe (e.g., Premiere Vision) and Asia (e.g., Hong Kong Fashion Week, TITAS) attract attendees from around the world.

The Selling Function

The selling function of apparel and home fashions companies is handled in one of the following ways:

- internal selling for private label merchandise and store brands
- corporate selling
- sales representatives and showrooms

Most apparel companies rely on sales representatives to perform the selling function, but a few rely on internal selling and corporate selling.

Internal Selling

With private label merchandise (e.g., JCPenney's Arizona brand) and store brands (e.g., Gap), the selling of merchandise to the retail buyers is handled internally. This is because merchandise is designed and produced for a particular retailer (see Chapter 7 for a description of private label and store brand product development). With **internal selling**, the design team presents seasonal lines to merchandisers within the company who select specific pieces of the line for production. Merchandisers also determine which items of the line will be sold at specific stores.

Corporate Selling

Corporate selling is typically used by some companies that manufacture designer price zone merchandise and sell to a limited number of retailers. Corporate selling is also used by very large companies that sell moderately priced merchandise to large corporate retailers. In these cases, selling processes are often conducted through their corporate headquarters without the use of sales representatives or showrooms.

Sales Representatives and Showrooms

The **sales representative** or *sales rep* is the individual who serves as the intermediary between the apparel manufacturer and the retailer, selling the apparel line to retail buyers (see Figure 8.10). Other names for sales representatives are *vendor representative, account executive,* and *manufacturer's representative.* **Showrooms** are the rooms used by sales representatives to show samples of an apparel line to retail buyers. Depending on the size of the company, showrooms can be elaborately decorated or very simple in decor. They always include display racks for the apparel samples and tables and chairs for the retail buyers.

Showrooms can be either permanent or temporary. Permanent showrooms are located in buildings in NYC's fashion center, in apparel marts, in buildings adjacent to marts, or within a company's headquarters or production facilities. During market weeks, sales representatives for companies that do not have permanent showrooms in that area use temporary showrooms or booths. Booths are set up and staffed by either the company's sales representative or a multiline representative. Some sales reps always use temporary showroom or booth space during market weeks. Some companies will use temporary showroom or booth space to "test the water" in a new region during a market week without having to commit to a sales rep or the mart on a permanent basis. Al-

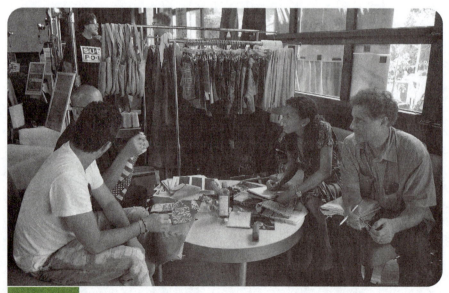

Figure 8.10 Sales representatives show seasonal lines to retail buyers.

though using temporary space can provide companies with a feel for the mart and the sales opportunities, there are also disadvantages. Because buyers are looking for long-term customer service from sales reps, they may seek assurance of continued service from reps who do not have a permanent showroom.

TYPES OF SALES REPS AND SHOWROOMS

One of the most important decisions made by apparel and home fashions marketers is whether to open an exclusive **corporate showroom** with company sales representatives or to use established independent **multiline sales representatives**. The primary difference between the two is that company sales reps work for a particular company and are housed in corporate showrooms owned by the company; independent multiline sales reps work for themselves and typically represent lines from several different, noncompeting but related, companies. For example, a multiline sales rep may offer a variety of noncompeting children's wear lines from several companies. In addition, this sales rep may also represent lines of children's toys and nursery accessories. Both company and multiline sales reps are assigned and work in a geographic territory (**regional sales territory**), which may be quite large (e.g., the West) or quite small (e.g., northern California), depending on the company and product line.

The main criteria used by an apparel company in deciding whether to use a corporate showroom or multiline sales rep are the type of product line and the amount of business the company expects to do. The corporate showroom is appropriate for a company with a large sales volume in a particular region of the country. For some marts, it is recommended that the company be capable of producing at least $1 million in sales at the mart in order to support a corporate showroom. Corporate showrooms are managed by company sales representatives who represent the lines of only that company. (It should be noted that because company sales reps generally represent large companies, most are based in a showroom.) Company sales reps may work on salary plus commission or on a straight commission basis, depending on the sales philosophy of the company. If the company pays the sales reps' expenses, which is often the case for company sales reps, then commission is lower than if expenses are not paid.

In addition to managing the showroom, company sales reps may travel to other marts' market weeks and trade shows. They may also visit retail accounts. Road travel is most typical for lines in the moderate price zone. For this type of merchandise, apparel manufacturers can often get sample lines (discussed in Chapter 7) to the sales rep prior to market weeks. This allows the sales reps to travel to accounts and sell outside of market weeks. Because of the costs associated with producing samples of designer and bridge lines, companies that produce these lines may only have one or two sets of sample lines per season. Thus, the sample line may travel from one city to another for their market weeks.

Corporate showrooms have advantages and disadvantages. With a corporate showroom, the staff can devote 100 percent of their time to the company's line(s) and the company's customers. In addition, the showroom can better portray the company's image and style of merchandise to retail buyers. However, a corporate showroom is an expensive investment. Space is leased from the mart; lease contracts should be evaluated in terms of services offered (e.g., janitorial services, utilities, mart-sponsored promotion activities, directory listings), as they can vary from mart to mart.

Rather than opening a corporate showroom, many companies choose to go with an independent multiline sales representative. Multiline sales representatives typically work for small manufacturers that cannot afford or do not want to hire their own sales representatives. The multiline sales rep works on straight commission, typically 5 to 10 percent of the wholesale price of goods that are shipped by the company. This means that if the company ships $100,000 (wholesale) in goods that are, in turn, sold by the sales rep, the sales rep would receive 5 to 10 percent of this amount ($5,000 to $10,000) as payment.

Independent multiline sales reps must pay all their own expenses, including the following:

- cost of leasing and furnishing showrooms (if they have them)
- travel expenses to market weeks or to visit retailers
- in some cases, the purchase of manufacturers' sample lines

For smaller companies, using an independent multiline sales representative can have several advantages. The main advantage is that no initial capital investment in the showroom is needed. In addition, established sales reps are familiar with local accounts and can promote the line with buyers. Although the initial costs of using an independent rep are less than with opening a corporate showroom, additional expenses to be expected include the following:

- fees for market week activities
- cooperative advertising expenses
- costs for hospitality service
- fashion shows

Some companies will begin with an independent multiline rep and then, as they grow, they will move into their own corporate showroom.

Finding the right fit between the product line and the sales representative is important to both the apparel company and the sales rep. Companies want to find a rep who has access to the types of retailers appropriate for the product line. Independent multiline sales reps should not represent competing lines. The company must be assured that the sales rep will spend the appropriate amount of time in promoting its line(s). Another consideration is whether the sales rep needs to travel to different retail accounts prior to market weeks. Table 8.2 compares the advantages and disadvantages of corporate showrooms and multiline sales representatives.

SAMPLE LINES

The manufacturer provides the sales representatives with a set of samples for the line(s) being presented to retail buyers. The samples include an example of each style included in the line in one colorway. The line catalog or brochure is used in conjunction with the samples to provide information about the line to the retail buyer. Some companies require the sales rep (usually independent multiline sales reps) to purchase the samples. In these cases, the sales reps are generally allowed to sell the samples at the end of the selling season. Other

Table 8.2 Comparisons between Corporate Showrooms and Multiline Sales Representatives

Type of Selling	Advantages for the Manufacturer	Disadvantages for the Manufacturer
Corporate showroom	Control over image of showroom possible	Capital investment necessary
	Staff can devote 100 percent of time to line	Lease agreements may vary from mart to mart
		In addition to commission, there may be other promotion expenses
Multiline sales representative	No initial capital investments needed	Determining right fit between sales rep and line may be difficult
	Established reps know local accounts	Rep may not devote adequate time to the line
	Buyers are exposed to related but noncompeting lines in the same showroom	Lack of control over image of the showroom

companies provide the samples to the sales rep (usually company sales reps). In these cases, the sales rep generally returns the samples at the end of the season. These companies may then allow employees to purchase samples at wholesale prices. Computer technology has made it possible for sales reps to use alternatives such as virtual samples and computer-generated buying instead of actually showing sample lines.

Virtual samples

As was mentioned in Chapter 6, the technology is in place to show a line with **virtual samples**, which are viewed on a computer screen. The intended fabric color and print of the style is shown, including fabric folds and shadows, so that it looks like a photograph of an actual prototype. However, nothing duplicates a buyer's ability to touch and feel samples of merchandise.

Computer-generated buying

Retail buyers and sales representatives can view the line and place orders without the manufacturer producing actual prototypes. Pieces of the line can be combined in a video presentation to show a variety of coordinating combinations. Video presentations can be customized for a specific customer.

An advantage of computer-generated buying is that key buyers can "forecast" the hot-selling styles. With design, development, and production software programs becoming more fully integrated, the time savings increase exponentially. The new style can be created by the designer on a three-dimensional CAD system, revised by the design team, shown to buyers (even in remote locations), and orders placed without the cost of developing a prototype.

Computer-generated buying systems that are part of an integrated computer-generated garment design, pattern, and material utilization system enhance the entire process of creating and marketing a new line. Linking the computer-aided design system to the computer-integrated manufacturing system provides the maximum cost efficiency, speed, accuracy, and quality. For example, it is possible to predict the efficiency of the fabric usage for a style and to revise the garment design with a more efficient fabric utilization without going through the patternmaking process. Chapters 9 and 11 discuss computer applications in the preproduction and production processes.

JOB FUNCTIONS OF THE SALES REPRESENTATIVE

The sales representative (whether a company sales rep or an independent multiline sales rep) performs a number of job functions, including selling activities, selling support activities, and nonselling activities. The most obvious of the functions that sales representatives perform are the selling functions. These include the following:

- showing lines to retail buyers and demonstrating product features
- negotiating terms of sale
- writing orders for merchandise

In negotiating the terms of sale, the sales representative and retail buyer focuses on several areas, including delivery date, cooperative advertising, and discounts (see the "Terms of Sale section," later in the chapter).

Order-writing software has reduced the amount of time that manufacturers' sales representatives spend on writing orders. Sales representatives use software systems whereby they can do the following:

- access up-to-date inventory information
- enter orders for next-day shipment
- analyze information from the order database

Sales representatives also perform a number of activities that support and expand the selling function, including the following:

- advising retail buyers regarding trends related to the target customer
- providing retailers with product and merchandising information
- training buyers and/or salespeople to promote and advertise the merchandise
- ordering and reordering merchandise for retailers to guarantee sufficient inventory
- dealing with complaints from retail customers regarding merchandise orders
- promoting customer relations

In addition, sales representatives perform many nonselling activities, including the following:

- making travel arrangements
- writing reports for the company
- keeping books of account
- attending sales meetings
- participating in market week activities, such as fashion shows
- managing and maintaining the showroom or trade booth (see Figure 8.11)

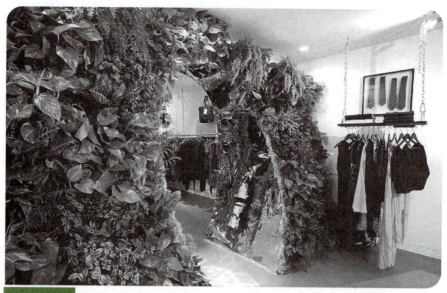

Figure 8.11 Temporary showrooms or booths are set up during market weeks as marketing tools to attract buyers and convey the company's image.

Although their career paths vary greatly, many sales representatives have retail buying experience before they become sales representatives. With this background, they understand the retail buying process and can address the needs of retail buyers.

Orders and Canceled Orders

The sales reps work with the retail buyers in placing orders for merchandise to be produced and delivered to the retailer. It is important to keep in mind that not every style in the line that is presented to buyers will be produced. Usually, only those styles that have a sufficient number of orders from retail buyers will be produced. Therefore, at the time the buyer places the order for a specific style, in specified colors and sizes, the order is tentative. Whether a specific style in a specific color will be produced is based on the cumulative orders from other retail buyers. The style will be produced only if the minimum number of orders for the style and color is achieved. The minimum number of items required to put a style into production is based on any of a number of factors. Sometimes a minimum order is based on the fabric manufacturer's minimum yardage requirement. Or the minimum order might be determined by the contractor who will sew the style. In some cases, a minimum of 300 units might be required, whereas with another company, the minimum order might be 3,000 units.

Thus, retail buyers place orders without knowing for certain whether every style they order in the preferred color will be produced. Orders can be canceled due to the following reasons:

- There are insufficient orders for a particular style or color.
- The fabric is not available from the textile manufacturer. The textile company will produce the fabric only if a sufficient number of yards have been ordered by various apparel companies to meet the textile manufacturer's minimum order. This creates a domino effect in these interrelated industries.
- A variety of production problems can occur, both with the textile manufacturer and with the apparel production facilities.
- Natural disasters and political crises in countries where the merchandise is being produced can make it impossible to meet retailers' orders.

When a retailer's order for a style cannot be filled by the apparel or home fashions manufacturer, the retailer may be willing to accept a substitute style or color. Or, the retailer may cancel the order, filling in any gaps in apparel style choices on the retail floor with merchandise from other companies.

Terms of Sale

A number of **terms of sale** are negotiated between the sales representative and retail buyer, including the following:

- delivery time for the goods to be delivered
- guarantees related to whether styles ordered will, in fact, be produced
- reorder capabilities and timing of the reorders (especially important for basic merchandise, such as jeans or hosiery, for which continuous inventory is essential to optimum sales)
- cooperative advertising allowances (will the manufacturer or retailer help pay for advertising?)
- discounts if bills are paid within a certain time period
- discounts if a certain quantity is purchased
- markdown allowances (is any credit given on goods that had to be marked down?)
- availability of promotion tools such as gift-with-purchase promotions or displays

As orders are placed by the retailer for styles in the new line, delivery dates and payment terms are arranged between the manufacturer and the retailer. If the manufacturer does not meet the delivery date, the manufacturer may be required to take a reduced payment for the shipment, or the retailer may be allowed to cancel the order. Late delivery may be the result of fabric arriving late from the textile mill, production delays with the contractor, or delays in transportation. With offshore production and the resulting time needed for communication and transportation, delays can be a problem. A manufacturer may have to pay the much greater cost of air shipment, instead of using sea transportation, to avoid a late penalty and the risk of losing the retailer's business.

The manufacturer needs to be aware of financial problems facing the retailer, especially in today's business environment of mergers, takeovers, and bankruptcies. For example, on the eve of a predicted announcement of bankruptcy by a major retailer, the management of a large apparel company faced the decision of whether to ship a large order to the retailer. If the retailer remained in business, the late shipment penalty would cost the apparel company substantially. However, if bankruptcy occurred, the apparel company would lose far more money by shipping the goods. These are difficult management decisions.

Marketing Strategies

Distribution Policies

The primary goal of a company's distribution policies is to make sure the merchandise is sold to stores that cater to the customers for whom the merchandise was designed and manufactured (the target customers). Thus, it is important for apparel and home fashions marketers to identify store characteristics and geographic areas that will optimize the availability of the merchandise to the target customers. For example, a manufacturer of designer price-zone men's suits may identify specialty stores in areas where residents have above-average incomes as its primary retail customers. A manufacturer of moderate-priced women's sportswear, on the other hand, may identify department stores as its primary retail customer. Once these basic criteria are established, apparel marketers must next decide on the company's policy regarding merchandise distribution. In general, there are two basic distribution policies: open-distribution policy and selected-distribution policy.

OPEN-DISTRIBUTION POLICY

With **open-distribution policy**, the manufacturer will sell to any retailer with whom they have satisfactory business experience and with whom they negotiate appropriate terms of sale.

SELECTED-DISTRIBUTION POLICY

With **selected-distribution policy**, manufacturers establish detailed criteria that stores must meet in order for them to carry the manufacturer's merchandise. Typically, the criteria focus on the following:

- expected sales volume
- geographic area
- retail image

For example, some manufacturers sell their merchandise to only one or two retailers within a certain geographic region; others sell only to retailers that portray an image that is consistent with the merchandise; others sell only to retail accounts that can purchase a specified amount of merchandise.

Based on these decisions, apparel and home fashions marketers focus on retail accounts that are consistent with their distribution policy. Distribution strategies are discussed further in Chapter 12.

International Marketing

As U.S. apparel and home fashions companies expand their businesses to include foreign markets, it is important to review the ways in which apparel is marketed internationally. There are four basic ways apparel and home fashions are marketed internationally:

1. *Selling through direct sales:* In some cases, U.S. manufacturers sell directly to foreign retailers through independent or company sales representatives.

2. *Selling through agents:* In some cases, U.S. manufacturers prefer to use international agents to handle the selling function in other countries. These agents have expertise in market demand, import/export issues, and international currency issues. Therefore, they can facilitate the establishment and processing of international accounts.

3. *Selling through exclusive distribution agreements:* In some cases, U.S. manufacturing companies have established agreements with specific international retailers for the exclusive distribution of their merchandise.

4. *Marketing through foreign licensees in a specific country or region:* In some cases, U.S. manufacturers license their lines to foreign companies. These licensing arrangements with foreign companies facilitate the marketing of the goods internationally.

Sales Promotion Strategies

Apparel and home fashions companies have essentially two groups of customers that need to know about their lines: retailers and consumers. Thus, sales promotion strategies developed by apparel and home fashions companies will focus on both of these groups. Apparel and home fashions companies use a number of promotion strategies to let retailers and consumers know about their merchandise. Decisions regarding promotion strategies are based on the following:

- company's advertising budget
- characteristics of its target customer
- characteristics of the product line
- area of distribution

Promotion strategies include advertising, publicity, and other promotion tools made available to retailers.

ADVERTISING

Through paid **advertising**, apparel and home fashions companies buy space or time in the print or broadcast media to promote their lines to retailers and consumers. Although some large companies may have in-house advertising departments, most companies hire advertising agencies to develop campaigns for them. Large companies that manufacture a brand name or designer merchandise (e.g., Nike, Ralph Lauren, Calvin Klein) can spend millions of dollars per year on advertising. Companies can also share the cost of the advertisement with a retailer, trade association, or another manufacturer through **cooperative advertising**, or **co-op advertising**. For example, a company and a retailer may share the cost of an advertisement that features both the merchandise and the retailer (see Figure 8.12).

The specific print, broadcast, or electronic media used in advertising campaigns depends upon the following:

- advertising budget
- target audience

- product line
- company image

For example, a company may rely on advertisements in trade publications such as *WWD* or *FN* when targeting retailers. When targeting consumers, designers such as Donna Karan or Calvin Klein may focus on slick print advertisements in fashion magazines; companies that manufacture national brand name merchandise (e.g., Levi's, Fruit of the Loom, or Nike) or store brands (e.g., Gap, Victoria's Secret) may use television ads to reach a wide audience.

PUBLICITY

Although the effect of positive publicity is the same as advertising (to promote lines to retailers and to consumers), unlike advertising, **publicity** is not controlled by the marketer. With publicity, the company or the company's line is viewed as "newsworthy" and thus receives coverage in print or electronic media or on television or radio. For example, media coverage of

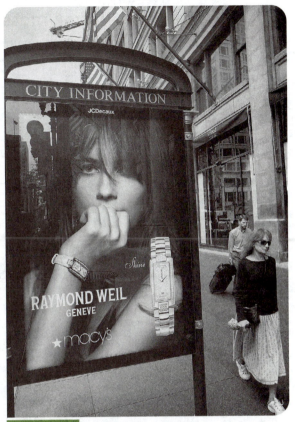

Figure 8.12 Cooperative advertisements are often used to connect a brand name with a retailer in the consumer's mind.

designers' runway shows often results in news stories and photographs or videos of the designers' collections in trade (e.g., *WWD*) or consumer newspapers, magazines, on television, or on the many fashion websites found on the Internet. Sometimes, the company will create news by sending out news releases about its company or lines. The primary advantage of publicity to the apparel or home fashions company is that the company does not have to pay the media source for communicating information about the company. In addition, consumers may respond positively to publicity that includes a third-party endorsement, since the endorsement may be perceived as more credible than a marketer-controlled advertisement. The primary disadvantage of publicity is that the company has little control over how the company or its merchandise will be portrayed.

OTHER PROMOTION TOOLS

A number of other tools are provided by apparel companies to promote their lines to retailers and to consumers:

- line catalogs or brochures
- media kits
- DVDs
- electronic communications
- social media websites
- direct mail

- visual merchandising tools
- trunk shows
- merchandise representatives
- style testing and participation promotions

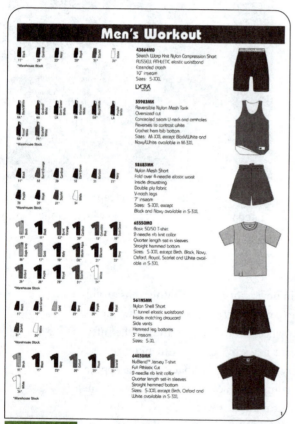

Figure 8.13 The line catalog, or line brochure, shows all of the styles, sizes, and colors available. Sales representatives and retail buyers use the line brochure to place orders.

Line catalogs or line brochures

Line catalogs or line brochures provide important information about the line to retail buyers (see Figure 8.13). They include photographs or drawings of the items in the line, along with style numbers, sizing information, colors (some may even include fabric swatches), and information regarding ordering procedures and guidelines.

Media kits

Photographs, media releases, television or radio spots, and other information are sometimes provided by manufacturers for publicity purposes or for retailers to use in advertisements.

DVDs

Manufacturers may provide DVDs for use by retailers in training their sales associates about the line or in promoting the line to consumers. For example, DVDs may be used to demonstrate visual displays, to demonstrate product usage, or to give fashion or styling information.

Electronic communications

A variety of communications technologies are used by apparel and home fashions manufacturers to promote goods to retailers, as well as to the ultimate consumer. Some companies use websites with virtual showrooms where retail buyers can "walk" through the showroom to view new seasonal lines. Other companies use private networks called *extranets* to communicate with their manufacturing and retail partners. Benefits include the ease of communication and simplification of order tracking. A number of companies use Web-based systems whereby retail buyers can place orders for merchandise online. Manufacturers and retailers have found the following advantages of these business-to-business (B2B) Web technologies (see Figure 8.14):

- No appointments are necessary.
- Paperwork is reduced.
- Because buyers need an ID and password to log on, security issues are resolved.

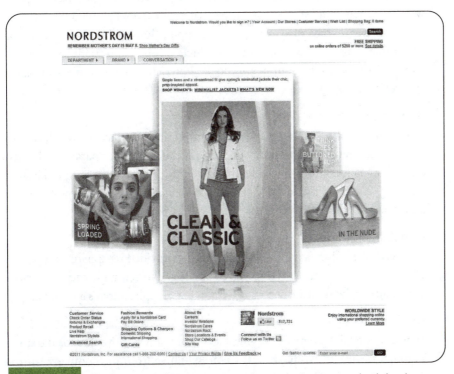

Figure 8.14   Websites are effective means of communications to both business clients and ultimate consumers.

Many companies also have websites designed as online stores for consumers to purchase goods (see additional discussion of e-commerce in Chapter 12). Indeed, some companies rely solely on online retail distribution. Over the past five years, technological advancements in website design have resulted in company websites that include increased abilities for consumers to visualize products, consumer blogs, customization of online shopping experiences, and consumer reviews.

Social media websites

Many companies also have social media websites such as Facebook, Twitter, or LinkedIn sites to create **brand communities** through advertising, sharing product information, providing promotional incentives and discounts to consumers, and providing opportunities for consumers to interact with each other and with company representatives. For example, according to *Apparel Magazine's* Top 50 Companies in Social Media approaches, as of July 2010, Victoria's Secret was ranked first with almost 4,750,000 "friends" on Facebook. Nike, American Eagle, and Abercrombie & Fitch each had approximately 1,300,000 Facebook friends. At that same time, Urban Outfitters and American Apparel were ranked first and second for Twitter with approximately 180,000 followers each. Companies have also expanded into applications or "apps" for Facebook sites and mobile phones to promote products through entertainment. For example, Target's application on Facebook allows customers to mix and match apparel items sold at Target.

Direct mail

Although e-mail and other electronic communications have grown in popularity, direct mail opportunities still exist. As a form of cooperative advertising, some manufacturers provide promotion inserts included with retail store mailings (e.g., credit card bills). Some companies also send out postcards or other mailings directly to consumers.

Visual merchandising tools

A variety of visual merchandising tools may be provided by apparel companies. These can range from providing posters and signs to setting up actual in-store shops and supplying all the necessary fixtures (e.g., Ralph Lauren's in-store shops).

Trunk shows

Typically, a retail buyer will not purchase a company's entire line for the store. Through the use of **trunk shows**, a representative from the company (or the designer himself or herself) will bring the entire line (or part of a line) to a store. Customers invited to attend the showing can purchase or order any piece in the line, whether or not it will be carried by the store (see Figure 8.15).

Designers often make appearances at their trunk shows to promote their collections. Trunk shows can benefit manufacturers, retailers, and consumers in the following ways:

- Manufacturers use trunk shows not only to promote their lines, but also to get consumers' reactions to their merchandise.

- For retailers, trunk shows provide an opportunity to offer an exclusive service to their customers. They also provide feedback from their customers about their tastes and preferences.

- Customers benefit because they have access to the full line of merchandise. "For shoppers who love fashion and want the luxury of reviewing and trying on a designer's entire collection in an uncrowded setting, but don't mind waiting a couple of months for their goods to arrive, trunk shows are a good bet" (Agins, 2001, p. B1).

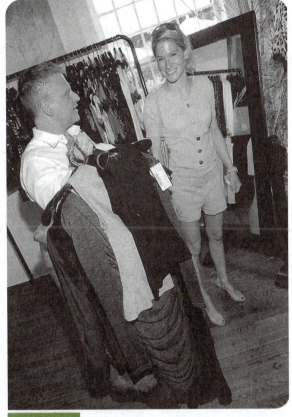

Figure 8.15 Trunk shows, such as this one for Dolce and Gabbana, are used to promote collections to prospective customers.

Merchandise representatives

Some companies use *specialists, merchandisers,* or *sales executives,* who are paid either partly by the apparel company and partly by the retailer or entirely by the apparel company, but who work in the retail store(s). These individuals may be based in one store or may travel to various stores within a region. Their role is to do the following:

- educate the retail sales staff and consumers about the merchandise
- demonstrate display procedures
- assist retailers in maintaining appropriate stock
- get feedback from the retailers and consumers for the apparel company

Style testing and participation promotions

Active sportswear companies often ask retail executives and athletes to test styles in a line or participate in sports activities as a way of promoting the line to retailers and ultimate consumers. For example, Columbia Sportswear invited selected retailers, sales reps, and skiers to test a new performance-oriented outerwear line on the slopes of Oregon's Mount Hood. The retailers could learn about the product, and Columbia Sportswear could hear suggestions from both retailers and ultimate consumers. Nike has invited retailers to go golfing, and Patagonia has sponsored kayaking trips for retailers. REI Adventures offers hiking, bicycling, backpacking, rafting, and climbing trips as a means of providing experiential opportunities for current and potential customers.

Summary

The marketing of apparel and home fashions products connects market research with the appropriate strategies for getting the right product to the target consumers at the right time, at the right price, and in the right place. Markets for apparel lines can be any city where apparel marts and showrooms are located. Large market centers such as New York City, Los Angeles, Dallas, Chicago, and Atlanta, are important to the manufacturing and retailing industries. All U.S. market centers except New York City have an apparel or merchandise mart that houses showrooms and exhibition halls used during market weeks. Marts and regional markets can also be found in a number of other cities throughout the United States. In New York City, showrooms are located in buildings throughout the fashion center in midtown Manhattan. During specific times of the year, known as *market weeks*, buyers visit apparel and home fashions markets to purchase merchandise for their stores. They may also attend trade shows sponsored by apparel marts or trade associations.

The selling function of apparel and home fashions companies is handled either through corporate selling or through sales representatives who work out of permanent or temporary showrooms. Sales representatives serve as liaisons between manufacturers and retailers. Some sales representatives work from a corporate showroom and focus on the line(s) of one company; others are multiline sales reps, representing a number of related but noncompeting lines. The job of sales representatives includes both selling and nonselling functions.

Apparel and home fashions marketers develop distribution and promotion strategies for their company. In general, there are two basic distribution policies: open distribution and selected distribution. These policies help determine which retail customers will be the focus of selling efforts. Sales promotion strategies of apparel and home fashions companies are directed to both retail customers and consumers. Strategies may include advertising, publicity, and other promotion tools.

The marketing of apparel and home fashions has career opportunities for individuals who manage apparel or merchandise marts, organize market weeks and trade shows, and serve as sales representatives, as well as those who perform promotion work such as advertising and public relations. For these careers, an understanding of the marketing process, product knowledge, creativity, organizational skills, analytical skills, and negotiation skills are important.

Field Sales Representative
Privately Owned Designer Hosiery Company

Position Description:
Sell basic stock and seasonal merchandise to the hosiery buyers for major department stores and specialty stores within a specific region; service the accounts that carry the merchandise within the sales territory.

Typical Tasks and Responsibilities:

- Prepare six-month merchandise plans in retail and cost dollars.
- Write orders.
- Obtain buyers' approvals for orders.
- Visit store accounts.
- Talk to sales associates about the merchandise.
- Entertain buyers and divisional merchandise managers.
- Make sure goods are shipped as planned.
- Keep in close contact with buyers and report on the status of orders.
- Plan and help with store promotions.
- Analyze sales using spreadsheets with sell-through and stock-to-sales ratios and stock turns for each stock-keeping unit by store.
- Plan model stocks (13-week supply) based on sales analysis (basic stock fill-in orders or automatic reorders are based on model stock plans).
- Hire and supervise merchandisers who also visit store accounts and conduct inventories.

CAREER PROFILES

Key Terms

advertising

brand community

co-op advertising

cooperative advertising

corporate selling

corporate showroom

internal selling

market

market center

market week

mart

multiline sales representative

open-distribution policy

open-to-buy

publicity

regional sales territory

retail relations program

sales representative

selected-distribution policy

showroom

terms of sale

trunk show

virtual sample

Discussion Questions and Activities

1. Interview a retail buyer in your community. Document the type of retailer (e.g., specialty store, department store) and the type of merchandise offered (e.g., children's wear, menswear). Ask which markets or trade shows the buyer attends and why. Compare your findings with those of your class-mates. Are there any patterns in market attendance related to geographic area, type of retailer, or type of merchandise?

2. Find two examples of co-op print advertisements in either a trade publica-tion, consumer publication, or online. What companies and/or associations joined forces for each advertisement? What are the advantages and disad-vantages for the companies in using co-op ads as part of their promotion strategy?

3. Locate the website of an apparel manufacturer/retailer. What type of infor-mation is provided on the site? Would this information be useful to retail-ers, to the target customer, or to both? Does the manufacturer also have social media sites? If so, how are they used? Evaluate the site's effectiveness.

References

Agins, Teri, (2001, February 5). Trunk show chic. *The Wall Street Journal*, pp. B1, B4.

AmericasMart (2010). AmericasMart—Atlanta Retrieved October 4, 2010, from http://www.americasmart.com

California Market Center (2010). California Market Center Retrieved October 4, 2010, from http:// www.californiamarketcenter.com

Dallas Market Center (2010). Dallas Market Center Retrieved October 4, 2010, from http://www.dallasmarketcenter.com

Design Trust for Public Space (2009). Made in Midtown Project Retrieved October 4, 2010, from http://www.designtrust.org/projects/project_09garment.html

The Fashion Center Business Improvement Center (2010) Retrieved October 4, 2010, from http://www.fashioncenter.com

Otis Report on the Creative Economy of the Los Angeles Region (2009) Retrieved October 3, 2010, from http://www.otis.edu/about/presidents_messages/creative_economy.html

PART 3

Apparel Production and Distribution

CHAPTER 9

Preproduction
Processes

In this chapter, you will learn the following:

- the role of financial agencies, called factors, in the apparel industry

- the process and timing used by apparel companies to order production fabrics and trims

- scheduling and management considerations in ordering production fabrics and trims

- the processes used to finalize a production pattern, grade the pattern, create a production marker, and to cut, spread, and bundle the fabric pieces

- ways in which grade rules, size range, styling, cost considerations, and grading processes influence pattern grading

- uses of new and related technologies in preproduction processes

Step 5: Preproduction

Step 1 Research and Merchandising

Step 2 Design

Step 3 Design Development and Style Selection

Step 4 Marketing the Apparel Line

Step 5 Preproduction

Order Production Fabrics, Trims, and Findings

Finalize Production Pattern and Written Documents

Grade Production Pattern into Size Range

Make Production Marker

Inspect Fabric

Spread, Cut, Bundle, and Manage Dye Lots for Production

Step 6 Sourcing

Step 7 Apparel Production Processes, Material Management, and Quality Assurance

Step 8 Distribution and Retailing

Production Orders

*T*he sales force has shown the new line to retailers during market week, and the retail buyers have placed their orders with the apparel or home fashions company. As discussed in Chapters 7 and 8, those styles in specific colors and sizes that meet the company's required minimum order will continue in the development process. Usually, styles that do not attain the minimum number of orders will be dropped from the line. Sometimes after a week or two of selling the line, a manufacturer will decide to drop a style that is not selling well. Let us imagine that, for the style we are following through the development process, a sufficient number of orders has been placed to warrant a production run (see Step 5 of the flowchart on the previous page).

Factoring

A company's financial credit line is an important consideration prior to the approval of any business transactions or approval of work orders. Therefore, apparel manufacturers, contractors, and retailers need to establish a credit line or cash advance so they can buy materials in advance of the season in which payment will be received.

Because of the nature of retailing fashion products, there is a high level of financial risk in the textile and apparel industries. Commercial banks are used by some textile and apparel businesses for their financial backing. However, their interest rates may be high, and some commercial banks are not willing to accept the degree of risk involved with fashion-related companies. Therefore, another type of financial agency called a **factor** is often used. **Factoring** is "the business of purchasing and collecting accounts receivable or of advancing cash on the basis of accounts receivable" (Young, 1996, p. 1). As an example, the factoring agency advances (loans) money to the apparel company so that the apparel company can pay the textile mill for the fabric that has been delivered. The loan allows the apparel company to pay for fabrics well in advance of the date that the apparel company receives its payment for the new styles that the retailer has purchased from the apparel company.

Factoring agencies are the companies that provide protection against bad debt losses, manage accounts receivable, and provide credit analysis in the apparel industry. The factor's procedures include the following:

- running a credit check on the company
- approving a credit line to the company
- approving the orders for shipping to the company
- receiving the invoices from the company's suppliers
- advancing the cash needed to pay the invoices to the company

The company pays interest on the money advanced until the company can repay the factor. Usually, a 60-day or 90-day payment period has been arranged between the factor and the company. The length of the time period is determined by the length of time the company usually waits to be paid by its customers. For example, based on the terms of agreement, the textile producer might need to wait 90 days after shipping the fabric to the apparel manufacturer to receive payment for the fabric. The factor's fees are similar to the interest paid on credit card debt. For example, a large apparel manufacturer might be charged the prime rate plus 1 percent of the value of each invoice.

Factoring has changed over the last decade. In the past, the textile mills that sold to apparel manufacturers were the major part of the factor's client base. As manufacturing moved overseas, the importer/manufacturer became the client and the retailer the client's customer. Harold Dundish (2009), Senior Vice president for IDB Factors, states that "the biggest concern among factors today is their customer base—the retailers." In the 1990's, large retailers were bought by venture capital firms and cash flow was good. However by 2009, there are large credit exposures by the consolidated retailers and factors are charging a premium for certain high risk retail customers (Dundish, 2009).

Small apparel companies often do not qualify for financial backing by a factor because their sales volume is lower than the factor's minimum. Therefore, such companies go to refactor agencies. Refactors are factors that give their credit, collection, and check-processing functions to larger, full-service factors and concentrate on acquiring new clients and businesses.

Before production can begin, the financial arrangements must be approved by the company's factoring firm or other lending institution. Examples of the credit checks that are done include the following:

- The textile producer checks the apparel manufacturer's credit before shipping fabric to the manufacturer.

- The manufacturer checks the contractor's credit before shipping fabric or cut goods to the contractor.
- The contractor may check the manufacturer's credit before deciding to accept the order.
- The manufacturer checks the retailer's credit before shipping finished goods to the retailer.
- The retailer may check the manufacturer's credit before deciding to place an order.

Keep in mind that the apparel manufacturer has paid the textile producer for the fabric and the contractor for the labor many months before the manufacturer is paid for the goods by the retailer. Some type of lending institution is used by all of these participants. After approval of credit, production can proceed. Some manufacturers will decide to take an account on their own without the factor's approval. For example, a manufacturer may decide to sell to a new retail account, such as a specialty store that has just opened and has not yet established credit. In this situation, the manufacturer carries the financial risk that the specialty store will pay the manufacturer for the merchandise delivered to the store.

Now that sufficient orders have been placed and the retailers' credit standings have been approved, the style is ready for the next step in development: preproduction.

Product Data (or Development) Management and Product Lifecycle Management

Some of the advantages of using computer systems such as PDM/PLM throughout the development process or throughout the lifecycle of a new style are discussed in previous chapters. Software provides seamless integration among all of these segments of a new style's development process (see Figure 9.1). A drawing created by the designer on a graphics program can be integrated into the garment specification sheet (spec sheet) used by design development, preproduction, and production personnel. Data from the garment specification sheet can be integrated with the bill of materials and other forms needed for production.

The first pattern created by the patternmaker using a pattern design system (PDS) is used for the production pattern. The PDS base pattern used for the new style can include the measurement dimensions and sizing standards (grade rules) coded into the base pattern, providing integration between design development and preproduction. In addition, some software programs

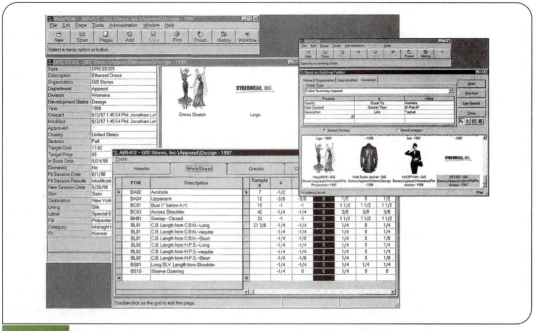

Figure 9.1 A PLM system, such as GalleryWeb software, enables a system server to provide authorized access to style information anywhere in the world by means of electronic communication.

are integrated so that a change on one form triggers that change to be made on all other forms in the database system. For example, changing the zipper length on a garment spec sheet will trigger a change on the bill of materials, the form used to order the zippers. While this system has many advantages, it can also mean that a mistake will be transmitted throughout the system, too.

Companies rely more and more on computer system integration, both internally (within the company) and externally (outside the company). Maintaining accurate and up-to-the-minute information about each style and every change in each style during design development in the line will increase the speed of work flow and increase accuracy within the system for all company personnel who need access to the data.

In his article "The Three Stages of Retail PLM Adoption," Rubman (2010) states that retailers who connect not only their internal product development with sourcing functions, but also include their external suppliers into their PLM systems will generate bigger reductions in costs and time and increase product quality and innovation. Providing electronic access to style information to external contacts, such as vendors and contractors, speeds information exchange and increases accuracy as well. Garment specifications can be shared instantly with contractors who intend to bid on production jobs. Web technology provides global exchange of product specifications and other pertinent information within companies and throughout contractor networks.

Cut Orders

A production **cut order** is issued in either of the following two situations:

- when a targeted number of orders for a style has been placed by retailers and received by the manufacturer
- when the apparel manufacturer decides to produce a style prior to receiving orders

The cut order specifies the number of items in each color and each size that will be included in the production run. A cut order for a specific style might include cutting fewer small sizes and more large sizes and may contain a mix of colors for each size. For example, a cut order for Style XXYY might include 80 items of size 6 divided into 24 of color A, 24 of color B, 16 of color C, and 16 of color D; 160 items of size 8 of the same style divided into 40 of color A, 60 of color B, 40 of color C, and 20 of color D; and so forth. The cut order includes the date when the goods must be delivered to each retailer. Thus, the production schedule is calculated from end to beginning—that is, backward from the retailer's delivery date, to the date when production of the goods must be finished, to the date production must begin, to the date when the fabrics, trims, and findings must be ordered.

Ordering Production Fabrics, Trims, and Findings

In an ideal situation, the apparel company would be able to wait until the majority of retail buyers had placed their orders before ordering the needed quantity of fabrics from the textile producers (a production run of one style might require 6,000 yards of fabric), as well as ordering the trims and findings for each style in the new line. Such a situation would eliminate any financial risk that would result from ordering fabric that might turn out not to be needed. If apparel companies were to wait to order fabrics until they knew exactly how much of each fabric in their lines would be needed, they would have to wait weeks for the fabrics to arrive from the textile producers.

If textile producers, not wanting to risk manufacturing excess fabric, were also to wait until the apparel companies had ordered fabric before beginning to produce the yardage to fill the manufacturers' orders, the apparel company would have to wait even longer, perhaps months, for the production yardage to be manufactured and delivered to the sewing facility. Producing the apparel goods would probably take several more weeks. As you can imagine, these cumulative delays would be so lengthy that the retailers would not receive the goods at the peak selling time. Thus, the apparel company is positioned between the textile producer and the retailer, with pressures from both sides. As one observer described it:

> In the middle of the supply chain, set against conflicting priorities, are apparel manufacturers. On one side are the retailers who ask for a variety of garments by size and color variation, delivered frequently in small lots, just in time for merchandising. On the other side, there are fabric mills that want to produce long runs and require advance commitments from manufacturers. (Gaffney, 1999, pp. 74–75)

Timing of Cut Orders

In reality, few apparel companies can afford to wait until all, or nearly all, of the buyers' orders are placed before ordering production fabric for the line. Therefore, apparel companies use a variety of means to determine how much yardage to order and when to order the yardage from the textile producers. Furthermore, some companies begin production on some styles before the buyers' orders have been received. This helps maintain an even work flow during production. These methods include the following:

- early production of proven sellers in basic colors
- the use of preline selling
- the use of early-season lines to predict sales
- the use of test markets
- the use of past sales figures

Some companies will project production estimates of some of the more "staple" styles and colors, especially if these are carryovers from a previous season. Some colors are known to sell especially well. For example, skiwear manufacturers know that black ski pants tend to sell well every year. Therefore, they may decide to begin early production on several styles of "proven sellers" in this basic color. Early production also allows the company to maintain a constant production flow in order to avoid times when the factories are overcommitted.

Preline selling is discussed in Chapter 7. Some apparel companies invite key retail accounts to place orders prior to market weeks. Early production of these styles can be advantageous to both retailers and apparel companies. Swimwear companies might use an early-season line to help predict which styles will sell well. An early January line of swimsuits sold at resorts in Florida could be used to help forecast production of the Spring line to be introduced to northern climates in April. Some of the hot-selling styles from Florida retail sales could be put into production for the main selling season before the line is sold at market to retailers in the rest of the country.

Sometimes a specific region is targeted as a test market, in which a small production run of the new line will be placed in key stores. Occasionally, an apparel company has its own test store(s), in which early sales help forecast production quantities. Levi Strauss & Co. also uses some of its stores as test markets for new styles. This "provides some sort of sell-through background [in order to give the retailers] some sort of data on whether it's a valuable new style" (DesMarteau, 2003, p. 35).

Past sales figures and the opinions of leading sales representatives and leading retail buyers might be used to determine which styles and colors might go into early production. For styles that are carryovers, production might be started prior to buyers' orders since management is fairly certain these styles will sell well.

Selection of Vendors

Using as much information as possible as early as possible, production yardage, trims, and findings are ordered from the various **vendors** (or **sources** or **suppliers**) of textiles, trims, and findings. Many variables influence the selection of vendors, including the following:

- lead time needed to secure the goods
- past history of on-time delivery
- the quality of goods
- whether the vendor uses supply chain management strategies
- the minimum yardage (or quantity) requirement for an order
- the financial stability of the vendor

Some manufacturers will ask for bids from several vendors as part of the decision-making process Software programs are available that provide cost comparisons based on inputting variables such as material costs from different vendors. Clearly, the selection of fabric and trim vendors is based on many important considerations. Sourcing is discussed in more detail in Chapter 10.

Production Fabric Considerations

During the process of planning production fabric orders, constant communication occurs between the apparel company and the fabric vendors. Vigilance is required to ensure that the production fabric matches the fabric used for the samples. Some of the fabric considerations include color control, lab dips, and strike offs (see Figure 9.2). Various requirements are also important considerations when ordering printed fabrics, staple fabrics, and trims and findings.

PREPRODUCTION COLOR MANAGEMENT

During preproduction processes, the apparel company needs to finalize a number of aspects regarding the fabrics that will be ordered for the new line. Chapter 7 discusses some of the aspects of color management; for example, one requirement is that all components of the prototype accurately match the intended color for the new style.

As discussed in Chapter 7, staff in the design development department might be responsible for working with the textile, trims, and findings vendors to develop and maintain exact color matching of all components of each style and to ensure that all products in the entire production run maintain the specified color match. Color management may begin at the prototype stage if a textile is to be dyed to match a color chip or swatch provided by the apparel company. If available, the specially dyed sample goods are used to make the prototype. Trim, findings, sample yardage, and production yardage will be ordered to match the prototype color.

It is important to the consumer, and thus to the retailer and the apparel company, that colors remain consistent throughout all the components that are used to make a garment style. First, the color of the garment style needs to match the color intended by the design team. This could require that the fabric vendor submit test samples until the "perfect" color is achieved. The trims and findings, such as buttons, zippers, and thread, must also match the garment color. If the color of the rib knit used for the sleeve band of a rugby shirt is not the same shade as the body of the shirt, the consumer will quite likely decide not to purchase the garment. Thus, when contractors supply the trims and findings for the products they make, it is important that they receive approval of the color match from the apparel company. An acceptable color match for contractor-provided matched goods is referred to as a **commercial match**.

STRIKE OFF/LAB DIP APPROVAL FORM

TO: KATHY SIMSES

CC: J. LEIBY, D. RAINEY, G. HUNTER, PRODUCT TECHS, PATTERNMAKERS, A. BEYMER

PATTERN NAME: URBAN LUAU

COLOR CODE: S31 OLIVE

PATTERN NUMBER: 35323-C

STYLES: Y2109, Y2020

VENDOR: A.G.X

SEASON: CRUISE 2011

PRINTED ON: COTTON SHEETING

SECTION: MAY COMPANY

APPROVAL A. BEYMER 8/17/10

COMMENTS: APPROVED PENDING PSO. SAND NEEDS TO BE A LITTLE
                 DARKER AND LESS RED—MATCH SWATCH TO ATTACHED.

Figure 9.2 Fabric color and design must be approved before the textile print is produced in large quantities.

When producing coordinated items in a line, color management can be a challenge. A fabric composed of one fiber might be selected for pants, and a fabric composed of another fiber or blend of fibers might be selected for the top. For example, rayon crepe pants might be planned to match a silk jersey tank. However, the color of the pants may not look like an exact color match to the tank because of the different reflective qualities of the fibers and fabrics. As another example of color management concerns, adjacent colors in plaid and print fabrics tend to affect their neighboring colors' hue, value, and intensity. Because of this optical effect, a color in a print or plaid may not look like it matches its solid-colored coordinate, even though when viewed by itself the color in the plaid or print does match the color standard. Thus, much time can be spent on perfecting the colors in a line.

LAB DIP

To ensure that color matching will be as perfect as possible, the vendor will supply a sample of the product (such as fabric, rib knit trim, or buttons) in the color requested (the apparel company might supply a fabric swatch or paint chip to the vendor that needs to be color matched). The sample the vendor supplies to the apparel company is called a lab dip because, in most cases, the fabric swatch (or trim or finding) was dipped in a specifically prepared dye bath in the "lab" to dye the sample. Vendors submit lab dips (called submits) for all the individual components required in a line. Since various blends of fabrics and other materials absorb dyestuffs differently, accurate color matching of all components may require multiple attempts by vendors.

The Lilly Pulitzer company is known for its easily identified colors and fabric prints. As explained by its vice president of production:

> Color matching is so important to us, but the sewing, as well as the fabric and trim dyeing processes take place in so many countries—including Peru, Columbia, Hong Kong, China, the Philippines, Turkey, Portugal, the United States, and Vietnam—that it requires a long timetable to ensure the lab dips from all these locations can be approved in one place and then compared. (Speer, 2004, p. 23)

Apparel companies usually have equipment to view colors to assess their match accuracy under controlled lighting conditions. Various lighting conditions can be simulated, such as daylight, fluorescent lighting, and incandescent lighting. The fabrics under consideration are placed into a cabinet and observed under controlled lighting conditions to assess the color accuracy.

The manufacturer may require that the vendor submit results of textile tests, such as color fastness and light fastness, performed by approved textile testing laboratories for each sample. These testing procedures are especially important for certain fabrics, such as nylon fabrics in neon bright colors. Each fabric, trim, and finding that is to match the line's color choice will require approval on a form supplied by the apparel company.

The approval process requires time and accurate record keeping. According to the vice president of production for Lilly Pulitzer, "it takes four to six weeks to complete two rounds of lab dip evaluations, and it requires two to four rounds to achieve approval. At the high end, that can mean an eight-to-twelve week color approval cycle" (Speer, 2004, p. 23). Therefore, if time can be saved in the lab dip approval process, the cycle time for style development can be shortened, thus resulting in a cost savings to the apparel company.

Enhanced computer software programs have decreased the time devoted to the color development and management processes. Datacolor's ENVISION software is one example. It includes "onscreen product simulations to eliminate the transportation of physical samples" (Cole, 2005, p. 22). Some of the software programs provide digital color communication via e-mail or the Web. Users can communicate digital color standards (for example, using the Pantone color system), send and receive color submissions, and keep records of color approvals. New computer technology can "see" beyond the human eye's color vision. The science of numeral spectral curves can be used for color management. The use of uniform digital standards allows global partners to communicate color standards electronically.

PRINTED FABRIC CONSIDERATIONS

Not all printed fabrics are printed by the textile mills that produce the fabrics. Sometimes the fabric is printed by a textile converter to the specific textile design requested by the apparel manufacturer (see Chapters 3, 6, and 7). Thus, many apparel companies work with textile converters as well as textile mills. The fabric might be purchased from the textile mill and then sent to a textile converter to print before it arrives at the cutting facility. For apparel companies that use textile converters, careful scheduling is required to ensure that the printed fabric is ready on time. Custom print fabrics require substantial lead time for orders; therefore, decisions about custom prints occur early in the design/production process. As mentioned in Chapter 6, some apparel companies create some or all of their textile designs in-house. This also requires careful planning for lead time, as well as the considerations discussed above.

New developments in digital printing have helped advance this technology into becoming a viable production option. Improvements in dyes and printing have overcome some of the earlier challenges of this technology. Digital printing provides for one-of-a-kind, exclusive items and is increasingly being evaluated to support customization scenarios and niche market opportunities. "Linking detail printing to the cut-and-sew process is the next step toward full integration into the sewn-product supply chain" (King, Garland, Pagan, Nienke, 2009, p. 33)

STRIKE OFF

A strike off is a fabric sample that is printed by the textile converter—the company printing the fabric (see Figure 9.3). Chapter 6 discusses strike offs in relation to samples of textile prints submitted by textile converters. Usually, a strike off consists of no more than a few yards of fabric. It shows the rendition of the textile print made from the artwork submitted to the textile converter by the apparel company (or textile company that develops the print). The strike off is examined carefully by the apparel company before approval is given to print production yardage. For screen prints composed of more than one color, each color requires a separate screen. The placement of each of the screens must be exact or the print will appear blurred. The accuracy of placement, or **registration**, of each of the color screens is checked (see Figure 9.4). The color match of each screened color is compared to color chips or fabric swatches submitted to the textile converter. The accuracy of the pattern repeat match is checked. Sometimes it is necessary for several strike offs to be made by the textile converter before approval is given.

STAPLE FABRIC ORDERS

Some staple fabrics, such as linings and interfacings, and some fashion goods, such as cotton poplin and cotton broadcloth and wool crepe and wool jersey in staple colors or piece dyed textiles, can be purchased closer to production (late-cycle ordering). Textile producers incorporate online technology using several automated sourcing services. The apparel manufacturer can view and order textiles using custom searches.

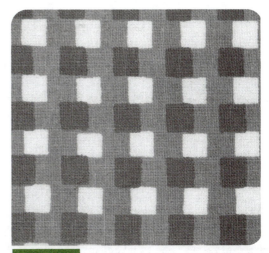

Figure 9.3 A strike off is a sample of the fabric provided by the textile vendor and sent to the apparel company for approval before the textile print is produced in large quantity.

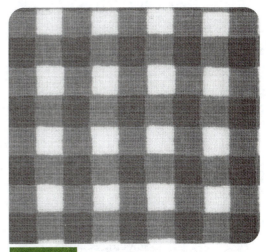

Figure 9.4 The strike off is sent from the textile mill or converter to the apparel manufacturer for approval. Sometimes it takes several attempts to gain approval.

In Figure 9.3, the strike off has poor registration—the screen printing of the two colors was not properly aligned. In Figure 9.4, the approved strike off has perfect registration.

For goods already produced and awaiting shipment at the textile producer, online sourcing is a viable option because it allows late-cycle ordering, which has advantages for the apparel manufacturer.

TRIMS AND FINDINGS

It may be necessary to order special trims very early in the planning process. For example, elastic for a waistband might be ordered in a three-color stripe to match the print colors used for pants. On the other hand, elastic in a standard width and color might be ordered just in time for production. Findings such as snaps, hooks, zippers, and thread tend to be kept in stock in large quantities at the production facility. Sometimes a new fashion color requires ordering thread or other findings that are not in stock. Thus, careful planning needs to take place to ensure that all the needed trims and findings are available for production at the appropriate time.

Decisions about findings, such as specifying the type of thread, may be more complex than one might imagine. Some of the issues to consider for thread selection include the following:

- capability of thread type to match fabric characteristics
- type of stitch or machine used for the operation
- wash procedures to be used
- degradation that will occur during washing

Thus, the selection process for findings may involve research and testing of some products in order to ensure a quality finished garment.

Pattern Finalization and Written Documents

The pattern for the style that has been approved for production needs to be finalized. Every detail needs to be perfect for production to run smoothly. Sometimes, minor pattern adjustments need to be made to improve ease of production. The production pattern, which has been made in the company's sample size, is then ready for **grading**; that is, each individual piece of the pattern in the sample size is remade in each of the sizes specified. Next, all the pattern pieces in all the sizes are arranged into a master cutting plan, called a **production marker**. The style is ready to move to the next stage, the production cutting and sewing operations. Each of these steps is discussed in more detail.

Finalizing the Production Pattern

A specialist called a **production engineer** or pattern engineer may be part of the team that is responsible for preparing the pattern for production. Production engineers are familiar with factory production processes and types of equipment. The pattern may need some minor changes to facilitate production. The production engineer is responsible for suggesting such changes in the pattern. He or she might also be responsible for suggesting the specific factory where production can best be accomplished.

All markings for factory production must be perfect, including the following:

- notches to ensure accurate matching of one piece to its mate
- drill holes to indicate dart tips (actually, the drill holes are marked at a specified distance from the dart tip to avoid creating a weakness in the fabric at the dart tip)
- placement for pockets or other details

One forgotten notch marking can cause production problems, especially since this notch marking will be missing on the pattern piece for the entire size range after the pattern has been graded. If the first pattern has been made on a computer pattern design system, any changes in the pattern needed at the preproduction stage can be accomplished very quickly because the pattern is already in the computer system (see Chapter 7).

Finalizing the Garment Specification Sheet

At the time the designer's sketch or drape of the style is delivered to design development, a garment specification sheet accompanies the design (see Chapter 7). The spec sheet lists all fabrics, trims, findings, and important construction details, such as logo placement, label type and placement, and color and weight of top-stitching thread (see Figure 9.5). Any changes that may have occurred during the development of the style must be transferred to the garment spec sheet. Any requested change not transferred to the spec sheet can cause difficulties in production. If a PDM/PLM software system is used to create and maintain the spec sheet, all changes can be made very easily as soon as they have been approved and will automatically be changed on any other necessary documents. Some computer systems include bilingual and multilingual flexibility, which is especially helpful when working with offshore sources.

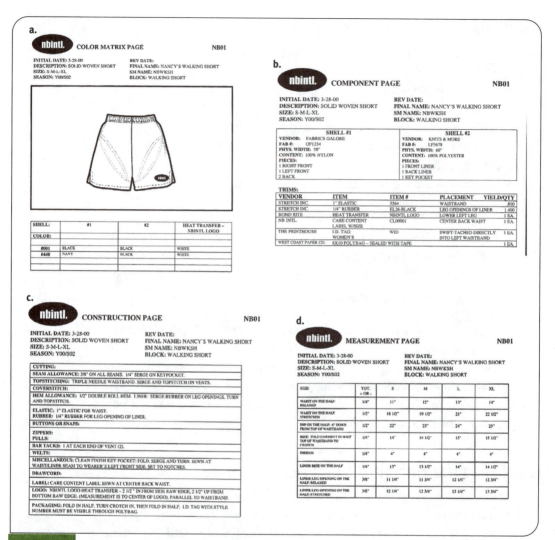

Figure 9.5 (a) The garment specification or spec sheet includes important information for producing the style, including the color matrix. (b) Fabric, trim, and findings are specified on the component page of the garment spec sheet. (c) This page of the garment spec sheet details construction-related instructions. (d) The measurement page details finished garment dimensions and allowable tolerances.

Another component of the garment specifications is the bill of materials (see Figure 9.6). It lists the fabrics, trims, and findings requirements for each color of a style in the line.

```
CUSTOM/BILST1        3/28/00  15 00 03    Style Bill Of Material       *** STANDARD COST ***                        PAGE   1
                                                                                          SEA-Y YR-00 Style- NB01
CO- 01                                DIV-01                           B-O-M TYPE-S SELLING Style  B-O-M
SEA-Y YR-00 Style-NB01        NANCY'S WALKING SHORT                    PRICE-       15.00     U/M-U          B-O-M U/M-U
Clr              Dim      SIZE   M PROCESS      Opt      PLANT    PART  LAST B-O-M MAINT. 3/28/00 STATUS-  OWNING DIV-
* C O M P O N E N T *     **** O P T I O N S ****                      ******** C U R R E N T /  S T A N D A R D ********
S   C                       Style *** ** MANUF. ***                   CURR/STD  CURR/STD   CURR/STD   CURR/STD  STD COST OWN
  SEA T NUMBER    Clr     SX Clr     Dim SIZE PR Opt  PL PA            PRICE UM  CONV FACT  QUANTITY UM      COST VARIANCE DIV S
                         1  FOR DEMONSTRATION PURPOSES ONLY - DATA IS FICTITIOUS
   D   A LF5678    001                                                 2.5000 YD            .3000 YD   .7500               01
       LINER FABRIC $5678                                              2.5000 YD  1.0000    .3000 YD   .7500
                  BLACK                                                                STD  3/28/00 LMT  0/00/00

   D   A OF1234    001     001                                         2.8000 YD            .4000 YD  1.1200               01
       OUTER FABRIC $1234                                              3.0000 YD  1.0000    .4000 YD  1.2000     .0800
                  BLACK                                                                STD  3/28/00 LMT  3/28/00

   D   A OF1234    440     440                                         2.9000 YD            .4000 YD  1.1600               01
       OUTER FABRIC $1234                                              3.0000 YD  1.0000    .4000 YD  1.2000     .0400
                  NAVY                                                                 STD  3/28/00 LMT  3/28/00

   D   E 1/4"ELASTC 001                                                2.0000 YD           1.4000 YD  2.8000               01
       1/4" ELASTIC FOR LINER                                         2.0000 YD  1.0000   1.4000 YD  2.8000
                  BLACK                                                                STD  3/28/00 LMT  0/00/00

   D   E 1"ELASTIC  100                                                2.0000 YD            .8000 YD  1.6000               01
       1" ELASTIC FOR WAIST                                          2.0000 YD  1.0000    .8000 YD  1.6000
                  WHITE                                                                STD  3/28/00 LMT  3/28/00

   D   H HTNBINTL   100                                                 .0500 EA           1.0000 EA   .0500               01
       HEAT TRANSFER NBINTL                                            .0500 EA  1.0000   1.0000 EA   .0500
                  WHITE                                                                STD  3/28/00 LMT  0/00/00

   D   T 8X10PB                                                         .0300 EA           1.0000 EA   .0300               01
       8 X 10 POLYBAG                                                  .0300 EA  1.0000   1.0000 EA   .0300
                                                                                      STD  3/28/00 LMT  3/28/00

   D   W CL00001                                                        .0500 EA           1.0000 EA   .0500               01
       CARE LABEL $1                                                   .0500 EA  1.0000   1.0000 EA   .0500
                                                                                      STD  3/28/00 LMT  3/28/00

   D   X WOMENSID                                                       .1000 EA           1.0000 EA   .1000               01
       WOMEN'S ID TAG WID                                             .1000 EA  1.0000   1.0000 EA   .1000
                                                                                      STD  3/28/00 LMT  0/00/00

GL$ C DESCRIPTION ******       PART PROC PLNT  Opt    ***** VARIABLE ******   ******* FIXED *******
                                             PCT      AMOUNT     PCT     AMOUNT
  00050 MFLAM LABOR COST CMT                           2.5000                        -CUR-    3/28/00
                                                       2.5000                        -STD-    3/28/00
        S02 CUT/MAKE/TRIM DEVO QUICK COST
  00051 MOOT  OTHER INVENTORY                           .2000                        -CUR-    3/28/00
                                                        .2000                        -STD-    3/28/00
        OVERHEAD ALLOWANCE

              * * * * * * * *  Style BILL-OF-MATERIAL COST SUMMARY * * * * * * * * * *
  Style    Clr
```

Figure 9.6 The bill of materials is used to order and track all components. Some garment styles require an extensive number of fabrics and trims.

Construction Specifications

Included with the written documentation that accompanies the style will be additional construction specifications related to the production sequence (see Figure 9.7). The production engineer or product technician often determines the sequence of steps (what will be sewn first, second, third, and so forth) required for factory production of the style. When the style is made in a factory owned by the apparel company, the production engineer is an employee of the apparel company. When the style is made by a contractor, the contractor's production engineer determines the production sequence. The sequence of production is related to the cost to manufacture the goods. Thus, the production sequence may have been determined at the time the final cost was calculated, as discussed in Chapter 7.

A GUIDE TO SEWING BLUE JEANS

Union Special

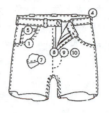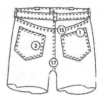

Sequence Of Operations For Traditional Blue Jeans

	OPERATION NUMBER	OPERATION	RECOMMENDED MACHINE STYLE	STITCH & SEAM TYPE
PRELIMINARY				
✔	1	Hem top of hip and watch pockets	56500R18 or FS311L51-2H72	401 EFb-2(inv.)
✔	2	Decorative stitch hip pockets	56500R18 or FS311L51-2H72	401 OSa-2
	3	Precrease hip and watch pockets	Pocket Creaser	
✔	4	Make belt loops	FS321J01-2A60Z	406 EFh-1
✔	5	Attach facings to front pockets	FS311L41-2H64CC1Z3	602 LSbj-1(mod.)
	6	Set watch pocket to right front facing	Juki LH2178	301 LSd-2
	7	Bag pockets	Juki MO3716	516 SSa-2
✔	8	Serge left and right fly pieces	39500CRU	504 EFd-1
✔	9	Attach zipper tape (continuous) to left fly piece	56400PZ16	401 SSa-2
✔	10	Attach zipper tape to right fly piece	56300G or FS311S01-1M	401 SSa-1
FRONTS & BACKS				
	11	Set left fly piece and edgestitch	Juki DLN5410	301 SSe-2
	12	Topstitch left fly	Juki LH2178	301 EFa-2 (inv.)
	13	Set right fly piece and cord fly	Juki DLN5410	301 LSq-2b
	14	Hang front pockets	Juki LH2178	301 LSd-2
✔	15	Attach risers to backs	FS315L63-3H36CC2PA1	401 LSc-3
	16	Set hip pockets to backs	Juki LH2178	301 LSd-2
✔	17	Join backs (seat seam)	FS315L63-3H36CC2PA1	401 LSc-3

✔ *(Union Special machine available)*

Figure 9.7 Union Special, an industrial sewing machine producer, distributes this guide, which illustrates a typical production sequence to manufacture jeans.

Experienced production engineers can examine a finished sample garment and quickly provide a reliable estimate of the number of minutes—and thus, the actual labor cost—required to sew a specific style. One of the reasons production engineers are often included in the development design team (see Chapter

7) is that their engineering and costing experience is highly valuable as a factor in style decisions. Computer software programs can be used to help analyze cost in comparing various production sequence options.

Measurement Specifications

The actual measurements at specific locations on the finished goods for each size specified for the style will be listed on the **measurement specification** chart. Measurement specs are part of the garment specifications. For example, for a jacket style, measurement specifications for each size to be produced would be recorded in chart form and might include the following:

- chest circumference
- waist circumference
- jacket hem circumference
- back length from neck to hem
- neck circumference
- sleeve length
- sleeve lower edge circumference

Since garments are measured flat, sometimes the circumferences are measured across just the front width or just the back width. These half-circumference measurements are listed as the *sweep*. This dimensional information is important to maintain accurate sizes, especially if several factories will be used to produce the same style for a large production order. Two jackets in the same style and size may fit differently if one factory is less accurate in sewing than another.

Some computer pattern design systems include a feature that allows the patternmaker to request the dimensions at specific points on the pattern. When this is the case, the patternmaker completes the measurement specifications on a separate computer screen during the patternmaking process. This saves considerable time in comparison to measuring each of the specified locations on the pattern pieces by hand. The software can provide the measurement specs in metric measurements as well as imperial (inches), since many offshore contractors use the metric system.

The measurement specifications also include a **tolerance**, usually listed as "+/−" a certain fraction of an inch that indicates a narrow range of acceptable dimension variations (see Figure 9.8). This means that a stated dimension on the measurement specifications may vary by the stated tolerance amount. The tolerance amount might be 1/2 inch (1.3 cm) for larger circumferences (such as the chest) or lengths (such as back length), and 1/4 inch (6 mm) for smaller circumferences (such as the neck). The stated dimensions, with allowable tolerance, serve as a contract between the apparel company and the sewing facility. If dimensional accuracy is not maintained within the tolerance range, the goods can be rejected by the apparel company.

The apparel company's quality assurance department is usually responsible for checking the finished dimensions of the delivered goods. Since it would be too time consuming to measure the specified dimensions of every garment in a production order, a sampling technique is used to measure a specified number of garments in specific sizes. If goods sewn by a contractor must be rejected due to size inaccuracy, the apparel company may miss the deadline for delivery of goods to the retailer. Therefore, it is important for apparel companies to select carefully the contractors with whom they do business, and it is critical for contractors to carefully adhere to the garment specifications.

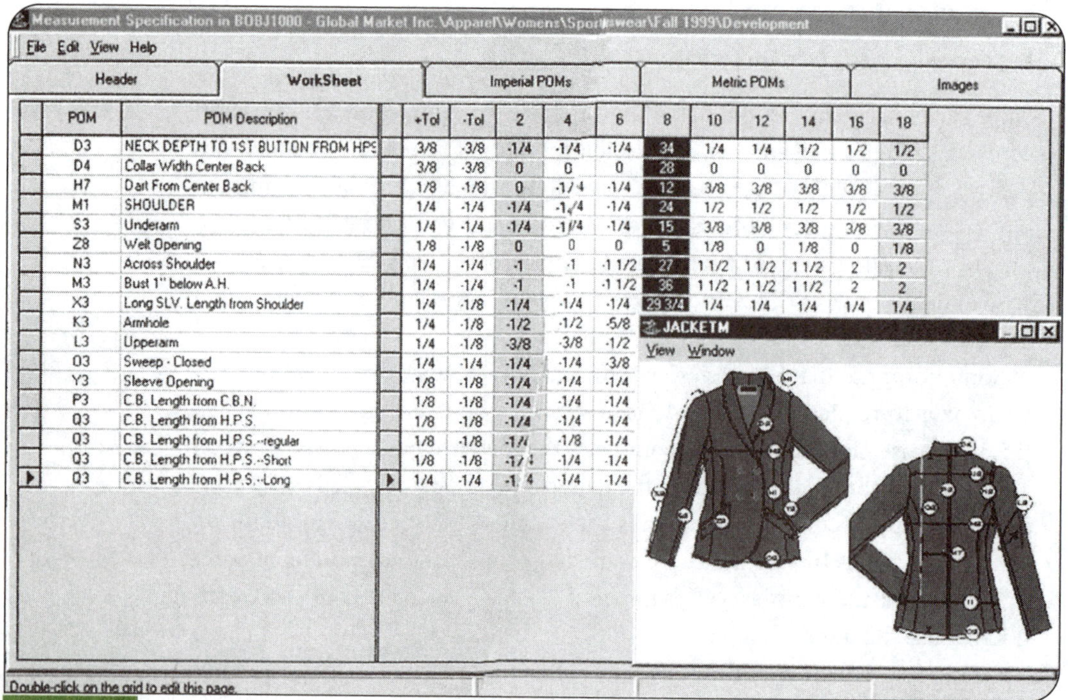

Measurement Specification in BOBJ1000 - Global Market Inc. \Apparel\Womens\Sportswear\Fall 1999\Development

File   Edit   View   Help

| Header | WorkSheet | Imperial POMs | Metric POMs | Images |

POM	POM Description	+Tol	-Tol	2	4	6	8	10	12	14	16	18
D3	NECK DEPTH TO 1ST BUTTON FROM HPS	3/8	-3/8	-1/4	-1/4	-1/4	34	1/4	1/4	1/2	1/2	1/2
D4	Collar Width Center Back	3/8	-3/8	0	0	0	28	0	0	0	0	0
H7	Dart From Center Back	1/8	-1/8	0	-1/4	-1/4	12	3/8	3/8	3/8	3/8	3/8
M1	SHOULDER	1/4	-1/4	-1/4	-1/4	-1/4	24	1/2	1/2	1/2	1/2	1/2
S3	Underarm	1/4	-1/4	-1/4	-1/4	-1/4	15	3/8	3/8	3/8	3/8	3/8
Z8	Welt Opening	1/8	-1/8	0	0	0	5	1/8	0	1/8	0	1/8
N3	Across Shoulder	1/4	-1/4	-1	-1	-1 1/2	27	1 1/2	1 1/2	1 1/2	2	2
M3	Bust 1" below A.H.	1/4	-1/4	-1	-1	-1 1/2	36	1 1/2	1 1/2	1 1/2	2	2
X3	Long SLV. Length from Shoulder	1/4	-1/8	-1/4	-1/4	-1/4	29 3/4	1/4	1/4	1/4	1/4	1/4
K3	Armhole	1/4	-1/8	-1/2	-1/2	-5/8						
L3	Upperarm	1/4	-1/8	-3/8	-3/8	-1/2						
O3	Sweep - Closed	1/4	-1/4	-1/4	-1/4	-3/8						
Y3	Sleeve Opening	1/8	-1/8	-1/4	-1/4	-1/4						
P3	C.B. Length from C.B.N.	1/8	-1/8	-1/4	-1/4	-1/4						
Q3	C.B. Length from H.P.S.	1/8	-1/8	-1/4	-1/4	-1/4						
Q3	C.B. Length from H.P.S.--regular	1/8	-1/8	-1/4	-1/8	-1/4						
Q3	C.B. Length from H.P.S.--Short	1/8	-1/8	-1/4	-1/4	-1/4						
Q3	C.B. Length from H.P.S.--Long	1/4	-1/4	-1/4	-1/4	-1/4						

JACKETM

View   Window

Double-click on the grid to edit this page.

Figure 9.8 The measurement specifications include the tolerances allowed at each specified garment location.

Grading the Production Pattern

Pattern grading involves taking the production pattern pieces that have been made in the sample size for the new style and creating a set of pattern pieces for each of the sizes listed on the garment spec sheet. Grading a garment pattern is much cheaper than developing a sample garment of each size. Therefore grading is a cost factor and does not assure the fit of the other sizes.

The written documents and production pattern are delivered to the pattern grading and marker making department if the apparel company is responsible for the grading and marker making operations. As mentioned in Chapter 7, when contractors are used for production, they will be responsible for one of the following scenarios:

- making the first pattern and production pattern, grading and making the marker, cutting and sewing (full-package contractor)

- making the production pattern (based on a first pattern developed by the apparel company), grading and making the marker, cutting and sewing

- grading and making the marker (based on a production pattern developed by the apparel company), cutting and sewing

- cutting and sewing (termed "CMT" for cut, make, and trim) only (based on a marker delivered by the apparel company). The fabric may be supplied by the apparel company, or it may be supplied by the contractor.

Chapter 10 discusses sourcing options in detail.

Some apparel companies that use contractors prefer to take responsibility for grading and marker making. For example, there are incentives in the U.S. trade laws for apparel companies that use offshore contractors located in specific countries. The trade laws require that U.S.-produced fabrics be used and that the garment pieces be cut in the United States. The cut pieces are then sent offshore for production.

Sending cut goods to the contractor minimizes the risk to the apparel company of grading and marker errors that could develop at the contractor's facility and ensures that the contractor is not responsible for any errors in pattern grading or marker making. However, if anything is not correct on the pattern or marker that the apparel company has provided, the contractor can blame the manufacturer for a late delivery or other related problems. For the manufacturer who provides the marker, maintaining an even work flow in the grading and marker making department is difficult, especially when the time frame for producing a season's line—determining that a style will be produced and having the marker ready for cutting—is very tight. Some contractors that have well-established partnerships with apparel companies communicate data such as patterns, markers, and garment specifications electronically. Although the contractor's initial investment in technology is high, the speed and accuracy provided may pay off quickly.

Grade Rules

Grading requires different amounts of growth (for a larger size) or reduction (for a smaller size) at various points on each pattern piece. Thus, it is not possible to place a pattern piece into a photocopy machine and enlarge or reduce the pattern piece uniformly. The amounts and locations of growth/reduction are called the **grade rules**. There is no industry standard for these grade rules, and some companies guard their grade rule standards carefully. The grade rule itself is the combination of a specific length and width that the pattern pieces need to increase or decrease at a specified point on the pattern. For example, the shoulder-neck point may need to increase for each subsequent larger size or decrease for each subsequent smaller size by ⅛ inch in height and 1/16 inch in width for each pattern size.

Pattern grading is more complex than it may appear. There are different grade rules for garments with set-in sleeves, raglan sleeves, kimono sleeves, and shirt sleeves. Style variations magnify the complexity of the different grade rules. For example, a raglan sleeve shirt could also include a front panel, so the grade rules would need to be modified for the extra style line added to the shirt front. Also, some companies use different grade rules for various sizes: for sizes 4, 6, and 8, a 1-inch width change increment per size may be used for the waist and hip dimensions; for sizes 10, 12, and 14, a 1½-inch width change increment per size may be used for the waist and hip dimensions; and for sizes 16, 18, and 20, a 2-inch width change increment per size may be used for the waist and hip dimensions.

Size Range and Style Cost Considerations

Depending on the style and the apparel company's policy, the size range might include a large number of sizes—for example, from size 4 to size 18 for a misses dress. Another apparel company might produce garments in a size range of small, medium, large, and extra large (designated S-M-L-XL). The cost to grade a pattern with many pattern pieces into a wide range of sizes may be more than the cost to grade a pattern with only a few pattern pieces in just four sizes. These cost differences are considered from the design stage onward. Another cost variation related to styling concerns designs that are asymmetrical—that is, different pattern pieces are required for the left and right halves of the body. An asymmetrical design might also require different left and right facing and interfacing patterns. Each separate pattern piece needs to be graded, multiplied by the number of sizes in the size range. Thus, asymmetrical designs can be more costly to grade if using noncomputer grading technology. For computerized grading, one can very quickly apply the same grade rules to a front facing pattern as was used for the front pattern.

The fabric selected may influence the size range in which the style will be produced. Some fabrics will look best in a narrow size range. Based on the scale of a plaid size and repeat, a plaid pleated skirt in misses sizes may look attractive only in certain mid-sizes—for example, sizes 8 through 16. It would be ideal to select a fabric that looks good in a wide size range, but this is not always possible. Some styles look best in certain sizes. Thus, the style may be offered in a limited size range.

Grading Processes

The pattern grading process can be accomplished by a variety of methods, and there are several approaches to these methods. Computer grading, combined with computer marker making, has gained widespread acceptance. It is the method of choice for apparel companies and contractors that can invest in a computer grading and marker making system. Other processes include hand grading and machine grading.

HAND GRADING

The hand grading process requires a ruler, pencil, and paper as the minimum tools. Using the production pattern pieces for the new style, the pattern grader (person grading the pattern) traces a copy of the pattern piece by moving the pattern piece the distance designated by the grade rules at specific points. Some hand graders use special grading rulers or graph paper as aids to grading. Most hand graders will develop a nested grade of the sizes so pattern shapes, such as armholes, can be maintained.

MACHINE GRADING

Pattern grading machines are used by some companies (see Figure 9.9). The grading machine is equipped with two dials—one for width increase/decrease, and the other for length increase/decrease. The pattern piece to be graded is clamped into or taped to the grading machine and paper is laid beneath. The pattern is traced in sequence by moving the dials on the grading machine to correspond to the grade rules at designated points on the pattern piece.

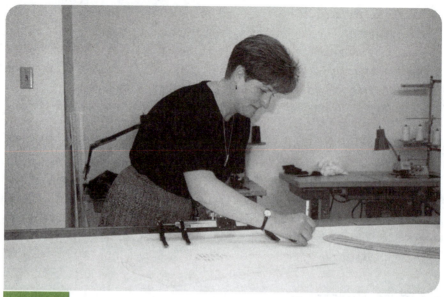

Figure 9.9 Some pattern graders use a grading machine to grade patterns into the entire size range.

COMPUTER GRADING

Computer grading is much faster than either hand or machine grading methods. Computer programs for pattern grading and marker making have been in use since the 1970s. The combined process is called **computer grading and marker making (CGMM)**. Companies that utilize computer systems to grade and make markers may refer to the department as the computer grading and marker making department. Many large apparel companies began their shift to computerization and formed CGMM departments early on. Computer use in patternmaking and design areas developed more recently. Although the investment in hardware, software, and employee training is substantial, the cost savings are quickly evident for companies that have a substantial quantity of work.

For companies that use a computer pattern design system for the production pattern, the pattern is ready for computer grading. Some companies, however, converted to computer grading before they began to use computers to make the patterns. For these companies, it is necessary to input the production pattern pieces into the computer before grading can be done. The process of inputting a pattern piece into the computer can be done by tracing the pattern piece or by scanning the piece. To trace a pattern piece, a table called a **digitizer** (also called a digitizing table) is used. The digitizer is sensitized at very small increments in both vertical and horizontal directions. These correspond to the *x* and *y* coordinates displayed on the computer monitor. The pattern piece is laid in place on the digitizer and traced using a handheld cursor (see Figure 9.10). The traced pattern piece appears on the computer monitor. During the tracing process, the pattern grader uses a keypad on the cursor to input the specific grade points and grade rules at the desired locations.

 GERBERdesigner™

Pattern Input - Digitizer

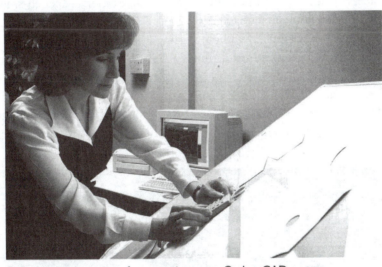

Easy, accurate inputting of patterns into your Gerber CAD system

You can quickly and efficiently input pattern pieces into your AccuMark™ system in several ways: through Silhouette 2000™, Pattern Design 2000™, or by digitizing. The digitizer workstation consists of a digitizing table with menu, and a cursor. The digitizer allows you to enter information that describes a pattern piece.

Using a predefined grade rule table as a reference, an entire range of sizes can be graded from a single base size pattern during digitizing.

Here are some of the types of information you can enter into the system:
• Grading information and data
• Piece outline and internals, such as stripe and plaid lines, and drill locations
• Piece identification
• Notch type and location, up to five different kinds per piece
• Piece labels and special point information, such as instructions for the GERBERcutter® system

You can use special digitizing techniques for a variety of pattern requirements, such as nested, copied, or mirrored pieces. All of the information entered into the digitizer is directly stored in the AccuMark system, where it is then ready for pattern modification and the marker making process.

⑤ GERBER TECHNOLOGY

Figure 9.10 A digitizer is used to input pattern pieces directly into a CAD system if the pattern was not made using a computer system.

Scanning equipment can be used to input the pattern piece information, including piece perimeters, grade points, and notches. Stripe lines, used to match pattern motifs on the fabric, and grainlines can be read from the pattern. The scanner will reorient a pattern piece as it is scanned if the pattern piece enters the scanner askew. Patterns can be scanned from a traced drawing, from a tagboard pattern, or from a plastic pattern piece.

The computer grading system not only calculates the graded dimensions for the entire size range, but it also develops smooth necklines, armholes, waistlines, and other curves. Each pattern piece can be viewed on the monitor as a "nest," with all of its sizes nested together (see Figure 9.11). This helps the grader decide if a grade rule is incorrect or a curve is not adequately smoothed. By using the horizontal and vertical coordinates for a specific point, corrections can be made quickly without starting over.

Some PDS programs include the option to select a grading function as the pattern is being made. These systems are integrated so that the pattern blocks used to begin making the style have specific grade rules "embedded" in them. Once the pattern has been completed, the grading is completed automatically. With the use of PDS, the operator can distribute the new measurements to all

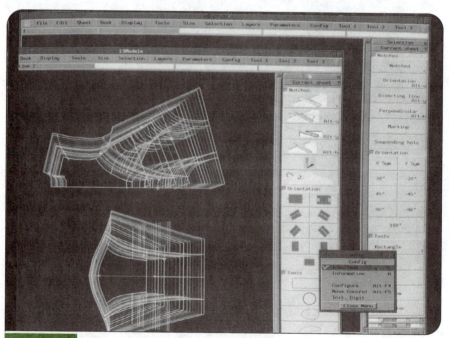

Figure 9.11   The computer screen shows a nested grade of the entire size range for this dress pattern piece.

affected pieces automatically without having to manually choose each pattern piece to be graded. For example, when a measurement change is made on the front shirt piece, the program automatically modifies the measurements of the opposite front, side, and back pieces, which will save patternmakers substantial time and effort (Figure 9.12).

Making the Production Marker

A costing marker, used to calculate the usage (yardage) required for one garment, is discussed in Chapter 7. At the preproduction stage, another type of marker is required. The production marker is the full-size cutting layout of all the pattern pieces for all the sizes specified for the style. The marker is drawn on paper, showing the outline of all the pattern pieces. Arranging all the pattern pieces into an efficient layout can be a challenge. The goal for the marker is a tightly arranged layout so that very little fabric is wasted. The waste, called **fallout**, represents fabric that cannot be used, and thus money lost to the apparel company. The efficiency of a marker's layout plan (marker efficiency) is measured in the percentage of fabric utilized. Thus, a high-utilization percentage represents a cost-effective marker. Highly efficient markers attain utilization with percentile figures in the high 80s and into the 90s (90 percent utilization means that there is about 10 percent fallout).

If a pattern for a style requires 10 pattern pieces, and 7 sizes are produced, the marker will include 70 pattern pieces. Sometimes, a marker is planned so that the layout will have two sets of pattern pieces in the most frequently purchased sizes—often those in the mid-size range. Therefore, the marker for a misses style could have two sets of sizes 10 and 12, for a total of 90 pattern pieces for the marker with 10 pattern pieces. For styles offered in the S-M-L-XL size range, it is fairly common to cut one set each of size S and size XL pattern pieces, and two sets each of size M and size L pattern pieces (or, one set of size S and two sets each of size M, L, and XL, especially in men's athletic wear). The cut order specifies the sizes and number of size sets in each of these sizes needed for the marker (as well as the colorway by size if various colors of fabrics will be stacked up for the cut order).

Marker Making by Hand

Prior to the development of computerized marker making, markers were typically made by hand. The layout is planned on a long sheet of paper (for example, 30 feet long), that is the width of the fabric to be cut. The tagboard pattern pieces are shifted into the tightest arrangement possible. The outlines of all the pattern pieces are traced by hand onto the paper beneath. Typically, the marker paper is of double thickness. The paper can be carbonless or have carbon between the layers, so that a copy of the original marker is made at the same time. Thus, after the original marker has been cut up, a reference copy remains. This copy can be traced again if another production order for the same style is received. If a similar style is produced later, the marker maker can refer to the file of markers to help guide the layout plan for the new style. After the pattern pieces have been traced, they are removed. The marker is laid onto the stacked layers of fabric. The cutter, using an industrial cutting knife, follows the drawn outlines of the pattern piece on the marker.

Other Marker Making Methods

Some apparel companies and contractors continue to make markers by hand. Other methods were developed years ago to increase the speed and efficiency of marker making. These methods include the following:

- the use of miniaturization of pattern pieces to create the marker in small scale, combined with enlargement photography to produce a full-size marker
- the use of light-sensitive paper in which the paper areas covered by the tagboard pattern pieces remain white, while exposed areas of the light-sensitive paper darken to show the silhouette of pattern pieces
- the use of water-soluble dye sprayed over the pattern pieces while they lie on the fabric, leaving the fabric uncolored in the areas covered by the pattern pieces

Computer Marker Making

While various marker-making methods are in use in today's industry, computer marker making is the most efficient and effective method. With CGMM, the marker-making function is tied to the pattern-grading function. Thus, a company that grades by computer also makes markers by computer. The CGMM system is purchased as a package, including the plotter that draws the marker. Once the pattern pieces have been graded by computer and stored in the computer's memory, the marker maker can retrieve all the pattern pieces needed in the size range. The fabric width is displayed on the monitor, along with markings for stripes, plaids, or prints that need to be matched, if applicable. With the use of the mouse, each pattern piece is moved one by one into the fabric area designated on the computer monitor, creating the layout plan. The computer is programmed to keep all pattern pieces aligned "on grain," to avoid skewing pattern pieces. Accidental overlapping of pattern pieces is avoided because the pattern piece blinks as a signal to the marker maker if one piece overlaps another, or the pattern piece cannot be set down if it would overlap another pattern piece. The marker making software calculates the usage, or fabric utilization, so the marker maker can continue to arrange pattern pieces until the utilization goal has been reached. After

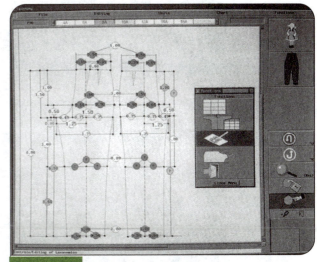

Figure 9.12 Some computer programs provide tools to allow faster grading processes and measurements of pattern dimensions.

the marker is completed, the system generates a letter-size printout of the layout. The small-scale marker can be analyzed for utilization and accuracy. It can also be used for reference during preproduction and production.

ADVANTAGES OF COMPUTER MARKER MAKING

As discussed earlier, the marker program calculates the fabric utilization, and this figure appears as a percentage on the monitor (see Figure 9.13). This helps the marker maker attain the highest utilization. Some manufacturers have estimated that the cost savings in better fabric utilization have paid for the computer equipment in less than two years. According to a study conducted at Clemson Apparel Research (Hill, 1994), a computer system used for grading and marking will result in a 2 percent fabric savings per year, quickly paying for the cost of the system for large manufacturers.

To save time, a marker from a previous similar style stored in the computer system might be studied by the marker maker to provide some guidance for creating a high-utilization marker on the first attempt. Some of the current marker software includes functions that will generate several possible marker layouts. Constraints such as plaid or stripe repeats can be accommodated by the software.

Multiple copies of the marker can be plotted whenever they are needed.

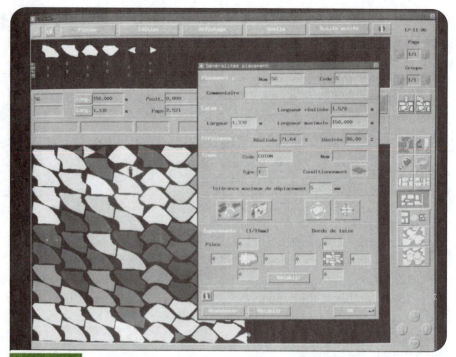

Figure 9.13 A production marker is displayed on the computer screen, showing the tight layout on the left and the utilization percentage on the right.

Accuracy is extremely high with CGMM, as each copy is exactly the same as the original. No accidental growth occurs as can happen when hand tracing markers.

Some companies that began their computerization with CGMM systems have integrated CGMM with other stages in design, development, and production using PDM/PLM software, as discussed earlier. Production integration is covered in Chapter 11. Complete integration of computer systems throughout the entire process provides advantages to all parties in the fiber-textile-apparel-retail supply chain.

As the cost of some CGMM systems decreases and their user friendliness increases, more companies are purchasing these systems. Some systems are in a price range affordable to small apparel companies. Other small companies might use the CGMM service of a larger company. Many contractors in foreign production centers as well as in the United States have CGMM equipment. As discussed in Chapter 7, the apparel company's PDS can be linked electronically to the contractor's CGMM system. This saves time and increases accuracy.

Fabric Inspection

The preproduction steps include ordering production fabrics and trims. A part of this process involves approving fabric and trim colors and the quality of components (discussed earlier in this chapter). Samples are submitted by suppliers and approved by the apparel company. It is assumed by the apparel company that the production fabrics and trims will accurately match the samples submitted and used for the production of the sample garments. As noted earlier, this is called a commercial match. The production fabrics are inspected to ensure that they match the samples.

The retailer's orders are written based on the materials, trims, and construction quality seen in the sample garment. If the quality or color match of any part of the production goods is inferior, the retailer may reject an entire order. Fabric inspection can be the responsibility of the apparel company or the textile producer.

Fabric Inspection by the Apparel Company

To avoid problems arising from inferior fabric quality, some apparel companies inspect fabrics on their arrival from the textile producers. Various types of machinery are used to speed this process, including computerized equipment that scans across the fabric along the entire length to note any shade variation from the beginning to the end of the fabric roll. Other equipment checks the density of the weave or knit. Some companies rely on visual inspection.

On occasion, it may be necessary to reject fabric orders because of color or quality problems. Ordering replacement fabric can delay production by weeks. At times, a textile producer may be unable to replace rejected goods. The production schedule for the contracted arrival date of the goods at the retailer can be jeopardized because of fabric problems. Therefore, every effort is made to ensure the arrival of satisfactory, on-time production fabrics.

If the apparel company is responsible for inspecting fabrics, the fabric goods must arrive at the cutting facility in time to allow for inspection before cutting begins. This requires a crew of workers paid by the apparel facility to inspect the goods. In addition, costs of production increase any time the fabric is in storage or in inventory and not being processed, such as when the fabric is waiting to be cut and sewn. As the apparel industry moved toward faster turnaround time, it became obvious that several processes would need to change. Among them is fabric inspection by the textile producer.

Fabric Inspection by the Textile Producer

Through Quick Response and supply chain management strategies, partnerships have been formed between the textile producer and the apparel manufacturer, ensuring that the textile producer inspected the goods and they were of the quality shown by the sample; and that the goods would arrive at the production facility just in time to cut and sew, as set forth by the apparel company's schedule. Therefore, the apparel company would not need to inspect fabric routinely. Instead, textile producers inspect the goods before they leave the textile facility. At the textile facility, any flaws in weaving or knitting are marked along the selvage edge of the fabric so that the apparel producer knows where the flaws are and can cut around them. Printed fabrics are inspected for color match and registration of motif placement when more than one color is printed. Once inspected, the fabric ordered for production is sent in large rolls from the textile producer, converter, or fabric wholesaler to the cutting facility.

Currently, many small apparel companies do not have the production volume to participate in this aspect of supply chain management. They continue to inspect the fabric and trims prior to sending them to cutting. Even with supply chain management participants, fabric flaws can occur. It is important for all workers to be alert to flaws, such as off-grain stripes, that could lead to the rejection of an order by the retailer.

For apparel companies that own their own factories, the fabric and trims are usually sent from the supplier either directly to the company's production plant or to the apparel company's warehouse (where inspection may occur), and then on to the production facility. For companies that use contractors for the cutting and sewing operations, the fabric might be ordered, received, and inspected by the apparel company, which then sends the fabric rolls to the cutting facility. Another option is that the fabric might be ordered by the contractor and sent directly to the production facility, in which case, the contractor assumes the responsibility for the quality of the fabrics and trims. This is typically done when the fabric is manufactured offshore and the cutting and sewing also occur offshore.

Production Spreading, Cutting, Fallout Disposal, Bundling, and Dye Lot Control

Several steps are involved in preparing the fabric for garment production. These steps include the following:

- spreading the fabric onto cutting tables
- cutting the fabric
- disposing of the excess fabric
- preparing the cut fabric pieces for production

These steps might be done at the production facility, such as at the contractor's facility. If the apparel company owns its production plants, then these steps might be done at one or more of the apparel company's facilities. Sometimes the apparel company is responsible for cutting and bundling. Then it ships the bundled pieces to a production facility. This might be done if the production facility is located in a country with trade incentives, as mentioned earlier in this chapter, if the apparel company wants to control the cutting of the goods, or if the selected contractor only makes and trims garments.

Spreading

Spreading (or laying up) is the process of unwinding the large rolls of fabric onto long, wide cutting tables. The fabric is stacked, layer upon layer, depending on the size of the cut order. For **production cutting**, the fabric is laid flat across its entire width from selvage to selvage (nothing is cut on a fold, as is frequently done in the home sewing industry). The length of each layer of fabric is determined by the specific style's marker length. For large cuts, thin sheets of paper may be laid between every 12 layers of fabric, in order to count the stacked layers of pieces quickly by dozens. This saves a great deal of time after cutting, when the stacks of cut pieces need to be assembled into different groups (bundles) for sewing. When a style will be produced in several colors, the fabric layers will reflect the correct number of layers for each color needed.

Fabrics that have a directional print or napped fabrics, such as corduroy and velvet, need to be laid so that all layers face the same direction (called *face-up*). This is a more time-consuming process than face-to-face spreading (two-directional), and is reflected in the labor cost for cutting. Fabrics such as stripes and plaids require matching, so they also take more time to lay up; therefore, these fabrics cost more to cut. Stretch fabrics, such as fabrics used for

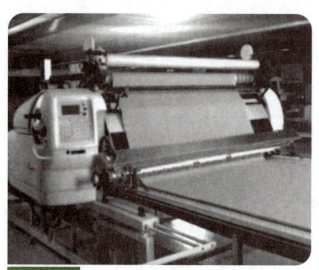

Figure 9.14 Fabric is spread carefully and stacked layer upon layer in preparation for production cutting. A spreading machine is used to roll the fabric onto the cutting table.

swimwear or intimate apparel, require great care during lay-up to avoid distorting the fabric. Stretch fabrics also require time to relax on the table after laying up and before cutting.

A variety of equipment speeds the fabric laying process. **Spreading machines** guided on tracks along the side edges of the cutting table carry the large rolls of fabric, spreading the fabric smoothly (see Figure 9.14). For face-up cutting, a cutting knife is sent across the fabric at the desired length that corresponds to the length of the marker, the spreading machine is returned to its origin, and another layer is spread on top of the previous layer. This process allows each layer to be laid face up. This process is also used if a print fabric is one directional, that is, if the motifs on the print all need to face in the same direction. For plaids and stripes, each layer is stacked so that the plaids or stripes match the layer beneath.

Other systems utilize spreading machines that roll along the floor beside the cutting table. Some spreading machines require operators, but automatic and robotic spreaders are an option. In 1995, Saber Industries introduced the first robotic, digitally controlled spreader in the apparel business ("Saber introduces," 1995).

Cutting

Either the apparel company or the contractor is responsible for making the production marker. The marker, whether drawn by hand or plotted by computer, is sent to the cutting facility or contractor for the cutting process. The marker made during preproduction is laid onto the top layer of fabric, serving as a cutting guide if the fabric will be cut by one of several hand processes. There are several types of specialized hand-guided electric knives and rotary cutters used for cutting the multiple thicknesses of fabric. Most electric knives look similar to a band saw, with a reciprocating blade that oscillates vertically to "saw" through the fabric layers.

Die cutting is another type of cutting process used for specific purposes. For very small pieces that will be cut repeatedly, season after season, it is more precise and more economical in the long run to use a die. The die is similar to a cookie cutter—a piece of metal with a sharp edge, tooled to the exact dimensions of the shape of the pattern piece. The die is positioned over several layers of fabric. Then, a pressurized plate is applied to the die to cut through the thicknesses of fabric. A fabric appliqué that might be used season after season is an example of a pattern piece that would be economical to cut using a die. The original cost of the die is expensive, but its continued use amortizes the initial cost and increases the cutting accuracy compared to hand cutting the same piece.

For facilities that have computerized cutting, special tables are required to accommodate the cutting equipment (see Figure 9.15). The table surface is covered with bristles that allow the cutting blade to slide between them. The fabric layers are compressed with air to provide a more compact cutting height, thereby increasing the accuracy of the cut. The table surface is designed to accommodate the required suction. The computer-generated marker is laid onto the top layer of fabric. The cutting equipment is guided by computer coordinates, not by

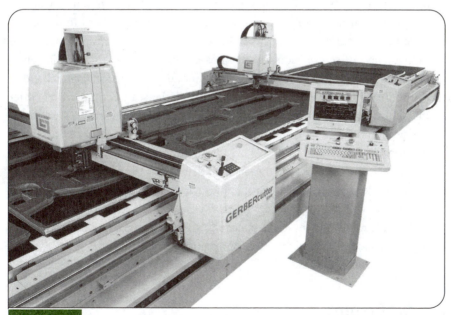

Figure 9.15 A computerized cutter requires a special table surface to accommodate the knife blade requirements. This Gerber cutter automatically conveys material from a spreading table to the cutting area, and then directly onto the bundling area.

"seeing" the pattern piece outlines on the marker. The plotted marker is used for the following two purposes: (1) to ensure that the marker is laid properly onto the fabric, especially when plaids or stripe notations must be aligned; and (2) to indicate the sizes of the pattern pieces and styles for the workers who will bundle the pieces after cutting. Computerized cutting is much faster and generally more accurate than hand cutting or even die cutting. Either a reciprocating knife blade or a rotary cutting blade is used for computerized cutting. The rotary cutting blade is effective for cutting very stretchy fabrics, such as swimwear fabrics. The rolling action of the blade minimizes fabric stretching and, thus, distortion of the fabric during cutting. However, notch marking with a rotary cutter is more limited.

Laser cutting is also driven by computer. It offers many of the same advantages as knife-blade computer cutting, including high speed and accuracy. Laser cutting can be done economically with one or several layers of fabric (called *single-ply* cutting and *low-ply* cutting), compared to the many stacked layers used with computer cutting. Several low-ply cutters can be purchased for about the same cost as one high-ply computerized cutting system. Since low-ply cutters offer the flexibility to produce small runs very quickly, there are additional benefits to consider as well. Several low-ply cutters can be working on different orders at the same time. They lend themselves well to the short-cycle manufacturing environment. Single-ply cutting systems are needed for individually customized cuts for the mass-customization manufacturing environment (see Chapter 11). On the other hand, if a production facility handles primarily large orders for mass production, a large-scale computerized cutter that cuts up to 300 dozen pieces per hour may be more efficient.

Computerized cutting and sewing facilities may be linked electronically to the apparel company's computer so that the marker file can be downloaded electronically. This increases the speed of delivery of the marker to the cutting facility or contractor. Often sewing contractors have CGMM equipment and may be responsible for making the marker. As mentioned earlier, the style's pattern file might be sent electronically from the apparel company to the sewing contractor, which will use CGMM equipment to grade the pattern, make the marker, and cut the style.

Fallout Disposal

Although the marker's layout utilizes the fabric in the most efficient plan possible, there is still a substantial quantity of fallout, or waste material. In the past, the waste goods commonly were delivered to landfills. This procedure has become more expensive, in part because of the reduction in available landfill space and the increase in transportation costs to disposal sites. Furthermore, today's society expects responsible recycling. Textile and apparel waste recyclers provide a market for most of this waste.

There are trade associations that promote the international trade of secondary and scrap textiles. These include Secondary Materials and Recycled Textiles (SMART), the Council for Textile Recycling, and the Textile Recycling Association (based in the U.K.). These associations help divert tons of textile waste from the solid waste stream.

Bundling

After cutting, the component pieces for each size and in each color must be grouped together in some way. **Bundling** is the process of disassembling the stacked and cut pieces and reassembling them, grouped by garment size, color dye lot, and number of units in which they will proceed through production. Bundling is done by hand, with one or more workers picking the required garment parts from the stacks and grouping them in bundles that are ready for production. The type of production process determines the number of garments to be included in each bundle. This varies from the cut fabric pieces for an individual unit (one garment) bundled together, to bundles of a dozen units (or sometimes specified parts of a dozen garments), usually in the same size and color (including same color dye lot) for all 12 garments. For some types of production, up to three dozen units might be bundled together.

Dye Lot Color Management

All coordinating pieces of an outfit, and those styles that are to coordinate in a line, need to be color matched exactly. Mismatching can occur if strict color management is not maintained. Even with adherence to color management, slight variations in shading can occur in the same dye lot of a production order. Therefore, it is important to code all fabric bolts with the dye lot number and to maintain accuracy in matching dye lots throughout spreading, bundling, production, and distribution processes.

Often an apparel company uses one sewing contractor for the suit pants production and another contractor for the suit jacket production. Each contractor receives a shipment of "matching" fabric from the textile producer. If dye lots are not matched, the suit pants might be a slightly different shade from the suit jacket. This discrepancy may not be noticed until the goods arrive at the apparel company's distribution center, the retailer's distribution center, or the retail selling floor, where the sale may be lost when the customer is trying on the jacket and pants and notices that the colors do not match exactly. The importance of maintaining dye lot consistency for pieces that are intended to match in color is critical to the success of the line.

Summary

Retail buyers' written orders in sufficient quantity to warrant production signal the chain of events that begins the process of producing a new style. The preproduction steps include ordering production fabrics, trims, and findings; maintaining color management, including the use of lab dips and strike offs; and finalizing the production pattern and written documents. To ensure quality production, the documents that accompany the pattern are as important as the pattern itself. These documents comprise the garment specification package. They include a tech drawing of the garment style; a list of all fabrics (with fabric swatches), trims, and findings in all colorways; construction specifications (construction details and sewing steps in sequence); and measurement specifications with stated tolerances. Accurate documentation is essential.

In company-owned production facilities, the production pattern is graded into the specified size range, and a production marker is made by the apparel company. For contracted production, either the apparel company or the contractor is responsible for the grading and marking procedures. Computer grading and marker making systems (CGMM) have gained widespread use in the apparel industry. The advantages of CGMM include increased speed and improved accuracy. Integrated computer systems provide product information management, including instantaneous electronic linkage between PDS (pattern design system) and CGMM, whether the two systems are separated by miles within a city (such as the design development department located at company offices, and the grading and marking department located at the company's factory) or by an ocean (such as the design development department located in the United States, and the contractor's grading and marking department located at the factory in Hong Kong).

Fabric inspection may be the responsibility of the textile producer, the apparel company, or the contractor. Spreading can be done by laying the fabric layers onto cutting tables by hand or by using spreading machines. Cutting can be done by hand-held cutting equipment, by computer knife blade, or by laser. After cutting, the fabric pieces are bundled into units ready for production.

The future promises continued developments in a "seamless" integration of all aspects of design, development, marketing, production, and distribution.

Possible career opportunities in preproduction processes include specification writing, production patternmaking, pattern and marker making, and materials management.

Purchasing Manager or Raw Materials Control Manager
Publicly Held Sportswear and Athletic Shoe Company

Position Description:

Manage raw materials buyers to ensure department goals are met. Manage the sales sample materials buyer to ensure timelines are met and all needed materials are ordered. Develop partnerships with vendors for the supply of necessary raw materials to ensure company needs are met. Develop partnerships with contractors to be sure the best possible services are provided for the company. Develop, monitor, and update systems to ensure efficiency in the department and to provide necessary information exchanges with other departments and liaison offices.

Typical Tasks and Responsibilities:

- Prepare annual department budget and action plans.

- Determine greige goods commitments and/or forecast company-developed styles. Have contracts issued. Work with offshore liaison offices to provide accurate and timely reports, updates, and information as requested to make ongoing greige goods commitments with vendors.

- Color sort and preorder raw materials as needed, keeping excess to a minimum and maintaining a program to dispose of excess raw materials.

- Monitor lab dip and first production. Submit information from the apparel lab to ensure materials will meet production timelines. Monitor deliveries to contractors. Troubleshoot quality problems.

- Generate computer reports using a variety of systems.

- Use telephone, fax, and electronic communications to communicate with vendors, contractors, other company departments, and offshore liaison offices.

- Perform constant ongoing "coaching" of buyers to meet department goals.

CAREER PROFILES

Trim Buyer
Publicly Held Suit and Dress Company

Position Description:
Write garment specifications and source vendors. Order trims, buttons, zippers, cording, snaps, interfacings, and lining fabrics. Work with designers and the production team on trim selection. Organize shipments to contractors in the United States and abroad.

Typical Tasks and Responsibilities:

- Make phone calls and send e-mails to vendors.
- Meet with sales representatives to review lines of trim, buttons, zippers, interfacings, and linings.
- Price and order trims and findings.
- Organize and oversee shipments of fabrics and trims to contractors.
- Meet with designers and the production team to select trims.
- Write the garment specifications for all styles in the line.

Key Terms

bundling	measurement specification
commercial match	pattern grading
computer grading and marker making (CGMM)	production cutting
	production engineer
cut order	production marker
die cutting	registration
digitizer	source
factor	spreading
factoring	spreading machine
fallout	supplier
grade rules	tolerance
grading	vendor
lab dip	

Discussion Questions and Activities

1. Describe orally or bring to class a product that provides an example of lack of color management, with one or more components not matching. How would you suggest that this mistake could have been avoided?

2. Give several examples of problems that may occur with fabric quality. Discuss options available to the apparel manufacturer to correct the problem, and explain how such problems—and their correction—affect production and delivery to the retailer.

3. Select a garment and determine how many pattern pieces were cut to assemble the garment. What findings or trims were used?

4. Discuss why garment specifications are important for the manufacturer. What areas of a garment might be very important to have as part of a specification sheet?

References

Cole, Michael D. (2005, November). Technology's next frontier on display at Tech Conference. *Apparel*, pp. 20–22.

DesMarteau, Kathleen. (2003, April). The potential for 3-D & e-collaboration. *Apparel*, pp. 33–36.

Dundish, H. (2009, August 18) The factoring business: how times have changed. *Apparel Magazine*. Retrieved September 9, 2010 from http://www.apparelmag.com

Gaffney, Gary. (1999, May). SCM: In reach for $5M to $25M firms? *Bobbin*, pp. 74–78.

Hill, Thomas. (1994, March). CAR Study: UPS, CAD provide 300%+ return on investment. *Apparel Industry Magazine*, pp. 34–40.

King, K.,Garland, G., Pagan, L., & Nienke, J. (2009, February) Moving digital printing forward for the production of sewn products. *AATCC Review*, pp.33–36.

Rubman, J. (2010, April 24) The three stages of retail PLM adoption (including five myth busters for better product development). *Apparel Magazine*. Retrieved September 9, 2010 from http://www.apparelmag.com

Saber introduces first truly robotic spreader. (1995, August). *Apparel Industry Magazine,* pp. 46–48.

Speer, Jordan K. (2004, June). Color profile: Examining processes. *Apparel*, pp. 22–26.

Young, Kristin. (1996, February 2–February 8). The F word. *California Apparel News*, pp. 1, 8–9.

CHAPTER **10**

Sourcing Decisions and Production Centers

In this chapter, you will learn the following:

- the criteria used by apparel, accessories, and home fashions manufacturers and retailers in their sourcing decisions

- the various sourcing options available to companies

- the advantages and disadvantages of these sourcing options

- current issues related to sourcing decisions

- the locations of the primary domestic and international production centers

Step 6: Sourcing

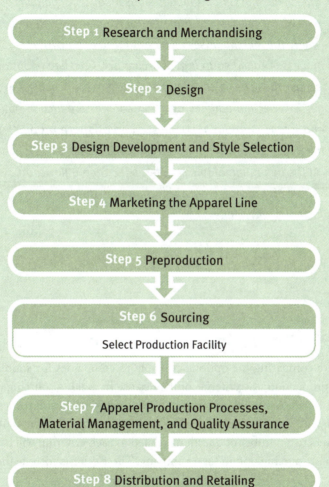

Step 1 Research and Merchandising

Step 2 Design

Step 3 Design Development and Style Selection

Step 4 Marketing the Apparel Line

Step 5 Preproduction

Step 6 Sourcing

Select Production Facility

Step 7 Apparel Production Processes, Material Management, and Quality Assurance

Step 8 Distribution and Retailing

Sourcing Decisions

Some of the most important decisions made by a company are how, when, and where fabrics and trims are purchased as well as how when, and where the merchandise will be produced and distributed. This decision-making process is called **sourcing**. Sourcing decisions are important to all companies because these decisions play an important role in achieving a competitive advantage. This section outlines decision criteria, production options for companies, and issues surrounding domestic and **offshore production** (producing outside the United States using production specifications furnished by U.S. companies). At the beginning of this chapter is the Step 6 flowchart, which summarizes the sourcing process. Figure 10.1 diagrams the sourcing options available to manufacturers and retailers.

Criteria Used in Sourcing Decisions

Before comparing the options available to companies for sourcing materials and production, the criteria companies use in making sourcing decisions will be outlined. A number of criteria are considered when companies decide how, when, and where materials will be purchased and products manufactured. The answers to a number of questions related to each criterion will help determine the best sourcing option for a company. These criteria include the following:

- *company and design criteria (internal to the company)*
  - the company's sourcing philosophy
  - labor requirements, costs, and productivity
  - fabric/materials quality and availability
  - quality assurance/control standards
  - equipment and skills requirements
  - required plant/factory capacities
  - social responsibility and environmental impact
- *political and geographical criteria (external to the company)*
  - trade agreements and other government regulations
  - shipping distance and expected turnaround time

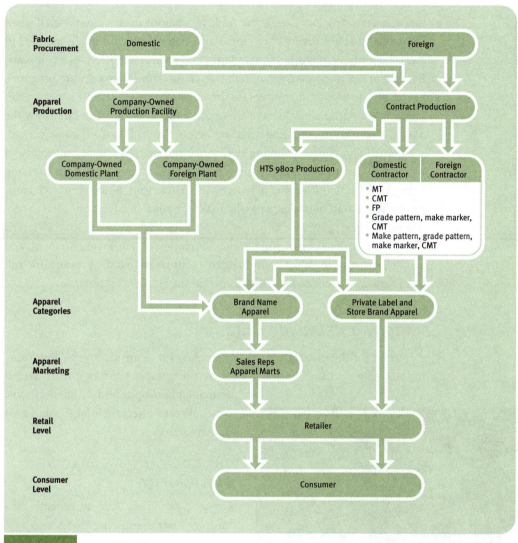

Figure 10.1   Sourcing options

– infrastructure of the country; availability of materials and supplies
– political and economic conditions of the country
– natural disasters

Because of the labor-intensive nature of the textile, apparel, and home fashions industries, labor costs have traditionally been a primary criterion for companies in their sourcing decisions. However, other factors such as geographical location, infrastructure needs, and trade regulations must be considered when companies make sourcing decisions. These criteria are continually assessed to meet the sourcing philosophy, standards, and production needs of a company. Because of the complexity of sourcing decisions, computer software programs have been developed that simulate the implications of various sourcing decisions for a company. Through these simulations, companies can assess the outcomes of varying sourcing decisions before the decisions are implemented.

In small companies, sourcing decisions are generally the responsibility of merchandisers. In larger companies, merchandisers may work with sourcing agents or sourcing managers in making these decisions. Some very large companies have a staff of individuals who make the sourcing decisions for a particular product category such as men's cotton trousers or women's wool sweaters. Those who work in design and product development, fabric procurement, and production sourcing must coordinate their efforts so that the product line will be successfully produced and distributed to the retailers on time.

Company and Design Criteria

A number of the criteria that must be taken into consideration when making sourcing decisions are controlled by the company through their overall sourcing philosophy and design decisions, which directly affect their fabrics and production needs.

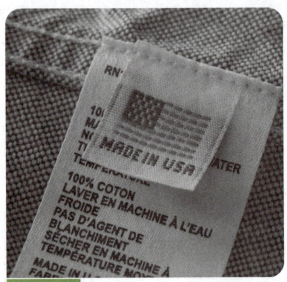

Figure 10.2   Being able to use the "Made in the USA" label on merchandise is an important criterion in some companies' sourcing decisions.

THE COMPANY'S SOURCING PHILOSOPHY

Often companies have a general philosophy toward sourcing that serves as a guideline or framework for sourcing decisions. For example, some companies are very committed to domestic production and want to be able to put "Made in the U.S.A." labels on their products (see Figure 10.2). Other companies have strong ties and positive working relations with contractors in other countries and, therefore, generally prefer offshore production.

Many companies also adopt a sourcing philosophy that incorporates **corporate**

responsibility, or **social responsibility**. For these companies, in addition to costs and profits associated with sourcing decisions, the decisions must also take human rights, labor conditions, and environmental implications of the decisions into account. This is often referred to as a **triple bottom line** for sourcing decisions; that is, people, planet, and profit factors are all considered. These philosophies are implemented in the selection of countries and factories and in the monitoring of factory conditions. Questions companies might ask include the following:

- How do we design, produce, and distribute the highest quality merchandise under the best factory and business conditions?

- How do we design, produce, and distribute products and services that are both sustainable and provide consumers with what they want and need?

These topics are discussed in greater detail later in the chapter.

LABOR REQUIREMENTS AND COSTS

Apparel and accessory production is very labor intensive, even though technological advances are increasingly automating the processes. Therefore, labor costs are an important consideration in sourcing decisions. Questions companies might ask include the following:

- How many workers will be required to produce the goods efficiently?

- What is the labor cost of domestic workers compared to workers in another country?

- What are the labor laws in a particular country? How are the workers treated?

- If the company owns the factories, what investments in technology and personnel training need to be made?

As discussed in Chapter 1, the U.S. and international textile and apparel industries have always been in search of cheaper labor—first within England; then within the United States; then in Japan, South Korea, and Hong Kong in the 1950s; in the Caribbean Basin from the 1960s to the 1980s; in Mexico, Canada, and the Caribbean Basin in the 1990s; in China and Southeast Asia after quotas were phased out for most World Trade Organization members in the early twenty-first century; and in South America and Africa as trade incentives with these regions became attractive for some product categories. Over the past 50 years, U.S. textiles, apparel, accessory, and home fashions companies and retailers have moved a great deal of production offshore where labor costs are considerably lower than in the United States. For example, in 2008, the average hourly compensation cost (in U.S. dollars, including social charges) for apparel production workers in the United States was $9.03, compared to $ 0.22 in Bangladesh, $0.38 in Vietnam, $0.51 in India, $1.08 in coastal China, $2.44 in Turkey, $2.54 in Mexico, and $3.35 in Costa Rica. Obviously, the labor costs in these other countries are much lower than in the United States. This is the primary reason why many manufacturers produce merchandise offshore. (See Table 10.1.) When comparing labor costs, companies must also take worker productivity into account. For example, since 2008, labor costs in China have steadily increased. However, when companies explore less costly alternatives, they must take into account the productivity of Chinese workers. Although many companies have left China for production facilities in Southeast Asian countries such as Vietnam, many have stayed with Chinese sourcing because of the Chinese workers' relatively high productivity.

It is important to note that simply because the labor costs are lower in a particular country, one cannot assume that overall production costs will also be lower. A number of other costs must be taken into consideration. These include:

- costs of fabrics, materials, and trims
- costs associated with support services and infrastructure
- cost of transportation and shipping
- costs associated with tariffs (taxes on imports)

Companies must examine both fixed and variable costs associated with manufacturing in the various options in order to accurately assess the financial benefits of any one option. (See Table 10.2.)

FABRIC/MATERIALS QUALITY AND AVAILABILITY

Tied closely with sourcing decisions about production are sourcing decisions about fabric and materials procurement. Typically, companies want to procure needed fabrics, materials, and trims as close as possible to where the finished product will be manufactured. This not only reduces shipping costs and lead time, but because less energy is used in shipping materials and merchandise, it contributes to a more environmentally sustainable product. For example, if a company is manufacturing premium denim jeans in the United States, they will most likely also be procuring the denim fabric in the United States. If they are manufacturing denim jeans in China, then the fabrics will also most likely be procured in China.

| Table 10.1 | Comparisons of Apparel Manufacturing Labor Costs (including Social Charges) in 2008 U.S. dollars |

Country	Labor Cost US$/Hour
Bangladesh	0.22
Cambodia	0.33
Pakistan	0.37
Vietnam	0.38
India	0.51
China III (Inland)	0.55–0.80
China II (Coastal 2)	0.86–0.94
Russia	1.01
China I (Coastal 1)	1.08
Guatemala	1.65
Honduras	1.72–1.82
Peru	1.78
Mexico	2.54
Costa Rica	3.35
Hungary	4.45

SOURCE: Jassin-O'Rourke Group, LLC, EmergingTextiles.com

| Table 10.2 | Comparison of Costs of Producing a 96% Cotton/4% Spandex Knit Skirt and Top in US$ |

	Garment Made In:		
	Mexico	Peru	China
Fabric cost per garment	10.70	10.30	9.35
Trim cost per garment	1.80	1.80	1.60
Cut/Make/Finish cost per garment	3.66	3.19	2.90
Average profit per garment	1.62	1.53	1.38
Average shipping cost per garment	0.09	0.11	0.12
Duty cost into United States (2005 level)	0.00	0.00	1.44
Total landed U.S. cost	**17.86**	**16.93**	**16.78**
Importers/brand owner price to retailer	21.97	20.82	20.64
Suggested retail price	59.00	59.00	59.00

SOURCE: EmergingTextiles.com (May 23, 2008)

Another important consideration when comparing options for sourcing fabric is trade agreements that have a **yarn forward rule of origin.** This stipulation to a trade agreement means that if a company produces apparel products in a country with whom the United States has such a trade agreement, in order to bring the apparel into the United States duty-free (i.e., without duties or tariffs on the product), the yarn and all manufacturing operations "forward" (e.g., textile production, apparel production) must occur either in the United States or in the country with whom we have the trade agreement. For example, The U.S.–Peru Trade Promotion Agreement, enacted in 2009, requires that for imported apparel from Peru to come into the United States duty-free, the yarn forward standard must be met; although the agreement outlines certain exceptions. This and other trade agreement issues are discussed later in the chapter.

QUALITY ASSURANCE/CONTROL STANDARDS

The importance of maintaining specific quality assurance/control standards is one criterion in a company's sourcing decision. Because quality is most effectively controlled in company-owned facilities, a company's response to the importance of quality control may be the primary reason for using company-owned factories for production or for selecting a contractor that the company knows produces high-quality products (although they may be at a higher cost). When using either a domestic or offshore contractor, companies will articulate (specify) quality standards that the contractor must meet and will also expect to see sample merchandise (see Figure 10.3).

EQUIPMENT AND SKILL REQUIREMENTS

Depending on the product category, equipment and skills needed to produce the product line will vary. Some products require specific types of equipment or sewing skills. For example, the manufacturing of brassieres requires specialized materials, equipment, and skills; and because of the importance of fit, it is typical for brassiere manufacturers to require that finished products be within 0.125 inches (0.3175 cm) of the specifications or standard pattern. Therefore, to assure quality standards, companies will ask the following questions:

- What equipment is needed to produce the goods efficiently?
- How specialized are these equipment needs?
- What specific skills are required to produce the product line?
- Will different equipment be needed next season or next year to produce goods for the company?

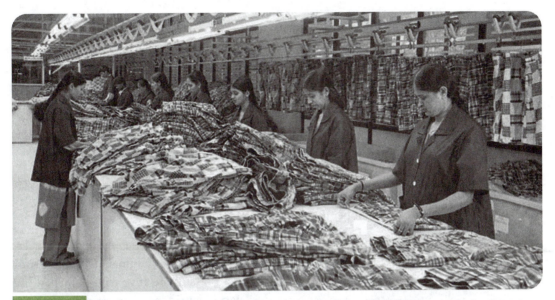

Figure 10.3   The ability to ensure that garments meet quality specifications can be an important criterion in sourcing decisions.

Companies will analyze the factory's equipment and the skills of sewing operators in terms of their production needs in their sourcing decisions (see Figure 10.4).

PLANT/FACTORY CAPABILITIES

Another criterion for sourcing decisions is what the factory capacities are relative to expected production needs. Companies will first estimate production needs and then assess the production capabilities of all factories (both company-owned and contractors) to determine whether these are sufficient. If they are found to be insufficient, the company may decide to hire (additional) contractors, expand current factories, or build new factories. Financial capacities to invest in new equipment will need to be analyzed. If factory capacities

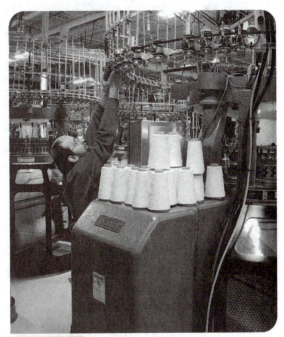

Figure 10.4   When specialized production equipment is required, companies will select contractors that have the required equipment.

are found to be greater than needed, then downsizing strategies are in order or subleasing their facilities may be considered. Facility costs will vary across countries, as will the terms of leasing. Some factories also require minimum orders. It is important for companies to read the fine print of lease contracts to determine what is included.

SOCIAL RESPONSIBILITY AND ENVIRONMENTAL IMPACT

Companies are increasingly using social responsibility and environmental impact factors in their sourcing decisions. Decreasing the environmental "footprint" of a company through their sourcing decisions can be accomplished through a number of practices including:

- *Procuring fabrics and trims that have a low environmental impact.* For example, Nike recently launched their Nike Environmental Design Tool, which is a public tool designed to assess the relative environmental impact of fabric and garment characteristics. Types of fabrics, marker efficiency, garment characteristics, and garment treatments are entered into the tool, and each garment is given a score that represents the garment's environmental impact. Procurement agents and designers can then compare garments' scores and their relative impact on the environment (see Figure 10.5).

- *Designing products that exhibit social responsibility.* **Socially responsible design** is achieved through inclusive design (i.e., inclusive based on age, physical ability, or socioeconomic status), physically and psychologically healthy design, design that promotes fair trade, and design decisions that facilitate efficient factory operations.

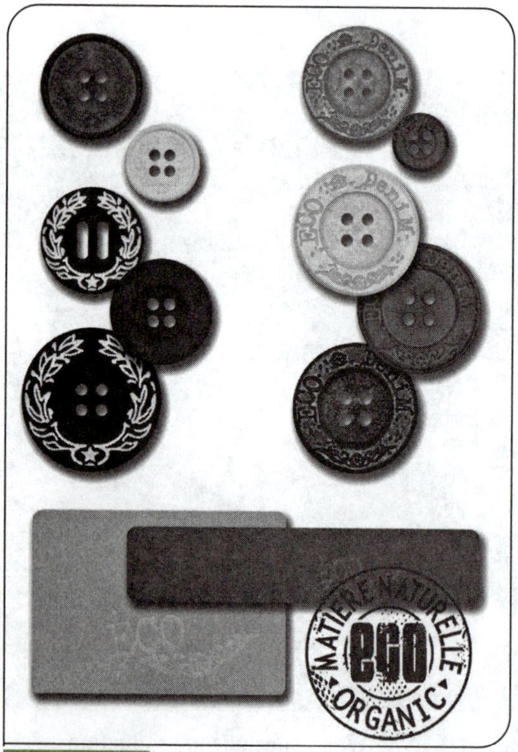

Figure 10.5 Environmentally responsible design decisions can include the selection of eco-friendly buttons such as these from Dorlet.

Political and Geographical Criteria

In addition to those factors that are internal to the company, a number of other considerations external to the company must be monitored and taken into account when making sourcing decisions.

TRADE AGREEMENTS AND OTHER GOVERNMENTAL REGULATIONS

Companies must continually monitor changes in trade agreements between the United States and other countries as they compare the advantages and disadvantages of sourcing in any particular country. Under current international trade policies, textile and apparel goods imported into the United States from many countries are subject to tariffs and, in limited cases, quotas. **Tariffs** are taxes assessed by governments on imports; **quotas** are limits on the number of units, kilograms, or square meters equivalent (SME) in specific categories that can be imported from specific countries. (The metric system for measurement is generally used for these numerical limits because of the predominant use of this system outside the United States). When producing offshore, the company must decide if and how these tariffs may affect importing the goods they produce into the United States or other countries. Because tariffs add to the overall cost of production, companies reflect on the relative advantage of the free-trade agreements that the United States has with a number of countries.

For example, the North American Free Trade Agreement (NAFTA) reduced trade barriers among the United States, Mexico, and Canada. Therefore, a number of companies selling to consumers in the United Staes moved their production from the United States to Mexico to take advantage of the lower labor costs in Mexico and the opportunities for importing the merchandising back into the United States duty-free.

Other government regulations that companies consider when making sourcing decisions include country-specific laws associated with government intervention regarding the following:

- industrial pollution
- the monitoring of air and water quality
- minimum wage requirements
- child labor laws
- other labor laws (e.g., terms of employment, unions)
- tax laws

When laws in other countries are less strict than U.S. companies believe is appropriate, or when enforcement of the laws is problematic, companies may establish their own **codes of conduct** (guidelines that address human resources, health and safety, and labor and environmental laws) that they require their contractors to follow. These codes of conduct are discussed later in the chapter.

SHIPPING DISTANCE AND EXPECTED TURNAROUND TIME

In an era when getting products to the consumer as quickly as possible is important to the success of a company, production, shipping, and distribution times need to be determined and compared. Questions asked by companies include:

- How fast can goods be produced, shipped, and distributed to retailers?
- Would turnaround time be faster if production location changed?
- Would shipping costs be reduced if production location changed?
- What are the energy costs associated with shipping and distribution options?

Companies should consider the distance and shipping time between the production factory/contractor and the company's distribution center. For example, a company with a distribution center in New York may choose a contractor in Mexico over a contractor in Thailand because of shipping time, costs, and environmental impact. In addition, improved supply chain management strategies such as enhanced communication and transaction technologies (e.g., e-mail, business-to-business Web technologies), information, business forms, and even money can be sent electronically and, therefore, reduce the time involved.

Turnaround time is particularly important for time-sensitive products such as swimwear. It is estimated that two-thirds of all swimwear is sold from May through July. Therefore, for reorders, swimwear companies need the fastest turnaround possible. Because of this, many swimwear companies manufacture their goods in locations close to where the goods will be distributed.

INFRASTRUCTURE OF THE COUNTRY—AVAILABILITY OF MATERIALS AND SUPPLIES

When making sourcing decisions, companies must also analyze the availability and reliability of each country's infrastructure and support areas. Questions asked by companies include:

- Are quality trims and threads readily available?
- Are sewing machine technicians and parts available?
- Are power sources, transportation methods, and shipping options reliable?

These questions are particularly important when exploring production in less developed countries such as Bangladesh, Cambodia, or Ecuador.

POLITICAL AND ECONOMIC CONDITIONS

Companies that source offshore continually monitor the political and economic conditions of countries where production is taking place. Political instability or economic problems can dramatically affect the availability of materials and the reliability of transportation and shipping alternatives. Safety of employees must also be taken into consideration when violence or terrorism may pose threats to employees.

NATURAL DISASTERS

Companies must also monitor the impact of natural disasters such as hurricanes or earthquakes on production capabilities. For example, the devastating earthquake that hit Haiti in 2010 had damaging effects on the country's infrastructure and consequently the country's apparel production industry. Whereas some companies decided to contract elsewhere, other companies believed in the economic development in Haiti. Indeed, it took less than a month for Superior Uniform Company, which contracts with One World Apparel in Haiti, to resume production after the earthquake because the earthquake spared one of their production facilities and equipment.

Options for Sourcing Production

Based on these factors, a number of options for sourcing production are available to companies. In general, major sourcing decisions focus on the following:

1. whether fabric and materials will procured and production will be
   - domestic
   - offshore
   - a combination of both
2. whether fabric and materials will be procured and production will be
   - in a company-owned facility
   - contracted to other companies
   - a combination of both

When using contractors, the decision must also be made about which of the following type of **contractor** is employed based on the services offered:

- *Cut, make, and trim services:* With the **cut, make, and trim** (CMT) option, the company provides the patterns, fabrics, and trims, and the contractor provides labor and supplies. The contractor cuts, makes, and trims. In some cases, the contractor receives pre-cut fabrics and only performs make and trim (MT) services.

- *Full-package services:* With the **full-package (FP)** option, the contractor provides preproduction services, fabrics, trims, supplies, and labor.
- *Other options:* For example, the apparel company provides the fabric, and cuts and bundles the fabric; the contractor sews and trims.

Advantages and disadvantages of each option must be weighed by companies in light of their product line, operation strategies, and organization philosophy. For some companies, the flexibility afforded by using contractors is necessary; other companies believe they have greater quality control by producing products in their own factories. Some companies produce offshore to take advantage of lower labor costs. However, just because labor costs are lower in another country does not necessarily mean that overall production costs are lower or that producing offshore is the right decision for a company. What follows are the basic sourcing alternatives available to companies. Tables 10.3 and 10.4 outline the primary advantages and disadvantages of these options for sourcing production.

Table 10.3   Advantages and Disadvantages of Domestic and Offshore Production

	Advantages	Disadvantages
Domestic production	Trade barriers not a concern Shipping time and costs may be lower Known infrastructure Known culture Supported by consumers who prefer products "made in the U.S.A."	Labor costs may be higher than in other countries Some types of fabrics may not be readily available
Offshore production	Labor costs may be lower than in the United States Can take advantage of trade agreement incentives Some types of fabrics are more readily available	Differences in cultural norms Monetary/currency differences Language barriers Possible trade barriers

Table 10.4	Advantages and Disadvantages of Company-Owned Facility Production and Contractor Production

	Advantages	Disadvantages
Company-owned facility production	Greater quality control Greater control over production timing Communication with textile suppliers and retailers optimized	Financial requirements associated with equipment and personnel Need to ensure continuous production Higher labor costs Foreign ownership creates additional financial risks
Contractor production	Greater flexibility to changing equipment or production needs No investment in factories, equipment, or training needed	Less control over quality or production timing

Domestic Fabric—Domestic Production in Company-Owned Facility

In this case, fabric produced in the United States is shipped to a company-owned factory in the United States for production. With vertically integrated companies, garment production facilities are in the same general location as where the fabric is produced. This option allows for the greatest control over quality and timing of production. Communication with textile suppliers and retailers is also optimized. To be competitive, companies that own their own facilities need to (and have the control to) invest in technology to increase productivity and reduce sewing costs. Companies that choose this option typically produce similar types of goods each year so that equipment requirements do not change drastically. Companies must also invest in training personnel and plan to maintain consistent and continuous production so that personnel are not continually laid off during slow periods and then rehired during busy periods. To maintain continuous production, these companies will sometimes serve as contractors for other companies during times of slow production. Labor costs are generally higher for companies that own their own factories, but many companies are dedicated to making domestic production competitive through increased productivity.

Generally, companies that have chosen this option are proud to put the "Made in the U.S.A." label on their products and are committed to domestic

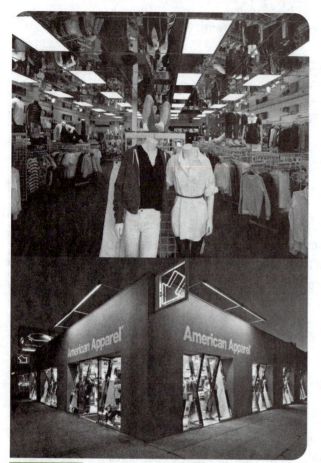

production. American Apparel is an example of a vertically integrated company that produces merchandise in its own facilities in the Los Angeles area, employing 7,500 there and 12,000 worldwide. American Apparel manufactures and retails men's, women's, and children's knitwear. Fabrics are knitted, dyed, and cut in-house. Garments are sewn in one of their three factories. Their first store opened in 2003 and by 2010 they operated more than 280 stores in 19 countries. This vertical integration allows American Apparel to control all aspects of production, thereby increasing the speed, quality control, and environmental impact of their operations (see Figure 10.6).

Figure 10.6 Headquartered in Los Angeles, American Apparel is one of the largest vertically integrated apparel company in the United States.

Domestic or Foreign Fabric—Domestic Contractor Production

Under this option, fabric is procured either domestically or from a foreign vendor, and production is contracted to a domestic company (contractor) that specializes in the type of production and services (CMT or FP) required. By using a contractor, the company may lose some control over quality and timing of production. However, with contractor production, the company does not have to invest in factories, equipment, or training personnel. This is important for small companies that may not have the financial resources to build or buy a production facility. By using contractors, companies have increased flexibility in production methods. This is important for companies with product lines—and, therefore, equipment needs—that vary from year to year. Sometimes manufacturers that typically produce in their own factories choose this option when orders outpace their production capacity. For those that believe producing in the United States is important, companies can still put "Made in the U.S.A." on their labels when they use domestic contractors. If the fabric is procured from another country, certain trade barriers (e.g., tariffs) need to be handled. Otherwise, trade barriers are not a concern, and shipping costs and production time may be advantageous.

An example of a successful domestic contractor is Koos Manufacturing, Inc., a Los Angeles-area high-end jeans manufacturer. Koos manufactures denim jeans for store brands such as J.Crew, Gap, The Buckle, and Abercrombie & Fitch. Its competitive advantages include its responsiveness to customers' needs, the specialty sewing and quality production expected in the designer price zone, and its proximity to denim laundry facilities where denim is given its faded or distressed appearance.

How do companies find the right contractor to produce their merchandise? Contractors can be located in the following ways:

- **Sourcing fairs** are trade shows that bring contractors and companies together. At these fairs, contractors have booths with samples of their merchandise and information regarding their expertise and capacities. Sourcing fairs are also held in conjunction with other trade shows, such as MAGIC (see Figure 10.7). Both domestic and foreign contractors use sourcing fairs to connect with companies, and companies use them to find appropriate

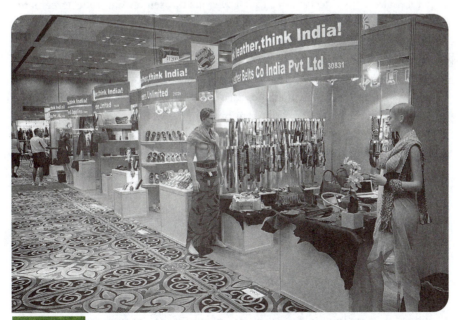

Figure 10.7 Sourcing at MAGIC trade show provides opportunities for companies to connect with contractors from around the world.

domestic and foreign contractors. Sourcing fairs can be face-to-face or through Web sites.

- Contractors and companies also use classified advertisements in trade papers such as *WWD* or *California Apparel News* to advertise their needs or availability.

- Headquartered in Atlanta, Georgia, the *American Apparel Producers' Network* is the primary trade association for contractors and other companies across the global supply chain that produce apparel for the U.S. consumer market. The association provides educational forums, research and data on sourcing effectiveness and on supply chain management technologies, and opportunities to build relationships among companies through networking events and travel.

Domestic or Foreign Fabric—HTS 9802 Production

Using fabric produced either in the United States or elsewhere, companies choosing this option combine domestic production (i.e., design and cut) with a special type of offshore production commonly known as **HTS 9802 production**. Under the Harmonized Tariff Schedule Section 9800 (including several subheadings under this section) of the U.S. tariff regulations, textiles and apparel that are produced under the provisions of preferential trade agreements such as the North American Free Trade Agreement or the Caribbean Basin Trade Partnership Act receive tariff reductions or eliminations. For example, if certain garment pieces are made of U.S. fabrics, cut in the United States, and shipped to contractors in specified countries for assembly, the goods can come into the United States tariff-free or tariffs are only on the "value added" to the garment (typically, the cost of assembly). For example, suppose the value of the cut garment pieces was $50,000 when they were shipped to Ecuador for assembly. After assembly, the garments were worth $150,000 when they were shopped back to the United States. Under this tariff regulation, the import tax would be calculated on $100,000, the value added to the garment pieces.

The passage of the North American Free Trade Agreement in 1994 and theDominican Republic–Central America–United States Free Trade Agreement (CAFTA-DR) in 2005 further solidified reciprocal reductions in tariffs among the United States and countries within North America and the Central America/Caribbean Basin region and, thus, fostered the use of contractors in these areas of the world. Miami has grown as a hub for numerous cutting operations for companies taking advantage of lower labor costs outside the United States and these various trade incentives.

This sourcing option allows the manufacturer to control the design and cut of the garments, while taking advantage of lower labor costs in other countries. Contractors that participate in this type of production offer a variation of CMT services—that is, the MT (make and trim) without the C (cut). With this option, however, companies must be able to handle possible language and cultural differences when working with contractors in other countries.

Domestic or Foreign Fabric—Foreign Contractor Production

This option is similar to the previous option, except that fabrics are generally not from the United States. Foreign contractors can provide both CMT and FP services to companies (see Figure 10.8). Advantages of this option can include lower labor costs found in other countries, fabric availability, and plant capacities. Disadvantages are similar to those for the previous option: possible trade restrictions, and language and cultural differences in other countries. When using domestic fabric, shipping time and costs may be higher than if fabrics were produced and procured closer to the production facilities.

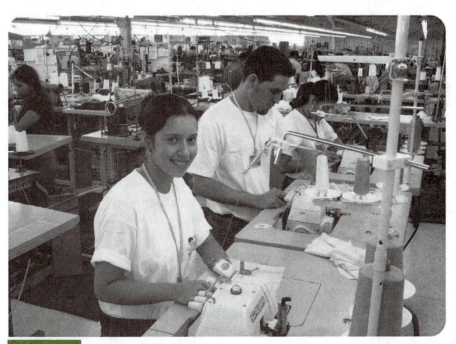

Figure 10.8 Foreign contractors such as this lingerie factory in Nicaragua provide CMT services for specific product categories.

Foreign Fabric—Foreign Production in Company-Owned Foreign Facility

In some cases, companies may own production facilities in other countries. For example, since the passage of NAFTA, there have been increased investments in production facilities by U.S. companies in Mexico. Although this option allows companies to have control over quality and timing of production while taking advantage of lower labor costs in other countries, the financial risks associated with building and running a production facility outside of the United States are great. Government policies, personnel expectations, and cultural norms regarding business operations in another country may be very different from those in the United States. In fact, under some countries' policies, foreign ownership of factories is prohibited. Companies that own their production facilities must abide by the laws governing international trade regarding tariffs and quotas, just as companies that contract offshore do.

Combination of Alternatives

Many companies diversify their sourcing; that is, they use a combination of options depending on their production requirements at any point in time. Using a variety of sourcing options provides companies with the flexibility needed to change production in response to consumer demand, production requirements, and international relations. Diversification of sourcing options also safeguards companies against natural disasters and political or economic crises that may occur within a country or region of the world.

Companies often combine domestic and offshore production. For example, Patagonia, headquartered in Ventura Beach, California, uses contractors located in the United States, China, Thailand, Vietnam, Japan, Turkey, Portugal, Mexico, Costa Rica, El Salvador, Israel, and the Philippines. To ensure product quality and that the contractors abide by environmental requirements, minimum wage, and minimum age standards set by Patagonia, Patagonia has a published code of conduct, and company representatives visit each contractor.

One of the most diverse contracting systems is that of Nike, Inc., the world's largest apparel and footwear company, headquartered near Beaverton, Oregon. In 2010, Nike contracted with 612 factories in 46 countries, including 136 factories in China, 56 in Thailand, 46 in the United States, 42 in Vietnam, and 40 in Indonesia (see Figure 10.9). The company also requires contractors to comply with a code of conduct and conducts faculty audits.

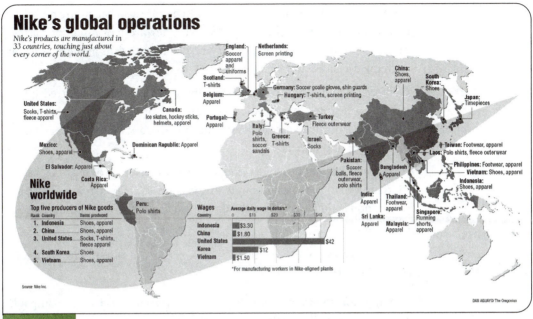

Figure 10.9 Nike produces merchandise through contractors around the world.

Trends in Sourcing

A number of factors are currently affecting sourcing decisions. These include:

- *Oil prices:* Rising oil prices have resulted in a rise in transportation and shipping costs, causing sourcing agents to adjust sourcing decisions in order to reduce distance between production and distribution facilities.

- *Availability and prices of raw materials:* Prices of natural fibers such as cotton are affected by both supply and demand. In 2010, worldwide cotton prices soared because of increased demand in countries such as China and India at the same time as decreased supply caused by droughts in other countries. Sourcing agents had to explore the use of alternative fibers and shift production accordingly.

- *Stakeholder concerns for corporate responsibility:* Consumers, shareholders, and other company stakeholders are demanding that companies be more aggressive in their corporate responsibility efforts. Companies have responded through a variety of initiatives and programs.

- *Increased threats of terrorism worldwide:* Companies strive to reduce disruptions in production and distribution. They are also becoming more vigilant in assuring employee safety. As such, they are becoming increasingly cautious of political issues that may result in terrorism and are adjusting sourcing decisions accordingly.

- *Increased demands by consumers to get products faster:* Spurred by fast fashion, consumers have come to expect new products on a regular basis. Sourcing agents must take delivery time into account for an increasing number of types of products.

- *Brand management:* The availability of counterfeit products has caused sourcing agents for name brands to focus on security services offered by production facilities and to make sourcing decisions based on the security of their brand.

As companies continually reevaluate their sourcing options, trends in sourcing decisions include:

- *Supply chain management orientation to sourcing decisions:* Companies are focusing on all aspects of materials procurement, production, and distribution in their sourcing decisions. This requires greater communication among decision makers throughout the supply chain. For example, designers must be aware of their decisions on both materials procurement and on production.

- *"Local" sourcing:* Local sourcing is a business strategy whereby companies procure materials within a specified radius of where the products will be produced and/or distributed. Whereas this strategy has achieved attention in food, restaurant, and building industries, it has not been as popular in the textile, apparel, and home fashions industries. This is because raw materials (e.g., cotton, wool, polyester, silk, etc.) are produced in limited areas of the world. However, some small companies who have a discerning target customer are identifying strategies whereby their materials and production are as close as possible. For example, Imperial Stock Ranch's production of wool and finished wool products are all carried out in central Oregon (see Figure 10.10).

Production Centers

Sourcing decisions are complex, and companies continually assess sourcing options to best meet their needs. In order to be competitive, production facilities—both domestic and offshore—must be responsive, flexible, efficient, and cost-effective.

U.S. Production Centers

Once one of the largest manufacturing industries in the United States, the domestic apparel industry has experienced continued decreasing employment over the past 20 plus years. According to the United States Bureau of Labor Statistics, in 2009, employment in apparel manufacturing nationwide was estimated at 180,780, down from 929,000 in 1990. Small pockets of employment in apparel production can be found in almost every state, although the states with the largest employment are California, New York, North Carolina, Texas, and Florida. This distribution reflects the historical concentration of apparel manufacturing in the New York City and Los Angeles areas and the lower wages found in the southern states in comparison to other states. Southern California has a pool of skilled labor, primarily from the Latino and Asian populations in the area. Southern states have benefited from trade agreements (NAFTA, CAFTA-DR), which have enhanced production activities such as garment cutting in these states, as well as from vertically integrated manufacturing facilities. U.S. production facilities pride themselves in offering flexibility, innovation, speedy turnaround time, and efficient delivery to retailers.

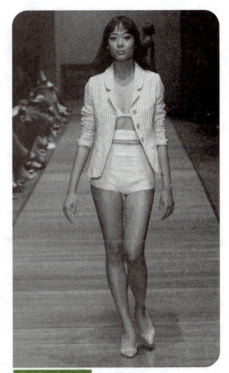

Figure 10.10 Local sourcing involves companies procuring materials as close to production facilities as possible. Wool garments in the Imperial Collection by Anna Cohen are an example.

Global Production Centers

Worldwide production of textiles and apparel has focused on providing the world's largest consumer markets (i.e., North America and Western Europe) with a steady supply of fashionable apparel, accessories, and home fashions. In the 1980s, Hong Kong, Taiwan, and South Korea were referred to as the "Big Three" Asian producers of textiles and apparel because of their importance in global trade of textiles and apparel. In the 1990s, China, India, Pakistan, Indonesia, and other Asian countries emerged as important worldwide producers. Asia continues to be the world's largest producer of textiles and apparel. It is expected to remain so for many years as investments in infrastructure, technology, and equipment over the past 20 years have resulted in efficient high-quality production processes.

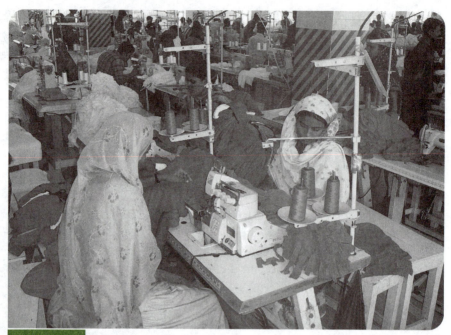

Figure 10.11 Developing countries such as Bangladesh rely on apparel manufacturing for their economic development.

From a U.S. perspective, since the mid-1980s, offshore contract production to Asia, Mexico, and Central and South America has steadily increased. Reasons for the increase in offshore contract production include the number of offshore contractors that have design and/or production capabilities (full-package services) and the progress that has been made in computer compatibility, which has led to an increased use in electronic transmission of information, such as garment specification sheets or patterns. Movement of production to China and other countries in Asia was spurred by the following:

- elimination of quotas for members of the World Trade Organization in 2005
- low labor costs
- specialization in certain types of fabrics and/or production processes that cannot be found elsewhere
- relatively fast production and worker productivity

Movement of production to Mexico and Central and South American countries was fueled largely by the following:

- favorable trade legislation (e.g., NAFTA and CAFTA-DR)
- competitive labor costs
- advantages of proximity to the U.S. market, which include
  - the ability to manage what are essentially nearby operations
  - lower shipping and transportation costs (compared to Asia)
  - the convenience of doing business in the same or close time zones

From a global perspective, apparel production facilities can be found in developed countries (highly industrialized countries) such as the United States, Canada, Australia, Brazil, and countries in Western Europe with large domestic consumer markets; developed Asian countries with historically strong textile and apparel industries including Japan, Hong Kong (administrative region of China), South Korea, and Taiwan (Chinese Taipei); and emerging and developing countries such as China, India, Bangladesh, Costa Rica, and Guatemala (see Figure 10.11).

Apparel industries in countries and world regions with large consumer markets, such as in North America, the European Union, Brazil, Australia, and Japan have typically focused on both domestic and export opportunities. Industries in countries and world regions without large consumer markets have typically focused on exporting merchandise. However, as consumer markets have grown in highly populated countries such as China and India, greater attention is being paid to both domestic and export production.

Worldwide, according to the World Trade Organization, the two largest textile exporters in 2009 were the European Union (29.5 percent share of world exports of textiles, not including their domestic market) and China (28 percent share of world exports of textiles, not including their domestic market). The United States, the Republic of Korea, India, Taiwan (Chinese Taipei), Turkey, and Pakistan accounted for a combined additional 20 percent share of world exports, not including their domestic market.

Also worldwide in 2009, according to the World Trade Organization, the two largest apparel exporters were China (34 percent share of world exports of apparel, not including their domestic market) followed closely by the European Union (31 percent share of world exports of apparel, not including their domestic market). Turkey, Bangladesh, India, and Vietnam combined accounted for another 13 percent share of world exports of apparel (see Table 10.5). As the world's largest consumer markets for apparel, the European Union in 2009 had a 48.5 percent share of world imports of apparel with the United States adding an additional 22 percent share of world imports and Japan an additional 8 percent share.

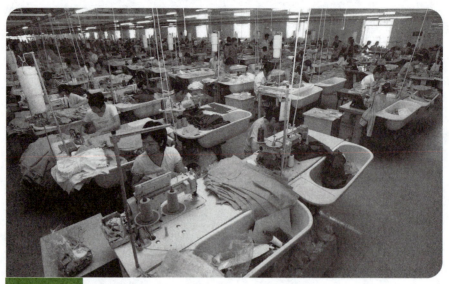

Figure 10.12 Apparel production in and exports from China have contributed to China's economic development.

According to the Department of Commerce Office of Textiles and Apparel, in 2009, the United States imported the most textiles and apparel (as measured in value in U.S. dollars) from the following countries (in order): China, Vietnam, India, Mexico, Indonesia, Bangladesh, and Pakistan. It should be noted that the value of imports from China (US$31.76 billion) were six times the value of the next country (Vietnam at a value of US$5.33 billion) (see Figure 10.12).

Many developing countries rely on textile and apparel manufacturing for their economic development and compete worldwide as low-wage production centers (see Table 10.6). Indeed, a significant proportion of these countries' exports are in textiles and apparel, as can be seen by the following statistics (2009):

- 86 percent of Haiti's total merchandise exports are apparel
- 71 percent of Bangladesh's total merchandise exports are apparel
- 71 percent of Cambodia's total merchandise exports are apparel
- 64.5 percent of Lesotho's total merchandise exports are apparel
- 46 percent of Honduras' total merchandise exports are apparel
- 41 percent of Sri Lanka's total merchandise exports are apparel
- 37 percent of Pakistan's total merchandise exports are textiles

Several characteristics of textile and apparel manufacturing account for the fact that apparel exports are important to the economies of many developing countries.

Table 10.5	Leading Exporters and Importers of Clothing, 2009

Exporters	Share of World Exports
China	34.0
European Union	30.7
Turkey	3.7
India	3.6
Bangladesh	3.4
Viet Nam	2.7
Indonesia	1.9
United States	1.3
Mexico	1.3
Thailand	1.2
Pakistan	1.1
Importers	
European Union	48.5
United States	21.8
Japan	7.7
Canada	2.3
Russian Federation	2.2
Switzerland	1.6
Australia	1.2

Because textile and apparel production is highly labor intensive, the industry provides work for many people. Compared with other manufacturing industries, apparel production is fairly inexpensive to establish. Essentially, all that is needed are industrial sewing machines, pressing equipment, and a building. In addition, because of continuously changing fashion trends, there is a constant demand for textile and apparel products. Therefore, developing countries in Southeast Asia, Africa, the Caribbean Basin, and South America greatly contribute to the global production of textiles and apparel.

International Trade Laws and Free Trade Agreements

International trade laws are constantly changing, and it is essential for apparel companies and retailers to stay on top of trade issues. Trade restrictions, including tariffs and quotas, must be taken into account in sourcing decisions. Several

Table 10.6	Textile and Clothing Exports' Percent Share in Country Economies' Total Merchandise Exports

Country	Textile Exports' Percent Share in Economy's Total Merchandise Exports
Nepal	29.9
Pakistan	36.8
Syrian Arab Republic	13.1
Turkey	7.6
Bangladesh	7.1
Macao, China	6.0
India	5. 6
China	5.0

Country	Clothing Exports' Percent Share in Economy's Total Merchandise Exports
Haiti	86.0
Bangladesh	71.1
Cambodia	70.8
Lesotho	64.5
Honduras	45.7
Sri Lanka	40.7
Mauritius	36.9
El Salvador	35.7

developments in international trade laws have affected apparel manufacturers' and retailers' decisions regarding offshore production.

World Trade Organization

Established in 1995, the World Trade Organization (WTO) is a global trade organization that deals with the "rules of trade" among member countries. As of 2010, 153 countries were members. The WTO's Agreement on Textiles and Clothing phased out quotas established by the Multi-Fiber Arrangement (MFA) and reduced tariffs on textiles and apparel over a 10-year period between 1995 and 2005. The quota phaseout (quotas remained for a few product categories after 2005 for China, Russia, Ukraine, and Vietnam) provided countries with more open access to consumer markets. This has been advantageous for the textile and apparel industries in some countries (e.g., China, India, Indonesia) that continue to have low wages and increased investments, and less advantageous for other countries (e.g., Costa Rica, Mauritius) that have relatively high wages.

Free Trade Agreements

The United States has a number of **free trade agreements (FTA)** negotiated with specific countries or world regions. The goals of these FTAs have been to reduce trade barriers among the countries, encourage economic development, and foster business relationships. These goals have been achieved through:

- elimination or reduction of tariff rates
- improvement of intellectual property regulations
- opening of government purchasing opportunities, and
- easing of investment rules

Country of origin rules and documentation have become very important with the implementation of FTAs. **Country of origin** of a product is defined as the country where the last step that added value (i.e., substantial change) to the product took place. Because FTAs are country-specific, country of origin documentation allows products from particular countries with whom we have negotiated FTAs to be imported into the United States with reduced or no tariffs. Thus, the U.S. Customs and Border Protection Office verifies country of origin documentation and collects the appropriate tariffs on the products.

Two of these FTAs (see Table 10.7 for a complete listing of U.S. FTAs) have had the most impact on the textile and apparel industries of the countries involved: the North American Free Trade Agreement (NAFTA) and the Dominican Republic–Central America–United States Free Trade Agreement (CAFTA-DR). NAFTA, which took effect on January 1, 1994, phased in duty-free trade between Canada, Mexico, and the United States. It is estimated that trade among the three countries has increased more than 200 percent since NAFTA's implementation. Prior to NAFTA, most of the U.S.-imported apparel from Mexico had been cut in the United States and imported under HTS 9802 trade regulations. In addition, at that time, quality and communications issues kept many U.S. companies from sourcing in Mexico. Since the implementation of NAFTA, the countries have done the following:

- developed specializations within the supply chain (with the United States and Canada focusing more on technology, design, and marketing, and Mexico focusing on production)
- improved communication and supply chain management strategies among the countries

Table 10.7	U.S Free Trade Agreements and Trade Preference Programs

U.S. Free Trade Agreements and implementation dates:

- Australia (2005)
- Bahrain (2006)
- Dominican Republic–Central America–United States Free Trade Agreement (CAFTA-DR, 2005): Costa Rica, El Salvador, Guatemala, Honduras, Nicaragua, the Dominican Republic, and the United States
- Chile (2004)
- Israel (1985)
- Jordan (2001)
- Morocco (2006)
- North American Free Trade Agreement (NAFTA, 1994): United States, Canada, and Mexico
- Oman (1985)
- Peru (2009)
- Singapore (2004)

U.S. Trade Preference Programs

- African Growth and Opportunity Act (AGOA
- Andean Trade Promotion and Drug Eradication Act (ATPDEA)
- Caribbean Basin Trade Partnership Act (CBTPA)
- Haitian Hemispheric Opportunity Through Partnership for Encouragement Act (HOPE Act)

Production in Mexico has become more technologically advanced, quality has improved, production has increased (particularly full-package contract production), and U.S. apparel companies are making more long-term financial commitments in Mexico.

CAFTA-DR was signed into law in 2005. Although most of the countries included in CAFTA-DR benefited from earlier trade initiatives implemented to boost economic development in Central America, CAFTA-DR further strengthened these relationships. Because developing countries in Central America, such as Honduras and El Salvador, compete with countries such as China and India as low-wage production centers, CAFTA-DR offered additional incentives (e.g., reduced tariffs on selected items) for U.S. companies to source in Central American countries.

Trade Preference Programs

The United States has also enacted several **trade preference programs** that have enhanced opportunities for trade and economic development with specific regions of the world. The African Growth and Opportunity Act (AGOA) supports 38 eligible nations (26 are eligible for the apparel provision) in sub-Saharan Africa. This program allows for tariff/duty-free and quota-free treatment for a number of eligible apparel products through 2015 including apparel made of U.S. yarns and fabric (yarn forward rule), apparel made of yarns and fabrics made in sub-Saharan Africa or not produced commercially in the United States, and certain hand-made or folklore products.

The Andean Trade Promotion and Drug Eradication Act supports nations in North and Central Western South America (ATPDEA). The Caribbean Basin Trade Partnership Act supports eligible nations that surround the Caribbean Sea (CBTPA). The Haitian Hemispheric Opportunity Through Partnership for Encouragement Act (HOPE Act) specifically supports economic development in Haiti. All of these Trade Preference Programs provide incentives for companies to source in these regions of the world through investments and infrastructure enhancements.

Sweatshops in Domestic and Offshore Production

What Is a Sweatshop?

Definitions of **sweatshops** vary depending upon the source of the definition. According to the U.S. General Accounting Office, a sweatshop is an employer that violates two or more federal or state labor, occupational safety and health, workers' compensation, or other laws regulating an industry. The International Labor Organization defines a sweatshop as an establishment where fundamental rights are denied, and the International Labor Rights Forum defines sweatshops as "workplaces where basic worker rights are not respected." Global Exchange's definition includes employees' inability to form independent unions and the absence of a wage that can support the basic needs of a small family (i.e., living wage). A review of the various definitions reveals a number of common characteristics. In general, a sweatshop is a workplace where workers are exploited including an absence of a living wage or benefits; excessively long hours of work required, often without overtime pay; poor working conditions; arbitrary discipline including verbal and/or physical abuse; and/or no ability to organize to negotiate better terms of work. Because of the highly decentralized nature of the industry, it is difficult to estimate the number of sweatshops in the United States and abroad. However, in the United States, the New York City and Los Angeles areas, where there are large concentrations of immigrants, are often cited as meccas for such establishments.

History of the Sweatshop Issue

Although sweatshops have been around since the turn of the twentieth century, after the Triangle Shirtwaist Co. factory fire of 1911, increased attention was paid to sweatshop conditions in the United States. Until the 1960s, a majority of U.S. apparel companies owned large factories where workers were usually unionized. Federal and state agencies could easily inspect the facilities and enforce labor, health, and environmental laws. However, in a highly competitive environment, many companies moved away from owning their own facilities to using contractors for the assembly phase of production. This resulted in a shift in apparel production from large, company-owned factories to a vast array of small, specialized contractors and subcontractors both within the United States and in other countries. Along with this shift, in the 1980s and 1990s, the industry saw a growth in and proliferation of sweatshops (Bonacich & Appelbaum, 2000). At the same time, there was a decrease in government agencies' ability to regulate working conditions. See Table 10.8 for a timeline of the sweatshop issue. Reminiscent of the early 1900s, stories emerged of lurid working conditions (see Figure 10.13), piecework pay below minimum wage, and children working and playing alongside their mothers in factories (Lii, 1995),

Table 10.8   A Timeline of the Sweatshop Issue

1851	Isaac Singer patents the sewing machine for factory use.
1900	International Ladies' Garment Workers Union (ILGWU) is formed to improve working conditions in the U.S. garment industry.
1911	146 garment workers die in a fire at the Triangle Shirtwaist Co. factory in New York's Greenwich Village. The tragedy stimulates a movement to end "sweatshop" conditions.
1917	The Amalgamated Clothing Workers of America union is formed as the primary union for the menswear industry.
1951	Employment in the apparel and knitwear industries in New York City peaks at 380,000.

Table 10.8	A Timeline of the Sweatshop Issue *(continued)*
1976	The Amalgamated Clothing Workers of America merges with the Textile Workers of America and the United Shoe Workers of America unions to form the Amalgamated Clothing and Textile Workers Union.
1991	Levi Strauss & Co. becomes the first multinational apparel company to establish a code of conduct for its contractors.
1995	The Amalgamated Clothing and Textile Workers Union and the International Ladies' Garment Workers Union merge to become the Union of Needletrades, Industrial, and Textile Employees (UNITE).
1996/April	The Kathie Lee Gifford sweatshop scandal: merchandise she endorsed is found to have been made in sweatshops in El Salvadoran maquiladoras (export-only factories).
1996/August	The White House forms the Apparel Industry Partnership (AIP), a voluntary partnership of apparel and shoe manufacturers, trade unions, and consumer and human rights organizations. The Partnership's task is to develop a plan of action to end sweatshops.
1997/April	The AIP releases a code of conduct for apparel producers.
1997/Fall	University of Notre Dame (South Bend, Indiana) becomes the first college or university in the country to adopt a code of conduct for companies producing licensed merchandise.
1998/July	Activists found the United Students Against Sweatshops (USAS).
1999	The Fair Labor Association (FLA) is created as a "collaboration effort of socially responsible companies, colleges and universities, and civil society organizations to improve working conditions in factories around the world" (www.fairlabor.org).
2000/January	Worldwide Responsible Accredited Production (WRAP) is established and is now the world's largest labor and environmental certification program for apparel manufacturers.
2000/April	The Workers Rights Consortium (WRC) is created as "an independent labor rights monitoring organization" (www.workersrights.org).
2001/January	The FLA approves seven companies for participation in their monitoring program and accredits its first independent external monitor (Verité).
2004	Hotel Employees and Restaurant Employees Union (HERE) and UNITE merge to create UNITE HERE.
2005	Nike becomes the first company in its industry to disclose its factory list.
2010	More than 200 colleges and universities have affiliated with the FLA; 180 have affiliated with the WRC.

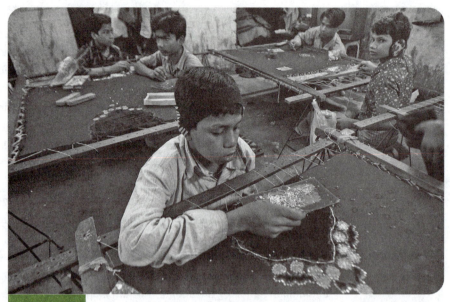

Figure 10.13 Use of child labor in textile and apparel factories is in violation of most companies' codes of conduct.

and of the notorious sweatshop in El Monte, California, where Thai immigrants were held in conditions of semi-enslavement (Bonacich & Appelbaum, 2000).

In the 1990s, many apparel manufacturers and retailers were admonished for using contractors in both the United States and abroad that violated human and labor rights by using child labor, tolerating poor working conditions, and accepting violence against union groups. Initially, the government as well as labor, human rights, and religious groups put pressure on apparel manufacturers and retailers to refrain from using foreign suppliers that violated human and labor rights, and hiring contractors in countries with political policies that violated human and labor rights. However, companies and organizations soon realized that simply boycotting such contractors or countries was not necessarily the answer to this complex problem. In many developing countries, apparel production was found to provide much-needed jobs for thousands of workers. In many cases, the wages of working children were essential for providing basic necessities for themselves and their families. Therefore, rather than punishing these individuals by boycotting the country or contractor and leaving them without needed jobs, apparel companies responded by attempting to reform working conditions and making sure that workers were not abused.

Company Responses—Codes of Conduct and Factory Monitoring/Auditing

Manufacturers and retailers have taken greater responsibility for monitoring the working conditions of their contractors and subcontractors. Many large retailers and mass manufacturers have adopted sourcing guidelines and regularly inspect contractors' facilities to ensure that workers are not being exploited. One of the first companies to implement such guidelines was Levi Strauss & Co. In 1991, it established guidelines for its hired contractors, covering issues such as the treatment of workers and the environmental impact of production (see Tables 10.9 and 10.10). Levi Strauss & Co., which works with contractors throughout the world, regularly inspects factories and will cancel contracts with companies that breach these rules.

In 1996, President Bill Clinton established the Apparel Industry Partnership (AIP), a task force of apparel companies, unions, and human rights groups to focus on sweatshop and human rights issues within the global apparel industry. Members of AIP included companies (e.g., Nike, Liz Claiborne, Nicole Miller, L.L.Bean, Reebok, Phillips-Van Heusen, Patagonia), unions (Union of Needletrades, Industrial, and Textile Employees, Retail Wholesale Department Store Union), and nonprofit organizations (e.g., National Consumers League, International Labor Rights Fund, Business for Social Responsibility). In 1997, the Apparel Industry Partnership presented its agreement and plan of action to end sweatshops. The agreement outlined a Workplace Code of Conduct and Principles of Monitoring that companies would voluntarily adopt and would require their contractors to adopt. The Workplace Code of Conduct includes the following:

- prohibitions against child labor, discrimination, and worker abuse or harassment
- recognition of workers' rights of freedom of association and collective bargaining
- a minimum or prevailing industry wage, a maximum 60-hour work week, and a cap on mandatory overtime
- a safe and healthful working environment

Most large companies, including Nike, Liz Claiborne, Gap, Columbia Sportswear, Reebok, JCPenney, Walmart, Nordstrom, and others, have established their own guidelines and codes of conduct (see Table 10.11 for an example of these guidelines).

Even as companies adopted guidelines, improvement of working conditions in factories was difficult, particularly if companies did not inspect factories and

Table 10.9   Levi Strauss & Co. Terms of Engagement, 2010

1. *Child Labor:* Use of child labor is not permissible. Workers can be no less than 15 years of age and not younger than the compulsory age to be in school. We will not utilize partners who use child labor in any of their facilities. We support the development of legitimate workplace apprenticeship programs for the educational benefit of younger people.

2. *Prison/Forced Labor:* We will not utilize prison or forced labor in contracting relationships in the manufacture and finishing of our products. We will not utilize or purchase materials from a business partner utilizing prison or forced labor.

3. *Disciplinary Practices:* We will not utilize business partners who use corporal punishment or other forms of mental or physical coercion.

4. *Legal Requirements:* We expect our business partners to be law abiding as individuals and to comply with legal requirements relevant to the conduct of all their businesses.

5. *Ethical Standards:* We will seek to identify and utilize business partners who aspire as individuals and in the conduct of all their businesses to a set of ethical standards not incompatible with our own.

6. *Working Hours:* While permitting flexibility in scheduling, we will identify local legal limits on work hours and seek business partners who do not exceed them except for appropriately compensated overtime. While we favor partners who utilize less than 60-hour work weeks, we will not use contractors who, on a regular basis, require in excess of a 60-hour week. Employees should be allowed at least one day off in seven.

7. *Wages and Benefits:* We will only do business with partners who provide wages and benefits that comply with any applicable law and match the prevailing local manufacturing or finishing industry practices.

8. *General Labor Practices and Freedom of Association:* We respect workers' rights to form and join organizations of their choice and to bargain collectively. We expect our suppliers to respect the right to free association and the right to organize and bargain collectively without unlawful interference. Business partners should ensure that workers who make such decisions or participate in such organizations are not the object of discrimination or punitive disciplinary actions and that the representatives of such organizations have access to their members under conditions established either by local laws or mutual agreement between the employer and the worker organizations.

9. *Discrimination:* While we recognize and respect cultural differences, we believe that workers should be employed on the basis of their ability to do the job, rather than on the basis of personal characteristics or beliefs. We will favor business partners who share this value.

10. *Community Involvement:* We will favor business partners who share our commitment to improving community conditions.

11. *Dormitories:* Business partners who provide residential facilities for their workers must provide safe and healthy facilities.

12. *Permits:* Factories must have all current permits as required by law (including business and operating permits, fire-safety and electrical certificates, permits for equipment such as boilers, generators, elevators, fuel and chemical storage tanks, etc. and building, emissions and waste-disposal permits).

SOURCE: Levi Strauss & Co.

Table 10.10	Levi Strauss & Co. Environment, Health, and Safety, 2010

Levi Strauss & Co. has prepared this Environment, Health and Safety (EHS) chapter to help our business partners meet our Social and Environmental Sustainability requirements. EHS requirements are no less important than meeting our quality standards or delivery time.

Safety Guidelines: including safety committees, emergency preparedness, checklists for physical inspections, noise management, temperature management, and asbestos management

Finishing Guidelines: including abrasive blasting and ozone information

Health Guidelines: including factory injuries and communicable disease

Environmental Guidelines: including hazardous materials storage, waste management, and emergency procedures

Sustainability Guidelines: including sustainability metrics and global effluent requirements

SOURCE: Levi Strauss & Co.

enforce their codes and if governments did not enforce certain standards. In many cases, countries resisted adopting certain guidelines, which they viewed as "Western standards" of business. Large companies that may contract in more than 50 countries and work with hundreds of different contractors also found it difficult to inspect and regulate working conditions in every factory. In addition, according to some critics, some companies were interested only in the public relations appeal of sourcing guidelines but did very little to enforce the rules.

Increased public attention was drawn to the sweatshop issue when, in 1996, merchandise endorsed by Kathie Lee Gifford for Walmart was found to have been made in sweatshops in El Salvador and the United States. The negative publicity surrounding this scandal led many manufacturers and retailers to take human rights issues more seriously. At this same time, student activists were waging protests and sit-ins on campuses throughout the United States, asking that colleges and universities provide assurances about how merchandise bearing the college or university name and/or logo was made. In 1998, student activists founded the United Students Against Sweatshops (USAS) as a vehicle for sharing information and organizing activities.

As an outgrowth of the Apparel Industry Partnership, in 1998, the Fair Labor Association (FLA) was established as a factory monitoring association. Members of the FLA must ensure that their factories and contractors comply with an established code of conduct. In 2001, the FLA began approving

Table 10.11	JCPenney Supplier Legal Compliance Program, 2010

Suppliers and Their Selection

In selecting suppliers, JCPenney tries to identify reputable companies that are willing and able to conduct their business in conformity with all applicable legal requirements and the high ethical standards espoused by JCPenney.

Contract Requirements

JCPenney's purchase contracts explicitly require our suppliers to comply with all applicable laws and regulations, including those of the United States and those of any foreign country in which the merchandise is manufactured or from which it is exported. Our contracts also require all suppliers to impose the same obligation on their contractors.

Foreign Sourcing Issues

To address issues of particular concern in the foreign sourcing area, we have stated in our *JCPenney Foreign Sourcing Requirement*s that we will not knowingly allow the importation into the United States of merchandise or knowingly accept merchandise that:

- Does not have accurate country-of-origin labeling;
- Was manufactured with convict, forced, or indentured labor;
- Was manufactured with illegal child labor; or
- Was manufactured in violation of any other applicable labor, workplace safety, or environmental law or regulation.

Labor Law Compliance

We require all domestic suppliers to certify that the merchandise in each shipment they make to JCPenney was produced in compliance with the Fair Labor Standards Act and applicable regulations and orders of the U.S. Department of Labor. Of suppliers of JCPenney brand merchandise we additionally require that they identify all factories and contractors, domestic or foreign, they plan to use to produce such merchandise and certify in writing that each factory will operate in compliance with all applicable labor laws.

Supplier Responsibility for Factory Compliance

We require all foreign and domestic suppliers of JCPenney brand merchandise, and all foreign suppliers of merchandise purchased and imported by JCPenney's sourcing subsidiary, J. C. Penney Purchasing Corporation, to participate in JCPenney's factory legal compliance survey program.

Investigative Procedures

As soon as JCPenney discovers or learns of a potential legal violation by a supplier or its contractors, we will notify the supplier, fully investigate the situation, and, if we determine that the allegations are supported by credible evidence, take corrective action. If the supplier does not cooperate in the investigation, we will terminate our relationship with the supplier.

Environmental Initiatives

In *Matters of Principle: JCPenney & Environmental Responsibility,* we state our commitment to continually review our operations to assess their potential impact on, and to take steps to eliminate or minimize significant threats to, the environment and human health and safety. We expect our suppliers, domestic and foreign, to make and keep the same commitment with respect to their operations, and to ensure that their contractors do the same.

SOURCE: JCPenney

company factory monitoring programs and accrediting independent external factory monitors for use by its member companies. Critics of the FLA voiced concerns over the organization's apparent industry focus. Therefore, in 1999, antisweatshop activists created an alternative system to the FLA, the Worker Rights Consortium (2010), "an independent labor rights monitoring organization" with the goal to "combat sweatshops and protect the rights of workers who make apparel and other products."

In 2000, the American Apparel and Footwear Association and counterpart manufacturers' associations from Mexico, South Africa, the Philippines, El Salvador, Honduras, the Dominican Republic, Nicaragua, Jamaica, and Sri Lanka endorsed their own core production principles of the (then called) Worldwide Responsible Apparel Production (WRAP) program. WRAP now stands for Worldwide Responsible Accredited Production. These production principles form the basis of WRAP's factory-based certification program "dedicated to the certification of lawful, humane, and ethical manufacturing throughout the world" (WRAP, 2010). The certification program focuses on compliance with 12 WRAP principles that focus on labor practices, workers' compensation, freedom of association, factory and environmental conditions, and customs compliance. During this same time period, the Clean Clothes Campaign (CCC) was being implemented in Europe. The CCC is a consortium of unions and nongovernmental organizations in fourteen European countries with the goal of improving working conditions in the worldwide apparel and footwear industries. Along with lobbying companies and government, the CCC has encouraged companies to adopt their Code of Labour Practices.

Organizational and company **codes of conduct** are guidelines that address human resources, health and safety, and labor and environmental laws. Codes of conduct typically include:

- *Corporate principles* or general statements that describe the company's values, objectives, and commitments to the rights of workers.

- *Management philosophy statements* that describe upper management's personal philosophy and their commitment to enforcing the code.

- *Compliance codes* that offer guidance about appropriate or prohibitive conduct. For example, a code of conduct may indicate that no child labor will be used by the contractor.

To be effective, codes of conduct must be credible, that is, taken seriously by governments, consumers, and all companies involved. Credibility, in turn, depends on the level of monitoring, enforcement, and transparency associated with the codes. Transparency is the extent to which the contractors, workers, organizations, governments, and consumers are aware of the codes and how they are enforced.

Thus, the need for effective enforcement of company codes of conduct resulted in the development of **factory monitoring/auditing programs** by companies and organizations. Many companies conduct their own factory monitoring or contract with an independent factory monitor to conduct periodic reviews of factories. The overall goal of these factory monitoring programs and organizations is to improve the working conditions in apparel factories in the United States and abroad. Factory audits typically include the following areas of evaluation:

- efficiency and capacity of the factory
- working conditions—safety, health, and hygiene.
- worker compensation including overtime
- opportunities for freedom of association and collective bargaining
- labor laws
- quality assurance
- security of brand name and merchandise
- subcontractor arrangements

Factory audits are conducted through visual observation of the factory, financial audits, management interviews, worker interviews, and review of government regulations/laws and reports. Factory audits conducted by companies and third-party auditing programs have had mixed results. In some cases, abuses, poor working conditions, and/or irregularities in worker compensation have been improved or corrected. In other cases, contractors have threatened workers, falsified documents, and/or coached workers to cover any problems that may lead to an unsatisfactory audit. However, reputable companies that effectively live up to their corporate responsibility philosophies have used factory audits as a fundamental strategy for improving the lives of and working conditions for individuals worldwide.

Summary

The term sourcing refers to the decision-making process companies use to determine how and where the textile and apparel products or their components will be procured and produced. In making sourcing decisions, companies take into consideration factors that are internal to the company: the company's sourcing philosophy; labor requirements, costs, and productivity; fabric/materials quality and availability; quality assurance/control standards; equipment and skills requirements; required plant/factory capacities; and social responsibility and environmental impact. Factors external to the company are also monitored and considered: trade agreements and other government regulations; shipping distance and expected turnaround time; infrastructure of the country; availability of materials and supplies; political and economic conditions of the country; and natural disasters. Based on these criteria, a number of sourcing options are available to apparel companies and retailers. Major sourcing decisions focus on whether production will be domestic or offshore and whether production will take place in a company-owned facility or will be contracted to others. When contracting, companies also must decide whether cut, make, and trim (CMT), full-package (FP) services, or other options will be used.

Worldwide production of textiles and apparel has focused on providing the world's largest consumer markets—North America and Western Europe—with a steady supply of fashionable apparel, accessories, and home fashions. As such, apparel production occurs in both developed and developing countries. Because of the labor-intensive nature of the apparel industry and the relatively high labor costs in the United States, apparel production within the United States has decreased dramatically over the past 20-plus years. China, India, and other Asian countries have emerged as large producers of both textiles and apparel. As factors such as rising oil costs, availability and cost of raw materials, consumer demand for faster product availability, worldwide threats of terrorism, and brand management emerge as growing concerns, companies are taking a full-supply management approach to sourcing decisions and, in some cases, exploring opportunities for more "local sourcing."

One of the current issues surrounding sourcing decisions is international trade laws that have reduced trade barriers among countries. These include the work of the World Trade Organization, free trade agreements implemented by the United States with other countries and world regions (e.g., NAFTA), and trade preference programs that provide incentives for economic development within certain world regions. As the use of contractors has increased, sweatshops in United States and abroad have re-emerged. Companies have strived to improve working conditions through the adoption and implementation of codes of conduct and factory monitoring/auditing. To be effective, codes of conduct must be credible, enforced, and transparent. Only then will factory audits result in needed improvements for workers worldwide.

To be successful in careers in sourcing, individuals should have an excellent knowledge of company goals, trade laws, production requirements, and available sourcing options. In addition, individuals should have excellent negotiation skills and cultural competency. Sourcing positions typically require travel worldwide.

Sourcing Analyst
Publicly Held Sportswear Company

Position Description:

Develop sourcing plans and costing worksheets, taking into consideration quotas, capacities, pricing, competitiveness, and quality of goods.

Typical Tasks and Responsibilities:

- Determine the source for garment production, and negotiate the terms of production with resources.
- Determine the effect of quotas, tariffs, freight, and other miscellaneous charges on the landed cost of garments.
- Conduct margins analyses.
- If needed, examine sample goods submitted by a source.
- Communicate with other departments (marketing, product development, forecasting and scheduling, customs, and cost accounting).
- Travel to inspect production facilities, examine samples, and negotiate terms.

Key Terms

code of conduct

contractor

corporate responsibility

country of origin

cut, make, and trim (CMT)
    contractor

factory monitoring/auditing program

free trade agreement (FTA)

full-package (FP) contractor

HTS 9802 production

offshore production

quota

social responsibility

socially responsible design

sourcing

sourcing fair

sweatshop

tariff

trade preference program

triple bottom line

yarn forward rule of origin

Discussion Questions and Activities

1. What does a sourcing philosophy of social/corporate responsibility mean for a company? How might a company implement this sourcing philosophy?

2. Over the past 20-plus years, most U.S. apparel companies have shifted from domestic production to offshore production, in many cases sourcing in multiple countries. What are the advantages and disadvantages of sourcing production in the United States? What are the advantages and disadvantages for a U.S. company to produce offshore? What are the advantages and disadvantages of sourcing in multiple countries?

3. Explore the website of a large apparel and/or footwear manufacturer. What is included in the company's code of conduct? How are these codes of conduct implemented? How are these codes of conduct beneficial to consumers?

4. Examine the labels on at least three garments or accessories in your closet. What country of origin is on the label of each item? Why do you believe the item was manufactured in that country?

References

American Apparel and Footwear Association (2010). Environmental standards and best practices guide. Retrieved December 20, 2010, from http://www.appareland-footwear.org/IndustryTools.asp

American Apparel and Footwear Association (2010). Trends: An annual compilation of statistics on the U.S. apparel and footwear industry. Retrieved December 30, 2010, from http:// www.apparelandfootwear.org/Statistics.asp

Bonacich, Edna, and Appelbaum, Richard P. (2000). *Behind the Label: Inequality in the Los Angeles Apparel Industry.* Berkeley: University of California Press.

Bureau of Labor Statistics, U.S. Department of Labor (2010). Career guide to industries, 2010-11 edition, textile, textile product, and apparel manufacturing. Retrieved June 27, 2010, from http://www.bls.gov/oco/cg/cgs015.htm

Clean Clothes Campaign (2010). Retrieved December 30, 2010, from http://www.cleanclothes.org/

EmergingTexiles.com (May 23, 2008). Apparel manufacturing labor costs. Retrieved November 28, 2010, from http://www.emergingtextiles.com/?q=art&s=080523-apparel-labor-cost&r=free

Fair Labor Association (2010). Retrieved November 15, 2010, from http://www.fairlabor.org/

International Labor Organization (2010). Retrieved December 15, 2010, from http://www.ilo.org/global/lang—en/index.htm

International Labor Rights Forum (2010). Creating a sweatfree world. Retrieved December 30, 2010 from http://www.laborrights.org/creating-a-sweatfree-world

Lii, Jane H. (1995, March 12). Week in sweatshop reveals grim conspiracy of the poor. *New York Times*, pp. 1, 40.

U.S. Department of Commerce (2010). International Trade Administration. Office of Textiles and Apparel. Trade Data. Retrieved November 30, 2010, from http://www.otexa.ita.doc.gov/msrpoint.htm

U.S. Trade Representative (2010). Trade Agreements. Retrieved November 1, 2010, from http://www.ustr.gov/trade-agreements

Worker Rights Consortium (2010). Retrieved December 1, 2010, from http://www.workersrights.org/

World Trade Organization (2010). International Trade Statistics 2010. Retrieved December 1, 2010, from http://www.wto.org/english/res_e/statis_e/statis_e.htm

Worldwide Responsible Accredited Production (2010). Retrieved December 30, 2010, from http://www.wrapcompliance.org/

CHAPTER 11

Production Processes
and Quality Assurance

In this chapter, you will learn the following:

- the manufacturing environments used for production

- the production processes used in manufacturing

- the components of quality assurance and the importance of quality assurance in delivering on-time, acceptable merchandise to the retailer

- the role of agents who assist manufacturers in bringing products produced offshore into the United States

**Step 7: Apparel Production Processes,
Material Management, and Quality Assurance**

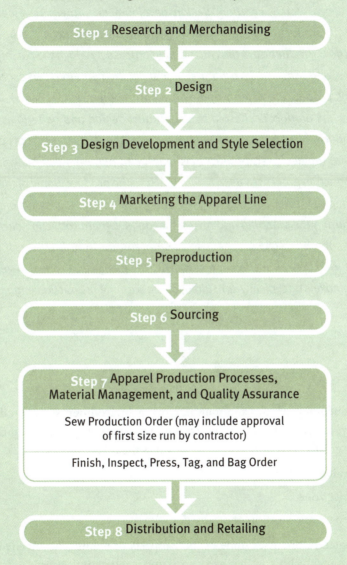

Step 1 Research and Merchandising

Step 2 Design

Step 3 Design Development and Style Selection

Step 4 Marketing the Apparel Line

Step 5 Preproduction

Step 6 Sourcing

Step 7 Apparel Production Processes,
Material Management, and Quality Assurance

Sew Production Order (may include approval
of first size run by contractor)

Finish, Inspect, Press, Tag, and Bag Order

Step 8 Distribution and Retailing

Production Considerations

*T*he previous chapters discuss the development of a product line from market research, creation, design development, pattern development, and preproduction through sourcing options. The product line is now ready for production. **Production** is the construction process by which the cut fabric pieces, findings, and trims are incorporated into a finished apparel, accessory, or home fashions product (see Step 7 of the flowchart on the previous page). The cost to produce the product is affected by the product design and pattern, as well as by the production process used. Therefore, it is essential to the success of the company that the designer, product developer, and patternmaker be well versed in the production processes used to manufacture the product. Some of the decisions regarding the relationship among the design, pattern, and production processes occur during the planning and review meetings. Other production decisions take place as the new style proceeds through preproduction. However, if difficulties arise during the production of a new style, the designer, product developer, and patternmaker are typically consulted, along with the production engineer.

Production processes and **manufacturing environments** (the production facility, location of production, choice of production process, and cycle time) vary greatly, depending on factors such as the following:

- available technology
- price zone
- geographic location of production

Chapter 10 discusses some of these aspects of manufacturing environments. Computer technology has had a great impact on manufacturing environments. In turn, changes continue to occur in the entire soft-goods pipeline, from the fiber producer to the consumer. Continual new developments in supply chain management and product lifecycle management (PLM) create great flexibility in production processes and manufacturing environments. This chapter provides an overview of the methods of producing, assuring product quality, and importing goods within three manufacturing environments.

Manufacturing Environments

The three manufacturing environments, or strategies, include mass production, fast fashion production, and mass customization. The product type as well as the strategy used for replenishment of the product will determine which of these three environments will be used for production. Each of these three manufacturing environments is discussed here.

Mass Production

The mass production manufacturing environment is suitable for cutting and sewing very large quantities of each product, using one of several possible mass production processes that are discussed later in this chapter. Mass production capitalizes on economies of scale. Basic staple products such as T-shirts, jeans, underwear, socks, and hosiery fit this manufacturing environment. These products have a low fashion risk, in part because they can remain on the retail floor longer than many fashion goods. The focus of mass production is on in-store replenishment of products (see Chapter 12). Seasonal goods include some staple products, such as turtlenecks, produced in seasonal colors. The selling time for seasonal goods falls between the selling time for staple goods and for fashion goods. Thus, some seasonal goods are manufactured in the mass-production environment, while other seasonal goods are manufactured in the short-cycle manufacturing environment, which is discussed in the next section.

The demand for staple goods and some seasonal goods tends to be easier to forecast than for fashion goods. This provides an opportunity for a slightly longer lead time for the mass-production manufacturing environment than the other manufacturing environments offer. Longer lead time means that production can be sourced globally, providing an opportunity for lower labor costs. With the relatively high labor costs for U.S. production, production of high-volume basic products is more cost efficient at vertically integrated factories or in factories in areas of the world where labor costs are lower. Because of its longer production time and retail selling time, the cost of carrying this inventory (both to the manufacturer and to the retailer) is greater than for goods that are manufactured closer to the time of their market demand.

Fast Fashion Production

To respond to the demands of fast fashion, retailers employ a variety of techniques, including strategic sourcing, production, and stocking. These practices accelerate the design-to-delivery cycle of their clothing by as much as 90 percent compared to the rest of the garment industry. They also cut costs throughout the design, delivery, and sales cycle. As the name implies, this manufacturing environment is well suited to products that are produced closer to the time of their market demand than mass-produced products. Fast fashion or **short-cycle production** is well suited for very high-fashion products, which are placed into the market for short selling seasons (six to eight weeks), with no intention of in-store replenishment.

Successful fast fashion retailers source labor and materials close to home and produce many small manufacturing runs to reduce cycle time. To accelerate the design process, these companies employ many in-house designers who can create thousands of designs based on upcoming trends. Due to the ever-increasing speed of production, a result of the application of computer technology to supply chain management, PDM/PLM, and the monitoring of consumer sales, **fast fashion production** (where products go from concept to retail stores in less than three weeks) is greatly reduced. The Spanish retailer Zara is particularly successful in reducing cycle time, claiming that some of their items go from concept to delivery in as little as two weeks. (Barry, 2004)

Mass Customization

A short-cycle manufacturing environment that is applied to an individual customer is called the mass-customization manufacturing environment. **Mass customization** involves the ultimate consumer in the customization of fit, design, or personalization of the product. Because the ultimate consumer is involved with design and/or fit choices, it may appear that mass customization can best be categorized as a design variation. However, mass customization deals with products that are already designed; the customer is simply customizing the product.

The emergence of new technology has provided a means to link the customer at the retail store to the apparel factory, resulting in mass customization. The cost efficiency of mass production is maintained. One key point in mass customization is that the customer selects and pays for the product before it is produced. Thus, the phrase *sell one, make one* is appropriate.

For the manufacturer and retailer, the advantages to mass customization include the following:

- reducing large inventories
- minimizing returns
- reducing distribution costs
- building strong customer relationships

- solidifying brand loyalty
- identifying customer preferences and buying habits

Mass customization requires electronically linked, seamless integration of components throughout the entire supply chain in order to operate. It requires a manufacturing environment suited to individualization, yet with a fast turn-around time and at a low cost. Custom tailors and dressmakers are not producing these goods; within the mass-customization manufacturing environment, agile manufacturing is required. This production process is discussed along with other production processes later in this chapter.

The mass-customization manufacturing environment utilizes all the newest computer technologies, supply chain management, PDM/PLM, and some level of customization of the product for the individual customer (see Figure 11.1).

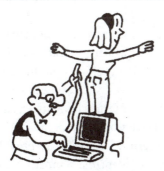

A sales clerk measures the customer using instructions from a computer as an aid.

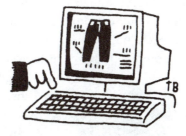

The clerk enters the measurements, and adjusts the data based on the customer's reaction to samples.

The final measurements are relayed to a computerized fabric-cutting machine at the factory.

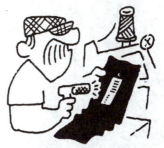

Bar codes are attached to the clothing to track it as it is assembled, washed and prepared for shipment.

Figure 11.1 Mass customization is made possible by computer technology.

Pattern alteration software allows customers to customize a garment for their specific size. The more traditional approaches to developing a design for a target market are discussed in previous chapters. The pattern is developed based on a company's target customer size standard. The "standard" size apparel fits some bodies better than others. With the development of new computer technology, PDM/PLM, and supply chain management, a type of custom apparel different from the custom-made apparel produced by personal tailors or dressmakers of the past is possible. Mass customization is a consumer-driven strategy that allows limited customization of a standard style, such as size, color, or trim choices. On the other hand, **made-to-measure** apparel is a fully customized process where a garment is made specifically for one individual based on his/her measurements and preferences. The difference between made-to-measure and mass customization is the degree of customization offered. However, the difference is blurring as technology provides tools to blend made-to-measure with mass customization (Figure 11.2).

Brooks Brothers, a retailer and manufacturer of men's and women's classic professional clothing, provides an example of mass customization with which customers can build their own dress shirt. Ordering shirts from the catalog is a simple process that gives customers basic choices, such as: neck size, sleeve length, choice of three body styles, choice of three cuff styles, and 17 top-end fabric selections. Patternmaking software provides the capability to adapt the standard pattern to specific design and sizes. Delivery takes two to three weeks.

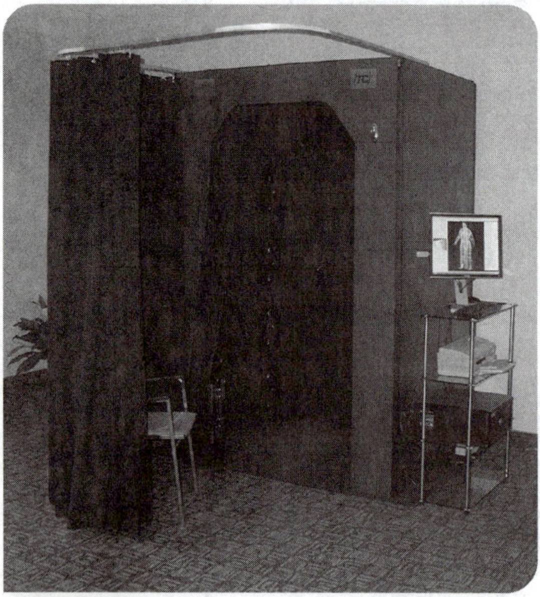

Early ventures in made-to-measure using mass production at the factory included men's tailored suits. The customer was measured at the tailor's retail store. With some systems, front, back, and side-view photographs of the customer standing in front of a measurement grid were also sent to the factory. The customer's measurements were input into the computer system that was linked electronically to the apparel factory's computer. The body dimensions were translated into specific differences between the "standard" pattern and the customer's needed adjustments. The pattern changes were made by computer

Figure 11.2 Body scanners capture precise body measurement data into a computer system.

calculations, and a customized pattern was plotted. Laser cutters allowed fast, single-ply computerized cutting of the garment pieces. With careful tracking through production, the cut pieces for each customized suit were sent through the mass-manufacturing process. The customer returned to the retail store for a final "fitting" for pant hemming and other minor adjustments handled by the retailer before the customer received the finished goods.

One of the challenges of made-to-measure apparel is the assessment of customer fit preferences, since some customers prefer a looser fit, while others prefer a more snug fit to their suits. The system "suggests a try-on size from the store's inventory, which is an integral part of the process" (Rabon, 2000, p. 40). Mass-customization options that include customizing the fit have expanded greatly with the continued development of electronically linked body measuring, patternmaking, cutting, and production technology.

Advances in computer pattern design systems have aided the implementation of mass customization (Figure 11.3). In some cases, once the customer's measurements have been input, the software analyzes the measurements and compares them to standard profiles to recommend a best size. Some made-to-measure software systems have built-in posture adjustments that can be requested, such as for round shoulders.

Another product well suited to mass customization is footwear. Each person's left foot is somewhat different in size from the right foot. By scanning each foot, the shoes can be customized to fit each foot precisely. The huge inventories of shoes stocked in varying lengths and widths, styles, and colors can be greatly reduced by mass customization, while the customer's shoe fit can be enhanced by scanning technology.

Production Sewing Systems

Although new production systems have been developed, older, traditional mass-manufacturing systems are still used in some facilities. It is important to understand the variety of production systems in order to make informed decisions about the production system most suitable for the garment style, price range, and sourcing option.

Single-Hand System

As discussed in Chapter 7, the prototype product is produced by a single individual. The sample maker (also called a *sample hand*) completes all the steps required in production, moving from one type of specialized equipment to another

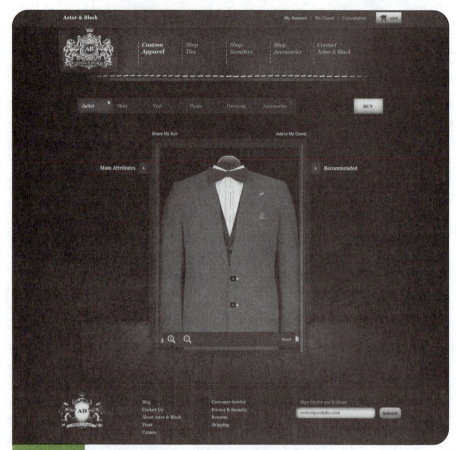

Figure 11.3   Mass customization links the customer's style preferences, selected at the retail store or through the Internet, to the production site.

as needed, based on the garment or product style's requirements. Some apparel and accessory goods are produced in limited quantities using a system similar to that used to sew the prototype. In a single-hand system, one individual is responsible for sewing an entire garment. The bundle for this production system would include all the garment or product parts for one style in one size. In today's market, the **single-hand system** is used for couture and for some very high-priced apparel produced in a limited quantity. This system is slower than mass-production systems, and it may include considerable detail or handwork during production.

While some apparel is still sewn one at a time in a single-hand system, most apparel is manufactured using one of several production systems of large-quantity or *mass manufacturing*. The most common categories of these production systems are **progressive bundle systems** and flexible manufacturing systems.

Progressive Bundle System

Before the implementation of Quick Response and supply chain management strategies, the progressive bundle system was the most common production system used by apparel manufacturers. With the progressive bundle system, garment parts for a specified number of garments (for example, a dozen garments) are bundled together and put in carts that are rolled from one sewing machine operator to another. Each machine operator is responsible for the following:

- opening the bundle of the garment parts
- performing one or two construction steps on each garment in the bundle
- rebundling the garment parts for transport to the next operator

The operator's pay is calculated based on the **piece-rate wage**, the number of pieces completed per day (see Figure 11.4).

The progressive bundle system is especially well suited to large bundles of work, usually from one dozen to three dozen units per bundle. At each operator's work station, one bundle is in process while one or several more bundles are waiting. Sometimes referred to as a *batch* or *push* system, the progressive bundle system tends to generate high levels of **work-in-process (WIP)**. Also, a considerable investment of inventory is tied up with the WIP.

With the progressive bundle system, equipment is selected and sometimes customized to perform one or several functions needed for the production of the specific style. Each piece of equipment is positioned on the floor in relation to the equipment and sewing sequence required before and

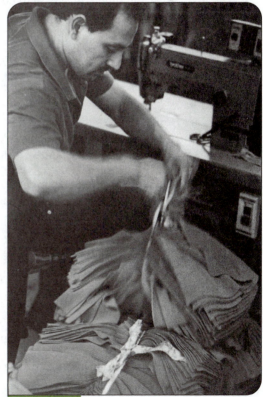

Figure 11.4 With the bundle system, a sewing operator performs one or several sewing steps on each garment in the bundle.

after each step in the production sequence. The machine operator is highly trained to perform one or several steps on specific equipment. Each sewing facility tends to specialize in certain types of products, such as backpacks or swimwear. This specialization is due in part to the fact that different types of equipment are needed for producing different categories of products.

Sometimes the facility is arranged so that the body of the jacket is assembled in one part of the facility, and the lining is assembled in another part of the facility. The two parts of each garment are united at the final assembly stage. This requires careful tagging to ensure that sizes and dye lots are matched correctly at the final assembly stage. Due to the nature of the progressive bundle system, it can be difficult to pinpoint where a quality problem originates.

A new style ready for production may differ from previous styles in its production sequence or equipment needs. Machine operators may need additional training, so it may take time to develop the expertise to run at full capacity. Equipment may have to be moved within the facility to prepare for a different production sequence.

Flexible Manufacturing Systems

For mass-manufactured products, the bottom line is cost containment. This is affected by the following:

- the length of time that is required to prepare the product for production
- the length of time that the product is in process (work-in-process or WIP)

Reduction in one or both of these will result in a lower production cost. Some companies focused on developing more **flexible manufacturing systems** involving one or all of the following:

- reorganization of existing equipment on the floor into a new systems approach
- development of new equipment
- reorganization of the way garments are routed through production
- reorganization of workers into teams who are cross-trained to handle a variety of operations using an assortment of equipment

Flexible manufacturing (FM) is defined as "any departure from traditional mass-production systems of apparel toward faster, smaller, more flexible production units that depend upon the coordinated efforts of minimally supervised teams of workers" (AAMA, Technical Advisory Committee, 1988, as cited in Hill, 1992). FM systems are known by many names, including the following:

- modular manufacturing
- self-directed work teams
- compact production teams
- flexible work groups

The emphasis of the strategy is on group effort, employee involvement, and employee empowerment.

In FM systems, manufacturing management makes a shift away from high individual productivity and low cost to short manufacturing cycles, small quantity of work-in-process, and quick delivery of the finished product. Flexible manufacturing is well suited to smaller production runs compared to large production runs that are efficient with the progressive bundle system. The term **modular manufacturing** is most often used in the U.S. apparel industry to describe flexible manufacturing.

With modular manufacturing, which is often referred to as a *pull system*, the sewing facility is organized into teams of seven to ten operators each. Operators are cross-trained in all areas of garment construction. Each operator might work on two or three machines. Operators might perform several tasks at each machine, or one machine might be used for a series of assembly operations. Every team is responsible for the production of entire garments, instead of one operator being assigned a single operation, such as setting in a sleeve or a zipper (as is done with the progressive bundle system). Equipment is arranged in modules so that work can be passed from one team member to another, who may work in either a standing or sitting position. The number of units within each operation may vary from only one to as many as ten.

Within a module, operators work as a team and solve problems, thus creating a more productive environment. Flaws in production are handled as a team; if a mistake is found, the entire garment is returned to the team, where the operators decide how best to fix it. Therefore, the traditional piece-rate wage is not applicable. The team is paid not only according to the quantity it produces, but also by the quality of its work. Pay is based on a collective effort. In theory, if an apparel factory was completely "modular," it would be redesigned into modular units, with each module producing complete garments in a few hours.

The following factors must be taken into consideration before a company decides to change to this system of manufacturing:

- Downtime is particularly critical with modular methods. With modular manufacturing, each minute a machine is down costs money, as it can slow down the entire team's work progress. A worker's absence can also slow down production.

* Converting to a modular manufacturing system requires the involvement of all employees, an investment in education and training, a shift of management responsibilities from a few people to the team as a whole, and support from management.

* The shift to modular manufacturing requires a cultural change within a company. The way employees think and perform has to create effective teams.

Some manufacturing facilities shifted to modular manufacturing in hopes of reducing manufacturing costs. For some companies, however, costs rose at first. Not only is there the cost involved if new equipment is purchased, cross-training employees costs money, and reduced productivity during training is an additional start-up cost. It may take months before a cost savings is realized (Abend, 1999).

For companies that commit to modular manufacturing, its cost benefits have been realized by containing costs through inventory reduction, a reduction in work-in-process, and for some facilities, an improvement in product quality.

Productivity has increased dramatically at some facilities that shifted to modular manufacturing. At Nygård International's Winnipeg manufacturing headquarters production capacity "jumped from 20,000 to approximately 75,000 units per week under the modular arrangement" (Winger, 1998, p. AS-16).

Another advantage of modular manufacturing is that production facilities can shift quickly from manufacturing one type of product category to another. For example, a manufacturer can change its production facilities to accommodate producing intimate apparel, backpacks, and swimwear. At one facility, "engineers swap out the equipment as the last items in one product go through the line. Overnight the facility is ready for the new line, and then it's a matter of training operators, which can take one to three weeks to reach full capacity" (Hill, 1998, p. AS-8).

Some companies that have tried modular manufacturing found it was not successful for them. Although Levi Strauss & Co. no longer has production facilities in the United States, its trial with modular manufacturing is worth reviewing. The company opened a new modular manufacturing facility in 1995. At the end of the first year, excess costs were astronomically high, attributed to exceptional start-up costs. By the end of the second year, the capacity had increased about 53 percent, but excess costs were over 31 percent. Halfway into the third year, capacity had increased 6 percent over the second year.

However, the excess costs had increased to 49 percent over standard (Dunagan, 1999). In an article about Levi's modular manufacturing attempt, consulting engineer Charles Gilbert stated, "Thirty-four months after start-up in modules, we converted the plant to the 'old' progressive bundle system" (Dunagan, 1999). Management at Levi Strauss & Co. did not have the answer regarding what went wrong with its attempt at modular manufacturing. A number of factors may have contributed to its lack of success. In some cases, companies do not completely convert all aspects of employee training, equipment needs, and management commitment to modular manufacturing. It is clear that the choice of manufacturing method is dependent on many variables.

UNIT PRODUCTION SYSTEMS

To achieve efficient manufacturing, some companies have invested in a computerized overhead transport system such as the **unit production system (UPS)**. With UPS, garment parts are fed on overhead conveyors, usually one garment at a time, to sewing machine operators (see Figure 11.5). Garment parts are delivered directly to the operators' ergonomically designed workstations. This dramatically reduces operator handling time during production.

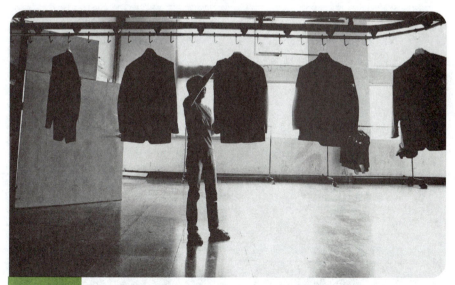

Figure 11.5 With a unit production system, the pieces of each garment are delivered to the sewing operator. The operator may not need to remove the garment from the conveyor while performing the sewing operation.

Workstations can be moved easily to accommodate different equipment needs for various garments. Operators are cross-trained in a number of procedures in the manufacturing cycle, similar to the way they are for modular manufacturing. The transport system is designed to include bar codes to track WIP.

A study by Clemson Apparel Research (Hill, 1994) determined that UPS would provide the hypothetical apparel manufacturing plant a 329 percent return on its investment and would pay for itself in 11 months. The primary savings to the company would be in the areas of reduced direct labor costs (shorter waiting periods, less overtime, improved ergonomics) and reduced work-in-process inventory levels. Figure 11.6 shows computerized tracking of WIP. Many production facilities have shown substantial increases in production with UPS. Other companies have found UPS to be less successful. As with modular manufacturing, many variables enter into the success of UPS.

AGILE MANUFACTURING

Agile manufacturing combines a variety of technologies that together form a totally integrated, seamless exchange of information linking retailers and sup-

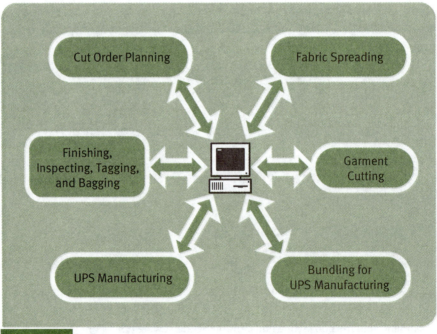

Figure 11.6 Computerized production systems permit computer tracking of work-in-process as well as increased efficiency compared with the bundle system.

pliers to the manufacturing facility. An example is mass customization. This manufacturing environment allows for individual changes in style, color, and fit, using a customer's body measurements and modifications of a pattern based on a style developed by the apparel company. The manufacturing facility cuts an individual customized style from a PDS and marker-making system linked electronically to a single-ply cutter. White fabric prepared for digital printing might be printed before or after cutting (see Chapter 6) to the customer's color and print specifications. After printing and cutting, the garment is manufactured using a production system that is designed to accommodate units of one (see Figure 11.7).

Rabon and Deaton (1999) contended that an overhead conveyor system for unit production (UPS) is a key to success of companies in the mass-customization arena. Modular

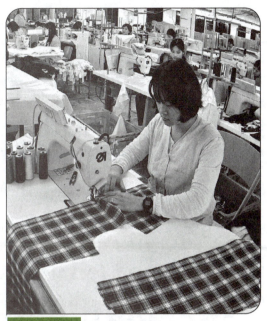

Figure 11.7 Manufacturing designed to accommodate units of one.

manufacturing teams of cross-trained operators sew the customized orders. Computer-based learning materials and interactive programs help provide the training that sewing operators need. After completion, the order is packaged and sent directly to the customer, eliminating warehouse inventories. It is the integration of these technologies that creates agile manufacturing.

Combination of Systems

Some production facilities utilize more than one type of production system. For example, a contractor may use UPS for certain garment styles that suit this production system, while using a progressive bundle system for other styles. As discussed earlier, the number of units to be made influences the production system. For example, modular manufacturing may be more economical for small production runs than the progressive bundle system.

Production Workers' Wage Rates

The progressive bundle system of production frequently uses a piece-rate wage system. Each operator's pay is based on individual productivity. The number of units the operator has completed at the end of each workday or week is the basis for the operator's pay for that time period. New developments in software provide a means to set accurate piece rates in a manufacturing environment that is constantly changing.

With modular manufacturing, some companies use a team wage calculation rate. Bonus incentives might be provided for exemplary productivity and/or a very low rate of errors or irregulars.

Some companies have decided that an hourly rate is most equitable. An hourly rate gives the flexibility to change production runs during the day, especially if a priority order has just been cut and needs to be produced immediately. Also, an hourly rate is fairer if production includes diverse products.

Developments in Production Equipment and Technology

The industrial machines used in production facilities are designed to sew much faster than home sewing machines. While home sewing machines are driven by motors, industrial machines have engines, with a clutch, a brake, and continuous oil feed. Home sewing machines can perform many different functions—sew straight stitch seams, zigzag, overcast, blind hem, and make buttonholes. Industrial machines perform very specialized functions—sew buttonholes or sew straight stitch (lockstitch) seams or blind stitch hems. The specialized equipment may be fitted with additional devices or guides to customize an operation further. For example, a metal plate can be added to the sewing bed to guide elastic evenly under the needle.

While many machines for production were developed so that operators sit during operation, standup sewing is another option (see Figure 11.8). It costs about $1,000 to convert a sewing machine to standup operation. Ergonomic analysis indicates that there are substantial advantages to stand-up sewing.

An example of a development in production technology is one that focused on reducing the puckering encountered when assembling wrinkle-resistant cotton and cotton/polyester-blend dress shirts, lightweight slacks, uniforms, and other casual wear. TAL Apparel of Hong Kong, one of the world's largest shirt makers, spent four years developing its TAL Pucker Free process. A bonding tape is inserted into the seam between two layers of fabric. The tape, which contains a thermal adhesive component, is melted during the manufacturing process. "The result is a strong, permanent bond along the seam that eliminates differential shrinkage between the thread and fabric, the primary cause of seam puckering" (DesMarteau, 1998). The company patented a seam

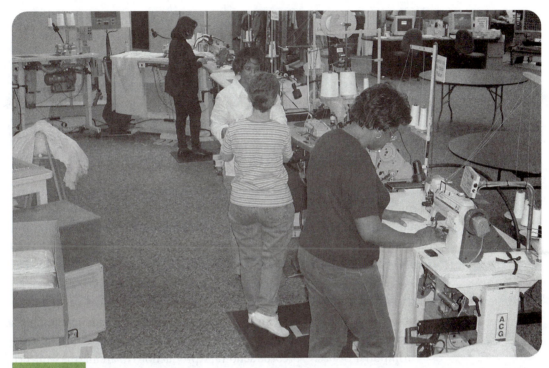

Figure 11.8 Sewing equipment has been developed to facilitate operation by workers who stand rather than sit while sewing.

sealing process in the United States and has licensed the technology to U.S. manufacturers. Licensees pay a royalty fee, a percent of the retail price of the garment, to TAL.

Equipment maintenance is a critical concern for production sewing. Any breakdown of equipment can stall production, which can be of great concern to an entire team on a production line. Maintenance personnel must be ready to troubleshoot, repair, or replace equipment rapidly. New developments have alleviated some of the maintenance concerns. For example, computerized systems have been developed to distribute power and electrical information to all sewing stations. In some countries, machine parts or technicians are not immediately available, causing delays in the production schedule.

The noise level and airborne fiber particles in sewing facilities are concerns, especially in some offshore facilities. In the United States, workers wear protective clothing, air filtration systems are used in factories, and other environmental controls have been implemented.

High-technology systems will continue to play an increasingly important role in cost reduction efforts. Regardless of the production system used, new equipment will be developed to enhance production. These developments include new types of computerized, programmable sewing machines; robotic sewing equipment; and continued improvements in cutting equipment. Just as the cost of personal computers has declined over time, high-tech equipment costs have also declined, making it more affordable to apparel manufacturers.

Production Sequence

Different categories of products may require very different processes and types of equipment. For example, men's tailored suits require many more steps in production than men's casual sportswear. In addition, the types of sewing and pressing equipment are quite different for tailored apparel as compared to sportswear. In Chapter 4, it was mentioned that different sewing processes and types of equipment are required for various classifications of apparel. Boys' and girls' clothing requires similar sewing processes and equipment and could be manufactured at the same facility, whereas men's tailored clothing and men's sportswear production need to be handled by different production facilities.

An important aspect of preproduction and production is planning the sequence of operations required to produce the garment style. Production includes the sewing sequence, as well as other tasks performed at the sewing facility that relate to completing the product. These tasks might include the following:

- fusing interfacing
- applying embroidery
- applying labels
- pressing
- attaching hangtags
- folding and packaging (or hanging and bagging) the finished product

These production steps and the time required for each step need to be determined for each garment style. This information is referred to as the *construction specifications* (see Chapter 9).

As discussed in Chapter 9, the sequence of sewing operations may have been determined at the time that the style's cost was calculated. The production sequence used to sew the sales representatives' samples, made to market the style to retail buyers, is frequently the same as the sequence used to sew the production orders. Any problems in production might be corrected during the production of the sales samples.

Determining the most efficient production sequence depends on many factors, such as the following:

- the equipment capabilities of the specific production facility (e.g., the availability of a pocket-setting machine can greatly speed production of a style with a welt pocket)

- the labor cost of the operators (in some factories where labor is very inexpensive, more work may be done by hand than with expensive equipment)

- whether certain steps should be subcontracted (e.g., a shirt with a pleated front inset might be less expensive to produce if the fabric for the front inset were sent to a pleating contractor and then returned to the production facility for cutting and sewing into the shirt)

Some operations may be performed prior to the sewing process, such as the following:

- Interfacing may be fused to garment sections prior to sewing. The pieces to be fused are laid on conveyor belts and moved through large fusing "ovens" to adhere the interfacing.

- Patch pockets, such as those sewn to the back of jeans, are prepared for sewing by prepressing the raw edges to the inside. By folding the edges over a metal template of the exact size of the finished pocket, accurate dimensions can be maintained. A fusing agent might be applied to help the seam allowances adhere to the inside of the pocket. Hundreds of pockets are prepared, then they are delivered to the site where they will be attached to the pants. Since garment pieces may be cut from dye lots with varying colors, care must be taken to match pocket pieces to garment sections from an identical dye lot. If the pockets were made in small, medium, and large sizes, care must be taken to attach the prepared pockets to the correct size pant.

- Belt loops might be made from very long strips prepared for the entire production run. Yards of the strips are wound onto holders attached to the sewing station. The belt loops are cut to length one at a time and sewn sequentially around the pant waistband.

Many processes are streamlined to provide the most labor-effective production.

Sometimes several different factories are used to produce a large order. In such cases, the production sequences may not be exactly the same at the different factories producing the same style. Each contractor submits a sample sewn at its factory to the apparel manufacturer for approval. For the samples sewn for sales representatives by contractors, the same process of submitting a sewn sample is used. The contractor's sample is called a **sew by** or a **counter sample**. After approval, this sample is used as the benchmark against which to check the sewn production goods.

Although great effort is expended to plan a smooth production run, many problems can stall production. Some problems that involve the procurement of materials have already been discussed. Production problems include complications due to delays in receiving a shipment of zippers or late arrival of subcontracted work. Troubleshooting is an integral part of production. When sourcing offshore, unexpected problems can be difficult to solve. A flood in Bangladesh, a hurricane in the Dominican Republic, or a rail workers' strike in France can cause production or delivery delays that could not be planned for or avoided. Management personnel of apparel manufacturers often travel to production facilities (whether company-owned or contractor-owned) to check on production or help solve production problems.

Finishing

At the end of the production line, the goods await various finishing steps. Pressing may occur only at this stage in production. Edge stitching or topstitching may be used to reduce the need to press during production, thereby reducing labor costs. Specialized pressing equipment produces excellent results on finished goods very quickly. For tailored jackets, a steam mannequin might be used to press the entire jacket while on a three-dimensional form. Other types of specialized equipment perform other functions, such as turning pant legs right-side-out (pants come off the production line inside out). Finishing operations include thread trimming, button and snap attachment, shoulder pad and lining tacking, pressing, and buttoning the garment.

Some labels are sewn in during production. These might include care labels, brand labels, and size labels. Printed care, fiber content, and size information can also be heat sealed directly onto the product. This method eliminates the potential for skin irritation from a woven label, as well as the bulk produced by one or more sew-in labels applied to a product. Called **tagless labels**, they debuted first on T-shirts, then underwear, performance wear, and children's wear—products where labels can be particularly annoying. The market trend is toward increased use of tagless labels (see Figure 11.9).

Other labels, as well as hangtags, might be attached during finishing operations. Hangtags can be used to provide additional product marketing information. For example, the water resistance or UV protective properties of a jacket's

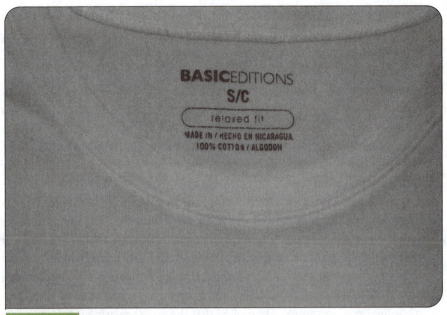

Figure 11.9 Finishing processes include the application of tagless labels.

fabric might be explained on the hangtag. Providing goods with floor-ready labels and hangtags takes place at this stage in production. Preparing floor-ready merchandise is discussed later in this chapter, as well as in Chapter 12. Labels might include identifying characteristics hidden to the eye. A bar code "fingerprint" visible to a scanning device can be included in the sew-in label to identify the product's production facility or retail destination. This technology can reduce the possibility of counterfeit goods and can also be used by the retailer to verify the origin of goods returned by customers.

One system uses a silicon chip tagging system. Called Radio Frequency Identification (RFID), the silicon chip is attached to an antenna made of thin, flexible silver ink that utilizes radio frequency identification technology. In addition to deterring hijacking and shoplifting, the tag can be used to sort laundry and to log the number of times a uniform has been laundered. The tag is about the size of a garment label and is coated with a plastic laminate to protect it from dry-cleaning chemicals. The tag can be sewn into a seam, hidden from view to deter removal by shoplifters or counterfeiters. (See also Chapter 1.) Another technology used to verify authenticity of products is the use of "metallic strips (similar to those in U.S. currency) that are woven into labels and covert yarns that are visible under certain wavelengths of light. Companies are also weaving serial numbers into labels, providing each garment with a unique identifier" (Speer, 2004, p. 29).

Other types of finishing operations include a variety of fabric treatments. Special finishes might be incorporated during finishing of the garments, rather than to the textile goods at the textile mill. For example, a wrinkle-resistant finish might be applied to apparel goods, such as 100 percent cotton trousers, after they are sewn. Technological developments will continue to improve garment-applied finishes.

Garments might be laundered before shipping. Laundering might be performed to enhance the hand or visual appeal of the fabric. For example, stone washing is used to soften denim fabric. Other treatments are used to "age" or distress denim. Another reason for laundering is to shrink a product prior to shipping. While we are familiar with purchasing some products large enough to "shrink to fit," many consumers find it advantageous to know that the garment has been preshrunk. They know that the way the garment fits when it is tried on at the retail store is the way it will fit after washing at home. For garments that will be laundered after production and before shipping, the pattern pieces for the garment have to be created very carefully with the exact shrinkage factor incorporated into each pattern piece.

Many apparel manufacturers produce dyed products in color allotments based on the quantity of orders for each color. Other manufacturers produce "colorless" garments, and then dye the garments during finishing. Such goods are referred to as **garment dyed**. Dyeing finished goods has several advantages. It can provide quick delivery of the goods to the retailer because production can begin on the colorless garments while the sales force is accumulating the sales totals by color. For the same reason, it represents a reduced risk to the manufacturer. Garment dyeing can be considered one of the Quick Response strategies. Care must be taken to select buttons and other findings and trims that can accommodate the dyeing operation.

Finishing operations can produce air pollutants or waste products that must be discarded. Since concern was first raised about the environmental consequences of some finishing operations, much has been done to minimize their negative environmental impact. New developments will continue to improve environmental protection.

Goods are prepared for shipping by being folded or hung. At some facilities, folding might be accomplished by hand, with cardboard, tissue, straight pins, and plastic bags. At other facilities, machines are used to fold the goods. For garments placed on hangers, overhead conveyors bring the garments to equipment that covers each item with a plastic bag. Some hanger and bagged garments are moved from a conveyor belt at the factory directly onto an overhead track on the truck that delivers the bagged garments to the manufacturer's distribution center, to the retailer's distribution center, or directly to the retail store (see Chapter 12).

Floor-Ready Merchandise

Floor-ready merchandise (FRM) is an aspect of Quick Response and supply chain management that results from an alliance between the apparel manufacturer and the retailer. FRM shifts certain steps from the retailer to the manufacturer, where they become part of the finishing process. The FRM policies generally require that the apparel manufacturer ship the goods to the retailer's distribution center or retail store with bar-coded price tickets, carton labels, shipping documents, and hanger applications. "If FRM can only remove two days of delay associated with a retailer's distribution center, and if the DC [distribution center] is typically receiving goods every two weeks, then it is possible to get 52 additional selling days per year" (Swank, 1995, p. 106). The use of floor-ready merchandise from the retailer's perspective is discussed in Chapter 12.

Quality Assurance

As discussed in Chapter 3, **quality assurance** involves making sure the product meets the standards of acceptance set forth by the contracting party. The contracting party might be the apparel manufacturer for goods produced by a contractor. The contracting party might be a retailer for private-label or store brand goods. Many of the fabrics and trims and sewing operations are specified in detail on the garment specification sheet and are an important part of quality assurance. Visual inspection after completion of production—for loose threads, for example—forms another important part of quality assurance.

The fabric inspection component of quality assurance was discussed in Chapters 3 and 9. The spreading and cutting operations include considerations such as on-grain garment parts and dye lot color matching. Quality assurance also takes place during the sewing and finishing operations. Garments are inspected during production to assure the specified quality standard. Inspectors can include machine operators, team quality auditors, plant supervisors, or quality auditors sent by the contracting party (apparel manufacturer or retailer).

Quality assurance includes the use of quality thread, buttons, zippers, snaps, elastic, hem tape, and other products; and the quality and accuracy of sewing operations such as stitch type and length, stitch tension, seam type, edge finish, top stitching, turned edges, buttonhole stitching, hem stitching, and plaid matching. Quality assurance personnel are well versed in evaluating all aspects of production quality and accuracy.

Another component of quality assurance is the consistency of the size specifications for all products produced in each size. All the finished products must conform to the specified tolerances (the amount the product can deviate, plus or minus, from the garment dimension) stated on the measurement spec sheet (see Chapter 9). Many apparel manufacturers check a specified number of garments in each shipment received from the contractor to determine whether the measurement specs have been met.

The difficulty lies in deciding what to do with any products that do not meet the quality standards. It may not be possible to cut and sew a replacement order of garments if a group of finished goods does not meet the specifications. The textile manufacturer may not have replacement fabric, or the time necessary to produce replacement garments may exceed the deadline established by the retailer. Some garments end up as seconds at company employee stores and outlet malls; they may be purchased by jobbers, or are given to charities. In addition to the loss to the apparel manufacturer and contractor, the retailer expecting the goods may suffer if an order cannot be filled. Therefore, it is to everyone's benefit to assure quality production.

In developing quality assurance programs, companies are relying less on after-the-fact inspection and more on building quality into the products during production. Through modular manufacturing methods, operators are responsible for the quality of the product throughout production.

Current emphasis in quality assurance focuses on actively monitoring the manufacturing methods, materials, work environment, and equipment to achieve the expected specifications on a continual basis. One such method is called statistical process control (SPC). SPC requires the in-line measurement of quality in a statistical sampling of consecutive garments—usually in small batches—as they come off a particular operation hour by hour. This is opposed to other commonly used methods, which tend to involve in-line and end-of-line inspections of large random samples. By in-process measurement and quality inspection, anomalies can be identified at a time when it is more likely that a correction can be made. Thus, quality assurance is a proactive rather than reactive approach to quality.

Export Agents, Freight Forwarders, and Customs Brokers

A substantial portion of the apparel and accessories industries relies on off-shore factory production. Thus, it is important to discuss some of the aspects related to shipping goods out of the country where they were produced and into the United States. Many foreign countries have export regulations for shipping goods out of the country. It can be helpful for the U.S. apparel manufacturer that contracted the goods (the *importer*) to appoint an **export agent** in the exporting country to assist with exporting the products.

A **freight forwarding company** arranges to move a shipment of goods from the country where the goods were produced to the United States. In Figure 11.10, a shipment of goods is off-loaded at its port of entry in the United States. Tariffs and quotas (regulations affecting apparel manufacturers that import apparel and textile products into the United States) are discussed in Chapters 2 and 10.

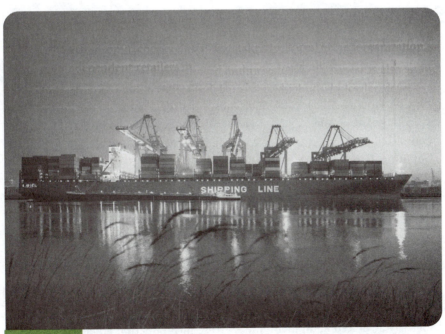

Figure 11.10 Container ships at the Port of Long Beach, California, unload their cargoes.

The Office of U.S. Customs and Border Protection, a part of the federal government, is the regulatory agency. A **customs broker** (licensed by the Office of U.S. Customs and Border Protection) in the United States is an agent hired by the U.S. apparel manufacturer to assist the company in importing the products produced for the company in another country. The customs broker is familiar with the complex U.S. customs regulations concerning importing textiles and apparel and will assist the apparel manufacturer to gain customs clearance. The manufacturer is charged a fee by the customs broker on a transaction basis, not by the number of items in a transaction. Although using a customs broker is optional, it can be very helpful to the apparel manufacturer. Sometimes, a shipment of goods is stalled by customs or sent back to the country of origin to correct the documentation. Not only does the apparel manufacturer face losing the retailer's business, but it may also face a fine by the shipping company that cannot unload the shipment. Of course, additional transportation costs are also involved. A consolidator might also be hired by the apparel manufacturer to serve as an intermediary for the freight forwarder and the customs broker.

Summary

This chapter examined some of the important aspects of production. With the background of the previous chapters, the interrelationship among research, design, pattern development, marketing, preproduction, sourcing, and production should be clear. All systems must work together for production to flow smoothly. Any problem along a style's path may slow production. Delays to the contracted delivery date may cost the manufacturer not only the style's profits, but future business from retailers.

A significant portion of the cost to produce apparel is consumed by the labor required to cut and sew the goods. Reducing labor costs can help retain reasonable prices for finished goods. Specialized equipment has been developed to speed production and improve accuracy. New technology in equipment and manufacturing systems has dramatically changed apparel production and provided a more efficient use of the labor team. Workers are more actively involved in providing an efficient production system and a team responsible for the quality of the goods produced. Even with the high cost of new, technologically advanced equipment, the increase in production efficiency can rapidly pay for the cash outlay to purchase new equipment.

Changes in production sewing systems have required changes in the manner in which employee compensation is determined. Pay based on the team's performance, group incentives for high performance and quality, and straight hourly wages have replaced traditional piece rates at many facilities. Workers are cross-trained on various types of equipment and in a variety of skills to provide greater flexibility to the workforce.

The number of different garment styles produced per season has increased for many production facilities. This makes it more difficult for production to flow smoothly. Flexibility in production systems will continue to be an important cornerstone of increased efficiency and decreased labor costs. Concern for workers' ergonomic needs is another trend that has changed the look of production facilities. We no longer see banks of seated sewers bent over sewing machines. Workers stand, walk from point to point, and sit on stools to provide better body positioning, circulation, and muscle relaxation.

Finishing operations performed at the end of production include laundering and applying garment finishes and garment dyeing, as well as packaging products ready for distribution. Providing floor-ready merchandise for the retailer with bar coded hangtags improves the efficiency of the entire flow of goods.

Quality assurance is an integral part of the product, from its inception to arrival in the customer's hands. Quality assurance includes meeting quality standards for all aspects of the product: the textile goods, component parts such as buttons and zippers, sewing, measurement specifications, and finishing.

With the growth in offshore apparel manufacturing, it is increasingly important to understand the various processes, agencies, and personnel involved in these complex business transactions. Changes in regulations, as well as in political and economic conditions and environmental considerations, can affect the production of goods.

CAREER PROFILES

Careers in production include positions as production cutters, sewing operators, production supervisors, plant managers, and quality assurance coordinators. If you are considering a career in the production area, what would your position description entail, and what would some of your typical tasks and responsibilities be?

Production Manager
Private-Label Manufacturer of Intimate Apparel

Position Description:

Manage the production of in-house sampling requirements (market, first fit, sew by, and photo samples); technical development; standards; quality control; price negotiations; place orders with suppliers and subcontractors; develop and implement production procedures and controls; and oversee production personnel. Manage contracted production in countries where the garments are produced.

Typical Tasks and Responsibilities:

- Serve as a liaison with design, sales, and the sample room, as well as with factories.
- Visit factories for a preproduction review of new styles and to check production in process, as well as approve production for shipment.
- Review samples from factories to check for specifications, and approve fabric, trims, and color.
- Organize labels and packaging.
- Prepare cost sheets.

Apparel Quality Analyst
Publicly Held Athletic Sportswear Company

Position Description:

Investigate and prepare reports on all apparel quality issues working toward a resolution. Recommend action and follow up with affected parties (development, marketing, sales, and promotion). Develop and maintain a strong working relationship with related departments. Conduct meetings with departments to inform and reach a joint decision. Arrange for components, fabric, and finished product tests and inspections as necessary. Communicate with quality assurance managers in the United States and throughout the world. The apparel quality analyst position functions as a global position.

Typical Tasks and Responsibilities:

- Communicate daily by e-mail and telephone with related departments throughout the life of the quality issue.

- Prepare weekly quality logs for the QA department.

- Investigate the scope, nature, probable cause, and resolution of quality issues. Samples from the field and distribution center come to this position.

- Prepare reports and submit samples to the textile testing lab when the quality issue involves fabric development.

- Perform inspection/audits at factories once a month. Being a field auditor is a small part of the apparel quality analyst's responsibility as there are other field auditors who inspect/audit factories.

Key Terms

agile manufacturing
counter sample
customs broker
export agent
fast fashion production
flexible manufacturing (FM)
flexible manufacturing system
floor-ready merchandise (FRM)
freight forwarding company
garment dyed
made-to-measure
manufacturing environment

mass customization
modular manufacturing
piece-rate wage
production
progressive bundle system
quality assurance
sew by
short-cycle production
single-hand system
tagless label
unit production system (UPS)
work-in-process (WIP)

Discussion Questions and Activities

1. Compare and contrast the advantages and disadvantages of the progressive bundle and flexible manufacturing systems of apparel production.
2. Describe a quality defect that you have encountered with an apparel/home fashions product or accessory. How might quality assurance have prevented this problem?
3. What are advantages and disadvantages of garment dyeing? What types of garments are more suitable for this process?

References

Abend, Jules. (1999, January). Modular manufacturing: The line between success and failure. *Bobbin*, pp. 48–52.

Barry, N. (2004). Fast fashion. *European Retail Digest*, 41, pp. 75–82.

DesMarteau, Kathleen. (1998, August). Wrinkle free now carefree. *Bobbin*, p. 188.

Dunagan, Evelyn. (1999, January). Another perspective on modular manufacturing: Levi's was right. *Apparel Industry Magazine*, pp. 96–98.

Hill, Ed. (1992, February). Flexible manufacturing systems, Part 1. *Bobbin*, pp. 34–38.

Hill, Suzette. (1998, December). VF's consumerization: A "right stuff" strategy. *Apparel Industry Magazine,* pp. AS-4–AS-12.

Hill, Thomas. (1994, March). CAR study: UPS, CAD provide 300 percent return on investment. *Apparel Industry Magazine*, pp. 34–40.

Rabon, Lisa. (2000, January). Mixing the elements of mass customization. *Bobbin*, pp. 38–41.

Rabon, Lisa, and Deaton, Claudia. (1999, December). Pre-production: Laying the cornerstones of mass customization. *Bobbin*, pp. 35–37.

Reda, Susan. (2004, March). Retail's great race. *Stores*, p. 38.

Swank, Gary. (1995, January). QR requires floor ready goods. *Apparel Industry Magazine*, p 106.

Speer, Jordan K. (2004, April). A label-conscious world. *Apparel*, pp. 24–29.

Winger, Rocio Maria. (1998, December). The Nygård vanguard: The way to chargebacks. *Apparel Industry Magazine*, pp. AS-14–AS-18.

CHAPTER 12

Distribution
and Retailing

In this chapter, you will learn the following:

- the strategies and processes for distributing apparel, accessory, and home fashions products to the ultimate consumer

- the nature of the alliances between manufacturers and retailers in carrying out supply chain management and product lifecycle management activities related to distribution

- the definitions and characteristics of the various categories of retailers

- the primary trade publications and trade associations involved in the distribution of apparel, accessory, and home fashions products

Step 8: Distribution and Retailing

Step 1 Research and Merchandising

Step 2 Design

Step 3 Design Development and Style Selection

Step 4 Marketing the Apparel Line

Step 5 Preproduction

Step 6 Sourcing

Step 7 Apparel Production Processes, Material Management, and Quality Assurance

Step 8 Distribution and Retailing

Send Retailer's Order to Manufacturer's Distribution Center

Pick Orders (may include quality assurance check)

Send to Retail Store Distribution Center or Directly to Retailer

Review Season's Sales Figures

Distribution Strategies

We have followed apparel, accessory, and home fashions products from their design through their production. The next stage is distribution to retailers and, finally, to the ultimate consumer (see Step 8 of the flowchart on the previous page). Companies must decide on the strategies they will use to distribute merchandise to their customers. Decisions regarding distribution strategies are based on a number of factors, which are examined in detail in this chapter.

Factors Affecting Distribution Strategies

Decisions around distribution strategies to be implemented by companies are based on a number of factors:

- *Type of marketing channel to which the company belongs:* Companies using **direct marketing channels** will sell directly to the ultimate consumer. Companies using **limited marketing channels** will sell merchandise through store or nonstore retailing venues. Companies using **extended marketing channels** will sell merchandise through a wholesaler, who then sells the merchandise to a retailer. (These channels—direct, limited, and extended—are described in Chapter 2.)

- *Buying characteristics of the target customer:* Certain target market customers will prefer certain distribution strategies. Questions a company might ask include: how and where does our target customer like to shop? What are the customer's decision-making processes in purchasing our merchandise? For example, a manufacturer of women's career apparel may focus on retail venues that are convenient to large office complexes and are service oriented. A manufacturer of men's golf accessories may focus on retailers including both large sports stores as well as small specialty stores such as golf club pro shops. Companies that sell merchandise targeted to a young customer may use strategies involving new technologies and social media.

- *Product type:* Categories of merchandise may lend themselves to certain retail distribution strategies. For example, socks, underwear, and other packaged merchandise lend themselves to retailers who include self-service fixtures in the retail venues.

- *National, private label, or store brand product:* National brands are generally found in many different retail stores, whereas private label merchandise and store brands are unique to particular stores or groups of stores.

- *Price zone of merchandise:* Budget-priced merchandise will more often be distributed through discount stores than through other types of retailers, whereas designer-priced merchandise will more often be distributed through boutiques or specialty stores than through other types of retailers.

Classifications of Distribution Strategies

Distribution strategies can be classified as mass distribution, selective distribution, or exclusive distribution.

- *Mass distribution:* With **mass distribution** (also called **intensive distribution**), products are made available to as many consumers as possible through a variety of retail outlets, including supermarkets, convenience stores, and mass merchandisers or discount stores. The Hanes hosiery, Jockey underwear, and Champion and Russell activewear brands use this distribution strategy.

- *Selective distribution:* With **selective distribution**, manufacturers allow their merchandise to be distributed only through certain stores. Some manufacturers require a minimum quantity to be purchased; others limit their products' distribution to retailers in noncompeting geographic areas. Some manufacturers also set criteria as to the image and location of stores in which their merchandise can be sold. Most national brands use this type of distribution strategy. For example, 7 for All Mankind premium denim is distributed through selected specialty and department stores based on criteria set by the manufacturer.

- *Exclusive distribution:* With **exclusive distribution**, manufacturers limit the stores in which their merchandise is distributed in order to create an image of exclusiveness. Companies that produce merchandise in the designer price zone (e.g., Chanel, Armani, Vera Wang) often use an exclusive distribution strategy by selling goods only through a few stores or boutiques. The distribution of private label merchandise (e.g., JCPenney's Arizona brand, Kmart's Jaclyn Smith brand, Target's xhilaration® brand, Macy's INC International Concepts brand), exclusive licensing brands (e.g., Target's Mossimo® and

Kohl's Simply Vera by Vera Wang), and store brands (e.g., Gap, The Limited, Ann Taylor) that are specific to a particular retailer is also considered to be exclusive because the brands are available only at specific stores and their websites.

Distribution Territories

Retailers must also determine how broad their distribution territories will be. Some retailers focus on a local target customer with retail establishments in a single community; others distribute more broadly, either regionally or nationally; and still others are global retailers, distributing merchandise in more than one country. With the retail saturation of the U.S. market, many companies have expanded their retail operations to other countries. For example, Walmart, the world's largest retailer, has retail operations in the United States, Argentina, Brazil, Canada, Chile, China, Costa Rica, El Salvador, Guatemala, Honduras, India, Japan, Mexico, Nicaragua, and the United Kingdom. JCPenney operates stores in the United States and Puerto Rico. Gap, Inc. has retail operations in the United States, Canada, the United Kingdom, France, Ireland, and Japan. In addition, with nonstore retailing, such as electronic retailing—**e-tailing,** for short—and television shopping, companies have expanded their distribution beyond local or even national markets. Before retailers expand their operations into other countries, it is imperative that they understand the demographics, decision-making orientation, and cultural norms of the consumers in the country.

Distribution Centers

For some apparel, accessory, and home fashions companies, shipments of finished merchandise to their retail accounts are made directly from the production facility. For other apparel, accessory, and home fashions companies, the flow of goods from production facilities to retailers involves the use of **distribution centers (DCs)**. Both manufacturers and retailers may utilize distribution centers as part of their distribution processes. Their decision to use distribution centers in their distribution processes is based on the following:

- the size of the company
- the number of products being distributed
- the number of retail stores being serviced
- the distance between where the merchandise was produced and where the retail accounts are located

The larger the company and the more products and retailers involved, the more likely distribution centers will be used.

Manufacturers' Distribution Centers

Apparel and home fashions manufacturers use distribution centers when shipments to retailers consist of goods produced in more than one location (especially when contractors are used). In these cases, merchandise from the various locations is brought to a central location for quality assurance, **picking** (selecting the appropriate assortment of goods to fill a specific retailer's order), packing the merchandise, and distributing to the retail store accounts (see Figure 12.1). Technology has become important in increasing the efficiencies of distribution centers. Robotics that pick orders and conveyor systems that move orders from one area to the next have been incorporated into distribution center processes.

No longer do distribution centers serve the purpose of warehousing inventory; in fact merchandise is typically stored at a distribution center for only short periods. Instead, **flow-through** facilities move merchandise from receiving to shipping with little, if any, time in storage. For example, Nike, Inc.'s 1.2 million-square-foot distribution center in Memphis, Tennessee, utilizes a combination of scanning and sorting technologies to achieve a 12-hour turnaround from the

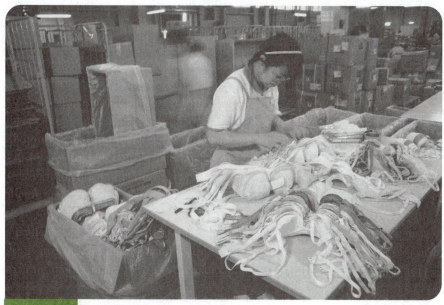

Figure 12.1   The distribution process includes inspecting, packing, and shipping merchandise to retail accounts.

time the product is received at the DC to the time it is shipped to the retailer.

In addition to being a centralized destination for merchandise flow-through, DCs also focus on adding value (doing something to a product to make it worth more to the manufacturer, retailer, or consumer) to the merchandise by affixing hangtags, labels, and price information in order to make the goods floor ready. When manufacturers pre-ticket merchandise, retailers do not have to spend extra time ticketing the items before the apparel hits the selling floor. This process, known as **vendor marking**, results in **floor-ready merchandise** (see also Chapter 11).

Even with greater efficiencies in distribution center operations, to speed up the process even more, some companies do not use distribution centers but ship merchandise to retailers directly from the production facility. In these cases, merchandise becomes floor-ready at the either the production facility or at the retail store.

Retailers' Distribution Centers

Retailers also use distribution centers to facilitate distribution of merchandise from a variety of apparel, accessory, and home fashions companies (vendors) to a number of stores. Goods are shipped from the manufacturers to a centralized retail distribution center, where merchandise for the retailer's stores is picked, combined, and shipped to the individual stores. If merchandise has not been vendor marked, hangtags, including **stock-keeping unit** (SKU) codes and price information, are affixed to the merchandise at the retailer's DC.

Retail distribution centers are often at geographical locations chosen to speed delivery to stores. For example, as of 2011, Target operated 27 distribution centers located throughout the United States; Walmart operated 147 distribution centers. A regional Walmart distribution center (2009) can have "twelve miles of conveyor belts, which can move hundreds of thousands of cases through the center each day."

In recent years, the productivity of distribution centers has been enhanced through warehouse management system (WMS) computer software programs, along with the use of bar coding and RFID tagging of pallets and cartons. These software programs and tracking devices assist retailers in the following:

- maximizing the space within the DC
- automating warehouse operations
- integrating data throughout the supply chain
- improving communication with vendors (manufacturers)
- improving shipping accuracy

Alliances between Manufacturers and Retailers: QR, PLM, and SCM

The primary goals of Quick Response (QR), product lifecycle management (PLM), and supply chain management (SCM) strategies are to increase the speed with which merchandise gets to the consumer, and to lower the costs of manufacturing and distributing merchandise through the sharing of data among companies throughout the production and distribution of the product. The establishment of alliances between manufacturers and retailers is imperative for these goals to be achieved.

The Foundations: UPC Bar Coding, Vendor Marking, EDI, and RFID

Alliances between manufacturers and retailers depend on several basic operation strategies that have been adopted by manufacturers and retailers. These include the use of the following:

- UPC bar coding on products and shipping containers
- vendor marking of merchandise
- electronic data interchange (EDI)
- the use of RFID tagging

UPC BAR CODING AND VENDOR MARKING

The **Universal Product Code (UPC)** system is one of several bar code symbologies used for the electronic identification of merchandise. The use of UPC bar coding is considered the foundation of many QR and SCM strategies because it is considered necessary for electronic communications between the manufacturer and retailer. A UPC is a 12-digit number that identifies manufacturer and merchandise items by stock-keeping unit: vendor, style, color, and size. It is represented by a bar code made up of a pattern of dark bars and white spaces of varying widths. A group of bars and spaces represents one character or digit.

UPC bar codes are electronically scanned and "read" by scanning equipment. The scanning equipment provides a source of intense light that illuminates the symbol. The dark bars absorb the light. The scanner collects the reflected pattern of light and dark and converts it into an electrical signal that is sent to a decoder. The decoder, which may be part of the scanner unit or may be a separate device, translates the electrical signal to binary numbers for use by the point-of-sale terminal or computer. Scanners can be categorized as one of the following:

- contact readers that must touch or come in close proximity to the symbol
- noncontact readers that can read the bar code when it is moved past a fixed beam or moving beam of light (see Figure 12.2)

UPC bar codes are attached to the merchandise by the manufacturer/vendor (vendor marking) or the retailer. Both vendor-marked merchandise and retailer-prepared bar codes are used to increase the speed of checkout and the accuracy of inventories. There are a number of benefits of UPC bar coding and point-of-sale (POS) scanning. One of the most obvious benefits of using bar codes is the reduction in time needed to complete a transaction at the point of sale. An even more important benefit of scanning bar codes is that accurate SKU information is retrieved at the point of sale. This means that product sales and retail inventory are automatically tracked. With this accurate and timely sales information, retailers and manufacturers can plan inventory needs to match sales or projected consumer demand more closely. For example, with accurate sales data, retailers are able to track sales trends. This helps retailers avoid overstocking merchandise and, thus, reduce markdowns. Correct point-of-sale information can also be used to reorder merchandise more efficiently and, thereby, reduce the possibility of a retailer being out of stock in a particular style, size, or color of merchandise. In addition, **replenishment**—automatic reordering of merchandise—is dependent upon the use of point-of-sale information provided by UPC bar codes. Replenishment strategies will be discussed later in this chapter.

In addition to using bar codes for these point-of-sale (POS) benefits, retailers also use them to scan inventory in their distribution centers and to facilitate the movement of shipping cartons in distribution centers. The bar codes identify each shipping container's contents and are used for tracking and sorting

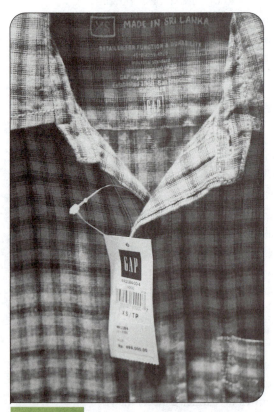

Figure 12.2 Benefits of UPC bar codes on merchandise hangtags include retrieval of accurate SKU information at point-of-sale.

merchandise at the DCs. While the UPC bar code is made up of only numbers, two other bar code formats—code 39 or code 128—can include both numbers and letters and are often used on shipping cartons.

ELECTRONIC DATA INTERCHANGE

Electronic data interchange (EDI) makes possible computer-to-computer communications between the manufacturer and retailer (see Figure 12.3). Prior to our current computer technology, purchase orders, invoices, and any other type of written communication generated by one company were sent to another company by mail or fax. The receiving company would then enter the data into its computer. With EDI technology, business data are transmitted electronically. In other words, computers from one company communicate directly to computers from other companies or through a third party's com-

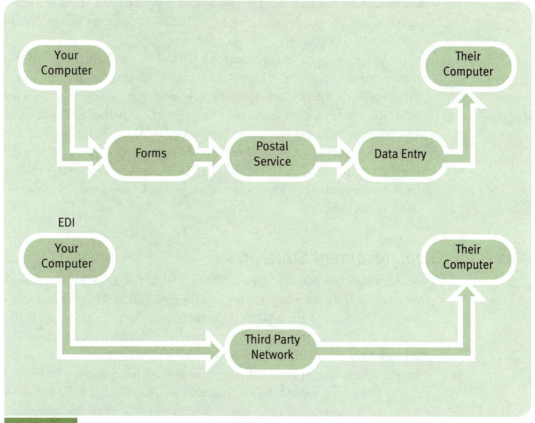

Figure 12.3 Electronic data interchange (EDI) improves efficiency by making possible computer-to-computer communications between manufacturers and retailers.

puter system called a **value-added network (VAN)**. Not only are paper documents replaced by electronic documents, but the time delays associated with using mail services and paper handling are eliminated. The most common EDI transactions in the apparel industry include the following:

- purchase orders, invoices, packing slips, and advance shipping notices (ASN)
- reports of inventory counts and changes in inventory, such as sales and returns data
- price/sales catalogs

In addition, through EDI, retail distribution centers can accommodate **cross-dockable shipments.** This means that goods are received from the manufacturer as floor-ready merchandise, so they can be sorted for store distribution without the need for additional processing. For cross-docking to happen, the retailer must request and receive advance shipping notices from the manufacturer, and the goods must arrive floor ready. This would not be possible without EDI technology.

In the age of supply chain management, the EDI capabilities of the manufacturer are the backbone of supply chain management through which retailer POS data feeds directly into apparel companies' manufacturing systems and by which manufacturers are directly linked to the suppliers of fabric, trims, and findings. With the increase of business-to-business (B2B) Internet, **Web EDI** has emerged as a viable option for both large and small companies located throughout the world to be part of an efficient and low-cost system of sharing data electronically. These systems have grown in popularity as security of websites has increased.

Replenishment Strategies

In the traditional manufacturer–retailer relationship, the retail buyer would order goods from the manufacturer, and the entire order for the season would then be delivered to the retailer at the beginning of the fashion season. The retailer would hope that the correct number of each style, color, and size had been ordered and delivered. However, with this arrangement, it was not uncommon for a customer to walk into a store knowing the style and size of a product he or she wanted, only to find that the store did not have the size in stock. Out-of-stock merchandise may have been a result of the desired product not being delivered on time, or it may be that the desired product had been purchased by another customer and a replacement product had not arrived at the store. Either way, a sale was lost. To help alleviate situations such as this, the retailer must be able to replenish merchandise in an accurate and timely manner. Several replenishment methods are used by manufacturers and retailers, including the following:

- The retailer initiates an electronic (EDI) order when it determines that the stock level warrants a reorder.

- Information about stock levels is automatically communicated to the manufacturer through EDI, and the manufacturer (vendor) automatically ships reorders when the merchandise stock at the retail store reaches a certain level.

- A specified percent of the retail buyer's order is delivered before the start of the fashion season, with the remainder of the order delivered either throughout the fashion season or as a single reorder. The mix of styles, colors, and sizes in the reorder(s) is based on POS data from the retail stores.

Replenishment strategies vary with the type of merchandise and size of retailer. For basic (staple) items, such as hosiery and jeans, replenishment may be an ongoing activity. For seasonal goods such as turtleneck sweaters and outerwear, replenishment may occur only within a particular fashion season. For fashion goods, merchandise may not be replenished during the fashion season. For companies engaged in fast fashion, replenishment rarely occurs as new merchandise is delivered on regular basis.

Manufacturers may use a variety of replenishment strategies depending upon their retail customers, and retailers may use a variety of replenishment strategies depending upon the capabilities of their vendors (manufacturers). One of the strategies most beneficial to improving the efficiency in the apparel supply pipeline between the manufacturer and retailer has been to establish programs whereby sales and **stockout data** (data on out-of-stock goods) are reviewed by the manufacturer, and replenishments are ordered as often as required. The strategy of having the manufacturer (vendor) automatically ship merchandise to the retail store based on POS data from the retailer is known as **vendor-managed inventory (VMI)** or vendor-managed replenishment. In some cases, data are reviewed daily rather than monthly or bimonthly, as was done in the past. Obviously, this type of strategy would not be possible without the retailer sending POS data to the manufacturer.

Vendor-managed inventory strategies are most commonly used with merchandise such as lingerie, hosiery, T-shirts, and basic jeans where style changes from season to season are minimal and it is important for retailers to have desired sizes and colors in stock (see Figure 12.4). For example, TAL Apparel, a

Hong-Kong based contractor, provides inventory stock replenishment services to L.L.Bean allowing L.L.Bean to manage the replenishment of polo knit shirts which includes over 2,000 SKU (stock-keeping units) across men's, women's and children's sizes with up to 20 colors.

Technologies are providing retailers with a variety of stock replenishment capabilities. For example, increased use of RFID to streamline inventory management is allowing sales associates to receive alerts when merchandise is delivered so that top-selling items are always in stock. **Data mining technology** can also be used to examine sales of products by style, size, and color. Data mining technology analyzes data information, searching for selling patterns or trends in the data and identifying correlations among data characteristics. When trends or patterns are found, producers can tailor assortment or replenishments for specific retailers or retail venues. For example, a company may discover that the selling season for shorts was longer in retail locations with higher median incomes and adjust assortment and replenishment accordingly.

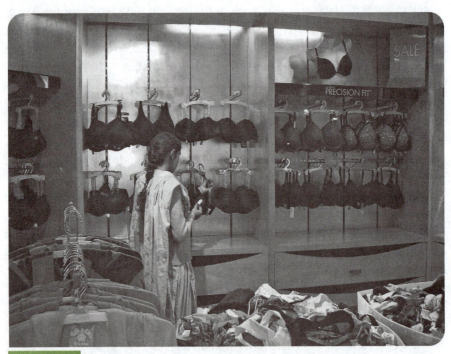

Figure 12.4   Vendor managed replenishment strategies are typical for products such as lingerie that are delivered to the retailer "floor ready."

Implementing Quick Response, Product Lifecycle Management, and Supply Chain Management

This book focuses on Quick Response (QR), product lifecycle management (PLM), and supply chain management (SCM) strategies implemented throughout the design, manufacturing, and retailing of apparel, accessory, and home fashions products. Recall that implementation of QR, PLM, and SCM includes:

- use of bar coding and EDI, which provide accurate sales data and speed communications
- replenishment strategy decisions, whereby retailers and suppliers jointly review sales data, develop forecasts for future demand, and reduce inventory while keeping stores fully stocked; decide that fashion merchandise will not be replenished; or a combination of both
- customized assortments and replenishment, not only for each retailer, but for each store unit in a retail chain
- private label, store brand, and/or fast fashion merchandise offerings, whereby merchandise is created jointly by the manufacturer and retailer or the manufacturer and retailer are one in the same

With SCM and PLM, either an order from a retailer or a retail sale electronically triggers the manufacturing process. Orders or sales data are tied to the apparel company's PDM/PLM systems and fabric and findings suppliers. At the retail level, the retailer's financial and merchandise plans are integrated. That is, the retailer's assortment plan is integrated with how much space each retail department will be allocated at each store, thus optimizing the store's merchandise mix. Integrated processes include:

- integration of an apparel company's patternmaking systems (PDS) with other product information through product information management (PIM) software (see Chapter 9)
- integration of an apparel company's various CAD/CAM systems, resulting in PDM/PLM (see Chapter 11)
- alliances between apparel companies and retailers, resulting in vendor-managed retail inventory
- integration of a retailer's merchandise assortment planning, financial planning, distribution processes, and store layout.

Retailing and Categories of Retailers

By definition, **retailing** is the process or business activity of selling goods or services to the ultimate consumer, and a **retailer** is the company or business that makes a profit by selling goods and services to the ultimate consumer (see Figure 12.5). Retailers range in size from small sole proprietorships that cater to a local market to large corporate store ownership groups. Table 12.1 lists some of the primary retail corporations and the stores owned and operated by these corporations. Retailers can be classified according to many of their characteristics, including their type of ownership, merchandise mix, size, location, and organizational and operational characteristics. One typical way of classifying

Table 12.1 Selected Major Retail Corporations	
Abercrombie & Fitch (www.abercrombie.com)	**Foot Locker Inc.** (www.footlocker-inc.com)
Abercrombie & Fitch	Foot Locker
abercrombie	Lady Foot Locker
Hollister	Kids Foot Locker
Gilly Hicks	Champs Sports
	Footaction
Bed Bath & Beyond Inc.	Eastbay
(www.bedbathandbeyond.com)	CCS
Bed Bath & Beyond	
Christmas Tree Shops	**Gap Inc.** (www.gap.com)
Harmon and Harmon Face Values	Gap
buybuy BABY	Banana Republic
	Old Navy
Burlington Coat Factory Warehouse Corporation	Piperlime
(www.coat.com)	Athleta
Burlington Coat Factory Stores	
Luxury Linens	**JCPenney Company, Inc.** (www.jcpenney.com)
Baby Depot	**Kohl's Department Stores** (www.kohls.com)
Cohoes Fashions	
	Limited Brands (www.limitedbrands.com)
Charming Shoppes, Inc.	Victoria's Secret
(www.charmingshoppes.com)	Henri Bendel
Lane Bryant	Bath and Body Works
Fashion Bug	La Senza
Catherines Plus Sizes	Pink
	C.O. Bigelow
Dillard's (www.dillards.com)	White Barn Candle Co.

Table 12.1 Selected Major Retail Corporations *(continued)*

Macy's Inc. (www.macysinc.com)
Macy's
Bloomingdale's

Neiman Marcus Group
(www.neimanmarcus.com)
Neiman Marcus
Bergdorf Goodman
Horchow
CUSP by Neiman Marcus

Nordstrom (www.nordstrom.com)
Nordstrom
Nordstom Rack
Last Chance
Jeffrey

Saks Incorporated (www.saksincorporated.com)
Saks Fifth Avenue
Saks Fifth Avenue OFF 5th

Sears Holdings Corporation
(www.searsholdings.com)
Sears, Roebuck & Co. (www.sears.com)
  Sears Full-Line Stores
  Sears Hometown Stores
  Sears Grand
  Sears Essentials
  The Great Indoors
  Orchard Supply Hardware
Kmart Corporation (www.kmart.com)
  Kmart
  Big Kmart
  Kmart Super Centers

Kmart Corporation LLC
Spiegel Brands Inc (www.spiegel.com)
  Spiegel
  Newport News
  Shape fx

Target Corporation (www.target.com)
Target
Target Commercial Interiors
SuperTarget

The TJX Companies, Inc. (www.tjx.com)
T.J. Maxx
Marshalls
Winners
HomeGoods
T.K. Maxx
HomeSense
StyleSense

Urban Outfitters Inc.
(www.urbanoutfittersinc.com)
Urban Outfitters
Anthropologie
Free People
BHLDN
Leifsdottir
Terrain

Wal-Mart Stores, Inc. (walmartstores.com/)
Walmart
Sam's Club

Williams-Sonoma, Inc.
(www.williams-sonoma.com)
Williams-Sonoma
Williams-Sonoma Home
Pottery Barn
Pottery Barn Kids
PBteen
West Elm

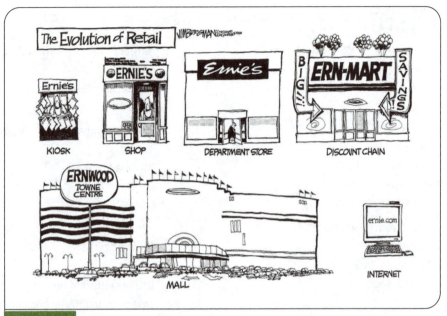

Figure 12.5   This illustration shows the evolution of retail.

retailers is on the basis of their merchandising and operating strategies, which results in the following categories:

- department stores
- specialty stores
- discount retailers
- off-price retailers
- supermarkets and hypermarkets
- warehouse retailers
- convenience stores
- contractual retailers
- chain stores
- nonstore retailers

Because of the diversity found among retailers, these categories are not mutually exclusive. For example, a specialty store retailer may also be a chain store operation; a department store may have both brick-and-mortar stores as well as a retail website (form of nonstore retailing). Indeed, **multichannel distribution** or **multichannel retailing** strategies involve offering merchandise through

| Table 12.2 | Number of Retail Establishments and Employment by Category |

	Number of Establishments	Total U.S. Employment
Furniture and home furnishings stores	64,590	562,698
Clothing stores	98,767	1,272653
Shoe stores	28,015	208,558
Jewelry stores	27,596	155,451
Luggage and leather goods stores	1,187	7,507
Department stores (not discount)	3,562	539,642
Discount department stores	4,991	689,847

SOURCE: U.S. Census Bureau. 2007 Economic Census, Retail Trade in the U.S.

more than one distribution channel. Most common is for companies to have brick-and-mortar stores along with mail order catalogs and/or websites. Examples of companies that focus on multichannel retailing include Coldwater Creek, J.Jill, Talbots, Pottery Barn, and Crate and Barrel. Table 12.2 lists the number of retailers in the United States by category of retailer.

Department Stores

Department stores are large retailers that divide their functions and their merchandise into sections or departments. Department stores have the following features:

- a fashion-oriented merchandise assortment
- a variety of services for customers (e.g., credit cards, wedding registry)
- merchandise offered at full markup price with seasonal sales
- at least 50 employees
- operate in stores large enough to be shopping center anchors (see Figure 12.6).

The category includes full-line department stores (which offer apparel, home fashions, housewares, and furniture), such as Macy's, JCPenney, Sears, Kohl's, and Dillard's, as well as limited-line department stores such as Nordstrom and Neiman Marcus. Multiunit department stores include department store chains as well as those that may have a flagship or primary store. For example, Macy's, Inc. includes 810 Macy's department stores and furniture galleries in 45 states, the District of Columbia, Guam, and Puerto Rico. Macy's flagship store is considered to be its Herald Square store in New York City. Table 12.3 is a list of the top 10 department stores based on retail sales.

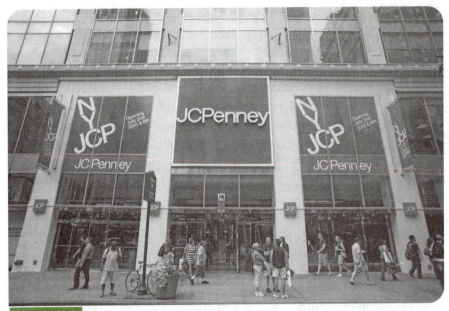

Figure 12.6 Full-line multiunit department stores such as JCPenney often serve as shopping center anchors.

With the goal of catering to a broad range of consumers, department stores carry a wide variety of merchandise lines with a reasonably wide selection within each category. Department stores usually carry national brands and private label merchandise, typically in the moderate and better price zones. Depending on their price assortment, they may also carry merchandise in the bridge and designer price zones.

Because of the fierce competition among department stores, visually appealing merchandise presentation, strong customer service, and offering private label and exclusive merchandise have been necessary strategies for success. Private label and exclusive brand merchandise have become important means for department stores to distinguish themselves from the competition. For example, in addition to their many private label brands, Macy's has a leased department relationship with Destination Maternity offering exclusive lines of A Pea in the Pod and Motherhood Maternity brand maternity wear brands in over 615 Macy's locations. Kohl's offers exclusive lines by Dana Buchman and Simply Vera by Vera Wang; JCPenney has an exclusive line of apparel by Liz Claiborne.

Many department stores also have **in-store shops** of designers and major brands. These in-store shops are merchandised according to the manufacturer's specifications and carry only the merchandise of the apparel company.

Table 12.3	Top Department Stores by Retail Sales

Company	2009 Retail Sales $US (000)
Macy's	23,489,000
JCPenney	17,556,000
Kohl's	17,178,000
Sears*	15,938,000
Nordstrom	8,258,000
Dillard's	5,890,000
Neiman Marcus	3,643,000
Belk	3,346,000
Bon-Ton	2,960,000
Saks	2,632,000

*Sears full-line department stores only

SOURCE: *STORES.* (2010, June). Top 100 Retailers.

Companies/brands such as Polo Ralph Lauren, Nautica, Tommy Hilfiger, Calvin Klein, Liz Claiborne, BCBG Max Azria, and Dockers have all had successful in-store shops. In-store shops benefit both the manufacturer and the retailer. For the manufacturer, they create brand awareness and make shopping easy for their customers. For the department stores, the in-store shops create a specialty store "feel" within the department store environment. Companies are expanding the in-store shop concept to their nonstore retailing venues. For example, Bloomingdales.com offers "designer shops" for a number of brands, including Elizabeth and James, MARC by MARC JACOBS, Nanette Lepore, and Theory.

Specialty Stores

A **specialty store** focuses on a specific type of merchandise in one of the following ways:

- by carrying one category of merchandise or a few closely related categories of merchandise (e.g., jewelry, footwear, eyeglasses, intimate apparel, housewares)

- by focusing on merchandise for a well-defined target market (e.g., men, women, bicyclists, plus-size consumers, individuals with small children)

- by carrying the merchandise of one manufacturer or brand (e.g., Liz Claiborne, Polo Ralph Lauren, Guess Kids)

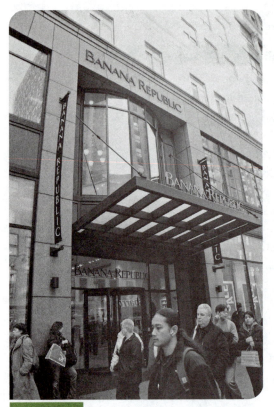

Figure 12.7 Banana Republic, a division of Gap Inc., is an example of a specialty store chain.

Specialty stores carry a limited but deep assortment (i.e., excellent selection of brands, styles, sizes) of merchandise. They may carry national brands or have their own store brand (e.g., Abercrombie & Fitch, Ann Taylor Stores, Crate and Barrel). Most specialty stores will carry merchandise in only one or two price zones. Two of the largest apparel specialty store chains in the United States are Gap (includes Gap, Old Navy, Banana Republic, Piperlime, and Athleta) and Limited Brands (includes Victoria's Secret, Pink, Bath & Body Works, La Senza, C.O. Bigelow, White Barn Candle Co., and Henri Bendel) (see Figure 12.7). See Table 12.4 for a listing of apparel specialty chains. Specialty stores that concentrate on designer price zone merchandise or unique merchandise distributed exclusively to only a few stores are typically referred to as **boutiques**. Specialty stores that are temporary or mobile in nature, focus on a new fad, or are associated with a live event are typically referred to as **pop-up retailers**.

Discount Retailers

A **discount store** sells brand name merchandise at less than traditional retail prices and includes apparel merchandise at the mass or budget price zone. Examples of discount chain department stores are Target, Kmart, and Walmart. An example of a discount chain specialty store is Bed, Bath & Beyond. In addition to national brands, discounters also carry private label merchandise (e.g., Kmart's Jaclyn Smith brand) and exclusive licensed brands (e.g., Liz Lange maternity for Target).

Through mass merchandising and supply chain management strategies, discounters are able to keep prices lower than other retailers. These strategies include the following:

- quantity discounts from manufacturers
- effective replenishment strategies to ensure that the merchandise customers want is in stock

Table 12.4	Top Apparel Specialty Chains by Retail Sales
Company	2009 Retail Sales $US (000)
TJX	15,845,000
Gap	10,491,000
Limited Brands	8,632,000
Ross Stores	7,184,000
Burlington Coat Factory	3,503,000
Abercrombie & Fitch	2,929,000
American Eagle Outfitters	2,716,000
Polo Ralph Lauren	2,263,000
Aéropostale	2,141,000
Charming Shoppes	2,064,000
Liz Claiborne	2,018,000
Urban Outfitters	1,834,000
Ann Taylor Stores	1,829,000

SOURCE: *STORES*. (2010, June). Top 100 Retailers.

- high turnover rates on products
- limiting brands and styles to only the most popular items
- self-service
- lower overhead costs
- promotions that cater to a broad target market

National and international discount chains such as Walmart (Figure 12.8), Kmart, and Target buy huge quantities of merchandise from manufacturers and can operate on smaller profit margins than can traditional department stores. Target is sometimes referred to as an **upscale discounter** because it has a department store feel and provides more fashion-forward merchandise. Table 12.5 lists the top discount stores.

Off-Price Retailers

Off-price retailers specialize in selling national brands, designer collections, or promotional goods at discount prices. Off-price retailers are characterized by their buying of merchandise at low prices, carrying well-established (including designer) brands, and having merchandise assortments that change quickly with inconsistent sizes and styles (sometimes referred to as broken

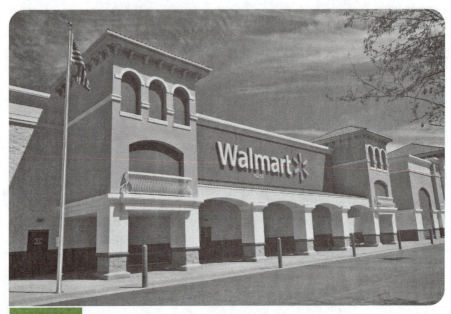

Figure 12.8 Walmart, an example of an international discount store chain, is the largest retailer in the world.

Table 12.5 Top Large Format Value/Discount/Warehouse Retailers by Retail Sales

Company	2009 $US Retail Sales (000)
Walmart	304,939,000
Target	63,435,000
Costco	56,548,000

SOURCE: *STORES*. (2010, June). Top 100 Retailers.

assortments). The following are types of off-price retailers: factory outlet stores, independent off-price retailers, retailer-owned off-price retailers, close-out stores, and sample stores.

FACTORY OUTLET STORES

Manufacturers' or **factory outlet stores** sell their own seconds, irregulars, or overruns (merchandise produced in excess of their orders), as well as merchandise produced specifically for the outlet stores. In some cases, manufacturers will use their outlet stores as test markets for styles, colors, or sizes of merchandise. Once located primarily near production or distribution centers, factory outlet stores comprising entire shopping centers are now common throughout the United States. They are typically located at a distance from full-price retailers that carry their goods (based on agreements with local full-price retailers).

OFF-PRICE RETAILERS

These stores buy irregulars, seconds, overruns, or leftovers from manufacturers or other retailers. Ross (Figure 12.9), T.J. Maxx, and Burlington Coat Factory are examples of independent off-price retailers.

RETAILER-OWNED OFF-PRICE RETAILERS

Some retailers operate their own off-price stores (e.g., Off 5th, Nordstrom Rack). In these off-price stores, retailers sell merchandise from their regular stores that had not sold within a specified time period, private label merchandise, or special orders purchased specifically for the off-price store.

CLOSEOUT STORES

Closeout stores specialize in buying a variety of merchandise through retail liquidations, bankruptcies, and closeouts. Then they sell this merchandise at bargain prices.

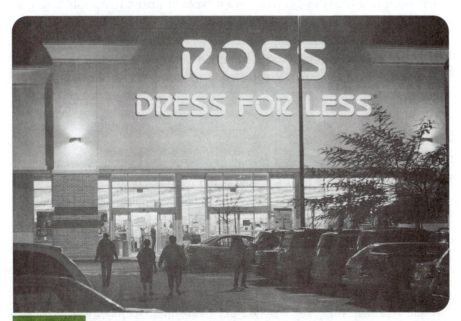

Figure 12.9   Independent off-price retailers such as Ross sell national brands and promotional goods at discount prices.

SAMPLE STORES

Sample stores specialize in selling apparel companies' sample merchandise at the end of the market selling period. These stores are located near major apparel marts, such as the California Market Center in downtown Los Angeles.

Supermarkets and Hypermarkets

Conventional **supermarkets** are large self-service grocery stores that carry a full line of foods and related products. Some supermarkets have broadened their merchandise and service offerings. **Superstores**, or **hypermarkets**, are upgraded supermarkets that combine the elements of a supermarket and a department store by offering a wide range of merchandise, including food, electronics, clothing and accessories, furniture, and garden items. These **big box stores** can be as large as 150,000 to 250,000 square feet.

At one time, only a limited number of apparel products (e.g., hosiery, packaged undergarments) or home fashions (e.g., kitchen towels) were distributed through supermarkets. However, with the growth of large discount retailer superstores/hypermarkets in the United States (e.g., Walmart Super Store, Super Kmart, SuperTarget) and internationally (e.g., Carrefour in Europe, South America, and Asia), more apparel, home fashions, and accessories are being sold through these types of stores. Items sold through supermarkets and superstores must accommodate a self-service merchandising strategy, so visual displays that assist consumers in selecting the right style and size are common. These items are also most likely to use an extended marketing channel that facilitates the supermarkets' buying of these goods.

Warehouse Retailers

Warehouse retailers offer goods at discount prices by reducing operating expenses and combining their warehouse and retail operations. In some cases, merchandise is obtained through an extended marketing channel. This category of retailers includes stores such as big box home improvement centers (e.g., The Home Depot, Lowe's) and warehouse clubs (e.g., Costco, Sam's Club).

Traditionally, apparel and home fashions products were not the primary merchandise sold through warehouse retailers. However, home improvement centers are now offering a larger array of home fashions goods (e.g., towels, bedding, carpets, rugs), and warehouse clubs are offering more styles and types of apparel and home fashions products. For example, Sam's Club offers a variety of apparel and footwear brands; Costco offers home fashion brands including Laura Ashley bedding. Generally, at warehouse retailers, apparel and home fashions are sold through self-service strategies with limited services (e.g., there are generally no fitting rooms).

Convenience Stores

Convenience stores are small stores that offer fast service at a convenient location (on a busy street or combined with a gas station), but they carry only a limited assortment of food and related items. 7-Eleven® is one of the most famous and largest international convenience store chains, with over 7,000 stores in the United States and Canada and another 32,000 in more than 15 other countries. The most typical apparel and accessory products carried by convenience stores are basic items such as mass-merchandised hosiery (e.g., L'eggs, Hanes), inexpensive novelty T-shirts or baseball caps, and inexpensive sunglasses, as well as fashion magazines.

Contractual Retailers

Retailers may enter into contractual agreements with manufacturers, wholesalers, or other retailers in order to integrate operations and increase market impact. Such contractual agreements include the following:

- retailer-sponsored cooperatives that take the form of an organization of small independent retailers
- wholesaler-sponsored voluntary chains, in which a wholesaler develops a program for small independent retailers
- franchises
- leased departments

The term **contractual retailers** covers all such arrangements. Franchises and leased departments are the most typical of the contractual retailers for the distribution of apparel.

FRANCHISES

In a **franchise** agreement, the parent company gives the franchisee the exclusive right to distribute a well-recognized brand name in a specific market area, as well as assistance with organization, visual merchandising, training, and management. In return, the franchisee pays the parent company a franchise payment. The franchisee agrees to adhere to standards regarding in-store design, visual presentation, pricing, and promotions specified by the parent company. Examples of franchises include Flip Flop Shops®, Apricot Lane Boutiques, and Kid to Kid Children's Resale franchise.

LEASED DEPARTMENTS

Some retailers will lease space within a larger retail store to a company that operates a specialty department. The larger retail store provides space, utilities, and basic in-store services. The specialty department operator provides the stock and expertise to run the department, and adds to the service or product mix of the larger store. Their lease or commission is typically based on square footage and sales.

Typical **leased departments** include beauty salons and spas; vision care and eyewear; florists and garden shops; books; restaurants; ticket offices; and fine jewelry, fur, and shoe shops. However, retailers may also offer leased departments for specialty merchandise. For example, Pea in the Pod leased departments in JCPenney stores offer maternity wear. In each of these cases, specific expertise and investment in stock are needed. With this arrangement, the primary advantage for the larger retailer is that it can offer its customers products and services that it might not be able to offer otherwise. The primary advantage for the specialty department is its association with the larger retailer and a convenient location for consumers to purchase their goods or services.

Chain Stores

Chain store organizations own and operate several retail store units that sell similar lines of merchandise with a standard method and function under a centralized organizational structure. Chain stores are characterized by the following features:

- centralized buying
- centralized distribution
- shared brands
- standardized store decor and layout

All management and merchandising decisions and policies are made by managers at a central headquarters or home office. Chain stores include:

- large chains (defined as 11 or more units), which may be national or international in scope, and include both department stores (e.g., JCPenney, Sears, Walmart), discount stores (e.g., Kmart, Target), and specialty stores (Aéropostale, Urban Outfitters, Men's Warehouse)
- small chains (two to ten retail units) within a local or regional area

Private label merchandise (e.g., JCPenney's Arizona, Worthington, and Stafford labels), exclusive brands (e.g., Kohl's Simply Vera by Vera Wang), and store brands (e.g., Gap, Polo Ralph Lauren) are important part of the merchandise mix for large chain store retailers. Franchises are always chain store operations. Although large chain stores benefit from the economies of scale that come with purchasing merchandise for a number of stores, they may carry merchandise that caters to the wants and needs of the local target markets. For example, a Kmart store in Athens, GA may carry University of Georgia licensed merchandise.

Nonstore Retailers

A **nonstore retailer** distributes products to consumers through means other than traditional brick-and-mortar retail stores. For apparel, accessories, and home fashions, the three most prevalent forms of nonstore retailing include **mail order/catalog**, **electronic/Internet** (e-tailing), and television selling. Other forms of nonstore retailing include at-home selling and vending machines. In the past 20 years, nonstore retailing, particularly mail order/catalog, electronic/Internet, and television selling, has grown tremendously. This trend is due to a number of social, economic, and lifestyle changes, including the following:

- the increased demand by consumers for convenience, product quality, and selection
- a highly fragmented market that demands products to fulfill special needs and interests
- the continued growth in the number of dual-income families, which creates increased time pressures for shopping among household members
- the expanding use and promotion of credit cards, such as those offered by Visa, Mastercard, American Express, and Discover, and store credit cards (e.g., Nordstrom)
- increased speed of delivery by package carriers (e.g., Federal Express, UPS, Priority Mail)
- technological advances in e-commerce, including improved security for sending credit card numbers electronically

In addition to selling merchandise, nonstore retailing, particularly mail order/catalog, electronic/Internet, and television retailing venues, are used by companies for a number of other purposes, such as the following:

- educating customers about the company and its product lines
- providing customers with fashion direction and style advice

- obtaining information from customers regarding product preferences
- building more traffic in their retail stores
- providing customers with a more convenient and/or more recreational form of shopping
- building relationships with customers through personalized customer service

Retailers selling apparel through mail order/catalog, electronic/Internet, and television retailing methods are faced with a unique set of challenges. Because the customer cannot physically evaluate the product, feel the fabric, or try on the merchandise, customer service and information about sizing, fabric, styling details, and color are important. For electronic/Internet retailers, advancements in Web technology allow customers to zoom in on photographs to see the details of products, to view the product from all sides, and to see the product in multiple colors and sizes. Many nonstore apparel, accessory, and home fashions retailers offer means for customers to connect with customer service representatives through the phone, online "chat rooms," or one-way video chat. Customers also have questions and concerns about shipping costs, timeliness of shipping, and returns. Because customers use nonstore retailing for its convenience, the ease in selecting styles, ordering, and returning merchandise is important.

Will nonstore retailing eventually put brick-and-mortar stores out of business? Most analysts believe that many consumers still want to touch and try on garments and accessories before purchasing them, and will still want the social experience of shopping in bricks–and-mortar stores. However, the growth in nonstore retailing has forced retailers to think about their retail environments in terms of better meeting customer needs. Retailers are merging technologies so that consumers reap the benefits of each of the retail formats. For example, many malls and brick-and-mortar stores provide kiosks whereby consumers can search products and stores online.

MAIL ORDER/CATALOG RETAILERS

Mail order/catalog retailers sell to the consumer through catalogs, brochures, or advertisements and deliver merchandise by mail or other carriers. Apparel is one of the top-selling items bought through catalogs. Customers can order by mail, phone, Internet, or fax. All types of retailers may operate mail order/catalog businesses. With the growth of e-tailing, virtually all large mail order companies also have Internet websites in addition to their catalogs. It is common for consumers to use catalogs for browsing and evaluating merchandise and then order and purchase merchandise online (see Figure 12.10).

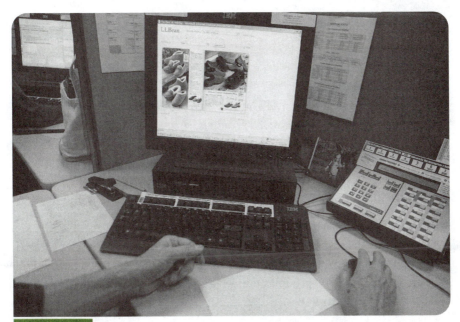

Figure 12.10 Mail order retailers such as L.L.Bean also provide customers with online catalogs and ordering services.

ELECTRONIC/INTERNET RETAILERS

Electronic/Internet retailers use **e-commerce**, the selling of goods over the Internet, to reach customers. Since the mid-1990s, e-commerce has grown consistently each year as more consumers have access to the Internet and as security issues related to sending credit card numbers electronically are being addressed by Internet retailers. Many apparel retailers and manufacturers have included e-commerce in their distribution strategy, offering goods only over the Internet or using the Internet as an addition to their stores and/or catalog retailing business as another aspect of their multichannel distribution strategy.

Although online apparel sales are a relatively small percentage of overall apparel retail sales, the number of "dot-com" websites devoted to apparel and accessories continues to grow. E-retailers generally fall into one or more of the following categories:

- exclusive e-retailers
- catalog retailers who have added websites
- department and specialty stores who have added websites
- apparel, accessory, and home fashions manufacturers' websites

- online fashion malls
- online auction/trade websites

Exclusive E-retailers

Some companies sell exclusively on the Web. These include designers of and merchants for specialized or niche products, such as organic cotton merchandise, and small retailers who may not be able to afford other forms of retail distribution. For example, Marianne Egan Custom Bridal offers bridal wear only through the company website. Websites such as ebay.com also provide opportunities for businesses to sell merchandise through these websites.

Catalog Retailers Who Have Added Web Sites

Companies that had been successful selling apparel through catalogs found they could make the transition to the Web fairly easily. In 1995, Lands' End offered fewer than 100 products online as an experiment. It is now one of the largest Internet apparel sites.

Department Stores and Stores Who Have Added Web Sites

Most large department stores and specialty stores have incorporated a multi-channel distribution strategy by adding e-commerce to their businesses. Online customers have gravitated to websites of well-known and trusted retailers such as Gap, Walmart, Target, Nordstrom, Sears, Macy's, and JCPenney. Because customers often use a retailer's website for information and comparison purposes and then will go to the retail store to try on the merchandise, integration of multiple distribution methods by the retailer is important.

Store retailers have found that access to new customers can be enhanced with online services. For example, many retailers sell certain merchandise exclusively online to attract a new or different customer than their brick-and-mortar retail store. For example, Old Navy offers its Women's Plus line only through Gap Inc. Direct, an online hub for all brands owned by Gap Inc.

Apparel, Accessory, and Home Fashions Corporate Web Sites

These websites may or may not include direct sales of merchandise to the ultimate consumer but provide corporate and investor information. For example, Liz Claiborne's corporate website, www.lizclaiborne.com, includes links to JCPenney's exclusive Liz Claiborne line, social media connections, and information about the Liz Claiborne Corporation, including the many brands owned by Liz Claiborne (e.g., Juicy Couture, Mexx, mac & jac). Nike's www.nikebiz.com website provides information about the corporation, careers with Nike, Nike's corporate responsibility initiatives, vendor information, and customer service. See Table 12.6 for a listing of the top mass merchant, apparel, and accessory Internet retailers.

Online Fashion Mall

One of the first Internet sites where apparel could be purchased online was Fashionmall.com, which was started in 1994. It provided a central location for a number of retailers, manufacturers, and magazines to offer fashion goods and services directly to customers (see Figure 12.11). Since that time, online fashion malls have served as destination websites that offer merchandise from a number of online stores. As such, consumers can go to a single website for products from multiple companies. Examples of online fashion malls and the companies/retailers that feature products for online purchase include the following:

Currently, fashionmall.com offers merchandise from approximately 50 companies/retailers, including babygap.com, Coldwater Creek, dELiAs.com, J.Crew.com, PacSun.com, and REI.

Amazon.com, another portal for apparel and accessories from multiple companies, features over 3,500,000 apparel and accessory products including brands such as Tommy Bahama, Ecko Unltd, Fossil, Nike, Patagonia, Reebok, and Southpole. Featured brands on Amazon.com for bed and bath products include Laura Ashley, Martex, Royal Velvet, Tommy Hilfiger, and DKNY.

Yahoo.com also offers "one-stop shopping" for name brand merchandise including Nike, Juicy Couture, L.A.M.B clothing, Sean John, and Phat Farm, to name only a few.

Table 12.6 Top Twelve Mass Merchant, Apparel, and Accessory Internet Retailers in order of Online Sales

Company	Category
Amazon.com Inc	Mass Merchant
Walmart.com	Mass Merchant
Sears Holdings Corp.	Mass Merchant
Liberty Media Corp. (QVC)	Mass Merchant
Costco Wholesale Corp.	Mass Merchant
JCPenney Co. Inc.	Mass Merchant
Victoria's Secret	Apparel/Accessories
Macy's Inc.	Mass Merchant
Target Corp.	Mass Merchant
Gap Inc. Direct	Apparel/Accessories
L.L. Bean Inc.	Apparel/Accessories
HSN Inc.	Mass Merchant

SOURCE: *Internet Retailer* (2010, May 18).

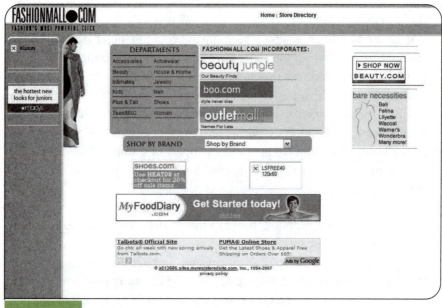

Figure 12.11 Fashiomall.com offers merchandise from over 50 companies/ retailers.

Online Auction/Trade Web Sites

Websites such as ebay.com offer opportunities for anyone worldwide to sell apparel, accessories, and home fashions online. Started in 1995 as an online auction website, eBay has grown into one of the largest websites, with more than 90 million active users worldwide and total worth of goods sold over $60 billion. Multitudes of new and previously worn apparel and accessories are offered for sale by individuals and companies throughout the world.

TELEVISION RETAILERS

Some retailers use television shopping channels to sell apparel, accessories, and home fashions products. With these formats, merchandise is presented on the television (and on accompanying websites), and customers order it over the telephone (usually using a toll-free number) or on the Web. Merchandise is delivered through the mail or by another carrier. Home shopping has become big business. QVC (see Figure 12.12), Home Shopping Network (HSN), and Shop at Home are three of the largest of these television shopping channels. TV shopping has expanded its merchandise assortment to include designer lines and a variety of product categories.

As with other retailers, the movement to multichannel strategies has also been found to be successful for those who started as nonstore retailers. HSN

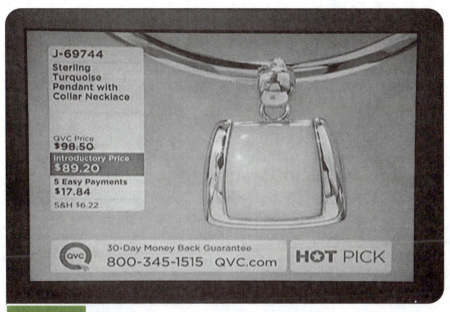

J-69744
Sterling
Turquoise
Pendant with
Collar Necklace

QVC Price
$98.50
Introductory Price
$89.20
5 Easy Payments
$17.84
S&H $6.22

30-Day Money Back Guarantee
800-345-1515 QVC.com   HOT PICK

Figure 12.12 QVC's multichannel retailing strategy includes TV, online, and brick-and-mortar stores.

offers customers shopping opportunities through TV (24 hours per day, seven days per week), online, through catalogs, and in brick-and-mortar stores. QVC has a very successful website and a flagship brick-and-mortar store (QVC @ The Mall) at Minnesota's Mall of America. The company also has six outlet stores throughout the United States. QVC, which stands for quality, value, and convenience, was founded in 1986. QVC showcases more than 1,000 products per week, televising 24 hours per day, 364 days per year. Approximately 60 million customers have shopped with QVC worldwide.

AT-HOME RETAILERS

At-home retailers (e.g., Doncaster, Polkadot Petals Home Parties) use the marketing strategy of making personal contacts and sales in consumers' homes. At-home retailing includes door-to-door sales or party plan selling methods. The party plan method involves a salesperson giving a presentation of merchandise at the home of a host or hostess who has invited potential customers to a "party." Accessories (e.g., handbags, jewelry), novelty items, and lingerie are typical apparel products sold using this retail method. The retailer Doncaster (owned by Tanner Companies) offers customers personalized attention and customer service through trained consultants. Merchandise is shown to customers on a periodic basis either in a home or in a pop-up retail studio.

VENDING MACHINES

Vending machines are coin-operated machines used to meet the needs of consumers when other retailing formats are unavailable or when space is limited for selling merchandise. Although vending machines are seldom used for the distribution of apparel products, they have been used to sell hosiery, T-shirts, and even men's dress shirts. One would most likely find such vending machines in locations such as airports or train stations.

Trade Associations and Trade Publications

As with other areas of textile and apparel industries, a number of trade associations and trade publications serve those involved in the distribution of apparel. See Table 12.7 for a list of selected retail trade associations. The National Retail Federation (NRF) is the largest trade association for retailers both within the United States and globally. It represents more than 1.6 million U.S. companies as well as companies in more than 45 other countries. The NRF Annual Convention and Expo is held in New York each January. The NRF has four divisions that focus on specific aspects of retailing:

- Association for Retail Technology Standards
- National Council of Chain Restaurants
- Retail Advertising and Marketing Association
- Shop.org (see Table 12.8).

Table 12.7   Selected Retail Trade Associations

Trade Association	Description
Electronic Retailing Association (www.retailing.org)	Leaders in direct-to-consumer commerce
International Council of Shopping Centers (www.icsc.org)	Serving the global retail real estate industry
National Retail Federation (www.nrf.com)	World's largest retail trade association and voice of retail worldwide
Shop.org of the NRF (www.shop.org)	National Retail Federation's digital division
National Shoe Retailers Association (www.nsra.org)	Represents independent footwear retailers
Retail Industry Leaders Association (www.retail-leaders.org)	Promotes consumer choice and economic freedom through public policy and industry operational excellence

The NRF publishes *STORES* magazine, a monthly trade publication that addresses the interests of those in the retailing industry. A number of other trade publications cater to those involved with distribution and retailing. Table 12.9 lists some of these publications.

Successes and Trends in Retailing

Change has become the norm in the textile, apparel, accessories, home fashions, and retailing industries. Faced with increased global competition, textile, apparel, accessories, home fashions, and retailing companies have made rapid changes in order to survive. The belief has been that the strongest advantage the U.S. industries could offer in this new, global marketplace was speed. If we could produce the goods faster, we could have them at market sooner. If we could produce goods closer to the delivery date, we could predict more accurately what would sell, and we would pay less interest on borrowed money needed for inventory and business operations. If we could automatically replenish goods sold by the retailer, then consumers would be more likely to find the goods they want when they want them.

How could we increase speed without decreasing product quality? How could we offer high quality merchandise produced in sustainable and socially responsible manners?

Table 12.8	Divisions of the National Retail Federation

Association for Retail Technology Standards (ARTS)
ARTS is an international membership organization dedicated to reducing the costs of technology through application standards exclusively to the retail industry. ARTS has four standards: The Standard Relational Data Model, UnifiedPOS, IXRetail, and the Standard RFPs.

National Council of Chain Restaurants (NCCR)
NCCR is the leading trade association exclusively representing chain restaurant companies.

Retail Advertising & Marketing Association (RAMA)
RAMA is a trade association of retail marketing and advertising professionals, plus their counterparts on the agency, media, and service-provider sides of the business.

Shop.org
Shop.org is the association for retailers online focusing on the evolving world of the Internet and multichannel retailing.

SOURCE: National Retail Federation (2011).

Table 12.9   Selected Trade Publications Related to Business, Distribution, and Retailing

Publication	Focus
Advertising Age (www.adage.com)	Focuses on advertising, marketing, and media news and information.
Bloomberg Business Week (businessweek.com)	Focuses on business news on Wall Street, media and advertising, international business, banking, interest rates, the stock market, and currencies and funds.
Chain Store Age (www.chainstoreage.com)	Focuses on information of interest to retail headquarters management, including trends and strategies in areas such as retail technology, store construction, marketing, physical support systems, finance, security, store design and visual merchandising, electronic retailing, payment systems, human resources, and supply chain.
Multichannel Merchant (multichannelmerchant.com)	For companies that sell goods through print catalogs and/or transactional Web sites including social media marketing
Retail Merchandiser (www.retail-merchandiser.com):	For executives and managers in the mass-merchandise, drug, club, and specialty retailing industries. Topics focus on merchandising and marketing issues, providing ideas and concepts that work within a retail environment.
Retailing Today.com (www.retailingtoday.com)	Focuses on mass-market retailing business news, trends, and research analysis.
STORES (www.STORES.org)	Print and online publication of the National Retail Federation with a focus on information of interest to retailers in general. Topics include retail technology, supply chain and logistics, credit and payment systems, online retailing, customer service, loss prevention, human resources, and other store operations.
Supermarket News (www.supermarketnews.com)	Weekly trade magazine for the food distribution industry. Executives use it as their information source for industry news, trends, and product features. Many large food retailers sell selected apparel, accessory, and home fashions products.
VM+SD (Visual Merchandising and Store Design) (www.visualstore.com)	Monthly magazine for retail designers and store display professionals with information on trends in store design and visual presentations, new products, merchandising strategies, and industry news.

A number of strategies for success in the ever-changing retail environment have focused on technology, consumer demand, and social responsibility. These include the following:

- knowledge about target consumers—their lifestyles, their wants, their needs, the limitations of their pocketbooks

- value associated with the product—consumers expect value for each and every dollar they spend

- building trust and establishing excellent relationships with vendors

- offering the highest quality product and service—successful companies make it easy to do business with them

- reviewing internal processes on a continual basis—exploring alternative ways of creating, manufacturing, and delivering merchandise is essential

- social/corporate responsibility in operations, vendor relations, and customer service

As multichannel distribution has become standard and as consumers seek and are comfortable with new ways of searching, evaluating, and purchasing apparel, accessories, and home fashions, a number of trends are being seen in the retail industry. These include fast fashion applications, mobile retailing, behavioral targeting, advanced merchandise management systems, and international retailing.

Fast Fashion Applications

With the success of Spanish apparel retailer Zara leading the way, followed by Mango, H&M, Topshop, and Uniqlo, many other types of retailers are seeking ways of getting fashion merchandise to consumers faster through increased demand for new ideas, shorter lead times, and increased deliveries. Although not all retailers will move entirely to a fast fashion strategy, elements of their operations will continue to be affected by the fast fashion phenomenon and resulting customer expectations.

Mobile Retailing

Mobile devices are offering both retailers and consumers with new ways of conducting business. For the retailer, mobile shopping assistance tools for sales staff allows sales associates to find product information and availability without leaving the customer. For the customer, mobile applications such as mobile self-checkout, which allows customers to purchase merchandise from their smart phones, are making the shopping experience integrated with their other mobile applications.

Behavioral Targeting

Behavioral targeting is the practice of collecting and analyzing customers' online consumer behavior activities to allow both manufacturers and retailers to personalize advertising and promotions. Automated integration of marketing research of online consumer behavior, use of retailer social media sites, and use of promotions will continue to facilitate the creation of these personalized marketing tools. Consumers are becoming more aware of privacy issues with this marketing practice, which may lead to changes in the legal aspects of this practice.

Advanced Merchandise Management Systems

Support for multichannel distribution and applications for optimizing inventory across all distribution channels have never been more important. A number of technological advances are now allowing companies to automate operations across brick-and-mortar and multiple online distribution channels.

International Retailing

With saturated markets in the United States, Japan, and Western Europe, growth in international retailing will be focused on emerging markets. Large companies will continue to invest in expanding operations globally, taking advantage of growing consumer markets in China, India, Brazil, and South Africa. According to *STORES* magazine's most recent report on global retailing (2011, January), success in global expansion will be dependent on companies focusing on the following:

- strategically aligning operations with their competitive advantage
- learning local tastes, aesthetics, customs, and consumer behavior
- utilizing managers locally
- developing local relationships with vendors
- investing on a relatively large scale to support efficiencies and build a strong consumer market

Apparel, accessory, and home fashions retailers will continue to be active in their global expansion. Indeed, in 2009, global fashion retailers sold their merchandise through brick-and-mortar stores, catalogs, and/or websites in an average of 17.5 countries, more than twice the average of other types of global retailers. Spurred by fast fashion retailers and strong brand name identification, this trend is expected to continue.

Summary

Apparel, accessory, and home fashions companies have a number of options with regard to the distribution of their merchandise to the ultimate consumer. Companies must decide how widely their merchandise will be distributed; some will choose mass distribution, whereas others will decide on a selective or exclusive distribution strategy. Many companies now have multichannel distribution strategies whereby merchandise is sold through a variety of retail formats. Apparel, accessory, and home fashions companies will distribute their goods either directly to their retail accounts or through distribution centers. Retailers with many stores may also use distribution centers as central locations for merchandise, from which it is then shipped to the various stores.

Quick Response, product lifecycle management, and supply chain management strategies are important in the distribution process, and alliances between apparel companies and retailers contribute greatly to the success of these strategies. The foundations for these strategies are to use Universal Product Code bar coding on product labels and shipping cartons; RFID tagging on shipping cartons; to have vendors (manufacturers) assuming responsibility for affixing labels and price information on products; and to use electronic data interchange for the electronic transmission of invoices, advance shipping notices, and other information. Replenishment of goods at the retail level is built on the foundation of these operations. In some cases, programs have been established whereby the vendor (manufacturer) manages retail inventory and automatically replenishes the retailer's stock when needed. RFID and data mining technology make possible even more sophisticated systems for making sure that the retailer has the right stock at the right time.

The retailing level of the marketing involves the selling of merchandise to the final consumer. Retailers are often classified according to merchandising and operating strategies into the following categories, which are not mutually exclusive: department stores, specialty stores, discount retailers, off-price retailers, supermarkets and hypermarkets, convenience stores, contractual retailers, warehouse retailers, chain stores, and nonstore retailing. Apparel, accessory, and home fashions manufacturers use a variety of retailers in the final distribution of their products to the ultimate consumer, although they use some (e.g., department stores, specialty stores, discount stores) more than others. Nonstore retailing, including mail order/catalog and electronic/Internet retailing, has experienced greater growth than traditional forms of retailing in recent years. Many companies are now focusing on multichannel retailing strategies whereby they distribute merchandise through both brick-and-mortar stores and nonstore retailing venues. Successful retailers rely on strategies that effectively incorporate technologies to better understand their customer, build relationships with vendors, manage inventories across distribution channels, and operate from a socially responsible framework. Trends in retailing include fast fashion applications, mobile retailing, behavioral targeting, advanced merchandise management systems, and international retailing.

Careers in retailing are as varied as the stores themselves. Some of the career possibilities include store management, merchandise buying, private label product development, catalog and nonstore retailing, and promotion and advertising, just to name a few.

Retail Store Manager
Women's Specialty Store Chain

Position Description:
Lead a management team of three to five assistant managers and oversee the performance of 25,000 to 30,000 square feet of store space. Identify key opportunities to increase sales, and manage payroll and expenses, as well as supervise and develop assistant managers.

Typical Tasks and Responsibilities:

- Ensure adherence to customer service policies and procedures.
- Oversee merchandise presentation activities on an ongoing basis.
- Motivate people to reach the store's goals.
- Manage payroll and operations.
- Oversee the development of assistant managers.

Merchandising Manager/Head Buyer
International Specialty Store

Position Description:
Ensure merchandise mix, availability, distribution to all stores, inventory management, pricing, market development, and trends for the future, and purchase target allocation for all stores.

Typical Tasks and Responsibilities:

- Select the merchandise mix to be carried throughout the stores.
- Work with local suppliers, and negotiate terms and conditions for each line of merchandise.
- Control inventory levels of merchandise (maximum three months inventory levels).
- Keep informed about the latest trends and developments (competitors, etc.).
- Set up a target purchase budget on a yearly basis.

Key Terms

big box store

boutique

chain store

contractual retailer

convenience store

cross-dockable shipments

data mining technology

department store

direct marketing channel

discount store

distribution center (DC)

e-commerce

electronic data interchange (EDI)

electronic/Internet retailer

exclusive distribution

extended marketing channel

e-tailing

factory outlet

floor-ready merchandise

flow-through

franchise

hypermarket

in-store shop

intensive distribution

leased department

limited marketing channel

mail order/catalog retailer

mass distribution

multichannel distribution

multichannel retailing

nonstore retailer

off-price retailer

picking

pop-up retail

replenishment

retailer

retailing

selective distribution

specialty store

stock-keeping unit (SKU)

stockout data

supermarket

superstore

Universal Product Code (UPC)

upscale discounter

value-added network (VAN)

vendor-managed inventory (VMI)

vendor marking

warehouse retailer

Web EDI

Discussion Questions and Activities

1. Describe the roles of distribution center for apparel, accessories, and home fashions manufacturers and retailers. How is valued added to the merchandise through these distribution centers?

2. Name and describe your favorite stores. What type of retail store is each? What are the characteristics of the types of retail stores you named? How does the store engage in multichannel distribution? What are the advantages and disadvantages of multichannel retailing strategies for this retailer?

3. Explore three websites that sell apparel, accessories, or home fashions on-line. What are the common features of these sites? What strategies do these retailers use to inform customers about product characteristics?

References

Amazon.com (2011). Clothing, Shoes, and Jewelry. http://www.amazon.com. Retrieved January 31, 2011.

Deloitte Touch Tohmatsu Limited and STORES Media, Leaving home: Global powers of retailing 2011. Section 2. (2011, January). http://www.deloitte.com/consumer-business

eBay (2011). Company Info. http://www.ebay.com. Retrieved January 31, 2011.

Home Shopping Network (2011). Company Overview. http://www.hsn.com. Retrieved January 31, 2011.

JCPenney (2011). About Us. http://www.jcpenney.com. Retrieved January 31, 2011.

Internet Retailer (2011). Portal to e-commerce Intelligence. http://internetretailer.com. Retrieved January 31, 2011.

Macy's (2011). About Us. http://macysinc.com. Retrieved January 31, 2011.

National Retail Federation (2011). About NRF. http://www.nrf.com. Retrieved January 31, 2011.

QVC (2011). About Us. http://www.qvc.com. Retrieved January 31, 2011.

Schulz, David P. (2010, July). Top 100 retailers. *STORES* http://www.STORES.org/stores-magazine-july-2010/top-100-retailers

7-Eleven (2011). The Company. http://www.7-eleven.com. Retrieved January 31, 2011.

Target (2011). About Target. http://www.target.com Retrieved January 31, 2011.

Walmart Corporate (2011). About Us. http://walmartstores.com. Retrieved January 31, 2011.

PART 4

Organization and Operation of the Accessories and Home Fashions Industries

CHAPTER 13

Accessories

In this chapter, you will learn the following:

- the relationship between fashion apparel and accessories

- the similarities and differences between the design and manufacturing of accessories and that of fashion apparel products

- the marketing and distribution strategies for fashion accessories

Relationship of Accessories to the Apparel Industry

*W*hat would a men's suit be without the right necktie? What would a new fashion look be without the right shoe style, belt, or jewelry? The accessories industries comprise a vital component of the total fashion industry and are integral to the success of the apparel industry. Primary accessory categories include footwear; hosiery and legwear; hats and headwear; scarves; belts, handbags, gloves; and jewelry. Other accessories not discussed in this chapter include sunglasses, handkerchiefs, hair accessories, watches, and umbrellas. Each season, changes occur in accessories that relate directly to the changes occurring in fashion apparel. For example, the styling, colors, textures, and scale of jewelry will correspond to the type of apparel with which it will be worn (see Figure 13.1). Fashion trends in apparel and accessories are so closely linked that one can purchase a sweater, belt, and shoes in the same hot new fashion color at the same time in the market. It is clear that these industries work together.

Yet fashion apparel products and accessories are distinctly different in some respects. Some accessories such as simple scarves can be manufactured very quickly when a new trend in apparel develops. In other cases, the accessories themselves are the fashion statement. This is often the case for sunglasses. Sunglass styles become very fashion forward as they are used by celebrities or seen in popular movies.

Other accessories take much longer to produce. The footwear industry needs time to design and produce the product, including time to procure materials. The design phase for shoes may begin before the design phase for an apparel product, especially if specialty leather materials are required. Therefore, forecasters in the shoe industry must be keenly aware of market and fashion trends in order to accurately predict appropriate shoe fashions that complement and coordinate with fashion apparel of upcoming seasons.

Accessories Categories

Accessories manufacturers are grouped into categories, including the following:

- footwear
- hosiery and legwear

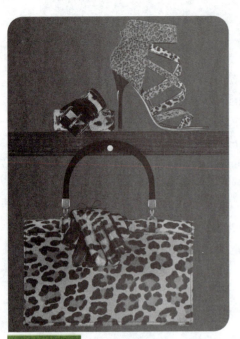

Figure 13.1 Fashion trends in apparel and accessories are closely linked.

- hats and headwear
- scarves
- belts
- handbags
- gloves
- jewelry

Many accessory companies specialize in manufacturing only one type of product; that is, some companies manufacture only shoes, and other companies produce only neckwear. Some companies prefer to diversify into more than one accessory category (see Figure 13.2). Dooney & Bourke and Coach, both traditionally handbag and small leather goods manufacturers, have diversified into footwear. Coach further diversified with a licensed apparel line.

The term **cross-merchandising** refers to the strategy used by both apparel companies and retailers to combine apparel and accessories in their product offerings. Some apparel manufacturers create their own accessories to coordinate with their apparel lines (e.g., Timberland, Eddie Bauer). Nike produces a line of backpacks and sports equipment bags in conjunction with its footwear and apparel lines. Other companies form agreements to produce coordinating apparel and accessories. In skiwear, for example, one apparel company may produce the outerwear apparel products, while another company produces the coordinating knit sweaters, headwear, and hand wear. Thus, the responsibility for manufacturing each type of product rests in the hands of the company with the required expertise and the best qualifications to produce it. Retailers employ cross-merchandising through displays that create a total fashion image and demonstrate to consumers how accessories might be worn with the apparel.

Licensing is a very important cross-merchandising strategy for coordinating apparel and accessory looks. In the typical licensing agreements, accessory manufacturers pay a royalty to the licensor company for the use of the brand, logo, or trademark on the merchandise. As discussed in Chapter 2, licensing agreements can be beneficial to both the accessory manufacturer and the designer. For the accessory manufacturer, the designer name provides immediate brand recognition among consumers. For the designer, he or she can expand into a variety of

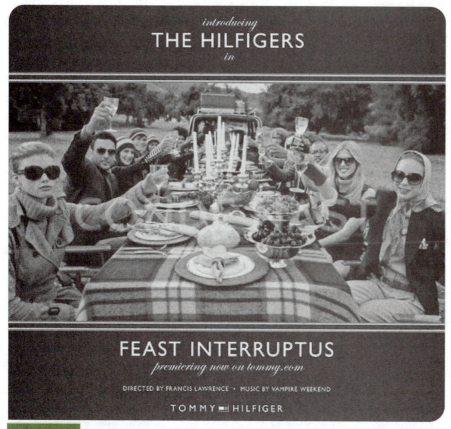

Figure 13.2 Some companies such as Tommy Hilfiger produce goods in more than one accessory category.

product lines bearing his or her name and become a total lifestyle brand by taking advantage of the manufacturer's product and market expertise.

Some accessories companies have licensed their names for apparel lines (e.g., Hush Puppies, Kenneth Cole). Many name designers of apparel use licensing agreements with accessory manufacturers to produce the specific styles of accessories that complete the total fashion looks they desire. Designers such as Tommy Hilfiger, Ralph Lauren, Liz Claiborne, Donna Karan, and Calvin Klein have their names linked to belts, hosiery, shoes, and eyewear. Kenneth Cole has successfully licensed a broad range of merchandise, including all of the company's non-footwear products except handbags. Depending on the licensing agreement, designers vary in their involvement and approval requirements with the licensee. Some designers, such as Kenneth Cole, are involved with design and approval. Others turn over design decisions to the licensee.

Athletic footwear companies often have unique licensing agreements with professional and collegiate sports leagues (e.g., Major League Baseball) or individual teams. In these agreements, footwear companies pay the leagues or teams for the right to sell merchandise with the league or team logo. In addition, they may also purchase the right to outfit the team with athletic footwear and/or uniforms bearing the company's logo.

Consumers' purchases of accessories are often impulse buying decisions; that is, the purchases are not planned. Therefore, to facilitate these impulse purchases, accessories are often sold on the main floor of department stores, included in displays throughout stores, and positioned near the checkout locations in stores.

As with other segments of the fashion industry, the accessories industries rely on trade associations for research, education efforts, marketing, public relations, and advertising. These trade associations may focus on several categories of accessories (e.g., Accessories Council) or on a single category of accessories (e.g., Neckwear Association of America). For example, the mission statement of the Accessories Council, founded in 1995, is to stimulate consumer awareness and demand for fashion accessory products, and to serve as the advocate of the accessory business in the United States.

Table 13.1 lists selected trade associations for accessories (see Chapter 4 for additional information). Trade publications are also essential to the dissemination of industry news and advertising to individuals in the accessories industry. Table 13.2 lists selected trade publications related to accessories.

Although there are differences in production processes within the accessories industries, most accessory lines are produced following procedures similar to the steps in the research, design, production, and distribution of apparel. These steps include the following:

- research, including color, material, trend, and market research
- design, including sketching and the use of CAD or graphics software
- patternmaking (or creating molds in the jewelry industry)
- developing prototypes
- costing and sourcing
- marketing, including presenting a minimum of two lines per year during market weeks and at trade shows (see Table 13.3)
- production
- distribution and retailing

Table 13.1	Selected Trade Associations for Accessories
Association	**Website**
Accessories Council	http://www.accessoriescouncil.org/
American Apparel and Footwear Association	http://www.apparelandfootwear.org/
Fashion Footwear Association of New York (FFANY)	http://www.ffany.org/
Headwear Association	http://www.theheadwearassociation.org/
International Fashion Jewelry and Accessory Group	http://www.jewelrytradeshows.com/
International Glove Association	http://www.iga-online.com/
Jewelers of America (JA)	http://www.jewelers.org/
National Fashion Accessories Association (NFAA)	http://www.accessoryweb.com/
National Shoe Retailers Association (NSRA)	http://www.nsra.org/
Sporting Goods Manufacturers Association (SGMA)	http://www.sgma.com/
The Hosiery Association (THA)	http://www.hosieryassociation.com/
United Shoe Retailers Association	http://www.usraonline.org/
World Shoe Association	http://www.wsashow.com/

Table 13.2	Selected Trade Publications for Accessories
Publication	**Description**
Accessories Magazine	Published six times a year by Bji Fashion Group; information for manufacturers and retailers of accessories including fashion trends, industry statistics, merchandising, and promotion. http://www.accessoriesmagazine.com/
California Apparel News	Published every Friday by MnM Publishing Corporation; covers fashion industry news with an emphasis on regional companies and markets on the West Coast. http://www.apparelnews.net/
FN-Footwear News	Published weekly by Fairchild Publications; includes footwear news, fashion trends, and business strategies targeted especially to manufacturers and retailers. http://www.wwd.com/footwear-news
Women's Wear Daily	Published weekdays by Fairchild Publications; includes special accessories supplements; Monday issues feature accessories, innerwear, and legwear industry news. http://www.wwd.com/

Table 13.3	Selected Trade Shows for Accessories
Show	**Held in:**
Accessories The Show	New York and Las Vegas
China International Clothing and Accessories Fair	Beijing, China
China International Footwear Fair	Hong Kong
Fashion Accessory Exposition	New York
Fashion Footwear Association of New York (FFANY) trade shows	New York
International Fashion Jewelry and Accessories Fair	Dubai
International Fashion and Accessories Show	New York
International Hosiery Exposition (IHE)	Charlotte, North Carolina
International Manufacturers of Fashion Jewelry and Accessories Fair	Madrid, Spain
International Shoe Fair (GDS)	Dusseldorf, Germany
JA International Jewelry Show	New York
JCK Fine Jewelry Show	New York and Las Vegas
Midec International Footwear Fashion Fair	Paris, France
Moda Accessories	Birmingham, UK
New York Accessories Market	New York
New York Shoe Expo	New York
Shoe Fair	Bologna, Italy

NOTE: Many apparel trade shows listed in Chapter 8 also include accessories.

Important aspects of research, design, production, marketing, distribution, and retailing of accessories for each of the major categories are discussed in the following sections.

Footwear

Footwear categories include the following:

- athletic footwear
- dress shoes and boots

- casual shoes

- sandals

- work shoes and boots

- western/casual boots

- hiking, hunting, and fishing boots

During the past few decades, the footwear industry has changed in a number of ways. First, as with apparel, footwear sold by U.S. manufacturers has shifted from domestic to global production. This is primarily because of the availability of raw materials and of rising labor costs in the United States; shoe production can be very labor intensive. Second, the production of leather footwear has been augmented by the production of footwear using a variety of manufactured materials. The types of shoes most frequently purchased have shifted as well. Athletic footwear has gained a tremendous market share of the footwear industry, with more athletic shoes sold than any of the other footwear categories. Shoe manufacturers have therefore developed styles that crossover

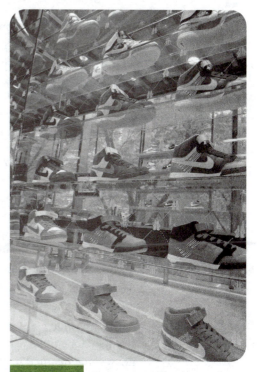

Figure 13.3 Crossover styling between athletic shoe styling and fashion shoe styling is seen in these shoes.

between athletic shoe styling and fashion shoe styling in which style components of each type of shoe are combined (see Figure 13.3).

Footwear Producers

The footwear industry in the United States is sometimes referred to as an *oligopoly* (see Chapter 2) in that several large shoe manufacturers produce the vast majority of shoes. The largest shoe manufacturers in the United States are no longer fashion shoe companies. Currently, Nike controls approximately one-third of the U.S. athletic shoe market. Both Nike and the adidas Group have diversified their footwear lines, with Nike acquiring Cole Haan and Converse, and the adidas Group acquiring Reebok. Several large companies also dominate the fashion footwear business. Among them are the United States Shoe Corporation and Brown Shoe Company.

From an international perspective, Nike and the adidas Group are two of the world's largest footwear companies. Italy, however, has a reputation for leading trends in fashion footwear. In addition to its design reputation, Italy has produced fine leathers for apparel as well as for footwear for centuries. The handcrafting of Italian leather products has maintained a worldwide reputation for centuries as well. Salvatore Ferragamo shoes and handbags, Bruno Magli shoes, and Gucci shoes and handbags epitomize quality Italian leather materials and workmanship.

Research, Design, and Production

The first steps in creating a footwear line and an apparel line are similar. Footwear companies begin their lines by conducting market research, including consumer research, product research, and market analysis. They examine demographic and consumer buying trends of their target customer, explore innovations in footwear styles and technology, and analyze trends in the footwear market in general. They develop a target customer profile describing the typical customer for their various lines of footwear.

Athletic shoe giants Nike and the adidas Group invest heavily in footwear research. One of Nike's early developments was the Nike air cushioning technology that debuted in 1979. Nike's Sports Research Lab employs a dozen researchers who study how feet and shoes function—from the way pressure dissipates each time a runner's foot strikes the ground to how women's toes flex and grip better than men's. In 2004, Nike introduced its Nike Free, based on creating a shoe that simulates how the foot performs while running barefoot. Nike is not alone in investing heavily in footwear research. For three years, the adidas Group worked to develop a computer-chip-embedded running shoe.

Fashion shoe designers research fashion trends in much the same way as do apparel designers. Many shoe designers throughout the world attend the Italian leather shows, as well as various shoe trade shows, to view the latest developments in leather and shoe design. Shoe designers work in conjunction with the company's merchandisers and production team to develop the shoe line each season. Designers work with the following shoe design components each season: materials, trims, style features, and heel height and shape. It is remarkable that shoe designers create such a variety of innovative styles each season given the small surface area of footwear. The fabrication of prototype shoe styles and patterns is performed using steps similar to those discussed for apparel products.

Shoes are made by forming the raw materials around a **last**. The last is a wood, plastic, or metal mold, shaped like a foot. In the United States, lasts are sized in widths as well as lengths. Historically, the width of the last for

European sizes has been different from that for U.S. sizes. Some U.S. footwear manufacturers produce shoes in Italy in order to take advantage of the Italian raw materials and craftsmanship. The shoes made in Italy for U.S. manufacturers are produced using U.S. lasts in order to fit the target customer's foot.

CAD technology has become an important part of the footwear industry. Computer software allows the shoe design to be viewed three-dimensionally on the screen. Some merchandisers for shoe companies consider computer images of the styles to be sufficient when selecting the shoes for the line. Thus, prototypes would be made only for those styles selected for production.

The sizes of pattern pieces for shoes are small compared to the sizes of most apparel pattern pieces. Accurate cutting is vitally important to the fit and craftsmanship of shoes. Therefore, cutting footwear often utilizes a die-cutting process (see Chapter 9) because of its accuracy. A metal die similar to a cookie cutter is made to duplicate the shape of each of the pattern pieces. Its very sharp edge cuts through the layer or multiple layers of materials. Computerized cutting and laser cutting are other options (see Chapter 9) that provide extremely accurately cut pieces.

Leather hides are used for much of the fashion footwear produced worldwide (see Chapter 3). The hides are irregular in shape, and they often have blemishes and thin areas, as is to be expected of this natural product. Thus, cutting hides for the production of shoes, handbags, belts, and other leather goods requires additional time and expertise, creates some waste of material due to the irregular shape of hides, and often necessitates single-ply cutting to avoid blemished areas.

Another factor to consider is that leather hides are a commodity traded on a market with a price that varies according to the supply. In this respect, the shoe industry is similar to the fur industry. Not only do prices vary based on supply, but since some of the hide sources are in other countries, the monetary exchange rate can affect the price of the raw materials.

Because shoe manufacturing involves a large number of steps that demand skilled workers, labor costs tend to be high (see Figure 13.4). Adding to the production time, and thus to the labor cost, is the difficulty of manipulating an awkwardly shaped product composed of many small pieces.

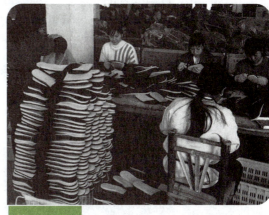

Figure 13.4 Shoe manufacturing involves a large number of steps that must be performed by skilled workers.

Examine the tiny material sections of a pair of toddler's athletic or hiking shoes to imagine what it would be like to assemble the shoe sections. The development of specialized machinery has helped to keep labor costs down for those manufacturers that can afford to invest in the equipment. Most of the domestic shoe production occurs in Pennsylvania, Maine, and Missouri. However, as labor costs have risen in the United States, more fashion shoes are being produced offshore. China has become the leading producer of shoes. South America (especially Brazil) and Asia also produce large quantities of the shoes sold in the United States.

Marketing and Distribution

New York City serves as the marketing center for footwear, with most companies having showrooms there. Domestic and international shoe trade shows, or markets, similar to the apparel market shows, are held two to four times a year. Fall/Winter shoe lines are typically shown in January or February, and Spring/Summer shoe lines are typically shown in August. The Fashion Footwear Association of New York (FFANY) sponsors footwear trade shows in New York City. Retail buyers as well as manufacturers and footwear producers attend these shows, just as the apparel trade shows are attended by people representing all aspects of the apparel industry.

The footwear industry utilizes similar promotional tools as the apparel industry in selling their lines to retail buyers. Sales representatives for footwear companies provide line catalogs to their retail customers. Some companies are currently using digital images of footwear in their presentations to retail buyers, thus creating a "virtual showroom."

Footwear is sold in many department stores, specialty shoe stores, specialty stores that offer footwear in addition to other products, sporting goods and athletic footwear stores, discounters, and by nonstore retailing venues (catalog, television, and Internet/Web). Some specialty shoe stores carry products from a range of manufacturers. Foot Locker and Lady Foot Locker stores, an athletic footwear chain, carry a variety of athletic footwear brands. In addition, the strategy of vertical integration is also common in the footwear industry, that is, some manufacturers own the shoe stores in which only their products are sold. Examples are Thom McAn, Redwing, and Stride Rite. Footwear companies such as Nine West and Easy Spirit have stores in outlet malls. Companies engaged in nonstore retailing of footwear include Lands' End, L.L.Bean, and Eddie Bauer, which offer shoes in addition to apparel products. The Nike.com website allows mass-customization, whereby customers may select colors and separate shoe sizes for left and right feet (see Figure 13.5).

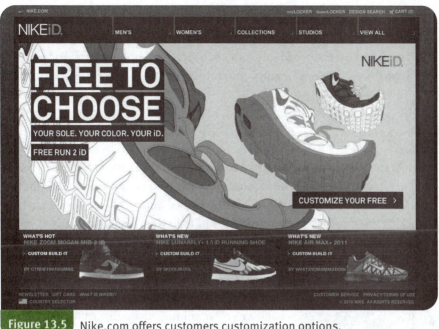

Figure 13.5 Nike.com offers customers customization options.

Private label and store brand apparel strategies are discussed in Chapter 7. In the footwear industry, store brand and private label business is also an important component. In 2005, Nike bought the Starter footwear brand and began to produce Starter sneakers for Walmart stores. This partnership provided an opportunity for Nike to enter a new channel of distribution. The discount retailers represent a very strong market segment, since consumers purchased about $1.5 billion worth of athletic shoes at discount stores.

Footwear retailing requires an immense inventory because of the large combination of shoe widths and lengths. When the range of seasonal colors is added to the size inventory, it is clear that shoe retailers have a challenging task to meet the consumer's need for the right product in the specific color and size. The footwear retailer must make a significant capital outlay and have large inventory space. This is one reason why some retailers lease their shoe departments to companies that specialize in shoe retailing (see Chapter 12).

The shift in location of footwear production from predominantly domestic, with some Western European production, to Asia and South America was discussed earlier in this chapter. The footwear industry has also shifted its customer market from domestic consumption to a global marketplace. Canadian, Mexican, and Japanese consumers have become major markets for U.S.

footwear. American athletic shoe brands are sought worldwide. The reputation for quality of the casual footwear produced by U.S. manufacturers, such as Timberland, has opened European markets for these products. For survival and expansion, footwear manufacturers must continue to seek a global market for their products.

Hosiery and Legwear

The hosiery and legwear industry comprises companies that produce men's, women's, and children's socks, stockings, pantyhose, and tights. This industry has a long and notable history in the United States. There is evidence that stocking knitting machines were in operation in New England as early as 1775. By 1875, the U.S. hosiery industry focused on the production of silk stockings, with an estimated worth of $6,000. By 1900, the industry had grown to a value of $186,413.

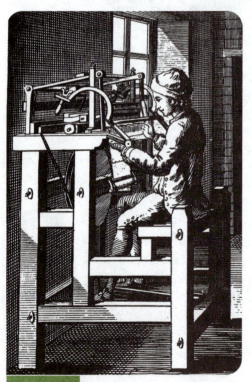

Figure 13.6 The development of framework knitting machines provided a faster way to produce hosiery.

For centuries, stockings were knit by hand using a circular knitting procedure so that no center back seam was required. The foot and leg shapes were produced by adding or subtracting stitches to increase or decrease the circumference of the stocking. The development of framework knitting machines (see Figure 13.6) in England at the end of the sixteenth century provided a way to produce stocking blanks ("The history of hosiery," 1974). However, the material was knit flat, or **flatknit**. This meant that a seam had to be sewn along the center back to create the tubular stocking. The **full-fashioned** technique provided the shaping of the knit goods to conform to the foot and leg shapes along the seam edges. The first full-fashioned hosiery factory in the United States was established by E. E. Kilbourn in the late 1860s.

The development of circular knitting machines in the nineteenth century provided a means to produce seamless (except for the seam used to close the toe) stockings, socks, and, later, tights and pantyhose. Early seamless stockings did not fit as well as full-fashioned seamed stockings. When women's hemlines were shortened during the 1920s, the better fit of seamed stockings was preferred. This is reflected in the increase in production of full-fashioned stockings from 26 percent of the market in 1919 to 60 percent of production in 1929 and more than 80 percent in the 1950s ("The history of hosiery," 1974).

The hosiery/legwear industry underwent major developments during the twentieth century. At the beginning of the twentieth century, hosiery consisted of primarily white, "nude," and black socks and stockings in cotton, wool, and silk (and later, rayon) knits. By 1928, technological advances in knitting allowed for the production of full-fashioned men's hosiery in argyle patterns, English ribs, and cable stitches. In 1939, stockings made of DuPont's nylon fiber were introduced. Women loved their sheerness. Just as the demand for "nylons" soared, they were removed from the market. Nylon was needed for the war effort during World War II, and women wore socks that coordinated creatively with their suits. An amusing anecdote survives regarding women's sense of loss during the war. Sixty women in Tulsa, Oklahoma, were asked what they missed most during the war. Twenty said they missed men the most; forty said they missed nylons the most! In 1946, when nylon stockings became available again, the crowds waiting to purchase them created a legendary sight.

Pantyhose were developed during the 1960s when very short hemline lengths required a product to replace stockings. As the name implies, the hose, or stocking, is joined to a panty, creating an all-in-one product. This eliminates the need for garters that are used to connect the stockings to a girdle or a garter belt. Nylon is the most prevalent fiber for pantyhose. Some pantyhose include a cotton-knit crotch piece. The pantyhose may include spandex fiber to provide some figure control. Since the 1980s, blending a small percentage of spandex with nylon in the leg portion of pantyhose has gained popularity. In the 1990s, microfiber (smaller-than-standard fiber diameter) nylon became popular, especially for opaque pantyhose or tights. Tights are similar to pantyhose, but they are made of a heavier material. Tights and pantyhose are either seamless or seamed along the center back.

Because pantyhose are made of manufactured fibers that are heat sensitive, the foot and leg shape can be built into the product during the finishing process. A heat setting process is used to mold the foot and leg shape by placing the hosiery over a leg-shaped board. Terms used for the application of heat to create the final shape in the finishing process are **blocking** or **boarding**.

Like textile production, hosiery production developed primarily in the Northeast. As with textile mills, however, production shifted to the South as labor costs increased in the Northeast. Hosiery/legwear is a dynamic, high-fashion industry for men's, women's, and children's products. Staple hosiery

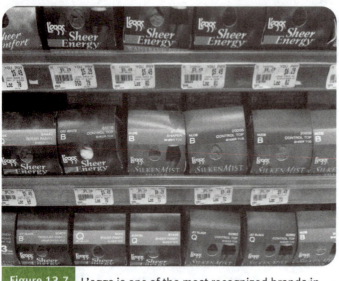

Figure 13.7 L'eggs is one of the most recognized brands in hosiery.

goods have been augmented with "fashion" socks, stockings, and pantyhose suitable for every holiday, to express one's personality, or to add extra punch to an outfit. As with apparel, hosiery/legwear can be found in all price zones, from mass/budget to designer. However, this product category has strong price appeal. The consumer can update an outfit inexpensively with accessories such as hosiery.

Hosiery and Legwear Producers

The hosiery/legwear industry is dominated by large firms that are often part of vertically integrated companies that produce knitted fabrics as well as the finished hosiery and legwear products. Most of the domestic hosiery/legwear producers are located in the Southeast, concentrated primarily in North Carolina, Alabama, Tennessee, and in Pennsylvania. Some of the largest U.S. hosiery manufacturers include Kayser-Roth (No nonsense, HUE, Calvin Klein), Gold Toe Brands, Inc. (Gold Toe, Silver Toe, Auro), and Hanesbrands, Inc. (Hanes, L'eggs, Just My Size) (see Figure 13.7).

Research, Design, and Production

Companies that produce hosiery and legwear analyze apparel style trends and consumer buying trends to make design decisions. In addition, color forecasting plays a very important role in determining the various colors in which hosiery and legwear will be produced. Designers also focus on new developments in textiles and knitting technology. For example, microfiber technology has provided consumers with softer and more sheer hosiery alternatives.

Socks are produced in varying lengths, including anklets, crew, mid-calf, and calf lengths. The most popular fibers for socks are cotton, wool, silk, acrylic, nylon, polypropylene, or blends of these fibers. Cotton and acrylic fibers are used frequently for ankle-length socks, while calf-length socks are often made of nylon, wool, silk, acrylic, or blends of two of these fibers. A small percentage of spandex might be added to provide some elasticity.

Sport socks or athletic socks continue to be a market growth area. Socks are at the forefront of textile innovation. Rick Rudinger, CEO of Next fiber technology LLC states "the hardest area to show added value is on the feet. If you can prove your technology in socks, the rest of the body is much easier." (Thiry, 2010. p. 32). Sports socks have become very specialized and sport-specific (see Figure 13.8).

The size range of hosiery varies according to the type of product. Sock and stocking sizes for men, women, and children are indicated with size numbers that correlate to shoe size. The consumer refers to a chart that shows the correct sock or stocking size based on the wearer's shoe size. There are fewer sock and stocking sizes than shoe sizes; each hosiery size fits a range of shoe sizes. For some products, the sock or stocking is available in only one size that fits the majority of shoe sizes. Pantyhose generally are sized to fit women who fall within categories based on their height and weight. Typical pantyhose sizes are *short, average*, and *tall. Queen size* and *plus size* are size categories for the larger or taller size market. Some pantyhose producers provide a petite size as well.

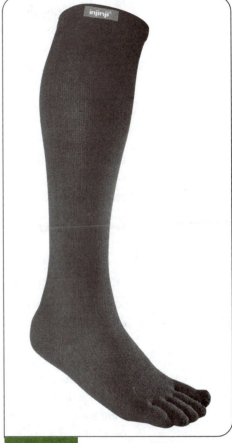

Figure 13.8 New developments in sport socks can be seen in Injinji toesocks.

One of the strengths of the hosiery industry is the impressive variety of innovative textures, colors, and patterns available for hosiery and legwear products. New technology continues to bring an ever-increasing array of materials for hosiery. Much of the machinery required to produce hosiery is automated or computerized, and some of it operates 24 hours a day. Computer software designed for hosiery includes a library of design components, including sock pattern templates, and a wide variety of knit stitch effects. Courtaulds Socks, a part of Sara Lee Courtaulds, is a leading sock supplier to British retail giant Marks & Spencer, as well as other department stores and supermarkets in the United Kingdom. At Courtaulds Socks, the design team is constantly creating new designs, as many as 30 per week. They rely on CAD. Images can be imported from other media such as sketches, photos, prints, and other CAD systems, or the designer may choose to draw the design directly on the system; the design is then quickly converted into stitch format and visualized on the sock template at the correct finished stitch tension.

Labor costs can be kept down by advanced technology. Thus, the hosiery industry is not threatened as much by inexpensive imports as some other industries. A strength of the hosiery industry is that many manufacturers are vertically integrated and, therefore, have enhanced supply chain management opportunities.

Although the hosiery industry will face challenges in the future, it is positioning itself for continued success. The hosiery industry relies on a close working partnership among the fiber producers, hosiery manufacturers, and retailers. By working together, the hosiery industry in the United States may be able to remain competitive with imported goods.

Marketing and Distribution

Market weeks for hosiery typically coincide with those for ready-to-wear apparel, although many hosiery and legwear products are marketed and distributed through extended distribution channels. The hosiery industry is a low-margin business. This means that the dollar amount of profit per item sold that the producer earns from the sale to the retailer is small. Similarly, the dollar amount of profit that the retailer garners from the sale to the customer is also small. Thus, the manufacturer and the retailer need high sales volume to compensate for the low margin. A number of strategies are used to create high sales volume. These strategies include vendor-managed inventory systems, distribution through discount stores, enhancing ease of shopping, and licensing.

VENDOR-MANAGED INVENTORY

To produce a large sales volume, it is important to maintain a complete stock of hosiery in the appropriate sizes, styles, and colors. Therefore, many large hosiery manufacturers use Quick Response and supply chain management strategies, including vendor marking and vendor-managed inventory. Through the sharing of sales data, stock is automatically replenished at the retail store to ensure a complete selection of products for the customer.

EASE OF SHOPPING

Most hosiery and legwear is sold through large discount chain stores (e.g., Walmart, Target, Kmart). Brands such as L'eggs, Hanes, and No nonsense are sold in this manner. The domination of discount store sales means that hosiery is extremely price competitive both at retail and at wholesale levels.

Because of the number of styles, colors, and sizes, selecting hosiery can be confusing for consumers. To allow for a self-service retailing strategy, package marketing is used by companies that sell hosiery in supermarkets, convenience stores, and discount retailers. This includes large-format sizing charts mounted on display racks, packaging that is color coded by style and size, and samples of the product available for consumers to touch and evaluate. Retail stores have adopted some of the same strategies to assist the consumer in selecting the right product. Because of the self-service approach to selling hosiery and legwear, companies have simplified packaging, improved signs, and enhanced display fixtures in an effort to assist the consumer.

Fashion trends also affect the sales volume of hosiery. In the 1990s, the trend toward more casual dressing at the office may have been a stimulus for the increase seen in the sales volume of socks. Promoting hosiery as a fashion accessory rather than a staple commodity can enhance sales volume. Hosiery departments in retail stores may feature bodywear in addition to the hosiery products. Many retailers have added cross-merchandising displays, displaying hosiery (as well as other accessories) with coordinating apparel.

Some retailers have narrowed the number of brands or have focused on private label hosiery to simplify options for consumers. In addition, private label hosiery can provide for greater markups for the retailer. Retailers such as JCPenney, Nordstrom, and Talbots, to name just a few, distribute private label hosiery.

LICENSING

Licensing products is another marketing strategy that has proved successful in the hosiery industry. As with footwear and other accessories, many name designers license their names for hosiery. Givenchy, Ralph Lauren, Calvin Klein, and Donna Karan are examples of designers who have licensing agreements with large hosiery companies for hosiery products.

Hats, Headwear, Scarves, and Neckwear

Accessories such as hats, headwear, scarves, and neckwear typically are manufactured by a company that specializes in the specific accessory item. These accessory categories are integrally connected with apparel fashions and social norms.

Hats and Headwear

For 2010, hats were projected to be 3 percent of the accessories market ("Accessories Census 2009," 2010). The popularity of hats follow fashion trends of the time and are no longer a social requirement as they were in the 1950s, when men and women would not think of going out without a properly matched hat. The popularity of wearing casual hats, sport hats, and sport caps (especially baseball caps) has increased, providing a growth area for the industry. Seventy percent of hat purchases in 2009 were made by 17- to 34-year-old consumers ("Accessories Census 2009," 2010).

Many hat and headwear producers specialize in one type of product. For example, a manufacturer (sometimes referred to as an **item house**) will specialize in producing only baseball caps. Soft-fabric hats and caps are usually sewn using construction techniques similar to those used for apparel. Handwork might be required for the more expensive hats, while less expensive hats and headwear are machine made. Traditionally styled wool felt hats and straw hats are usually formed over a hat block, using steam to mold the hat into shape (see Figure 13.9).

Men's hats are produced in sizes, from 6½ to 7½ (in ⅛-inch intervals), that correspond to head circumference, or, for less structured hats, in sizes *small, medium, large*, and *extra large*. Caps may be produced in one size. Most women's hats are made in one size; however, some designer hats are produced in several sizes. Small children's caps and hats may be sized by age,

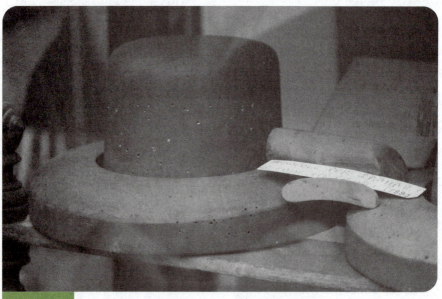

Figure 13.9 Felt hats are molded into shape over hat blocks such as the one seen here.

while older children's hats may be produced in sizes *extra small, small, medium*, and *large*.

Baseball caps are used extensively as promotional items for many businesses. They can be manufactured quickly with technologically advanced equipment. A large number of baseball caps with a company logo might be ordered for a special event. Quick delivery of the product is a necessity to meet this need. The New Era Cap Co. of Buffalo, New York, is a business built on speedy production in large quantities through flexible manufacturing. It is a licensed official supplier of caps to Major League Baseball, the National Basketball Association, and the National Hockey League, as well as a supplier to many colleges and universities and hundreds of Little League teams.

Millinery is a term that refers specifically to women's hats and usually denotes that handwork is involved in the hat-making process. Until the late 1960s to early 1970s, most large department stores had millinery departments with millinery specialists. However, very few retailers have retained millinery departments. The hats sold in most retail stores are machine made and moderately priced. Only a small market for fine millinery continues to exist. Most of the fine milliners are located in New York City, although milliners can also be found in Los Angeles and other major metropolitan areas.

Scarves and Neckwear

Scarves (preferred industry spelling) represent another product for which styles follow fashion cycles, and sales rise and fall with fashion trends. At times, large square scarves, perhaps even in shawl sizes, are popular; at other times, small square or oblong scarves might be fashionable. The scarf business is very specialized. A scarf manufacturer may specialize in only silk scarves or only woolen (or wool-blend, acrylic, or cotton) scarves. The printing processes used to apply the fabric design to silk are different from those used for woolen materials; thus, it is common for companies to specialize in one of these materials to ensure a quality product.

The cost of producing scarves is tied to the fabrics, designs, and printing methods used. The Italian design house of Emilio Pucci is well known for scarves in the designer price zone. Pucci's silk scarves in brightly colored prints became famous in the 1960s and have been instantly recognizable ever since. The scarf prints are very carefully silk-screened, so that the narrow black outlines around each motif are perfectly aligned (registered).

Many item houses in the United States produce scarves in a wide variety of materials, from silk chiffon to cashmere, in an array of textures, colors,

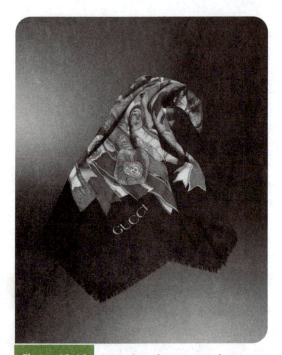

Figure 13.10 Many item houses produce scarves.

and prints (see Figure 13.10). Echo is one of the best-known U.S. manufacturers in the moderate-to-bridge price zones. Echo produces scarves, neckties, and bedding under its own label, as well as private label goods for stores such as Saks Fifth Avenue and Ann Taylor, and licensed scarves for Ralph Lauren. Many name designers, such as Ralph Lauren, Liz Claiborne, Oscar de la Renta, and Bill Blass, license their names for scarves and neckties.

Many scarf manufacturers use fabric manufactured in Asia and use Asian contractors for the printing as well. The material cost and labor cost related to printing may be lower in Asia, thereby making it more profitable to source offshore. The actual scarf-construction process can be very rapid, with machine-rolled hemming for moderate- and mass-priced goods, or time consuming, with hand-rolled hemming for some scarves in the designer price zone.

Necktie manufacturers are usually specialists that produce only neckties. Finer-quality neckties are made of silk, while lower-priced neckties are polyester. Wool, linen, cotton, leather, and other specialty materials comprise a small segment of production. Most necktie materials are woven; a small percentage of neckties are made of knit fabric. For neckties made of woven fabrics, the material is usually cut on the **bias**, or diagonal, to provide a more attractive knot and contour around the curve of the neck. Because a large amount of fabric is required to cut neckties on the bias, this practice increases the cost. The bias cut also produces the diagonal angle of the stripe seen on neckties as they are worn (see Figure 13.11).

The fabric design for neckties is either a print, applied to the surface of the woven fabric, or a stripe, plaid, or motif woven into the fabric. Typical necktie stripes are called **regimental stripes** because they are derived from various historical military regiments. These stripes are spaced with wider widths for the background and narrower widths for the various stripes. Many private secondary schools, military schools, colleges, and universities have their own regimental stripes with unique combinations of colors and spacing that denotes the specific institution. The regimental stripe tie is considered a classic choice for conservative business attire.

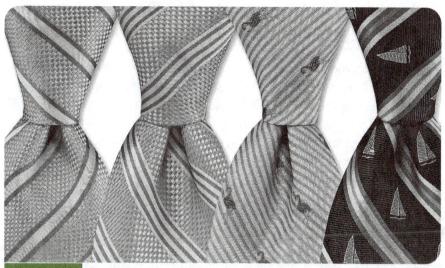

Figure 13.11   Men's ties are usually cut on the bias, producing the diagonal angle of the stripe on the necktie.

The construction process for neckties involves machine processes; some higher-priced goods require handwork as well. The price reflects the amount of time required to produce the necktie, as well as the cost of the materials. Computer-aided textile design processes and new computer printing technologies provide additional ways to reduce costs for the scarf and necktie industries in the United States.

The market for neckties reflects fashion cycles. The fashion pendulum moves from narrow ties to wide ties, from bow ties to no ties, from bright prints to subtle stripes. With the trend toward casual business dress, neckties are no longer required at some offices that traditionally had required that neckties be worn. This change may have had some impact on the necktie business. On the other hand, specialty tie shops in retail malls provide consumer awareness, interest, and offer shopping convenience. Conversational or theme necktie prints have provided an impetus to sales. Whether the necktie displays one's profession or hobby or promotes a seasonal holiday, the consumer can use his necktie to "speak" to observers.

In addition to neckties, other types of neckwear for men include neck scarves, or **mufflers**, often wool or silk, worn as an accompaniment to a wool overcoat for more formal occasions or worn with a casual jacket or coat to provide neck warmth or a fashion statement. An **ascot**, a long neck scarf worn looped at the neck, is another item of men's neckwear. While neck scarves and ascots are not purchased as frequently as neckties, retailers such as Brooks Brothers include such items as a necessary component of a well-stocked classic men's retail store.

Scarves, neckties, and other neckwear are sold to consumers through a variety of retail venues: department stores, specialty stores, discount stores, boutiques, and nonstore retailers (e.g., catalog companies). The merchandising of scarves and neckwear often requires instruction to consumers on how to tie the scarf or necktie effectively. Retailers often use promotion tools provided by the manufacturer to educate the consumer. These might include point-of-sale videos, booklets, and demonstrations.

Belts, Handbags, and Gloves

Belts, handbags, gloves, and other small leather accessories add elements to project one's personal style. These items, too, reflect fashion trends seen in apparel and other accessories. When pants are cut with a low rise, contour belts that shape to fit the body contour are fashionable. When the waist is a fashion focus, wide belts are an important accessory. Some of the unique aspects of each of the accessories categories of belts, handbags, and gloves are discussed separately in the following section.

Belts

The belt industry is divided into the following two segments: **cut-up trade** and **rack trade**. The cut-up trade includes manufacturers that produce the belts that apparel companies add to their pants, skirts, and dresses and supply as a component of the products that apparel companies ship to retailers. The rack trade is made up of manufacturers that design, produce, and market belts to retailers.

Manufacturers in the cut-up trade specialize in low-cost, high-volume items. These garment belts might be made with less expensive materials and processes, such as gluing rather than stitching the backing material to the belt. Self-belts made from the same fabric as the garment might be produced by a belt contractor or the apparel manufacturer at the same time that the garment is produced.

Belts for the rack trade often provide an important component of a fashion look; therefore, this part of the accessories industry works closely with the apparel segment. U.S. belt production is centered in New York City's fashion district. Typical materials include leather as well as numerous other materials, from cording to beaded fabrics. The type of material used determines the construction techniques and manufacturing processes.

For leather belts, cutting can be performed by hand or by the use of a strap cutting machine that cuts even-width strips. Some leather belts are curved or contoured, in which case the leather can be die cut for speed and accuracy. A myriad of decorative effects can be used to enhance belts (see Figure 13.12). Belt designers add creativity with the use of buckles, stitching, jewels, chains, metal pieces, plastics, stones, nailheads, and other embellishments. Belt backings are attached by stitching or gluing.

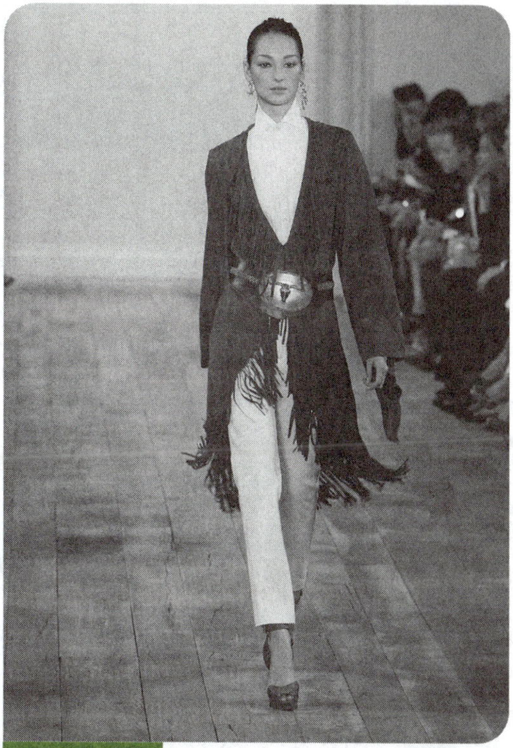

Handbags

Although this category of accessories is referred to as *handbags*, a variety of products is retailed within the classification. Handbags are also called *purses*. Many of the purses produced and sold today are actually shoulder bags rather than handbags. Women's briefcases are included in the *handbag*

Figure 13.12 Buckles, stamping, and other decorative effects add lively interest to belts.

category, as are wallets, coin purses, and eyeglasses cases. (Men's briefcases are typically sold with luggage.)

Handbags are made from a variety of materials. Many of the handbags sold in the United States are made of leather, reptile (such as snakeskin), or eel skin. Other materials include a variety of fabrics, plastics (vinyl is the most common), and straw. Judith Leiber is well known for beaded and metal evening bags, with retail prices beginning at approximately $500.

Structured handbags are supported by a frame that provides a distinctive shape and to which hardware, such as the closure, is attached. Soft handbags, such as pouch styles, may not use a frame. Handles or straps are attached to carry the handbag. **Clutch** bags are designed to be held in the hand (the term is derived from the fact that the bag is clutched in the hand) and may have a strap that can be stored inside the bag. Most handbags are lined in materials such as leather, suede, cloth, or vinyl. Structured bags may also have an interlining made from a stiff material to provide a firm shape.

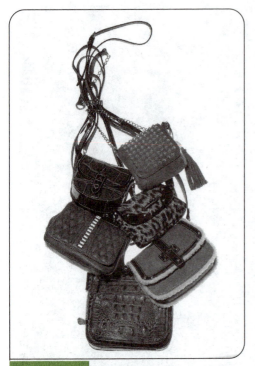

Figure 13.13 Designers use new shapes, colors, textures, and hardware for bags to create new styles each season.

Handbag styles range from large satchels to tiny clutches. While fashion trends play an important role in handbag styling, personal choice plays a role as well. Some women prefer a very functional bag, designed to hold everything, either in a roomy tote or a compartmentalized style. Other women prefer a compact style that could range from a wallet-on-a string to a decorative evening bag to hold only a few essentials. Many European men carry bags, and some American men have adopted this practice, particularly to store personal electronic devices.

Designing handbags requires the same steps as many other products. Ideas are sketched, and decorative trims, handles, hardware, and materials are researched. Materials and trims, and size and shape of a bag are some of the design parameters (Figure 13.13). A myriad of possible design details contributes to the design inspiration. Colored piping is considered "classic" for some handbags, but new color combinations add a fresh look. After ideas and sketches have been generated, prototypes are made, and then the line is finalized.

Leather handbags follow manufacturing procedures similar to other leather products discussed in this chapter. Fabric handbags may use die cutting and other processes similar to garment and shoe production. Computerized cutting equipment is used by the factory in Sainte Florence, France, to produce Louis Vuitton's "Alma" bag made from the famous monogram fabric. Plant director Pascale Tinozzi commented, "There is absolutely no allowance for error in cutting; the maximum permissible tolerance is half a millimeter" ("Louis Vuitton: 15 Vectors meet exacting production demands," 2001, p. 10).

For all handbags, some of the assembly processes, especially adding the hardware, require handwork. Thus, labor costs are an important part of the costing structure. For leather goods, the price and availability of hides is another cost consideration. There are a number of small companies that produce many of the handbags produced in the United States. Most of these companies are centered in the mid-Manhattan area of New York City. New York City is also the primary market center for handbags and small leather goods. Since most handbags and small leather goods sold in the United States are imported, offshore production sites in Asia, Spain, Italy, and South America are important production centers.

Because many of the production processes are similar for various leather goods, shoe manufacturers might also make handbags and belts. For example, Ferragamo produces coordinated handbags for some of its shoes, and Coach produces belts and other small leather goods as well as handbags. The handbag trade shows, generally four per year, coincide with the apparel markets.

In the 1970s, several designer names became sought after by consumers. The Louis Vuitton vinyl handbags with the "LV" logo appeared everywhere and sold at a premium price. Gucci bags became a status symbol. French fashion designer names such as Pierre Cardin and Christian Dior appeared on the outside of handbags. Since then, the licensing of designer and well-known brand names for handbags has become a major component of this business.

Handbags and small leather goods are sold through department stores, specialty stores, discount stores, boutiques, and nonstore venues. Some department stores have established in-store shops to feature the leather products of a specific manufacturer. Coach bags and belts often have a designated retail space, distinctively styled with shelf units and signage that the customer associates with Coach. We also see vertical integration within this industry. For example, Coach also operates its own retail stores (see Figure 13.14).

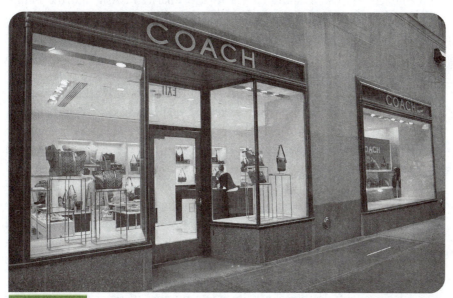

Figure 13.14   Coach handbags might be sold through in-store shops in department stores or through Coach specialty stores.

Gloves

Gone are the days when a well-dressed man, woman, or child did not leave home without both hat and gloves. The popularity of dress gloves rises and falls with fashion trends, while functional gloves and mittens, such as those worn for cold winter weather, remain a steady part of the industry. Sport gloves are a rising segment of the glove industry, with gloves specially designed for skiing, snowboarding, bicycling, weightlifting, golf, and many other sports. Women's dress gloves are produced in a variety of lengths, from wrist-length "shorties" to shoulder-length 16-button gloves for bridal and evening wear. (The term *button* is used to designate each inch of length.)

The two primary categories of the glove industry are leather gloves and fabric gloves. The difference in the handling of these two types of materials results in substantial differences in production. The majority of fabric gloves are made of knit fabric. Production is similar to that of other knit items and is located primarily in the Southeast, where many knitting mills are located. Knit gloves and mittens are produced quickly by using a circular knitting machine (see "Hosiery and Legwear" earlier in this chapter).

The production of leather gloves, however, still requires many hand operations. Automating the processes is difficult, and skilled operators are required. Because of the labor-intensive nature of the industry, many glove manufacturers use offshore contractors, primarily in Asia and the Philippines, to reduce labor costs. In the United States, a large portion of glove manufacturing is located in the state of New York. Two of the glove industry's largest companies, Fownes Brothers and Co. and Grandoe Corporation, are headquartered there.

The types of leather used for gloves need to be strong, yet thin and supple. Leather gloves are produced in a variety of lengths and from many different leathers (see Figure 13.15). Typical glove leathers include kidskin, lambskin (*cabretta* is a type of lambskin), pigskin, deerskin, and sueded leathers. Among the steps in the production of better-quality gloves is a process to dampen and then stretch the leather in order to improve suppleness. Some leather glove manufacturers specialize in only one part of the production process, such as cutting. This step requires careful assessment of the hide for quality and most efficient utilization. Cutting might be accomplished entirely by hand, called **table cutting**, for the top-quality gloves, or by less time-consuming die cutting, or **pull-down cutting**, for less expensive gloves.

Higher-quality leather gloves include a number of separate sections that provide flexibility for hand movement. These sections include the following:

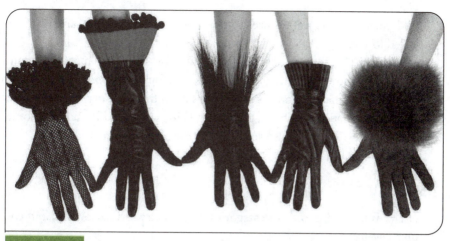

Figure 13.15   Gloves are made from different types of leathers and other materials.

- a thumb section
- a **trank** piece for the palm and another piece for the face of the hand
- **fourchettes**, which are rectangular strips between the second/third, third/fourth, and fourth/fifth fingers to provide width
- three **quirks**, tiny triangular gussets at the base of the second, third, and fourth fingers.

Each of these pieces requires painstaking care in construction in order to fit the pieces together properly.

Woven-fabric gloves require pattern pieces and steps similar to those for leather gloves. Less expensive gloves may have fewer pattern pieces and, therefore, may not provide as much hand mobility and comfort as gloves made with more pattern pieces. The seams may be stitched so the raw edges are to the inside or may be sewn with raw edges to the outside, depending on the style of glove. Gloves can be made of a combination of leather and fabric. For example, a sport glove might have leather tranks and knit fourchettes. Some leather gloves are lined with knit fabric or fur.

Knit gloves may be manufactured in one size if the fabric stretches sufficiently to fit a wide range of hand sizes. Leather gloves usually are produced in sizes *small, medium, large*, and *extra-large*, or they are sized numerically, in ¼-inch intervals, corresponding to the circumference in inches around the palm and forehand (sizes 7 to 10 for men and sizes 5 ½ to 8 for women). For children, gloves and mitten sizes (often sized *as small, medium,* and *large*) are related to age.

New York City is the primary market center for gloves, and most glove companies have showrooms there. Specialists called glove buyers in retail stores are from a bygone era. Today's gloves are sold in the accessory departments of department or specialty stores, along with belts, scarves, handbags, and sometimes jewelry. Gloves are also sold by specialty accessory retailers.

Jewelry

Jewelry is divided into three categories: fine jewelry, bridge jewelry, and costume jewelry.

Fine Jewelry

Fine jewelry is the most expensive jewelry category. This category includes pieces made from precious metals, such as silver, gold, and platinum, either alone or with precious and semiprecious gemstones (see Figure 13.16). Because gold is too soft to be used by itself, it is usually combined with other metals for jewelry. The gold content of a piece of jewelry is expressed in *karats*, or k, with 24k referring to solid gold; 18k and 14k gold are most often used in fine jewelry. Any alloy less than 10 karats cannot be labeled *karat gold*. Platinum, which is heavier and more expensive than gold, is often used for rings, particularly diamond rings. Silver is the least expensive of the precious metals. Silver is often combined with other metals, usually copper. To be labeled sterling silver, the metal must be at least 925 parts silver to 1000 total parts.

Precious gemstones include diamonds, emeralds, sapphires, and rubies. All are measured in karats, with 1 karat equaling 100 points. Pearls are also included in this category, even though they are not a stone per se. Semiprecious stones include amethyst, garnet, opal, lapis, jade, topaz, and aquamarine. In recent years, semiprecious stones have gained popularity as consumers' preference for colored gemstones has increased.

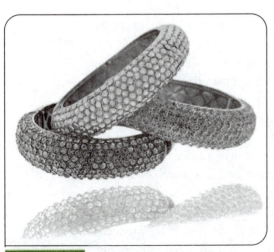

Figure 13.16 Fine jewelry is made from precious metals and precious and semiprecious gemstones.

Fine jewelry companies are often vertically integrated organizations, with the designer, producer, and retailer under one roof. Fine jewelry is sold through specialty jewelry stores and the fine jewelry departments of upscale department stores. Many consumers have turned to nonstore retailers, particularly television retailers such as QVC, to purchase fine jewelry.

Bridge Jewelry

Similar to the bridge price zone for ready-to-wear apparel, which falls between designer and better price zones, **bridge jewelry** falls between fine and costume jewelry. Bridge jewelry serves as an umbrella term for several types of jewelry, including ones that involve the use of silver, gold (typically of 14, 12, or 10 karats), and less expensive "stones," such as onyx, ivory, coral, or freshwater pearls. One-of-a-kind jewelry designed by artists using a variety of materials is also considered bridge jewelry. Bridge jewelry is sold in the same stores or departments within stores as fine jewelry and costume jewelry.

Costume Jewelry

Costume jewelry is the least expensive of the jewelry categories. In the 1920s and 1930s, Coco Chanel was the first prominent designer to accessorize her couture garments with costume jewelry, thus legitimizing the wearing of less expensive jewelry by women everywhere. This type of jewelry is mass produced using plastic, wood, brass, glass, Lucite, and other less expensive materials. Although there are large companies in the costume jewelry industry, including Monet and Trifari, the industry is dominated by small companies that produce jewelry sold through a variety of retail outlets, including nonstore retailers (see Figure 13.17).

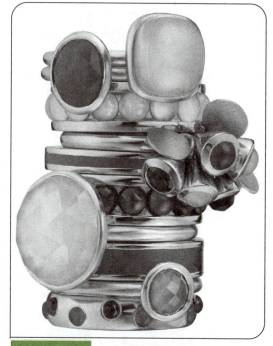

Figure 13.17 Costume jewelry is produced using plastic, glass, and inexpensive metals.

Summary

Accessories comprise important segments of the fashion industry. Changes in accessories complement changes found in the ready-to-wear apparel industry. Therefore, the apparel and accessories markets work together in creating total fashion looks. Accessories are grouped into the following categories: footwear; hosiery and legwear; hats and headwear; belts, handbags, gloves; and jewelry. Although production processes vary, most accessory lines are created according to the following steps: research, designer's sketches, patternmaking, development of prototypes, costing, marketing, production, distribution, and retailing. These steps mirror the steps used for the creation of apparel.

The footwear industry produces men's, women's, and children's dress shoes and boots, athletic shoes, casual shoes, and other footwear. The main raw materials used for footwear include leather, fabrics, and plastics. Shoes are produced by forming raw materials around a last or mold shaped like a foot. To reduce labor costs, shoe production has shifted from domestic to primarily offshore venues. New York City serves as the primary market center for footwear.

The hosiery/legwear industry produces men's, women's, and children's socks, stockings, and hosiery. The hosiery industry is dominated by large firms that are often part of vertically integrated companies. Most of the domestic hosiery producers are currently located in the Southeast. Production of hosiery is highly automated and, therefore, is not threatened by imports as much as are other industries. Hosiery companies are very involved with Quick Response and supply chain management strategies, including vendor-managed retail inventory.

Although hats and headwear companies currently comprise a much smaller segment of the accessories industries than they did decades ago, they are still important. Item houses that produce specialty merchandise, such as baseball caps, have grown as the popularity of this type of accessory has increased. The belt industry includes the rack trade (manufacturers that design, produce, and market belts to retailers) and the cut-up trade (manufacturers that produce belts for apparel companies). The handbag industry produces small leather goods as well as handbags. Leather gloves and fabric gloves are the two primary categories in the glove industry.

Jewelry is divided into three categories: fine jewelry, bridge jewelry, and costume jewelry. New York City serves as the market center for virtually all accessories. Trade shows and trade associations play an important role in promoting all components of the accessories industries.

As with the ready-to-wear industry, the accessories industries include a wide variety of career possibilities, from design to production to marketing and distribution.

Accessories Pattern Maker/Sample Maker
Publicly Held Sportswear and Athletic Shoe Company

Position Description:
Support the design prototype process for the accessories team, including drafting patterns; interpreting design and constructing prototypes; and creating specifications, technical drawings, and construction details.

Typical Tasks and Responsibilities:

- Draft accessories patterns from design sketches.
- Construct, build, and/or sew accessories samples, such as bags, hats, or gloves.
- Create product specifications and ensure accuracy.
- Create product technical drawings, complete with construction details, to facilitate more accurate samples from the field.
- Review accessory samples for accuracy, color matching, durability, and function.
- Review construction details to ensure that specifications are correct.
- Collaborate with accessory designers, developers, and engineers to ensure that the best product is produced, and work out construction problems.
- Calculate fabric utilization data and other costing factors in collaboration with engineers, designers, and developers.
- Evaluate new equipment with the sample room supervisor and technology services manager.
- Cut fabrics and trim.
- Purchase and maintain inventory of materials, supplies, and notions.

CAREER PROFILES

Key Terms

ascot
bias
blocking
boarding
bridge jewelry
clutch
costume jewelry
cross-merchandising
cut-up trade
fine jewelry
flatknit
fourchette

full-fashioned
item house
last
millinery
muffler
pull-down cutting
quirk
rack trade
regimental stripe
table cutting
trank

Discussion Questions and Activities

1. Think about the accessories you are currently wearing. How do they complement the fashion apparel you are wearing? How are the design, production, and distribution of these accessories similar to and different from that of fashion apparel?

2. If you were a shoe designer, before starting your next line of shoes, what sources of information would you turn to for market and trend research? Why would this information be important in your design decisions?

3. Study the ads for accessories in a current fashion magazine. Note how many ads there are for shoes, jewelry, and purses. How do the number of accessories ads compare to the number of apparel advertisements? Can you think of some reasons for the ratio of accessories to apparel ads?

4. Visit a fine jewelry store and have a jeweler explain the different stones and materials used in their products. How does the jeweler obtain their merchandise?

References

Accessories Census 2009 (2010, March) *Accessories*, pp. 18–42.

The history of hosiery: Early industry developed slowly. (1974, November 8). *Hosiery Newsletter*, pp. 3–9.

Louis Vuitton: 15 Vectors meet exacting production demands. (2001). *Lectra Mag* number 2, pp. 8–10.

Thiry, M.C. (2010, July/August). Best foot forward: Socks and hosiery leading innovation. *AATCC Review*, pp. 32–38.

CHAPTER 14

Home Fashions

In this chapter, you will learn the following:

- the similarities, differences, and relationships between the home fashions and the ready-to-wear apparel and accessories industries

- the design, marketing, production, and distribution processes of textile products, such as upholstery fabrics, window coverings, area floor coverings, towels, and bedding

- the steps the industry has taken to ensure sustainable design in home fashions

What Are Home Fashions?

*P*revious chapters in this book have primarily examined the design, marketing, production, and distribution of ready-to-wear apparel and accessories. Because of the growth and increased relationship between apparel and home fashions, this chapter focuses specifically on the home fashions industry. **Home fashions** are textile products, such as towels, bedding, upholstery fabrics, area floor coverings, draperies, and table linens for home end uses that have styles that change over time in response to evolving fashion trends. Therefore, home fashions include the upholstery; window treatments; soft floor coverings; and bed, bath, and tabletop categories of the broader home furnishings industry. The home fashions industry consists of companies that design, produce, market, and distribute these home fashions products.

This chapter examines the similarities, differences, and relationships among the design, production, marketing, and distribution of home fashions and ready-to-wear apparel and accessories. An understanding of the organization and operation of the home fashions industry in the broader context of apparel fashions is important for several reasons. Home fashions companies are important customers for many companies that also cater to the apparel industry, such as trend forecasting companies, textile mills, and textile converters. Also, the ready-to-wear industry and the home fashions industry have become increasingly interconnected as a growing number of apparel companies are now designing, producing, marketing, and distributing home fashions.

As we examine the home fashions industry, it is important to keep in mind that the average **product turn** (the frequency rate at which a product is sold and replaced at the retail store) in home fashions is less than two per year, compared to the apparel industry where the average turn is four to six times a year (or with fast fashion up to 12 times per year). This difference in product turn has implications for the design, manufacture, distribution, and retail sales of home fashions.

Categories for Home Fashions

In general, the home fashions industry is divided into the following four primary end-use categories (Yeager, 1988):

- upholstered furniture coverings and fillings
- window treatments and wall coverings

- soft floor coverings, including area rugs, scatter rugs, runners, and cushions (room and wall-to-wall carpeting are beyond the scope of this chapter)
- bed, bath, tabletop, and other home textile accessories and accents

Later in this chapter, these end-use categories are discussed in greater detail. First, an overall context for the design, marketing, and production of these end-use products is provided in the following sections:

- a general discussion of some overarching trends in the home fashions industry
- the organization and operation of the home fashions industry
- the marketing of home fashions

Home Fashions Industry Trends

A number of trends in the home fashions industry affect the design, production, and distribution of home fashions. These trends include the following:

- strong consumer demand for home fashions
- crossover between apparel and home fashions
- growth of private label and store brand products
- multichannel distribution of home fashions
- increased social responsibility and sustainability initiatives in the production of home fashions (discussed later in the chapter)

Consumer demand for home fashions has been strong, and analysts predict continued strong demand. Although this industry was negatively affected by the severely slowed housing industry in 2009–2010, a growing remodeling industry, consumers' desire to spend more time at home, and the growing selection of home fashions available to consumers forced companies to reexamine their product categories and distribution methods. Even with this slowing housing market, analysts continue to predict a growing demand for home fashions, as evidenced by the increasing number of **home fashions centers,** which bring together a variety of home improvement and decorating retailers, such as furniture, tile, carpeting, and lighting. With this continued growth, the design, production, marketing, and distribution of home fashions encompasses a large potential market for exciting and rewarding careers for individuals who have expertise in textiles, design, and marketing.

The crossover between apparel and home fashions continues to be a strong trend. Since the early 1980s when Laura Ashley and Ralph Lauren started licensing their brand names to home fashions items, numerous apparel designers and ready-to-wear manufacturers have added home fashions to their licensing mix, including the following:

- Giorgio Armani
- Tommy Bahama
- Tommy Hilfiger
- Calvin Klein
- Michael Kors
- Nautica
- Sigrid Olsen
- Pendleton Woolen Mills
- Lilly Pulitzer
- Sean John
- Vera Wang

Retailers have found that these well-known designer and manufacturer brand names attract customers who purchase home fashions through their various retail venues (see Figure 14.1).

Another trend in home fashions has been the growth of private label and store brand merchandise. A number of stores have introduced their own lines and collections of home fashions under brand names unique to the stores. Macy's offers private label brands, including Charter Club and Barbara Berry (see Figure 14.2). Kmart offers Jacyln Smith Today and Jaclyn Smith Traditions Bed and Bath lines. Target offers private label brands such as Thomas O'Brien and Simply Shabby Chic by Rachel Ashwell through exclusive licensing agreements. Pottery Barn, Crate and Barrel, and Pier 1 offer home fashions as store brands. For example, Pottery Barn's in-house designers create a variety of store brand collections (e.g., PB Essential, Matine Toile Collection) that are exclusive to Pottery Barn.

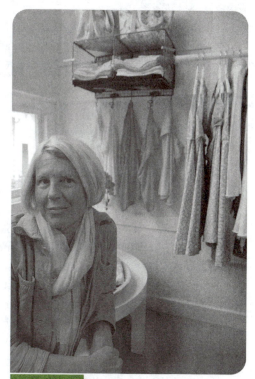

Figure 14.1 Designers such as Sigrid Olsen often add home fashions to the product categories of their licensed merchandise.

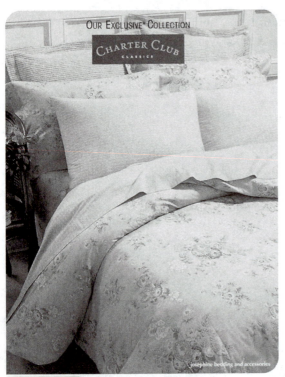

Figure 14.2 Charter Club is one of Macy's private label store brands for home fashions.

Home Fashions and the Textile Industry

The textile industry forms the base for the structure of the home fashions industry. The design and performance of the textiles used in home fashions play a very important role in the success of the end-use product. For many home fashions, the design of the fabric is as important as the design of the end-use product itself. As mentioned in Chapter 3, some textile companies focus entirely on home fashions end uses (e.g., Springs Global) whereas others produce fabrics for both apparel and home fashions (e.g., International Textile Group, Milliken). The general organization and structure of textile companies that produce textiles primarily for the home fashions industry are the same as for those companies that produce textiles for the apparel industry (see Chapter 3 about the organizational structure of the U.S. textile industry).

The home fashions industry is dominated by vertically integrated textile companies that produce both fabrics and home fashions end-use products (see Figure 14.3). These include home fashions powerhouses such as WestPoint™ Home and Springs Global. This is because production of home fashions is often highly automated and can be accomplished very efficiently within a vertical operation. In many cases, the fabric may not need to be cut and sewn to complete the product (e.g., towels and rugs), or minimal sewing, such as sheet hemming, is performed at the textile facility. For example, a single facility owned by WestPoint™ Home performs all production processes, from cleaning cotton to creating the finished products (e.g., sheets and pillowcases) that are ready for distribution.

Because of this vertical integration and automation of production, many large production facilities still exist in the United States. Home fashions fabric companies have also expanded production internationally. For example, Springs Global has operations in the United States, Canada, Mexico, Brazil,

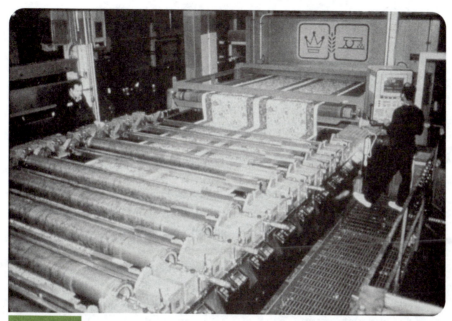

Figure 14.3 Vertical integration and automation are typical characteristics of major producers of home fashions.

Argentina, Turkey, India, China, and other Asian countries. According to their website (www.springs.com), each area of the world offers unique and important contributions to their global production and distribution:

- USA: critical distribution, brand building, design expertise, marketing, and access to U.S. retailers
- Mexico: low cost/high volume manufacturing
- South America: low cost/high volume manufacturing; access to the growing Brazilian cotton market
- Euro-Asia: low cost/high volume manufacturing; added-value sewing and fashion embellishment

Licensing in Home Fashions

Licensing agreements involve the manufacturer purchasing the rights to use an image, design, or name on its products (see Chapter 2 for a complete discussion of licensing). As in the apparel industry, licensing agreements have become an important component of the home fashions industry. Licensing agreements in home fashions are classified in the same categories as apparel, including the following:

- designer name licensing
- character licensing
- corporate licensing
- nostalgia licensing
- sports licensing

Well-known ready-to-wear apparel designers have moved into the world of home fashions through licensing agreements with textile mills and home fashions manufacturers. One of the first apparel designers to license home fashions was Laura Ashley, who now has licensing agreements with Hollander Home Fashions, for bedding and other sleep items; with Kravet, for upholstery and other home fashions fabrics; and Mohawk Home, for area rugs. In 1983, Ralph Lauren became the first fashion designer to establish an entire home fashions licensed collection, including bedding, towels, area rugs, wall coverings, and tabletop accessories (see Figure 14.4). Today, some of the best-known designer brand names with home fashions licensing agreements include Giorgio Armani, Ralph Lauren, Liz Claiborne, Laura Ashley, and Calvin Klein.

In addition to name designers, companies with well-known brand names are also entering into licensing agreements for home fashions. West-Point™ Home produces bedding under the Harley-Davidson®, Rachel Ray®, and Lauren Ralph Lauren® brand names. Historic reproductions and historically inspired fabrics have a strong market appeal. Licensing is also big business for home fashions geared to children. As with apparel, licensing has been successful for cartoon and movie characters (e.g., Disney, Warner Brothers), sports teams (e.g., St. Louis Rams), and toys (e.g., Barbie). Whereas Beatrix Potter, Winnie the Pooh, and Disney are timeless and endearing character licenses for juvenile home fashions, *Harry Potter*, *Twilight*, and Justin Bieber licensed bedding and home décor have emerged as recent favorites.

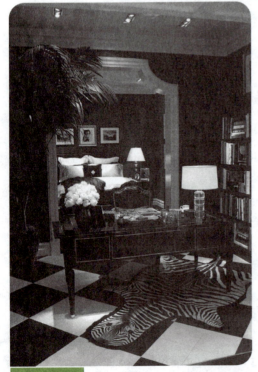

Figure 14.4 Ralph Lauren Home collection includes a variety of licensed home fashion products.

What makes these licensing agreements successful? As discussed in Chapter 2, a successful licensing agreement, whether in ready-to-wear or home fashions, depends on a well-recognized brand name with a distinct image and a licensed product that reflects that image. Successful licensed home fashions collections that follow this strategy include Ralph Lauren Home Collection, Laura Ashley Home, Tommy Bahama Home Furnishings, and the myriad sports, movie, and character licenses.

Home Fashions Design

During the design phase of developing home fashions products, textile and trim designers create exciting materials, and product designers determine the form of the final end-use product. As previously discussed, some home fashions products roll out of the textile production facility as finished products. For other types of products, the product designer works with new textiles, trims, and findings to create exciting pillows, comforters, tabletop accents, and accessories for the home. In general, designers in the home fashions industry create designs for two fashion seasons: Spring/Summer and Fall/Winter. Because fashion trends do not change as quickly for home fashions as for apparel, home fashions designs may stay on the market longer than apparel designs.

Research

Designers must take into account many factors (influences and constraints) in order to develop new and exciting products successfully season after season. Inspiration can come from numerous sources when creating new shapes, textures, and color combinations. New fiber and fabric developments are a part of the design inspiration. In addition, important functional needs must be met. Performance criteria are important to the consumer. A towel must be absorbent, soft, easily laundered, and durable, as well as look attractive while displayed in the bathroom. As with apparel, fabrics used for home fashions are designed and tested for performance characteristics. Some home fashions products (e.g., rugs, fabrics for upholstered furniture) must meet specific safety standards (e.g., flammability) set by law.

The designer strives to be aware of emerging social, political, economic, and consumer trends. Anticipating and meeting customer needs are critical components of the design and production aspects of the industry. Two key elements of current home fashions trends are self-expression and individuality. These are evidenced by the increased customization of products to meet a consumer's individual wants and needs. The research conducted on home fashions products and consumer trends is similar to the research for apparel products. For example, Thinsulate, an insulative material manufactured by 3M with an established name in apparel, also has attributes suited to the bedding market. However, the fiber composition needed for bedding differs from Thinsulate's specifications for apparel products. In order to apply this fiber to a new end use in the home fashions market, 3M needed to conduct research and development procedures specific to home fashions.

Color Forecasting

As in the apparel industry, color forecasting is an important component of home fashions product development. Some of the color forecasting services mentioned in Chapters 3 and 5 provide research and trend forecasting for home fashions, as well as for apparel products.

Historically, changes in the color palette for home fashions were based on a 10-year cycle. Who can forget the following color palettes?

- pink, salmon, cerise, turquoise, and gray of the 1950s
- avocado and orange of the 1960s
- beige, yellow (harvest gold), and brown of the 1970s
- mauve, forest green, slate blue, and gray of the 1980s
- the neutrals and jewel tones of the 1990s
- the oranges, greens, and purples of the early twenty-first century

However, that 10-year color cycle appears to be accelerating as consumers are interested in updating their home décor (interior decoration) more frequently, and companies are providing consumers with more alternatives. Designers are often inspired by colors of the past and reintroduce them with a contemporary feel.

Home textile sample books might be used to market home textiles for several years. Therefore, accurate color forecasting is necessary for the fashion colors to appear as up-to-date as possible. In addition, substantial lead time is needed to produce coordinated home fashions products. Therefore, on-target color forecasting is critical for success. Some of the color forecasting services discussed in Chapters 3 and 5 provide color forecasts specifically for the home fashions industry.

Based in Alexandria, Virginia, the Color Marketing Group (CMG) is an international not-for-profit color forecasting association of color professionals located in over 20 countries. One of its purposes is to forecast color directions for all industries, manufactured products, and services. CMG sponsors two international conferences each year, during which members meet and come to a consensus on future color trends (19 months or more in advance) for a variety of consumer products, including home fashions.

Many interrelated factors and influences are considered during the selection process for the seasonal color palette for a new home fashions line. According to the CMG website, "these 'influences' run the gamut from social issues to politics, the environment, the economy, and cultural diversity. It is an understanding of the influences that provides the most useful information, and it is the input of so many Color Designers that gives each Forecast its tremendous validity" (CMG, 2011).

Textile Processes

A number of textile processes are involved with the creation of home fashions including textile design, printing, weaving, and finishing (through textile converters).

TEXTILE DESIGN AND PRINTING

Textile design for home fashions includes the design of the fabric structure (e.g., weave pattern) as well as the surface design (e.g., printing, napping, glazing). Although woven fabrics are more common than other fabric structures for home fashions products, the industry has seen an increased use of knits and nonwoven fabrics, primarily for less costly products.

Textile designers for home fashions often work with a variety of computer-aided design (CAD) programs to develop their designs. Textile designers also create original painted artwork for fabric prints that are later scanned into a CAD system. Once the textile design is in the CAD system, details of the design are refined. The various colors used in the print design can be separated by computer for the printing process. Each color of the print requires a separate roller for rotary printing or a separate screen if screen printed.

CAD systems greatly speed the work pace in rug design studios (see Figure 14.5). The textile designer creates a new rug design on a CAD system in hours or scans an image into the system in minutes. CAD/CAM technology provides the means to design exclusive patterns for private label programs rapidly and easily.

Using traditional print methods (e.g., roller printing, screen printing), prints with a larger number of colors (13 to 15) are more costly to produce than prints with a few colors (1 to 3). Therefore, some companies set a limit on the number of colors that can be included in their print designs. The cost of developing the new print is more economical if the print can be produced in several color combinations, or **colorways**. Therefore, several colorways, or color variations, are typically created for each print design. When designing a

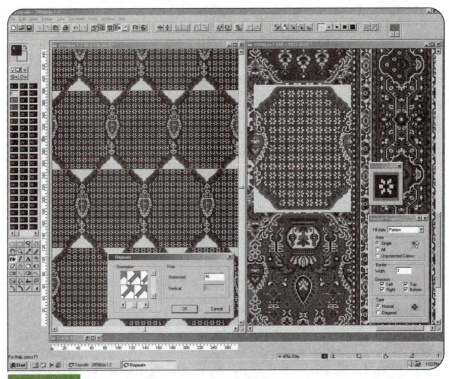

Figure 14.5 CAD software increases the efficiency of carpet and rug designers.

print, textile designers must take into consideration the repeat of the print so that the design can be printed efficiently (see Chapters 3, 6, and 9 for additional discussion of textile design).

Digital printing used in the apparel industry is discussed in Chapters 3, 6, and 11. With technological advancements, digital printing of textiles for home fashion end uses has also become more common. For example, converters can now digitally print curtain and upholstery fabrics to the specifications of the company using millions of colors.

WEAVING

Weaving looms for products such as rugs are controlled by sophisticated computer-aided manufacturing programs. Computers are used in the production of woven, tufted, and printed rugs. For example, carpets and rugs manufactured by Shaw Industries, one of the largest carpet manufacturers in the world, are produced on state-of-the art computerized looms that are integrated with the CAD system. This allows for immediate communications of designs to the weaving floor where the design is loaded into the computerized loom. Rugs are produced as orders are received, thus greatly reducing inventory.

CONVERTERS

As in the apparel and textile industries, textile **converters** play an important role in the production of textiles for specific home fashions end uses. These end uses include upholstery fabrics, table linens, and other fabrics that are printed or finished to improve the aesthetics and performance of the end-use product. For example, soil-hiding and soil-resistant finishes are often applied to fabrics used for upholstery or table linens.

As with the apparel and textile industries, many home fashions textile print converters such as Covington Fabric and Design and Richloom Fabrics Group are based in New York. The Robert Allen Group, another home textile converter, is headquartered in Foxboro, Massachusetts, with operations also in Canada and the UK. Alexander Henry Fabrics, a leader in conversational print design for both home and apparel is headquartered in Burbank, CA.

In most cases, converters provide either original painted fabric print designs or CAD designs to a finishing company that incorporates the design into a computer system, develops pigments for printing, and prints and finishes the fabric. The textile converter is also heavily involved in the marketing of the textiles and promotion of the home textile brands. For example, Richloom Fabrics Group markets the Liz Claiborne Home® and Better Homes and Garden® lines of decorative home fabrics.

Marketing Home Fashions

Marketing components for home fashions are similar to those used in the apparel industry, including manufacturers' showrooms, company sales representatives, trade shows, and advertising and promotion. However, the home fashions industry relies on textile converters and jobbers to perform marketing and distribution functions more often than does the apparel industry.

As with apparel, the establishment of well-respected brand names is important in the marketing of home fashions. Consumers often rely on brand names in their decisions to purchase goods. WestPoint™ Home is well known for its Martex®, Utica®, Vellux®, Lauren Ralph Lauren®, EcoPure™, and Patrician® brands. Springs Global is known for its Springmaid®, Wamsutta®, and Court of Versailles® brands. As discussed earlier, retailers have developed private label brands of home fashions to further distinguish their merchandise (e.g., Macy's Charter Club, Target's Thomas O'Brien, and Simply Shabby Chic by Rachel Ashwell).

Manufacturers' Showrooms and Sales Representatives

Marketing headquarters and manufacturers' showrooms for many home fashions companies are located in New York City. Companies use showrooms to provide enticing visual displays of new home textiles as well as finished products for their interior design, manufacturing, and retail customers. Most companies display new fabrics made into end-use products to show customers how the new fabrics can be used. Coordinated ensembles of products for bed and bath, kitchen, living room, and dining areas are presented. Companies also distribute sample books to interior design and manufacturing customers and include similar information on their websites. These sample books and websites include either real or virtual swatches of home textiles that are available as well as pictures of finished products using the textiles.

Decorative Fabric Converters and Jobbers

In addition to manufacturers' showrooms, **decorative fabric converters** and jobbers also play an important role in the marketing of home fashions. As mentioned earlier, textile converters in the home fashions industry design and sell finished textiles to jobbers, designers, and manufacturers, who use the textiles in home fashions end-use products. Some converters also produce end-use products such as bed linens and window treatments. Similar to manufacturers, converters also create and distribute sample books. They also have showrooms in New York City or elsewhere where they display and sell their goods to jobbers, as well as to interior design, manufacturing, and retailing customers.

The Robert Allen Group, one of the largest residential woven-fabric converters in the United States, has showrooms in over 40 countries in North America, Europe, the Middle East, Africa, Asia, and Australia. In each fabric category (e.g., upholstery, drapery), teams of designers work to create new fabrics for their customers under the following four distinct brands: Robert Allen, Beacon Hill, Robert Allen Contract, and Robert Allen@Home. The Robert Allen Group markets its products through showrooms and showroom boutiques, where finished products are shown using exclusive fabrics. In addition to fabrics, these showrooms have displays of wall coverings and finished products, such as bed coverings and draperies. Other well-known converters include Covington Fabrics and Design, Richloom Fabrics, F. Shumacher & Co., and Kravet.

Decorative fabric jobbers are also involved in the marketing and distribution of home textile piece goods, particularly upholstery and drapery fabrics.

Traditionally, jobbers have served a warehousing and distribution function within the industry. In the past, regional jobbers would visit New York twice a year, where they would buy large quantities of fabrics from a number of mills and converters. They would then sell smaller quantities to interior designers, furniture manufacturers, and retail customers.

Over the years, the jobber market has evolved into a year-round market, with a number of jobbers providing nationwide distribution. Jobbers continue to select colors, designs, and fabrics that best meet their customers' needs. Similar to manufacturers and converters, jobbers put together sample books for their customers. In recent years, the jobber market has changed as jobbers have started providing a number of services, such as importing fabrics, creating exclusive in-house fabric designs, converting fabrics, and marketing fabrics through showrooms. Thus, the differences between the functions of textile mills, converters, and jobbers are less distinct than in the past. In fact, as some jobbers have turned to converting, some top converters have begun to perform jobbing/distribution functions.

Marketing Tools

As in the apparel industry, companies in the home fashions industry use a variety of marketing tools to advertise and promote their products to their customers and to the ultimate consumers. These marketing tools include the following:

- sample books (for home textiles)
- catalogs
- print advertisements in trade and popular press publications
- websites
- television advertisements
- social media sites including Facebook and Twitter

Co-op advertising (see Chapter 8) helps to provide the links in consumers' minds between brand names, end-use products, and retailers. The use of web technology will continue to expand and open new marketing possibilities for the entire soft-goods pipeline. Business-to-business communication and web-based commerce provide numerous opportunities for marketing home fashions. Textile converters generally have *to the trade* links on corporate websites where commercial customers can contact sales representatives and preview and purchase goods.

Trade Associations, Trade Shows, and Trade Publications

As with other fashion-related industries, the home fashions industry is supported by a number of industry-specific trade associations, trade shows, and trade publications.

TRADE ASSOCIATIONS

In both the ready-to-wear and the home fashions industries, there are trade associations for various textiles, general categories of merchandise, and specific aspects of the industry. Textile trade associations for home fashions are the same as those for fashion apparel. These include the National Council of Textile Organizations, Cotton Incorporated, and the Wool Council (see Chapter 3 for a description of these trade associations). For example, Cotton Incorporated promotes the use of cotton in home fashions products (see Figure 14.6). Cotton Incorporated's research department develops new products that are adopted and produced by textile mills. Cotton Incorporated has also developed cotton fabrics that can be used for upholstery, window treatments, wall coverings, table linens, and area rugs.

Some trade associations promote home furnishings or home fashions in general. Other trade associations focus on specific aspects of the industry, such as the Carpet and Rug Institute (CRI) and the National Home Furnishings Association. These trade associations assist in conducting market research, connecting suppliers with customers, and promoting specific end uses or areas of the industry. Table 14.1 lists selected trade associations in the home fashions industry.

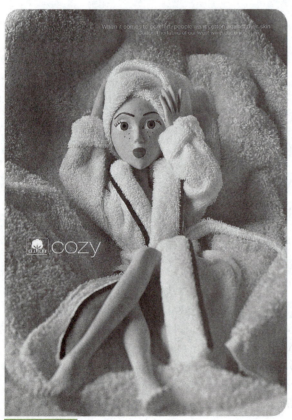

Figure 14.6 Cotton Incorporated, a trade association, promotes the use of cotton for home fashions.

TRADE SHOWS

Trade shows that showcase products from the home fashions industry often cover a variety of other related markets

Table 14.1	Selected Trade Associations for the Home Fashions Industry
Association	**Website**
American Home Furnishings Alliance (AFHA)	www.ahfa.us
Carpet and Rug Institute (CRI)	www.carpet-rug.com
International Furnishings and Design Association (IFDA)	www.ifda.com
International Home Furnishings Representatives Association (IHFRA)	www.ihfra.org
International Sleep Products Association (ISPA)	www.sleepproducts.org
National Association of Decorative Fabrics Distributors (NADFD)	www.nadfd.com
National Home Furnishings Association (NHFA)	www.nhfa.org
Upholstered Furniture Action Council (UFAC)	www.ufac.org
Window Coverings Association of America (WCAA)	www.wcaa.org

as well. In addition, home fashions may be displayed in trade shows that focus primarily on other industries. For example, textile trade shows such as Fabric at MAGIC may include textiles for home fashions, although the primary focus is on apparel. Gift markets also include home fashions products. For example, the Atlanta International Gift and Home Furnishings Market includes home accents, fine linens, and area rugs, in addition to tabletop accessories, fine home furnishings, and fine gifts. The New York Home Textiles Show runs concurrently with the New York International Gift Fair. Design trade shows are attended by interior designers and architects, as well as some professionals in the home fashions industry. One example is the Fine Design Residential Furnishings Show at NeoCon World Trade Fair, which is geared toward furniture, lighting, kitchen cabinets, and wall coverings, as well as textiles, carpets, and bath products. Other trade shows focus on decorator fabrics, such as Heimtextil in Frankfurt, Germany.

In addition to housing most manufacturers' showrooms for home fashions, New York City is also the home of the New York Home Textiles Show. During market weeks, companies show samples of home textiles to jobbers, designers, manufacturers, and retailers (see Figure 14.7). Some of the home fashions markets are held in the same merchandise marts that house the apparel trade shows, such as the Chicago Merchandise Mart (where the Fine Design Residential Furnishings Show is held), and Dallas Market Center (where the Dallas International Gift and Home Accessories Show is held). On the other hand, the High Point Market, held in High Point, North Carolina, is the largest home furnishings market in the world. High Point Market shows upholstery fabrics, as well as furniture, with 2,500 exhibitors and 80,000 attendees from over 100

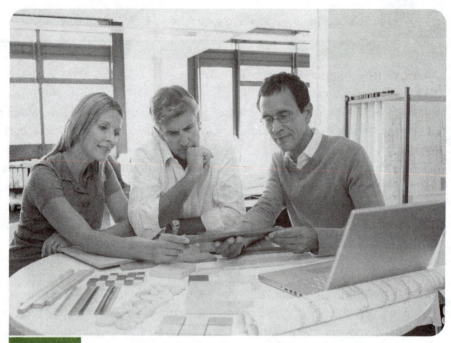

Figure 14.7   Home textiles are shown to designers, manufacturers, and retailers through showrooms and at trade shows.

countries. Most of the markets for the home fashions industry are held twice a year. Table 14.2 lists selected trade shows for the home fashions industry.

TRADE PUBLICATIONS

Trade publications are an important source of information for professionals in the home fashions industry (see Figure 14.8). As with the apparel industry, some trade publications cover the entire industry, whereas others focus on specific aspects of the industry. See Table 14.3 for a listing of selected trade publications in the home fashions industry.

Production of Home Fashions

Price, value, and quality are key features sought by home fashions consumers. These features are related to the production of the product. Fast, efficient production can help to control costs. Chapter 11 discusses how quality must be built into the product throughout the production processes in the apparel industry. This is also true for home fashions. Quality assurance programs are an integral part of home fashions production facilities.

Table 14.2	Selected U.S. and International Trade Shows for the Home Fashions Industry

Atlanta International Gift and Home Furnishings Market
AmericasMart, Atlanta
  home accents, fine linens, fine furnishings, tabletop, fine gifts, area rugs
	High Point Market
	High Point, NC
	  comprehensive exhibition of residential home furnishings

Dallas Total Home and Gift Market
Dallas Market Center, Dallas
  Home accessories, furniture, holiday and seasonal items, floral, and jewelry/fashion accessories
	Interior Lifestyle, Japan
	Tokyo
	  high-end bedding, kitchen and bath textiles, decorative and furnishing fabrics, window and tabletop products

Decorex International
London, UK, various locations
  Design-led interior products including fabrics, wallcoverings, furniture, lighting, accessories, kitchen, and bath
	L.A. Mart Gift & Home Market
	L.A. Mart, Los Angeles
	  Gifts, tabletop, home textiles

Fine Design Show at NeoCon World's Trade Fair
The Merchandise Mart, Chicago
  Luxury furnishings, fabrics, wall and floor coverings, casual/outdoor furnishings, art, antiques, accessories
	Maison et Objet
	Paris, France
	  furniture, rugs, decorative lighting, home textiles

	MoOD Brussels, Belgium Upholstery, window and wall coverings

Heimtextil International Trade Fair for Home and Contract Textiles
Heimtextil, Frankfurt, Germany
Heimtextil Russia, Moscow
Heimtextil Japan, Tokyo
  Home and contract textiles
	New York International Gift Fair: At Home and Home Textiles Market Week in New York
	Javits Center, NYC
	  Comprehensive college of home furnishings and home textiles

As indicated earlier, the home fashions industry includes a number of vertically integrated companies that produce not only the fabric but also the end-use product. To avoid increasing costs, some vertically integrated companies have ceased production of their own yarns. For example, a mill might save money by outsourcing yarn production rather than investing in new yarn facilities. Some domestic apparel manufacturers turned to offshore production as a cost-saving procedure years ago. This trend has repeated itself in the home

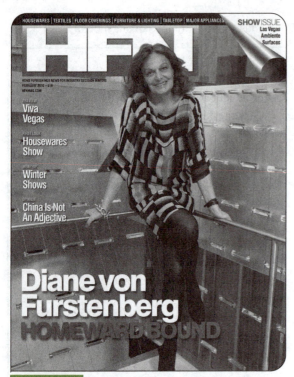

Figure 14.8 Trade publications for the home fashions industry are important sources of information for manufacturers and retailers of home fashions.

fashions industry. Many home fashions manufacturers have also elected to cease domestic production, sourcing production in other parts of the world. Increased global competition in home textiles has forced U.S. companies to develop new competitive strategies. In some cases, factories have been closed. In other cases, companies have expanded international operations.

Quick Response strategies, supply chain management, and product lifecycle management, which were discussed in previous chapters, are applicable to the home fashions industry as well. Home fashions companies continue to upgrade their operations with product information management and computer integrated manufacturing. Whether companies are vertically integrated or focus on specific design, production, or marketing aspects of the home fashions industry, integrating computer design and information systems has been crucial for remaining competitive in the global home fashions industry. Internet communication provides immediate access for fiber, fabric, trim, and findings suppliers; manufacturers and contractors; retailers; and consumers.

As in the apparel industry, fast delivery of raw goods from suppliers and quick turnaround time on production help speed the product to the retailer and ultimate consumer. Continued reduction in the lead time needed to produce goods has provided additional cost savings. Faster delivery of products has also resulted from the following:

- increased vertical integration
- partnerships among segments of the industry
- UPC bar coding and use of RFID
- floor-ready merchandise

For example, Oriental Weavers, a multinational corporation that produces woven carpets and rugs, incorporates companies that integrate all stages of

Table 14.3	Selected Trade Publications for the Home Fashions Industry
Bed Times (www.bedtimesmagazine.com)	business journal of the sleep products industry
Floor Covering Weekly (www.floorcoveringweekly.com)	focuses on topics of interest to the flooring and interior surfacing product industry; reports news to floor covering retailers, contract dealers, distributors, and manufacturers
Furniture Today (www.furnituretoday.com)	news, trends, research and operations information for furniture store retailers
HFN (www.hfnmag.com)	features in-depth news and analysis of products and retail trends in the home furnishings industry
Home Accents Today (www.homeaccentstoday.com)	focuses on merchandising and fashion news for the home accent industry; aimed at decorative accessory, specialty home accent, and gift buyers
Home Textiles Today (www.hometextilestoday.com)	focuses on marketing, merchandising, and retailing of home textile products
Interior Design (www.interiordesign.net)	for professional interior designers of office, commercial, and residential interiors

the design and production, from raw material to finished product. This vertical integration allows them to deliver machine-made rugs to retailers quickly and efficiently (Oriental Weavers, 2011). Capel Rugs, a vertically integrated rug manufacturer headquartered in Troy, North Carolina, integrates spinning, dyeing, weaving, braiding, sewing, and selling operations to increase speed of delivery (Capel, 2011).

End-Use Categories

As stated earlier, the home fashions industry is divided into the following four general end-use categories:

- upholstered furniture coverings and fillings
- window and wall coverings
- soft floor coverings, including area rugs, scatter rugs, and runners
- bed, bath, tabletop, and other textile accessories and accents

Coordinated ensembles among categories have become popular. The same or coordinated textiles produced by one textile manufacturer might be used for the upholstered furniture, window treatments, bedding, and wall coverings for an entire room. Examples include the following:

- Waverly, a division of F. Schumacher & Co., has been at the forefront of providing consumers with a coordinated, total home look by producing coordinated bed linens, bath rugs, shower curtains, laminated fabrics, lamp shades, and other products.

- Coordinated prints, stripes, plaids, and monochrome cotton fabrics are produced by Laura Ashley, in addition to coordinating wallpaper, lamp shades, ceramic tile, and tableware.

Upholstered Furniture Coverings and Fillings

Upholstery fabrics for home fashions are used primarily for sofas, love seats, chairs, and ottomans (see Figure 14.9). Textiles used for upholstery fabrics are made from many natural and manufactured fibers. Before the development of manufactured fibers, wool, cotton, and linen were the most prevalent fibers used in upholstered home fashions. Silk has been used less frequently for upholstery due to its cost, care requirements, and delicate structure. Manufactured fibers, particularly nylon and polyester, are commonly used in today's market. Fiber companies in the United States known for producing fibers for upholstery fabrics include FiberVisions, Inc.(maker of bicomponent and performance polyolefin fibers) and INVISTA (maker of brands of polyester and nylon include Antron® carpet fiber and Tactesse® carpet fiber).

Advances in olefin (also known as polypropylene or polyolefin) have made it a popular fiber in the

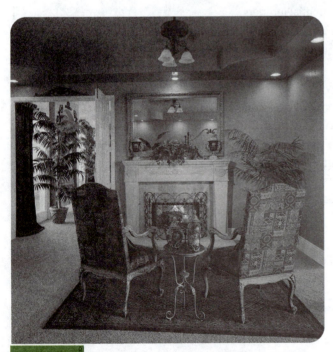

Figure 14.9 Upholstery fabrics play an important role in creating the look and atmosphere of the home.

upholstery market, and cotton has regained some of its importance. Rayon blends for upholstery fabrics are experiencing growth in sales.

The performance characteristics of wool and cotton fibers are highly valued for some types of upholstered home fashions. The rising cost of these natural fibers lowered their market share in comparison to the less expensive manufactured fibers. Currently, the high-end market uses a higher percentage of natural fibers than the moderate and mass markets.

Fabric structure is another important consideration for upholstery. The durability of a fabric is affected by its fabric structure. For example, twill weaves are very durable, whereas satin weaves are less durable for upholstery. Although both pile and nonpile fabrics are used for upholstery, nonpile fabrics are preferred for heavy-use upholstered items, such as family room sofas.

Some upholstery fabrics are coated with a backing substance to enhance end-use properties, such as durability. Protective and soil-resistant or soil-release finishes are often applied to upholstery fabrics. Many of these, such as 3M's Scotchgard™ upholstery fabric protector can be applied by the manufacturer or by the consumer (see Figure 14.10).

The price range for upholstery fabrics is broad, from budget to designer price zones. Low-cost upholstery fabric made from manufactured fibers or blends is the mainstay for most furniture manufacturers and retailers. Some upholstery fabrics are created and sold to the high-end market segment. For example, Larsen, the company founded by textile designer Jack Lenor Larsen, is known for creating innovative high-end textile designs for upholstery and other home fashions end uses. This company is now part of Colefax and Fowler, a British home fashions company.

Over-the-counter upholstery fabrics (sold at fabric stores) provide a source for individuals who want to create their own home fashions. Consumers enjoy the opportunity to coordinate their home fashions from the broad choice of materials offered over the counter. Textile converter F. Schumacher & Co.'s Waverly brand of

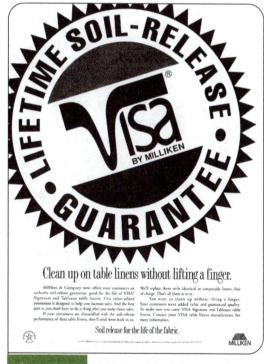

Clean up on table linens without lifting a finger.

Milliken & Company now offers your customers an exclusive soil-release guarantee, good for the life of VISA® Signature and Tableaux table linens. This value-added promotion is designed to help you increase sales. And the best part is, you don't have to do a thing after you make those sales.

If your customers are dissatisfied with the soil-release performance of these table linens, they'll send them back to us.

We'll replace them with identical or comparable linens, free of charge. That's all there is to it.

You want to serve up without lifting a finger. Your customers want added value and guaranteed quality. So make sure you carry VISA Signature and Tableaux table linens. Contact your VISA table linens manufacturer for more information.

Soil release for the life of the fabric.

MILLIKEN

Figure 14.10 Soil-release finishes are often applied to fabrics used for table linens and upholstery.

decorator fabrics and Robert Allen fabrics are sold over the counter to individuals as well as to manufacturers. Thus, individuals who want to create their own home fashions have access to some of the same fabrics used in manufactured home fashions.

Window and Wall Coverings

Window treatments consist of draperies, curtains, and fabric shades, as well as decorative treatments such as valances, cornices, and swags. **Curtains** are typically described as "sheer, lightweight coverings that are hung without linings" (Yeager & Teter-Justice, 2000, p. 261), whereas **draperies** are described as "heavy, often opaque, and highly patterned coverings usually hung with linings" (Yeager & Teter-Justice, 2000, p. 261). Curtains might be combined with draperies for home use, providing both decorative and functional purposes. During the day, sheer curtains allow diffused light into a room while providing some privacy. At night, opaque draperies can be drawn for total privacy and increased warmth. Fabric valances, cornices, and swags are popular window treatments.

Customers feel more confident about changing window treatments than about changing more expensive items of home décor. Thus, the category of window treatments is a very popular segment of home fashions. However, the display of window treatments in retail stores is a challenge because window treatments require substantial floor space. Department stores and mass merchants have developed creative ways of displaying window treatments with small-scale versions of the window treatments and the use of photographs that show the items on actual windows.

The fibers and fabrics used for curtains and draperies must withstand more exposure to heat and sunlight than many other textile products. Some manufactured fibers, such as nylon and polyester, withstand environmental exposure better than natural fibers, such as silk and cotton. Linen and wool, at one time quite commonly used for window coverings, are now used only occasionally. Manufactured fibers such as rayon, acrylic, nylon, and polyester fibers are typically used in blends with other fibers for window treatments. The ease of care of manufactured fibers and blends that combine natural with manufactured fibers is another important consideration for many consumers. Figure 14.11 gives a sense of the wide variety of fabrics available for home fashions.

There are many similarities in the design, development, and production processes of apparel products and home fashions. However, one of the differences is the length of time that the home fashions producers want fabric lines to be available for reorders compared to the time wanted by apparel produc-

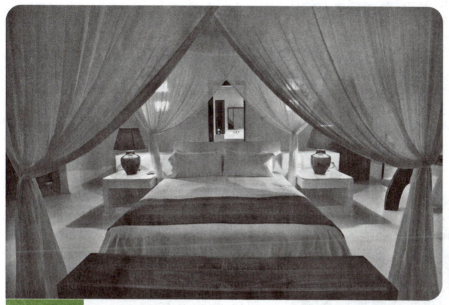

Figure 14.11 A wide variety of fabrics are used for home fashions such as bedding and window coverings.

ers. Home fashions producers want the fabric lines to be available for several seasons, whereas many of the fabric lines used by apparel producers change every season. For those home fashions producers, such as window treatment companies, who use some of the same fabrics used by the apparel industry, this presents a problem. Therefore, selection of fabric lines that will remain in production for several seasons is critical to the window treatment producers.

A variety of textiles is used for wall coverings and vertical panels and partitions. Fabric used as a wall covering can provide a room with a cozy ambiance or an elegant distinctiveness. There are various techniques for applying fabrics to wall surfaces. A tightly woven material with a sturdy fabric structure will withstand the tension needed to provide a smooth fabric surface. Cotton is one of the easiest and most versatile fabrics for use as a wall covering. Luxurious visual statements can be made with velvet or moiré fabrics; however, these fabrics are more challenging to mount. Silk fabrics function best as wall coverings if they are first quilted or laminated to a backing fabric to stabilize them.

Soft Floor Coverings

Soft floor coverings include wall-to-wall carpeting, area rugs, runners, and scatter rugs. The discussion of this end-use category will focus on area floor

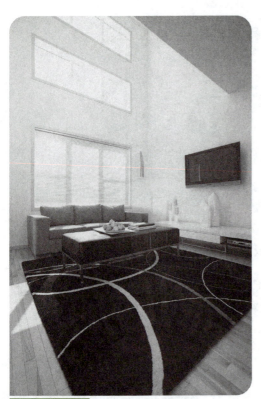

Figure 14.12 The soft floor covering category includes area rugs and runners in a variety of shapes and sizes.

coverings (area rugs, runners, and scatter rugs). Area floor coverings are produced in a wide variety of fibers and blends. For kitchens and bathrooms, cotton, polyester, and nylon fibers are most typical. Ease of cleaning is an important consideration to the consumer for bath and kitchen area rugs. Bedroom area floor coverings might consist of natural fibers, including wool and cotton, manufactured fibers, or blends of fibers. For other areas of the home, such as the living room, family room, and dining room, a wide variety of fibers is available. Fibers used for area floor coverings include nylon, polyester, olefin, wool, and cotton, as well as sisal, jute, and other natural plant materials. Companies in the United States that produce manufactured fibers used in carpets and rugs include INVISTA and FiberVisions, Inc.

Area floor coverings might be laid atop a hardwood floor or carpeting. A variety of sizes for area rugs and runners provides many home fashions options (see Figure 14.12). Scatter rugs are usually small, for example, 2 by 3 feet or 3 by 5 feet. Area rugs tend to be larger, in sizes such as 8 by 11 feet or 11 by 14 feet. Runners are long and narrow because they are designed for hallways or entries.

A number of companies in the United States produce area floor coverings, including the following:

- The Dixie Group, headquartered in Chattanooga, Tennessee, produces carpets and rugs through its Fabrica International, Masland Carpets and Rugs, and Dixie Home divisions.

- Mohawk Industries, headquartered in Calhoun, Georgia, produces carpets and rugs under the Aladdin®, Horizon®, WundaWeve®, and Karastan® brands.

- Shaw Industries, headquartered in Dalton, Georgia, manufactures residential carpets and rugs under the Cabin Crafts Carpets, Philadelphia Carpets, Queen Carpets, ShawMark Carpets, Shaw Rugs, Sutton Carpets, and Tuftex brands. They also produce Kathy Ireland® Home carpets.

- Milliken & Company, headquartered in Spartanburg, South Carolina, produces residential carpets and area rugs in addition to commercial applications.

Some area floor coverings are made by machine, in a process similar to that used for carpet manufacturing. The design and texture of an area rug is often determined during the production stage by varying the colors and types of yarns used, or by the weaving or fabrication techniques. Multicolor effects can be achieved by applying the same dye color to a yarn composed of different fibers, producing a heather effect.

Continual improvements in technology for carpet and rug production have increased the variety of patterns and textures available to the consumer. Computerized systems allow companies to create different multilevel surfaces, colors, and textures in rugs ranging from basic bath rugs to high-fashion accent rugs. Several other production methods are used to create handwoven, braided, hooked, crocheted, knotted, or embroidered area floor coverings. Many ethnic floor coverings are produced by hand processes. Both the ethnic design and hand processes add an exotic flavor to home fashions.

As with other types of home textiles, carpets and rugs are often developed or finished to enhance their performance. For example, the INVISTA Stainmaster® brand of carpet and area rugs are manufactured with a specified nylon 6.6, which has a unique fiber structure that is stain resistant and crush resistant.

Bed, Bath, Table, and Other Home Textile Accessories and Accents

Textile accessories and accents include the following:

- textile bedding products, including sheets and pillowcases, blankets, bedspreads, quilts, comforters, and pillows (see Figure 14.13)
- textile products for the bath, including towels, bath rugs and mats, and shower curtains
- textile accessories for tabletops, including tablecloths, napkins, table runners, and place mats
- textile products for the kitchen, including towels, dishcloths, hot pads, and aprons
- textile accents, such as textile wall hangings, tapestries, quilts, needlework accents, and lace accents

The term **linens** refers to towels, sheets, tablecloths, napkins, and other home textiles once made almost exclusively from linen. Although these products are rarely made from linen anymore, they are commonly still referred to as linens.

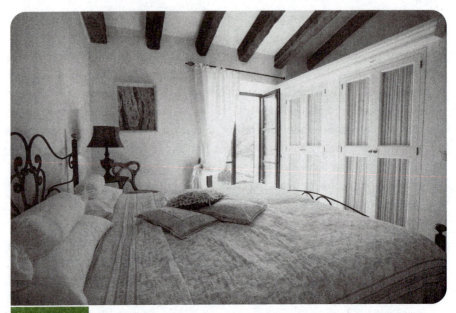

Figure 14.13 Bedding category of home fashions includes sheets and mattress covers as well as top-of-the-bed items such as comforters and pillow shams.

BEDDING AND BATH

Cotton fiber has an estimated 60 percent share of the sheet industry. Most sheets are made from a blend of cotton and polyester (often 50 percent of each fiber). A number of companies also offer 100 percent cotton sheets. Recently, rayon and bamboo rayon have been introduced as fabrics for sheets. Wrinkle-free, all-cotton sheets have also become popular. Several luxury producers offer linen and silk sheets.

Percale and flannel are the most typical fabric structures for sheets. Satin, sateen, and jacquard weaves are available for the specialty market. Knit fabric, especially cotton jersey knit, is another option for sheets. Eyelet trims, contrast piping, and scalloped edging are used as embellishments.

Besides fiber content and fabric structure, woven sheets are distinguished by their thread count and their size. **Thread count** refers to the total number of threads or yarns in one square inch of fabric. Typical thread counts range from 200 to 400. A higher thread count tends to signify a softer fabric. Sheets are available in crib, twin, double, queen, and king sizes, corresponding to standard bed sizes.

The **top-of-the-bed category** includes comforters, duvet covers, blankets, bedspreads, dust ruffles, pillow shams, and throws. This category has been growing in recent years as consumers strive for a coordinated look in bed and bath decoration. Bedspreads are made from a variety of fabrics and in a variety of styles, including quilted fabrics. Quilts and comforters typically are made from multicomponent fabrics and filled with down, feathers, fiberfill, or other materials.

The infant and juvenile bedding category has grown in recent years. Licensed printed goods are spurring the market. Examples include Disney products, featuring characters from recent films (e.g., *Harry Potter*, *Twilight*) or classic Disney characters (see Figure 14.14), as well as Looney Tunes products, with characters such as Bugs Bunny. There are specialty trade shows and associations for the juvenile market. The International Juvenile Products Manufacturers Show, sponsored by the Juvenile Products Manufacturers Association, is the largest U.S. trade event for specialty baby-to-teen retailers. The show includes furniture, bedding, and decorative accessories.

In the bath market, cotton is by far the dominant fiber, with an estimated 95 percent share (see Figure 14.15). Terry cloth is by far the most popular fabrication for towels. The yarns forming the loops of terry cloth are generally all cotton to enhance moisture absorbency for drying purposes. The warp and weft yarns that form the base weave structure that holds the loops in place might consist of a blend of cotton with a small percentage of polyester for increased durability. When the loops have been sheared on one side or both sides, the terry cloth fabric is called *velour*.

Towel size is a product feature that can provide market appeal. For years, towel sizes were standardized. Then, longer towels became

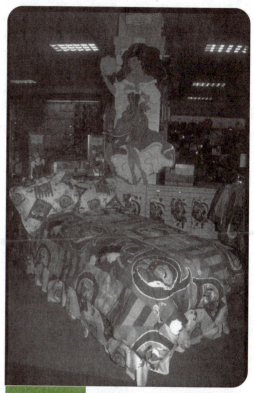

Figure 14.14 Licensed characters are common for bedding and other home fashions.

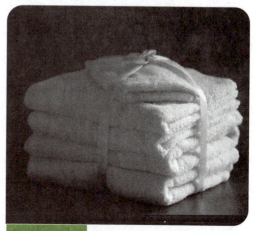

Figure 14.15 Cotton is by far the dominant fiber used for products in the bath category of home fashions.

popular at luxury hotels and spas. Soon manufacturers began to offer a variety of towel lengths at various price points for the retail market.

Market research on customer preferences contributes valuable information to both producers and retailers. What are the factors customers consider to be the most important for their towel purchasing decisions? A survey conducted by Cotton Incorporated's Lifestyle Monitor™ (2006) found that the three most important, desirable features of bath towels were as follows:

- softness (83 percent)
- absorbency (83 percent)
- durability (76 percent)

However, the following features were also important influences for bath towel purchases:

- size (73 percent)
- life of the bath towel (67 percent)
- price (66 percent)
- color (61 percent)

More than 25 percent of the women surveyed purchased bath towels more than once per year, and nearly 40 percent purchased new bath towels because their current towels were worn out.

A wide variety of coordinating bath mats contributed to an increase in sales in the bath category. The surge in the bath market coincided with a similar increase in popularity of coordinated kitchen towels, dishcloths, oven mitts, pot holders, and aprons.

TEXTILE ACCESSORIES FOR TABLETOP AND KITCHEN

Textile accessories for the tabletop include tablecloths, napkins, place mats, and table runners. The terms **napery** and **table linens** are both used to refer to tablecloths and napkins. Tabletop accessories can protect the finish of fine wood tables and can enhance the warmth and visual theme of a dining room (see Figure 14.16). Therefore, many fibers and fabrics that provide visual appeal are used in tabletop accessories.

One especially important feature for tabletop accessories is that they be easy to care for. For example, Milliken applies a soil release finish to table linens to increase their performance. Tabletop accessories are available in a variety of sizes to fit a wide range of table shapes and sizes. Labeling laws require that the "cut size" given on labels on tablecloths must be the dimensions of the finished product.

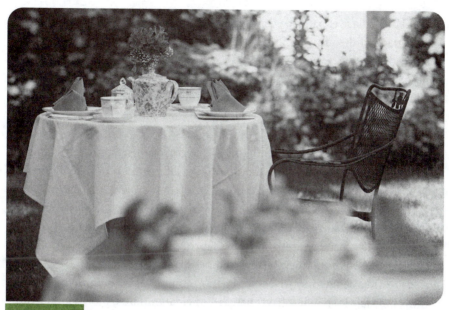

Figure 14.16 Tabletop category in home fashions includes table linens, place mats, and table runners.

Textile accessories for the kitchen include towels, dishcloths, pot holders, oven mitts, and aprons. As with other textile accessories, both appearance and performance characteristics are important determinants for fiber and fabric choices.

Distribution and Retailing of Home Fashions

Home fashions constitute an important segment of the retail industry. Discount retail stores (e.g., Walmart, Target, and Kmart), which carry budget and moderate-priced floor and window coverings, bed and bath fashions, and products for kitchens and bathrooms, are the dominant players in the retailing of home fashions. Bed and bath accessories, window and wall coverings, floor coverings, and upholstered furniture also provide substantial sales for department stores such as JCPenney, Macy's, and Dillard's. Specialty stores, including Bed, Bath & Beyond, Pottery Barn, Williams Sonoma, and Crate and Barrel, offer a mix of home fashions with other merchandise related to home activities and lifestyles. Direct marketing companies such as Lands' End, Linens 'n Things, Domestications, The Linen Source, and The Company Store fill another market niche. Home improvement stores such as The Home Depot and Lowe's have expanded their home fashions offerings as they strive to take advantage of the growing number of customers involved with do-it-yourself home decorating. Even apparel and accessory retailers, such as Nordstrom, offer home fashions items. As with other areas of the fashion industry, nonstore and multichannel retailing has created multiple purchasing venues for consumers. QVC and other television shopping networks consistently sell bedding, tabletop accessories, and area rugs.

Consumers are currently updating the décor of their home environments more frequently by changing the decorative fabrics used in their homes. In light of this trend, the retailing of home fabrics has grown in recent years (see Figure 14.17).

Some stores, such as Calico Corners, headquartered in Kennett Square, Pennsylvania, focus entirely on home fabrics. For other fabric stores, an increasing percentage of their business comes from home fabrics. In response to this growing demand for over-the-counter home fabrics, a number of home furnishing fabric suppliers have increased their attention to the over-the-counter home textiles business. Jo-Ann Fabric and Craft Stores, Inc., based in Hudson, Ohio, is the largest fabric and craft retailer in the United States, with 746 stores in 48 states and an online division (joann.com).

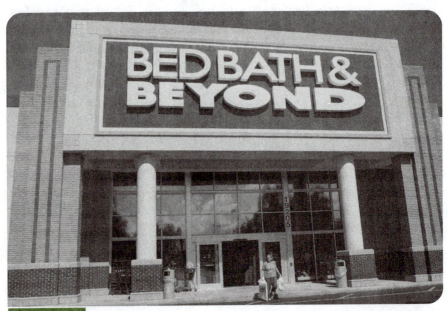

Figure 14.17 Retailing of home fashions includes department stores and specialty stores, as well as nonstore retailing venues.

Social and Environmental Responsibility

The soft-goods industry thrives on change at a fast pace. This can lead to a public perception that it is an industry that encourages waste. As a society, we discard many products long before their full potential for use is exhausted. In recent years, the industry has focused on social and environmental responsibility in all phases of the product use cycle. The home fashions industry has been a leader in efforts to promote **sustainable design** (also called **environmental design** or **green design**), a term used to encompass the concept that the decisions related to the creation, use, and discarding of a product should preserve the ecosystem.

Sustainable design efforts include the following examples from the fiber stage through the discard stage:

- naturally grown fibers such as organic cotton
- humanely sheared, free-range sheep
- yarn blended for user comfort and compostability
- environmentally compatible dyes and chemicals
- elimination of pollutants used in textile manufacturing
- use of recycled components (e.g., fibers) in textile manufacturing
- elimination of toxic vapors emitted during production or product use (such as formaldehyde on fabric wall coverings)
- biodegradability or reuse of postconsumer products (see Figure 14.18)

One of the first companies to focus on sustainable design in home fashions was DesignTex, based in New York City. In the early 1990s, through a collaboration with William McDonough and Michael Braungart, they created an environmentally responsible line of textiles for upholstered furniture that met sustainability guidelines. Their first collections utilized fabrics made from a blend of wool and ramie, both natural fibers. Working with an independent environmental research institute in Germany and an environmental

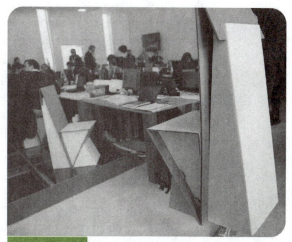

Figure 14.18   Sustainable design, such as these chairs and tables made from recycled cardboard, are an important trend in the home fashions industry.

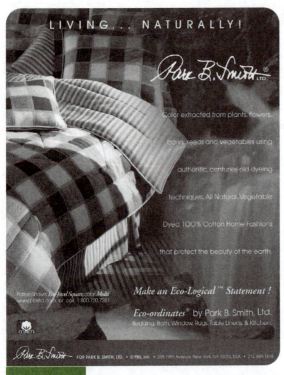

Figure 14.19 The home fashions industry has been a leader in environmentally responsible business practices.

chemist, DesignTex selected dyes that used no toxins. The textile mill selected to manufacture the fabric improved its manufacturing processes to conform to McDonough's design principles and criteria, referred to as Cradle to Cradle. Since that time, DesignTex's commitment to sustainability has continued through their use of nontoxic chemical dyes, organically grown renewable resources, and environmentally responsible polyester and nylon (DesignTex, 2011).

Many other companies in the home fashions industry have adopted a variety of environmentally responsible business practices in the development, production, and marketing of their products (see Figure 14.19). Examples include Shaw Rugs Eco Solution Q nylon fiber, EcoWorx Broadloom sustainable carpet backing, and Milliken's Earthwise Ennovations process to encourage customers to reuse carpet tile.

The home fashions industry provides many other examples of sustainable design. Local, regional, and national network directories offer databases of references to locate product manufacturers that utilize recycled materials.

The retailer may play an additional part in a product's lifecycle. Some retailers offer convenient home pickup and recycle options for discarded products for consumers who have purchased a new product. At the time a new mattress is delivered to the consumer, the old mattress might be picked up by the retailer's delivery crew and recycled.

Lifecycle evaluation of products from the producer's, the retailer's, and the consumer's points of view will continue to be an important component in the home fashions industry. It may add complexity and cost to the design-manufacture-market-consume process, but sustainable design is important to future success in business.

Other forms of socially responsible behavior in the industry include community development efforts by local and national companies. Companies such as The Home Depot and Lowe's sponsor community-focused initiatives that assist individuals, nonprofit organizations, and environmental programs throughout the United States. In addition, our global marketplace provides opportunities to support socially responsible practices throughout the world. GoodWeave International is an international nongovernment organization whose goal is to end child labor in the handmade rug industry. The Good-Weave certification program, formerly known as RugMark, allows manufacturers to join as licensees and adhere to standards of production set by Good-Weave International.

New York-based Tufenkian Artisan Carpets sells carpets made by weavers using traditional design and weaving techniques. The carpets are produced in partnership with designers and workers in Nepal and Armenia. By providing a marketing outlet for these beautiful products, the company helps ensure that traditional carpets can continue to be produced. The weavers earn a livelihood with satisfactory working and living conditions, and Tufenkian provides schooling for children at the factory site to ensure that children are not involved in the production. To avoid pollution of the environment, the carpet washing is not done in Nepal, since pollution controls there are inadequate. This collaboration of producer/weaver and marketer provides an example of social, economic, political, and environmental responsibility (Tufenkian, 2011).

Summary

This chapter has focused on the home fashions industry, which includes four end-use categories: upholstered furniture coverings and fillings; window and wall coverings; soft floor coverings; and bed, bath, tabletop, and other home textile accessories and accents. The design and performance of the textiles used for home fashions play a very important role in the success of the end use. That being the case, the textile industry is the base for the home fashions industry, which is dominated by vertically integrated textile companies that produce both fabrics and home fashions products. Production of home fashions is often highly automated and can be accomplished very efficiently within a vertical operation. Some home fashions, such as towels and rugs, come off the production line as finished goods, not needing further cutting and sewing to complete the product.

An understanding of the organization and operation of the home fashions industry in the broader context of apparel fashions is important for several reasons. In recent years, the apparel and home fashions industries have become more interrelated. Many apparel companies also market home fashions, and well-known apparel designers have licensing agreements with textile mills and home fashions manufacturers. Other licensing agreements for children's home fashions include ones for cartoon and movie characters, sports teams, and toys.

Consumer demand for home fashions continues to be strong despite a slowing housing industry. Home fashions constitute an important segment of the retail industry. Discount retailers such as Walmart, Target, and Kmart are dominant competitors in the retailing of home fashions. Other important home fashions merchants include department stores, specialty stores, direct marketing companies, and home improvement retailers. Sales of over-the-counter fabrics for the home sewing industry are also strong.

Market research and color forecasting are conducted prior to developing the seasonal collections. The textile and trim designers, who create innovative materials, and the product designers, who determine the form of the final end-use product, consider many factors and work within many constraints. Important functional needs and performance criteria must be met. Some products must also meet safety standards set by law. Converters that print or finish fabrics to improve their performance play an important role in the production of textiles for home fashions. Often the converter contracts for specific finishing work with a variety of finishing plants.

The marketing process for home fashions is similar to the process used in the apparel industry that includes the use of manufacturers' showrooms, company sales representatives, trade shows, and advertising and promotion. However, the home fashions industry relies on converters and jobbers to perform marketing and distribution functions more frequently than does the apparel industry. The establishment of well-respected brand names is important in the marketing of home fashions. Trade associations, trade shows, and trade publications form an important network for promoting the home fashions industry.

In recent years, the industry has focused on social and environmental responsibility for all phases of the product use cycle. The home fashions industry has been a leader in efforts to promote sustainable design, encompassing the concept that the creation, use, and discard of a product should preserve the ecosystem. Efforts to practice sustainable design include procedures from the fiber stage through discarding of the product. In addition, some retailers have entered the arena by providing consumers with recycling services when new products are delivered to their homes.

As with the ready-to-wear and accessories industries, the home fashions industry includes a wide variety of career possibilities, from design to production to marketing and distribution.

Design Manager, Woven Bedding
Home Fashions Products Company

Position Description
Supervise the design team for woven bedding products overseeing product development, color direction, and finished product design for all channels of retail distribution.

Typical Tasks and Responsibilities

* Provide leadership in color direction, design, and product development for top-of-the-bed and sheeting products.

* Coordinate decisions with colleagues in design, sales, product development, and sourcing to achieve goals and meet deadlines for delivery to retail venues.

* Be responsible for the creation of prints for top-of-the-bed and sheeting products.

Stylist, Product Development
Home Fashions Product Company

Position Description
Be responsible for assisting the design manager in the development of concepts, finished art, colorways, concept boards, and vendor specification packages for sourced top-of-the-bed and sheeting products.

Typical Tasks and Responsibilities

* Assist the design manager to develop concept boards.

* Utilize CAD and graphics software programs to create finished art for textile prints.

* Be responsible for providing vendor specification packages for top-of-the-bed and sheeting products.

Key Terms

colorway	linens
converter	napery
curtains	product turn
decorative fabric converter	soft floor coverings
decorative fabric jobber	sustainable design
draperies	table linens
environmental design	thread count
green design	top-of-the-bed category
home fashions	upholstery fabric
home fashions center	window treatment

Discussion Questions and Activities

1. Designers and ready-to-wear brands often have licensed home fashions products. Name three examples of home fashions that are licensed. What are the advantages and disadvantages of these licensing agreements?

2. Select a home fashions product (e.g., towel, rug, sheets). Outline the process used in the design, production, marketing, and distribution of the product. Describe three effective multichannel retailing strategies for home fashions products. What makes these strategies effective?

3. Select a home fashions product in your home that will need replacement in the future. Discuss sustainable design criteria that might be used in the selection of the replacement product and the disposal of the used textile product.

References

Capel (2011). Capel Rugs: America's Rug Company™. Retrieved January 30, 2011, from http://www.capelrugs.com January 30, 2011

Color Marketing Group (2011). About CMG. Retrieved April 28, 2007, from http://www.colormarketing.org

Cotton, Incorporated (2006, July 6). The bath towel: More than just fluff. Retrieved April 29, 2007 from http://www.cottoninc.com/lsmarticles/?articleID=498

DesignTex, Inc. (2011). Corporate sustainability. Retrieved January 10, 2011, from http://www.designtex.com

HFN/Home Furnishing News (2011). About HFN. Retrieved January 15, 2011, from http:www.hfnmag.com

Oriental Weavers (2011). Social responsibility. http://www.orientalweavers.com

Tufenkian Artisan Carpets (2011). A sense of humanity—No child labor. Retrieved January 30, 2011, from http://www.tufenkiancarpets.com

Yeager, Jan. (1988). *Textiles for Residential and Commercial Interiors.* New York: HarperCollins.

Yeager, Jan, and Teter-Justice, Lara. (2000). *Textiles for Residential and Commercial Interiors* (2nd ed.). New York: Fairchild Publications.

Glossary

A

advertising Strategy by which companies buy space or time in print, broadcast, or electronic media to promote their lines to retailers and consumers.

agile manufacturing Use of a combination of technologies that form an integrated, seamless exchange of information linking retailers and suppliers to the manufacturing facility ([TC]^2, 1993; see Chapter 11).

articles of association see articles of incorporation.

articles of incorporation or **articles of organization** or **articles of association** Legal document that outlines the nature and scope of ownership and operations of a corporation.

articles of organization see articles of incorporation.

articles of partnership Written contracts to form a partnership between two individuals or among three or more individuals.

ascot A long neck scarf worn looped at the neck.

atelier de couture Workrooms of haute couture designers and staff.

B

bar codes A series of black-and-white bars that encodes a universal product code (UPC), which enables a retailer or manufacturer to track products.

base pattern or **block** or **sloper** Basic pattern in the company's sample size, without any style features, used as the starting point for creating a pattern for a new style.

bias The diagonal cut of fabric, or 45 degrees to the length or width of the fabric, used to produce better shaping of the fabric than a straight-grain cut.

big box stores Stores that can be as large as 150,000 to 250,000 square feet, which usually contain elements of a supermarket and a department store by offering a wide range of merchandise, including food, electronics, clothing and accessories, furniture, and garden items such as outdoor furniture and accessories, equipment, and gardening tools.

bilateral trade agreement Trade agreements between two countries.

block see base pattern.

blocking or **boarding** The application of heat to create the final shape in the finishing process for knit goods.

board of directors Chief governing body of a corporation elected by the corporation's stockholders.

boarding see blocking.

boutique Specialty store that concentrates on designer price zone merchandise or unique merchandise distributed to only a few stores.

brand community A community formed on the basis of attachment to a product. For example, Harley-Davidson motorcycle owners/riders or Barbie doll owners.

brand extension   Expanding the use of a well-known brand name to a variety of merchandise; e.g., decorative pillows and throw rugs manufactured by WestPoint Stevens with the Harley-Davidson logo.

brand merchandise   Apparel, accessories, or home fashions whose brand or label is well recognized by the public.

brand name or **trade name**   Distinctive name given to a product or service for the purpose of making the product or service readily identifiable to consumers.

brand tier   Strategy by which a manufacturer or retailer offers brands in two or more price zones, with each brand focusing on a specific price zone.

bridge jewelry   Umbrella term for several types of jewelry, including those made from silver, gold (14K, 12K, 10K), and less expensive stones; jewelry designed by artists using a variety of materials.

bundling   The process of disassembling stacked cut fabric pieces and reassembling them grouped by garment size, color dye lot, and quantity of units ready for production.

business-to-business (B2B)   Business operations that are conducted between companies through web-based technologies.

C

C corporation or **regular corporation**   Type of corporation whereby profits of the corporation are distributed to shareholders in the form of dividends.

capital   Funds or resources needed to start or expand a business.

cashmere   A soft, luxury fiber that comes from the undercoat wool of the cashmere or Kashmir goat, mainly from China, Mongolia, and Tibet.

carryover   Item in a line or collection that is carried over from one season to the next.

catalog retailer   see mail order/catalog retailer.

chain store   Retail organization that owns and operates several retail outlets that sell similar lines of merchandise in a standardized method, and function under a centralized form of organizational structure.

classification   The process by which apparel manufacturers are categorized (classified) by the type of merchandise produced, by the wholesale prices of the products or brands, or by an industry classification system for government tracking.

close corporation   see private corporation.

closely held corporation   see private corporation.

clutch   Handbag designed to be held (clutched) in the hand, but may have a strap that can be stored inside the bag.

co-branded apparel   Product development strategy whereby a retailer partners with an apparel manufacturer in the creation of the retailer's private label line.

code of conduct   Guidelines for contractors and subcontractors regarding workplace environment and operations; generally focus on safeguards for workers' health and rights.

collection A group of apparel items presented together to the buying public, usually by high-fashion designers.

color control Color matching requirement for all like garments in a line and for all their components, such as knit collars and cuffs, buttons, thread, and zippers.

color forecasting Process of predicting consumers' future color preferences for merchandise for a specific fashion season. Predictions are based on research conducted by color forecasters for companies and trade associations.

color forecasting service A company that predicts consumers' future color and trend preferences in textiles, apparel, accessories, and home fashions.

color management Process of maintaining an acceptable color match for all like garments in a line, including all their components, such as knit collars and cuffs, buttons, thread, and zippers.

color palette A selected group of colors, often represented by color chips. Each new line will be composed of a group of selected colors.

color story Color palette identified for each group's fashion season.

colorway The variety of three or four seasonal color choices for the same solid or print fabric available for each garment style.

commercial match Contractor-provided acceptable match of color for fabric, trim, or finding to a control color chip or fabric provided by the apparel company.

computer-aided design (CAD) Both the hardware and software computer systems used to assist with the design phase of the fabric design or garment design.

computer grading and marker making (CGMM) The computer hardware and software systems that process the pattern grading and marker making segments of the pattern for production.

concept garment End-use garment created by a textile company to promote its new fibers to textile mills.

concept shop A company's in-store shop when applied to a nonstore retail venue, such as the Ralph Lauren concept shop on Bloomingdales.com.

conglomerate Diversified company involved with significantly different lines of business.

consolidation The combining of two companies to form a new company.

consumer research Information gathered about consumer characteristics and consumer behavior, including broad trends in the marketplace as well as more specific information about a target group of consumers.

contractor Company that specializes in the sewing and finishing of goods or that specializes in a specific part of the production process (such as pleating piece goods).

contractual retailer Retailer that has entered into a contractual agreement with a manufacturer, wholesaler, or other retailers in order to integrate operations and increase market impact.

controlled brand name program or **licensed brand name program**   Marketing strategy whereby minimum standards of fabric performance for trademarked fibers are determined and promoted.

convenience store   Retailer that offers fast service and convenient location.

conventional manufacturer   A company that performs all functions of creating, marketing, and distributing an apparel line on a continual basis.

conventional marketing channel   Independent companies that separately perform the manufacturing, distribution, and retailing functions.

converted goods or **finished goods**   Fabrics that have been dyed, printed, or finished.

converter or textile converter   Company that specializes in finishing fabrics (including printing).

co-op advertising   A type of advertising strategy whereby companies share the cost of the advertisement that features all of the companies.

cooperative advertising   see co-op advertising.

copyright   The exclusive right of the copyright holder to use, perform, or reproduce written, pictorial, and performed work.

corporate social responsibility (CSR)   A philosophy whereby a company takes into consideration human rights, labor conditions, and environmental implications when making business decisions.

corporate selling   Strategy by which apparel companies sell their merchandise directly to retailers without the use of sales representatives.

corporate showroom   Showroom owned and operated by a single company to market its lines of merchandise; generally managed by company sales representatives.

corporation   Company established by a legal charter that outlines the scope and activity of the company. Corporations are legal entities regardless of who owns stock in the company.

cost or **cost to manufacture** or **wholesale cost**   The total cost to manufacture a style, including materials, findings, labor, and auxiliary costs such as freight, duty, and packaging.

cost to manufacture   see cost.

costume jewelry   Mass-produced jewelry made from plastic, wood, brass, glass, Lucite, and other less expensive materials.

cotton   Natural fiber obtained from the fibers surrounding the seeds of the cotton plant.

cotton gin   Machine that cleans cotton seed from the cotton fibers; invented in 1794 by Eli Whitney.

counter sample or **sew by**   A sample garment sewn by a contractor and submitted to the apparel manufacturer for approval. This sample is then used as a benchmark to compare the sewn production goods.

counterfeit goods   Products that incorporate unauthorized use of registered trade names or trademarks.

country of origin   This term is defined as the country where last step that added value (i.e., substantial change) to the product happened.

couture   A French term that literally means "sewing," it refers to the highest-priced apparel produced in small quantities, made of high-quality fabrics utilizing considerable hand-sewing techniques, and sized to fit individual clients' bodies.

couture house   Name for each designer's business, thus, there is the House of Dior, the House of Givenchy, and the House of Chanel.

couturier (couturière)   Designer of haute couture (couturier = masculine; couturière = feminine).

croquis or **lay figure**   A French term that refers to a figure outline used as a basis to sketch garment design ideas.

cross-dockable shipments   Goods are received from the manufacturer as floor-ready merchandise, so they can be sorted for store distribution without the need for additional processing.

cross-merchandising   Strategy by which apparel companies and retailers combine apparel and accessories in their product offerings.

curtains   Type of fabric window covering that provides both screening and decorative functions.

customs broker   A person in the United States, licensed by the Office of Customs and Border Protection, to assist manufacturers in gaining customs clearance to import goods produced offshore.

cut, make, and trim (CMT)   Apparel contractors who cut, make, and trim the garments for the apparel manufacturer.

cut order   Instructions for production cutting that include the specific number of items in each color and each size that will be included in the production run.

cut-up trade   Belt manufacturers who produce belts for apparel manufacturers to add to their pants, skirts, and dresses.

D

data mining technology   Technology used by companies to analyze purchasing data to determine selling patterns or trends and identify correlations among data characteristics.

décor   The interior decoration that creates a room's ambiance.

decorative fabric converter   Company that designs and sells finished textiles to jobbers, designers, and manufacturers who use the textiles in home fashions end-use products.

decorative fabric jobber   Company involved in the marketing and distribution of home textile piece goods, particularly upholstery and drapery fabrics.

demographics   Information about consumers that focuses on understanding characteristics of consumer groups, such as age, gender, marital status, income, occupation, ethnicity, and geographic location.

department store   Large retailer that departmentalizes its functions and merchandise.

design and product development The process by which a new style moves from concept sketch to prototype.

die cutting A piece of metal with a sharp edge similar to a cookie cutter tooled to the exact dimensions of the shape of the pattern piece (the die). The die is positioned over the fabric to be cut; then a pressurized plate is applied to the die to cut through the fabric layers.

diffusion line A designer's less expensive line (e.g., A/X Armani Exchange, DKNY).

digital printing Method of direct fabric printing that utilizes digital artwork.

digitizer A table embedded with sensors that relate to the X and Y coordinates (horizontal and vertical directions) that allow the shape of the pattern piece to be traced and converted to a drawing of the pattern in the computer.

direct market brand or **store brand** Brand name on merchandise that is also the name of the retailer, e.g., Gap, L.L.Bean.

direct marketing channel Marketing channel by which manufacturers sell directly to the ultimate consumer.

discount store Retailer who sells brand name merchandise at below traditional retail prices, including apparel at the budget/mass wholesale price zone.

distribution center (DC) Centralized location used by manufacturers and retailers for quality assurance, tagging, picking, packing of merchandise, and distribution to retail stores.

distribution strategy Business strategy to assure that merchandise is sold in stores that cater to the target market for whom the merchandise was designed and manufactured.

dividend Corporate profits paid to its stockholders; dividends are taxed as personal income.

double taxation Situation with a C or regular corporation whereby earnings of the corporation are taxed twice—once at the corporate level and again at the individual level.

draperies Type of fabric window covering (long curtains) made with heavy fabrics designed to cover the full window.

draping A process of creating the initial garment style by molding, cutting, and pinning fabric to a mannequin.

dual distribution Distribution strategy whereby manufacturers sell their merchandise through their own stores as well as through other retailers.

duplicate or **sample** A copy of the prototype or sample style used by the sales representatives to show and sell styles in the line to retail buyers.

E

e-commerce Buying and selling of goods and services conducted over the Internet.

e-market Companies that "enable trading partners to conduct business over the Internet eliminating the need for more costly paper and custom EDI methods" (eMarkets, 2001, p. 4; see Chapter 12).

e-tailing Term for electronic retailing.

electronic data interchange (EDI) Computer-to-computer communications between companies.

electronic/Internet retailer Company that offers goods and/or services over the Internet or uses the Internet in addition to its stores and/or catalog retailing business.

eMarket Community of companies that conduct business primarily through B2B websites.

entrepreneur see sole proprietor.

environmental design Design decisions related to the creation, use, and discarding of a product in ways that preserve the ecosystem.

exclusive distribution Strategy whereby manufacturers limit the stores in which their merchandise is distributed in order to create an image of exclusiveness.

export agent A person located in the country that produced the goods who assists the (U.S.) manufacturer with exportation of the products.

extended marketing channel Marketing channel in which wholesalers acquire products from manufacturers and sell them to retailers, or jobbers buy products from wholesalers and sell them to retailers.

F

fabric construction Methods used to make fabrics from solutions, directly from fibers, and from yarns; weaving and knitting are the most common methods.

fabrication see fabric construction.

factor An agency that provides protection against bad debt losses, manages accounts receivable, and provides credit analysis in the apparel industry.

factoring The business of purchasing and collecting accounts receivable or of advancing cash on the basis of accounts receivable ("The F word," 1996, p. 1; see Chapter 9).

factory monitoring/auditing program In a factory, a monitoring system could include at-a-glance information about what machines are being used, whether machines are cleared to be used, and who is on duty at a particular station.

factory outlet A type of off-price retailer that sells its own seconds, irregulars, or overruns (merchandise produced in excess of its orders), as well as merchandise produced specifically for the outlet stores.

fallout The fabric that remains in the spaces between pattern pieces on the marker, representing the amount of fabric that is wasted.

fashion color Color used in a seasonal line that reflects the current color trends, determined by the apparel company for the target customer.

fashion forecasting service A company that predicts consumers' future style preferences and trends in textiles and apparel. Predictions are based on research conducted by its staff and other associations.

fashion magazine Magazine sold over-the-counter as well as by subscription whose primary focus is on the latest fashion trends.

fashion season Name given to lines or collections that correspond to seasons of the year when consumers would most likely wear the merchandise; e.g., Spring, Summer, Fall, Holiday, and Resort.

fast fashion Ultra-fast supply chain operations that focus on consumer demand of fashion goods.

fast fashion production Manufacturing of fast fashions in which products go from concept to retail store in less than three weeks.

fiber The basic unit in making textile yarns and fabrics.

filament yarn Yarn created by spinning together long continuous fibers.

findings Also called notions or sundries, the garment components other than fabrics, such as fasteners, elastic, stay tape, and hem tape.

fine jewelry Jewelry made from precious metals alone, and with precious and semiprecious stones.

finish Application to a fiber, yarn, or fabric that changes the appearance, hand, or performance of the fiber, yarn, or fabric.

finished goods see converted goods.

finishing "Any process that is done to fiber, yarn, or fabric either before or after fabrication to change the appearance (what is seen), the hand (what is felt), or the performance (what the fabric does)"

(Kadolph & Langford, 2002, p. 270, see Chapter 3).

first adoption meeting Gathering when a new line is presented (often as sketches and fabric swatches), and each style in the line is reviewed by the design team.

fit model The live model whose body dimensions match the company's sample size and who is used to assess the fit, styling, and overall look of new prototypes.

flat or **flat sketch** Also called a tech drawing, this technical sketch of a garment style represents how the garment would look lying flat, as on a table. Garment details are clearly depicted.

flatknit Goods that are knit flat, as compared to goods knit in a tube (tubular knit).

flat pattern The patternmaking process used to make a pattern for a new style from the base pattern (or block or sloper).

flat sketch see flat.

flexible manufacturing (FM) Production that focuses on optimizing equipment, flow of goods, and teams of workers to produce the product as efficiently as possible.

flexible manufacturing system "Any departure from traditional mass production systems of apparel toward faster, smaller, more flexible production units that depend upon the coordinated efforts of minimally supervised teams of workers" (AAMA Technical Advisory Committee, 1988, as cited in Hill, 1992, p. 34; see Chapter 11).

floor-ready merchandise (FRM) Merchandise shipped by the manufacturer or distribution center affixed with hangtags, labels, and price information so that the retailer can place the goods immediately on the selling floor.

flow-through Facilities that move merchandise from receiving to shipping with little, if any, time in storage.

fourchette On gloves, a strip of material located between the second/third, third/ fourth, and fourth/baby fingers to provide depth for the thickness of the finger.

franchise A type of contractual retail organization whereby the parent company provides the franchisee with the exclusive distribution of a well-recognized brand name in a specific market area, as well as assistance in running the business in return for a franchise payment.

free trade agreement (FTA) Reciprocal reductions in tariffs among the United States and countries. This sourcing option allows the manufacturer to control the design and cut of the garments, while taking advantage of lower labor costs in other countries.

freight forwarding company A company that moves a shipment of goods from the country where the goods were produced to the United States.

full-fashioned Goods knit with shaping along the edges to conform to the body contour.

full-package contractor (FP) A type of service option whereby the apparel contractor provides preproduction services, fabrics, trims, supplies, and labor.

G

garment dyed Apparel produced as white or colorless goods and then dyed during the finishing process.

garment spec sheet see garment specification sheet.

garment specification sheet or garment spec sheet A listing of vital information for the garment style including garment sketch, fabric swatches and/or specifications, and specifications for findings, sizes, construction, and finished garment measurements.

general partner Co-owner of a company who shares responsibilities with other owners in the running of a company under a partnership agreement.

general partnership Form of ownership in which co-owners of a company share in the liability as well as the profits of the company according to the conditions of the partnership contract.

generic family Classification of fibers according to chemical composition and characteristics.

globalization Process whereby the economies of nation states become integrated.

grade rules The amounts and locations of growth or reduction for pattern pieces to create the various sizes.

grading or pattern grading Using the production pattern pieces made in the sample size for a style to develop a set of pattern pieces for each of the sizes listed on the garment spec sheet.

green design   See environmental design.

greige goods   Fabrics that have not received finishing treatments, such as bleaching, shearing, brushing, embossing, or dyeing; unfinished fabrics.

group   Coordinated apparel items using several colors and fabrics within an apparel line.

H

hand   How a fabric feels to the touch.

haute couture   Also sometimes referred to as couture, apparel in the highest price zone. This apparel is produced in small quantities, utilizes hand-sewing techniques, is sized to fit an individual's body dimensions, and uses very expensive fabrics and trims.

hide   An animal pelt weighing more than 25 pounds when shipped to the tannery.

home fashions   Textile products for home-end uses such as towels, bedding, upholstery fabrics, area floor coverings, draperies, and table linens.

home fashions centers   Business centers that bring together a variety of home improvement and decorating retailers, such as furniture, tile, carpeting, and lighting companies.

horizontally integrated   Business strategy whereby a company focuses on a single stage of production/distribution but with varying products or services.

HTS 9802 production   The Harmonized Tariff Schedule Section 9800 of the U.S. tariff regulations, textiles and apparel are produced under the provisions of preferential trade agreements such as the North American Free Trade Agreement or the Caribbean Basin Trade Partnership Act receive tariff reductions or eliminations.

hypermarket   see superstore.

I

importer/packager   Company that develops full lines of apparel with contractors in other countries and sells them to retailers as complete packages for use as private-label merchandise.

information flow   Communication among companies within the marketing channel pipeline.

initial cost estimate   The preliminary estimate of the cost of a new style based on materials, trims, findings, labor, and other components such as duty and freight.

initial public offering (IPO)   When a company wants to become a publicly traded corporation, or "go public" it sells shares to public investors in an initial public offering.

in-store shop   Area within a department store that is merchandised according to manufacturers' specifications and carries only the merchandise of the manufacturer.

intensive distribution or **mass distribution** Strategy whereby products are made available to as many consumers as possible through a variety of retail venues.

internal selling Process used for private label merchandise whereby a company's design team will present seasonal lines to merchandisers within the company who will select specific pieces of the line for production.

interindustry partnership Partnerships between companies in different industries that share common target customers.

intraindustry partnership Partnering with companies that are in the same sector of the industry but have different target customers.

item house Contractor that specializes in the production of one type of product such as baseball caps.

J

jobber An intermediary in the apparel industry who carries inventories of apparel for ready shipment to retailers.

K

kip Animal pelt weighing 15 to 25 pounds when shipped to the tannery.

knockoff A facsimile of an existing garment that sells at a lower price than the original. The copy might be made in a less expensive fabric and might have some design details modified or eliminated.

L

lab dip The vendor-supplied sample of the dyed-to-match product such as fabric, zipper, button, knit collar or cuff, or thread.

last A wood, plastic, or metal mold, shaped like a foot and used to form shoes.

lay figure see croquis.

leased department Contractual retail agreement whereby a retailer leases space within a large department store to run a specialty department. Typical leased departments are fine jewelry, furs, and shoes.

licensed brand name program see controlled brand name program.

licensing An agreement whereby the owner (licensor) of a particular image or design sells the right to use the image or design to another party, typically a manufacturer (licensee), for payment of royalties to the licensor.

licensor Company that has developed a well-known image (property) and sells the right to use the image to manufacturers to put on merchandise.

lifestyle brand A term used to describe brands that are associated with a particular target customer's activities and way of life. Tommy Bahama is a good example of a lifestyle brand as the merchandise is associated with the lifestyle of individuals who live or vacation in tropical locations.

lifestyle merchandising Use of the appeal of the target customer's lifestyle choices, especially in product advertising.

limited liability Arrangement whereby owners of a company are liable only for the amount of capital they invested in the company but are not personally liable beyond that for debts incurred by the business.

Limited Liability Company (LLC) Form of company ownership that provides owners with the tax advantages of a partnership, along with the limited liability of a corporation.

limited marketing channel Marketing channel in which manufacturers sell their merchandise to consumers through retailers.

limited partnership A specialized type of partnership in which a partner is liable only for the amount of capital invested in the business, and any profits are shared according to the conditions of the limited partnership contract.

line One large group or several small groups of apparel items developed with a theme that links the items together.

line catalog or **line sheet** A brochure or catalog of all the styles and colorways available in the line, used to market the line to retail buyers.

line-for-line copy A garment made as an exact replica of an existing garment style, produced in a similar fabric.

line sheet see line catalog.

linens Towels, sheets, tablecloths, napkins, and other home textiles once made almost exclusively from linen. The term linens continues to be used, even though these products are rarely made from linen anymore.

long-range forecasting Research focusing on general economic and social trends related to consumer spending patterns and the business climate.

M

made-to-measure "A fully customized process where a garment is made specifically for one individual based on his/her measurements and preferences" (Made to measure or mass customization: Is it for you?," 1998, vol. 18, no. 1 *Cuttings*, p. 3, see Chapter 11).

mail order/catalog retailer Retail company that sells merchandise to consumers through catalogs, brochures, or advertisements, and delivers the merchandise by mail or other carrier.

manufacturer A company that performs all functions of creating, marketing, and distributing an apparel, accessory, or home fashions line on a continual basis. These companies may use outside contractors to perform the manufacturing function.

manufacturing environment Production circumstances including choice of production facility, location of production, production process, and cycle time to produce goods.

margin The difference between the cost to manufacture a style and the wholesale price the retailer will pay the manufacturer for the style. Margin can also refer to the difference between the cost the retailer paid the manufacturer for the goods and the selling price for the goods.

marker A master cutting plan for all the pattern pieces in the sizes specified on the cut order to manufacture the style.

market 1) consumer demand for a product or service; 2) location where the buying and selling of merchandise takes place; 3) to promote a product or service through media or public relations efforts.

market analysis Information about general market trends.

market center Name given to cities that not only house marts and showrooms, but also have important manufacturing and retailing industries, e.g., New York, Los Angeles, Dallas, Atlanta, Chicago.

market niche Specific segment of the retail trade determined by a combination of product type and target customer.

market research Process of providing information to determine what the customer will need and want, and when and where the customer will want to make purchases.

market week Time of the year in which retail buyers come to showrooms or exhibit halls to see the seasonal fashion lines offered by apparel companies.

marketing Process of identifying a target market and developing appropriate strategies for product development, pricing, promotion, and distribution.

marketing channel Sequence of companies that perform the manufacturing, wholesaling, and retailing functions to get merchandise to the ultimate consumer.

marketing channel integration Process of connecting the various levels of the marketing channel so that they work together in getting the right product to the right customer at the right price and the right place.

marketing pipeline see marketing channel.

mart Building or group of buildings that house showrooms in which sales representatives show merchandise lines to retail buyers.

mass customization The use of computer technology to customize a garment style for the individual customer, by individualizing the fit to the customer's measurements, by offering individualized combinations of fabric, garment style, and size options, or by personalization of a finished product.

mass distribution see intensive distribution.

mass fashion Originally developed for the teenage market, mass fashion focused on simplified styling and sizing, mass production sewing in large factories, with distribution through retail chain stores.

master calendar A calendar which indicates when each step of the design and distribution of a season's line must be completed.

measurement specification The actual garment measurements at specific locations on the finished goods for each of the sizes specified for a style.

merchandiser 1) An apparel company employee who is responsible for planning and overseeing to ensure that the company's needs for a line are met. This person often coordinates several lines presented by the company; 2) one who visually displays merchandise within a retail store (visual merchandiser).

merchandising 1) The process of buying and selling goods and services; 2) area of an apparel company that develops strategies to have the right merchandise, at the right price, at the right time, at the right locations to meet the wants and needs of the target customer.

merger Blending of one company into another company.

millinery Women's hats, and especially hat making that requires hand work.

modular manufacturing A term often used in the U.S. apparel industry to describe flexible manufacturing (Hill, 1992, p. 34; see Chapter 11).

mohair Natural fiber obtained from the wool of the Angora goat.

monopolistic competition Competitive situation in which many companies compete in terms of product type, but the specific products of any one company are perceived as unique by consumers.

monopoly Competitive situation in which there is typically one company that dominates the market and can thus price its goods and/or services at whatever scale its management wishes.

muffler Long oblong scarf, often wool or silk and often worn wrapped around the neck to provide added warmth.

multichannel distribution Distribution strategy whereby a manufacturer offers merchandise through varying retail venues: bricks-and-mortar stores, catalogs, and/or Web sites.

multichannel retailing Retail strategy whereby merchandise is offered through bricks-and-mortar stores, catalogs, and/or websites

multilateral trade agreement Trade agreements among multiple countries usually negotiated by the World Trade Organization

multiline sales representative Individual who sells lines from several noncompeting but related companies to retail buyers.

multinational corporation Private or publicly traded corporation that operates in several countries.

muslin An inexpensive fabric, usually unbleached cotton, often used to develop the first trial of a new garment style.

N

nanotechnology Technology that functions in the range of nanometers, one-billionth of a meter, with applications in enhanced manufacturing and the development of "smart" fibers.

napery or **table linens** Home fashions products that include tablecloths and napkins.

national/designer brand Brand name that is distributed nationally and to which consumers attach a specific image, quality level, and price.

nonstore retailer Distributor of products to consumers through means other than bricks-and-mortar retail stores.

North American Industry Classification System (NAICS) U.S. Department of Commerce categories and subcategories based on the company's chief industrial activity.

O

off-price retailer Retailer who specializes in selling national brands or designer apparel and home fashions lines at discount prices.

offshore production Production outside the United States using production specifications provided by U.S. companies.

oligopoly Competitive situation in which a few companies dominate and essentially have control of the market, making it very difficult for other companies to enter.

oligopsony Competitive situation that involves a large number of sellers offering goods and services to a small number of buyers.

open-distribution policy Policy by which a company will sell to any retailer who meets basic characteristics.

open to buy The process of planning merchandise sales and purchases. Merchandise is budgeted for purchase during a certain time period.

ownership flow or **title flow** Transfer of ownership or title of merchandise from one company to the next.

P

partnership Company owned by two or more persons; operation of partnerships is outlined in a written contract or "articles of partnership."

patent "Publicly given, exclusive right to an idea, product, or process" (Fisher & Jennings, 1991, p. 595; see Chapter 2).

pattern design system (PDS) A computer hardware and software system that is used by the patternmaker to create and store new garment (pattern) styles.

pattern grading see grading.

payment flow Transfer of monies among companies as payment for merchandise or services rendered.

PDM/PLM A term used when combining product data management and product lifecycle management. This approach requires all computer systems in the pipeline to be compatible in order to share product data.

pelt The unshorn skin of an animal used in making leather and fur.

perfect competition see pure competition.

personalization The process of customizing a product for an individual consumer.

physical flow Movement of merchandise from the manufacturer to the ultimate consumer.

picking The process of selecting the appropriate assortment of goods to fill a specific retailer's order.

piece-rate wage Method of compensation whereby each production operator's pay is based on individual productivity, that is, specified task completed by the operator on the total number of units in a given time period.

popular fashion magazine Magazine available for individual purchase or by subscription to consumers and typically read by the target customer.

pop-up retail Specialty stores that are temporary or mobile in nature, focus on new fads, or are associated with a live event.

precosting see initial cost estimate.

preline A preview of the line shown to key retail buyers prior to its introduction at market. These accounts may place orders in advance of market.

prêt-à-porter French term for ready-to-wear; in the United Kingdom, this merchandise is called *off-the-peg*; and in Italy, it is called *moda pronto*.

price averaging A price strategy whereby one style will be priced to sell for less than the company's typical profit margin while another style in the same line will be priced to sell for more than the typical profit margin. The margin's gain and loss of the two styles are averaged.

price point A price range that relates to the merchandise available in a given price range; designer, bridge, better, moderate, or mass.

price zone see price point.

private corporation Type of corporation whereby there is not a public market for the stock in the corporation and stock has not been issued for public purchase.

private label brand Brand name that is owned and marketed by a specific retailer for use in its stores. Private label merchandise bears the retailer's label; the retailer has partial or full control over the manufacture of the product.

private label product development or **store brand product development** Development of new styles by retailers to sell in their retail stores under a store brand label or private label.

privately held corporation See private corporation.

product data management (PDM) or **product development management (PDM)** The integration of computer systems that link style information among departments within a company, and/or among external contacts such as vendors and contractors.

product development management (PDM) see product data management (PDM).

product lifecycle management (PLM) Electronic access to style information throughout the design, development, production, and distribution processes within a company and by external contacts such as vendors and contractors.

product research Information gathered by a company regarding preferred product design and product characteristics desired by a specific customer group.

product turn   The frequency rate at which a product is sold and replaced at the retail store.

product type   The specific category or categories of apparel the company specializes in producing.

production   The construction process by which the materials, trims, findings, and garment pieces are merged into a finished apparel product, accessory, or home fashion.

production cutting   Process in which the production fabric, laid open across its entire width and many feet in length, is stacked in multiple layers with the marker resting on the top, and cut by computer or by using hand-cutting machines.

production engineer   A specialist who is responsible for the production pattern and/or for planning the production process, facilities, and final costing.

production marker   The full-size master cutting layout for all the pattern pieces for a specific style, for all the sizes specified for production.

progressive bundle system   Groups of a dozen (usually) garment pieces placed in bundles and moved from one sewing operator to the next. Each operator performs one or several construction steps on each garment in the bundle and then passes the bundle on to the next operator.

promotion flow   Flow of communication to promote merchandise either to other companies or to consumers in order to influence sales.

proprietary   A contractual agreement between two parties (such as a textile company and an apparel manufacturer) that allows exclusive rights to the use of a product or process for a specified period of time.

prototype   The sample garment for a new style in the company's base size made in the intended fashion fabric or a facsimile fabric. If made in muslin, the prototype is usually called a toile.

psychographics   Information gathered about a target group's buying habits, attitudes, values, motives, preferences, personality, and leisure activities.

publicly held corporation   Type of corporation whereby stock has been issued for public purchase and at least some of the shares of stock are owned by the general public.

publicly traded corporation   see publicly held corporation.

publicity   Promotional strategy whereby the company's activities are viewed as newsworthy and thus are featured or are mentioned in print, television, electronic, or other news media.

pull-down cutting   The process of cutting gloves by die cutting the pieces.

pure competition or **perfect competition**   Competitive situation in which there are many producers and consumers of similar products, so that price is determined by market demand.

pull system   Demand-side strategies that are based on the flow of timely and accurate information about consumers' wants and needs from consumers to the manufacturers.

push system   Supply-side strategies used to push the products produced on the consumer.

Q

quality assurance   Area of a company that focuses on quality control issues but also takes into consideration satisfaction of consumer needs for a specific end use; standards of acceptance set forth by the contracting party (the apparel manufacturer, for example) for the product being produced.

quality control   Area of a company that focuses on inspecting finished products and making sure they adhere to specific quality standards.

Quick Response (QR)   Comprehensive business strategy that promotes responsiveness to consumer demand, encourages business partnerships, and shortens the business cycle from raw materials to the consumer.

quirk   Tiny triangular gusset in gloves at the base of the second, third, and fourth fingers.

quota   Limits on the number of units, kilograms, or square meters equivalent in specific categories that can be imported from specific countries.

R

rack trade   Belt manufacturers who design, produce, and market belts to retailers.

radio-frequency identification (RFID)   Tagging technology that utilizes a silicon computer chip. The chip is incorporated into containers, pallets, merchandise packaging, or individual items, and is used for purposes of accurate tracking of merchandise through production processes and the supply chain or to deter counterfeiting and shoplifting.

ready-to-wear (RTW)   Apparel made with mass production techniques using standardized sizing; sometimes referred to as "off-the-rack."

regimental stripe   Fabric used for men's ties with wide and narrow stripes that were used originally to signify the various historical military regiments.

registration   For printed textiles with more than one color screen, specified placement for each of the screens to produce the multi-color print.

regional sales territory   Geographic area assigned to be covered by a corporate or multiline sales representative.

regular corporation   see C corporation.

regular tannery or tannery   Tannery that buys skins and hides, performs tanning methods, and sells finished leather.

relationship merchandising   An emphasis of retail stores on presentation, personal customer service, and having the right products for their target market that are different from the merchandise carried by other stores.

replenishment   Automatic reordering of merchandise.

retail relations program Programs run by merchandising marts, which include a number of services designed to assist retail buyers during market weeks and trade shows.

retail store/direct market brand A retail store whose merchandise carries the retail store name as its exclusive label.

retailer "Any business establishment that directs its marketing efforts toward the final consumer for the purpose of selling goods and services" (Lewison, 1994, p. 5; see Chapter 12).

retailing The "business activity of selling goods or services to the final consumer," (Lewison, 1994, p. 5, see Chapter 12).

retro The return to the fashion look of recent decades (abbreviated use of the word retrospective).

S

S corporation Type of corporation that is given special status by the Internal Revenue Service in that earnings of the corporation are taxed only at the individual level.

sales representative Individual who serves as the intermediary between the manufacturer and the retailer, selling the apparel, accessories, or home fashions lines to retail buyers.

sales volume The actual level of sales, expressed as either the total number of units of a style that sold at retail or the total number of dollars consumers spent on the style.

salon de couture Haute couture designer's showroom.

sample see duplicate.

sample cut A three- to five-yard length of fabric ordered from a textile mill by the apparel manufacturer to use for making a prototype garment.

sample sewer A highly skilled technician who sews the entire prototype (sample) garment using a variety of sewing equipment and production processes similar to those used in factories.

selected-distribution policy Policy by which a company establishes detailed criteria that stores must meet in order to carry the company's merchandise.

selective distribution Strategy whereby manufacturers allow their merchandise to be distributed only through certain stores.

sell through The percentage computed by the number of items sold at retail compared to the number of items in the line the retailer purchased from the manufacturer.

servicemark Trade name, symbol, or design used to identify a service that is offered for sale.

sew by see counter sample.

shopping the market Looking for new fashion trends in the retail markets that may influence the direction of an upcoming line.

short-cycle production Mass production of goods that can be produced quickly. It is especially suited to high-fashion products that are produced close to their market demand.

short-range forecasting Researching specific fashion trends and new styles for an upcoming season and determining the level of demand and timing for these styles (also referred to as what, when, and how much to manufacture).

showroom Facility used by sales representatives to show samples of a line to retail buyers; may be permanent or temporary.

single-hand system A garment production method in which an individual sewer is responsible for sewing an entire garment. It is used primarily for couture or very high-priced, limited-production apparel and for sewing prototypes.

size standards Proportional increase or decrease in garment measurements for each size produced by a ready-to-wear apparel company.

skin Animal pelt weighing 15 pounds or less when shipped to the tannery.

SKU (stock-keeping unit) A number or code used to identify each distinct product and service that can be purchased, thus enabling the company to systematically track its inventory or product availability,

sloper see base pattern.

slops Less expensive clothes from scrap material left over from sewing custom-made suits. The term later became a standard term for cheap, ready-made clothing.

"smart" fiber Optical fiber with integrated electronics that allow the fiber to sense, process, and store data, and which can be woven into fabric; applications include medical devices, high performance and protective fabrics, and military uniforms.

social responsibility see corporate responsibility.

socially responsible design Achieved through inclusive design (i.e., inclusive based on age, physical ability, or socioeconomic status), physically and psychologically healthy design, design that promotes fair trade, and design decisions that facilitate efficient factory operations.

socially responsible distribution The intermediaries responsible for bringing goods to market. These intermediaries deliver goods from producers to end users in a manner that takes into consideration human rights, labor conditions and environmental implications.

socially responsible marketing An organization shows concern for the people and environment in which it transacts business.

socially responsible production Production that balances the environmental, ethical and community needs with costs needed to produce a product.

socially responsible supply chain management Supply chain management (SCM) is the oversight of materials, information, and finances as they move in a process from supplier to manufacturer to wholesaler to retailer to consumer. Socially responsible companies consider employee training, philanthropy, environment, workplace diversity, health and safety, and community issues as part of this management.

soft floor covering Area rugs, runners, and scatter rugs, as well as wall-to-wall carpeting.

sole proprietorship Company owned by a single individual.

source or **supplier** or **vendor** Company from which textile producers, apparel manufacturers, or retailers purchase components or products necessary in their production and distribution operations (e.g. fiber sources, fabric sources, apparel product sources).

sourcing Decision process of determining how and where a company's products or their components will be produced.

sourcing fair Trade shows that bring contractors and companies together. At these fairs, contractors have booths with samples of their merchandise and information regarding their expertise and capacities.

specialty store Retailer who focuses on a specific type of merchandise.

specification buying Retailer-initiated design and manufacturing of apparel goods in which the retailer may work directly with the sewing contractors (or their agents) to produce store brand or private label goods. Sometimes the retailer works with an apparel manufacturer to produce store brand or private label goods.

spreading The process of unwinding the large rolls of fabric onto long, wide cutting tables, stacked layer-upon-layer, in preparation for cutting.

spreading machine Equipment designed to carry the large rolls of fabric, guided on tracks along the side edges of the cutting table or rolled along the floor next to one side of the cutting table, to spread the fabric smoothly, and quickly onto the cutting table.

spun yarn Yarn created by the spinning together of short staple fibers.

staple color Color such as black, navy, white, gray, or tan that is used in a line that appears frequently, season after season.

stockout data Data on out-of-stock goods are reviewed by the manufacturer, and replenishments are ordered as often as required. The strategy of having the manufacturer (vendor) automatically ship merchandise to the retail store based on stock data.

stockholder Owner of stock or shares in a corporation; each share of stock owned by a stockholder represents a percentage of the company.

store brand Concept whereby the store offers only merchandise with the store name as its brand, for example The Limited, Gap, Banana Republic, and Old Navy.

See direct market brand.

store brand product development see private label product development.

strike off A length of sample yardage of a printed fabric, used to proof the colors and quality of the print.

style number   A number (usually four to six digits) assigned to each garment style that is coded to indicate the season/year for the style and other style information.

subcontractor   A subcontractor is hired by a main contractor to perform a specific task as part of the overall project.

supermarket   Retailer who carries a full line of foods and related products using a self-service strategy.

superstore or **hypermarket**   Upgraded large supermarkets that offer a wide range of merchandise including food, electronics, clothing and accessories, furniture, sporting goods, and garden items.

supplier   see source.

supply chain management (SCM)   "Collection of actions required to coordinate and manage all activities necessary to bring a product to market, including procuring raw materials, producing goods, transporting and distributing those goods and managing the selling process" (Abend, 1998, p. 48; see Chapter 1).

sustainable design   A term used to designate the "awareness of the full short- and long-term consequences of a transformation of the environment" (DesignTex, 1995, p. 53; see Chapter 14).

swatch   A small sample of the fabric intended to be used for a garment style.

sweatshop   Originally referred to the system of contractors and subcontractors whereby work was "sweated off."

Later, the term became associated with the long hours, unclean and unsafe working conditions, and low pay of contract sewing factories, as well as with the dismal conditions of home factories, where contract workers sewed clothing. Currently used to refer to a company that violates labor, safety and health, and/or worker compensation laws, or that has work environments that are unsafe, inhumane, or abusive without providing opportunities for workers to organize or negotiate better terms of work.

T

table cutting   The process of cutting gloves entirely by hand, on a work table.

table linens   see napery.

tagboard   A heavy-weight paper (also called oaktag or hard paper) used for pattern pieces instead of pattern paper.

tagless label   Printed information such as care instructions, fiber content, and size, heat sealed directly onto the product.

takeover   The result of one company or individual gaining control of another company by buying a large enough portion of the company's shares; can be either a merger or consolidation.

tannery   see regular tannery.

tanning   The process of finishing leather, making the skins and hides pliable and water resistant.

target costing   A pricing strategy in which the fabric cost and styling features are manipulated in order to provide a new style for a predetermined cost.

target customer   Description of the gender, age range, lifestyle, geographic location, and price zone for the majority of the company's customers for a specific line.

tariff   Tax assessed by governments on imports.

tawning   The process of finishing furs, making the pelts pliable and water resistant.

tech drawing   A drawing of the garment style as viewed flat rather than depicted three-dimensionally on a fashion figure (an abbreviation of the term technical drawing). It could include drawings of close-up details of the garment. A tech drawing might also be called a flat or a flat sketch.

terms of sale   Negotiated agreements between the manufacturer and retailer regarding the sale of merchandise; may include discounts, terms of delivery, availability of cooperative advertisements and other promotional tools.

textile   "Any product made from fibers" (Joseph, 1988, p. 347; see Chapter 3).

textile accessory and accent   Includes a wide variety of textile products for bedding, bath, tabletop accessories, kitchen, and textile accents such as wall hangings, tapestries, quilts, needlework, and lace accents.

Textile/Clothing Technology Corporation ([TC]^2)   Nonprofit corporation that develops, tests, and teaches advanced apparel technology.

textile converter   see converter.

textile jobber   Company that buys fabrics from textile mills, converters, and large manufacturers, and then sells to smaller manufacturers and retailers.

textile mill   Company that specializes in the fabric construction stage of production (e.g., weaving, knitting).

textile stylist   Individual who has expertise in the design and manufacturing of textiles as well as an understanding of the textile market and works directly with manufacturers and retailers in creating textile designs.

textile testing   "Process of inspecting, measuring and evaluating characteristics and properties of textile materials" (Cohen, 1989, p. 165; see Chapter 3).

thread count   Total number of yarns (warp plus weft) in one square inch of fabric.

throwster   Company that modifies filament yarns for specific end uses.

title flow   see ownership flow.

toile   A French term whose literal translation means "cloth"; refers to the muslin trial or sample garment.

tolerance   The stated range of acceptable dimensional measurements as a (+) or (−) in inches (or metric dimensions) of the size specifications.

top-of-the-bed   Home fashions products that includes comforters, duvet covers, blankets, bedspreads, dust ruffles, pillow shams, and throws.

trade association   Nonprofit association made up of member companies designed to research, promote, or provide educational services regarding an industry or a specific aspect of an industry.

trade dress   Subset of trademark law; protects the overall look or image of a product or the packaging of a product.

trade name   see brand name.

trade preference program   Agreements that provide incentives for companies to source in these regions of the world through investments and infrastructure enhancements.

trade publication   A publication such as a newspaper or magazine that is targeted to the trade, such as retailers, manufacturers, or textile producers, and generally is available by subscription or at some specialty book and magazine sellers.

trade show   Event sponsored by trade associations, apparel marts, and/or promotional companies, to allow companies to promote their newest products to prospective buyers who have the opportunity to review new products of a number of companies under one roof.

trademark   "Distinctive name, word, mark, design, or picture used by a company to identify its product" (Fisher & Jennings, 1991, p. 595; see Chapter 2).

trademark infringement   Illegal use of a trademark or servicemark; use without the permission of the owner of the trademark or servicemark.

trank   The section of a glove that covers the palm and the face of the hand.

trend research   Information on future directions of consumer behavior, color, fabrics, and fashion styling obtained by reading trade publications and/or fashion magazines, making observations, or other data collection methods.

triple bottom line   For companies, in addition to costs and profits associated with sourcing decisions, the decisions must also take the following into account human rights, labor conditions, and environmental implications of the decisions. For sourcing decisions; people, planet, and profit factors are all considered.

trunk show   Marketing strategy by which a company will bring an entire line to a retail store as a special event to show and sell to customers.

U

unit production system (UPS)   Production system whereby the parts for each garment are transported as a unit on a conveyor track, one garment at a time, to the sewing operator who performs one or several sewing operations, and then releases the garment for transport to the next work station.

Universal Product Code (UPC)   One of several bar-code symbologies used for electronic identification of merchandise. A UPC is a 12-digit number that identifies the manufacturer and merchandise item by stockkeeping unit.

unlimited liability Situation in which owners of a company are personally liable for debts incurred by the business; often the case in sole proprietorships and in some partnerships.

upholstery fabric Textiles used primarily for covering sofas, love seats, chairs, and ottomans.

upscale discounter Discount retail store with department store feel and provides more fashion-forward merchandise (e.g., Target).

usage The number of yards (yardage) of fabric(s) required to make the garment style. It usually denotes the most economical layout to use the least amount of fabric.

V

vendor see source.

vendor-managed inventory (VMI) Programs whereby retail sales/stockout data are reviewed by the manufacturer and replenishments are ordered as often as required.

vendor marking Affixing hangtags, labels, and price information to merchandise by the vendor (manufacturer).

vertical integration Business strategy whereby a company handles several steps in production and/or distribution.

vertical marketing channel see vertical integration.

vertically integrated see vertical integration.

virtual draping Computer-created simulation of a fabric draped three-dimensionally over an image of a garment as shown on a body or mannequin.

virtual sample Digital images of merchandise samples that are viewed on the computer screen.

W

warehouse retailer Retailer who reduces operating expenses and offers goods at discount prices by combining showroom, warehouse, and retail operations.

Web EDI An efficient and low-cost system of sharing data electronically and is a viable option for both large and small companies located throughout the world.

wholesale cost see cost.

wholesale price The price of the style that the retailer will pay the apparel manufacturer for the goods. The price is based on the manufacturer's cost to produce the style plus the manufacturer's profit.

window treatment Draperies, curtains, and fabric shades as well as decorative treatments such as valances, cornices, and swags.

wool Natural fiber derived from the fleece of sheep, goats, alpacas, and llamas.

work-in-process (WIP) The quantity of goods in the process of assembly in the sewing factory at a given time.

Y

yarn Collection of fibers or filaments laid or twisted together to form a continuous strand strong enough for use in fabrics.

yarn forward rule of origin This stipulation to a trade agreement means that if a company produces apparel products in a country with whom the United States has such a trade agreement, in order to bring the apparel into the United States duty-free (i.e., without duties or tariffs on the product), the yarn and all manufacturing operations "forward" (e.g., textile production, apparel production) must occur either in the United States or in the country with whom the United States has the trade agreement.

Z

zeitgeist The general social spirit and popular culture of of a given time period.

Photo Credits

7.4: (no credit)
7.5: (no credit)
7.6: Courtesy of Optitex
7.7: (no credit)
7.8: Daniel Acker/Bloomberg via Getty Images
7.9: Courtesy of Nancy Bryant
7.10: (no credit)
7.11: Courtesy of Nancy Bryant
7.12: (no credit)
7.13: Courtesy of International Concepts

8.1: Illustration by Mike Miranda
8.2: Illustration by Mike Miranda
8.3: Courtesy of WWD/Ronda Churchill
8.4: Courtesy of WWD
8.5: Courtesy of WWD/Steve Eichner
8.6: Courtesy of WWD/George Chinsee
8.7a: Courtesy of WWD/Tyler Boye
8.7b: Courtesy of WWD
8.8: Raymond Boyd/Michael Ochs Archives/Getty Images
8.9: Courtesy of WWD
8.10: Courtesy of WWD/Stefanie Keenan
8.11: Courtesy of WWD/Robert Mitra
8.12: Scott Olson/Getty Images
8.13: (no credit)
8.14: Courtesy of Nordstrom
8.15: Courtesy of WWD/Steve Eichner

9.1: (no credit)
9.2: (no credit)
9.3: Courtesy of Nancy Bryant
9.4: Courtesy of Nancy Bryant
9.5: Courtesy of Kristen Sandberg
9.6: Courtesy of Kristen Sandberg
9.7: Courtesy of Union Special Technical Training Centre
9.8: © Gerber Technology, Inc.
9.9: Courtesy of Nancy Bryant
9.10: © Gerber Technology, Inc.
9.11: (no credit)
9.12: (no credit)
9.13: (no credit)
9.14: © Gerber Technology, Inc.
9.15: © Gerber Technology, Inc.

10.1: Illustration by Mike Miranda
10.2: David Engelhardt/Getty Images
10.3: Courtesy of WWD
10.4: Courtesy of WWD
10.5: Courtesy of WWD
10.6: Courtesy of WWD
10.7: Courtesy of WWD/Bryan Haraway
10.8: Courtesy of WWD
10.9: Courtesy of Nike, Inc.
10.10: © 2009 Edward Kavishe FASHIONWIREPRESS.COM
10.11: Courtesy of WWD
10.12: Courtesy of WWD/Jason Lee
10.13: Reuters/Rupak De Chowdhuri/Landov

11.1: Illustration by Mike Miranda
11.2: Provided by the authors
11.3: Courtesy of Astor & Black

11.4: Provided by the authors
11.5: Guang Niu/Getty Images
11.6: Illustration by Mike Miranda
11.7: Provided by the authors
11.8: Images courtesy of [TC]^2, Gary, NC, USA (www.tc2com)
11.9: Provided by the authors
11.10: © EschCollection/Getty Images

12.1: © TWPhoto/Corbis
12.2: Dimas Ardian/Getty Images
12.3: Illustration by Mike Miranda
12.4: Courtesy of WWD
12.5: Borgman © 1999 The Cincinnati Enquirer. Reprinted by permission of Universal Press Syndicate. All Rights Reserved.
12.6: Courtesy of WWD/Kyle Ericksen
12.7: Courtesy of WWD/Kyle Ericksen
12.8: Courtesy of WWD
12.9: David McNew/Getty Images
12.10: Joe Raedle/Getty Images
12.11: Courtesy of FashionMall.com
12.12: © Jeff Greenberg/Alamy

13.1: Courtesy of WWD/David Sawyer
13.2: Courtesy of Tommy Hilfiger
13.3: Courtesy of WWD/Yukie Kasuga
13.4: © Andrew Holbrooke/Corbis
13.5: Courtesy of Nike, Inc.
13.6: © Bettman/Corbis
13.7: Photo by Sarah Silberg
13.8: Courtesy of WWD/Jean E. Palmieri
13.9: Ron Mullet @2010
13.10: Courtesy of WWD/Alessio Cocchi
13.11: Courtesy of WWD
13.12: Courtesy of WWD/John Aquino
13.13: Courtesy of WWD/Robert Mitra
13.14: Courtesy of WWD/Talaya Centeno
13.15: Courtesy of Condé Nast Publications
13.16: Courtesy of WWD
13.17: Courtesy of WWD/Paul Hartley

14.1: Courtesy of WWD/Meghan Colangelo
14.2: Courtesy of Charter Club
14.3: Virgil Smithers/Fieldcrest Cannon
14.4: Courtesy of WWD/Robert Mitra
14.5: Image from Vision Carpet Studio ™ by NedGraphics BV.
14.6: Courtesy of Cotton, Inc.
14.7: Robert Daly / Alamy
14.8: Courtesy of Home Furnishings News
14.9: © Emeraldlight/Corbis
14.10: Courtesy of Milliken
14.11: © Scott Stulberg/Corbis
14.12: Veer
14.13: © Norbert Schafer/Corbis
14.14: © Trapper Frank/Corbis Sygma
14.15: Huw Jones/Alamy
14.16: © Jack Hollingsworth/Corbis
14.17: Jeff Greenberg/Alamy
14.18: Vincenzo Pinto/AFP/Getty Images
14.19: Courtesy of Cotton, Inc.

Index